Fifth Edition
MEDICAL PHARMACOLOGY &THERAPEUTICS

Dedication

To our families

Fifth Edition
MEDICAL PHARMACOLOGY & THERAPEUTICS

Derek G. Waller
BSc (HONS), DM, MBBS (HONS), FRCP

Consultant Cardiovascular Physician, University Hospital Southampton,
Senior Clinical Lecturer, University of Southampton,
Southampton, United Kingdom
Senior Medical Adviser to the British National Formulary

Anthony P. Sampson
MA, PhD, FHEA, FBPhS

Associate Professor in Clinical Pharmacology, Faculty of Medicine,
University of Southampton, Southampton, United Kingdom

ELSEVIER

Edinburgh   London   New York   Oxford   Philadelphia   St Louis   Sydney   Toronto   2018

ELSEVIER

First edition 2001
Second edition 2005
Third edition 2010
Fourth edition 2014
Fifth edition 2018

The rights of Derek G. Waller and Anthony P. Sampson to be identified as authors of this work have been asserted by them in accordance with the Copyright, Designs and Patents Act 1988.

Notices

Knowledge and best practice in this field are constantly changing. As new research and experience broaden our understanding, changes in research methods, professional practices, or medical treatment may become necessary.

Practitioners and researchers must always rely on their own experience and knowledge in evaluating and using any information, methods, compounds, or experiments described herein. In using such information or methods they should be mindful of their own safety and the safety of others, including parties for whom they have a professional responsibility.

With respect to any drug or pharmaceutical products identified, readers are advised to check the most current information provided (i) on procedures featured or (ii) by the manufacturer of each product to be administered, to verify the recommended dose or formula, the method and duration of administration, and contraindications. It is the responsibility of practitioners, relying on their own experience and knowledge of their patients, to make diagnoses, to determine dosages and the best treatment for each individual patient, and to take all appropriate safety precautions.

To the fullest extent of the law, neither the Publisher nor the authors, contributors, or editors, assume any liability for any injury and/or damage to persons or property as a matter of products liability, negligence or otherwise, or from any use or operation of any methods, products, instructions, or ideas contained in the material herein.

ISBN: 978-0-7020-7167-6
Printed in China
Last digit is the print number: 9 8 7 6 5 4 3 2 1

Senior Content Strategist: *Pauline Graham*
Content Development Specialist: *Carole McMurray*
Project Manager: *Dr. Atiyaah Muskaan*
Design: *Amy Buxton*
Illustration Manager: *Karen Giacomucci*
Marketing Manager: *Deborah Watkins*

your source for books,
journals and multimedia
in the health sciences

www.elsevierhealth.com

Working together
to grow libraries in
developing countries

www.elsevier.com • www.bookaid.org

The
publisher's
policy is to use
**paper manufactured
from sustainable forests**

Contents

SECTION 8 THE IMMUNE SYSTEM

SECTION 9 THE ENDOCRINE SYSTEM AND METABOLISM

SECTION 10 THE SKIN AND EYES

SECTION 11 CHEMOTHERAPY

SECTION 12 GENERAL FEATURES: DRUG TOXICITY AND PRESCRIBING

Preface

The fifth edition of *Medical Pharmacology and Therapeutics* has been extensively revised and updated while preserving the popular approach of the fourth edition. We particularly wish to acknowledge here the contributions made to previous editions of this book by Emeritus Professor Andrew Renwick OBE BSc PhD DSc and Dr Keith Hillier BSc PhD DSc, Senior Lecturer in Pharmacology, formerly our colleagues in the University of Southampton Faculty of Medicine. As before, a disease-based approach has been taken to explain clinical pharmacology and therapeutics and the principles of drug use for the management of common diseases. *Medical Pharmacology and Therapeutics* provides key information on basic pharmacology and other relevant disciplines sufficient to underpin the clinical context. It provides information suitable for all healthcare professionals who require a sound knowledge of the basic science and clinical applications of drugs.

The text is structured to reflect the ways that drugs are used in clinical practice. The chapters covering generic concepts in pharmacology and therapeutics include sections on how drugs work at a cellular level, drug metabolism and pharmacokinetics, pharmacogenetics, drug development and drug toxicity. The basic principles of prescribing have been emphasized and new information provided on preparing for the Prescribing Safety Assessment (PSA) in the UK. New sections have been included on pharmacovigilance, on so-called 'legal highs' and in all other areas, and the sections on clinical management have been thoroughly revised and updated.

Each chapter in this fifth edition retains the following key features:

- An up-to-date and succinct explanation of the major pathogenic mechanisms of disease and consequent clinical symptoms and signs, helping the reader to put into context the actions of drugs and the consequences of their therapeutic use.
- A structured approach to the principles of disease management, outlining core principles of drug choice and planning a therapeutic regimen for many common diseases.
- A comprehensive review of major drug classes relevant to the disease in question. Basic pharmacology is described with clear identification of the molecular targets, clinical characteristics, important pharmacokinetic properties and unwanted effects associated with individual drug classes. Example drugs are used to illustrate the common pharmacological characteristics of their class and to introduce the reader to drugs currently in widespread clinical use.
- To complement the information provided within each chapter, a drug compendium is included describing the main characteristics of all drugs in each class listed in the British National Formulary.
- A revised section of self-assessment questions for learning and revision of the concepts and content in each chapter, including one best answer (OBA), extended matching items (EMI), true-false and case-based questions.

It is our intention that the fifth edition of this book will encourage readers to develop a deeper understanding of the principles of drug usage that will help them to become safe and effective prescribers and to carry out basic and clinical research and to teach. As medical science advances these principles should underpin the life-long learning essential for the maintenance of these skills.

DGW
APS

Drug dosage and nomenclature

DRUG NOMENCLATURE

In the past, the nonproprietary (generic) names of some drugs have varied from country to country, leading to potential confusion. Progressively, international agreement has been reached to rationalise these variations in names and a single recommended International Non-proprietary Name (INN) given to all drugs. Where the previously given British Approved Name (BAN) and the INN have differed, the INN is now the accepted name and is used throughout this book.

A special case has been made for two medicinal substances: adrenaline (INN: epinephrine) and noradrenaline (INN: norepinephrine). Because of the clinical importance of these substances and the widespread European use and understanding of the terms *adrenaline* and *noradrenaline*, manufacturers have been asked to continue to dual-label products adrenaline (epinephrine) and noradrenaline (norepinephrine). In this book, where the use of these agents as administered drugs is being described, dual names are given. In keeping with European convention, however, adrenaline and noradrenaline alone are used when referring to the physiological effects of the naturally occurring substances.

DRUG DOSAGES

Medical knowledge is constantly changing. As new information becomes available, changes in treatment, procedures, equipment and the use of drugs become necessary. The authors and the publishers have taken care to ensure that the information given in the text is accurate and up to date. However, readers are strongly advised to confirm that the information, especially with regard to drug usage, complies with the latest legislation and standards of practice.

1

General principles

1 Principles of pharmacology and mechanisms of drug action

STUDYING PHARMACOLOGY

Drugs are defined as active substances administered to prevent, diagnose or treat disease, to alleviate pain and suffering, or to extend life. Pharmacology is the study of the effects of drugs on biological systems, with medical (or clinical) pharmacology concerned with the drugs that doctors, and some other healthcare professionals, prescribe for their patients. The prescribing of drugs has a central role in therapeutics, and gaining a good knowledge of pharmacology is essential for health professionals to become safe and effective prescribers.

Drugs may be chemically synthesised or purified from natural sources with or without further modification, but their development and clinical use are based on rational evidence of efficacy and safety derived from controlled experiments and randomised clinical trials. Drugs can be contrasted with placebos (*placebo* is Latin for 'I will please'), defined as inactive substances administered as though they are drugs, but which have no therapeutic effects other than potentially pleasing the patient, providing a sense of security and progress. Pharmacology evolved on the principle of studying known quantities of purified, active substances to identify their specific mechanisms of action and to quantify their effects in a reproducible manner, usually compared with a placebo or other control substance.

Much of the success of modern medicine is based on pharmacological science and its contribution to the development of safe and effective pharmaceuticals. This book is confined to pharmacology as it relates to human medicine and aims to develop knowledge and understanding of medical pharmacology and its application to therapeutics. The objectives of learning about medical pharmacology and therapeutics are:

- to understand the ways that drugs work to affect human systems, as a basis for safe and effective prescribing;
- to appreciate that pharmacology must be understood in parallel with related biological and clinical sciences, including biochemistry, physiology and pathology;
- to develop numerical skills for calculating drug doses and dilutions, and to enable accurate comparison of the relative benefits and risks of different drugs;
- to comprehend and participate in pharmacological research advancing the better treatment of patients.

The answer to the frequently asked question 'What do I need to know?' will depend upon the individual requirements of the programme of study being undertaken and the examinations that will be taken. The depth and type of knowledge required in different areas and topics will vary when progressing through the programme; for example, early in the course it may be important to know whether a drug has a narrow safety margin between its wanted and unwanted effects, and in the later years this may translate into detailed knowledge of how the drug's effects are monitored in clinical use. Personal enthusiasm for medical pharmacology is important and should be driven by the recognition that prescribing medicines is the most common intervention doctors (and increasingly other health professionals) use to improve the health of their patients.

FINDING DRUG INFORMATION

Learning about medical pharmacology is best approached using a variety of resources in a range of learning scenarios and preferably in the context of basic science and therapeutics, not from memorising lists of drug names. The following provides a useful structure to organise the types of information that you should aim to encounter:

- the nonproprietary (*generic*) drug name (not the *proprietary* or *trade name*);
- the *class or group* to which the drug belongs;
- the way the drug works (its *mechanism of action* and its *clinical effects*), usually shared to variable extents by other drugs in the same class;
- the main clinical reasons for using the drug (its *indications*);
- any reasons why the drug should not be used in a particular situation (its *contraindications*);
- whether the drug is a *prescription-only medicine* (PoM) or is available without prescription (over-the-counter [OTC]);
- how the drug is given (*routes of administration*);
- how its effects are quantified and its doses modified if necessary (*drug monitoring*);
- how the drug is absorbed, distributed, metabolised and excreted (ADME; its *pharmacokinetics*), particularly where these show unusual characteristics;
- the drug's *unwanted effects*, including any interactions with other drugs or foods;
- whether there are nonpharmacological treatments that are effective alternatives to drug treatment or will complement the effect of the drug.

The **Appendix** at the end of this chapter provides a formulary of core members of each major drug class to give students in the early stages of training a manageable list of the drugs most likely to be encountered in clinical practice. At the end of later chapters, the **Compendium** provides a classified listing and key characteristics of those drugs discussed within the main text of each chapter and also other drugs listed in the corresponding section of the *British National Formulary* (BNF).

The BNF (www.evidence.nhs.uk) contains monographs for nearly all drugs licensed for use in the United Kingdom and is the key drug reference for UK prescribers. Students should become familiar at an early stage with using the BNF for reference. More detailed information on individual drugs (the Summary of Product Characteristics [SPC]), patient information leaflets (PIL) and contact details for pharmaceutical companies is available from the electronic Medicines Compendium (eMC; www.medicines.org.uk/emc/).

RECEPTORS AND RECEPTOR-MEDIATED MECHANISMS

Pharmacology describes how the physical interaction of drug molecules with their macromolecular targets ('receptors') modifies biochemical, immunological, physiological and pathological processes to generate desired responses in cells, tissues and organs. Drugs have been designed to interact with many different types of macromolecules that evolved to facilitate endogenous signalling between cells, tissue and organs, or to play key roles in the normal cellular and physiological processes that maintain controlled conditions (homeostasis). Drugs may also target macromolecules produced by pathogens, including viruses and bacteria. While the term 'receptor' was originally applied in pharmacology to describe any such drug target, more commonly a receptor is now defined in biochemical terms as a molecule on the surface of a cell (or inside it) that receives an external signal and produces some type of cellular response.

The function of such a receptor can be divided typically into three main stages:

1. **The generation of a biological signal.** Homeostasis is maintained by communication between cells, tissues and organs to optimise bodily functions and responses to external changes. Communication is usually by signals in the form of chemical messengers, including neurotransmitter molecules, local mediators or endocrine hormones. The signal molecule is termed a *ligand*, because it ligates (ties) to the specialised cellular macromolecule. The cellular macromolecule is a *receptor* because it receives the ligand.
2. **Cellular recognition sites (receptors).** The signal is recognised by responding cells by its interaction with a site of action, binding site or receptor, which may be in the cell membrane, the cytoplasm or the nucleus. Receptors in the cell membrane react with extracellular ligands that cannot readily cross the cell membrane (such as peptides). Receptors in the cytoplasm often react with lipid-soluble ligands that can cross the cell membrane.
3. **Cellular changes.** Interaction of the signal and its site of action in responding cells results in functional changes within the cell that give rise to an appropriate biochemical or physiological response to the original homeostatic stimulus. This response may be cell division, a change in cellular metabolic activity or the production of substances that are exported from the cell.

Each of these three stages provides important targets for drug action, and this chapter will outline the principles underlying drug action mainly in stages 2 and 3.

ACTIONS OF DRUGS AT BINDING SITES (RECEPTORS)

For very many drugs, the first step in producing a biological effect is by interaction of the drug with a receptor, either on the cell membrane or inside the cell, and it is this binding that triggers the cellular response. Drugs may be designed to mimic, modify or block the actions of endogenous ligands at that receptor. The classified list of receptors at the end of this chapter shows that cell-membrane and cytosolic receptors tend to occur in different families (receptor types), reflecting their evolution from common ancestors. Within any one family of receptors, different receptor subtypes have evolved to facilitate increasingly specific signalling and distinct biological effects. As might be expected, different receptor families have different characteristics, but subtypes within each family retain common family traits.

In pharmacology, the perfect drug would be one that binds only to one type or subtype of receptor and consistently produces only the desired biological effect without the unwanted effects that can occur when drugs bind to a related receptor. Although this ideal is impossible to attain, it has proved possible to develop drugs that bind avidly to their target receptor to produce their desired effect and have very much less (but not zero) ability to bind to other receptors, even ones within the same family, which might produce unwanted effects.

Where a drug binds to one type of receptor in preference to another, it is said to show *selectivity of binding* or *selectivity of drug action*. Selectivity is never absolute but is high with some drugs and lower with others. A drug with a high degree of selectivity is likely to show a greater difference between the dose required for its biological action and the dose that produces unwanted actions at other receptor types. Even a highly selective drug may produce unwanted effects if its target receptors are also found in tissues and organs other than those in which the drug is intended to produce its therapeutic effect.

MAJOR TYPES OF RECEPTORS

Despite the great structural diversity of drug molecules, most act on the following major types of receptors to bring about their pharmacological effects:

- **Transmembrane ion channels.** These control the passage of ions across membranes and are widely distributed.
- **Seven-transmembrane (7TM) (heptahelical) receptors.** This is a large family of receptors, most of which signal via guanine nucleotide-binding proteins (G-proteins). Following activation by a ligand, second messenger substances are formed inside the cell, which can bring about cellular molecular changes, including the opening of transmembrane ion channels.
- **Enzyme-linked transmembrane receptors.** This is a family of transmembrane receptors with an integral or associated enzymic component, such as a kinase or phosphatase. Activation of these enzymes produces changes in cells by phosphorylating or dephosphorylating intracellular proteins, including the receptor itself, thereby altering their activity.
- **Intracellular (nuclear) receptors.** These receptors are found in the nucleus or translocate to the nucleus from the cytosol to modify gene transcription and the expression of specific cellular proteins.

Transmembrane ion channels

Transmembrane ion channels that create pores across phospholipid membranes are ubiquitous and allow the transport of ions into and out of cells. The intracellular concentrations of ions are controlled by a combination of two types of ion channel:

- ion pumps and transporters, which transport specific ions from one side of the membrane to the other in an energy-dependent manner, usually against their concentration gradient;
- ion channels, which open to allow the selective, passive transfer of ions down their concentration gradients.

Based on concentration gradients across the cell membrane:

- both Na^+ and Ca^{2+} ions will diffuse into the cell if their channels are open, making the electrical potential of the cytosol more positive and causing depolarisation of excitable tissues;
- K^+ ions will diffuse out of the cell, making the electrical potential of the cytosol more negative and inhibiting depolarisation;
- Cl^- ions will diffuse into the cell, making the cytosol more negative and inhibiting depolarisation.

The two major families of ion channel are the *ligand-gated ion channels* (*LGICs*) and the *voltage-gated ion channels* (*VGICs*; also called *ionotropic receptors*). LGICs are opened by the binding of a ligand, such as the neurotransmitter acetylcholine, to an extracellular part of the channel. VGICs in contrast are opened at particular membrane potentials by voltage-sensing segments of the channel. Both channel types can be targets for drug action. Both LGICs and VGICs can control the movement of a specific ion, but a single type of ion may flow through more than one type of channel, including both LGIC and VGIC types. This evolutionary complexity can be seen in the example of the multiple types of K^+ channel listed in Table 8.1.

LGICs include nicotinic acetylcholine receptors, γ-aminobutyric acid (GABA) receptors, glycine receptors and serotonin (5-hydroxytryptamine) 5-HT$_3$ receptors. They are typically pentamers, with each subunit comprising four transmembrane helices clustering around a central channel or pore. Each peptide subunit is orientated so that hydrophilic chains face towards the channel and hydrophobic chains towards the membrane lipid bilayer. Binding of an active ligand to the receptor causes a conformational change in the protein and results in extremely fast opening of the ion channel. The nicotinic acetylcholine receptor is a good example of this type of structure (Fig. 1.1). It requires the binding of two molecules of acetylcholine for channel opening, which lasts only milliseconds because the ligand rapidly dissociates and is inactivated. Drugs may modulate LGIC activity by binding directly to the channel, or indirectly by acting on G-protein-coupled receptors (GPCRs; discussed later), with the subsequent intracellular events then affecting the status of the LGIC.

VGICs include Ca^{2+}, Na^+ and K^+ channels. The K^+ channels consist of four distinct peptide subunits, each of which has between two and six transmembrane helices; in Ca^{2+} and Na^+ channels there are four domains, each with six transmembrane helices, within a single large protein. The pore-forming regions of the transmembrane helices are largely responsible for the selectivity of the channel for a particular ion. Both Na^+ and K^+ channels are inactivated after opening; this is produced by an intracellular loop of the channel, which blocks the open channel from the intracellular end. The activity of VGICs may thus be modulated by drugs acting directly on the channel, such as local anaesthetics which maintain Na^+ channels in the inactivated site by binding at an intracellular site (Chapter 18). Drugs may also modulate

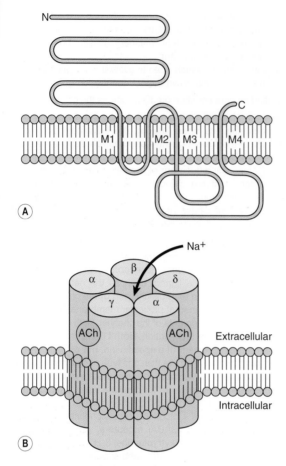

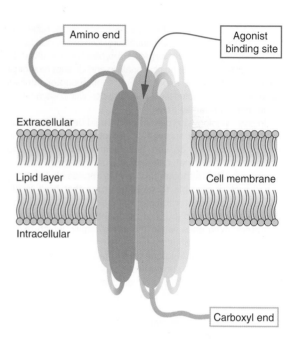

Fig. 1.1 The acetylcholine nicotinic receptor, a typical ligand-gated transmembrane ion channel. (A) The receptor is constructed from subunits with four transmembrane regions (M1–M4). (B) Five subunits are assembled into the ion channel, which has two sites for acetylcholine binding, each formed by the extracellular domains of two adjacent subunits. On acetylcholine binding, the central pore undergoes conformational change that allows selective Na^+ ion flow down its concentration gradient into the cell. *N*, amino terminus; *C*, carboxyl terminus.

Fig. 1.2 Hypothetical seven-transmembrane (7TM) receptor. The 7TM receptor is a single polypeptide chain with its amino (N-) terminus outside the cell membrane and its carboxyl (C-) terminus inside the cell. The chain is folded such that it crosses the membrane seven times, with each hydrophobic transmembrane region shown here as a thickened segment. The hydrophilic extracellular loops create a confined three-dimensional environment in which only the appropriate ligand can bind. Other potential ligands may be too large for the site or show much weaker binding characteristics. Selective ligand binding causes conformational change in the three-dimensional form of the receptor, which activates signalling proteins and enzymes associated with the intracellular loops, such as G-proteins and nucleotide cyclases.

VGICs indirectly via intracellular signals from other receptors. For example, L-type Ca^{2+} channels are inactivated directly by calcium channel blockers, but also indirectly by drugs which reduce intracellular signalling from the β_1 subtype of adrenoceptors (see Fig. 5.5).

The ability of highly variable transmembrane subunits to assemble in a number of configurations leads to the existence of many different subtypes of channels for a single ion. For example, there are many different voltage-gated Ca^{2+} channels (L, N, P/Q, R and T types).

Seven-transmembrane receptors

Also known as 7TM receptors, heptahelical receptors and serpentine receptors, this family is an extremely important group, as the human genome has about 750 sequences for 7TM receptors and they are the targets of over 30% of current drugs. The function of over a hundred 7TM receptors is still unknown. The structure of a hypothetical 7TM receptor is shown in Fig. 1.2; the N-terminal region of the polypeptide chain is on the extracellular side of the membrane, and the polypeptide traverses the membrane seven times with helical regions, so that the C terminus is on the inside of the cell. The extracellular loops provide the receptor site for an appropriate agonist (a natural ligand or a drug), the binding of which alters the three-dimensional conformation of the receptor protein. The intracellular loops are involved in coupling this conformational change to the second messenger system, usually via a heterotrimeric G-protein, giving rise to the term GPCR.

The G-protein system

The heterotrimeric G-protein system (Fig. 1.3) consists of α, β and γ subunits.

- **The α-subunit.** More than 20 different types have been identified, belonging to four families (α_s, α_i, α_q and $\alpha_{12/13}$). The α-subunit is important because it binds guanosine

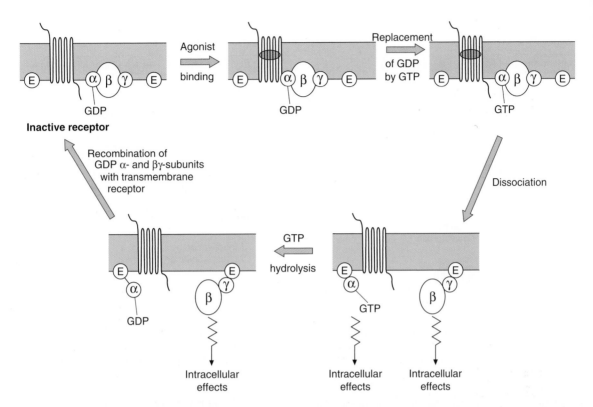

Fig. 1.3 **The functioning of G-protein subunits.** Ligand (agonist) binding results in replacement of GDP on the α-subunit by guanosine triphosphate (GTP) and the dissociation of the α- and βγ-subunits, each of which can affect a range of intracellular systems (shown as E in the figure) such as second messengers (e.g. adenylyl cyclase and phospholipase C), or other enzymes and ion channels (see Figs 1.4 and 1.5). Hydrolysis of GTP to GDP inactivates the α-subunit, which then recombines with the βγ-dimer to reform the inactive receptor.

diphosphate (GDP) and guanosine triphosphate (GTP) in its inactive and active states, respectively; it also has GTPase activity, which is involved in terminating its own activity. When an agonist binds to the receptor, GDP (which is normally present on the α-subunit) is replaced by GTP. The active α-subunit–GTP dissociates from the βγ-subunits and can activate enzymes such as adenylyl cyclase. The α-subunit–GTP complex is inactivated when the GTP is hydrolysed back to GDP by the GTPase.

- **The βγ-complex.** There are many different isoforms of β- and γ-subunits that can combine into dimers, the normal function of which is to inhibit the α-subunit when the receptor is unoccupied. When the receptor is occupied by a ligand, the βγ-complex dissociates from the α-subunit and can itself activate cellular enzymes, such as phospholipase C. The α-subunit–GDP and βγ-subunit then recombine with the receptor protein to give the inactive form of the receptor–G-protein complex.

Second messenger systems

Second messengers are the key distributors of an external signal, as they are released into the cytosol as a consequence of receptor activation and are responsible for affecting a wide variety of intracellular enzymes, ion channels and transporters. There are two complementary second messenger systems: the cyclic nucleotide system and the phosphatidylinositol system (Fig. 1.4).

Cyclic nucleotide system

This system is based on cyclic nucleotides, such as:

- Cyclic adenosine monophosphate (cAMP), which is synthesised from adenosine triphosphate (ATP) by adenylyl cyclase. cAMP induces numerous cellular responses by activating protein kinase A (PKA), which phosphorylates proteins, many of which are enzymes. Phosphorylation can either activate or suppress cell activity.
- Cyclic guanosine monophosphate (cGMP), which is synthesised from GTP by guanylyl cyclase. cGMP exerts most of its actions through protein kinase G, which, when activated by cGMP, phosphorylates target proteins.

There are 10 isoforms of adenylyl cyclase; these show different tissue distributions and could be important sites of selective drug action in the future. The cyclic nucleotide second messenger (cAMP or cGMP) is inactivated by hydrolysis by phosphodiesterase (PDE) isoenzymes to give AMP or GMP. There are 11 different families of PDE isoenzymes (Table 1.1), some of which are the targets of important drug groups, including selective PDE4 inhibitors used in respiratory disease and PDE5 inhibitors used in erectile dysfunction.

The phosphatidylinositol system

The other second messenger system is based on inositol 1,4,5-triphosphate (IP$_3$) and diacylglycerol (DAG),

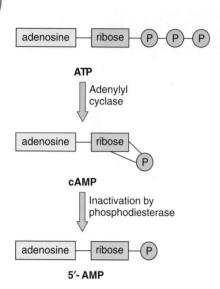

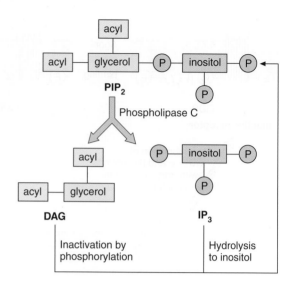

Fig. 1.4 **Second messenger systems.** Stimulation of G-protein-coupled receptors produces intracellular changes by activating or inhibiting cascades of second messengers. Examples are cyclic adenosine monophosphate (cAMP), and diacylglycerol (DAG) and inositol triphosphate (IP$_3$) formed from phosphatidylinositol 4,5-bisphosphate (PIP$_2$). See also Fig. 1.5.

which are synthesised from the membrane phospholipid phosphatidylinositol 4,5-bisphosphate (PIP$_2$) by phospholipase C (see Fig. 1.4). There are a number of isoenzymes of phospholipase C, which may be activated by the α-subunit–GTP or βγ-subunits of G-proteins. The main function of IP$_3$ is to mobilise Ca^{2+} in cells. With the increase in Ca^{2+} brought about by IP$_3$, DAG is able to activate protein kinase C (PKC) and phosphorylate target proteins. IP$_3$ and DAG are then inactivated and converted back to PIP$_2$.

Which second messenger system is activated when a GPCR binds a selective ligand depends primarily on the nature of the Gα-subunit, as illustrated in Fig. 1.5:

- G$_s$: Stimulation of adenylyl cyclase (increases cAMP), activation of Ca^{2+} channels
- G$_{i/o}$: Inhibition of adenylyl cyclase (reduces cAMP), inhibition of Ca^{2+} channels, activation of K$^+$ channels
- G$_{q/11}$: Activation of phospholipase C, leading to DAG and IP$_3$ signalling
- G$_{12/13}$: Activation of cytoskeletal and other proteins via the Rho family of GTPases, which influence smooth muscle contraction and proliferation

The βγ-complex also has signalling activity: it can activate phospholipases and modulate some types of K$^+$ and Ca^{2+} channels.

Activation of these second messenger systems by G-protein subunits thus affects many cellular processes such as enzyme activity (either directly or by altering gene transcription), contractile proteins, ion channels (affecting depolarisation of the cell) and cytokine production. The many different isoforms of G$_α$, G$_β$ and G$_γ$ proteins may represent important future targets for selective drugs.

It is increasingly recognised that GPCRs may assemble into dimers of identical 7TM proteins (homodimers) or into heterodimers of different receptor proteins; the functional consequences of GPCR dimerisation and its implications for drug therapy are unclear.

Protease-activated receptors

Protease-activated receptors (PARs) are GPCRs stimulated unusually by a 'tethered ligand' located within the N terminus of the receptor itself, rather than by an independent ligand. Proteolysis of the N-terminal sequence by serine proteases such as thrombin, trypsin and tryptase enables the residual tethered ligand to bind to the receptor within the second extracellular loop (Fig. 1.6). To date, four protease-activated receptors (PAR 1–4) have been identified, each with distinct N-terminal cleavage sites and different tethered ligands. The receptors appear to play roles in platelet activation and clotting (Chapter 11), and in inflammation and tissue repair. Most of the actions of PAR are mediated by G$_i$, G$_q$ and G$_{12/13}$.

Enzyme-linked transmembrane receptors

Enzyme-linked receptors, most notably the receptor tyrosine kinases, are similar to the GPCRs in that they have a ligand-binding domain on the surface of the cell membrane; they traverse the membrane; and they have an intracellular effector region (Fig. 1.7). They differ from GPCRs in their extracellular ligand-binding domain, which is very large to accommodate their polypeptide ligands (including hormones, growth factors and cytokines), and in having only one transmembrane helical region. Importantly, their intracellular action requires a linked enzymic domain, most commonly an integral kinase which activates the receptor itself or other proteins by phosphorylation. Activation of enzyme-linked receptors enables binding and activation of many intracellular signalling proteins, leading to changes

Table 1.1 Isoenzymes of phosphodiesterase

Enzyme	Main substrate	Main site(s)	Examples of inhibitors	Therapeutic potential
PDE1	cAMP + cGMP	Heart, brain, lung, lymphocytes, vascular smooth muscle	–	Atherosclerosis?
PDE2	cAMP + cGMP	Adrenal gland, brain, heart, lung, liver, platelets, endothelial cells	–	Involved in memory?
PDE3	cAMP + cGMP	Heart, lung, liver, platelets, adipose tissue, inflammatory cells, smooth muscle	Aminophylline Enoximone Milrinone Cilostazol	Asthma (Chapter 12) Congestive heart failure (Chapter 7) Peripheral vascular disease (Chapter 10)
PDE4	cAMP	Sertoli cells, endothelial cells, kidney, brain, heart, liver, lung, inflammatory cells	Aminophylline Roflumilast	Asthma, COPD (Chapter 12) Inflammation IBD?
PDE5	cGMP	Smooth muscle, endothelium, neurons, lung, platelets	Sildenafil Tadalafil Vardenafil Dipyridamole	Erectile dysfunction (Chapter 16) Pulmonary hypertension (Chapter 6)
PDE6	cGMP	Photoreceptors, pineal gland	Dipyridamole Sildenafil (weak)	Undefined
PDE7	cAMP	Skeletal muscle, heart, kidney, brain, pancreas, spinal cord, T-lymphocytes	–	Inflammation (combined with PDE4 inhibitor)? Spinal cord injury?
PDE8	cAMP	Testes, eye, liver, skeletal muscle, heart, kidney, ovary, brain, T-lymphocytes	–	Undefined
PDE9	cGMP	Kidney, liver, lung, brain	–	Undefined
PDE10	cAMP + cGMP	Testes, brain, thyroid	–	Schizophrenia?
PDE11	cAMP + cGMP	Skeletal muscle, prostate, kidney, liver, pituitary and salivary glands, testes	Tadalafil (weak)	Undefined

cAMP, Cyclic adenosine monophosphate; *cGMP*, cyclic guanosine monophosphate; *COPD*, chronic obstructive pulmonary disease; *IBD*, inflammatory bowel disease, *PDE*, phosphodiesterase.

in gene transcription and in many cellular functions. There are five families of enzyme-linked transmembrane receptors:

- **Receptor tyrosine kinase (RTK) family.** Ligand binding causes receptor dimerisation and transphosphorylation of tyrosine residues within the receptor itself and sometimes in associated cytoplasmic proteins. Up to 20 classes of RTK include receptors for growth factors, many of which signal via proteins of the mitogen-activated protein (MAP) kinase cascade, leading to effects on gene transcription, apoptosis and cell division. Constitutive overactivity of an RTK called Bcr-Abl causes leucocyte proliferation in chronic myeloid leukaemia, which is treated with imatinib, a drug that blocks the uncontrolled RTK activity. Several other RTKs are also the targets of anticancer drugs.
- **Tyrosine phosphatase receptor family.** These dephosphorylate tyrosines on other transmembrane receptors or cytoplasmic proteins; they are particularly common in immune cells.
- **Tyrosine kinase-associated receptor family (or nonreceptor tyrosine kinases).** These lack integral kinase activity but activate separate kinases associated with the receptor; examples include inflammatory cytokine receptors and signalling via the JAK/Stat pathways to affect inflammatory gene expression.
- **Receptor serine-threonine kinase family.** Activation of these phosphorylates serine and threonine residues in target cytosolic proteins; everolimus is a serine-threonine kinase inhibitor used in renal and pancreatic cancer.
- **Receptor guanylyl cyclase family.** Members of this family catalyse the formation of cGMP from GTP via a cytosolic domain.

Intracellular (nuclear) receptors

Many hormones act at intracellular receptors to produce long-term changes in cellular activity by altering the genetic expression of enzymes, cytokines or receptor proteins. Such hormones are lipophilic to facilitate their movement across the cell membrane. Examples include the thyroid hormones and the large group of steroid hormones, including glucocorticoids, mineralocorticoids and the sex steroid hormones. Their actions on DNA transcription are mediated by interactions with intracellular receptors (Table 1.2) located either in the cytoplasm (type 1) or the nucleus (type 2).

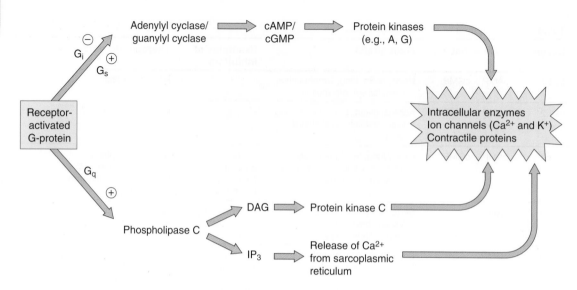

Fig. 1.5 **The intracellular consequences of receptor activation.** The second messengers cyclic adenosine monophosphate (cAMP), cyclic guanosine monophosphate (cGMP), diacylglycerol (DAG) and inositol 1,4,5-triphosphate (IP_3) produce a number of intracellular changes, either directly or indirectly via actions on protein kinases (which phosphorylate other proteins) or by actions on ion channels. The pathways can be activated or inhibited depending upon the type of receptor and G-protein and the particular ligand stimulating the receptor. The effect of the same second messenger can vary depending upon the biochemical functioning of cells in different tissues.

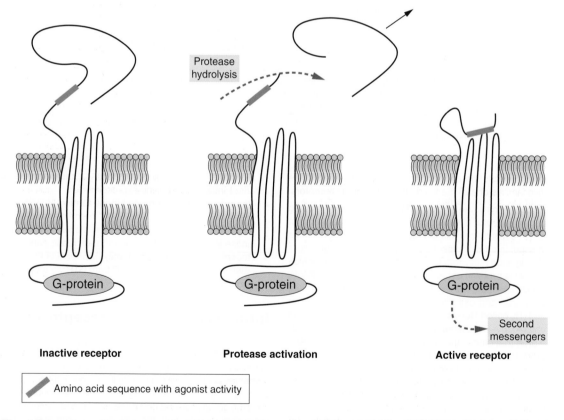

Fig. 1.6 **Protease-activated receptors.** These G-protein-coupled receptors are activated by proteases such as thrombin which hydrolyse the extracellular peptide chain to expose a segment that acts as a tethered ligand (shown in red) and activates the receptor. The receptor is inactivated by phosphorylation of the intracellular (C-terminal) part of the receptor protein.

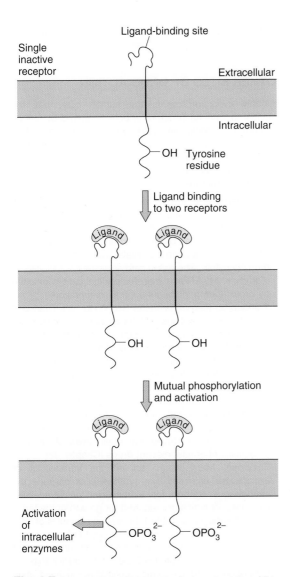

Fig. 1.7 Enzyme-linked transmembrane receptors. This receptor tyrosine kinase has a large extracellular domain, a single transmembrane segment and an integral kinase domain. Ligand binding causes phosphorylation of tyrosine residues on the receptor and on other target proteins, leading to intracellular changes in cell behaviour. Other enzyme-linked receptors have tyrosine phosphatase, serine-threonine kinase or guanylyl cyclase enzymic activity.

Table 1.2 Some families of intracellular receptors

	Subtypes
Type 1 (cytoplasmic)	
Oestrogen receptors	ER (α, β)
Progesterone receptors	PR (A, B)
Androgen receptors	AR (A, B)
Glucocorticoid receptor	GR
Mineralocorticoid receptor	MR
Type 2 (nuclear)	
Thyroid hormone receptors	TR (α_1, β_1, β_2)
Vitamin D receptor	VDR
Retinoic acid receptors	RAR (α, β, γ)
Retinoid X receptors	RXR (α, β, γ)
Liver X (oxysterol) receptors	LXR (α, β)
Peroxisome proliferator-activated receptors	PPAR (α, β/δ, γ)

Table 1.3 The structure of steroid hormone receptors

Section of protein	Domain	Role
A/B	N-terminal variable domain	Regulates transcriptional activity
C	DNA-binding domain (DBD)	Highly conserved; binds receptor to hormone response element in DNA by two zinc-containing regions
D	Hinge region	Enables intracellular translocation to the nucleus
E	Ligand-binding domain (LBD)	Moderately conserved; enables specific ligand binding; contains nuclear localisation sequence (NLS); also binds chaperone proteins and facilitates receptor dimerisation
F	C-terminal domain	Highly variable; unknown function

The intracellular receptor typically includes a highly conserved DNA-binding domain with zinc-containing loops and a variable ligand-binding domain (Table 1.3). The sequence of hormone binding and action for type 1 intracellular receptors is shown in Fig. 1.8. Type 1 receptors are typically found in an inactive form in the cytoplasm linked to chaperone proteins such as heat-shock proteins (HSPs). Binding of the hormone induces conformational change in the receptor; this causes dissociation of the HSP and reveals a nuclear localisation sequence (or NLS) which enables the hormone–receptor complex to pass through nuclear membrane pores into the nucleus. Via their DNA-binding domain, the active hormone–receptor complexes can interact with hormone response elements (HRE) at numerous sites in the genome. Binding to the HRE usually activates gene transcription, but sometimes it silences gene expression and decreases mRNA synthesis.

Translocation and binding to DNA involves a variety of different chaperone, co-activator and co-repressor proteins, and the system is considerably more complex than indicated

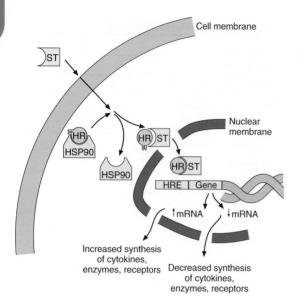

Fig. 1.8 **The activation of intracellular hormone receptors.** Steroid hormones (ST) are lipid-soluble compounds which readily cross cell membranes and bind to their intracellular receptors (HR). This binding displaces a chaperone protein called heat-shock protein (HSP90) and the hormone–receptor complex enters the nucleus, where it can increase or decrease gene expression by binding to hormone response elements (HRE) on DNA. Intracellular receptors for many other ligands are activated in the nucleus itself.

in Fig. 1.8. Co-activators are transcriptional cofactors that also bind to the receptor and increase the level of gene induction; an example is histone acetylase, which facilitates transcription by increasing the ease of unravelling of DNA from histone proteins. Co-repressors also bind to the receptor and repress gene activation; an example is histone deacetylase, which prevents further transcription by tightening histone interaction with the DNA.

Type 2 intracellular receptors, such as the thyroid hormone receptors (TR) and the peroxisome proliferator-activated receptor (PPAR) family (see Table 1.2), are found within the nucleus bound to co-repressor proteins, which are liberated by ligand binding without a receptor translocation step from the cytoplasm. PPAR nuclear receptors function as sensors for endogenous fatty acids, including eicosanoids (Chapter 29), and regulate the expression of genes that influence metabolic events.

Intracellular receptors are the molecular targets of 10–15% of marketed drugs, including steroid drugs acting at type 1 receptors and other drugs acting at type 2 receptors. Steroids show selectivity for different type 1 intracellular receptors (ER, PR, AR, GR, MR; see Table 1.2), which determine the spectrum of gene expression that is affected (Chapters 14, 44, 45 and 46). Steroid effects are also determined by the differential expression of these receptors in different tissues. Intracellular hormone–receptor complexes typically dimerise to bind to their HRE sites on DNA. Steroid receptors form homodimers (e.g. ER–ER), while most type 2 receptors form heterodimers, usually with RXR (e.g. RAR–RXR). The thiazolidinedione drugs used in diabetes mellitus and the

fibrate class of lipid-lowering drugs act on specific members of the PPAR family of type 2 receptors.

OTHER SITES OF DRUG ACTION

Probably every protein in the human body has the potential to have its structure or activity altered by foreign compounds. Traditionally, all drug targets were described pharmacologically as 'receptors', although many drug targets would not be defined as receptors in biochemical terms; in addition to the receptor types discussed previously, drugs may act at numerous other sites.

- **Cell-membrane ion pumps.** In contrast to passive diffusion, primary active transport of ions against their concentration gradients occurs via ATP-dependent ion pumps, which may be drug targets. For example, Na^+/K^+-ATPase in the brain is activated by the anticonvulsant drug phenytoin, whereas in cardiac tissue it is inhibited by digoxin; K^+/H^+-ATPase in gastric parietal cells is inhibited by proton pump inhibitors such as omeprazole.
- **Transporter (carrier) proteins.** Secondary active transport involves carrier proteins, which transport a specific ion or organic molecule across a membrane; the energy for the transport derives not from a coupled ATPase but from the co-transport of another molecule down its concentration gradient, either in the same direction (symport) or in the opposite direction (antiport). Examples include:
  - Na^+/Cl^- co-transport in the renal tubule, which is blocked by thiazide diuretics (Chapter 14);
  - the reuptake of neurotransmitters into nerve terminals by a number of transporters selectively blocked by classes of antidepressant drugs (Chapter 22).
- **Enzymes.** Many drugs act on the intracellular or extracellular enzymes that synthesise or degrade the endogenous ligands for extracellular or intracellular receptors, or which are required for growth of bacterial, viral or tumour cells. Table 1.4 provides examples of drug groups that act on enzyme targets. The PDE isoenzymes that regulate second messenger molecules are important drug targets and are listed in Table 1.1. In addition to being sites of drug action, enzymes are involved in inactivating many drugs, while some drugs are administered as inactive precursors (pro-drugs) that are enzymatically activated (Chapter 2).
- **Adhesion molecules**. These regulate the cell-surface interactions of immune cells with endothelial and other cells. Natalizumab is a monoclonal antibody directed against the α_4-integrin component of vascular cell adhesion molecule (VCAM)-1 and is used to inhibit the autoimmune activity of lymphocytes in acute relapsing multiple sclerosis. Other monoclonal antibody-based therapies are targeted at cellular and humoral proteins, including cytokines and intracellular signalling proteins to suppress inflammatory cell proliferation, activity and recruitment in immune disease.
- **Organelles and structural proteins.** Examples include some antimicrobials that interfere with the functioning of ribosomal proteins in bacteria, and some types of anticancer drugs that interrupt mitotic cell division by blocking microtubule formation.

The sites of action of some drugs remain unknown or poorly understood. Conversely, many receptors have

Table 1.4 Examples of enzymes as drug targets

Enzyme	Drug class or use	Examples
Acetylcholinesterase (AChE)	AChE inhibitors (Chapter 27)	Neostigmine, edrophonium, organophosphates
Angiotensin-converting enzyme (ACE)	ACE inhibitors (Chapter 6)	Captopril, perindopril, ramipril
Antithrombin (AT)III	Heparin anticoagulants (*enhancers* of antithrombin III) (Chapter 10)	Enoxaparin, dalteparin
Carbonic anhydrase	Carbonic anhydrase inhibitors (Chapters 14, 50)	Acetazolamide
Cyclo-oxygenase (COX)-1	Nonsteroidal anti-inflammatory drugs (NSAIDs) (Chapter 29)	Ibuprofen, indometacin, naproxen
Cyclo-oxygenase (COX)-2	Selective COX-2 inhibitors (Chapter 29)	Celecoxib, etoricoxib
Dihydrofolate reductase	Folate antagonists (Chapters 51, 52)	Trimethoprim, methotrexate
DOPA decarboxylase	Peripheral decarboxylase inhibitors (PDIs) (Chapter 24)	Carbidopa, benserazide
Coagulation factor Xa	Direct inhibitors of Factor Xa (Chapter 11)	Rivaroxaban
HMG-CoA reductase	Statins (HMG-CoA reductase inhibitors) (Chapter 48)	Atorvastatin, simvastatin
Monoamine oxidases (MAOs) A and B	MAO-A and MAO-B inhibitors (Chapters 22, 24)	Moclobemide, selegiline
Phosphodiesterase (PDE) isoenzymes	PDE inhibitors (Chapters 12, 16)	Theophylline, sildenafil (see Table 1.1)
Reverse transcriptase (RT)	Nucleos(t)ide and nonnucleoside RT inhibitors (Chapter 51)	Zidovudine, efavirenz
Ribonucleotide reductase	Ribonucleotide reductase inhibitor (Chapter 52)	Hydroxycarbamide (hydroxyurea)
Thrombin	Direct thrombin inhibitors (Chapter 11)	Dabigatran
Viral proteases	HIV/hepatitis protease inhibitors (Chapter 51)	Saquinavir, boceprevir
Vitamin K epoxide reductase	Coumarin anticoagulants (Chapter 11)	Warfarin
Xanthine oxidase	Xanthine oxidase inhibitors (Chapter 31)	Allopurinol

been discovered for which the natural ligands are not yet recognised; these orphan receptors may represent targets for novel drugs when their pharmacology is better understood.

PROPERTIES OF RECEPTORS

Receptor binding

The binding of endogenous ligands and most drugs to their receptors is normally reversible; consequently, the intensity and duration of the intracellular changes are dependent on repeated ligand–receptor interactions that continue for as long as the ligand molecules remain in the local environment of the receptors. The duration of activity of a reversible drug therefore depends mainly on its distribution and elimination from the body (pharmacokinetics), which typically requires hours or days (Chapter 2), not on the duration of binding of a drug molecule to its receptor, which may last only a fraction of a second. For a reversible drug, the extent of drug binding to the receptor (receptor occupancy) is proportional to the drug concentration; the higher the concentration, the greater the occupancy. The interaction between a reversible

ligand and its receptor does not involve covalent chemical bonds but weaker, reversible forces, such as:

- ionic bonding between ionisable groups in the ligand (e.g. NH_3^+) and the receptor (e.g. COO^-);
- hydrogen bonding between amino-, hydroxyl-, keto- and other groups in the ligand and the receptor;
- hydrophobic interactions between lipid-soluble sites in the ligand and receptor;
- van der Waals forces, which are very weak interatomic attractions.

The receptor protein is not a rigid structure: binding of the ligand alters the conformation and biological properties of the protein, enabling it to trigger intracellular signalling pathways. There is growing recognition that different ligands may stabilise different conformational states of the same receptor that are distinct from those produced by the endogenous ligand. Rather than simply switching a receptor between inactive and active states, a 'biased' ligand may produce preferential receptor signalling via specific G-protein pathways or by non-G-protein effectors, such as the family of arrestin proteins, leading to different cellular behaviours. Drugs may therefore be developed with functional selectivity to generate different cell responses from the same receptor, in contrast to the classical concept of different responses being generated by drugs acting at different receptors.

Receptor selectivity

There are numerous possible extracellular and intracellular signals produced in the body, which can affect many different processes. Therefore a fundamental property of a useful ligand–receptor interaction is its *selectivity*; that is, the extent to which the receptor can recognise and respond to the correct signals, represented by one ligand or group of related ligands. Some receptors show high selectivity and bind a single endogenous ligand (e.g. acetylcholine is the only endogenous ligand that binds to N_1 nicotinic receptors; see Chapter 4), whereas other receptors are less selective and will bind a number of related endogenous ligands (e.g. the β_1-adrenoceptors on the heart will bind noradrenaline, adrenaline and to some extent dopamine, all of which are catecholamines).

The ability of receptors to recognise and bind the appropriate ligand depends on the intrinsic characteristics of the chemical structure of the ligand. The formulae of a few ligand families that bind to different receptors are shown in Fig. 1.9; differences in structure that determine selectivity of action between receptors may be subtle, such as the those illustrated between the structures of testosterone and progesterone, which nevertheless have markedly different hormonal effects on the body due to their receptor selectivity. Receptors are protein chains folded into tertiary and quaternary structures such that the necessary arrangement of specific binding centres is brought together in a small volume – the receptor site (Fig. 1.10). Receptor selectivity occurs because the three-dimensional organisation of the different sites for reversible binding (such as anion and cation sites, lipid centres and hydrogen-bonding sites) corresponds better to the three-dimensional structure of the endogenous ligand than to that of other ligands.

There may be a number of subtypes of a receptor, all of which can bind the same common ligand but which differ in their ability to recognise particular variants or derivatives of that ligand. The different characteristics of the receptor subtypes therefore allow a drug (or natural ligand) with a particular three-dimensional structure to show selective actions by recognising one receptor preferentially, with fewer unwanted effects from the stimulation or blockade of related receptors. For example, α_1-, α_2-, β_1-, β_2- and β_3-adrenoceptors all bind adrenaline, but isoprenaline, a synthetic derivative of adrenaline, binds selectively to the three β-adrenoceptor subtypes rather than the two α-adrenoceptor subtypes (Chapter 4). As the adrenoceptor subtypes occur to a different extent in different tissues, and produce different intracellular changes when stimulated or blocked, drugs can be designed that have highly selective and localised actions. The cardioselective β-adrenoceptor antagonists such as bisoprolol are selective blockers of the β_1-adrenoceptor subtype that predominates on cardiac smooth muscle, with much less binding to the β_2-adrenoceptors that predominate on bronchial smooth muscle. Although ligands may have a much higher affinity for one receptor subtype over another, this is never absolute, so the term *selective* is preferred over *specific*.

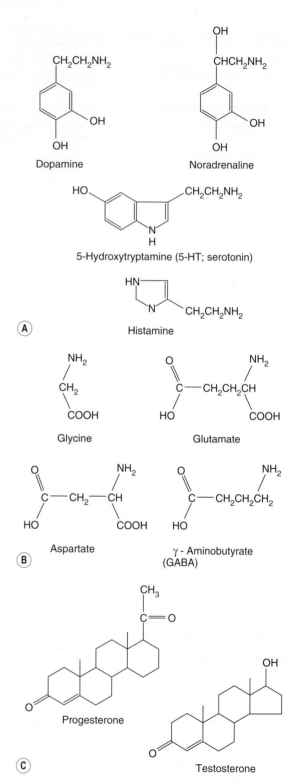

Fig. 1.9 **Groups of related chemicals that show selectivity for different receptor subtypes in spite of similar structure.** (A) Biogenic amines; (B) amino acids; (C) steroids.

Adrenoceptor

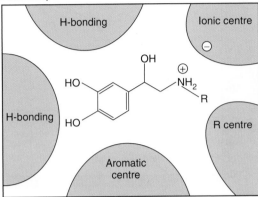

Muscarinic receptor

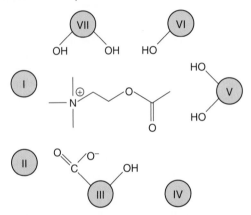

Fig. 1.10 Receptor ligand-binding sites. The coloured areas are schematic representations of the regions of the adrenoceptor (top) and muscarinic receptor (bottom) responsible for binding their respective catecholamine and acetylcholine ligands. In the muscarinic receptor, cross-sections of the seven transmembrane segments are labelled I–VII. Different segments provide different properties (hydrogen bonding, anionic site, etc.) to make up the active binding site.

Traditionally, receptor subtypes were discovered pharmacologically when a new agonist or antagonist compound was found to alter some but not all of the activities of a currently known receptor class. Developments in molecular biology, including the Human Genome Project, have accelerated the recognition and cloning of new receptors and receptor subtypes, including orphan receptors for which the natural ligands are unknown. These developments are important in guiding development of new drugs with greater selectivity and fewer unwanted effects. Based on such information it is recognised that there are multiple types of most receptors, and that there is genetic variation among individuals in the structures, properties and abundance of these receptors, which can lead to differences in drug responses (pharmacogenetic variation; discussed later). Greater understanding of genetic differences underlying human variability in drug responses offers the potential for individualisation of the mode of treatment and selection of the optimal drug and dosage (personalised medicine).

Drug stereochemistry and activity

The three-dimensional spatial organisation of receptors means that the ligand must have the correct configuration to fit the receptor, analogous to fitting a right hand into a right-handed glove. Drugs and other organic molecules show stereoisomerism if they contain four different chemical groups attached to a single carbon atom, or one or more double bonds, with the result that compounds with the same molecular formula can exist in different three-dimensional configurations. If a drug is an equal (racemic) mixture of two stereoisomers, the stereoisomers may show different receptor binding characteristics and biological properties. Most often, one stereoisomer is pharmacologically active while the other is inactive, but in some cases the inactive isomer may be responsible for the unwanted effects of the racemic mixture. Alternatively the two isomers may be active at different receptor subtypes and have synergistic or even opposing actions. The different isomers may also show different rates of metabolism. As a consequence, there has been a trend for the development of single stereoisomers of drugs for therapeutic use; one of the earliest examples was the use of levodopa, the levo-isomer of dihydroxyphenylalanine (DOPA) in Parkinson's disease (Chapter 24).

Receptor numbers

The number of receptors present in, or on the surface of, a cell is not static. There is usually a high turnover of receptors being formed and removed continuously. Cell-membrane receptor proteins are synthesised in the endoplasmic reticulum and transported to the plasma membrane. Regulation of functional receptor numbers in the membrane occurs both by transport to the membrane (often as homo- or heterodimers) and by removal by internalisation. The number of receptors within the cell membrane may be altered by the drug being used for treatment, with either an increase in receptor number (*upregulation*) or a decrease (*downregulation*) and a consequent change in the ability of the drug to effect the desired therapeutic response. This change may be an unwanted loss of drug activity contributing to tolerance to the effects of the drug (e.g. opioids; Chapter 19). As a result, increased doses may be needed to maintain the same activity. Alternatively, the change in receptor number may be an important part of the therapeutic response itself. One example is tricyclic antidepressants (Chapter 22); these produce an immediate increase in the availability of monoamine neurotransmitters, but the therapeutic response is associated with a subsequent, adaptive downregulation in monoamine receptor numbers occurring over several weeks.

PROPERTIES OF DRUG ACTION

Drug actions can show a number of important properties:

- dose–response relationship,
- selectivity,
- potency,
- efficacy.

DOSE–RESPONSE RELATIONSHIPS

Using a purified preparation of a single drug, it is possible to define accurately and reproducibly the relationship between the doses of drug administered (or concentrations applied) and the biological effects (responses) at each dose. The results for an individual drug can be displayed on a dose–response curve. In many biological systems, the typical relationship between an increasing drug dose (or concentration in plasma) and the biological response is a hyperbola, with the response curve rising with a gradually diminishing slope to a plateau, which represents the maximal biological response. Plotting instead the logarithm of the dose (or concentration) against the response (plotted on a linear scale) generates a sigmoid (S-shaped) curve. The sigmoid shape of the curve provides a number of advantages for understanding the relationship between drug dose and response: a very wide range of doses can be accommodated easily on the graph, the maximal response plateau is clearly defined, and the central portion of the curve (between about 15% and 85% of maximum) approximates to a straight line, allowing the collection of fewer data points to delineate the relationship accurately.

Fig. 1.11 shows the log dose–response relationship between a drug and responses it produces at two types of adrenoceptors. In each case, the upward slope of the curve to the right reflects the chemical law that a greater number of reversible molecular interactions of a drug (D) with its receptor (R), due in this case to increasing drug dose, leads to more intracellular signalling by active drug–receptor complexes (DR) and hence a greater response of the cell or tissue (within biological limits). This principle is diametrically opposed to the principle of homeopathy, which argues that serially diluting a drug solution until essentially no drug molecules remain enhances its activity, a belief that is not supported theoretically or experimentally.

Selectivity

As drugs may act preferentially on particular receptor types or subtypes, such as β_1- and β_2-adrenoceptors, it is important to be able to quantify the degree of selectivity of a drug. For example, it is important in understanding the therapeutic efficacy and unwanted effects of the bronchodilator drug salbutamol to recognise that it is approximately 10 times more effective in stimulating the β_2-adrenoceptors in the airway smooth muscle than the β_1-adrenoceptors in the heart.

In pharmacological studies, selectivity is likely to be investigated by measuring the effects of the drug in vitro on different cells or tissues, each expressing only one of the receptors of interest. Comparison of the two log dose–response curves in Fig. 1.11 shows that for a given response, smaller doses of the drug being tested are required to stimulate the β_1-adrenoceptor compared with those required to stimulate the β_2-adrenoceptor; the drug is therefore said to have selectivity of action at the β_1-adrenoceptor. An example might be dobutamine, which is used to selectively stimulate β_1-adrenoceptors on the heart in heart failure. The degree of receptor selectivity is given by the ratio of the doses of the drug required to produce a given level of response via each receptor type. It is clear from Fig. 1.11 that the ratio is highly dose-dependent and that the selectivity disappears at extremely high drug doses,

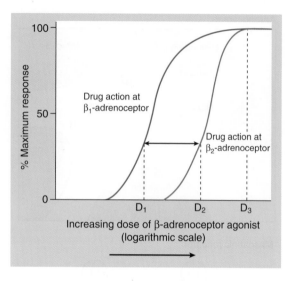

Fig. 1.11 Dose–response relationship and receptor selectivity. Each curve shows the responses (expressed as percentage of maximum on a linear vertical axis) produced by a hypothetical β-adrenoceptor agonist drug at a range of doses shown on a logarithmic horizontal axis. Plotting the logarithmic dose allows a wide range of doses to be shown on the same axes and transforms the dose–response relationship from a hyperbolic curve to a sigmoid curve, in which the central portion is close to a straight line. The two curves illustrate the relative selectivity of the same drug for the β_1-adrenoceptor compared with the β_2-adrenoceptor. At most doses the drug produces β_1-adrenoceptor stimulation with less effect on β_2-adrenoceptors. If dose D_1 is 10 times lower than dose D_2, the selectivity of the drug for the β_1-adrenoceptor is 10-fold higher. This selectivity diminishes at the higher end of the log dose–response curve and is completely lost at a dose (D_3) that produces a maximum response on both β_1- and β_2-adrenoceptors.

because the dose then produces the maximal response of which the biological tissue is capable.

Potency

The potency of a drug in vitro is largely determined by the strength of its binding to the receptor, which is a reflection of the receptor affinity, and by the inherent ability of the drug/receptor complex to elicit downstream signalling events. The more potent a drug, the lower the concentration needed to give a specified response. In Fig. 1.12, drug A_1 is more potent than drug A_2 because it produces a specified level of response at a lower concentration. It is important to recognise that potencies of different drugs are compared using the doses required to produce (or block) the *same response* (often chosen arbitrarily as 50% of the maximal response). The straight-line portions of log dose–response curves are usually parallel for drugs that share a common mechanism of action, so the potency ratio is broadly the same at most response values – for example, 20%, 50% or 80%, but not at 100% response. A drug concentration sufficient to produce half of the greatest response achievable by that

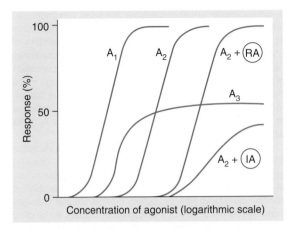

Fig. 1.12 **Concentration–response curves for agonists in the absence and presence of competitive and noncompetitive antagonists.** Responses are plotted at different concentrations of two different full agonists (A_1 being more potent than A_2) and also a partial agonist (A_3), which is unable to produce a maximal response even at high concentrations. Responses are also shown for the full agonist A_2 in the presence of a fixed concentration of a competitive (reversible) antagonist (RA) or a fixed concentration of a noncompetitive (irreversible) antagonist (IA). The competitive antagonist reduces the potency of agonist A_2 (the curve is shifted parallel to the right), but high concentrations of A_2 are able to surmount the effects of the competitive antagonist and produce a maximal response. A noncompetitive antagonist reduces agonist activity either by irreversibly blocking the agonist binding site, or by changing its conformation by binding reversibly or irreversibly at an allosteric site. Unlike competitive antagonists, a noncompetitive antagonist reduces the maximal response even at high agonist concentrations, as shown in the curve A_2 + IA compared with A_2 alone.

drug is described as its EC_{50} (the effective concentration for 50% of the maximal response). The EC_{50} (or ED_{50} if drug *dose* is considered) is a convenient way to compare the potencies of similar drugs; the lower the EC_{50} (or ED_{50}), the more potent the drug.

In vivo the potency of a drug, defined as the dose of the drug required to produce a desired clinical effect, depends not only on its affinity for the receptor, the receptor number and the efficiency of the stimulus–response mechanism, but also on pharmacokinetic variables that determine the delivery of the drug to its site of receptor action (Chapter 2). Therefore the relative potencies of related drugs in vivo may not directly reflect their in vitro receptor-binding properties.

Efficacy

The efficacy of a drug is its ability to produce the maximal response possible for a particular biological system and relates to the extent of functional change that can be imparted to the receptor by the drug, based on its affinity for the receptor and its ability to induce receptor signalling (discussed later). Drug efficacy is arguably of greater clinical importance than potency because a greater therapeutic benefit may be

obtained with a more efficacious drug, while a more potent drug may merely allow a smaller dose to be given for the same clinical benefit. In turn, efficacy and potency need to be balanced against drug toxicity to produce the best balance of benefit and risk for the patient. Drug toxicity and safety are discussed in Chapters 3 and 53.

TYPES OF DRUG ACTION

Drugs can be classified by their receptor action as:

- agonists,
- antagonists,
- partial agonists,
- inverse agonists,
- allosteric modulators,
- enzyme inhibitors or activators,
- nonspecific,
- physiological antagonists.

AGONISTS

An agonist, whether a therapeutic drug or an endogenous ligand, binds to the receptor or site of action and changes the conformation of the receptor to its active state, leading to signalling via second messenger pathways. An agonist shows both *affinity* (the strength of binding for the receptor) and *intrinsic activity* (the extent of conformational change imparted to the receptor leading to receptor signalling). Drugs differ in their affinity and intrinsic activity at the same receptor, as well as between different receptors.

Agonists are traditionally divided into two main groups (Fig. 1.12):

- full agonists (curves A_1 and A_2), which give an increase in response with an increase in concentration until the maximum possible response is obtained for that system;
- partial agonists (curve A_3), which also give an increase in response with increase in concentration, but cannot produce the maximum possible response in the system.

The reasons for this difference, and also a third group of agonists (inverse agonists), are described as follows.

Affinity and intrinsic activity

The affinity of a drug is related to the aggregate strength of the atomic interactions between the drug molecule and its receptor site of action, which determines the relative rates of drug binding and dissociation. The higher the affinity, the lower the drug concentration required to occupy a given fraction of receptors. Affinity therefore determines the drug concentration necessary to produce a certain response and is directly related to the potency of the drug. In Fig. 1.12, drug A_1 is more potent than drug A_2, but both are capable of producing a maximal response (they have the same efficacy as they are full agonists).

Intrinsic activity describes the ability of the bound drug to induce the conformational changes in the receptor that induce receptor signalling. Although affinity is a prerequisite for binding to a receptor, a drug may bind with high affinity but have low intrinsic activity. A drug with zero intrinsic activity is an antagonist (as discussed later).

It should be noted that the rate of binding and rate of dissociation of a reversible drug at its receptor are of negligible importance in determining its rate of onset or duration of effect in vivo, because these depend mainly on the rates of delivery of the drug to, and removal from, the target organ; that is, on the overall absorption, distribution and elimination rates of the drug from the body (Chapter 2).

Spare receptors

Some full agonists that have relatively low intrinsic activity may have to occupy all of the available receptors to produce a maximal response. However, many full agonists have sufficient affinity and intrinsic activity that the maximal response can be produced even though many receptors remain unoccupied; that is, there may be *spare receptors* (or a *receptor reserve*). The concept of spare receptors does not imply a distinct pool of permanently redundant receptors, only that a proportion of the receptor population is unoccupied at a particular point in time. Spare receptors may function to enhance the speed of cellular response, because an excess of available receptors reduces the distance and therefore the time that a ligand molecule needs to diffuse to find an unoccupied receptor; an example is the excess of acetylcholine nicotinic N_2 receptors that contributes to fast synaptic transmission in the neuromuscular junction (Chapter 27).

The concept of spare receptors is also helpful when considering changes in receptor numbers during chronic treatment, particularly receptor downregulation. As maximal responses are often produced at drug concentrations that do not attain 100% receptor occupancy, the same maximal response may still be produced when receptor numbers are downregulated, but only with higher percentage occupancy of the reduced number of receptors. If receptors are downregulated still further, the number remaining may be insufficient to generate a maximal response. Receptor downregulation may therefore contribute to a decline in responsiveness to some drugs during chronic treatment (drug tolerance).

ANTAGONISTS

Pharmacological antagonists (often called 'blockers') reduce the activity of an agonist at the same receptor, and can be contrasted with physiological antagonists (discussed later) that act at another type of receptor or at other sites of action to oppose the physiological response to the agonist. Pharmacological antagonists can be competitive (surmountable) or noncompetitive (nonsurmountable).

A *competitive* antagonist binds reversibly to the ligand binding site of a receptor, either alone or in competition with a drug agonist or natural ligand. It therefore must have affinity for the ligand binding site (which may be as high as that of any agonist), but it has zero intrinsic activity. It therefore cannot cause the conformational change that converts the receptor to its active state and induces intracellular signalling. The antagonist will, however, competitively impair access of agonist molecules to the ligand binding site and thereby reduce receptor activation. The presence of a competitive antagonist may only be detectable by its impairment of agonist activity, and the extent of antagonism will depend on the relative amounts of agonist and antagonist. For example,

β_1-adrenoceptor antagonists lower the heart rate markedly only when it is already elevated by endogenous agonists such as adrenaline and noradrenaline. The reversible binding of competitive antagonists means that the receptor blockade can be overcome (surmounted) by an increase in the concentration of an agonist. Therefore competitive antagonist drugs move the dose–response curve for an agonist in a parallel fashion to the right but do not alter the maximum possible response at high agonist concentrations (as shown in curve A_2 + RA when compared with A_2 alone in Fig. 1.12).

Noncompetitive antagonists either bind to the receptor irreversibly (covalently) at the ligand binding site, denying access to the agonist, or they change the conformation of the receptor by binding reversibly or irreversibly at another (allosteric) site, producing conformational changes that impede the ability of the agonist to access its binding site or block the conformational changes in the receptor needed for intracellular signalling. In either case, the effects of noncompetitive antagonists cannot be negated (surmounted) by competition from the agonist, so they reduce the magnitude of the maximum response that can be produced by any concentration of agonist (as shown by curve A2 + IA in Fig. 1.12). A noncompetitive antagonist will also cause a rightward shift of the agonist log dose–response curve if there is no reserve of spare receptors.

Like agonists, antagonists exhibit varying degrees of selectivity of action. For example, phenoxybenzamine is an antagonist which blocks the ligand binding site of α-adrenoceptors, but not that of β-adrenoceptors. Conversely, propranolol is an antagonist of β-adrenoceptors, but not α-adrenoceptors. Bisoprolol is further selective for the β_1-adrenoceptor subtype, and has less blocking action at β_2-adrenoceptors (or α-adrenoceptors).

PARTIAL AGONISTS

An agonist that is unable to produce a maximal response is a partial agonist (e.g. drug A_3 in Fig. 1.12). Even maximal occupancy of all available receptors produces only a submaximal response due to low intrinsic activity of the partial agonist, for example because of incomplete amplification of the receptor signal via the G-proteins. Despite their name, partial agonists can be considered to have both agonist and antagonist properties, depending on the presence and type of other ligands. A partial agonist usually shows weak agonist activity in the absence of another ligand, and such partial agonism can be blocked by an antagonist. But in the presence of a full agonist, a partial agonist will behave as a weak antagonist because it prevents access to the receptor of a molecule with higher intrinsic ability to initiate receptor signalling; this results in a reduced response. Partial agonism is responsible for the therapeutic efficacy of several drugs, including buspirone, buprenorphine, pindolol and salbutamol. These drugs can act as stabilisers of the variable activity of the natural ligand, as they enhance receptor activity when the endogenous ligand levels are low or zero, but block receptor activity when endogenous ligand levels are high.

INVERSE AGONISTS

The previously provided definitions of agonists, partial agonists and antagonists reflect the classical model of drug–receptor interactions, in which an unoccupied receptor has no signalling activity. It is now recognised that many GPCRs show constitutive signalling independently of an agonist. Inverse agonists were first recognised when some compounds were found to show negative intrinsic activity: they acted alone on unoccupied receptors to produce a change opposite to that caused by an agonist. Inverse agonists shift the receptor equilibrium towards the inactive state, thereby reducing the level of spontaneous receptor activity. An inverse agonist can be distinguished from the typical antagonists discussed previously, which, on their own, bind to the receptor without affecting receptor signalling, as they have zero intrinsic activity ('neutral' or 'silent' antagonists). The action of a neutral antagonist depends on depriving the access of agonists to the receptor; a neutral antagonist can therefore block the effects of either a positive or inverse agonist at a receptor with spontaneous signalling activity.

The role of inverse agonism in the therapeutic effects of drugs remains to be fully elucidated, but a number of drugs exhibit this type of activity (Table 1.5). The same drug may even show a mixed pattern of full or partial agonism, inverse agonism or antagonism at different receptors. Some drugs (e.g. some β-adrenoceptor antagonists) can act as neutral antagonists at a receptor in one tissue and as inverse agonists when the same receptor is expressed in a different tissue, probably due to association of the receptor with different G-proteins.

ALLOSTERIC MODULATORS

Allosteric modulation has been described previously in the context of one type of noncompetitive antagonist, which does not compete directly with an agonist for access to the ligand binding site (also called the orthosteric site), but binds to a different (allosteric) site. Allosteric modulation changes receptor activity by altering the conformation of the orthosteric binding site or of sites involved in intracellular signalling. Allosteric modulators can also enhance the binding of the natural ligand or other drugs to the receptor or enhance their propensity to induce receptor signalling. In some cases,

Table 1.5 Examples of drugs with inverse agonist activity

Receptor	Drugs
α_1-Adrenoceptor	Prazosin, terazosin
β_1-Adrenoceptor	Metoprolol, carvedilol, propranolol
Angiotensin II receptor (AT$_1$)	Losartan, candesartan, irbesartan
Cysteinyl-leukotriene (CysLT$_1$)	Montelukast
Dopamine (D$_2$)	Haloperidol, clozapine, olanzapine
Histamine (H$_1$)	Cetirizine, loratadine
Histamine (H$_2$)	Cimetidine, ranitidine, famotidine
Muscarinic (M$_1$)	Pirenzepine
Opioid (μ, MOR)	Naloxone

an allosteric modulator may not bind to the allosteric site (or only bind poorly) in the absence of the agonist, but its allosteric binding increases when binding of the agonist to the orthosteric site alters receptor conformation. An example of allosteric modulators is the family of benzodiazepine anxiolytic drugs, which allosterically alter the affinity of chloride channels for the neurotransmitter ligand GABA and enhance its inhibitory activity on neurons (Chapter 20).

ENZYME INHIBITORS AND ACTIVATORS

The site of action of many drugs is an enzyme, which may be an intracellular or cell-surface enzyme or one found in plasma or other body fluids. Such drugs act reversibly or irreversibly either on the catalytic site or at an allosteric site on the enzyme to modulate its catalytic activity; most often the effect is inhibition, and important examples of enzyme inhibitors are shown in Table 1.4. An example of an enzyme activator is heparin, which enhances the activity of antithrombin III, a protease that regulates the activity of the coagulation pathway.

NONSPECIFIC ACTIONS

A few drugs produce their desired therapeutic outcome without interaction with a specific site of action on a protein; for example, the diuretic mannitol exerts an osmotic effect in the lumen of the kidney tubule, which reduces reabsorption of water into the blood (Chapter 14).

PHYSIOLOGICAL ANTAGONISTS

Physiological antagonism is said to occur when a drug has a physiological effect opposing that of an agonist but without binding to the same receptor. The increase in heart rate produced by a β_1-adrenoceptor agonist, an effect which mimics the action of the sympathetic autonomic nervous system, can be blocked pharmacologically with an antagonist at β_1-adrenoceptors or physiologically by a muscarinic receptor agonist, which mimics the opposing (parasympathetic) autonomic nervous system. The site of action of the physiological antagonist may be on a different cell, tissue or organ than that of the agonist.

TOLERANCE TO DRUG EFFECTS

Tolerance to drug effects is defined as a decrease in response to repeated doses, often necessitating an increase in dosage to maintain an adequate clinical response. Tolerance may occur through pharmacokinetic changes in the concentrations of a drug available at the receptor or through pharmacodynamic changes at the drug receptor. Pharmacokinetic effects are discussed in Chapter 2; some drugs stimulate their own metabolism, so they are eliminated more rapidly on repeated dosing, and lower concentrations of the drug are available to produce a response.

Most clinically important examples of tolerance arise from pharmacodynamic changes in receptor numbers and in concentration–response relationships. Desensitisation is used to describe both long-term and short-term changes arising from a decrease in response of the receptor. Desensitisation can occur by a number of mechanisms:

- decreased receptor numbers (downregulation), due to decreased transcriptional expression or receptor internalisation;
- decreased receptor binding affinity;
- decreased G-protein coupling;
- modulation of the downstream response to the initial signal.

GPCRs can show rapid desensitisation (within minutes) during continued activation, which occurs through three mechanisms:

- **Homologous desensitisation.** The enzymes activated following selective binding of an agonist to its receptor–G-protein complex include G protein-coupled receptor kinases (GRKs), which interact with the βγ-subunit of the G-protein and inactivate the occupied receptor protein by phosphorylation; a related peptide, arrestin-2, enhances the GRK-mediated desensitisation of the GPCR and may itself activate distinct cell signalling pathways.
- **Heterologous desensitisation.** Also known as cross-desensitisation, this occurs when an agonist at one receptor causes loss of sensitivity to other agonists. The agonist increases intracellular cAMP which activates protein kinase A or C; these phosphorylate the cross-desensitised receptors (whether occupied or not), and members of the arrestin family prevent them from coupling with G-proteins. Other mechanisms of heterologous desensitisation exist.
- **Receptor internalisation.** Internalisation can occur within minutes when constant activation of a GPCR makes the receptor unavailable for further agonist action by uncoupling the G-protein from the receptor.

The phosphorylated receptor protein is endocytosed and may undergo intracellular dephosphorylation prior to re-entering the cytoplasmic membrane.

Downstream modulation of the signal may also occur through feedback mechanisms or simply through depletion of some essential cofactor. An example of the latter is the depletion of the thiol (-SH or sulphydryl) groups necessary for the generation of nitric oxide during chronic administration of organic nitrates (Chapter 5).

GENETIC VARIATION IN DRUG RESPONSES

Biological characteristics, including responses to drug administration, vary among individuals, and genetic differences can contribute to these inter-individual variations. For most drugs, the nature of the response is broadly similar in different individuals, but the magnitude of the response to the same dose can differ markedly, at least partly due to genetic factors. Such variability creates the need to individualise drug dosages for different people.

Drug responses may follow a unimodal (Gaussian) distribution, reflecting the sum of many small genetic variations in receptors, enzymes or transporters that respond to or handle the drug (Fig. 1.13A). Genetic variation may also give rise to discrete subpopulations of individuals in which a drug shows distinctly different responses (see Fig. 1.13B), such that some individuals may have no response to a standard dose, while others show toxicity. Understanding genetic variation is of increasing importance in drug development (see Chapter 3) because it allows the possibility of genetic

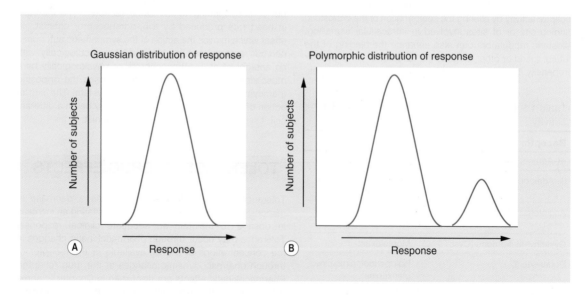

Fig. 1.13 **Inter-individual variation in response.** The graphs show the numbers of individual subjects in a population plotted against their varying levels of response to a single dose of a drug. (A) In the unimodal distribution most individuals show a middling response and the overall shape is a normal (Gaussian) distribution. Part of this variability may result from polymorphism in multiple genes encoding drug receptors and proteins involved in the drug's absorption and elimination. (B) The bimodal distribution shows discrete responder and nonresponder subgroups, possibly due to a single genetic polymorphism in a drug receptor or drug-metabolising enzyme.

screening to optimise drug and dosage selection (personalised or individualised medicine).

Pharmacogenetics has been defined as the study of genetic variation that results in differing responses to drugs. Such variation may arise from genetic factors that alter the structure, expression or regulation of drug targets (pharmacodynamic effects) or that change the metabolic fates of drugs in the body, usually by altering proteins involved in their absorption, distribution or elimination (pharmacokinetic effects, discussed in Chapter 2). Pharmacogenetic research has been undertaken for many decades, largely in relation to variability in vivo, and has often used classic genetic techniques such as studies of patterns of inheritance in twins.

Pharmacogenomics has been defined as the investigation of variation in DNA and RNA characteristics related to drug response, and the term refers mainly to genome-wide approaches that define the presence of single-nucleotide polymorphisms (SNPs) which affect the activity of the gene product. Molecular biological techniques have predicted more than 3 million SNPs in the human genome. SNPs can be:

- in the upstream regulatory sequence of a coding gene, which can result in increased or decreased expression of the gene product (this product remains identical to the normal or 'wild-type' gene product);
- in the coding region of the gene resulting in a gene product with an altered amino acid sequence (this may have higher activity, although this is unlikely; similar activity; lower activity or no activity at all, compared with the wild-type protein);
- inactive, because they are in noncoding or nonregulatory regions of the genome, or, if in a coding region, because the base change does not alter the amino acid encoded, due to the redundancy of the genetic code.

There is still a major challenge in defining the functional consequences of the large numbers of identified SNPs (functional genomics), particularly in the context of combinations of genetic variants (haplotypes). Such studies often require very large numbers of subjects to allow comparison of function in multiple, small haplotype subgroups.

Rapid advances in molecular biology have allowed analysis of interindividual differences in the sequences of many genes encoding drug receptors and proteins involved in drug metabolism and transport. Polymorphism in the latter is likely to have the greatest impact on dosage selection (Chapter 2), while polymorphism in drug targets may be more important in determining the optimal drug for a particular condition. For example, genetic variation in angiotensin AT_1 receptors, β_1-adrenoceptors and Ca^{2+} ion channels may determine the relative effectiveness of angiotensin II receptor antagonists, β-adrenoceptor antagonists (β-blockers) and calcium channel blockers in the treatment of essential hypertension.

In practice, although genetic polymorphism has been reported in many receptor types and these have been a major focus of research in relation to the aetiology of disease, relatively few studies to date have demonstrated a clear influence on drug responses. Common polymorphisms have been identified in the human β_2-adrenoceptor gene *ADRB2*, and certain variants have been associated with differences in receptor downregulation and loss of therapeutic response in people with asthma while using β_2-adrenoceptor agonist inhalers (Chapter 12). The clinical response in people with asthma to treatment with leukotriene modulator drugs is influenced by genetic polymorphism in enzymes of the leukotriene (5-lipoxygenase) pathway. Variants in the epidermal growth factor receptor (EGFR), an RTK, have been reported to predict tumour response to the EGFR inhibitor gefitinib in individuals with nonsmall-cell lung cancer. Such examples may support genotyping to target drug treatments to those individuals most likely to respond.

Conversely, pharmacogenetic information may be used to avoid a particular treatment in people likely to experience serious adverse reactions to a specific drug. Variation in human leucocyte antigen (HLA) genes has been associated with adverse skin and liver reactions to several drugs, including abacavir, an antiretroviral drug used in HIV infection.

Compared with pharmacodynamic targets, genetic variation has been more extensively characterised in drug-metabolising enzymes, particularly in cytochrome P450 isoenzymes and others involved in glucuronidation, acetylation and methylation. Gene variations in drug-metabolising enzymes are discussed at the end of Chapter 2. Detailed information on human genotypic variation can be found in the Online Mendelian Inheritance in Man (OMIM) database (www.ncbi.nlm.nih.gov/omim). Therapeutic exploitation of genotypic differences will require specific information about individuals based on detailed genetic testing. Until such genetic information is routinely incorporated in clinical trials, careful monitoring of clinical response will remain the best guide to successful treatment.

SUMMARY

The therapeutic benefits of drugs arise from their ability to interact selectively with target receptors, most of which are regulatory molecules involved in the control of cellular and systemic functions by endogenous ligands. Drugs may also cause unwanted effects; judging the balance of benefit and risk is at the heart of safe and effective prescribing. Increasing knowledge of the complexity of receptor pharmacology and improvements in drug selectivity offer the promise of safer drugs in the future, especially when information on genetic variation is more routinely available.

SELF-ASSESSMENT

True/false questions

1. Clinical pharmacology is the study of drugs that doctors use to treat disease.
2. Drugs act at receptors only on the external surface of cells.
3. Diluting drugs enhances their pharmacological effects.
4. Drugs produce permanent biochemical changes in their receptors.
5. Plotting drug dose (or plasma concentration) against response usually produces a sigmoid curve.
6. The EC_{50} is the concentration of drug that produces a half-maximal response.
7. On a log dose–response plot, the drug with a curve to the right is more potent than a drug with a curve on the left.

8. A receptor antagonist is defined as a drug with zero affinity for the receptor.
9. A competitive antagonist shifts the log dose–response curve of an agonist to the right, without affecting the maximal response.
10. A partial agonist is one that, even at its highest dose, cannot achieve the same maximal response as a full agonist at the same receptor.
11. A full agonist achieves a maximal response when all its receptors are occupied.
12. Changes in receptor numbers can cause tolerance to drug effects.

ANSWERS

True/false answers

1. **True**. Clinical pharmacology also deals with drugs used in disease prevention and diagnosis, and in the alleviation of pain and suffering.
2. **False**. While many types of receptors are found in cell membranes, including ion channels, GPCRs and tyrosine kinase receptors, other drug targets, including steroid receptors and many enzymes (e.g. cyclo-oxygenase, PDE), are intracellular and others are humoral, such as thrombin in plasma.
3. **False**. The relationship between the dose or concentration of a drug and the response may be complex but is typically dependent on the number of interactions between the drug molecules and their molecular target, a consequence of the Law of Mass Action, and so are usually greater at higher drug concentrations, within biological limits.
4. **False**. Molecular interactions between most drugs and their receptors are typically transient, and the conformational changes induced in the receptor are reversible; irreversible drugs may act by covalent chemical bonding.

5. **False**. Plotting drug dose or plasma concentration against response typically produces a hyperbola; a sigmoid (S-shaped) curve is produced by plotting the logarithm of dose or concentration against the response.
6. **True**. The EC_{50} (or ED_{50}) is the concentration (or dose) effective in producing 50% of the maximal response and is a convenient way of comparing drug potencies.
7. **False.** A drug with its log dose–response curve to the left is the more potent, as it produces a given level of response at a lower dose.
8. **False**. A full ('neutral' or 'silent') antagonist must have affinity to bind to its receptor, but it has zero intrinsic ability to activate the receptor. Partial agonists can also have an antagonist effect in the presence of a full agonist. Receptors with inherent signalling activity, even when unoccupied, can be antagonised by inverse agonists.
9. **True**. A fixed dose of a competitive antagonist shifts the log dose–response curve of the agonist to the right in a parallel fashion; it can be surmounted by increasing the dose of agonist, so that the same maximal response can be achieved.
10. **True**. A partial agonist has low intrinsic ability to induce conformational change in the receptor so it does not elicit a maximal response even with full receptor occupancy.
11. **False**. Many full agonists are able to elicit a maximal response when less than 100% of receptors are occupied; the unoccupied receptors are termed 'spare receptors'.
12. **True**. Tolerance may be caused by desensitisation, internalisation or downregulation of receptors, requiring higher drug doses to maintain the same response. Tolerance also often results from enhanced drug elimination that alters the concentrations of drugs available to interact with the receptor.

FURTHER READING

Alexander, S.P.H., Davenport, A.P., Kelly, E., et al., 2015. IUPHAR/BPS concise guide to pharmacology 2015–16. Br. J. Pharmacol. 172, 5729–6202.

Baker, E.H., Pryce Roberts, A., Wilde, K., et al., 2011. Development of a core drug list towards improving prescribing education and reducing errors in the UK. Br. J. Clin. Pharmacol. 71, 190–198.

Katritch, V., Cherezov, V., Stevens, R.C., 2012. Diversity and modularity of G protein-coupled receptor structures. Trends Pharmacol. Sci. 33, 17–27.

Kenakin, T., 2004. Principles: receptor theory in pharmacology. Trends Pharmacol. Sci. 25, 186–192.

Keravis, T., Lugnier, C., 2012. Cyclic nucleotide phosphodiesterase (PDE) isozymes as targets of the intracellular signalling network: benefits of PDE inhibitors in various diseases and perspectives for future therapeutic developments. Br. J. Pharmacol. 165, 1288–1305.

Khilnani, G., Khilnani, A.J., 2011. Inverse agonism and its therapeutic significance. Indian J. Pharmacol. 43, 492–501.

Luttrell, L.M., 2014. More than just a hammer: ligand 'bias' and pharmaceutical discovery. Mol. Endocrinol. 28, 281–294.

Maxwell, S., Walley, T., 2003. Teaching safe and effective prescribing in UK medical schools: a core curriculum for tomorrow's doctors. Br. J. Clin. Pharmacol. 55, 496–503.

Rosenbaum, D.M., Rasmussen, S.G.F., Kobilka, B.K., 2009. The structure and function of G-protein-coupled receptors. Nature 459, 356–363.

Schöneberg, T., Kleinau, G., Brüser, A., 2016. What are they waiting for? – Tethered agonism in G protein-coupled receptors. Pharmacol. Res. http://dx.doi.org/10.1016/j.phrs.2016.03.027.

Wang, L., McLeod, H.L., Weinshilboum, R.M., 2011. Genomics and drug response. N. Engl. J. Med. 364, 1144–1153.

Examples of cell surface receptor families and their properties

This is a reference list of members of important families of GPCRs, LGICs and VGICs, many of which are therapeutic drug targets. Examples of agonists and antagonists are also shown; these include endogenous ligands and some drugs not currently in clinical use. For further information see the relevant sections of Alexander, S.P.H., et al., 2015. IUPHAR/BPS concise guide to pharmacology 2015–16. *Br. J. Pharmacol.* 172, 5729–6202 (available at http://guidetopharmacology.org). For examples of important intracellular receptors and enzymes targeted by therapeutic drugs, see Tables 1.2 and 1.4.

Type	Typical location(s)	Principal transduction mechanism	Major biological actions	Agonists	Antagonists
G-protein-coupled receptors (GPCRs)					
Cholinergic					
Muscarinic					
M_1	CNS, salivary, gastric; minor role in autonomic ganglia	G_q	Neurotransmission in CNS, gastric secretion	*Nonselective for all M receptors:* carbachol	Pirenzepine *Nonselective for all M receptors:* atropine, ipratropium, oxybutynin, tolterodine
M_2	Heart, CNS	G_i	Bradycardia, smooth muscle contraction (GI tract, airways, bladder)		
M_3	Smooth muscles, secretory glands, CNS	G_q	Contraction, secretion	I	Darifenacin, tiotropium
M_4	CNS	G_i	Unclear		
M_5	CNS	G_q	Unclear		
Adrenergic					
α-Adrenoceptors					
α_1 (α_{1A}, α_{1B}, α_{1D})	CNS, postsynaptic in sympathetic nervous system, human prostate (α_{1A})	G_q	Contraction of arterial smooth muscle, decrease in contractions of gut, contraction of prostate tissue	Phenylephrine, methoxamine, NA $\geq$ Adr	Prazosin, indoramin (tamsulosin α_{1A})
α_2 (α_{2A}, α_{2B}, α_{2C})	Presynaptic (in both α- and β-adrenergic neurons)	G_i	Decreased NA release	Clonidine, Adr > NA (oxymetazoline α_{2A})	Yohimbine
β-Adrenoceptors					
β_1	CNS, heart (nodes and myocardium), kidney	G_s	Increased force and rate of cardiac contraction, renin release	Dobutamine, NA > Adr	Atenolol, metoprololol
β_2	Bronchial smooth muscle, also widespread	G_s	Bronchodilation, decrease in contraction of gut, glycogenolysis	Salbutamol, salmeterol, terbutaline, Adr > NA	Butoxamine
β_3	Adipocytes, bladder	G_s	Lipolysis, bladder emptying	Adr = NA	–
Cannabinoids					
CB_1	Cortex, hippocampus, amygdala, basal ganglia, cerebellum	$G_{i/o}$	Behaviour, pain, nausea, stimulation of appetite, addiction, depression, hypotension	Tetrahydrocannabinol, anandamide, 2-arachidonylglycerol	Rimonabant

Examples of cell surface receptor families and their properties (cont'd)

Type	Typical location(s)	Principal transduction mechanism	Major biological actions	Agonists	Antagonists
CB$_2$	Leucocytes, osteocytes	G$_{i/o}$	Immunity, bone growth	Tetrahydrocannabinol	
Dopamine					
D$_1$	CNS (N, O, P, S – *see footnote for key to CNS areas*), kidney, heart	G$_s$	Vasodilation in kidney	Fenoldepam	Chlorpromazine
D$_2$	CNS (C, N, O, SN), pituitary gland, chemoreceptor trigger zone, gastrointestinal tract	G$_i$	Cognition (schizophrenia), prolactin secretion, nigrostrial control of movement, memory	Cabergoline, pramipexole, ropinirole, rotigotine	Butyrophenones, chlorpromazine domperidone, metoclopramide, sulpiride
D$_3$	CNS (F, Me, Mi) (limbic system)	G$_i$	Cognition, emotion	Cabergoline, pramipexole, ropinirole, rotigotine	Chlorpromazine, sulpiride
D$_4$	CNS, heart	G$_i$	Cognition (schizophrenia)	Cabergoline, ropinirole, rotigotine	Chlorpromazine, clozapine
D$_5$	CNS (Hi, Hy)	G$_s$	Similar to D$_1$		
5-Hydroxytryptamine (5-HT, serotonin)					
5-HT$_{1A}$	CNS, blood vessels	G$_i$	Anxiety, appetite, mood, sleep	Buspirone	
5-HT$_{1B}$	CNS, blood vessels	G$_i$	Vasoconstriction presynaptic inhibition	Sumatriptan, eletriptan	
5-HT$_{1D}$	CNS, blood vessels	G$_i$	Anxiety, vasoconstriction	Sumatriptan, eletriptan	Metergoline
5-HT$_{1E}$	CNS, blood vessels	G$_i$			
5-HT$_{1F}$	CNS	G$_i$		Sumatriptan, eletriptan	
5-HT$_{2A}$	CNS, GI tract, platelets, smooth muscle	G$_q$	Schizophrenia, platelet aggregation, vasodilation/ vasoconstriction	LSD, psilocybin	Ketanserin, atypical antipsychotics, e.g. olanzapine
5-HT$_{2B}$	CNS, GI tract, platelets	G$_q$	Contraction, morphogenesis		
5-HT$_{2C}$	CNS, GI tract, platelets	G$_q$	Satiety		
5-HT$_4$	CNS, myenteric plexus, smooth muscle	G$_s$	Anxiety, memory, gut motility	Metoclopramide, renzapride	
5-HT$_{5a}$	CNS	G$_i$	Anxiety, memory, mood		
5-HT$_6$	CNS	G$_s$	Anxiety, memory, mood		
5-HT$_7$	CNS, GI, blood vessels	G$_s$	Anxiety, memory, mood	LSD	
Histamine					
H$_1$	CNS, endothelium, smooth muscle	G$_q$	Sedation, sleep, vascular permeability, inflammation		Cetirizine, desloratadine

Examples of cell surface receptor families and their properties (cont'd)

Type	Typical location(s)	Principal transduction mechanism	Major biological actions	Agonists	Antagonists
H_2	CNS, cardiac muscle, stomach	G_s	Gastric acid secretion	Dimaprit	Cimetidine, ranitidine
H_3	CNS (presynaptic), myenteric plexus	G_i	Appetite, cognition		Thioperamide
H_4	Eosinophils, basophils, mast cells	G_i		4-Methylhistamine	

Gamma-aminobutyric acid receptor type B (GABA$_B$)

Type	Typical location(s)	Principal transduction mechanism	Major biological actions	Agonists	Antagonists
$GABA_B$	Brain neurons, glial cells, spinal motor neurons and interneurons	G_i	Inhibition of neurotransmission in brain and spinal cord	Baclofen	

Peptides

Angiotensin II

Type	Typical location(s)	Principal transduction mechanism	Major biological actions	Agonists	Antagonists
AT_1	Blood vessels, adrenal cortex, brain	G_q/G_o	Vasoconstriction, salt retention, aldosterone synthesis, increased noradrenergic activity, cardiac hypertrophy		Candesartan, losartan, valsartan
AT_2	Blood vessels, endothelium, adrenal cortex, brain	$G_{i/o}$, tyrosine and ser/thr phosphatases	Weak vasodilation (endothelial nitric oxide release), foetal development, vascular growth		

Bradykinin

Type	Typical location(s)	Principal transduction mechanism	Major biological actions	Agonists	Antagonists
B_1 (induced)	Widespread (induced by injury, cytokines)	G_q	Acute inflammation; stimulates nitric oxide synthesis	ACE inhibitors (indirect, by blocking bradykinin breakdown)	
B_2 (constitutive)		G_q	Chronic inflammation. Most kinin actions (vasodilation, pain)		Icatibant

Endothelin

Type	Typical location(s)	Principal transduction mechanism	Major biological actions	Agonists	Antagonists
ET_A	Endothelium	G_q	Vasoconstriction, angiogenesis		Bosentan
ET_B	Endothelium	G_q, G_i	Indirect vasodilation (nitric oxide release), direct vasoconstriction, natriuresis		Bosentan

Opioids

Type	Typical location(s)	Principal transduction mechanism	Major biological actions	Agonists	Antagonists
DOP (δ), KOP (κ), MOP (μ), nociception	Brain, spinal cord, peripheral sensory neurons	G_i	Analgesia, sedation, respiratory depression	Endogenous opioids, opioid drugs (morphine)	Naloxone, naltrexone

Protease-activated receptors

Type	Typical location(s)	Principal transduction mechanism	Major biological actions	Agonists	Antagonists
PAR_1, PAR_2, PAR_3, PAR_4	Platelets, endothelial cells, epithelial cells, myocytes, neurons	G_q, G_i	Activated by proteolytic cleavage	Trypsin, thrombin, tryptase	

Examples of cell surface receptor families and their properties (cont'd)

Type	Typical location(s)	Principal transduction mechanism	Major biological actions	Agonists	Antagonists
Vasopressin and oxytocin					
Vasopressin V_{1a}	Brain, uterus, blood vessels, platelets	G_q	Vasoconstriction, platelet aggregation	Desmopressin	Conivaptan, demeclocycline
Vasopressin V_{1b}	Pituitary, brain	G_q	Modulates ACTH secretion	Desmopressin	Conivaptan, demeclocycline
Vasopressin V_2	Kidney	G_s	Antidiuretic effect on collecting duct and ascending limb of loop of Henle	Desmopressin	Conivaptan demeclocycline, tolvaptan
Oxytocin OXT	Brain, uterus	G_q, G_i	Lactation, uterine contraction, CNS actions (mood)	Oxytocin > arginine-vasopressin	Atosiban
Purinergic receptors (purinoceptors)					
Adenosine A_1	Heart, lung	G_i	Cardiac depression, vasoconstriction, bronchoconstriction		Methylxanthines
Adenosine A_{2A}	Widespread	G_s	Vasodilation, inhibition of platelet aggregation, bronchodilation	Regadenoson	Methylxanthines
Adenosine A_{2B}	Leucocytes	G_s	Bronchoconstriction		Methylxanthines
Adenosine A_3	Leucocytes	G_i	Inflammatory mediator release		Methylxanthines
Purinergic P2Y family ($P2Y_1$, $P2Y_2$, $P2Y_4$, $P2Y_6$, $P2Y_{11}$–$P2Y_{14}$)	Widespread	G_q, G_s or G_i	Depends upon G-protein coupling	ATP, ADP, UTP, UDP, UDP-glucose	$P2Y_{12}$: clopidogrel, ticlopidine
Ligand-gated ion channels (LGICs)					
Nicotinic N_1	Autonomic ganglia	LGIC	Ganglionic neurotransmission	Carbachol, nicotine	Trimetaphan, mecamylamine
Nicotinic N_2	Neuromuscular junction	LGIC	Skeletal muscle contraction	Nicotine, suxamethonium (depolarising)	Gallamine, vecuronium, atracurium
Serotonin $5\text{-}HT_3$	CNS (A), enteric nerves, sensory nerves	Ligand-gated Na^+/K^+ channel	Emesis		Granisetron, ondansetron, metoclopramide
$GABA_A$	Brain neurons, spinal motor neurons and interneurons	Ligand-gated Cl^- channel (open)	Inhibition of neurotransmission in brain and spinal cord	Muscimol, barbiturates, benzodiazepines, zolpidem	Picrotoxin, flumazenil (benzodiazepine antagonist)
Glycine GlyR	Brain neurons, spinal motor neurons and interneurons	Ligand-gated Cl^- channel (open)	Inhibition of neurotransmission in brain and spinal cord	Intravenous anaesthetics, alanine, taurine	Strychnine, caffeine, tropisetron, endocannabinoids
Ionotropic glutamate (NMDA) receptor	CNS (B, C, sensory pathways)	Ligand-gated Ca^{2+} channel (slow)	Synaptic plasticity, excitatory transmitter release; excessive amounts may cause neuronal damage	NMDA	Ketamine, phencyclidine, memantine

Examples of cell surface receptor families and their properties (cont'd)

Type	Typical location(s)	Principal transduction mechanism	Major biological actions	Agonists	Antagonists
Ionotropic glutamate (kainate) receptor	CNS (Hi)	Ligand-gated Ca^{2+} channel (fast)	Synaptic plasticity, transmitter release	Kainate	Topiramate
Ionotropic glutamate (AMPA) receptor	CNS (similar to NMDA receptors)	Ligand-gated Ca^{2+} channel (fast)	Synaptic plasticity, transmitter release	AMPA	Topiramate
Purinergic P2X family (P2X$_1$–P2X$_7$)	CNS, autonomic nervous system (P2X$_2$), smooth muscle (P2X$_1$), leucocytes	LGICs (Na$^+$, Ca^{2+}, K$^+$)	Neuronal depolarisation, influx of Na$^+$ and Ca^{2+}, efflux of K$^+$	ATP	Suramin
Voltage-gated ion channels (VGICs)					
Epithelial sodium channel (ENaC)	Renal tubule, airways, colon	Na$^+$ channel, tonically open	Sodium reabsorption in aldosterone-sensitive distal tubule and collecting duct	Expression upregulated by aldosterone	Amiloride, triamterene
L-type calcium channels (Ca$_v$1.1–1.4)	Widespread	Voltage-gated Ca^{2+} channels (dihydropyridine-sensitive)	Vascular and cardiac smooth muscle contraction, prolong cardiac action potential		Nifedipine, amlodipine, diltiazem, verapamil
Ryanodine (RyR1, RyR2, RyR3)	Skeletal muscle (RyR1), heart (RyR2), widespread (RyR3)	Ca^{2+} channels	Calcium-induced Ca^{2+} release (CICR)	Cytosolic Ca^{2+}, ATP, ryanodine, caffeine	Dantrolene

Abbreviations: ACE, Angiotensin-converting enzyme; ACTH, adrenocorticotropic hormone (corticotropin); Adr, adrenaline; AMPA, α-amino-3-hydroxy-5-methyl-4-isoxazole propionic acid; CNS, central nervous system; GI, gastrointestinal; LSD, lysergic acid diethylamide; NA, noradrenaline; NMDA, N-methyl D-aspartate.
Key to CNS areas: A, Area postrema; B, basal ganglia; C, caudate putamen; F, frontal cortex; Hi, hippocampus; Hy, hypothalamus; Me, medulla; Mi, midbrain: N, nucleus accumbens; O, olfactory tubercle; P, putamen; S, striatum; SN, substantia nigra.

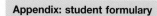

Appendix: student formulary

This student formulary used for educational purposes at Southampton University Faculty of Medicine is adapted from the formulary originally described by Maxwell and Walley (*Br. J. Clin. Pharmacol.* 2003; 55:496–503). See also the lists of commonly prescribed drugs in Baker et al. (*Br. J. Clin. Pharmacol.* 2011; 71:190–198) and the World Health Organisation (WHO) Model List of Essential Medicines (www.who.int/medicines/publications/essentialmedicines/en/).

Therapeutic problem	Core drugs
Gastrointestinal system	
Emergency treatment of poisoning	Adsorbant: activated charcoal Paracetamol antidotes, e.g. acetylcysteine, methionine Opioid antagonist, e.g. naloxone Organophosphate antidote, e.g. pralidoxime
Dyspepsia, GORD and gastric ulcer healing	Antacids, e.g. magnesium salts Compound alginates, e.g. Gaviscon Proton pump inhibitors, e.g. omeprazole, lansoprazole H_2 receptor antagonists, e.g. ranitidine, cimetidine *Helicobacter pylori* antibiotics: clarithromycin, amoxicillin, metronidazole Motility stimulants, e.g. metoclopramide Others: misoprostol, sulcralfate
Inflammatory bowel disease (ulcerative colitis, Crohn's disease)	Corticosteroids, e.g. prednisolone Aminosalicylates, e.g. sulfasalazine, mesalazine Cytokine inhibitors, e.g. infliximab
Antibiotic-associated colitis	Antibiotics for *Clostridium difficile*, e.g. metronidazole, vancomycin
Diarrhoea	Oral rehydration therapy Opiate antimotility drugs, e.g. loperamide
Constipation	Bulk-forming laxatives, e.g. ispaghula, methylcellulose Stimulant laxatives, e.g. senna, docusate Osmotic laxatives, e.g. magnesium hydroxide, lactulose
Antispasmodics	Antimuscarinics, e.g. atropine, hyoscine Others: mebeverine
Cardiovascular system	
Hypertension	β-Adrenoceptor antagonists, e.g. atenolol α-Adrenoceptor antagonists, e.g. doxazosin Centrally acting drugs, e.g. clonidine Angiotensin-converting enzyme (ACE) inhibitors, e.g. captopril, ramipril, perindopril Angiotensin receptor antagonists, e.g. candesartan, losartan Thiazide diuretics, e.g. bendroflumethazide, indapamide Loop diuretics, e.g. furosemide Potassium-sparing diuretics, e.g. amiloride, spironolactone Compound potassium-sparing diuretic: co-amilofruse Calcium channel antagonists, e.g. nifedipine verapamil Potassium channel openers, e.g. minoxidil, nicorandil
Heart failure	Many of the above plus the following positive inotropic drugs: Cardiac glycosides, e.g. digoxin PDE inhibitors, e.g. milrinone β-Adrenoceptor antagonist: bisoprolol
Acute coronary syndrome (angina, myocardial infarction)	Many drugs listed under hypertension plus the following: Inhibitors of platelet aggregation, e.g. low-dose aspirin, dipyridamole, clopidogrel, abciximab Thrombolytics, e.g. streptokinase, tenecteplase Heparin (unfractionated) Heparins (low molecular weight), e.g. enoxaparin Oral anticoagulants, e.g. warfarin
Hyperlipidaemia	Statins, e.g. simvastatin, atorvastatin, pravastatin, rosuvastatin Fibrates, e.g. gemfibrozil, fenofibrate
Arrhythmias	Antiarrhythmic drugs, e.g. digoxin, adenosine, amiodarone, lidocaine, β-adrenoceptor antagonists, calcium channel blockers

Appendix: student formulary (cont'd)

Therapeutic problem	Core drugs
Respiratory system	
Asthma, COPD, respiratory failure	Oxygen β_2-Adrenoceptor agonists, e.g. salbutamol, salmeterol Antimuscarinics, e.g. ipratropium, tiotropium Methylxanthines, e.g. theophylline, aminophylline PDE type 4 inhibitor, e.g. roflumilast Leukotriene antagonists, e.g. montelukast Antiallergic drugs, e.g. cromoglicate, nedocromil Magnesium sulphate Inhaled corticosteroids, e.g. beclometasone, fluticasone Oral corticosteroid, e.g. prednisolone β_2-Agonist/corticosteroid coformulations, e.g. Seretide
Allergy, anaphylaxis	Antihistamines, e.g. cetirizine, loratadine Adrenaline, e.g. Epipen
Cough suppression	Dextromethorphan, codeine
Central nervous system	
Insomnia, anxiety	Benzodiazepines, e.g. temazepam, diazepam Z-drugs, e.g. zopiclone, zolpidem Others, e.g. buspirone, propranolol
Schizophrenia, mania	Classical antipsychotics, e.g. chlorpromazine, haloperidol, flupentixol Atypical antipsychotics, e.g. olanzapine, risperidone, quetiapine Depot preparations, e.g. fluphenazine decanoate Mood stabilisers, e.g. lithium
Depression	Tricyclic antidepressants (TCAs), e.g. amitriptyline Selective serotonin reuptake inhibitors (SSRIs), e.g. fluoxetine, citalopram, sertraline Serotonin-noradrenaline reuptake inhibitors, e.g. venlafaxine Monoamine oxidase-B inhibitors, e.g. moclobemide Others, e.g. mirtazepine
Analgesia	Nonsteroidal anti-inflammatory drugs (NSAIDs): see section on musculoskeletal disease Compound analgesics, e.g. co-codamol, co-dydramol Moderately potent opioid analgesics, e.g. tramadol Potent opioid analgesics, e.g. codeine, morphine, fentanyl
Nausea and vertigo	Dopamine antagonists, e.g. metoclopramide Serotonin receptor antagonists, e.g. ondansetron Muscarinic receptor antagonists, e.g. hyoscine Others: betahistine
Migraine	*Acute*: 5-HT$_1$ receptor agonists, e.g. sumatriptan *Prophylaxis*: β-adrenoceptor antagonists, e.g. propranolol
Epilepsy	Anticonvulsant drugs, e.g. diazepam, carbamazepine, clonazepam, ethosuximide, gabapentin, lamotrigine, phenytoin, tiagabine, valproate
Parkinson's disease	Levodopa/DOPA decarboxylase coformulations, e.g. co-careldopa, co-beneldopa Dopamine receptor agonists, e.g. ropinirole COMT inhibitors, e.g. entacapone MAO-B inhibitors: selegiline, rasagiline Antimuscarinic drugs, e.g. procyclidine
Dementia (Alzheimer's)	Anticholinesterases, e.g. donepezil NMDA receptor antagonists, e.g. memantine

Appendix: student formulary (cont'd)

Therapeutic problem	Core drugs
Infectious diseases	
Community- and hospital-acquired infections	Penicillins, e.g. benzylpenicillin
	Penicillinase-resistant penicillins, e.g. flucloxacillin
	Broad-spectrum penicillins, e.g. amoxicillin, co-amoxiclav
	Cephalosporins, e.g. cefalexin, cefuroxime
	Tetracyclines, e.g. oxytetracycline
	Folate inhibitors, e.g. trimethoprim
	Aminoglycosides, e.g. gentamicin
	Vancomycin (for *C. difficile*)
	Macrolides, e.g. erythromycin
	Chloramphenicol
	Quinolones, e.g. ciprofloxacin
	Metronidazole (for anaerobes and protozoans)
	Antituberculosis drugs, e.g. isoniazid, rifampicin, ethambutol
	Antifungal drugs, e.g. amphotericin, fluconazole, miconazole, terbinafine
	Viral DNA polymerase inhibitors, e.g. aciclovir (herpes), ganciclovir (CMV)
	Neuraminidase inhibitors, e.g. zanamivir (influenza)
	Nucleoside reverse transcriptase inhibitors, e.g. zidovudine, abacavir
	Nonnucleotide reverse transcriptase inhibitors, e.g. efavirenz
	HIV protease inhibitors, e.g. saquinavir
	Antimalarial drugs, e.g. mefloquine, proguanil, malarone
Endocrine system	
Diabetes mellitus, thyroid disease and hypothalamo pituitary hormones	Insulins (long- and short-acting)
	Secretagogues
	Sulfonylureas, e.g. gliclazide
	Meglitinides, e.g. repaglinide
	DPP4 inhibitors, e.g. saxagliptin
	GLP agonists, e.g. exenatide
	Sensitisers:
	Biguanides, e.g. metformin
	Thiazolidinediones, e.g. pioglitazone
	Thyroid disease, e.g. levothyroxine, carbimazole
	ADH mimetics, e.g. desmopressin
	LHRH, e.g. gonadorelin
	Human growth hormone, e.g. somatropin
Osteoporosis	Calcium, vitamin D, calcitonin, parathyroid hormone, teriparatide
	Bisphosphonates, e.g. alendronic acid, risedronate
	Selective estrogen receptor modulators (SERMs), e.g. clomifene
Genitourinary system	
Urinary retention, benign prostatic hypertrophy and prostate cancer	α_1-Adrenoceptor antagonists, e.g. doxazosin
	5α-Reductase inhibitors, e.g. finasteride
	Antiandrogens, e.g. flutamide
Urinary frequency/incontinence	Antimuscarinic drugs, e.g. darifenacin, fesoterodine
Erectile dysfunction	PDE5 inhibitors, e.g. sildenafil, tadalafil
Obstetrics and gynaecology	
Steroidal contraception	Combined hormonal contraceptives (oral, transdermal patch)
	Progestogen-only contraceptives (oral, subdermal implant)
	Progestogen-containing intrauterine device
	Emergency contraception, e.g. levonorgestrel, ulipristal
	Injectable contraception, e.g. medroxyprogesterone acetate
Dysmenorrhoea`	Combined oral hormonal contraceptives
	NSAIDs, e.g. mefenamic acid
Menorrhagia	Antifibrinolytic agent, e.g. tranexamic acid
	Progestogen-containing intrauterine device
Endometriosis	Progestins
	Gonadorelin analogues, e.g. goserelin
	Danazol

Appendix: student formulary (cont'd)

Therapeutic problem	Core drugs
Induction of labour	Oxytocics, e.g. oxytocin Prostaglandin analogues, e.g. gemeprost
Prevention of pre-term labour (tocolysis)	Calcium channel blockers, e.g. nifedipine β-Adrenoceptor agonists, e.g. terbutaline
Induction of abortion	Oxytocics, mifepristone Antiprogestogen, e.g. mifepristone Prostaglandin analogues, e.g. gemeprost
Postpartum haemorrhage	Oxytocics, ergometrine
Menopause	Oestrogens (with progestins) Others: tibolone, raloxifene

Malignant disease and immunosuppression

Cancer and immunosuppression	Alkylating agents, e.g. cyclophosphamide Cytotoxic antibiotics, e.g. doxorubicin Antimetabolites, e.g. methotrexate, fluorouracil Vinca alkaloids, e.g. vinblastine Taxanes, e.g. paclitaxel Tyrosine kinase inhibitors, e.g. gefitinib, imatinib Topoisomerase I and II inhibitors, e.g. irinotecan, etoposide Other cytotoxic drugs, e.g. crisantaspase, cisplatin Antioestrogens, e.g. tamoxifen, anastrazole Immunosuppressant drugs, e.g. azathioprine, corticosteroids, ciclosporin Immunobiologicals, e.g. rituximab (anti-B-lymphocyte CD20), interferon alfa, bevacizumab (anti-VEGF), trastuzumab (anti-HER2)

Musculoskeletal disease

Rheumatoid arthritis	NSAIDs, e.g. indometacin, diclofenac Corticosteroids, e.g. prednisolone Immunosuppressants, e.g. methotrexate, azathioprine, leflunomide Cytokine (TNFα) modulators, e.g. adalimumab, etanercept, golimumab, infliximab Others: gold, penicillamine, sulfasalazine, hydroxychloroquine
Myasthenia gravis	Anticholinesterases, e.g. pyridostigmine
Spasticity	Skeletal muscle relaxants, e.g. baclofen, dantrolene
Gout	*Acute*: colcichine; *chronic*: allopurinol

Ophthalmology

Glaucoma	β-Adrenoceptor antagonists, e.g. timolol Prostaglandin analogues, e.g. latanoprost Sympathomimetics (α_2-agonists), e.g. brimonidine Carbonic anhydrase inhibitors, e.g. acetazolamide Miotics, e.g. pilocarpine
Conjunctivitis	Topical antibiotics, e.g. chloramphenicol
Tear deficiency	Ocular lubricants, e.g. hypromellose
Others	Mydriatics, e.g. phenylephrine Mydriatics/cycloplegics, e.g. atropine, tropicamide Topical formulations (eye drops) of many drugs, including anti-inflammatory corticosteroids (e.g. betamethasone), antivirals and local anaesthetics (e.g. tetracaine)

Surgery, anaesthetics and intensive care

Surgery, anaesthetics and intensive care	Many drugs used are listed in other sections, including opioid analgesics, sympathomimetics and antiemetics, plus the following: Intravenous (induction) anaesthetics, e.g. thiopental, propofol Inhalation (maintenance) anaesthetics, e.g. isoflurane Muscle relaxants, e.g. suxamethonium, atracurium Antimuscarinics, e.g. atropine, glycopyrronium Anticholinesterases, e.g. neostigmine Local anaesthetics, e.g. lidocaine, bupivacaine

Abbreviations: *ADH*, Antidiuretic hormone; *CMV*, cytomegalovirus; *COMT*, catechol-O-methyltransferase; *COPD*, chronic obstructive pulmonary disease; *DPP4*, dipeptidyl peptidase 4; *GLP*, glucagon-like peptide; *GORD*, gastro-oesophageal reflux disease; *HER2*, human epidermal growth factor receptor 2; *LHRH*, luteinising hormone-releasing hormone; *MAO-B*, monoamine oxidase B; *NMDA*, N-methyl D-aspartate; *NSAID*, nonsteroidal anti-inflammatory drug; *PDE*, phosphodiesterase; *TNFα*, tumour necrosis factor alpha; *VEGF*, vascular endothelial growth factor.

2 Pharmacokinetics

Pharmacokinetics refers to the movement of drugs into, through and out of the body. The type of response of an individual to a particular drug depends on the inherent pharmacological properties of the drug at its site of action. However, the speed of onset, the intensity and the duration of the response usually depend on parameters such as:

- the rate and extent of uptake of the drug from its site of administration;
- the rate and extent of distribution of the drug to different tissues, including the site of action;
- the rate of elimination of the drug from the body.

Overall, the response of an individual to a drug depends upon a combination of the effects of the drug at its site of action in the body called *pharmacodynamics* (or 'what the drug does to the body') and the way the body influences drug delivery to its site of action (*pharmacokinetics*, or 'what the body does to the drug'; Fig. 2.1). Both pharmacodynamic and pharmacokinetic aspects are subject to a number of variables, which affect the dose–response relationship. Pharmacodynamic aspects are determined by processes such as drug–receptor interaction and are specific to the class of the drug (see Chapter 1). These aspects are determined by general processes, such as transfer across membranes, metabolism and renal elimination, which apply irrespective of the pharmacodynamic properties.

Pharmacokinetics may be divided into four basic processes, sometimes referred to collectively as 'ADME':

- **Absorption.** The transfer of the drug from its site of administration to the general circulation
- **Distribution.** The transfer of the drug from the general circulation into the different organs of the body
- **Metabolism.** The extent to which the drug molecule is chemically modified in the body
- **Excretion.** The removal of the parent drug and any metabolites from the body; metabolism and excretion together account for drug *elimination*.

This chapter will first describe each of these processes qualitatively in biological terms, and then in mathematical terms, which determine many of the quantitative aspects of drug prescribing.

THE BIOLOGICAL BASIS OF PHARMACOKINETICS

Most drug structures bear little resemblance to normal dietary constituents such as carbohydrates, fats and proteins, and they are handled in the body by different processes. Drugs that bind to the same receptor as an endogenous ligand rarely resemble the natural ligand sufficiently closely in chemical structure to share the same carrier processes or metabolising

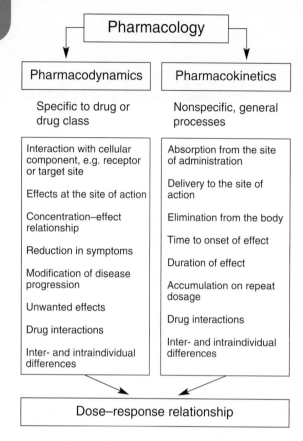

enzymes. Consequently, the movement of drugs in the tissues is mostly by simple passive diffusion rather than by specific transporters, whereas metabolism is usually by enzymes of low substrate specificity that can handle a wide variety of drug substrates and other xenobiotics (foreign substances).

GENERAL CONSIDERATIONS

Passage across membranes

With the exception of intravenous or intra-arterial injections, a drug must cross at least one membrane in its movement from the site of administration into the general circulation. Drugs acting at intracellular sites must also cross the cell membrane to exert an effect. The main mechanisms by which drugs can cross membranes (Fig. 2.2) are:

- passive diffusion through the lipid layer,
- diffusion through pores or ion channels,
- carrier-mediated processes,
- pinocytosis.

Passive diffusion

All drugs can move passively down a concentration gradient. To cross the phospholipid bilayer directly (see Fig. 2.2), a drug must have a degree of lipid solubility, such as ethanol or steroids. Eventually a state of equilibrium will be reached in which equal concentrations of the diffusible form of the drug are present in solution on each side of the membrane. The rate of diffusion is directly proportional to the concentration gradient across the membrane, and to the area and permeability of the membrane, but inversely proportional to its thickness (Fick's law). In the laboratory, transient water-filled pores can be created in the phospholipid

Fig. 2.1 **Factors determining the response of an individual to a drug.**

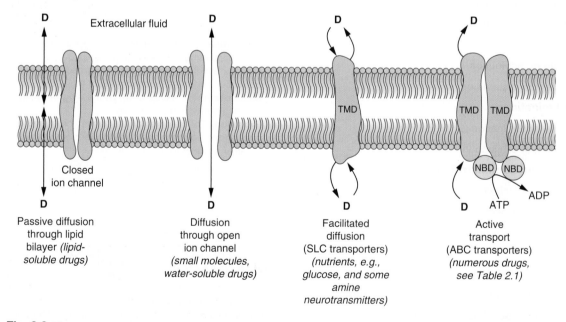

Fig. 2.2 **The passage of drugs across membranes.** Molecules can cross the membrane by simple passive diffusion through the lipid bilayer or via a channel, or by facilitated diffusion, or by ATP-dependent active transport. *ABC*, ATP-binding cassette superfamily of transport proteins; *D*, drug; *NBD*, nucleotide-binding domain; *SLC*, solute carrier superfamily of transporters; *TMD*, transmembrane domain (see Table 2.1).

bilayer by applying a strong external electric field, and this process (electroporation) is used to introduce large or charged molecules, such as DNA, drugs and probes into live cells in suspension.

Passage through membrane pores or ion channels

Movement through channels occurs down a concentration gradient and is restricted to extremely small water-soluble molecules (<100 Da), such as ions. This is applicable to therapeutic ions such as lithium and also to radioactive iodine. Water itself crosses membranes rapidly via a ubiquitous family of aquaporins.

Carrier-mediated processes

Two carrier-mediated processes are of widespread importance in the transport of drugs, particularly those with low lipid solubility, across membranes.

Active transport utilises energy (adenosine triphosphate [ATP]) and transports drugs into or out of cells against their concentration gradient. It is performed particularly by a family of nonspecific carriers termed the ATP-binding cassette (ABC) superfamily of membrane transporters (see Fig. 2.2 and Table 2.1). In humans, the ABC active-transporter superfamily contains 49 members organised into seven subfamilies (A–G) based on their relative sequence homology. Interest in this area has expanded rapidly since the discovery of P-glycoprotein (P-gp), also known as multidrug resistance 1 (MDR1) or ABCB1 transporter. P-gp transports a wide range of drug substrates, including anticancer drugs, steroids and immunosuppressive agents, from the cytoplasm to the extracellular side of the cell membrane, and therefore acts as an efflux transporter. Verapamil increases the concentrations of anticancer drugs at their intracellular sites of action by inhibiting P-gp (see Chapter 52). ABCB transporter proteins contain two hydrophobic transmembrane domains, which consist of different numbers of membrane-spanning α-helices (12 in P-gp), and two hydrophilic nucleotide (ATP)-binding domains, which bind and hydrolyse intracellular ATP. The transporter is on the apical surface and acts as an efflux pump that transports substrates from the cell into the interstitial fluid, plasma, bile, urine or gut lumen. Examples of other ABC transporters are given in Table 2.1.

Facilitated transport of a molecule by a carrier either aids its passive movement down its own concentration gradient, or uses the electrochemical gradient of a co-transported solute to transport the molecule against its own concentration gradient; in neither case is the use of ATP required. The major examples are members of the solute carrier (SLC) superfamily of transporters (see Fig. 2.2 and Table 2.1). The SLC superfamily comprises over 300 types of organic anion transporters (OATs), organic anion-transporting polypeptides (OATPs), organic cation transporters (OCTs), organic cation/carnitine transporters (OCTNs), and members of other transporter families (see Table 2.1). OAT1 to OAT4 are present in various tissues; OAT1 is the classic organic anion transporter in the kidney, which secretes urate and penicillins and is blocked by probenecid (see Chapter 31). Organic cation transporters (OCT1, OCT2 and OCT3) effect facilitated diffusion and can transport cations in both directions across the membrane. Substrates common to all three OCT transporters are serotonin (5-hydroxytryptamine,

5-HT), noradrenaline, histamine and agmatine; although some drugs are substrates for the transporters (see Table 2.1), many basic drugs act as inhibitors of the transporters.

Members of the ABC and SLC transporter families are therefore important in many of the processes by which drugs are absorbed in the gut, distributed into tissues and eliminated in the liver or kidney. Interactions between drugs at the same transporter, or between drugs and the natural substrates of the transporter, may contribute to variation in kinetic parameters for individual drugs between patients and over time. Genetic variation in the expression and functioning of transporters may also contribute to drug toxicity.

Pinocytosis

This can be regarded as a form of carrier-mediated entry into the cell cytoplasm. Pinocytosis is normally concerned with the uptake of endogenous macromolecules and may be involved in the uptake of recombinant therapeutic proteins; drugs can also be incorporated into a lipid vesicle or liposome for pinocytotic uptake (e.g. amphotericin and doxorubicin; see Chapter 51).

Drug ionisation and membrane diffusion

Ionisation is a fundamental property of most drugs that are either weak acids, such as aspirin, or weak bases, such as propranolol. The presence of an ionisable group(s) is essential for the mechanism of action of most drugs, because ionic forces represent a key part of ligand–receptor interactions (see Chapter 1). The extent of ionisation may also influence the extent of absorption of a drug, its distribution into organs such as the brain or adipose tissue, and the mechanism and route of its elimination from the body.

Drugs with ionisable groups exist in equilibrium between charged (ionised) and uncharged (un-ionised) forms (Fig. 2.3). The extent of ionisation of a drug depends on the strength of the ionisable group and the pH of the solution. The extent of ionisation is given by the acid dissociation constant, K_a.

$$K_a = \frac{[\text{conjugate base}][\text{H}^+]}{[\text{conjugate acid}]} \tag{2.1}$$

The term *conjugate acid* refers to a form of the drug able to release a proton, such as:

- an un-ionised acidic drug (Drug–COOH), or
- an ionised basic drug (Drug–NH$_3^+$).

The *conjugate base* is the corresponding equilibrium form of the drug that has lost a proton, such as:

- an ionised acidic drug (Drug–COO$^-$), or
- an un-ionised basic drug (Drug–NH$_2$).

The value of K_a is normally much less than 1, so it is easier to compare compounds using the negative logarithm of K_a, which is called pK_a. For example, a K_a of 10^{-5} becomes pK_a 5, and a K_a of 10^{-10} becomes pK_a 10. Based on the equation given previously, a strong acid (such as an –SO$_3$H functional group) that readily donates its H$^+$ ion will have a relatively high K_a value (e.g. 10^{-1} or 10^{-2}) and hence a low pK_a (i.e. 1 or 2), whereas weakly acidic groups, which donate their H$^+$ ion less readily, have a pK_a of 4–5. Conversely, for basic functional groups, the stronger the base, the greater

Table 2.1 Examples of carrier molecules involved in drug transport

Transporter	Typical substrates	Sites in the body
ABC superfamily	ATP-binding cassette superfamily of transport proteins. All use ATP hydrolysis and function as active efflux or uptake transporters. Although there are a number of transporters in each family, the four ABC transporters listed here can explain multidrug resistance in most cells analysed to date.	
MDR1 or P-glycoprotein (ABCB1)	Hydrophobic and cationic (basic) molecules; numerous drugs, including anticancer drugs	Apical surface of membranes of epithelial cells of intestine, liver, kidney, blood–brain barrier, testis, placenta and lungs
MRP1 (ABCC1)	Numerous, including anticancer drugs, glucuronide and glutathione conjugates	Basolateral surface of membranes of most cell types with high levels in lung, testis and kidney and in blood–tissue barriers
MRP2 (ABCC2)	Numerous, including anticancer drugs, glucuronide and glutathione conjugates	Apical surface of membranes; mainly in liver, intestine and kidney tubules
BCRP (ABCG2) Breast cancer resistance protein	Anticancer, antiviral drugs, fluoroquinolones, flavonoids	Apical surface of breast ducts and lobules, small intestine, colon epithelium, liver, placenta, brain barrier and lung
SLC superfamily	Solute carrier superfamily of transporters. Comprises organic anion transporters (OATs), organic anion-transporting polypeptides (OATPs), organic cation transporters (OCTs), organic cation/carnitine transporters (OCTNs) and many other families. Solute carriers do not use ATP hydrolysis and most function as uptake transporters	
OAT1 (SLC22A6)	Anionic drugs, acyclovir, adefovir, NSAIDs, penicillins, diuretics and phase 2 drug metabolites	Kidney (basolateral), brain, placenta, smooth muscle
OAT2 (SLC22A7)	Anionic drugs, acyclovir, salicylate, acetylsalicylate, PGE_2, dicarboxylates	Kidney (basolateral), liver
OAT3 (SLC22A8)	Similar to OAT1	Kidney (basolateral), liver, brain, smooth muscle, testis
OAT4 (SLC22A11)	Methotrexate, pravastatin, sulfated sex steroids	Kidney (apical), placenta
OATP1B1 (SLCO1B1)	Pravastatin, rosuvastatin	Liver
OATP1B3 (SLCO1B3)	Methotrexate, rosuvastatin	Liver
OCT1 (SLC22A1)	Cationic drugs, serotonin, noradrenaline, histamine, agmatine, aciclovir, ganciclovir, metformin	Mainly in the liver, but also in kidney, small intestine, heart, skeletal muscle and placenta
OCT2 (SLC22A2)	Cationic drugs, serotonin, noradrenaline, histamine, agmatine, amantadine, metformin, cimetidine	Mainly in the kidney, but also in placenta, adrenal gland, neurons and choroid plexus
OCT3 (SLC22A3)	Cationic drugs, serotonin, noradrenaline, histamine, agmatine, metformin	Liver, kidney, intestine, skeletal and smooth muscle, heart, lung, spleen, neurons, placenta and the choroid plexus
OCTN1 (SLC22A4)	Carnitine, acetylcholine	Kidney, intestine
OCTN2 (SLC22A5)	Carnitine, choline	Kidney, skeletal muscle

ABC, ATP-binding cassette; *NSAIDs*, nonsteroidal anti-inflammatory drugs; *PGE₂*, prostaglandin E₂; *SLC*, solute carrier.
For details of other ABC and SLC transporters, see Nigam, S.K., 2015. What do drug transporters really do? Nat. Rev. Drug. Discov. 14, 29–44.

its ability to retain the H^+, resulting in low K_a and high pK_a values. Thus strongly basic groups have a pK_a of 10–11, while weakly basic groups have a pK_a of 7–8.

Drugs are 50% ionised when the pH of the solution equals the pK_a of the drug. Acidic drugs (low pK_a values) are least ionised in acidic solutions (low pH) and most ionised in alkaline solutions (high pH). Conversely, basic drugs (high pK_a values) are least ionised in alkaline solutions (high pH), and most ionised in acid solutions (low pH). In either case, the ionised form of the molecule can generally be regarded as the water-soluble form and the un-ionised form as the lipid-soluble form. The ease with which an ionisable drug can diffuse across a lipid bilayer is determined by the lipid solubility of its un-ionised form (Fig. 2.4).

The pH of body fluids is controlled by the buffering capacity of the ionic groups present in endogenous molecules

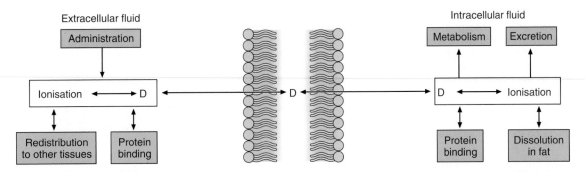

Fig. 2.3 The effect of pH on drug ionisation. Acidic conditions (low pH, high H⁺ concentrations) push the equilibrium of acidic drugs towards their un-ionised (protonated) form, and basic drugs towards their ionised form. Basic conditions (high pH) have the opposite effect.

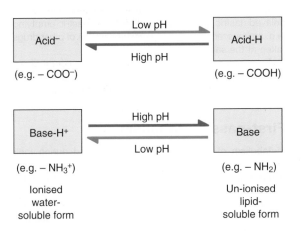

Fig. 2.4 Passive diffusion and the factors that affect drug concentrations in equilibrium between un-ionised and ionised forms. In this case, the pH is assumed to be the same on each side of the membrane; see Fig. 2.5 for drug partitioning when there is a pH gradient across the membrane.

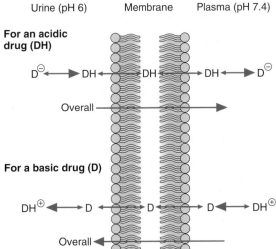

Fig. 2.5 Partitioning of acidic and basic drugs across a pH gradient. Only the un-ionised forms (DH and D) are able to diffuse across the membrane. In urine (pH 6), the un-ionised acidic drug (DH) can be readily reabsorbed into the plasma, where its ionised form (D⁻) becomes concentrated, while the ionised basic drug (D⁺) is trapped within the urine. Alkalinising the urine would reduce reabsorption of the acid drug and enhance that of the basic drug.

such as phosphate ions and proteins. When the fluids on each side of a membrane have the same pH value, there will be equal concentrations of both the diffusible (un-ionised) form and the nondiffusible (ionised) form of the drug on each side of the membrane at equilibrium (see Fig. 2.4).

When the fluids on each side of a membrane are at different pH values, the concentrations of the un-ionised form on each side of the membrane at equilibrium will remain equal, as it can diffuse reversibly across the membrane, but the concentrations of the ionised form will be determined by the pH of the solution. This results in pH-dependent differences in total drug concentration on each side of a membrane (pH trapping or partitioning), with the total drug concentration being higher on the side of the membrane on which it is most ionised. This is exemplified by the pH difference between urine (pH 5–7) and plasma (pH 7.4), which can influence renal elimination of drugs (Fig. 2.5). The relatively low pH of the urine forces an acidic drug to become predominantly un-ionised, allowing its reabsorption into the plasma, while the higher pH in plasma (7.4) converts the drug to the ionised form, preventing it diffusing back and trapping (partitioning)

it in the plasma. The opposite situation prevails with basic drugs, which are enabled to diffuse from the plasma into urine, where they become trapped.

After drug overdose, when the aim is to enhance drug elimination, alkalinisation of the urine (using intravenous sodium bicarbonate) can be used to reduce reabsorption of acidic drugs, such as aspirin, leading to their faster elimination in the urine. Acidification of the urine (with oral ammonium chloride) can enhance ionisation and renal elimination of basic drugs, such as dexamfetamine.

The pH difference between gastric contents (pH 1–2) and plasma (pH 7.4) affects the absorption of many oral drugs. The acidity of stomach contents means that an acidic drug is present largely in its un-ionised (protonated) form, allowing it to pass into plasma where its ionised form becomes partitioned. In contrast, basic drugs are highly ionised in the stomach, and absorption is negligible until the stomach empties and the drug can be absorbed from the more alkaline lumen of the duodenum (pH ~8).

Drugs that are fixed in their ionised form at all pH values, such as the quaternary amine compound suxamethonium (see Chapter 27), cross cell membranes extremely slowly or not at all; they are given by injection (because of lack of absorption from the gastrointestinal tract) and have limited effects on the brain (because of lack of entry).

ABSORPTION

Absorption is the process of transfer of the drug from the site of administration into the general or systemic circulation.

ABSORPTION FROM THE GUT

The easiest and most convenient route of administration of medicines is orally by tablets, capsules or syrups. The large surface area of the small intestine combined with its high blood flow can give rapid and complete absorption of oral drugs. However, this route presents a number of obstacles for a drug before it reaches the systemic circulation.

Drug structure

Drug structure is a major determinant of absorption. Drugs need to be lipid-soluble to be absorbed from the gut. Highly polar acids and bases tend to be absorbed only slowly and incompletely, with much of the unabsorbed dose being voided in the faeces. High polarity may, however, be useful for delivery of the drug to a site of action in the lower bowel (see Chapter 34). The structures of some drugs can make them unstable either at the low pH of the stomach (e.g. benzylpenicillin) or in the presence of digestive enzymes (e.g. insulin). Such compounds have to be given by injection, but administration by other routes may be possible (e.g. inhalation for insulin).

Drugs that are weak acids or bases undergo pH partitioning between the gut lumen and mucosal cells. Acidic drugs will be least ionised in the stomach lumen, and most absorption would be expected at this site, but absorption in the stomach is limited by its relatively low surface area (compared with the small intestine) and the presence of a zone of neutral pH on the immediate surface of the gastric mucosal cells (the mucosal bicarbonate layer; see Chapter 33). As a consequence, the bulk of the absorption of drugs, even weak acids such as aspirin, occurs in the small intestine.

Drug formulation

A drug cannot be absorbed when it is taken in a tablet or capsule until the vehicle disintegrates and the drug is dissolved in the gastrointestinal contents to form a molecular solution. Most tablets disintegrate and dissolve quickly and completely, and the whole dose rapidly becomes available for absorption. However, some formulations are designed to disintegrate slowly so that the rate of release and dissolution of drug from the formulation determines the rate of absorption. In modified-release (i.e. slow-release) formulations the drug is either incorporated into a complex matrix from which it diffuses slowly or in a crystallised form that dissolves slowly. Dissolution of a tablet in the stomach can also be prevented by coating it in an acid-insoluble layer, producing enteric-coated formulations. This is useful for drugs such as omeprazole (see Chapter 31), which is unstable in an acid environment, and allows delivery of the intact drug to the duodenum.

Gastric emptying

The rate of gastric emptying determines how soon a drug taken orally is delivered to the small intestine, the major site of absorption. Delay between oral drug ingestion and the drug being detected in the circulation is usually caused by delayed gastric emptying. Drugs that slow gastric emptying (e.g. antimuscarinics) can delay the absorption of other drugs taken at the same time.

Food has complex effects on drug absorption; it slows gastric emptying and delays drug absorption, and it can also bind drugs and reduce the total amount of drug absorbed.

First-pass metabolism

Metabolism of drugs can occur before and during their absorption, and this can limit the amount of parent compound that reaches the general circulation. Drugs taken orally have to pass four major metabolic barriers before they reach the general circulation. If there is extensive metabolism of a drug at one or more of the sites listed in the sections that follow, only a fraction of the original oral dose reaches the general circulation as the parent compound. This process is known as first-pass metabolism because it occurs at the first passage through the organ.

Intestinal lumen

The intestinal lumen contains digestive enzymes secreted by the mucosal cells and pancreas that are able to split peptide, ester and glycosidic bonds. Intestinal proteases prevent the oral administration of peptide drugs, such as insulin and other products of molecular biological approaches to drug development. In addition, the lower bowel contains large numbers of aerobic and anaerobic bacteria that are capable of performing a range of metabolic reactions on drugs, especially hydrolysis and reduction.

Intestinal wall

The walls of the upper intestine are rich in cellular enzymes such as monoamine oxidase (MAO), aromatic L-amino acid decarboxylase, cytochrome P450 isoenzymes (e.g. CYP3A4) and the enzymes responsible for phase 2 conjugation reactions described later. In addition, the luminal membrane of the intestinal cells (enterocytes) contains efflux transporters such as P-gp (noted previously), which may limit the absorption of a drug by transporting it back into the intestinal lumen. Drug molecules that enter the enterocyte may thus undergo three possible fates – that is, diffusion into the hepatic portal circulation, metabolism within the cell or transport back into the gut lumen (by P-gp). The substrate specificities of CYP3A4 and P-gp overlap, and for common substrates their combined actions can prevent most of the oral dose of some drugs reaching the hepatic portal circulation.

Liver

Blood from the intestine is delivered by the splanchnic circulation directly to the liver, which is the major site of drug metabolism in the body. Hepatic first-pass metabolism can be avoided by administering the drug to a region of the gut from which the blood does not drain into the hepatic portal vein (e.g. the buccal cavity or rectum); a good example of this is the buccal administration of glyceryl trinitrate (see Chapter 5).

Lung

Cells of the lungs have high affinities for many basic drugs and are the main site of metabolism for many local hormones via monoamine oxidase or peptidase activity.

ABSORPTION FROM OTHER ROUTES

Percutaneous (transcutaneous) administration

The human epidermis (especially the stratum corneum) is an effective permeability barrier to water loss and to the transfer of water-soluble compounds. Although lipid-soluble drugs are able to cross this barrier, the rate and extent of entry are very limited. As a consequence, this route is only effective for use with potent, nonirritant drugs, such as glyceryl trinitrate (see Chapter 5) or fentanyl (see Chapter 19), or to produce a local effect. The slow and continued absorption from dermal administration (e.g. via adhesive patches) can be used to produce low but relatively constant blood concentrations of some drugs (e.g. nicotine replacement therapy; see Chapter 54).

Intradermal and subcutaneous injection

Intradermal or subcutaneous injection avoids the barrier presented by the stratum corneum, and entry into the general circulation is limited mainly by the rate of blood flow to the site of injection. However, these sites generally only allow the administration of small volumes of drugs and tend to be used mostly for local effects, such as local anaesthesia, or to deliberately limit the rate of drug absorption (e.g. insulin; see Chapter 40). Subdermal implants are increasingly used for long-term hormonal contraception; the implants are flexible polymer rods or tubes inserted under the skin of the upper arm that slowly release the hormone for up to 3 years, with contraception being reversible by removal of the implant (see Chapter 45).

Intramuscular injection

The rate of absorption from an intramuscular injection depends on two variables: the local blood flow and the water solubility of the drug. An increase in either of these factors enhances the rate of removal from the injection site. Absorption of drugs from the injection site can be prolonged intentionally by incorporation of the drug into a lipophilic vehicle, such as flupentixol decanoate (see Chapter 21), creating a depot formulation from which the drug is released over days or weeks.

Intranasal administration

The nasal mucosa provides a good surface area for absorption, combined with low levels of proteases and drug-metabolising enzymes compared with the gastrointestinal tract. As a consequence, intranasal administration is used for the administration of some drugs, such as triptan drugs for migraines (see Chapter 26) and desmopressin (see Chapter 43), as well as drugs designed to produce local effects, such as nasal decongestants and topical corticosteroids (see Chapter 39).

Inhalation

Although the lungs possess the characteristics of a good site for drug absorption (a large surface area and extensive blood flow), inhalation is rarely used to produce systemic effects. The principal reasons for this are the difficulty of delivering nonvolatile drugs to the alveoli and the potential for local toxicity to alveolar membranes. Therefore drug administration by inhalation is largely restricted to:

- volatile compounds, such as general anaesthetics (see Chapter 17);
- locally acting drugs, such as bronchodilators and corticosteroids used in the treatment of airway disease such as asthma and chronic obstructive pulmonary disease (see Chapter 12).

Drugs in the latter group are not volatile and have to be given either as aerosols containing droplets of dissolved drug or as fine particles of the solid drug (dry powder; see Chapter 12). Particles greater than 10 μm in diameter settle out in the pharynx and upper airways, which are poor sites for absorption, and the drug then passes back up the airways via ciliary motion and is eventually swallowed. Particles less than 1 μm in diameter are not deposited in the airways and are immediately exhaled. It was shown some years ago that only 4–6% of an inhaled dose is deposited in the small airways, although the percentage of deposited drug may be higher with modern inhaler devices delivering particle sizes closer to the optimum for airways deposition (2–5 μm).

Minor routes

Drugs may be applied to any body surface or orifice to produce a local effect. Absorption from the site of administration may be important in limiting the duration of local action and the production of unwanted systemic actions.

DISTRIBUTION

Distribution is the process by which the drug is transferred reversibly from the general circulation into the tissues as the concentrations in blood increase, and then returns from the tissues into blood when the blood concentrations decrease. For most lipid-soluble drugs this occurs by passive diffusion across cell membranes (see Fig. 2.2). Once equilibrium is reached, any process that removes the drug from one side of the membrane results in movement of drug across the membrane to re-establish the equilibrium (see Fig. 2.4). Drugs that are less lipid-soluble can penetrate tissues by diffusing through intercellular junctions.

After an intravenous injection of the drug, there is a high initial plasma concentration and the drug may rapidly enter well-perfused tissues such as the brain, liver and lungs (Table 2.2). This may be so rapid that these tissues can be assumed to equilibrate instantaneously with plasma and represent part of the 'central' compartment (described later). However, the drug will continue to enter poorly perfused tissues, and this will lower the plasma concentration. The high concentrations in the rapidly perfused tissues then decrease in parallel with the decreasing plasma concentration, resulting in a transfer of drug back into the plasma (Fig. 2.6). This redistribution is important for terminating the action of some drugs given as a rapid intravenous injection or bolus. For example, intravenous thiopental produces rapid anaesthesia, but effects in the brain are short-lived because continued uptake into muscle lowers the concentrations in the blood and therefore indirectly in the brain (see Figs 2.6 and 17.2).

The processes of elimination (such as metabolism and excretion) are of major importance and are discussed in detail in the upcoming sections. Elimination results in a net transfer of the drug from other tissues via the circulation to the organ(s) of elimination (see the dashed lines in Fig. 2.6).

REVERSIBLE PROTEIN BINDING

Many drugs show an affinity for sites on nonreceptor proteins, resulting in reversible binding:

$$\text{Drug} + \text{protein} \rightleftharpoons \text{Drug–protein complex}$$

Such binding occurs with plasma proteins, most commonly with albumin, which binds many acidic or steroidal drugs, and α_1-acid glycoprotein, which binds many basic or neutral drugs (Table 2.3). Drugs may also bind reversibly with intracellular

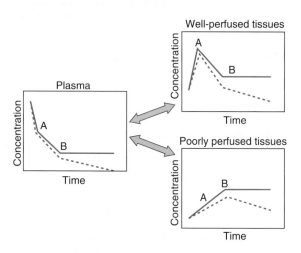

Fig. 2.6 A simplified scheme for the redistribution of drugs between tissues. The initial decrease in plasma concentrations results from uptake into well-perfused tissues, which essentially reaches equilibrium at point A. Between points A and B, the drug continues to enter poorly perfused tissues, resulting in a decrease in the concentrations in both plasma and well-perfused tissues. At point B all tissues are in equilibrium. The additional presence of an elimination process would produce a decrease from point B (shown as a dashed line), which would be parallel in all tissues.

Table 2.2 Relative organ perfusion rates in a typical adult at rest

Organ	Proportion of cardiac output (%)	Blood flow (mL/min per 100 g of tissue)
Well-perfused organs		
Lung	100	1000
Adrenals	0.5	200
Kidneys	15	350
Thyroid	1.5	500
Liver	27	110
Heart	4	100
Gastrointestinal tract	15	300
Brain	12	56
Placenta (full term)	—	10–15
Poorly perfused organs		
Skin	5	12
Skeletal muscle	12	4
Bone, connective tissue	3	3
Adipose (fat)	4	3

Table 2.3 Examples of drugs that undergo extensive binding to plasma protein

Bound to albumin	Bound to α_1-acid glycoprotein
Dexamethasone	Chlorpromazine
Digitoxin	Erythromycin
Furosemide	Lidocaine
Ibuprofen	Methadone
Indometacin	Propranolol
Phenytoin	Quinine
Salicylates	Tricyclic antidepressants
Sulphonamides	
Thiazides	
Tolbutamide	
Warfarin	

proteins. The drug–protein binding interaction resembles the drug–receptor interaction since it is rapid, reversible and saturable, and different ligands can compete for the same site. It does not result in a pharmacological effect but lowers the free concentration of the drug available to act at receptors; the amounts of drug remaining available may be only a minute fraction of the total body load. Proteins such as albumin can therefore act as depots, rapidly releasing the bound drug when the free drug is distributed to other compartments or eliminated.

Competition for binding to proteins in plasma or inside cells can occur between different drugs (drug interaction; see Chapter 56) and between drugs and endogenous ligands. A highly protein-bound drug such as aspirin can displace other drugs such as warfarin from their binding sites on plasma proteins; the increase in unbound drug concentration can increase the biological activity of the displaced drug. Relatively few such interactions have important clinical consequences, although an example of drug interaction with an endogenous ligand is the displacement of bilirubin from albumin by sulphanilamide drugs, causing a potentially dangerous increase in the bilirubin concentration in plasma, leading to kernicterus.

IRREVERSIBLE PROTEIN BINDING

Certain drugs, because of chemical reactivity of the parent compound or a metabolite, undergo covalent binding to plasma or tissue components such as proteins or nucleic acids. When the binding is irreversible (e.g. the interaction of some cytotoxic drugs with DNA), this can be considered as equivalent to elimination, because the parent drug cannot re-enter the circulation. In contrast, some covalent binding may be slowly reversible, such as the formation of disulphide bridges by captopril with its target (angiotensin-converting enzyme [ACE]) and with plasma proteins (see Chapter 6); the covalently bound drug will not dissociate rapidly in response to a decrease in the concentration of unbound drug, and such binding represents a slowly equilibrating reservoir of drug.

DISTRIBUTION TO SPECIFIC ORGANS

Two systems require more detailed consideration of drug distribution: the brain, because of the difficulty of drug entry, and the fetus, because of the potential for drug toxicity.

Brain

Lipid-soluble drugs readily pass from the blood into the brain, and for such drugs the brain represents a typical well-perfused tissue (see Table 2.2). In contrast, the entry of water-soluble drugs into the brain is much slower than into other well-perfused tissues, giving rise to the concept of a blood–brain barrier as a highly selective permeability barrier that separates the blood from the extracellular fluid of the brain. The functional basis of the barrier to water-soluble drugs (Fig. 2.7) is reduced permeability of brain capillaries owing to:

- tight junctions between adjacent endothelial cells (capillaries are composed of an endothelial layer a single cell thick, with no smooth muscle),
- smaller size and lower number of pores in the endothelial cell membranes,
- the presence of a contiguous surrounding layer of astrocytes.

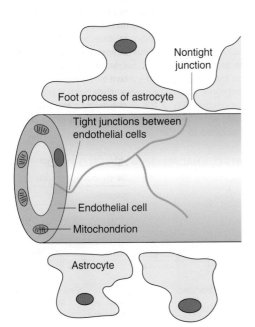

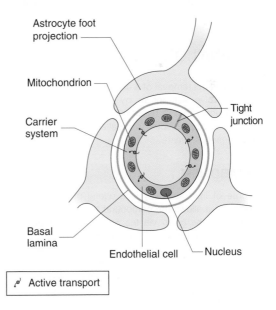

Fig. 2.7 **The blood–brain barrier.** The barrier arises from the low number of membrane pores, the tight junctions between adjacent cells and the presence of efflux transporters that remove any drug that enters the endothelial cell. The presence of astrocytes is the stimulus for these changes in endothelial structure and function. Astrocytes are one of the several types of cells found in the central nervous system that make up the glia; they have numerous sheet-like processes and may provide nutrients to neurons.

In addition, efflux transporters in the endothelial cells are an important part of the blood–brain barrier and return drug molecules back into the circulation, thereby preventing their entry into the brain and reducing effects in the central nervous system.

Water-soluble endogenous compounds needed for normal brain functioning, such as carbohydrates and amino acids, enter the brain via specific uptake transporters of the SLC superfamily (see Table 2.1). Some drugs (e.g. levodopa) may enter the brain using these transport processes, and in such cases the rate of transport of the drug will be influenced by the concentrations of competitive endogenous substrates.

There is limited drug-metabolising ability in the brain, and drugs leave by diffusion back into plasma, by active transport processes in the choroid plexus or by elimination in the cerebrospinal fluid. Organic acid transporters of the SLC superfamily (see Table 2.1) are important in removing polar neurotransmitter metabolites from the brain.

Fetus

Lipid-soluble drugs can readily cross the placenta and enter the fetus. The placental blood flow is low compared with that in the liver, lung and spleen (see Table 2.2); consequently, the fetal drug concentration equilibrates slowly with that in the maternal circulation. Highly polar and very large molecules (such as heparin; see Chapter 11) do not readily cross the placenta. The fetal liver has only low levels of drug-metabolising enzymes, so it is mainly the maternal elimination that clears the fetal circulation of drugs.

After delivery, the neonate may show effects from drugs given to the mother close to delivery (such as pethidine for pain control; see Chapter 19). Such effects may be prolonged because the neonate now has to rely on his/her own immature elimination processes (see Chapter 56).

ELIMINATION

Elimination is the removal of a drug's activity from the body and may involve metabolism, by which the drug molecule is transformed into a different molecule, and/or excretion, in which the drug molecule is expelled in the body's liquid, solid or gaseous 'waste'.

METABOLISM

A degree of lipid solubility is a useful property of most drugs, since it allows the compound to cross lipid barriers and hence to be given via the oral route. Metabolism is necessary for the elimination of lipid-soluble drugs from the body because it converts a lipid-soluble molecule into a water-soluble species capable of rapid elimination in the urine. A lipid-soluble molecule filtered into the kidney tubule would otherwise be reabsorbed from the tubule into the circulation (discussed later).

Metabolism of the drug produces one or more new chemical entities, which may show different pharmacological properties from the parent compound:

- **Decrease in biological activity.** The most common result of drug metabolism, arising from reduced receptor binding due to the changed molecular structure.

- **Increase in activity.** Sometimes metabolites may be more potent than the parent drug; for example a prodrug is an inactive compound that is converted by metabolism into an active molecular species.
- **Change in the nature of the activity.** The metabolite shows qualitatively different pharmacological or toxicological properties.

Drug metabolism can be divided into two phases (Fig. 2.8). Although many compounds undergo both phases of metabolism, it is possible for a drug to undergo only a phase 1 or a phase 2 reaction, or for a proportion of the drug to be excreted unchanged. Phase 1 metabolism (often an oxidation, reduction or hydrolysis reaction) is sometimes described as preconjugation, because it produces a molecule that is a suitable substrate for a phase 2 or conjugation reaction. The enzymes involved in these reactions have low substrate specificities and can metabolise a wide range of drug substrates and other xenobiotics.

Phase 1

Cytochrome P450 is a superfamily of membrane-bound haemoprotein isoenzymes (Table 2.4). They are present in the smooth endoplasmic reticulum of cells (Fig. 2.9), particularly in the liver, which is the major site of drug oxidation; the amounts in other tissues are low in comparison. The cytochrome P450 families CYP1 to CYP4 are involved in drug metabolism; the specific isoenzymes CYP2C9, CYP2D6 and CYP3A4 are involved in the phase 1 metabolism of approximately 10%, 24% and 55% of drugs, respectively.

Oxidation reactions (Table 2.5) are the most important of the phase 1 reactions and can occur at carbon, nitrogen or sulphur atoms within the drug structure. In most cases, an oxygen atom is retained in the metabolite, although some reactions, such as dealkylation, result in loss of the oxygen atom in a small fragment of the original molecule. Oxidation reactions are catalysed by a diverse group of enzymes, of which the cytochrome P450 system is the most important. The cytochrome P450 isoenzyme binds both the drug and molecular oxygen (Fig. 2.10), and catalyses the transfer of one oxygen atom to the substrate, while the other oxygen atom is reduced to water:

$$RH + O_2 + NADPH + H^+ \rightarrow ROH + H_2O + NADP^+$$

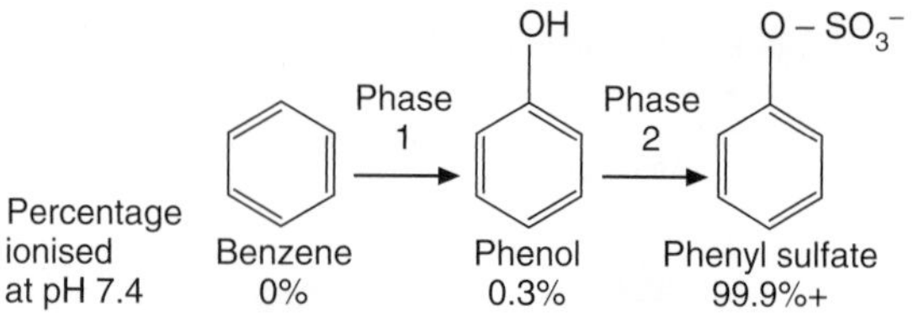

Fig. 2.8 The two phases of drug metabolism. Benzene is shown as a simple example of a lipid-soluble substance undergoing phase 1 and phase 2 metabolism. In Phase 1 benzene is oxidised to phenol and in Phase 2 the phenol metabolite is conjugated with sulfate to produce a highly hydrophilic metabolite-conjugate (phenyl sulfate).

Table 2.4 Cytochrome P450 superfamily

Isoenzyme	Comments
CYP1A	Important for methylxanthines and paracetamol; induced by smoking
CYP2A	Limited number of substrates; significant interindividual variability
CYP2B	Limited number of substrates
CYP2C	CYP2C9 is an important isoform; CYP2C19 shows genetic polymorphism
CYP2D	Metabolises numerous drugs; CYP2D6 shows genetic polymorphism
CYP2E	Metabolises alcohol
CYP3A	Main isoform in liver and intestine; metabolises 50–60% of current drugs
CYP4	Metabolises fatty acids

Human liver contains at least 20 isoenzymes of cytochrome P450. Families CYP1–4 are involved in drug metabolism.

Table 2.5 Examples of oxidation, reduction and hydrolytic reactions

Oxidation	
Alkyl groups	$RCH_3 \rightarrow RCH_2OH \rightarrow RCHO \rightarrow RCOOH$
Deamination	$RCH_2NH_2 \rightarrow RCHO + NH_3$
Amines	$R'\text{-}NH\text{-}R \rightarrow R'\text{-}N(OH)\text{-}R$
Reduction	
Aldehydes	$RCHO \rightarrow RCH_2OH$
Disulfides	$R\text{-}S\text{-}S\text{-}R' \rightarrow RSH + HSR'$
Hydrolysis	
Esters	$RCO{\cdot}OR' \rightarrow RCOOH + HOR'$
Amides	$RCO{\cdot}NHR' \rightarrow RCOH + H_2NR'$

R, R', Aliphatic groups.

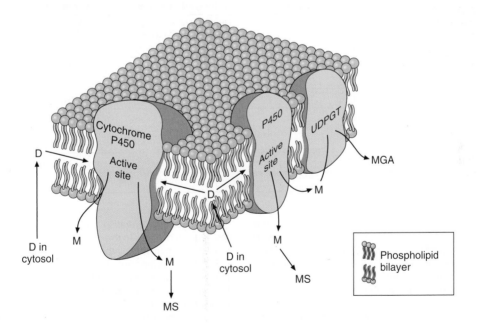

Fig. 2.9 Drug metabolism in the smooth endoplasmic reticulum. The lipid-soluble drug (D) partitions into the lipid bilayer of the endoplasmic reticulum. The cytochrome P450 oxidises the drug to a metabolite (M) that is more water-soluble and diffuses out of the lipid layer. The metabolite may undergo a phase 2 (conjugation) reaction catalysed by UDP-glucuronyl transferase (UDPGT) in the endoplasmic reticulum to give a glucuronide conjugate (MGA) or with sulfate in the cytosol to give a sulfate conjugate (MS).

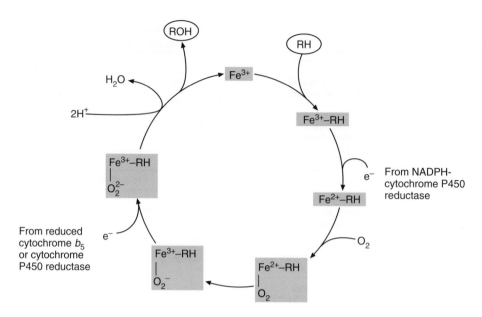

Fig. 2.10 **The oxidation of substrate (RH) by cytochrome P450.** Fe^{3+}, the active site of cytochrome P450 in its ferric state; *RH*, drug substrate; *ROH*, oxidised metabolite. Cytochrome b_5 is present in the endoplasmic reticulum and can transfer an electron to cytochrome P450 as part of its redox reactions. *NADPH*, nicotinamide adenine dinucleotide phosphate.

Table 2.6 Major conjugation reactions

Reaction	Functional group	Activated species	Products
Glucuronidation	–OH –COOH –NH$_2$	Uridine-diphosphate glucuronic acid (UDPGA)	Glucuronide conjugates
Sulfation	–OH –NH$_3$	3'-Phosphoadenosine-5'-phosphosulfate (PAPS)	–O–SO$_3$H –NH–SO$_3$H
Acetylation	–NH$_2$	Acetyl-CoA	–NH–COCH$_3$
Methylation	–OH –NH$_2$ –SH	S-Adenosyl methionine	–OCH$_3$ –NHCH$_3$ –SCH$_3$
Amino acid conjugation	–COOH	Drug-CoA	CO-NH·CHR·COOH
Glutathione conjugation	Various	–	Glutathione conjugates

The reaction involves initial binding of the drug substrate to the ferric (Fe^{3+}) form of cytochrome P450, followed by reduction (via a specific cytochrome P450 reductase) and then binding of molecular oxygen. Further reduction is followed by molecular rearrangement, with release of the reaction products (drug metabolite and water) and regeneration of ferric cytochrome P450.

Oxidations at nitrogen and sulphur atoms are frequently performed by a second enzyme of the endoplasmic reticulum, the flavin-containing mono-oxygenase, which also requires molecular oxygen and NADPH. A number of other enzymes, such as alcohol dehydrogenase, aldehyde oxidase and MAO, may be involved in the oxidation of specific functional groups.

Reduction reactions (see Table 2.5) are less common than oxidation reactions, but occur at unsaturated carbon atoms and at nitrogen and sulfur centres by the actions of cytochrome P450 and cytochrome P450 reductase (and also by the intestinal microflora).

Hydrolysis and hydration reactions (see Table 2.5) involve the addition of water to the drug molecule. In hydrolysis, the molecule is then split by the addition of water. A number of ubiquitous enzymes are able to hydrolyse ester and amide bonds in drugs. Intestinal bacteria are also important for the hydrolysis of esters and amides, and of drug conjugates eliminated in the bile (discussed later). In hydration reactions, the water molecule is retained in the drug metabolite. Hydration of an epoxide ring by epoxide hydrolase is an important reaction in the metabolism and toxicity of a number of aromatic drugs (e.g. carbamazepine; see Chapter 23).

Phase 2

Phase 2 (conjugation) reactions involve the formation of a covalent bond between the drug, or its phase 1 metabolite, and an endogenous substrate. Table 2.6 shows the types of phase 2 reactions, the functional group necessary in the drug molecule and the activated species needed for the reaction. The products of conjugation reactions are usually highly water-soluble and lack biological activity.

The activated endogenous substrate for glucuronide synthesis is uridine-diphosphate glucuronic acid (UDPGA). UDP-glucuronyl transferases in the endoplasmic reticulum close to the cytochrome P450 system (see Fig. 2.9) transfer glucuronate to the drug. Glucuronide conjugation in the gut wall and liver is important in the first-pass metabolism of substrates such as simple phenols.

Sulfate conjugation is performed by a cytosolic enzyme, which utilises high-energy sulphate (3′-phosphoadenosine-5′-phosphosulfate or PAPS) as the rate-limiting endogenous substrate. Saturation of sulfate conjugation contributes to the hepatotoxic consequences of overdose with paracetamol (acetaminophen; see Chapter 53).

Acetylation and methylation reactions often decrease polarity because they block an ionisable functional group (see Table 2.6), but they mask active groups such as amino and catechol moieties. These reactions are primarily involved in inactivation of neurotransmitters such as noradrenaline and local hormones such as histamine.

The conjugation of drug carboxylic acid groups with amino acids is unusual because the drug is converted to a high-energy form (a Coenzyme A derivative) prior to the formation of the conjugate bond by transferase enzymes. Conjugation with the tripeptide glutathione (GSH or L-α-glutamyl-L-cysteinylglycine) is catalysed by a family of transferases which covalently bind the drug to the thiol group in the cysteine (Fig. 2.11). The substrates are often reactive drugs or activated metabolites, which are inherently unstable (see Chapter 53), and the reaction can also occur nonenzymatically. The glutathione conjugate then undergoes further metabolic reactions.

Glutathione conjugation is a detoxification process in which glutathione acts as a scavenging agent to protect the cell from toxic damage. Glutathione conjugates and endogenous cysteine conjugates, such as the cysteinyl-leukotriene (LT) C_4, are transported out of cells by the MRP1 transporter (see Table 2.1).

The complex array of biotransformation reactions typically involved in drug metabolism is illustrated by the anxiolytic drug diazepam (see Chapter 20), which is metabolised to biologically active intermediates before undergoing conjugation with glucuronide (Fig. 2.12).

Factors affecting drug metabolism: inducers and inhibitors

The liver is the main site of drug metabolism; the large surface area of the sinusoids, combined with high levels of enzyme activity in hepatocytes, can result in very rapid drug uptake and metabolism as the blood flows through the liver (see Chapter 56 for normal sinusoid architecture and the effects of liver disease on hepatic drug uptake). Environmental influences including chemical contaminants and therapeutic drugs may induce or inhibit the activity of hepatic drug-metabolising enzymes, particularly cytochrome P450 (Table 2.7). This can affect both the bioavailability and the elimination of other drugs undergoing hepatic elimination (discussed later).

Inducing agents increase the cellular expression of cytochrome P450 enzymes. This occurs over a period of a

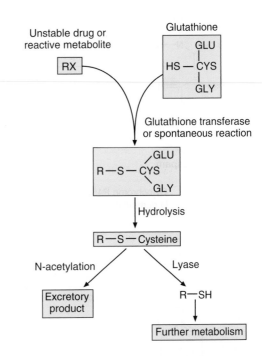

Fig. 2.11 **The formation and further metabolism of glutathione conjugates.** There are multiple types of glutathione transferase that detoxify substances by glutathione conjugation.

few days, during which the inducer interacts with nuclear receptors to increase mRNA transcription of genes coding for cytochrome P450. The increased amounts of the enzyme last for a few days after the removal of the inducing agent, and are removed by normal protein turnover. Environmental contaminants such as organochlorine compounds (e.g. dioxins) and polycyclic aromatic hydrocarbons (e.g. benzo[a] pyrene in cigarette smoke) induce CYP1A. Therapeutic drugs can induce members of the CYP2 and CYP3 families. Chronic consumption of alcohol induces CYP2E.

In contrast, inhibition of cytochrome P450 by drugs occurs by direct reversible competition for the enzyme site, not a change in enzyme expression, so the time course closely follows the absorption and elimination of the inhibitor substance. Examples of inhibitors are the histamine H_2 receptor antagonist cimetidine (see Chapter 33) and components of grapefruit juice (see Table 2.7).

The activity of drug-metabolising enzymes is also dependent on the delivery of their drug substrates by the circulation. The metabolism of many drugs is affected significantly by lower hepatic blood flow in the very young and in the elderly (see Chapter 56). Genetic variation in drug-metabolising enzymes is discussed at the end of this chapter.

EXCRETION

Drugs and their metabolites may be eliminated via circulation by various routes:

- **In fluids (urine, bile, sweat, tears, breast milk, etc.).** Important for low-molecular-weight polar compounds;

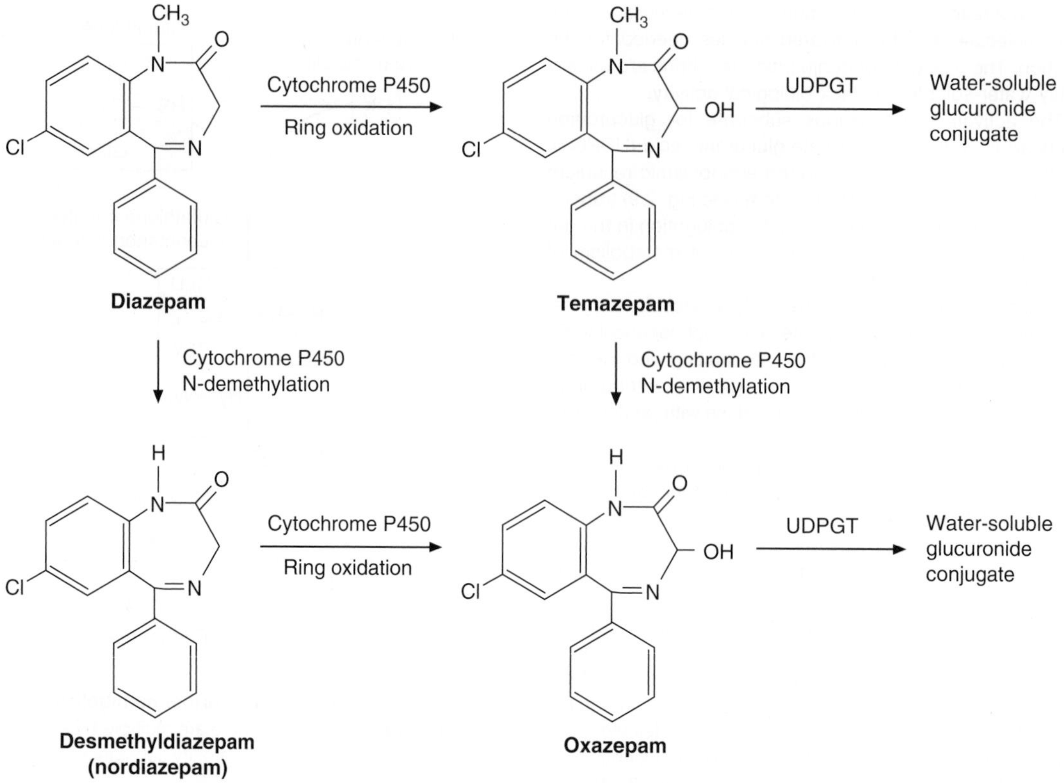

Fig. 2.12 **Complex pathways of metabolism in humans.** This figure illustrates that a single drug, in this case diazepam, may generate a number of active metabolites before phase 2 conjugation terminates the activity of the parent drug and metabolites.

urine is the major route; milk is important because of the potential for exposure of the breastfed infant.

- **In solids (faeces, hair, etc.).** Faecal elimination is most important for high-molecular-weight compounds excreted in bile; the sequestration of drugs into hair is not quantitatively important, but the distribution of a drug along the hair shaft can indicate the history of drug intake during the preceding weeks.
- **In gases (expired air).** Important only for volatile compounds

Excretion via the urine

There are three processes involved in the handling of drugs and their metabolites in the kidney: glomerular filtration, reabsorption and tubular secretion. The total urinary excretion of a drug depends on the balance of these three processes:

$$\text{Total excretion} = \text{glomerular filtration} \\ + \text{tubular secretion} - \text{reabsorption}$$

Glomerular filtration

All molecules less than about 20 kDa undergo filtration under positive hydrostatic pressure through pores of 7–8 nm diameter in the glomerular membrane. The glomerular filtrate comprises about 20% of the flow of plasma to the glomeruli, and hence about 20% of all water-soluble, low-molecular-weight compounds free in the plasma enter the filtrate on each pass. Plasma proteins and protein-bound drugs are not filtered, so the efficiency of glomerular filtration for a drug is influenced by the extent of plasma protein binding.

Reabsorption

The glomerular filtrate contains numerous constituents that the body cannot afford to lose. Most of the water is reabsorbed, and there are specific tubular uptake processes for carbohydrates, amino acids, vitamins and so on (see Chapter 14). A few drugs also pass from the tubule back into the plasma, as they are substrates for these specific uptake processes. The urine is concentrated on its passage down the renal tubule; as the tubule-to-plasma concentration gradient increases, only the most polar molecules remain in the urine. Because of extensive reabsorption, lipid-soluble drugs are not eliminated via the urine, but are returned to the circulation until they are metabolised to water-soluble products, which are then efficiently removed from the body by renal excretion. The pH of urine is usually less than that of plasma; consequently, pH partitioning between urine (pH 5–6) and plasma (pH 7.4) may increase or decrease the tendency of the compound to be reabsorbed (see Fig. 2.5).

Tubular secretion

The renal tubule also has secretory transporters (see Table 2.1) on both the basolateral and apical membranes

Table 2.7 Examples of common substrates, inhibitors and inducers of cytochrome P450 isoenzymes

Isoenzyme	Substrates	Inhibitors	Inducers
CYP1A2	Caffeine, clozapine, haloperidol, naproxen, olanzapine, paracetamol, theophylline, verapamil	Amiodarone, cimetidine, efavirenz, grapefruit juice	Carbamazepine, chargrilled meat, cigarette smoke, rifampicin
CYP2A6	Coumarin, halothane, nicotine	Grapefruit juice, ketoconazole, tranylcypromine	Dexamethasone, phenobarbital, rifampicin
CYP2B6	Bupropion, cyclophosphamide, efavirenz, ifosfamide, ketamine, methadone, propofol, selegiline	Orphenadrine, ticlopidine, voriconazole	Artemisinin, carbamazepine, phenobarbital, phenytoin, rifampicin
CYP2C8	Montelukast, repaglinide	Gemfibrozil, montelukast	Phenobarbital, rifampicin
CYP2C9	Celecoxib, diclofenac, glibenclamide, glipizide, ibuprofen, losartan, tolbutamide, S-warfarin	Amiodarone, efavirenz, fluconazole, isoniazid, metronidazole, paroxetine, voriconazole	Carbamazepine, phenobarbital, rifampicin, St John's wort
CYP2C19	Citalopram, clopidogrel, diazepam, omeprazole, pantoprazole, phenytoin, proguanil	Cimetidine, fluoxetine, fluvoxamine, ketoconazole, lansoprazole, moclobemide, omeprazole, oral contraceptives, pantoprazole, voriconazole	Efavirenz, rifampicin, ritonavir, St John's wort
CYP2D6	Amitriptyline, bisoprolol, codeine, desipramine, encainide, many SSRIs, metamfetamine, metoprolol, ondansetron, propranolol, risperidone	Amiodarone, bupropion, cimetidine, duloxetine, fluoxetine, paroxetine, quinidine	Carbamazepine, phenobarbital, phenytoin, rifampicin
CYP2E	Chlorzoxazone, ethanol, halothane (and other inhalation anaesthetics), paracetamol	Disulfiram	Ethanol
CYP3A4	Numerous drugs of many different classes, e.g. amlodipine, alfentanil, atorvastatin, carbamazepine, ciclosporin, diazepam, diltiazem, erythromycin, fluconazole, lidocaine, midazolam, nifedipine, saquinavir, sildenafil, tamoxifen, terfenadine	Antivirals (indinavir, nelfinavir, ritonavir), clarithromycin, erythromycin, grapefruit juice, itraconazole, ketoconazole	Carbamazepine, efavirenz, phenobarbital, phenytoin, pioglitazone, rifampicin, St John's wort

SSRIs, Selective serotonin re-uptake inhibitors.
Information taken mainly from Flockhart, D.A., 2007. Drug interactions: cytochrome P450 drug interaction table. Indiana University School of Medicine. <http://medicine.iupui.edu/clinpharm/ddis/clinical-table> (accessed 16.04.2016).

for compounds that are acidic (OATs) or basic (organic cation transporters [OCTs]). Drugs and their metabolites, especially the glucuronic acid and sulphate conjugates, may undergo an active carrier-mediated elimination, primarily by OATs but also by multidrug-resistance-associated proteins (MRPs). Because tubular secretion rapidly lowers the plasma concentration of unbound drug, there will be a rapid dissociation of any drugs bound to proteins in the plasma. As a result, even highly protein-bound drugs may be cleared almost completely from the blood in a single passage through the kidney.

Excretion via the faeces

Uptake into hepatocytes and subsequent elimination in bile is the principal route of elimination of larger molecules (molecular weight >500 Da). Conjugation with glucuronic acid increases the molecular weight of the substrate by almost 200 Da, so bile is an important route for eliminating glucuronide conjugates. Once the drug or its conjugate has entered the intestinal lumen via the bile (Fig. 2.13), it passes down the gut and may eventually be eliminated in the faeces. However, some drugs may be reabsorbed from the lumen of

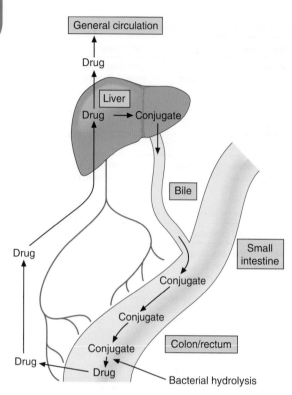

Fig. 2.13 Enterohepatic circulation of drugs. Drug molecules may circulate repeatedly between the bile, gut, portal circulation, liver and general circulation, particularly if the drug conjugate is hydrolysed by the gut flora.

the gut and re-enter the hepatic portal vein. As a result, the drug is recycled between the gut lumen, hepatic portal vein, liver, bile and back to the gut lumen; this is described as *enterohepatic circulation*. Some of the reabsorbed drug may escape hepatic extraction and proceed into the hepatic vein, maintaining the drug concentrations in the general circulation.

Highly polar glucuronide conjugates of drugs or their oxidised metabolites that are excreted into the bile undergo little reabsorption in the upper intestine. However, the bacterial flora of the lower intestine may hydrolyse the conjugate, so the original, lipid-soluble drug or its metabolite is liberated and can be reabsorbed and undergo enterohepatic circulation.

THE MATHEMATICAL BASIS OF PHARMACOKINETICS

The use of mathematics to describe the fate of a drug in the body can be complex and daunting for undergraduates. Nevertheless, a basic knowledge is essential for understanding many aspects of drug handling and the rational prescribing of drugs:

- why oral and intravenous treatments may require different doses,
- the calculation of dosages and dose intervals during chronic therapy,
- why a loading dose may be needed,

- the dosage adjustment that may be necessary in hepatic and renal disease,
- the calculation of dosages for vulnerable patient groups.

Calculation of drug doses may be required in the UK Prescribing Safety Assessment (PSA) (see Chapter 55).

GENERAL CONSIDERATIONS

The processes of drug absorption, distribution, metabolism and excretion (ADME) are described in this section in mathematical terms, as it is important to quantify the rate and extent to which the drug undergoes each process.

For nearly all physiological and metabolic processes, the rate of reaction is not uniform but proportional to the amount of substrate (drug) available: this is described as a *first-order reaction*. Diffusion down a concentration gradient, glomerular filtration and enzymatic hydrolysis are examples of first-order reactions. At higher concentrations, more drug diffuses or is filtered or hydrolysed than at lower concentrations. Protein-mediated reactions, such as metabolism and active transport, are also first order, because if the concentration of the substrate is doubled, then the rate of formation of product is also doubled. However, as the substrate concentration increases, the enzyme or transporter can become saturated with substrate, and the rate of reaction cannot respond to a further increase in concentration. The process then occurs at a fixed maximum rate independent of substrate concentration, and the reaction is described as a *zero-order reaction*; rare examples are the metabolism of ethanol (see Chapter 54) and phenytoin (see Chapter 23). When the substrate concentration has decreased sufficiently for protein sites to become available again, then the reaction will revert to first order.

Zero-order reactions

If a drug is being processed (absorbed, distributed or eliminated) according to zero-order kinetics, then the change in concentration with time (dC/dt) is a fixed *amount* (mass) of the drug per time, independent of concentration:

$$\frac{dC}{dt} = -k \qquad (2.2)$$

The units of k (the reaction rate constant) are therefore a mass per unit time (e.g. mg/min). A graph of concentration against time will produce a straight line with a slope of $-k$ (Fig. 2.14A).

First-order reactions

In first-order reactions, the change in concentration at any time (dC/dt) is proportional to the concentration present at that time:

$$\frac{dC}{dt} = -kC \qquad (2.3)$$

The rate of change will be high at high drug concentrations but low at low concentrations (see Fig. 2.14B), and a graph of concentration against time will produce an exponential

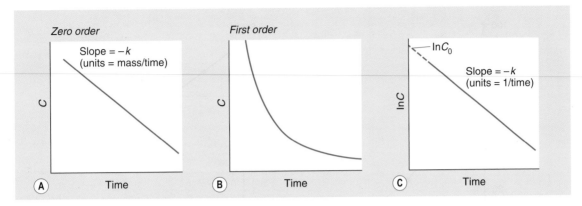

Fig. 2.14 Zero- and first-order kinetics. (A) The zero-order reaction is a uniform change in concentration C over time, representing the same *amount* (mass) of drug being removed per unit of time. (B) The first-order reaction is an exponential curve in which concentrations fall fastest when they are highest; the curve reflects the same *proportion* of drug being removed per unit of time. (C) Plotting the natural logarithm of the concentration (ln$C$) in a first-order reaction against time generates a straight line with slope $-k$ (where k is the rate constant) and the intercept gives the concentration at time zero, C_0.

decrease. Such a curve can be described by an exponential equation:

$$C = C_0 e^{-kt} \qquad (2.4)$$

where C is the concentration at time t and C_0 is the initial concentration (when time = 0). This equation may be written more simply by taking natural logarithms:

$$\ln C = C_0 - kt \qquad (2.5)$$

and a graph of ln$C$ against time will produce a straight line with a slope of $-k$ and an intercept of lnC_0 (see Fig. 2.14C).

The units of the rate constant k (1/time, e.g. per hour) may be regarded as the proportional change per unit of time but are difficult to use practically, so the rate of a first-order reaction is usually described in terms of its half-life ($t_{1/2}$), which is the time taken for a concentration to decrease by one-half. In the next half-life, the drug concentration falls again by one-half, to a quarter of the original concentration, and then to one-eighth in the next half-life, and so on. The half-life is therefore independent of concentration and is a characteristic for a particular first-order process and a particular drug. The intravenous drug shown in Fig. 2.15 has a $t_{1/2}$ of 1 hours.

The relationship between the half-life and the rate constant is derived by substituting $C_0 = 2$ and $C = 1$ into the previous equation, when the time interval t will be one half-life ($t_{1/2}$), giving:

$$\ln 1 = \ln 2 - kt_{1/2}$$
$$0 = 0.693 - kt_{1/2} \qquad (2.6)$$
$$t_{1/2} = 0.693/k \text{ or } k = 0.693/t_{1/2}$$

(Note: 0.693 = ln2.)

A half-life can be calculated for any first-order process (e.g. for absorption, distribution or elimination). In practice, the 'half-life' normally reported for a drug is the half-life for the elimination rate from plasma (the slowest, terminal phase of the plasma concentration–time curve; discussed later).

ABSORPTION

The mathematics of absorption apply to all nonintravenous routes (e.g. oral, inhalation, percutaneous) and are illustrated by absorption from the gut lumen.

RATE OF ABSORPTION

The rate of absorption after oral administration is determined by the rate at which the drug is able to pass from the gut lumen into the systemic circulation. Following oral doses of some drugs, particularly lipid-soluble drugs with very rapid absorption, it may be possible to see three distinct phases in the plasma concentration–time curve, which reflect distinct phases of absorption, distribution and elimination (Fig. 2.16A). However, for most drugs slow absorption masks the distribution phase (see Fig. 2.16B). A number of factors can influence this pattern.

- **Gastric emptying.** Basic drugs undergo negligible absorption from the stomach, so there can be a delay of up to an hour between drug administration and the detection of drug in the general circulation.
- **Food.** Food in the stomach slows drug absorption and also slows gastric emptying.
- **Decomposition or first-pass metabolism before or during absorption.** This will reduce the *amount* of drug that reaches the general circulation but will not affect the *rate* of absorption, which is usually determined by lipid solubility.
- **Modified-release formulation.** If a drug is eliminated rapidly, the plasma concentrations will show rapid fluctuations during regular oral dosing, and it may be necessary to take the drug at very frequent intervals to maintain a therapeutic plasma concentration. The frequency with which a drug is taken can be reduced by giving a modified-release formulation that releases drug at a slower rate. The plasma concentration then becomes more dependent on the rate of absorption than the rate of elimination.

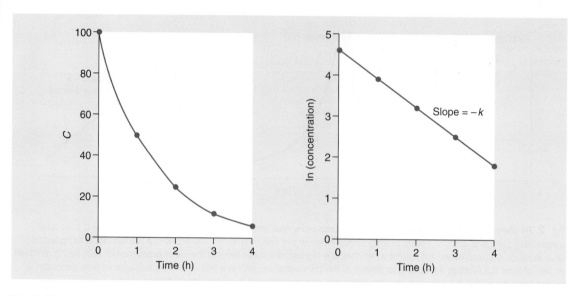

Fig. 2.15 The elimination half-life of a drug in plasma. Here the drug concentration C decreases by 50% every hour (i.e. the half-life is 1 hour).

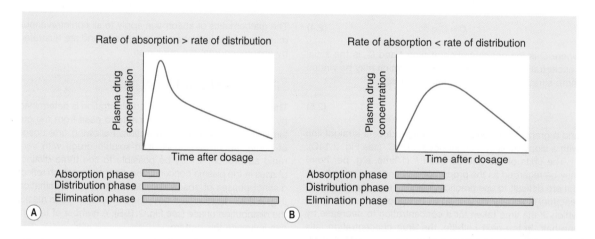

Fig. 2.16 Plasma concentration–time profiles after oral administration of drugs with different rates of absorption. The processes of distribution and elimination start as soon as some of the drug has entered the general circulation. (A) A clear distribution phase is seen if the rate of absorption is so rapid as to be essentially complete before distribution is finished. (B) For most drugs, the rate of absorption is slower and masks the distribution phase.

EXTENT OF ABSORPTION

Bioavailability (F) is defined as the fraction of the administered dose that reaches the systemic circulation as the parent drug (unaltered, not as metabolites). For intravenous administration the bioavailability (F) is therefore 1, as 100% of the parent drug enters the general circulation. For oral administration, incomplete bioavailability (F < 1) may result from:

■ incomplete absorption and loss in the faeces, because either the molecule is too polar to be absorbed or the tablet did not release all of its contents;
■ first-pass metabolism in the gut lumen, during passage across the gut wall or by the liver before the drug reaches the systemic circulation.

The bioavailability of a drug has important therapeutic implications, because it is the major factor determining the drug dosage for different routes of administration. For example, if a drug has an oral bioavailability of 0.1, the oral dose needed for therapeutic effectiveness will need to be 10 times higher than the corresponding intravenous dose.

The bioavailability is a characteristic of the drug and independent of dose, providing that absorption and elimination are not saturated. Bioavailability is normally determined by comparison of plasma concentration data obtained after oral administration (when the fraction F of the parent drug enters the general circulation) with data following intravenous administration (when, by definition,

$F = 1$). The amount in the circulation cannot be compared at a single time point, because intravenous and oral dosing show different concentration–time profiles, so instead the total area under the plasma concentration–time curve (AUC) from $t = 0$ to $t =$ infinity is used, as this reflects the total amount of drug that has entered the general circulation. If the oral and intravenous (iv) doses administered are equal:

$$F = \frac{AUC_{oral}}{AUC_{iv}} \qquad (2.7)$$

or if different doses are used:

$$F = \frac{AUC_{oral} \times Dose_{iv}}{AUC_{iv} \times Dose_{oral}} \qquad (2.8)$$

This calculation assumes that the elimination is first order.

An alternative method to calculate F is to measure the total urinary excretion of the parent drug (Aex) following oral and intravenous administration of identical doses:

$$F = \frac{Aex_{oral}}{Aex_{iv}} \qquad (2.9)$$

DISTRIBUTION

Distribution concerns the rate and extent of movement of the parent drug from the blood into the tissues after administration and its return from the tissues into the blood during elimination.

RATE OF DISTRIBUTION

Because a distinct distribution phase is not usually seen when a drug is taken orally (see Fig. 2.16B), the rate of distribution is normally measured following an intravenous bolus dose. Some intravenous drugs reach equilibrium between blood and tissues very rapidly, and a distinct distribution phase is not apparent. In Fig. 2.17A the slope of plasma concentration against time therefore mainly reflects elimination of the drug; this is described as a *one-compartment model*.

Most intravenous drugs, however, take a finite time to distribute into the tissues; the initial distribution out of the plasma, combined with underlying elimination, produces a steep initial slope (slope A–B in Fig. 2.17B), followed by a slower terminal phase (slope B–C) in which distribution has been largely completed and elimination predominates. Back-extrapolation of this terminal elimination phase to

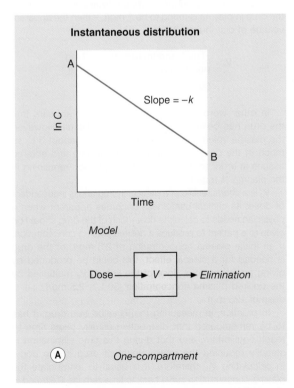

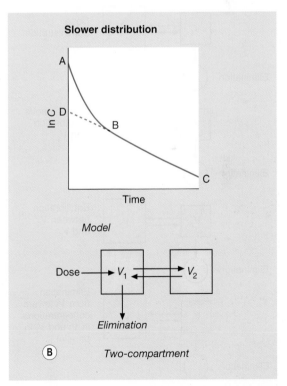

Fig. 2.17 **Plasma concentration–time curves for the distribution of intravenous drugs into one- and two-compartment models.** (A) When distribution of an intravenous drug bolus into tissues is so rapid as to be essentially instantaneous, the slope of the plasma concentration–time curve mainly reflects the rate of elimination (one-compartment model). (B) When distribution is slower, the initial fall in concentration (slope A–B) is due to simultaneous distribution and elimination followed by the terminal elimination phase (two-compartment model; slope B–C). Back-extrapolating to D at time zero allows the contribution of distribution during A–B to be distinguished from the underlying contribution of elimination.

time zero gives an initial value (D), which is the theoretical concentration that would have been obtained if distribution had been instantaneous. The actual rate of distribution can therefore be estimated by the difference between the rapid initial fall in concentration (distribution plus elimination, A–B) and the underlying rate of elimination alone (D–B). In practice, knowing the rate of drug distribution is rarely of clinical importance.

Such a two-compartment model in which the drug in one compartment (e.g. blood) equilibrates more slowly with a second compartment (e.g. poorly perfused tissues; or a fetus) is also shown in Fig. 2.18. The rate of distribution into the second compartment is dependent on the solubility of the drug:

- For *water-soluble drugs*, the rate of distribution depends on the rate of passage across membranes (i.e. the diffusion characteristics of the drug).
- For *lipid-soluble drugs*, the rate of distribution depends on the rate of delivery (the blood flow) to those tissues, such as adipose tissue, that accumulate the drug.

The plasma concentration–time curves of some drugs show three or more distinct phases, due to distribution of the drug from the central compartment into two or more peripheral compartments at different rates; such *multicompartment models* are of limited clinical importance.

EXTENT OF DISTRIBUTION

The *extent* of distribution of a drug from plasma into tissues is more important clinically than the rate, because it determines the total amount of a drug that has to be administered to produce a particular plasma concentration (and therapeutic effect). In humans only the concentration in blood or plasma can be measured easily, so the extent of distribution has to be estimated from the amount remaining in blood, or more usually plasma, after completion of distribution.

The parameter that describes the extent of distribution is the *apparent volume of distribution* (V_d). In general terms, the concentration of a drug solution is the amount (or dose) of drug dissolved in a volume; rearranging this gives:

$$V_d = \frac{\text{Total amount (dose) of drug in the body}}{\text{Plasma concentration}} \quad (2.10)$$

If an intravenous dose of 50 mg of a particular drug is injected – and after an appropriate interval to allow time for distribution to reach equilibrium, the total concentration of the drug in plasma is found to be 1 mg/L – then the apparent volume of distribution (V_d) is:

$$V_d = \frac{\text{Total amount (dose)}}{\text{Plasma concentration}} = \frac{50\,\text{mg}}{1\,\text{mg/L}}$$
$$= 50\,\text{L}$$

In other words, after giving the dose, it appears that the drug has been dissolved in 50 L of plasma. However, the plasma volume in adult humans is only about 3 L; so much of the drug must have left the plasma and entered tissues in order to give the low concentration remaining in the plasma (1 mg/L).

V_d is a characteristic of a particular drug and is independent of dose; its clinical usefulness becomes apparent when a physician needs to calculate how much of the drug should be given to a patient to produce a desired plasma concentration. If an initial plasma concentration of 2.5 mg/L of the drug is needed for a clinical effect, this could be produced by giving an intravenous dose of the known V_d multiplied by the desired plasma concentration (50 L × 2.5 mg/L; i.e. a dose of 125 mg).

In practice, in measuring the V_d value of a drug, it has to be remembered that distribution usually takes time to reach equilibrium, and that during this time elimination is steadily reducing the total amount of drug in the body. In calculating V_d, therefore, it is usual to extrapolate the plasma-concentration curve back to time zero (as illustrated in Fig. 2.17B) to find the theoretical concentration as if the drug has distributed instantaneously and significant elimination has not yet occurred:

$$V_d = \frac{\text{Total amount (dose)}}{\text{Extrapolated plasma concentration at time zero}} \quad (2.11)$$

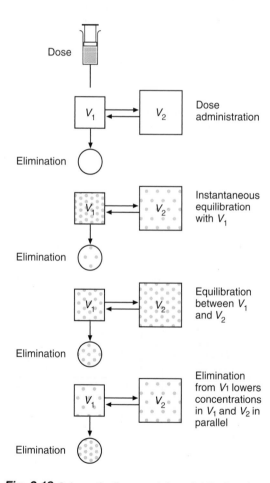

Dose

V_1 → V_2 Dose administration

Elimination

V_1 → V_2 Instantaneous equilibration with V_1

Elimination

V_1 → V_2 Equilibration between V_1 and V_2

Elimination

V_1 → V_2 Elimination from V_1 lowers concentrations in V_1 and V_2 in parallel

Elimination

Fig. 2.18 **Schematic diagram of drug distribution.** A drug injected instantly into the circulation (V_1) distributed slowly into the tissues (V_2). At equilibrium, the drug concentrations are transiently the same in volumes V_1 and V_2. Distribution into the tissues is then reversed as the drug in the circulation is gradually eliminated.

It is important to recognise that V_d may not be a true physiological volume. If the V_d calculated for a drug is 2.5–3 L, this might indicate that it has been confined within the circulatory volume, while a V_d value of about 40 L might mean it has been able to pass into tissues and is distributed uniformly into the total volume of body water, which is about 40 L in adults. However, V_d is only a theoretical measure based on how much the concentration of drug remaining in the plasma has been diluted by its distribution in the body. While a large V_d may indeed occur when the drug is distributed at uniform concentrations into a large body compartment (such as total body water), the same high V_d may also occur if the drug has been highly bound or sequestered by a tissue component within one or more smaller compartments. For example, binding tightly to tissue proteins in a single organ, or sequestration of a lipophilic drug at high concentrations into adipose (fat) cells, may reduce the plasma drug concentration to the same extent (and produce the same large V_d). Identifying such effects can be achieved only by measuring drug concentrations in tissues, which is rarely practicable in humans.

The V_d of a drug is nevertheless an important concept. It indicates the theoretical volume that has to be cleared of the drug by the organs of elimination, such as the liver and kidneys, which extract the drug from the plasma for metabolism and excretion. Together with clearance (the volume of plasma from which the drug can be cleared in a certain time), it determines the overall rate of elimination and therefore the half-life of the drug. In turn, the rate of elimination equals the rate of dosing required to maintain a steady plasma concentration and the half-life determines the duration of action of a single dose and hence the optimal interval between repeated doses of the drug (discussed later).

ELIMINATION

The rate at which the drug is eliminated is important because it usually determines the duration of response, the time interval between doses and the time to reach equilibrium during repeated dosing.

RATE OF ELIMINATION

The rate of elimination of a drug from the circulation (and its associated plasma half-life) is usually indicated by the terminal slope of the plasma concentration–time curve (slope B–C in Fig. 2.17B). The elimination half-lives of drugs range from a few minutes to many days (and, in rare cases, weeks).

The activity of the organ of elimination

The main organs of elimination (the liver and kidneys) can only remove drugs delivered to them via the blood. A key concept in understanding drug elimination is that as long as the elimination process is not saturated, a constant *proportion* (not a constant amount) of the drug carried in the blood will be removed on each passage through the organ of elimination, whatever the drug concentration in the blood. In effect, this is equivalent to a constant proportion of the blood flow to the organ being cleared of drug. For example, if 10% of the drug carried to the liver by the plasma (at a flow rate of 1000 mL/minute) is cleared by uptake and metabolism, this is equivalent to a clearance of 10% of the plasma flow (100 mL/minute); if the drug is metabolised more efficiently such that 20% of the drug is cleared, this gives a clearance of 200 mL/minute.

Clearance is therefore the *volume* of blood or plasma cleared of drug per unit time, not the *amount* of drug cleared in that time, which will also depend on the drug concentration in the blood. If the drug concentration in the blood is high, there is a greater amount of the drug in the volume that is cleared per unit time, resulting in a greater rate of elimination; if the drug concentration is low, the same clearance will eliminate a smaller amount of the drug per unit time. Overall, the rate of drug elimination from the body is therefore the product of plasma concentration of the drug (Cp) and its plasma clearance (CL), a relationship which can be rearranged to:

$$CL = \frac{\text{Rate of elimination from the body}}{\text{Drug concentration in plasma}} \quad (2.12)$$

The plasma clearance is a characteristic value for a particular drug (Table 2.8); it is a constant for first-order reactions and is independent of dose or concentration. The units of clearance are volume per time, such as mL/minute or L/hour.

Reversible passage of drug from the blood into tissues

The organs of elimination can only act on a drug that is delivered to them via the blood supply, and the amount of drug eliminated depends on its concentration within the volume of plasma being cleared per unit time. By definition,

Table 2.8 Pharmacokinetic parameters of selected drugs (in a 70-kg adult male)

Drug	Clearance (CL), (mL/min)	Apparent volume of distribution (V_d) (L)	Half-life ($t_{1/2}$) (h)
Warfarin	3	8	37
Digitoxin	4	38	161
Diazepam	27	77	43
Valproic acid	76	27	5.6
Digoxin	130	640	39
Ampicillin	270	20	1.3
Amlodipine	333	1470	36
Nifedipine	500	80	1.8
Lidocaine	640	77	1.8
Propranolol	840	270	3.9
Imipramine	1050	1600	18

Half-life ($t_{1/2}$) = $0.693 V_d$/CL. A long half-life may result from a high V_d (e.g. amlodipine), a low CL (e.g. digitoxin), or both.

a drug that is distributed at equilibrium into a large apparent volume of distribution has a low plasma concentration; hence the rate of elimination is inversely proportional to apparent V_d:

$$\text{Elimination} \propto \frac{1}{V_d} \qquad (2.13)$$

The overall rate constant of elimination (k) can therefore be related directly to the volume of plasma cleared per minute (CL) and inversely to the total apparent volume of plasma that has to be cleared (V_d):

$$k = \frac{CL}{V_d} \qquad (2.14)$$

Since also (from Eq. 2.6):

$$k = \frac{0.693}{t_{1/2}}$$

Therefore:

$$t_{1/2} = \frac{0.693\, V_d}{CL}$$

The relationship between elimination, volume of distribution and clearance is illustrated in Fig. 2.19. The elimination rate constant (k) or half-life ($t_{1/2}$) are the best indicators of a fall in drug concentration with time, and for most drugs this will be accompanied by a decrease in therapeutic activity.

Clearance is the best measure of the ability of the organs of elimination to remove the drug and determines the average plasma concentrations (and therefore therapeutic activity) at steady state (discussed later). Clearance is usually determined using the AUC extrapolated to infinity after an intravenous dose. Clearance and the AUC of a given dose of drug are inversely related; if clearance was zero, the drug would not be eliminated and its plasma concentration would remain at equilibrium indefinitely (the AUC would be infinitely large). Conversely, if the clearance was infinite, the AUC would be zero, as the drug would be eliminated instantly. The ratio of an intravenous drug dose to the AUC (note: not the logarithm of plasma concentration) is therefore a measure of clearance:

$$CL = \frac{Dose}{AUC} \qquad (2.15)$$

If an oral drug is used instead, the dose in this equation would be corrected by its bioavailability (i.e. $F \times$ Dose).

The two equations for clearance (2.14 and 2.15) can be combined to derive Eq. 2.16, which is used to calculate V_d more reliably than the extrapolation method given in Eq. 2.11 and Fig. 2.17B:

$$CL = \frac{Dose}{AUC} = k \cdot V_d$$
$$V_d = \frac{Dose}{AUC \times k} \qquad (2.16)$$

The plasma clearance of a drug is the sum of all possible clearance processes (metabolism + renal excretion + biliary excretion + exhalation + etc.). Measurement of its component processes is only really possible for renal clearance, performed by relating the rate of urinary excretion to the midpoint plasma concentration. Subtracting renal clearance from the total plasma clearance gives a reasonable estimate of metabolic (mainly hepatic) clearance, which cannot be measured directly. Being able to estimate both renal and hepatic clearance values can be useful in predicting the impact of renal or liver disease.

EXTENT OF ELIMINATION

The extent of elimination is of limited value because eventually all of the drug will be removed from the body. Measurement of the parent drug and its metabolites in urine and faeces can give useful insights into the extent of renal and biliary elimination.

CHRONIC ADMINISTRATION

Repeated drug doses are used to maintain a constant concentration of the drug in the blood and at the site of action for a persistent therapeutic effect. In practice, a perfectly stable concentration can only be achieved by maintaining a constant intravenous infusion that has reached a steady-state balance between drug input and drug elimination (Fig. 2.20).

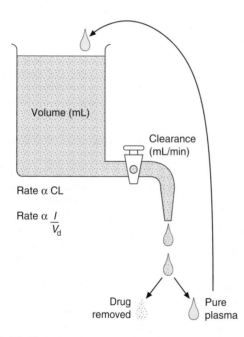

Fig. 2.19 **The relationship between clearance, apparent volume of distribution and overall elimination rate.** The drug is eliminated by the clearance process, which removes whatever amount of the drug is present in a fixed volume of plasma, per unit time. The drug is then separated and the pure plasma added back to the reservoir to maintain a constant volume (the apparent volume of distribution, V_d). The fluid, therefore, continuously recycles via the clearance process and the concentration of drug decreases exponentially.

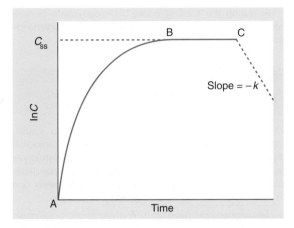

Fig. 2.20 **Constant intravenous infusion (between points A and C).** A steady-state concentration (C_{ss}) is reached at point B and can be used to calculate clearance (CL = rate of infusion/C_{ss}). Conversely, knowing a drug's clearance means that a doctor using this equation can calculate the rate of intravenous infusion required to produce a desired C_{ss} in a patient. Clearance can also be calculated from the total dose infused between A and C and the area under the total curve (AUC). The negative slope after ending the infusion gives the terminal elimination phase (k). The rate of elimination determines the time taken to reach C_{ss}, approximately four to five half-lives.

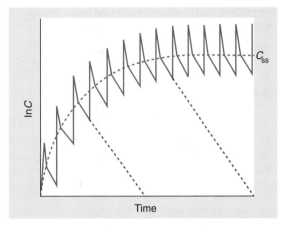

Fig. 2.21 **Chronic oral therapy** *(solid line)* **compared with intravenous infusion** *(dashed red line)* **at the same dosage rate.** Each oral dose shows rapid absorption and distribution to reach a peak, followed by a slower elimination phase in which concentrations fall to a trough. Successive peaks (or successive troughs) align with the dose interval. Cessation of therapy after any dose would produce the lines shown in blue. The dose rate (D/t) corrected for oral bioavailability (F) equals clearance (CL) × steady-state plasma concentration (C_{ss}), so knowing a drug's clearance and bioavailability means a doctor can calculate the dose and the dose interval to produce a desired C_{ss} in a patient.

TIME TO REACH STEADY STATE

During constant infusion, the time to reach steady state is dependent on the elimination half-life; as a rule of thumb, about 93–96% of steady state is approached after four or five times the elimination half-life. A drug with slow elimination takes a long time to reach its steady state, as it will accumulate to high plasma concentrations before its elimination rate rises to match the rate of drug infusion (because the elimination rate depends on plasma concentration; Eq. 2.12). Since the elimination half-life is also dependent on volume of distribution (Eq. 2.14), a high V_d can also contribute to delay in achieving steady state. It is easy to envisage the slow 'filling' of such a high volume of distribution during regular administration.

PLASMA CONCENTRATION AT STEADY STATE

Once steady state has been reached, the plasma and tissues are in equilibrium and the distribution rate and V_d will no longer affect the plasma concentration. The key insight is that a steady-state concentration (C_{ss}) is achieved when the rate of elimination equals the rate of infusion. From Eq. 2.12 the rate of elimination equals CL × C_{ss}, so at steady state the rate of infusion also equals CL × C_{ss}, or:

$$C_{ss} = \frac{\text{Rate of infusion}}{\text{CL}} \qquad (2.17)$$

Alternatively, the rate of an intravenous infusion and the C_{ss} achieved can be used to calculate plasma clearance:

$$CL = \frac{\text{Rate of infusion}}{C_{ss}} \qquad (2.18)$$

Clearance and volume of distribution can also be calculated using the AUC between zero and infinity and the terminal slope after cessation of the infusion (see Fig. 2.20).

ORAL ADMINISTRATION

Most chronic administration of drugs is by the oral route, and the rate and extent of absorption affect the shape of the plasma concentration–time curves. Because oral therapy is by intermittent doses, there will be a series of peaks and troughs matching the intervals between repeated doses (Fig. 2.21). The rate of absorption will influence the profile, since very rapid absorption will exaggerate fluctuations, while slow absorption will dampen down the peaks. As not all the administered dose (D) will be absorbed, the rate of dosage during chronic oral therapy is corrected for bioavailability (F):

$$\frac{D \times F}{t} \qquad (2.19)$$

where t is the *interval* between doses. When steady state is achieved, the rate of administration is equal to the rate of elimination, which is the clearance (CL) multiplied by the drug concentration averaged between the peaks and troughs (C_{ss}), so:

$$\frac{D \times F}{t} = CL \times C_{ss} \qquad \textbf{(2.20)}$$

Therefore:

$$C_{ss} = \frac{D \times F}{t \times CL} \qquad \textbf{(2.21)}$$

This important equation means it is possible to alter plasma C_{ss} by altering either the dose (D) or the dose interval (t). For example, the plasma C_{ss} could be doubled by giving twice the dose at the same intervals, or by giving the same dose twice as frequently. The bioavailability (F) depends largely on the drug formulation, and clearance (CL) is usually constant unless there is a change in hepatic or renal function.

LOADING DOSE

A problem may arise when a rapid onset of effect is required for a drug that has a very long half-life; for example, if the half-life of the drug is 24 hours, the steady-state conditions will not be reached until 4–5 days, and if the half-life is 1 week, reaching a steady state will take over 4–5 weeks. Increasing the dose rate (by increasing the dose or shortening the dose interval) would accelerate the rise in plasma concentrations, but if the higher dose-rate were sustained, it would lead to a higher steady-state concentration being achieved than desired.

Delay between starting treatment and reaching the steady-state therapeutic concentration can be avoided by administering a *loading dose*. This is a high initial dose that 'loads up' the body to shorten the time to steady state. The key principle is that the loading dose is the single dose required to produce the desired concentration in the apparent volume of distribution (i.e. C_{ss} = loading dose/V_d; see Eq. 2.10), so:

$$\text{Loading dose} = C_{ss} \times V_d \qquad \textbf{(2.22)}$$

The loading dose is equivalent to the total body load of drug that would be achieved more slowly by the chronic dosage regimen (Eq. 2.21).

In cases where C_{ss} or V_d are not known, the loading dose can be calculated based on the parameters of the proposed maintenance regimen by replacing C_{ss} with Eq. 2.21 and V_d by Eq. 2.14:

$$\begin{aligned} \text{Loading dose} &= \frac{D \times F}{t \times CL} \times \frac{CL}{k} \\ &= \frac{D \times F}{t \times k} \qquad \textbf{(2.23)} \\ &= \frac{D \times F \times 1.44 \times t_{1/2}}{t} \end{aligned}$$

This last equation shows that the magnitude of a loading dose is proportional to the half-life.

If a drug has a very long half-life such that a very large loading dose is required, it may be given in divided doses over 24–36 hours, as local variations in the rate of distribution to different tissues may otherwise cause high localised concentrations and hence toxicity.

Following the loading dose, the steady-state plasma concentration can be sustained indefinitely by the *maintenance* dosage regimen given by Eq. 2.21.

PHARMACOKINETICS OF BIOLOGICAL DRUGS

The first recombinant protein drug was human insulin, marketed in 1982, and there are now hundreds of biological drugs available, including monoclonal antibodies, cytokines, growth factors and blood products. Such biopharmaceuticals can create special pharmacokinetic problems, mainly due to their protein structures, as follows:

- **Absorption.** pH-dependent and enzymatic breakdown of proteins in the gastrointestinal tract (>99%) precludes oral administration. Administration of biopharmaceuticals is by parenteral routes (intravenous, subcutaneous, intramuscular), including, occasionally, intranasal and inhaled routes. Bioavailability of protein drugs may be low due to local proteolysis, such as at subcutaneous or intramuscular injection sites. Larger molecules (>30 kDa) cross the capillary endothelium poorly and may enter the systemic circulation by the lymphatic system.
- **Distribution.** Biological drug distribution may be confined to the blood and extracellular tissues. Protein drugs may bind extensively to albumin and other plasma proteins, affecting their distribution and rate of metabolism.
- **Elimination.** Biological drugs are not excreted unchanged but undergo extensive proteolysis in the blood, liver, kidneys and other tissues to small peptides and amino acids, which enter the general pool of amino acids used in endogenous protein synthesis. Degradation depends on molecular weight, charge and the extent of glycosylation. Recombinant drug molecules may be designed to lack common sites of proteolytic cleavage, or coated with polyethylene glycol (pegylated) to improve solubility and resistance to proteolysis. The elimination kinetics of biopharmaceuticals can be variable and complex; concentrations of monoclonal antibodies in plasma fall initially as they bind tightly to their targets, but their terminal elimination half-life may be as slow as that of endogenous immunoglobulins (14–28 days), enabling long dosing intervals.
- **Toxicity and clinical use.** Biopharmaceuticals are often highly species-specific, and their toxicity is usually receptor-dependent or immunogenic in origin. Immunogenicity is reduced in drugs based on human protein sequences, but these are more difficult to develop, as they may lack efficacy in animal models. The complex tertiary structure of recombinant proteins makes them more vulnerable to degradation by heat, pH effects and shear forces during manufacture, storage and handling.

GENETIC VARIATION AND PHARMACOKINETICS

The effects that variation in the genes encoding drug targets can have on drug action are discussed in Chapter 1. Genetic variation may also affect drug responses by altering proteins involved in the absorption, distribution and elimination of the drug. The earliest pharmacogenetic studies were on enzymes involved in drug metabolism. N-Acetyltransferase (NAT) was one of the first drug metabolism pathways found to show genetic polymorphism that influenced both the plasma concentrations of a drug (isoniazid) and its therapeutic response. Individuals with low enzyme activity, so-called slow acetylators, had higher blood concentrations and a better response to isoniazid but a greater risk of toxicity than fast acetylators.

Because N-acetylation is a minor pathway of drug metabolism, pharmacogenetics remained of largely academic interest until the late 1970s, when it was found that the cytochrome P450 isoenzyme CYP2D6, which is involved in the phase 1 metabolism of 20–25% of all drugs, showed functionally important genetic polymorphism. CYP2D6 activity can be tested phenotypically by monitoring a plasma metabolite of debrisoquine, a CYP2D6 substrate, or the CYP2D6 genotype, identified by genetic tests. Genotyping may be useful in guiding the prescribing of a number of drugs to optimise their efficacy and reduce adverse effects, including tetrabenazine used in Huntington's disease and the oestrogen receptor modulator tamoxifen. Developments in genotyping have allowed the identification of polymorphism in a number of other cytochrome P450 isoenzymes, with consequences for the phase 1 metabolism and elimination of many drugs; examples are listed in Table 2.9. Polymorphism has also been identified in a number of phase 2 metabolic enzymes; notable among these is the *28 variant in UDP glucuronyl transferase (UGT1A1*28), which results in impaired metabolism of the topoisomerase inhibitor irinotecan and greater adverse effects when the drug is used for treatment of colon cancer. Genetic tests for the UGT1A1 allele are available. Another example is thiopurine-S-methyltransferase (TPMT), which detoxifies 6-mercaptopurine used in treating inflammatory bowel disease and leukaemia. Genetic variation in TPMT influences the efficacy and toxicity of mercaptopurine, and individuals can be phenotyped for TMPT activity in blood or genotyped for variant TMPT alleles.

The prevalence of gene variants may differ between ethnic groups; people from the Indian subcontinent have a lower systemic clearance of nifedipine (a CYP3A4 substrate) compared with Europeans, and intolerance to alcohol ingestion associated with polymorphism in alcohol dehydrogenase (ADH) and acetaldehyde dehydrogenase (ALD) is common in people of Chinese and Japanese origin (see Table 2.9).

Polymorphism that affects the metabolism of drugs may influence their efficacy and safety by altering plasma concentrations of the active drug, or by modifying the amounts of active or toxic metabolites. It may also alter the enzymatic conversion of prodrugs into their active metabolites. Polymorphism in transporter molecules may affect the absorption, distribution or elimination of drugs by altering their transport across cell membranes in the gut, liver, renal tubule and other sites. Functional polymorphism is apparent in some ABC transporter proteins, including the MDR1 gene which codes for P-gp, and in OATs in the kidney, although the consequences of these for drug transport are unclear. Genetic polymorphism is likely of greatest clinical significance when the polymorphic protein is in the main or exclusive pathway affecting bioavailability and/or elimination and when the drug has a narrow therapeutic index (see Chapter 53).

The influence of genetic variation must be set against environmental factors, including age, pregnancy, interactions with other drugs (including alcohol and constituents of tobacco) and concurrent conditions including impairment of renal or hepatic function, which may be of greater importance in predicting drug efficacy and unwanted effects (see Chapter 56). A number of commercial tests have been marketed for specific polymorphic alleles in drug-metabolising enzymes, including some of those listed in Table 2.9. There are nevertheless formidable obstacles to the widespread use of genetic testing, including issues of cost and privacy. In most cases, individual gene variants have limited predictive value, and testing for haplotypes of multiple variants in the same gene or in other genes within the same metabolic pathways may be more predictive, but also more costly and difficult to interpret. A major hurdle to genetic testing at present is that reliable clinical trial data are not often available in people with diverse genotypes to guide prescribers in making appropriate alterations in drug regimens. Regulatory bodies including the FDA and EMA (see Chapter 3) are nevertheless increasingly recommending that genetic data are included in drug information.

SELF-ASSESSMENT

True/false questions

1. Un-ionised molecules cross phospholipid membranes more readily than their ionised forms.
2. Weak acidic drugs are mostly ionised in acid solutions.
3. Weak acidic drugs, such as aspirin, are mostly absorbed in the stomach.
4. Basic drugs may bind reversibly to α_1-acid glycoprotein in the plasma.
5. The plasma clearance of a drug usually decreases with increases in the dose prescribed.
6. First-pass metabolism may limit the bioavailability of oral drugs.
7. Drugs with high first-pass hepatic metabolism also have a high systemic clearance.
8. The half-life of many drugs is longer in babies than in children or adults.
9. A decrease in renal function affects oral bioavailability.
10. Depot injections of drugs have a prolonged half-life because their renal clearance is reduced.
11. Nifedipine is eliminated more rapidly in cigarette smokers.
12. Chronic treatment with phenobarbital can increase the plasma concentrations of co-administered drugs.
13. A loading dose is not necessary for drugs that have short half-lives.
14. An obese subject is likely to require higher doses of drugs than a nonobese subject during chronic therapy.
15. Alcohol intolerance due to genetic polymorphism is common in some ethnic groups.

One-best-answer (OBA) questions

1. What is the clearance of a drug?
   A. The drug volume from which plasma is removed per unit of time.
   B. The proportion of drug cleared from the blood per unit of time.

Table 2.9 Pharmacogenetic differences in drug-metabolising enzymes

Enzyme	Incidence of deficiency or slow-metaboliser phenotype in Caucasians	Typical substrates	Consequences of deficiency or slow-metaboliser status
Phase 1 reactions			
Pseudocholinesterase (butyrylcholinesterase, plasma cholinesterase)	1 in 3000	Suxamethonium (succinylcholine)	Prolonged paralysis and apnoea for up to 3 h after a dose
Alcohol dehydrogenase, acetaldehyde dehydrogenase	5–10% (>50% in Asians)	Ethanol and acetaldehyde	Profound vasodilation on ingestion of alcohol
CYP1A1	10%?	Polycyclic aromatic hydrocarbons	Increased risk of low birth weight with maternal smoking
CYP2A6	15%	Nicotine, coumarin	Reduced nicotine metabolism
CYP2B6	3–4% (15–40% in Asians, 20% in African Americans)	Ifosfamide, efavirenz	Increased efavirenz toxicity
CYP2C9	About 10% (3% in Africans)	Tolbutamide, diazepam, warfarin	Increased response if parent drug is active, e.g. increased risk of haemorrhage with warfarin
CYP2C19	3–6% (13–23% in Asians, 40–80% in Polynesians)	Clopidogrel, omeprazole, diazepam,	Variable efficacy of diazepam, omeprazole; reduced conversion of clopidogrel to active metabolite
CYP2D6	6%–10% (higher in African populations, <2% in Asians)	Codeine, nortriptyline, tamoxifen, tetrabenazine	Increased response if parent drug is active, but reduced response if oxidation produces the active form, e.g. codeine
Dihydropyrimidine dehydrogenase (DPD)	2–8%	Fluorouracil, capecitabine	Enhanced drug response
Phase 2 reactions			
N-Acetyltransferase	40–70% (10–20% in Asians, 80% in Egyptians)	Isoniazid, hydralazine, procainamide	Enhanced drug response and/or toxicity in slow acetylators
UDP glucuronyl transferase (UGT1A1)	10% (1–4% Asians)	Irinotecan	Enhanced effect (Gilbert's syndrome; increased bilirubin)
Glutathione transferase family	Various	Reactive compounds or metabolites	Increased risk of cancer from environmental carcinogens; therapeutic implications unclear
Thiopurine-S-methyl transferase (TPMT)	Low activity in 10%, absent in 0.3%	Mercaptopurine, azathioprine	Increased risk of toxicity (because the doses normally used are close to toxic)
Catechol-O-methyltransferase	25%	Levodopa	Slightly enhanced drug effect
Transporters			
ABCB1 (P-gp)	A number of SNPs identified in MDR1 gene (incidences vary with ethnic origin)	Digoxin, anticancer drugs, dihydropyridine calcium channel blockers	Possibly higher drug levels with some SNPs, but lower drug levels due to increased activity with other SNPs

P-gp, P-glycoprotein; *SNP*, single nucleotide polymorphism.

C. The rate of elimination of drug from the body by the liver and kidneys.

D. The time it takes to eliminate all of a drug from the body.

E. The volume of plasma from which drug is removed per unit of time.

2. Which statement about cytochrome P450 (CYP) isoenzymes is the most accurate?

A. CYP enzymes do not catalyse drug conjugation reactions.

B. CYP isoenzyme activity is not affected by diet.

C. The major site of CYP-mediated drug metabolism is the gut wall.

D. The activity of CYP enzymes is consistent among individuals.

E. Most drugs induce their own metabolism by CYP.

3. Identify the most accurate statement concerning apparent volume of distribution (V_d).

A. The V_d will be high if the drug is highly bound to plasma proteins.

B. The V_d is the dose of intravenous drug divided by the plasma concentration extrapolated back to time zero.

C. The V_d is proportional to the dose of drug administered.

D. The elimination half-life of a drug depends only on the V_d.

E. The V_d is used to calculate the maintenance dosage of a drug.

Descriptive question

Fig. 2.22 shows the changes in plasma levels of two drugs, A and B, each given to an adult man as 10-mg doses by the oral and intravenous routes (at time zero) on separate occasions. From the plasma concentration–time curves, compare drugs A and B for the following properties:

1. Absorption from the gut
2. Oral bioavailability
3. Distribution to tissues
4. Elimination half-life
5. Extent of accumulation with once-daily administration of each drug.

Case-based questions

Case 1

Meghan is a 7-year-old girl (weighing 31 kg) admitted to the emergency department with acute asthma. She is to be given aminophylline (a soluble form of theophylline) by slow intravenous injection. She has not had oral theophylline within the previous 24 hours. The target plasma concentration initially is 10 μg/mL. The apparent volume of distribution (V_d) of theophylline is 0.5 L/kg, and it comes in an injection solution containing 25 mg/mL of the drug.

1. What would be a suitable intravenous loading dose (in mg)?
2. What volume of the injection solution should be administered?
3. The British National Formulary for Children (BNFC) advises following the intravenous injection by a continuous intravenous infusion at a rate of 1 mg/kg/hour. Some hours after starting the infusion, the plasma theophylline concentration was only 7.5 μg/mL (which is subtherapeutic), and it was decided to raise this to 15 μg/mL for optimal benefit. What should be the new infusion rate?

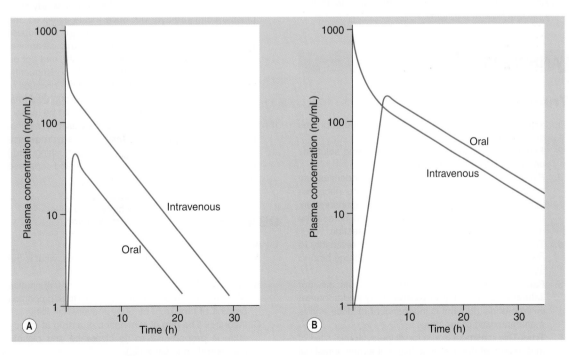

Fig. 2.22 **Plasma concentration–time curves for oral and intravenous doses of drugs A and B.** This figure accompanies the descriptive question in the self-assessment section.

Case 2

A man weighing 70 kg was admitted to hospital with a serious infection and was treated with two antibacterials. Gentamicin is given by intravenous administration, and cefalexin is given orally with bioavailability of 90% ($F = 0.9$).

	Gentamicin	Cefalexin
Volume of distribution (V_d) (L)	18	18
Clearance (CL) (L/h)	5.4	18
Half-life (h)	2–3	0.9

Gentamicin is very toxic, and its therapeutic plasma concentrations should not exceed 5 mg/L, since higher concentrations can lead to ototoxicity and nephrotoxicity.

1. You have been asked to give him 900 mg of gentamicin by injection as a bolus (single) dose. Is this a safe dose?
2. Because of the short half-life of gentamicin, you decide that it will be best to give him a continuous intravenous infusion to maintain a steady-state plasma concentration of 2.5 mg/L. What rate of infusion should be given?
3. What maximum plasma concentration of cefalexin would be obtained if a single oral loading dose of 500 mg was given?

Case 3

Mrs J. (body weight 70 kg) was diagnosed with congestive heart failure and atrial fibrillation. Treatment was started with digoxin, which has an apparent volume of distribution (V_d) of 9 L/kg and a half-life ($t_{1/2}$) of 42 hours. The plasma concentrations for therapeutic effectiveness are 0.8–2 ng/mL, and toxic effects occur above 2 ng/mL.

1. Approximately how long would it take to reach a steady-state concentration in plasma?
2. What dose should be given as a loading dose to achieve a plasma level of 0.8 ng/mL?

ANSWERS

True/false answers

1. **True.** Ionisation reduces lipid solubility and improves solubility in water.
2. **False.** Weak acids are least ionised in acid solutions and most ionised in basic solutions.
3. **False.** Although low pH in the stomach renders aspirin into its un-ionised, lipid-soluble form, the low surface area of the stomach wall limits the extent of drug absorption; the bulk of most oral drugs is absorbed across the much larger surface area of the small intestine.
4. **True.** Basic (or neutral) drugs may bind reversibly to α_1-acid glycoprotein, while many acidic drugs bind to albumin.
5. **False.** Provided the elimination processes are not saturated, clearance (like bioavailability and apparent volume of distribution) is independent of dose and is a characteristic of the drug.
6. **True.** This statement is true for all 'presystemic' sites of metabolism of the oral dose (e.g. gut lumen, intestinal wall and liver). Low bioavailability may also arise from poor absorption from the gut.

7. **True.** If the liver is able to clear a high proportion of the drug on first pass, then the drug fraction that survives to enter the general circulation will experience further rapid clearance on subsequent passes through the liver.
8. **True.** Infants under 12 months have relatively low hepatic metabolism and renal excretion, so many drugs are cleared more slowly and have longer half-lives than in older children and adults.
9. **False.** A decrease in renal function could affect systemic clearance, but bioavailability is simply the fraction of the oral dose that reaches the general circulation unaltered, and the kidneys are not part of the route between gut lumen and general circulation.
10. **False.** Using a depot injection of a drug prolongs its apparent elimination half-life due to slower, sustained release from the site of injection. Once absorbed into the blood, the circulating drug is handled by the kidneys as normal; the volume of plasma cleared of the drug per unit time (clearance) is unaltered.
11. **False.** From Table 2.7, nifedipine is metabolised by CYP3A4, while smoking induces CYP1A2, so no interaction is likely to occur.
12. **False.** Phenobarbital is a potent inducer of several cytochrome P450 isoenzymes (e.g. CYP2C9, CYP3A4), and this would *reduce* plasma concentrations of co-administered drugs that are substrates for the same CYP isoenzymes.
13. **True.** Drugs with short elimination half-lives reach therapeutic concentrations relatively rapidly, and a loading dose is usually unnecessary.
14. **False.** A lipid-soluble drug would have a higher apparent V_d in an obese person due to greater distribution into adipose tissue. It will therefore take longer (or require a larger loading dose) to achieve the desired steady-state plasma concentration, but once this is achieved, the maintenance dose rate will be the same as in a nonobese person because it depends on systemic clearance, which is unlikely to be different in obesity, and not on apparent V_d (see Eq. 2.21). There would consequently be no need to modify chronic drug dosage because of an increase in V_d in an obese person, although the total body load of a drug at steady state would be higher.
15. **True.** Genetic variations that alter the activity of alcohol dehydrogenase and acetaldehyde dehydrogenase underlie the alcohol intolerance (facial flushing, etc.) experienced by many people of Chinese and Japanese ancestry.

OBA answers

1. **Answer E** is the best definition.
   A. Incorrect. This statement is meaningless; what is the volume of a drug?
   B. Incorrect. A drug has first-order (exponential) kinetics when its plasma concentration falls by a fixed proportion per unit of time (e.g. by 50% in every half-life).
   C. Incorrect. The rate of elimination of a drug at steady state is proportional to its clearance and plasma concentration ($= CL \times C_{ss}$).
   D. Incorrect. The time it takes to eliminate a drug from the body is inversely proportional to clearance.

E. **Correct**. Clearance is therefore expressed in units of volume (of plasma) cleared of the drug per unit of time e.g. mL/minute or L/hour.

2. **Answer A** is the most accurate statement.
   A. **Correct**. CYP enzymes perform many types of reaction (oxidation, reduction, hydrolysis, hydration) during phase 1 drug metabolism, but phase 2 (conjugation) reactions usually require additional enzymes such as UDPGT and glutathione transferases.
   B. Incorrect. CYP isoenzymes can be inhibited or induced by dietary items such as grapefruit juice or charred meat.
   C. Incorrect. The liver has higher levels of CYP isoenzymes than other tissues.
   D. Incorrect. Pharmacogenetic variation between individuals is particularly marked for CYP2C19 and CYP2D9.
   E. Incorrect. Most drugs do not induce (or inhibit) CYP isoenzymes.

3. **Answer B** is the most accurate statement.
   A. Incorrect. Drugs confined within the circulation (e.g. by plasma protein binding) have a *low* apparent V_d. (The total drug concentration in plasma, both free and bound, is used when calculating V_d. Extensive binding of the drug to proteins in tissues *outside* the circulation could inflate the apparent V_d.)
   B. Incorrect. Extrapolation of the plasma concentration to time zero estimates the apparent V_d before elimination reduces the total amount of drug in the body.
   C. **Correct**. Apparent V_d is a characteristic of a particular drug, but is independent of dose.
   D. Incorrect. The half-life is proportional to V_d and inversely proportional to clearance.
   E. Incorrect. The loading dose is $C_{ss} \times V_d$.

Descriptive answers

1. The rate of absorption is determined by the rate of increase after oral dosing. Drug A is absorbed rapidly, while drug B takes about 6 h to reach a peak concentration.
2. Bioavailability (F) is determined by the ratio of the area under the oral and intravenous curves (AUC_{oral}/AUC_{iv}). For drug A, bioavailability (F) is visibly much less than 1, while for drug B the AUC_{oral} approximately equals the AUC_{iv}, so F is about 1, suggesting it is completely absorbed after oral dosing.
3. The rate of distribution is given by the steep initial slope of the *intravenous* drug curve from time zero to the establishment of the slower, terminal elimination phase, which is at about 1 hour for drug A and 3–4 hours for drug B, so drug A distributes more rapidly. Extrapolating the gentle slope of the terminal elimination phase back to time zero gives similar intercepts (apparent V_d) for both drugs, indicating they have a similar extent of distribution.
4. The slope of the elimination phase is greater for drug A than for B, so its elimination rate (k) is greater and its half-life is therefore shorter ($t_{1/2} = 0.693/k$). This must be due to a lower clearance (CL) of drug B, since it was shown previously that the volume of distribution is similar for both drugs. This is also apparent from the greater AUC for intravenous drug B, as the doses were the same (10 mg).

5. The potential for accumulation depends on the difference between the half-life and the dose interval (once-daily = 24 hours). It is clear that after 24 hours nearly all of drug A has been removed from the plasma, but considerable amounts of B remain, so drug B would show significant accumulation.

Case-based answers

Case 1

1. Note that the apparent V_d of theophylline is given as 0.5 L/kg of the child's bodyweight (31 kg), so it needs to be expressed as total V_d in litres, and also that the desired plasma concentration (10 µg/mL) should be expressed as 10 mg/L for consistency in units. The loading dose ($= C_{ss} \times V_d$) will therefore be:

$$10\ \text{mg/L} \times (0.5\ \text{L/kg} \times 31\ \text{kg}) = 155\ \text{mg}$$

2. The volume of a 25 mg/mL solution required for a dose of 155 mg is $(155/25) = 6.2$ mL. This is given slowly (over 20 minutes).
3. If the desired plasma concentration is now 15 µg/mL, twice as high as the concentration actually achieved by the infusion (7.5 µg/mL), then the infusion rate should be doubled (from 1 mg/kg/hour to 2 mg/kg/hour). The latter is equivalent to 62 mg/hour in this 31 kg patient or about 2.5 mL/hour of the 25 mg/mL solution. The simple linear relationship that steady-state plasma concentration is directly proportional to the infusion rate (assuming that clearance is unchanged) is shown by Eq. 2.17. In practice, the plasma theophylline concentration would continue to be monitored and the infusion rate titrated up or down accordingly.

Case 2

1. The maximal recommended dose is given by maximal plasma concentration (C_{ss}) × volume of distribution (V_d), so 5 mg/L × 18 L = 90 mg. The advice to give a bolus dose of 900 mg is therefore not safe, as it would give a plasma concentration 10 times higher than recommended.
2. At steady state, the rate of infusion = the rate of elimination = CL (clearance) × C_{ss} (Eq. 2.17), so for a plasma concentration of 2.5 mg/L, you will need to give an infusion rate of 5.4 L/hour × 2.5 mg/L = 13.5 mg/h.
3. For a single oral dose, the peak concentration is approximately equal to the *absorbed* dose divided by the apparent volume of distribution (V_d) (Eq. 2.10). Including a correction for the bioavailability ($F = 0.9$) of the oral dose ($D = 500$ mg), the concentration is:

$$C = (D \times F)/V_d = (500\ \text{mg} \times 0.9)/18\ \text{L} = 25\ \text{mg/L}$$

Due to some elimination occurring before the peak concentration is reached, the peak concentration achieved would be lower than 25 mg/L, but this could be ignored in clinical practice.

Case 3

1. It takes about four to five times the elimination half-life for a drug to approach its steady-state plasma concentration on repeated dosing. For digoxin ($t_{1/2}$ = 42 hour) this is 168–210 hours, or about 7–9 days; hence the need for a loading dose.

2. Using Eq. 2.22 and adjusting V_d (9 L/kg) for the patient's body weight (70 kg) gives:

   Loading dose = $C_{ss} \times V_d$ = 0.8 µg/L × (9 L/kg × 70 kg) = 504 µg

   In practice, a rounded dose of 500 µg would be given, and from the BNF this could be two 250 µg tablets.

FURTHER READING

Backmann, J.T., Filppula, A.M., Niemi, M., et al., 2016. Role of cytochrome P450 2C8 in drug metabolism and interactions. Pharmacol. Rev. 68, 168–241.

Batchelor, H.K., Marriott, J.F., 2015. Paediatric pharmacokinetics: key considerations. Br. J. Clin. Pharmacol. 79, 395–404.

Baumann, A., 2006. Early development of therapeutic biologics—pharmacokinetics. Curr. Drug Metab. 7, 15–21.

Daly, A.K., 2010. Pharmacogenetics and human genetic polymorphisms. Biochem. J. 429, 435–449.

Feero, W.G., Guttmacher, A.E., Collins, F.S., 2010. Genomic medicine—an updated primer. N. Engl. J. Med. 362, 2001–2011.

Flockhart, D.A., 2007. Drug interactions: cytochrome P450 drug interaction table. Indiana University School of Medicine. <http://medicine.iupui.edu/clinpharm/ddis/clinical-table> (Accessed 16 April 2016).

Gabrielsson, J., Green, A.R., 2009. Quantitative pharmacology or pharmacokinetic-pharmacodynamic integration should be a vital component in integrative pharmacology. J. Pharmacol. Exp. Ther. 331, 767–774.

Holland, I.B., 2011. ABC transporters, mechanisms and biology: an overview. Essays Biochem. 50, 1–17.

Nigam, S.K., 2015. What do drug transporters really do? Nat. Rev. Drug Discov. 14, 29–44.

Pirmohamed, M., 2011. Pharmacogenetics: past, present and future. Drug Discov. Today 16, 852–861.

Shah, R.R., Shah, D.R., 2015. Personalised medicine: is it a pharmacogenetic mirage? Br. J. Clin. Pharmacol. 74, 698–721.

Tannenbaum, C., Sheehan, N.L., 2014. Understanding and preventing drug–drug and drug–gene interactions. Expert. Rev. Clin. Pharmacol. 7, 533–744.

Tucker, G.T., 2012. Research priorities in pharmacokinetics. Br. J. Clin. Pharmacol. 73, 924–926.

Verkmann, A.S., 2009. Aquaporins: translating bench research to human disease. J. Exp. Biol. 212, 1707–1715.

Wang, L., McLeod, H.L., Weinshilboum, R.M., 2011. Genomics and drug response. N. Engl. J. Med. 364, 1144–1153.

3

Drug discovery, safety and efficacy

Historically, most medicines were of botanical or zoological origin, and most had dubious therapeutic value. A handful of medicines with real therapeutic efficacy have been known for many centuries, such as preparations of opium used more or less successfully for the treatment of pain and diarrhoea (i.e. dysentery) for thousands of years, but others were often misused, such as the antimalarial drug quinine being prescribed for fevers of nonmalarial origin.

Early medicines consisting of crude extracts of plants or animal tissues usually contained a mixture of many organic compounds, of which one, more than one or none may have had useful biological applications. The active constituents of some plant-derived preparations are bitter-tasting organic molecules known as alkaloids. For example, opium contains high but variable concentrations of analgesic alkaloids including morphine, codeine and other compounds. Foxglove extracts (which contain cardiac glycosides) were used successfully for the treatment of 'dropsy' (fluid retention); however, there was also considerable toxicity, because the plant preparations contained highly variable amounts of the active glycoside, as well as other compounds that may produce harmful effects. Similarly, for centuries, extracts of white willow bark were used to ease joint pain and reduce fever, although their active ingredient, salicylic acid, also carries substantial toxicity and the extracts contained a range of unrelated compounds with biological activity, such as flavonoids and plant oestrogens.

During the 19th and 20th centuries there were major advances in inorganic and organic chemistry, allowing the synthesis of huge arrays of small organic molecules to be screened systematically for pharmacological activity. Improved laboratory techniques also allowed the generation of libraries of compounds purified from bacterial, fungal and botanical materials, which were prolific sources of novel molecules with biological activity. A major advance in the safety of plant-derived medicines was therefore the isolation, purification and chemical characterisation of the active component. The first purification of a compound from a plant source was the isolation of morphine from opium by Friedrich Serturner around 1805. The use of purified compounds in pharmaceutical research and testing has three main advantages:

- The administration of controlled amounts of the purified active compound removed biological variability in the potency of the crude plant preparation.
- The administration of the active component removed the unwanted and potentially toxic effects of contaminating substances in the crude preparations.
- The identification and isolation of the active component allowed the mechanism of action to be defined, leading to the synthesis and development of chemically related compounds based on the structure of the active component but with greater potency, higher selectivity, fewer unwanted effects, altered duration of action and better bioavailability. For example, chemical modification of salicylic acid by acetylation produced acetylsalicylic acid, first marketed as aspirin in 1899, with greater analgesic and antipyretic activity and lower toxicity than the parent compound.

Advances in drug development for the treatment of disease are illustrated most dramatically with antimicrobial chemotherapy, which revolutionised the chances of people surviving severe infections such as lobar pneumonia, the mortality from which was 27% in the pre-antimicrobial era, but fell to 8% (and subsequently lower) following the introduction of sulphonamides and then penicillins in the 1930s and 1940s. Latterly, advances in molecular biology have enabled the development of a growing number of 'biological' drugs (biopharmaceuticals) based on the structures of antibodies, receptors and other human proteins. Meanwhile, the Human Genome Project, and the growth of technologies that allow systematic study of the entire range of cellular RNAs, proteins, lipids and other small molecules (known as transcriptomics, proteomics, lipidomics and metabolonomics, respectively), have expanded knowledge of the range of gene products and processes that might present targets for novel drugs. Increasingly, pharmacogenomic research is describing the genetic factors that predict variations in drug efficacy and safety in individual patients, holding out the promise of personalised medicine.

Thus, although drug therapy has natural and humble origins, it is the application of scientific principles, particularly the use of controlled experiments and clinical trials of known quantities of pure compounds to generate reliable knowledge of drug actions, which has given rise to the clinical safety and efficacy of modern medicines. In the age of 'scientific reason' it is surprising that many people believe that 'natural' medicinal products, sometimes diluted beyond the point of disappearance of the last molecule of the product, offer equivalent therapeutic effectiveness or inherently carry no risk of unwanted effects.

A major advantage of modern drugs is their ability to act selectively – that is, to affect only certain body systems or processes. For example, a drug that both lowers blood glucose and reduces blood pressure may not be suitable for the treatment of someone with only diabetes mellitus (because of unwanted hypotensive effects) or a person with only hypertension (because of unwanted hypoglycaemic effects), or even of those with both conditions (because different doses may be needed for each effect).

DRUG DISCOVERY

The discovery of a new drug can be achieved in several different ways (Fig. 3.1). At the heart of the process is subjecting new chemical entities (novel compounds not previously synthesised) to a battery of screening assays designed to detect different types of biological activity. These include in vitro studies on isolated tissues, as well as in vivo studies of complex and integrated systems, such as animal health and behaviour. Novel compounds for screening may be produced by direct chemical synthesis or isolated from biological sources, then purified and characterised in relevant assays. The process of screening has been revolutionised in recent years by developments in high-throughput screening (HTS), which takes advantage of laboratory robotics for liquid handling of tiny (microlitre) reaction volumes in microplates containing hundreds or thousands of reaction wells. These are used for biochemical assays or with cell lines expressing cloned target proteins. Active compounds, which may be derived from small-molecule libraries of bacterial or fungal origin, or proteins derived from solid-phase peptide synthesis, can then be selected based on interactions with molecules and cells that express a range of possible sites of action, such as G-protein-coupled or nuclear receptors or enzymes important in drug metabolism. HTS methods allow the screening in some cases of hundreds of thousands of microplate wells each week; a positive result ('hit') in more than one HTS assay may define a 'lead' candidate, which is subjected to more labour-intensive and detailed investigation, including preclinical tests in laboratory animals (usually rodents).

A second, but not mutually exclusive, approach involves the synthesis and testing of chemical analogues and modifications of existing pharmaceuticals; generally, the products of this approach (the study of structure–activity relationships or SAR) show incremental advances in potency, selectivity and bioavailability. However, additional or even new properties may become evident when the compound is tested in animals or trialled in humans; for example, minor modifications of the sulfanilamide antimicrobial molecule gave rise to the thiazide diuretics and the sulfonylurea hypoglycaemics.

Drug development programmes usually attempt to identify substances to target a particular biological or pathological mechanism. This may entail the purification, adaptation or synthesis of a relevant endogenous substance, or a structural analogue, precursor or antagonist of it. Examples of targeted drug development include levodopa, used in the treatment of Parkinson's disease; the histamine H_2 receptor antagonists; and omeprazole, the first proton pump inhibitor. Logical drug development of this type depends on a detailed understanding of human physiology both in health and disease. Identification of putative drug targets may begin with a bioinformatics approach to 'mine' existing data in scientific publications and patents. Genetic polymorphism associated with human disease may provide clues as to pathological mechanisms. The validation of putative drug targets requires techniques ranging from in vitro biochemical, cell or tissue culture models up to whole animal models. Antisense oligonucleotides can be used to observe the effects of blocking the synthesis of individual proteins in cells and tissues, and transgenic technology that inserts or deletes specific genes can be used similarly at the whole animal level. Appropriate assays to identify molecules with the required action at the designated target may arise naturally from these models, or require the development of specialist assays to which HTS can be applied.

A limiting factor in rational drug design is often the lack of detailed knowledge of the three-dimensional structure of the putative binding site on a specific enzyme, receptor or other protein target, which usually requires complex analyses by X-ray crystallography or nuclear magnetic resonance (NMR) spectroscopy. The modelling of ligand–receptor interactions may also be attempted by homology with the known structures of related proteins. In silico (computer-aided) approaches to the virtual modelling of drug binding to receptor sites ('molecular docking' studies) have facilitated the development of ligands with high binding affinities and, often, high selectivity.

Recent advances in molecular biology have led to the increasing use of genomic techniques to identify genes associated with pathological conditions. An example of

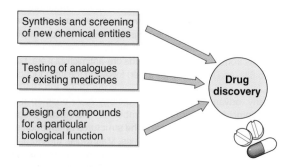

Fig. 3.1 **Approaches to drug discovery.**

drug development arising from this approach is the drug imatinib (see Chapter 52), developed to inhibit the Bcr-Abl receptor tyrosine kinase, which was implicated in chronic myeloid leukaemia cells by molecular biological methods; imatinib is a nonprotein organic molecule with a high oral bioavailability. A growing number of new drugs described in many chapters in this book are themselves proteins that directly mimic or otherwise interfere with the activity of the target gene product. Include recombinant antibodies or antibody fragments that block cell-surface receptors or humoral proteins, and soluble receptors that can neutralise cytokines. Being proteins, such biopharmaceuticals present particular problems of drug delivery to the relevant tissue and to the site of action (which may be intracellular; see Chapter 2), and also issues related to safety testing (discussed later).

Drug development is a long and costly process, with estimates of approximately 14 years and over GB£500 million to bring one new drug to market. Much of this cost lies in gaining the preclinical and clinical evidence required for approval of a new drug by regulatory bodies.

DRUG APPROVAL

Each year, many thousands of new chemical entities and compounds purified from plant and microbial sources are screened for useful and novel pharmacological activities. Potentially valuable compounds are then subjected to a sequence of in vitro studies, in vivo animal testing and clinical trials in humans, which provide essential information on safety and therapeutic benefits (Fig. 3.2).

All drugs and formulations licensed for sale in the United Kingdom have to pass a rigorous evaluation of:

- safety,
- quality,
- efficacy.

In the European Union (EU), new drugs are approved under a harmonised procedure of drug regulation. The European Medicines Agency (EMA; www.ema.europa.eu/ema) is a decentralised body of the EU with its headquarters in London and is responsible for the regulation of medicines within the EU. It is broadly comparable to the Food and Drug Administration (FDA; www.fda.gov) in the United States. The EMA receives advice from the Committee for Medicinal Products for Human Use (CHMP), which is a body of international experts who evaluate data on the safety, quality and efficacy of medicines. Other EMA committees are involved in evaluating paediatric medicines, herbal medicines and advanced therapies such as gene therapy. Under the current EU system, new drugs are evaluated by the CHMP, and national advisory bodies have an opportunity to assess the data before a final CHMP conclusion is reached.

The UK Commission on Human Medicines (CHM) was established in 2005 to replace both the Medicines Commission (MC) and the Committee on Safety of Medicines (CSM), which previously had evaluated medicines regulated in the UK under the Medicines Act (1968). The CHM is one of a number of committees established under the Medicines and Healthcare products Regulatory Agency (MHRA; www.mhra.gov.uk). The CHM provides advice on human medicines to the UK Secretary of State for Health and other government ministers.

SAFETY

Historically, the introduction of new drugs has been bought at a price of significant toxicity, and regulatory systems have arisen as much to protect patients from drug toxicity as to ensure benefit. In the United States, the FDA was established in 1937, following a dramatic incident in which 76 people died of renal failure after taking an elixir of sulfanilamide containing the solvent diethylene glycol. Similarly, some 30 years later, the occurrence of limb malformations (phocomelia)

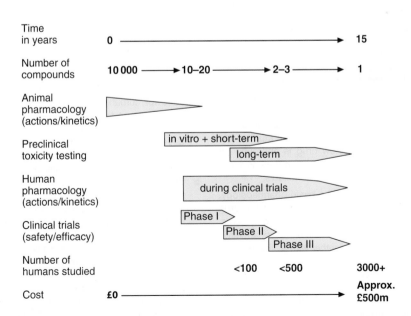

Fig. 3.2 **The development of a new drug to the point at which a licence is approved.** Postmarketing surveillance will continue to add data on safety and efficacy.

and cardiac defects in infants born to mothers who had taken thalidomide for the treatment of nausea in the first trimester of pregnancy led to the establishment of the precursor of the CHM in the United Kingdom.

Today, major tragedies are avoided by a combination of in vitro studies and animal toxicity tests (preclinical testing) and by careful observation during clinical studies on new drugs (discussed later). The development and continuing refinement of preclinical toxicity testing has increased the likelihood of identifying chemicals with direct organ toxicity. During clinical trials, immunologically mediated effects are likely to be seen at the lower end of the dose ranges that are used in such trials (see Chapter 53).

QUALITY

An important function of regulatory bodies is to ensure the consistency of prescribed medicines and their manufacturing processes. Drugs have to comply with defined criteria for purity, and limits are set on the content of any potentially toxic impurities. The stability and, if necessary, sterility of the drug also have to be established. Similarly, licensed formulations must contain a defined and approved amount of the active drug, released at a specified rate. There have been a number of cases in the past in which a simple change to the manufactured formulation affected tablet disintegration, the release of drug and the therapeutic response. The quality of drugs for human use is defined by the specifications in the European Pharmacopoeia (Ph.Eur.) and the British Pharmacopoeia (BP).

EFFICACY

All medicines, apart from homeopathic products, must have evidence of efficacy for their licensed indications. Efficacy (i.e. the ability to produce a predefined level of clinical response) can be established only by trials in people with the disease, for whom the medicine is intended, and therefore the demonstration of efficacy is a major aim of the later phases of clinical research (see Fig. 3.2).

ESTABLISHING SAFETY AND EFFICACY

Regulatory bodies such as the CHMP and CHM require supporting data from in vitro studies, animal studies and clinical investigations before a new drug is approved for use in a specific clinical indication. Although there is some overlap, the basic aims and goals are as follows:

- **Preclinical studies.** Establish the basic pharmacology, pharmacokinetics and toxicological profile of the drug and its metabolites, using animals and in vitro systems.
- **Phase I clinical studies.** Establish the human pharmacology and pharmacokinetics, together with a simple safety profile.
- **Phase II clinical studies.** Establish the dose–response relationship and develop the dosage protocol for clinical use, together with more extensive safety data.
- **Phase III clinical studies.** Establish the efficacy and safety profile of the drug in people with the proposed disease for which the drug will be indicated.

- **Phase IV (pharmacovigilance or post-marketing surveillance).** Monitor adverse events following approval and marketing of the drug.

PRECLINICAL STUDIES

Preclinical studies must be carried out before a compound can be administered to humans. These studies investigate three areas:

- **Pharmacological effects.** In vitro effects using isolated cells, tissues or organs; receptor-binding characteristics; in vivo effects in animals and/or animal models of human diseases; prediction of potential therapeutic use;
- **Pharmacokinetics.** Identification of metabolites (since these may be the active form of the compound); evidence of bioavailability (to assist with the design of both clinical trials and in vivo animal toxicity studies); establishment of principal route and rate of elimination;
- **Toxicological effects.** A battery of in vitro and in vivo studies undertaken with the aim of identifying toxicity as early as possible, and before there is extensive in vivo exposure of animals or, subsequently, humans.

TOXICITY TESTING

Toxicity testing has two primary goals: identification of hazards and prediction of the likely risk of that hazard occurring in humans receiving therapeutic doses of the new medicine. A wide range of doses is studied: high doses are required to increase the ability to detect hazards, and lower doses are needed to analyse dose–response relationships to predict the risk at doses producing the anticipated therapeutic effect. Toxicity tests include the following:

- **Mutagenicity.** A variety of in vitro tests using bacterial cells (such as the Ames test) and cell lines from rodents are employed at an early stage to define any damage to DNA or chromosomal structures that may be linked to carcinogenicity or teratogenicity; in vivo studies may be undertaken to investigate the mechanism of genotoxicity.
- **Acute toxicity.** A single dose is given to animals by the route proposed for human use; this may reveal a likely site for toxicity and is essential in defining the initial dose for human studies. Acute toxicity data, including information on the doses causing lethality, are essential for safe manufacture; the LD_{50} (a precise estimate of the dose required to kill 50% of an animal population) has been replaced by simpler and more humane methods that define the dose range associated with acute toxicity.
- **Subacute toxicity.** Repeated doses are given to animals for 14 or 28 days; this will usually reveal the target for toxic effects, and comparison with single-dose data may indicate the potential for accumulation.
- **Chronic toxicity.** Repeated doses are given to animals for up to 6 months; this reveals the target for toxicity (except cancer). The aim is to define dose regimens associated with adverse effects and a 'no observed adverse effect level' (NOAEL; the 'safe' dose).
- **Carcinogenicity.** Repeated doses are given throughout the lifetime of the animal (usually 2 years in a rodent).
- **Reproductive toxicity.** Repeated doses are given to animals from before mating and throughout gestation

to assess any effect on fertility, implantation, fetal growth, the production of fetal abnormalities (teratogenicity) or neonatal growth.

The extent of animal toxicity testing required prior to the first administration to humans is related to the proposed duration of human exposure and the population to be treated. All drugs are subjected to an initial in vitro screen for mutagenic potential. If satisfactory, this is followed by acute and subacute studies for up to 14 days of administration to two animal species. Doses studied are usually a low dose sufficient to cause the pharmacological/therapeutic effect, a high dose sufficient to cause target organ toxicity and an intermediate dose, together with a control group of untreated animals. Teratogenicity and reproductive toxicity studies are required if the drug is to be given to women of childbearing age; since the thalidomide tragedy, rabbits have been used for teratogenicity studies because, unlike rodents, they show fetal abnormalities when treated with thalidomide. Carcinogenicity testing is necessary for drugs that may be used for long periods (e.g. longer than 1 year).

An international review of the extent of in vivo animal testing necessary prior to phase I and phase II clinical trials concluded that the duration of animal toxicity tests should be the same as proposed human exposure (Table 3.1). In Japan and the United States, the same advice applies for phase III studies, but the EU recommends more extensive animal toxicity studies to support phase III trials. Dogs are the 'nonrodent species' usually studied.

The use of animals for the establishment of chemical safety is an emotive issue, and there is extensive current research to replace animal studies with in vitro tests based on known mechanisms of toxicity. The UK government policy published a delivery plan in February 2014 for the replacement, reduction and refinement of the use of animals in research (the '3Rs'). However, toxicology as a predictive science is still in its infancy, and at present it is impossible to replicate the complexity of mammalian physiology and biochemistry by in vitro systems. In vivo studies remain essential to investigate interference with either integrative functions or complex homeostatic mechanisms. Carefully controlled safety studies in animals are an essential part of the current procedures adopted to prevent extensive human toxicity, which would inevitably result from the use of untested compounds. Although toxicology has failed in the past to prevent some tragedies (discussed previously), these have led to improvements in methods and current tests provide an effective predictive screen. Nevertheless, there have been examples of approved drugs being withdrawn because of reactions that were not detected in preclinical studies (e.g. the high rate of rhabdomyolysis produced by cerivastatin, which was withdrawn worldwide in 2001). This may be increasingly important in the future because drugs developed using molecular biological methods to act specifically at human proteins may show limited or no activity at the analogous rodent receptors; however, animal studies will still provide a useful screen for nonspecific, nonreceptor-mediated effects.

Students should recognise that not all hazards detected at high doses in experimental animals are of relevance to human health. An important function of expert advisory bodies such as the CHMP is to assess the relevance to human health of effects detected in experimental animals at doses that may be two orders of magnitude (or more) above human exposures. Many drug 'scare stories' in the media are based on a hazard detected at experimental doses in animals much higher than the relevant doses for humans.

CLINICAL TRIALS: PHASES I–III

The purposes of premarketing clinical studies are:

- to establish that the drug has a useful action in humans,
- to define any toxicity at therapeutic doses in humans,
- to establish the nature of common (type A) unwanted effects (see Chapter 53).

Subjects in clinical studies give informed consent to participate, and the trials are approved by ethics committees and regulatory agencies. Traditionally, premarketing clinical studies have been subdivided into three phases. Although the distinction between these is blurred, the following classification system provides a useful framework.

Phase I studies

Phase I is the term used to describe the first trials of a new drug in humans, with typically between 20 and 100 volunteers. A principal aim of these studies is to define basic properties, such as route of administration, pharmacokinetics and tolerability. The studies are usually carried out by the pharmaceutical company, often using a specialised contract research organisation. Subjects taking part in phase I studies are often healthy volunteers recruited by open advertisement, especially when the compound is of low predicted toxicity and has wide potential use (e.g. an antihistamine). In some cases, people suffering from the condition in which the drug will be used may be studied, such as cytotoxic agents used for cancer chemotherapy.

The first few administrations are usually in a very small number of subjects ($n < 10$) who receive an oral dose that may be as low as one-fiftieth or one-hundredth of the minimum required to produce a pharmacological effect in animals (after scaling for differences in body weight). Such a 'microdose' study may be termed a phase 0 trial. The dose may then be built up incrementally in larger subject groups until a pharmacological effect is observed or an unwanted

Table 3.1 European Medicines Agency guidelines for the length of animal toxicity studies necessary to support phase I and phase II studies in humans

Duration of proposed phase I or II clinical trials	MINIMUM RECOMMENDED DURATION OF REPEAT-DOSE ANIMAL TOXICITY STUDIES	
	Rodents	**Nonrodents**
Single dose	2–4 weeks	2 weeks
Up to 2 weeks	2–4 weeks	2 weeks
Up to 1 month	1 month	1 month
Up to 3 months	3 months	3 months
More than 3 months	6 months	9 months

Support of phase III clinical studies may require longer animal toxicity studies than shown here.

action occurs. During these studies, toxic effects are sought by routine haematology and biochemical investigations of liver and kidney function; other tests, including an electrocardiogram, will be performed as appropriate.

It is also usual to study the disposition, metabolism and main pathways of elimination of the proposed new drug in humans at this stage. Such studies help identify the most suitable dose and route of administration for future clinical studies. Investigations of drug metabolism and pharmacokinetics often necessitate the use of radioactively labelled compounds containing carbon-14 or tritium (^{3}H) as part of the drug molecule.

Peptide drugs have to be given intravenously in clinical trials to mimic the route of proposed clinical use. Very low doses are studied in the first instance, especially with peptides that are designed to interact specifically with human homeostatic or signalling systems, because studies in animals may not reveal the full biological activities. Despite these safeguards, TGN 1412, a monoclonal antibody directed against CD28, a co-stimulatory molecule for T-cell receptors, caused multiple organ dysfunction in its first phase I trial in six human volunteers in March 2006. The severe toxicity occurred at a dose 500 times lower than the dose found to be safe in animals, including nonhuman primates.

Phase II studies

During phase II studies, the detailed clinical pharmacology of the new compound is determined, typically in groups of 100–300 individuals with the intended clinical condition. A principal aim of these studies is to define the relationship between dose and pharmacological/therapeutic response in humans. Evidence of a beneficial effect may emerge during phase II studies, although a placebo control is not always used. Additional studies may be undertaken at this stage in special groups such as elderly people, if it is intended that the drug will be used in that population. Other studies may investigate the mechanism of action, or test for interactions with other drugs. Phase II studies normally define the optimum dosage regimen, and this is then used in large clinical trials to demonstrate the efficacy and safety of the drug.

Phase III studies

Phase III studies are the main clinical trials, usually performed in 300–3000 people with the condition that the drug is intended to treat, in multiple centres, in comparison with a placebo that looks (and tastes) the same as the active compound. The allocation to active compound or placebo requires randomisation, which reduces selection bias in the assignment of treatments and facilitates the blinding (masking) of the identity of treatments from the investigators. The advantages and disadvantages of the new compound may also be compared with the best available treatment or the leading drug in the class. It may be ethically impossible to justify the use of a placebo if an effective form of treatment has been established for the condition being studied, as substituting the novel drug for the established treatment in the trial could result in significant risk to those participating in both the placebo and treatment groups. The drug under evaluation may therefore be used in addition to the established treatment and compared with the established treatment plus a placebo.

Clinical trials are of two main types: within-subject and between-subject comparisons (Fig. 3.3). In within-subject trials, an individual is randomly allocated to commence treatment either with the new compound or with a placebo (or comparator drug) before 'crossing over' to the alternative therapy, usually with a washout period in between. In contrast, between-subject comparisons involve randomisation of subjects to receive only one of two (or more) treatments for the duration of the study.

Within-subject comparisons (also called crossover trials) can usually be performed on a smaller number of subjects, since the individuals act as their own controls and most nontreatment-related variables are eliminated. However, such studies often require a longer involvement of each individual. Also, there may be carry-over effects from one treatment that affect the apparent efficacy of the second treatment, although statistical analysis should be able to deal with this problem. Studies of this type may be difficult to interpret when there is a pronounced seasonal variation in the severity of a condition, such as Raynaud's phenomenon or hay fever. Crossover studies (see Fig. 3.3) cannot be used if the treatment is curative (e.g. an antimicrobial for treating acute infections).

Between-subject comparisons (also called parallel-group studies) require roughly twice as many participants as within-subject trials, but have the advantage that each subject will usually be studied for a shorter period and carry-over effects are avoided. Although it is not possible to provide a perfect match between subjects entering the two (or more) different treatment groups, this approach to the evaluation of new drugs is preferred by many drug regulatory authorities.

Whichever form of comparison is made, measurements of benefits (and adverse effects) are made at regular intervals using a combination of objective and subjective techniques (Table 3.2). Throughout these studies, careful attention is paid to detecting and reporting both unwanted effects (type A reactions) and unpredictable (type B) reactions (see Chapter 53). Rare type B reactions are not usually seen prior to the marketing of a new drug, because they may occur only once in every 1000–10,000 or more individuals treated with the drug. It is salutary to note that by the time a new medicine is marketed, only 2000–3000 people may have taken the drug,

Table 3.2 Examples of response measurements during clinical trials

New drug type	MEASUREMENT TECHNIQUES	
	Objective	**Subjective**[a]
Antianginal	Exercise tolerance	Fatigue
	Blood pressure Heart rate	Frequency of anginal attacks
	Glyceryl trinitrate use	Pain intensity
Antiarthritic	Grip strength	Duration of morning stiffness
	Joint size	—
	Paracetamol use	Pain intensity

[a]Subjective effects are often scored on a numerical scale, e.g. 0 = no pain at all, 10 = the worst imaginable pain.

Within-subject trial

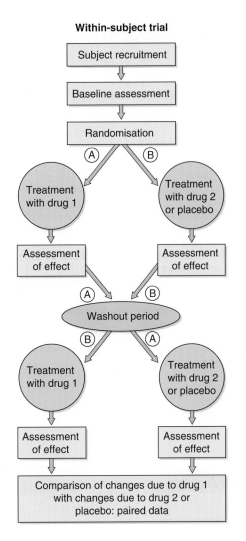

Between-subject trial

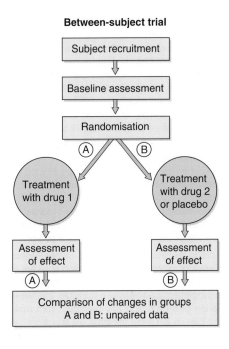

Fig. 3.3 **The design of clinical trials.** Subjects are randomly allocated to group A or group B.

often for relatively short periods such as 6 months, amounting to only a few hundred patient-years of drug exposure.

POSTMARKETING SURVEILLANCE: PHASE IV (PHARMACOVIGILANCE)

The full spectrum of benefits and risks of medicines may not become clear until after they are marketed. Reasons for this include the low frequency of certain adverse drug reactions, and the tendency to avoid the inclusion of children, the elderly and women of childbearing age in premarketing clinical trials. Another factor is the widespread use of other medicines in normal clinical practice, which could produce an unexpected interaction with the new drug. Phase IV studies involve postmarketing surveillance of efficacy and adverse reactions, sometimes in clinical indications additional to those licensed. Pharmacovigilance is the identification of risk/benefit issues for authorised medicines arising from their use in clinical practice, and includes the effective dissemination of information to optimise the safe and effective use of medicines.

Pharmacovigilance reports across the EU are coordinated by the EudraVigilance network (http://eudravigilance.ema.europa.eu/human/). Within the United Kingdom, a number of systems of postmarketing surveillance are in use. The most important is known as the Yellow Card system; it depends on doctors reporting suspected serious adverse reactions to the MHRA, either online (see the MHRA website, www.mhra.gov.uk) or using postage-prepaid cards included in the British National Formulary (BNF) and the Monthly Index of Medical Specialties (MIMS). In addition to reporting suspected serious adverse effects of established drugs, doctors are asked to supply information about all unwanted effects of medicines that have been marketed recently. Each year the MHRA receives some 20,000 yellow cards/slips. In return, doctors are supplied regularly with information about current drug-related problems.

A second form of pharmacovigilance involves systematic postmarketing surveillance of recently marketed medicines. This may be organised by the pharmaceutical company responsible for the manufacture of the new drug. (Companies also receive information via their representatives.) The MHRA administers the Clinical Practice Research Datalink (CPRD; www.cprd.eu), formed in 2012 from the General Practice Research Database, which collects anonymised, longitudinal patient records from participating UK general practices. It is used in conjunction with the Yellow Card scheme to provide a warning system for approved medicines.

Prescription event monitoring (PEM) provides a further method for detailed study of possible associations provided by pharmacovigilance programmes. This involves:

- identification of a possible health problem associated with an approved medicine;
- identification by the UK Prescription Pricing Authority of individuals who have been prescribed a drug of interest;
- the subsequent distribution of 'green cards' to those individuals' GPs, with a request that they complete all details about the person and events that occurred.

The cards are returned to the Drug Safety Research Unit (DSRU; www.dsru.org), which collates and analyses the data. PEM has the advantage that it does not require doctors to make a judgement concerning a possible link between the prescription of a drug and any medical event that occurs while the person is taking the drug. At first sight, a broken leg may be thought an unlikely drug-related adverse effect, but it could be the result of drug-induced hypotension, ataxia or metabolic bone disease.

Finally, detailed monitoring of adverse reactions to drug therapy takes place in some hospitals. These data contribute further to our overall knowledge.

When assessing efficacy and associated toxicity, combining the data from a number of clinical trials (meta-analysis) can provide an overview of the validity and reproducibility of clinical findings. Meta-analysis is complex, and only well-designed trials should be combined. The Cochrane Library (www.thecochranelibrary.com) provides a regularly updated collection of evidence-based meta-analyses.

The National Institute for Clinical Excellence was established in 1999 and became the National Institute for Health and Care Excellence (NICE; www.nice.org.uk) in 2005, following its merger with the Health Development Agency. Since 2013, NICE has been a nondepartmental public body under the Health and Social Care Act 2012, providing guidance for people using the National Health Service (NHS) in England, with decisions on implementation in Wales, Scotland and Northern Ireland determined by the devolved administrations. It provides advice on the clinical value and cost-effectiveness of new treatments, but also on existing treatments if there is uncertainty about their use. NICE produces guidance on:

- Health technology – specific medicines, treatments and procedures;
- Clinical practice – how health professionals should treat diseases and conditions;
- Public health – preventing illness and health promotion;
- Social care – services to help people with daily life at home, in care homes or day centres;
- Quality standards statements designed to drive quality improvements within a particular area of care.

SELF-ASSESSMENT

One-best-answer (OBA) questions

1. In which phase of drug development is a placebo most likely to be used?
   A. Phase 0
   B. Phase I
   C. Phase II
   D. Phase III
   E. Phase IV

2. Which is the best description of a phase III crossover trial?
   A. Randomisation is not required in a crossover trial.
   B. People with the most severe disease are allocated to receive the active drug first.
   C. The second treatment period starts as soon as the first treatment period ends.
   D. Crossover trials are preferred for trials of curative drugs.
   E. Participants receive two or more treatments in a random sequence.

3. Which is the organisation directly responsible for advising UK government ministers on human medicines?
   A. CHM
   B. CPRD
   C. DSRU
   D. MHRA
   E. NICE

ANSWERS

OBA answers

1. **Answer D** is correct. A drug is most likely to be compared with a placebo in large-scale (phase III) trials, although a placebo may also be used in phase II trials. The drug (and placebo) may be added to the existing best treatment, or compared with a leading drug for the same condition.

2. **Answer E** is correct. Randomisation is designed to produce treatment groups that match in all important characteristics, including disease severity. In a within-subject (or crossover) trial, randomisation of the sequence of treatments that each subject receives reduces the probability of confounding by an effect of one treatment persisting into the second treatment period; an interval between treatments (washout) helps ensure this. Crossover trials are generally not used to test curative drugs for acute conditions (e.g. antimicrobials), as the condition may not persist through both treatment periods.

3. **Answer A** is correct. The CHM (Commission on Human Medicines) advises UK government ministers on the safety, efficacy and quality of medicinal products.

FURTHER READING

Adams, C.P., Brantner, V.V., 2006. Estimating the cost of new drug development: is it really $802 million? Health Aff. 25, 420–428.

Fox, S., Farr-Jones, S., Sopchak, L., et al., 2006. High-throughput screening: update on practices and success. J. Biomol. Screen. 11, 864–869.

Hughes, J.P., Rees, S., Kalindjian, S.B., et al., 2011. Principles of early drug discovery. Br. J. Pharmacol. 162, 1239–1249.

Kerwin, R., 2004. The National Institute for Clinical Excellence and its relevance to pharmacology. Trends Pharmacol. Sci. 25, 346–348.

Layton, D., Hazell, L., Shakir, S.A., 2011. Modified prescription-event monitoring studies: a tool for pharmacovigilance and risk management. Drug Saf. 34 (12), e1–e9.

Relling, M.V., Evans, W.E., 2015. Pharmacogenomics in the clinic. Nature 526, 343–350.

Schneider, G., Fechner, U., 2005. Computer-based de novo design of drug-like molecules. Nat. Rev. Drug Discov. 4, 649–663.

Wagner, B.K., 2016. The resurgence of phenotypic screening in drug discovery and development. Exp. Opin. Drug. Discov. 11, 121–125.

4

Neurotransmission and the peripheral autonomic nervous system

This chapter deals with the peripheral autonomic nervous system; the central nervous system and the somatic nervous system are discussed in Section 5 and Chapter 27, respectively.

THE CENTRAL AND PERIPHERAL NERVOUS SYSTEMS

There are two principal neuronal control systems in the body. Functionally they are highly integrated and should be considered holistically, but for clarity they are introduced separately:

- The *central nervous system* (CNS) comprises neuronal networks of the brain, brainstem and spinal cord (see Section 5).
- The *peripheral nervous systems* interconnect the CNS to the organs of the body; these include:
    - the *autonomic* (automatic or involuntary) nervous system, which comprises the sympathetic and parasympathetic nervous systems, and also includes the nervous system of the gut (enteric system),
    - the *somatic* (voluntary) nervous system, which innervates skeletal muscle (see Chapter 27).

The CNS integrates, processes and responds to sensory messages. It receives sensory information from all parts of the body, including visceral sensory afferent nerves (e.g. from viscera, smooth muscle and cardiac muscle) and somatic sensory afferents (e.g. from skeletal muscle). It then responds by sending instructions via the autonomic efferent nerves of the sympathetic and parasympathetic systems (e.g. to glands, smooth muscle and cardiac muscle) and via somatic motor efferents to skeletal muscle.

PRINCIPLES OF NEUROTRANSMISSION

Action potentials (APs) passing along neuronal axons signal to other neurons or nonneuronal cells (e.g. smooth muscle cells). Signals are transferred by the release of chemical neurotransmitters from the presynaptic endings of the neuron, which diffuse across the synaptic cleft and stimulate the receiving (postsynaptic) cells via receptor proteins (Fig. 4.1). The binding of the transmitter to the receptors may instruct the receiving cells to increase or reduce their activity.

Neurotransmitters can be either synthesised within the presynaptic axon terminal (e.g. noradrenaline) or transported from the cell body to the synaptic region (e.g. peptides). The neurotransmitter is taken up from the cytosol by specific vesicular transporters within the nerve ending and stored within membrane vesicles. The release of the neurotransmitter

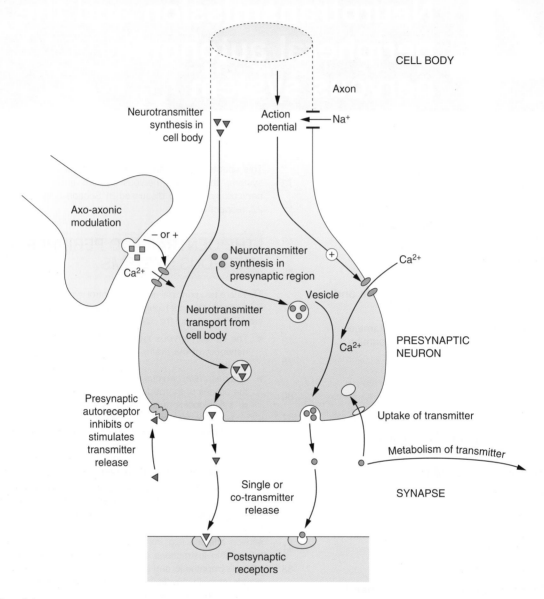

Fig. 4.1 **Principles of neurotransmission at a synapse.** Basic pathways of synthesis, storage, release, action and inactivation of a typical neurotransmitter are shown, as described in the text. At many synapses, co-transmission of different neurotransmitters occurs.

can be 'fine-tuned' by axo-axonic connections and by presynaptic receptors (discussed later). A generalised scheme for neurotransmission is as follows (see Fig. 4.1):

1. The cell body (or soma) responds to an appropriate stimulus by generating an AP.
2. The AP is conducted along the axon by the opening of voltage-gated Na^+ channels and the influx of Na^+; when the AP reaches the presynaptic nerve terminal, it results in an influx of Ca^{2+} through voltage-dependent channels.
3. Ca^{2+}-dependent processes result in fusion of neurotransmitter-containing vesicles with the presynaptic membrane and the release of stored neurotransmitter into the synaptic cleft.
4. The released neurotransmitter binds to the appropriate receptors in the postsynaptic membranes and generates

biochemical changes in the recipient cells; these may be functional changes (e.g. smooth muscle contraction) or excitation or inhibition of another neuron (e.g. transmission of the AP to postsynaptic nerve fibres).

5. The released neurotransmitter may also stimulate autoreceptors in the presynaptic membranes, and thereby modulate the further release of the neurotransmitter.
6. The transmitter is degraded by enzymes or taken back into the presynaptic neuron for reuse.

Neurons may release a single transmitter, but often more than one transmitter is released; there are many examples of *co-transmission*, which are described later in this book.

Table 4.1 The control of transmitter release by presynaptic receptor mechanisms

Neurotransmitter	Presynaptic receptors inhibiting release	Presynaptic receptors facilitating release
ACh	M_2, α_2, D_2/D_3, 5-HT_3	N_1, NMDA
Dopamine	D_2/D_3, M_2	N_1, NMDA
GABA	$GABA_B$	—
Histamine	H_3	—
5-HT	5-HT_{1D}, α_2	5-HT_3
Noradrenaline	α_2, H_3, M_2, D_2, opioid	β_2, N_1, angiotensin II

5-HT, Serotonin (5-hydroxytryptamine); *ACh,* Acetylcholine; *GABA,* γ-Aminobutyric acid; *NMDA,* N-methyl-D-aspartate.

PRESYNAPTIC RECEPTORS AND MODULATION OF TRANSMITTER RELEASE

An important characteristic of neurons is the presence of presynaptic receptors (see Fig. 4.1 and Table 4.1). Presynaptic receptors may increase or, more typically, decrease the release of the neurotransmitter, and are described as facilitatory and inhibitory, respectively. Inhibition of transmitter release is usually achieved by limiting Ca^{2+} entry through voltage-gated ion channels into the neuron. There are two functional categories of presynaptic receptors:

- autoreceptors respond to neurotransmitter released from the neurons upon which the receptor sits,
- heteroceptors respond to neurotransmitters released from other neurons, usually by axo-axonal synapses (see Fig. 4.1).

The first recognition of a clinically important presynaptic receptor came with the discovery that the antihypertensive agent clonidine lowers blood pressure via stimulation of presynaptic α_2-adrenoceptors, with subsequent inhibition of the release of vasoconstricting noradrenaline. Presynaptic receptors (see Table 4.1) are increasingly recognised as playing important roles in the clinical effects produced by many drugs.

THE PERIPHERAL AUTONOMIC NERVOUS SYSTEM

The peripheral autonomic nervous system (ANS) is an important site for the action of many drugs because:

- the ANS either controls or contributes to the control of the functioning of nearly all of the major organ systems of the body;
- ANS dysfunction is present in many diseases;
- ANS dysfunction can occur as an unwanted effect of drug treatment;
- the ANS utilises two major different neurotransmitters and a number of receptor subtypes; these provide a variety of sites for drug action (Box 4.1), which allows modification of particular body functions with some degree of selectivity.

The peripheral ANS is subdivided into two main branches (Fig. 4.2, Box 4.2):

- the *parasympathetic nervous system (PNS)*, which utilises acetylcholine (ACh) as the final transmitter at muscarinic

Box 4.1　Targets for drug action within the autonomic nervous system

- Muscarinic receptors at postganglionic nerve endings in the parasympathetic nervous system (M–M_3 receptor subtypes)
- Adrenoceptors in the sympathetic nervous system (α- and β-adrenoceptor subtypes)
- Presynaptic receptors in the parasympathetic and sympathetic nervous systems
- Modification of the synthesis, storage, release and inactivation of acetylcholine and noradrenaline

receptors on the cells being stimulated (called the innervated or effector cells or organs);

- the *sympathetic nervous system (SNS)*, which utilises noradrenaline as the transmitter at adrenoceptors on most, but not all, effector organs; the release of adrenaline and noradrenaline from the adrenal medulla during SNS stimulation is also an important and integral part of the SNS response.

Anatomically, in both branches of the ANS, the efferent neurons innervating effector organs are linked to neurons in the CNS via ganglia. The distribution and neuronal interconnections differ between the two branches (see Fig. 4.2):

- The parasympathetic efferents give more discrete innervation of organs; the ganglia are close to the innervated organs, and they therefore have long preganglionic fibres and short postganglionic fibres; there are few or no interconnections between ganglia, so that innervated organs can be controlled independently.
- The sympathetic efferents are classically described as being involved in the fight-or-flight response and affect many body systems simultaneously. Many of the ganglia are in the paravertebral sympathetic ganglion chain that lies close along each side of the spinal column, so these nerves have short preganglionic fibres and long postganglionic fibres. All neurons in the sympathetic system can be activated simultaneously because of numerous neuronal interconnections within the paravertebral chain; also, axons passing through the chain without synapsing can interconnect with ganglia such as the inferior mesenteric ganglion and then diversify to innervate several organs (see Fig. 4.2).

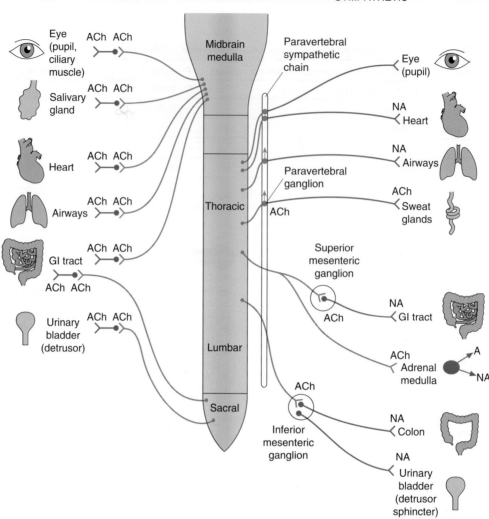

PARASYMPATHETIC

Eye (pupil, ciliary muscle) — ACh ACh

Salivary gland — ACh ACh

Heart — ACh ACh

Airways — ACh ACh

GI tract — ACh ACh

ACh ACh

Urinary bladder (detrusor) — ACh ACh

Midbrain medulla

Thoracic

Lumbar

Sacral

Paravertebral sympathetic chain

Paravertebral ganglion

ACh

ACh

Superior mesenteric ganglion

ACh

ACh

Inferior mesenteric ganglion

SYMPATHETIC

Eye (pupil)

NA Heart

NA Airways

ACh Sweat glands

NA GI tract

ACh Adrenal medulla → A, → NA

NA Colon

NA Urinary bladder (detrusor sphincter)

Fig. 4.2 Organisation of the parasympathetic and sympathetic autonomic nervous systems. Activation of the sympathetic nervous system leads to widespread neuronal release of noradrenaline, supplemented by release into the circulation of adrenaline (and noradrenaline) from the adrenal medulla; these act at α- and β-adrenoceptors (see Table 4.2). Stimulation of the parasympathetic nervous system produces more localised effects at particular organs, mediated by acetylcholine acting at muscarinic receptors (see Table 4.3). Some tissues, such as airways, have sparse sympathetic innervations, and sympathetic effects are mainly a result of circulating adrenaline. Sympathetic innervation of sweat glands is mediated, unusually, by acetylcholine. The ganglia innervating some organs are not part of the paravertebral chain but grouped together to form the coeliac, superior mesenteric or inferior mesenteric ganglia; the transmitter at all ganglia is acetylcholine acting at nicotinic N_1 (ganglion type) receptors. A, Adrenaline; ACh, acetylcholine; GI, gastrointestinal; NA, noradrenaline.

Box 4.2	Organisation of the autonomic nervous system (see also Figs 4.2 and 4.7)

- ACh and NA are the principal neurotransmitters in the autonomic nervous system, but other substances also have neurotransmitter roles.
- The neurotransmitters are released into synapses in response to depolarisation and Ca^{2+} influx caused by an action potential.
- Parasympathetic and sympathetic efferent nerves from the spinal cord synapse at intermediate ganglia, where the transmitter is ACh acting on nicotinic N_1 receptors to elicit action potentials in the postganglionic fibres.
- Stimulation of the sympathetic nervous system has a widespread effect in the body because of paravertebral

chain connections between efferent pathways, whereas the parasympathetic nervous system is more organ-specific.
- Parasympathetic postganglionic fibres release ACh that acts at muscarinic receptors on the end-organs.
- Sympathetic postganglionic fibres release NA that acts on α- and β-adrenoceptors on the end-organs, except for sympathetic cholinergic innervation of sweat glands and hair follicles.
- Adrenaline and NA are synthesised and released in the adrenal medulla in response to sympathetic stimulation, and enhance the effects of local NA release.

ACh, Acetylcholine; *NA*, noradrenaline.

Many organs are innervated by both the parasympathetic and SNSs, which act in concert and may have opposite effects on the organ function. Physiological functions therefore often require inverse coordination of sympathetic and parasympathetic activities; for example, urination is brought about by a decreased sympathetic activity on the sphincter muscle and increased parasympathetic activity on the bladder wall (detrusor) muscle (see urinary bladder, Tables 4.2 and 4.3, and Chapter 15).

The concept of opposing actions, although imperfect, can be useful in remembering the effects that each part of the autonomic nervous system has on organ function, and hence the effects of drugs that modulate SNS and PNS activity. Tables 4.2 and 4.3 show the effects that stimulation of the sympathetic or PNSs have on major tissues and the primary receptors that are involved. Under resting conditions, the predominant drive to many organs is from the PNS, with the SNS producing more transient but highly coordinated responses.

THE SYMPATHETIC NERVOUS SYSTEM AND NORADRENERGIC TRANSMISSION

Noradrenaline and adrenaline are members of the catecholamine family of amine transmitters (Fig. 4.3A). Both the catechol ring and the amino group are important for receptor binding. Noradrenaline and adrenaline stimulate adrenoceptors, and their effects at these receptors are described as noradrenergic and adrenergic, respectively.

The approved European names of noradrenaline and adrenaline, when formulated as medicines, are

Table 4.2 Effects of sympathetic nervous system activity via adrenoceptor subtypes in major tissues

Tissue	Effect	Main receptor type
Heart rate	Increase	β_1 (β_2 in heart disease)
Contractility	Increase	β_1 (β_2 in heart disease)
Atrioventricular conduction	Increase	β_1
Blood vessels in skin/gut	Constriction	α_1
Blood vessels in skeletal muscle	Dilation[a]	β_2
Bronchial smooth muscle	Dilation[a]	β_2
Gastrointestinal motility	Relaxation	α_1, β_2
Gastrointestinal sphincter tone	Contraction	α_1
Uterine smooth muscle	Contraction	α_1
	Relaxation	β_2
Bladder detrusor	Relaxation	β_2, β_3
Bladder sphincter	Constriction	α_1
Penis	Ejaculation	α_1
Pilomotor muscles	Constriction	α_1
Sweat glands	Secretion	Muscarinic
Pupil (radial muscle)	Contraction dilates pupil	α_1
Hepatic glycogenolysis	Increase	β_2, α
Skeletal muscle glycogenolysis	Increase[a]	β_2
Fat cell lipolysis	Increase[a]	β_1, α, β_3
Pancreas insulin secretion	Decrease	α_2
Platelets	Aggregation	α_2
Presynaptic nerve terminal (noradrenergic)	Inhibition of NA release	α_2
	Increased NA release	β_2
Presynaptic nerve terminal (muscarinic)	Inhibition of ACh release	α_2
Kidney (juxtaglomerular) renin release	Increase	β_1

[a]Respond to circulating adrenaline; little noradrenergic innervation.
ACh, Acetylcholine; *NA,* noradrenaline.

Table 4.3 Effect of stimulation of parasympathetic nerves (via muscarinic M_1–M_3 receptor subtypes) in major tissues[a]

Tissue	Effect	Main receptor type
Heart rate	Decrease	M_2
Contractility of atria	Decrease	M_2
Atrioventricular conduction velocity	Decrease	M_2
Vascular smooth muscle	Constriction	M_3
Vascular endothelium	Nitric oxide release (vasodilator)	M_3, M_1
Bronchial smooth muscle	Constriction	M_3, M_2
Gut motility	Contraction, relaxation	M_3, M_2
Gut sphincter tone	Increased	M_3
Gut secretions	Increased	M_3, M_1
Bladder detrusor	Contraction	M_3
Bladder sphincter	Relaxation	M_3
Penis	Erection	M_3
Eye pupil circular muscle	Contraction (miosis)	M_3
Eye: Ciliary muscle	Contraction (lens accommodates for near vision)	M_3
Pancreatic insulin secretion	Increased	M_1, M_3
Salivary glands	Secretion	M_3, M_1
Emesis	Increased	M_3

[a]Muscarinic M_1 and M_3 receptors are typically excitatory on smooth muscle and glandular tissues. M_2 receptors are typically inhibitory, notably in the heart, and also as inhibitory autoreceptors in many tissues. M_4 and M_5 receptor subtypes occur predominantly in the central nervous system.

norepinephrine and *epinephrine*, respectively; however, when their physiological actions are being described, the terms noradrenaline and adrenaline are retained. Most preparations of adrenaline and noradrenaline in Europe are dual-labelled with both terms. In the United States, the terms epinephrine and norepinephrine are used for both therapeutic and physiological descriptions.

SYNTHESIS AND STORAGE OF CATECHOLAMINES: NORADRENALINE, ADRENALINE AND DOPAMINE

Catecholamine neurotransmitters are synthesised from phenylalanine or tyrosine, which are aromatic amino acids derived from the diet (see Fig. 4.3B). The sequence of synthesis of adrenaline (via dopamine and noradrenaline) is shown in Fig. 4.3B. The oxidation of tyrosine to levodopa by tyrosine hydroxylase, which occurs within the neuron, commits the molecule to become a neurotransmitter. This step is subject to negative feedback by the catecholamines that are subsequently produced, thereby regulating supply. The conversion of levodopa to dopamine is catalysed by a cytosolic enzyme, aromatic L-amino acid decarboxylase (also known as dihydroxyphenylalanine [DOPA] decarboxylase). The amine product, dopamine, is taken up by vesicles via a specific transporter termed the vesicular monoamine transporter 2 (VMAT2). In neurons that use dopamine as their primary transmitter, this is the end of the synthetic pathway. Dopamine is a neurotransmitter in some parts of

the peripheral nervous system and also in important pathways in the CNS (see Chapters 7, 21 and 24).

The vesicles in noradrenergic neurons contain dopamine-β-hydroxylase, largely within the vesicle membrane, and this enzyme generates noradrenaline. Noradrenaline and its precursor dopamine are stored in the vesicles complexed with adenosine triphosphate (ATP) and proteoglycans.

The chromaffin cells of the adrenal medulla contain an additional cytosolic enzyme (phenylethanolamine-N-methyl transferase), which converts noradrenaline to adrenaline by the addition of a methyl group (see Fig. 4.3B). Adrenaline is then transferred into chromaffin cell granules by vesicular monoamine transporter 1 (VMAT1), where it is stored, ready for release.

NORADRENALINE RELEASE

Release in response to a nerve impulse occurs following Ca^{2+} influx and Ca^{2+}-mediated fusion of the noradrenaline-containing vesicle with the cytoplasmic membrane.

Noradrenaline in the presynaptic neuron may also be released by so-called indirectly acting sympathomimetic amines, which are low-molecular-weight basic compounds, including food constituents (such as tyramine), therapeutic drugs (such as ephedrine) and some drugs of abuse (such as amphetamine and metamphetamine). These compounds are taken into the presynaptic cytosol, where they interact with vesicular monoamine transporters to cause displacement of noradrenaline from the vesicles into the cytosol and

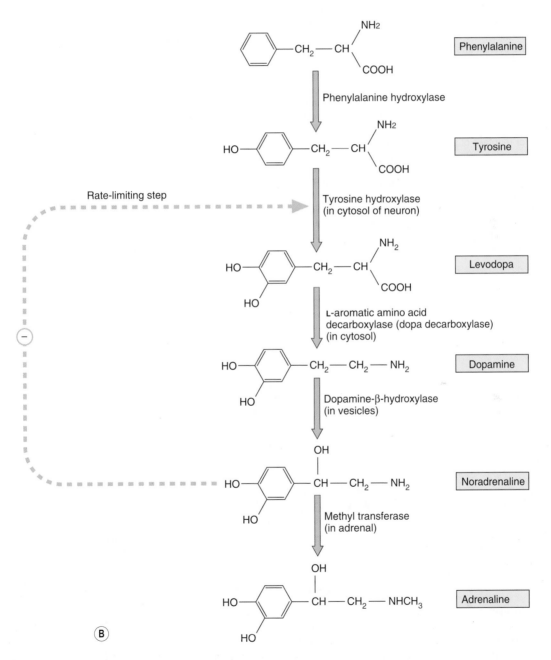

Fig. 4.3 **The structure of the main physiological catecholamines (A) and their synthesis from amino acid precursors (B).** The catecholamine synthetic pathway is described in the text.

thence into the synaptic cleft, leading to biological effects at postsynaptic adrenoceptors.

UPTAKE AND METABOLISM OF RELEASED NORADRENALINE

The principal mechanism for the removal of noradrenaline from the synapse is uptake (approximately 70–90%) into the presynaptic neuron via a specific high-affinity carrier called uptake 1 (or the norepinephrine transporter, NET); it also takes up dopamine but not adrenaline (Fig. 4.4). Both noradrenaline and dopamine can then be transferred from the cytosol into the vesicles by VMAT2. Some of the noradrenaline remaining in the synapse is taken up into nonneuronal tissues by a low-affinity carrier called uptake 2 (or the extraneuronal monoamine transporter), which can also transport adrenaline. The rest of the remaining noradrenaline and the majority of any adrenaline released into the circulation as a co-transmitter is metabolised. Separate transporters exist for reuptake of serotonin (5-hydroxytryptamine, 5-HT) and dopamine from their respective neurons, termed the serotonin transporter (SERT) and dopamine transporter (DAT), respectively. Therapeutic agents that block NET, SERT, DAT or permutations of these transporters increase the amount of monoamine neurotransmitters in the synaptic cleft and are used in treating depression (see Chapter 22). The uptake of noradrenaline by NET is also blocked by cocaine and amfetamine.

There are two main enzymes involved in the initial steps in the catabolism of noradrenaline: monoamine oxidase (MAO) and catechol-O-methyltransferase (COMT).

Monoamine oxidase

MAO is present on the surface of the mitochondria of the presynaptic neuron, where it oxidises free cytoplasmic noradrenaline, and also in many other sites such as the gastrointestinal epithelium and liver. There are two main MAO isoenzymes, MAO-A and MAO-B, which differ in their organ distribution and substrate affinities (Table 4.4). Oxidative removal of the amino group by MAO is the major pathway of catabolism of noradrenaline and other amine neurotransmitters. Loss of the amino group prevents binding to the postsynaptic receptor and therefore inactivates the transmitter. Metabolism of noradrenaline by MAO and COMT results in the formation of vanillylmandelic acid, which is the main urinary metabolite. The use of inhibitors of MAO-A and/or MAO-B isoenzymes in depression and Parkinson's disease is discussed in Chapters 22 and 24.

Catechol-O-methyltransferase

COMT occurs only at low levels in noradrenergic neurons, but is present in many other tissues, including the adrenal gland and liver. The enzyme catalyses the transfer of a methyl

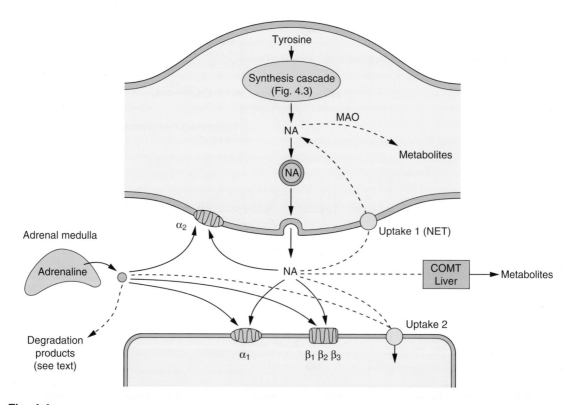

Fig. 4.4 **A noradrenergic nerve terminal (varicosity) showing the synthesis and sites of action of noradrenaline and adrenaline.** Dashed lines show how the actions of the catecholamines are curtailed. *COMT*, Catechol-O-methyltransferase; *MAO*, monoamine oxidase; *NA*, noradrenaline; *NET*, norepinephrine transporter (uptake 1).

Table 4.4 Monoamine oxidase and its inhibitors

Isoenzyme	Location in human tissues	Main substrates	EXAMPLES OF DRUG INHIBITORS	
			Irreversible	Reversible
MAO-A	Gastrointestinal tract, placenta	Serotonin, noradrenaline		Moclobemide
MAO-B	Brain,[a] liver,[a] platelets	Phenylethylamine, tyramine	Selegiline, rasagiline	
MAO-A or MAO-B		Tyramine, dopamine, adrenaline	Isocarboxazid, phenelzine, tranylcypromine	

[a]Both isoenzymes are present, but in humans the amount of MAO-B exceeds that of MAO-A.
MAO, Monoamine oxidase.

group onto the aromatic ring, which prevents binding to the postsynaptic receptor. COMT is a minor route of inactivation of both dopamine and noradrenaline. Inhibitors of COMT are used as an adjunct to levodopa therapy for Parkinson's disease (see Chapter 24).

SYMPATHETIC NERVOUS SYSTEM RECEPTORS

All autonomic ganglia utilise ACh as a neurotransmitter, acting predominantly on nicotinic type 1 (N_1) receptors (also known as 'ganglion-type' nicotinic receptors) to elicit an AP in the postganglionic axon. The receptors at most, but not all, postganglionic nerve endings in the SNS are adrenoceptors.

Based on the effects of a number of agonists and antagonists, adrenoceptors are divided into two types, α and β, and further into α-subtypes (α_1 and α_2) and β-subtypes (β_1, β_2 and β_3; see Table 4.2 and the drug receptor list at the end of Chapter 1). The endogenous catecholamines, noradrenaline and adrenaline, show modestly different affinities for the adrenoceptor subtypes:

α_1: noradrenaline $\geq$ adrenaline
α_2: adrenaline $\geq$ noradrenaline
β_1: noradrenaline $\geq$ adrenaline
β_2: adrenaline > noradrenaline
β_3: adrenaline = noradrenaline

Selective stimulation or blockade of individual adrenoceptor subtypes forms the basis of significant areas of pharmacology and therapeutics, and is discussed in later chapters. It is further understood that there are multiple forms of the α_1- and α_2-adrenoceptor subtypes (namely α_{1A}, α_{1B} and α_{1D}, and α_{2A}, α_{2B} and α_{2C}), and these are also discussed where clinically relevant.

THE PARASYMPATHETIC NERVOUS SYSTEM AND CHOLINERGIC TRANSMISSION

SYNTHESIS OF ACETYLCHOLINE

ACh is synthesised within the cytosol of the cholinergic neuron from choline and acetyl-CoA (Fig. 4.5). Choline is a highly polar, quaternary amino compound that is also present in phosphatidylcholine; it is obtained largely from the diet. Because of its fixed positive charge, it does not readily cross cell membranes; there are specific transporters to allow uptake into the presynaptic neuron (see Fig. 4.5) and from the gastrointestinal tract and across the blood–brain barrier (see Chapter 2). Acetylation of choline to form ACh is catalysed by choline acetyltransferase. The rate of synthesis of ACh is closely controlled and related to ACh turnover, so that rapid release of ACh stores is associated with enhanced synthesis.

STORAGE OF ACETYLCHOLINE

Cytosolic ACh is taken up into membrane vesicles by a specific transmembrane transporter (the vesicular ACh transporter, VAChT) and stored in the vesicles in association with ATP and acidic proteoglycans. Each vesicle contains 1000–50,000 ACh molecules, and neuromuscular junctions (see Chapter 27) contain about 300,000 vesicles.

RELEASE OF ACETYLCHOLINE

Release occurs by Ca^{2+}-mediated fusion of the vesicle membrane with the cytoplasmic membrane and exocytosis (see Fig. 4.5). This process can be inhibited by botulinum toxin from *Clostridium botulinum* bacteria and stimulated by latrotoxin from the black widow spider (*Latrodectus* spp.). The number of vesicles released depends on the site of the synapse, with between 30 and 300 vesicles undergoing exocytosis, releasing from 30,000 to over 3 million ACh molecules into the synaptic cleft. Neurons within the CNS are more sensitive to ACh release, and require fewer ACh molecules to be released to stimulate a recipient axon compared with the neuromuscular junction, which requires millions of ACh molecules for skeletal muscle contractility to occur.

METABOLISM AND INACTIVATION OF RELEASED ACETYLCHOLINE

Both presynaptic and postsynaptic membranes are rich in acetylcholinesterase (AChE); hence the released ACh is hydrolysed very rapidly (usually <1 ms) to give choline and acetate. This rapid hydrolysis, and the rapid equilibration between ACh bound to the receptor and free in the synapse, means that the 'receptor phase' of the transmission process only lasts for 1–2 ms (the postsynaptic changes may be more prolonged, as discussed later).

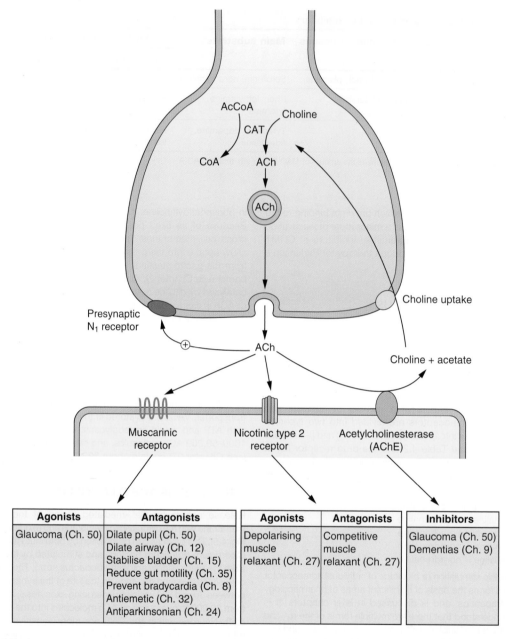

Fig. 4.5 The mechanisms involved in the synthesis, release and inactivation of acetylcholine. The actions of agonists and antagonists of muscarinic and nicotinic N_2 receptors and inhibitors of acetylcholinesterase are shown with the relevant chapters dealing with their pharmacology. *AcCoA*, Acetyl-CoA; *ACh*, acetylcholine; *CAT*, choline acetyltransferase.

AChE is an important target for drug action and for the toxic effects of some chemicals; the active site of the esterase has two critical features involved in the metabolism of ACh (Fig. 4.6):

- an anionic site, which forms an ionic bond with the quaternary nitrogen of the choline part of ACh;
- a hydrolytic site, which contains a serine moiety; the hydroxyl group of the serine accepts the acetyl group from ACh and very rapidly transfers it to water to complete the hydrolysis reaction.

Inhibition of AChE will prevent the breakdown of ACh and lead to prolonged receptor occupancy, the consequences of which depend on the nature of the receptor and the innervated cell/tissue.

AChE inhibitors can be divided into three types:

- AChE inhibitors that bind reversibly to the anionic site (e.g. edrophonium; see Chapter 28).
- AChE inhibitors that carbamylate the serine group. These bind to the anionic site and transfer a carbamoyl group (instead of an acetyl group) to the serine hydroxyl group

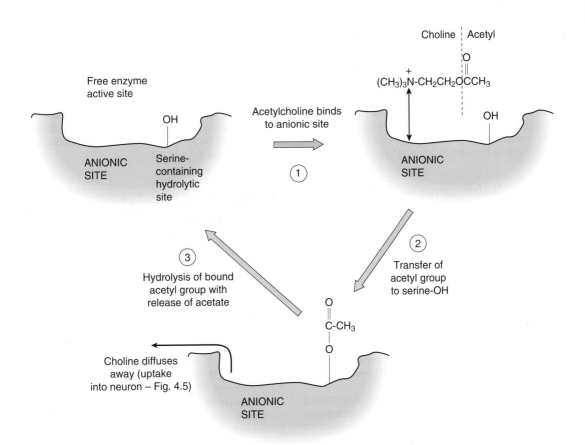

Fig. 4.6 **The mechanism of hydrolysis of acetylcholine by acetylcholinesterase.** The choline moiety of acetylcholine binds to the anionic site of the acetylcholinesterase active site, allowing transfer of the acetyl group to the serine hydroxyl moiety at the enzyme's hydrolytic site, with subsequent release of choline and acetate.

at the enzyme hydrolytic site. The carbamoyl group is hydrolysed more slowly from the serine than an acetyl group, resulting in prolonged and profound (but reversible) inhibition of the enzyme; examples include neostigmine and pyridostigmine, which are used for reversal of neuromuscular block (see Chapter 27) and in the treatment of myasthenia gravis (see Chapter 28). Reversible AChE inhibitors such as donepezil and rivastigmine are used in the treatment of Alzheimer's disease (see Chapter 9).

■ AChE inhibitors that phosphorylate the serine group. Inhibitors such as the organophosphates react with the serine hydroxyl group at the hydrolytic site (with or without binding to the anionic site) to produce a phosphorylated enzyme, which is resistant to hydrolysis. These inhibitors therefore cause inhibition, which is irreversible (or very slowly and partially reversible). Such changes in enzyme activity are of limited clinical use, although ecothiopate irreversibly phosphorylates AChE and is used in ophthalmology. Irreversible AChE inhibition may also be encountered clinically in people suffering accidental poisoning with organophosphate compounds, such as some agricultural pesticides (e.g. malathion), or even after exposure to some nerve gases used for chemical warfare (e.g. sarin). The active serine hydroxyl group of AChE may be reactivated soon after organophosphate exposure by administration of

pralidoxime (2-PAM), although its efficacy as an antidote is contentious. A few hours after organophosphate exposure, the phosphorylated enzyme undergoes changes known as ageing, and pralidoxime cannot then reactivate the enzyme.

Unlike many other neurotransmitters, there is no reuptake process for ACh, but after it is hydrolysed into choline and acetate by AChE, there is a specific reuptake of choline into the presynaptic neuron. Choline is a limited resource and reuptake allows its reincorporation into ACh, while no reuptake occurs for acetate because it is readily available from intermediary metabolism. Presynaptic uptake of choline can be inhibited by structural analogues, such as hemicholinium, but such drugs are not useful clinically because of the widespread and nonspecific consequences of impairment of ACh uptake, synthesis and release.

CHOLINERGIC RECEPTORS

The cholinergic receptors can be divided into nicotinic receptor types, all of which are coupled to cation channels, and muscarinic receptor types, which are G-protein-coupled receptors (see the drug receptor table at the end of Chapter 1). The receptors were originally named after nitrogen-containing basic compounds (alkaloids) present in plants (*nicotine*) or fungi (*muscarine*) that act as selective agonists at these receptors. Fig. 4.5 outlines the effects of agonists and antagonists at muscarinic and nicotinic receptors, and also of AChE inhibitors, listing key chapters covering the clinical relevance of these drugs.

Nicotinic receptors of more than one subtype are found in the CNS, where they are often presynaptic and modulate release of neurotransmitters such as dopamine. In the autonomic nervous system, two nicotinic receptor types are distinguished: N_1 (ganglion receptors) and N_2 (muscle type receptors).

Nicotinic N_1 (or ganglion type) receptors

Nicotinic N_1 receptors occur on the postsynaptic membranes of all ganglia of both the sympathetic and PNSs, and are activated by ACh released from preganglionic fibres. They are also responsible for the cholinergic stimulation of adrenaline release from adrenal glands.

Nicotinic N_2 (or muscle type) receptors

Nicotinic N_2 receptors occur at the junction between the somatic motor nerves and skeletal muscles (the neuromuscular junction; see Chapter 27).

Nicotinic receptors are ligand-gated ion channels of five subunits (see Fig. 1.1), with disulfide cross-linking between adjacent subunits; there are different types of subunits, classified into α, β, γ, δ and ε subfamilies, and different permutations of subunits give rise to the different nicotinic receptor types in the CNS, autonomic ganglia and neuromuscular junction. The differences between nicotinic N_1 and N_2 receptors in their agonist/antagonist binding characteristics are clinically very important, because they allow neuromuscular blockade (paralysis) without major effects on the ANS.

Muscarinic receptors

These are G-protein-coupled receptors (GPCRs) widely distributed in the CNS and in pre- and postganglionic fibre/effector organ junctions of the parasympathetic branch of the ANS. They are also present on most sweat glands (other than the palms of the hands), which are, however, innervated by the *sympathetic* branch of the ANS. Table 4.3 shows the effect of stimulation of the muscarinic (M) receptors in major tissues and the principal muscarinic receptor subtype that is involved. There are five subtypes of muscarinic receptor (M_1–M_5; see the drug receptor table at the end of Chapter 1). All five subtypes are found in the CNS; the distribution and functions of M_1, M_2 and M_3 receptors have also been well characterised at parasympathetic effector sites (see Table 4.3). M_2 receptors are particularly associated with inhibition of cardiac activity, and M_3 receptors with stimulating smooth muscle and glandular tissues.

It should be appreciated that AChE inhibitors increase the concentrations of ACh at all nicotinic and muscarinic receptor sites, and therefore produce a diverse array of effects. For example, when an AChE inhibitor is used to overcome reversible neuromuscular blockade (see Chapter 27), it increases ACh-mediated effects produced via the PNS, such as on the gastrointestinal tract and heart. These unwanted effects of ACh can be blocked by co-administration of an antimuscarinic agent (see the drug receptor list at the end of Chapter 1).

The distribution of the key neurotransmitters and receptors of the somatic and autonomic nervous systems is summarised in Fig. 4.7, which should be understood in association with the activities of the sympathetic and PNSs on specific tissues shown in Tables 4.2 and 4.3.

OTHER TRANSMITTERS IN THE PERIPHERAL NERVOUS SYSTEM

In addition to ACh and noradrenaline, there are other transmitters with roles in neurotransmission and functions in the peripheral nervous system. Many of these are also of considerable importance in the CNS. The different transmitters are dealt with in the chapters that describe their clinical importance, and include:

- amines (e.g. dopamine, histamine, serotonin),
- amino acids (e.g. glutamate, glycine, γ-aminobutyric acid [GABA]),
- peptides (e.g. opioids, substance P),
- purines (e.g. adenosine, ATP).

Nitric oxide (NO), calcitonin gene-related peptide (CGRP), vasoactive intestinal peptide (VIP), neuropeptide Y (NPY), ghrelin and others are described later in this book.

AMINES

Dopamine

Dopamine is an important neurotransmitter in both the CNS and the periphery, and subsequent chapters cover its actions (see Chapters 7, 21, 24 and 32).

Synthesis and storage of dopamine

The synthesis and storage of dopamine have been described previously in the section on noradrenaline.

Release of dopamine

Nerve stimulation causes the release of preformed dopamine present in vesicles (see the section on noradrenaline). Dopaminergic neurons are not important in the clinical responses to indirectly acting sympathomimetics, although certain behavioural responses to amfetamines are linked to dopamine D_2 receptor activity. The antiviral drug amantadine, which is of some value in Parkinson's disease, causes release of dopamine among other actions (see Chapter 24).

Removal of activity of released dopamine

Dopamine is removed by similar mechanisms to those described previously for noradrenaline, with reuptake by the DAT representing the major pathway.

Dopamine receptors

There are a number of types of dopamine receptors, and relatively selective therapeutic agents are available for some

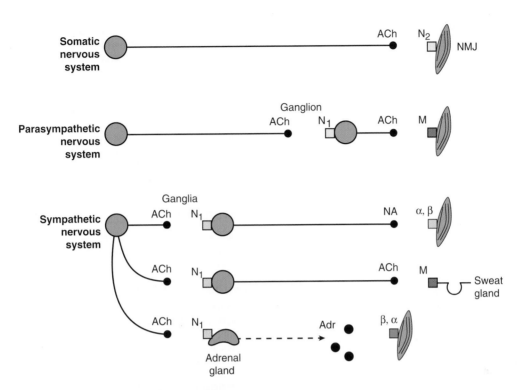

Fig. 4.7 Schematic diagram of the distribution of the main neurotransmitters and receptors of the somatic, parasympathetic and sympathetic nervous systems. *ACh*, Acetylcholine; *Adr*, adrenaline; *M*, muscarinic receptor; *N₁*, *N₂*, nicotinic receptors; *NA*, noradrenaline; *NMJ*, neuromuscular junction; *α*, *β*, adrenoceptors.

of these (see the drug receptor list at the end of Chapter 1). Dopamine receptors are classified into those that increase cyclic adenosine monophosphate (cAMP) (D_1 and D_5) and those that decrease cAMP (D_2, D_3 and D_4). The D_4 receptor shows polymorphic expression. Dopamine receptor subtypes D_2 and D_4 are associated with schizophrenia, and relatively selective antagonists of each are valuable antipsychotic drugs (see Chapter 21).

Serotonin (5-hydroxytryptamine)

Serotonin (or 5-HT; Fig. 4.8A) is a neurotransmitter in the CNS and periphery that has properties similar to the catecholamines.

Synthesis of serotonin

Serotonin is synthesised from the amino acid tryptophan by two reactions that are similar to those involved in the conversion of tyrosine to dopamine. The first reaction forms 5-hydroxytryptophan and is catalysed by tryptophan hydroxylase, which is the rate-limiting step and only found in serotonin-producing cells. Conversion to serotonin is catalysed by aromatic L-amino acid decarboxylase (see the previous discussion of noradrenaline synthesis).

Serotonin is present in the diet but undergoes essentially complete first-pass metabolism by MAO-A in the gut wall and liver. Serotonin is not synthesised by blood platelets, but they accumulate high concentrations of serotonin from the

circulation which can be released when platelets aggregate and during migraine episodes.

Storage of serotonin

The major site of serotonin storage in the body (>90%) is the enterochromaffin cells of the gastrointestinal tract. Platelets accumulate serotonin, and neurons utilising serotonin are widely distributed in the brain. In presynaptic neurons serotonin is stored in vesicles as a complex with ATP, and there is an active uptake process which transfers cytoplasmic serotonin into the storage vesicle.

Release of serotonin

The release of serotonin vesicles is by Ca^{2+}-mediated exocytosis. A rise in intraluminal pressure in the gastrointestinal tract stimulates the release of serotonin from the chromaffin cells. Release of serotonin from chromaffin cells contributes to nausea following cancer chemotherapy with cytotoxic drugs by stimulation of the chemoreceptor trigger zone (see Chapter 32) and of sensory receptors within the gastrointestinal tract. There is a significant release of platelet serotonin in migraine (see Chapter 26).

Metabolism and removal of serotonin activity

The principal mechanism of inactivation of released serotonin is via its reuptake into the presynaptic nerve by the SERT,

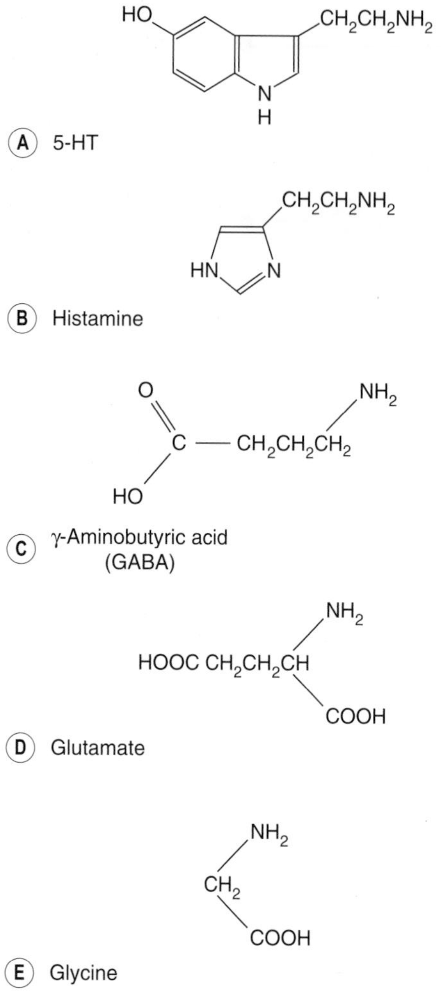

(A) 5-HT

(B) Histamine

(C) γ-Aminobutyric acid (GABA)

(D) Glutamate

(E) Glycine

Fig. 4.8 Diverse structures of important amine and amino acid neurotransmitters. **(A)** 5-HT; **(B)** histamine; **(C)** γ-aminobutyric acid (GABA); **(D)** glutamate; **(E)** glycine.

which shows a high affinity for serotonin and is distinct from the NET. Dual inhibitors of serotonin and noradrenaline reuptake (SNRIs) and selective serotonin reuptake inhibitors (SSRIs) are important antidepressants (see Chapter 22). Serotonin reuptake is also carried out by a low-affinity plasma membrane monoamine transporter (PMAT), which is insensitive to SSRIs and also transports noradrenaline and dopamine.

Metabolism of serotonin within the neuron is by MAO, which generates the excretory product 5-hydroxyindoleacetic acid (5-HIAA). There is a considerable turnover of serotonin in the chromaffin and nerve cells, and 5-HIAA is a normal constituent of human urine.

Serotonin receptors

There is a large family of serotonin receptors (see the drug receptor list at the end of Chapter 1), with 13 different G-protein-coupled seven-transmembrane (7TM) receptors

and one ligand-gated ion channel so far identified. These are divided into seven classes (5-HT$_1$ to 5-HT$_7$) on the basis of their structural and functional characteristics. Not all of the subtypes of receptors have recognised physiological roles. Receptors in the 5-HT$_1$ group are mostly presynaptic and inhibit adenylyl cyclase, whereas those in the 5-HT$_2$ group are mostly postsynaptic in the periphery and activate phospholipase C. 5-HT$_3$ receptors are ligand-gated ion channels. Identification of receptor subtype functions and selective inhibitors or stimulants has facilitated progress in the treatment of diseases, including depression (see Chapter 22) and migraines (see Chapter 26).

Histamine

Histamine (see Fig. 4.8B) is an important transmitter both in the CNS and in the periphery, as well as being an allergic mediator released from mast cells and basophils.

Synthesis of histamine

The amino acid histidine is decarboxylated to histamine by histidine decarboxylase. In addition to the synthesis and storage of histamine by mast cells and basophils, there is continual synthesis, release and metabolic inactivation by growing tissues and in wound healing.

Storage of histamine

Most attention has focused on the storage of histamine in mediator-releasing cells such as mast cells and basophils (see Chapter 12). In these cells, it is present in granules associated with heparin. The presence of histidine decarboxylase and the synthesis of histamine in neurons in the CNS, although less well explored, appear to be associated mainly with the hypothalamus, from where projections run to many parts of the brain. Histamine plays a role in wakefulness, memory, appetite and many other functions.

Release of histamine

The release of histamine from mast cells and basophils has been studied extensively in relation to allergic reactions (see Chapters 12 and 39). In chromaffin cells in the gut and enterochromaffin-like (ECL) cells in the gastric mucosa, histamine is synthesised rapidly when required (see Chapter 33). The release of histamine from neurons may be similar to the release of other amine neurotransmitters, but this has not been demonstrated unequivocally.

Removal of histamine activity

Histamine is rapidly inactivated by oxidation to imidazole acetic acid. Histamine is not a substrate for MAO, and the oxidation is catalysed by diamine oxidase (or histaminase). A second, minor route of metabolism is methylation by histamine-N-methyltransferase, and the product is then a substrate for MAO. Histamine is also eliminated as an N-acetyl conjugate.

Histamine receptors

There are four receptors for histamine (see the drug receptor list at the end of Chapter 1). H$_1$ receptors have been studied extensively in relation to inflammation and allergy (see Chapters 12 and 39). Histamine-containing neurons are found in the brain, particularly in the brainstem, with pathways projecting into the cerebral cortex. H_1 receptors are probably important in these pathways, because sedation is a serious problem with H_1 receptor antagonists that are able to cross the blood–brain barrier (see Chapter 2). Later generations of H_1 antihistamines produce less sedation. H_1 receptors are also involved in emesis (see Chapter 32).

The discovery of H_2 receptors affecting the release of gastric acid led to the development of important H_2-selective antagonists that reduce acid secretion and contribute to the treatment of dyspepsia and to ulcer healing (see Chapter 33). H_2 receptors are also present in the brain and are probably responsible for the confusional state associated with the use of the H_2 receptor antagonist cimetidine. H_3 receptors are found in the CNS and other sites, and H_4 receptors are localised mainly to leucocytes, but their functions are poorly understood.

AMINO ACIDS

γ-Aminobutyric acid

GABA is an important inhibitory neurotransmitter responsible for about 40% of all inhibitory activity in the CNS (see Fig. 4.8C).

Synthesis and storage of γ-aminobutyric acid

GABA is formed by the decarboxylation of glutamate by glutamate decarboxylase in GABAergic neurons. GABA is stored in membrane vesicles in the brain and in interneurons in the spinal cord (particularly laminae II and III).

Release of γ-aminobutyric acid

GABA is released by Ca^{2+}-mediated exocytosis. Co-transmitters such as glycine, metenkephalin and neuropeptide Y are stored in GABA vesicles and released with GABA.

Removal of γ-aminobutyric acid activity

Uptake by the GABA transporter (GAT) family of transporters is the principal mechanism for the removal of GABA from the synaptic cleft. The antiepileptic drug tiagabine acts as an inhibitor of GABA uptake by GABA transporter-1 (GAT-1) (see Chapter 23).

GABA is metabolised by transamination with α-ketoglutarate, which forms the corresponding aldehyde (succinic semialdehyde) and amino acid (glutamic acid). The antiepileptic drug vigabatrin may inhibit GABA transamination.

γ-Aminobutyric acid receptors

There are two main types of GABA receptor, with different mechanisms of action (see the drug receptor list at the end of Chapter 1). The stimulation of both receptors produces hyperpolarisation of the cell membrane, with $GABA_A$ causing rapid inhibition and $GABA_B$ producing a slower and more prolonged response. The $GABA_A$ receptor comprises a number of subunits. There are multiple forms of each subunit and numerous possible combinations (see Fig. 20.1); consequently, the $GABA_A$ receptor should be regarded as a family of receptors. Hyperpolarisation following $GABA_A$ receptor stimulation results from the opening of Cl^- channels and influx of Cl^- ions. $GABA_B$ receptors are G-protein-linked receptors that hyperpolarise the cell indirectly by closing Ca^{2+} channels and opening K^+ channels. A subtype of $GABA_A$ receptor ($GABA_A$-ρ) is found in the retina, where its significance remains unclear. Both $GABA_A$ and $GABA_B$ receptors are found presynaptically and inhibit neurotransmitter release by hyperpolarising the cell (by opening Cl^- or K^+ channels) and reducing release of the vesicles of the innervating cell (by closing Ca^{2+} channels). Many important drugs act by altering GABA synthesis or breakdown, or by enhancing GABA activity at its receptors, including drugs used for anxiety (see Chapter 20) and epilepsy (see Chapter 23).

Glutamate

Glutamate (see Fig. 4.8D) is an important excitatory amino acid neurotransmitter with wide-reaching actions in physiological and pathological conditions. The functions of glutamate are described in later chapters. Aspartate (which is similar to glutamate but has only one CH_2 group) acts at the same receptors. Administration of glutamate or aspartate causes CNS excitation, tachycardia, nausea and headache, and convulsions at very high doses. Hyperactivity at glutamate receptors has been proposed as a factor in the generation of epilepsy (see Chapter 23).

Synthesis and storage of glutamate

Glutamate (glutamic acid) is found in most cells and is widely distributed within the CNS. Glutamate is stored in presynaptic vesicles in the neurons.

Release of glutamate

Exocytosis of vesicles is mediated via the influx of Ca^{2+} into the presynaptic nerve terminal, as occurs for other neurotransmitters. Some antiepileptic drugs (e.g. lamotrigine and valproate; see Chapter 23) inhibit glutamate release.

Removal of glutamate activity

The action of glutamate in the synapse is terminated by excitatory amino acid transporters (EAATs), which take up glutamate (and aspartate) into the neuron and surrounding glial cells.

Glutamate receptors

There are two major types of glutamate receptor, the ionotropic family, comprising AMPA (α-amino-3-hydroxy-5-methyl-4-isoxazole propionic acid) receptors, kainate receptors and NMDA (*N*-methyl-D-aspartate) receptors, and the metabotropic glutamate receptor (mGluR) family, which have a range of biological actions (see the drug receptor list at the end of Chapter 1). The glutamate NMDA receptor antagonist memantine is used in treating Alzheimer's disease (see Chapter 9), and the AMPA receptor antagonist perampanel is used in epilepsy (see Chapter 23).

Glycine

Glycine (see Fig. 4.8E) is a widely available amino acid that acts as an inhibitory neurotransmitter. It is released in response to nerve stimulation and acts in the spine, lower brainstem and retina.

Synthesis and storage of glycine

Glycine is present in all cells and is accumulated by neurons within vesicles.

Release of glycine

Vesicle release accompanies an AP, as described previously for other neurotransmitters. The tetanus toxin prevents glycine release, and the decrease in glycine-mediated inhibition results in reflex hyperexcitability.

Removal of glycine activity

Released glycine undergoes cellular uptake via the high-affinity glycine transporters GLYT-1 and GLYT-2 in glial and neuronal cells.

Glycine receptors

Glycine receptors (GlyR) are ligand-gated Cl⁻ channels similar in structure to GABA$_A$ channels; they are present mainly on interneurons in the spinal cord. Strychnine produces convulsions through the blockade of glycine receptors. Glycine is important for the activity of NMDA receptors (see the drug receptor table at the end of Chapter 1).

Imidazoline receptor ligands

Studies of the centrally acting α_2-adrenoceptor agonists clonidine, moxonidine and rilmenidine showed their antihypertensive effects could not be interpreted wholly by actions on the α_2-adrenoceptor. These imidazoline compounds are thought to act at least partly at imidazoline (I)-binding sites, of which there are three main types (I_1, I_2, I_3), with the I_1 site mediating the sympatho-inhibitory actions on blood pressure in the brainstem. The putative natural ligand for I receptors, agmatine, is a decarboxylated derivative of arginine; it also binds to α_2-adrenoceptors and activates nitric oxide synthase, but its role in disease is unclear.

PEPTIDES

The importance of peptides as neurotransmitters has been highlighted in recent years, largely because of the development of sensitive immunohistochemical probes, which have allowed for their detection and measurement in tissues. Unlike other classes of neurotransmitter, peptides are synthesised in the cell body as precursors, which are transported down the axon to the site of storage. There are specific receptors for different peptides (see the drug receptor table at the end of Chapter 1). An AP causes the release of the peptide from its precursor; inactivation is probably via hydrolysis by a local peptidase.

Peptide neurotransmitters are often found stored in the same nerve endings as other transmitters (described previously) and undergo simultaneous release (co-transmission).

Peptides do not cross the blood–brain barrier readily. A major problem for exploiting our increasing knowledge of the importance of peptides is devising ways to deliver the novel products derived from molecular biology to the sites within the brain where they can have an effect.

Substance P is released from C-fibres (see Chapter 19) by a Ca^{2+}-linked mechanism and is an important neurotransmitter for sensory afferents in the dorsal horn. It is also present in the substantia nigra, associated with dopaminergic neurons, and may be involved in the control of movement.

Opioid peptides are a range of endogenous peptides that are the natural ligands for opioid receptors; opioid receptors were recognised in the brain and gastrointestinal tract for many years before the natural ligands were identified. These are discussed in Chapter 19.

A number of other peptides are detectable in the CNS particularly in the hypothalamus and/or pituitary gland (e.g. neurotensin, oxytocin, somatostatin, vasopressin; see Chapters 43 and 45) or in the gastrointestinal tract (e.g. cholecystokinin and vasoactive intestinal peptide).

PURINES

Adenosine and guanosine are endogenous purines and exist in the body in the free form, attached to ribose or deoxyribose (as nucleosides), and as mono-, bi- or triphosphorylated nucleotides. Purines within cells are usually incorporated into nucleotides, which are involved in the energetics of biochemical processes (e.g. ATP), act as intracellular signals (e.g. cAMP and cyclic guanosine monophosphate [cGMP]; see Chapter 1) and are involved in the synthesis of RNA and DNA. ATP is present in the presynaptic vesicles of some other neurotransmitters and is released along with the primary neurotransmitter, following which it may act on postsynaptic receptors (co-transmission). Extracellular ATP is rapidly hydrolysed via adenosine diphosphate (ADP) to adenosine. Adenosine itself is very rapidly metabolised and inactivated.

There is a family of purine receptors that show individual selectivity for different purines and give different responses (see the drug receptor list at the end of Chapter 1). G-protein-coupled purinergic receptors (P2Y) are specific for the adenosine and uridine phosphates, and ADP causes platelet aggregation via P2Y$_{12}$-type receptors. This effect of ADP can be inhibited with clopidogrel and ticagrelor, which have important antiaggregatory actions (see Chapter 11). Ligand-gated P2X receptors for ATP are widely distributed in the brain. The adenosine receptors A$_1$–A$_3$, formerly called P1 receptors, show very high selectivity for adenosine itself. Adenosine is used therapeutically to terminate supraventricular tachycardia.

SELF-ASSESSMENT

True/false questions

1. The sympathetic division of the autonomic nervous system utilises adrenaline as its primary transmitter substance.
2. The parasympathetic and sympathetic nervous systems have opposite effects in every organ.
3. Sympathetic nervous stimulation to the gut inhibits gut motility and sphincter tone.
4. Acetylcholine is metabolised by plasma cholinesterase in the synaptic cleft.
5. Dopamine and noradrenaline are synthesised from levodopa.
6. Dopamine is a transmitter in the peripheral autonomic nervous system.
7. Tyramine is metabolised by both isoenzymes of neurotransmitter oxidase (MAO-A and MAO-B).

8. Both α_1- and α_2-adrenoceptor antagonists can be used to lower blood pressure.
9. Botulism is caused by poisoning with a bacterial toxin.
10. Botulinum toxin enhances acetylcholine release from all cholinergic neurons.
11. There are two subtypes of β-adrenoceptor.
12. Drugs that alter GABA activity are important in treating epilepsy.
13. The actions of synaptic serotonin and noradrenaline are curtailed mainly by metabolism by MAO and COMT.
14. The synaptic uptake of noradrenaline and serotonin can be inhibited selectively.
15. The vagal cranial nerve to the eye decreases pupil size.
16. Blockade of H_1 histamine receptors reduces gastric acid secretion.
17. Glutamate and glycine are inhibitory amino acid transmitters.
18. Substance P is a transmitter in the dorsal horn of the spinal cord.

One-best-answer (OBA) question

1. Which of the following is the *most accurate* statement about neurotransmission?
   A. Neurotransmitters are synthesised in the presynaptic nerve terminal.
   B. Monoamine transmitters are taken up into the presynaptic neuron by passive diffusion.
   C. Acetylcholine release is modified by receptors on the presynaptic membrane.
   D. Each postganglionic sympathetic neuron releases a single neurotransmitter.
   E. Fusion of vesicles with the presynaptic membrane is facilitated by K^+ influx triggered by the action potential.

ANSWERS

True/false answers

1. **False.** Noradrenaline is the main transmitter substance at postganglionic nerve endings. Adrenaline is released only from the adrenal medulla, while acetylcholine is the transmitter in sympathetic ganglia and in sympathetically innervated sweat glands and hair follicles.
2. **False.** While the two autonomic systems have broadly opposing actions on many organs, other organs may be controlled by only one system (e.g. the lens of the eye). The kinetics of the two systems also vary, with the PNS fine-tuning organ activity at rest, while the SNS produces rapid coordinated responses of many organs in a physiological emergency.
3. **False.** Sympathetic nervous stimulation releases noradrenaline and inhibits gut motility but increases the tone of the sphincters.
4. **False.** Within the synaptic cleft, acetylcholine is mainly broken down by acetylcholinesterase.
5. **True.** Levodopa is converted into dopamine by dopa decarboxylase and then to noradrenaline by dopamine-β-hydroxylase.

6. **True.** Dopamine is predominantly an important transmitter in the CNS but also in some peripheral sites (e.g. the renal vascular smooth muscle).
7. **True.** This is important, as selective inhibitors of MAO-A used in the treatment of depression leave MAO-B unaffected, so it is available to metabolise tyramine in food, thereby avoiding the 'cheese reaction'.
8. **False.** Antagonism of α_1-adrenoceptors on peripheral resistance vessels causes relaxation and lowers blood pressure, but presynaptic α_2-adrenoceptors reduce noradrenaline release. Blockade of these autoreceptors would increase noradrenaline release and tend to raise vascular resistance.
9. **True.** Botulinum toxin from the anaerobic bacterium *C. botulinum* can cause fatal poisoning.
10. **False.** Botulinum toxin inhibits acetylcholine release and causes skeletal muscle paralysis; it can be used locally where there is muscle spasm or excessive sweating.
11. **False.** A third type, the β_3-adrenoceptor, is found in adipocytes, the heart, colon, bladder and some other tissues, but is less widespread than the β_1- and β_2-adrenoceptors.
12. **True.** As well as drugs that act at $GABA_A$ receptors, such as benzodiazepines, others that alter GABA uptake or breakdown are of growing importance in epilepsy treatment.
13. **False.** The actions of serotonin and noradrenaline are curtailed mainly by reuptake into the presynaptic neuron by their respective transporters, SERT and NET.
14. **True.** The SERT and NET uptake transporters can be inhibited by SSRIs and other selective antidepressant drugs.
15. **True.** Vagal (parasympathetic) stimulation causes miosis of the pupil and also accommodates the lens for near vision.
16. **False.** Gastric acid secretion is promoted by histamine released from enterochromaffin-like (ECL) cells acting at H_2 receptors, and is reduced by H_2 receptor antagonists such as ranitidine.
17. **False.** Glycine is an inhibitory transmitter, but glutamate is excitatory.
18. **True.** Substance P in the dorsal horn is an important transmitter in sensory afferents.

OBA answer

1. **Answer C** is correct.
   A. Incorrect. Catecholamines are synthesised in the terminal, but peptides are synthesised in the cell body and transported to the postganglionic nerve ending.
   B. Incorrect. Active transporters such as NET, SERT and DAT transfer monoamine neurotransmitters back into the presynaptic neuron.
   C. **Correct.** On parasympathetic nerve endings, stimulation of presynaptic N_1 autoreceptors increases acetylcholine release, whereas stimulation of presynaptic M_2 receptors decreases acetylcholine release.
   D. Incorrect. Co-transmission is common, such as noradrenaline and vasoactive intestinal polypeptide released from sympathetic nerve endings to the gut.
   E. Incorrect. An influx of Ca^{2+} is associated with neurotransmitter release.

FURTHER READING

Abrams, P., Andersson, K.-E., Buccafusco, J., et al., 2006. Muscarinic receptors: their distribution and function in body systems, and the implications for treating overactive bladder. Br. J. Pharmacol. 48, 565–578.

Alexander, S.P.H., Davenport, A.P., Kelly, E., et al., 2015. The concise guide to pharmacology 2015/16: G protein-coupled receptors. Br. J. Pharmacol. 172, 5744–5869.

Baker, J.G., Hill, S.J., Summers, R.J., 2011. Evolution of β-blockers: from anti-anginal drugs to ligand-directed signalling. Trends Pharmacol. Sci. 32, 227–234.

Beaulieu, J.M., Gainetdinov, R.R., 2011. The physiology, signaling, and pharmacology of dopamine receptors. Pharmacol. Rev. 63, 182–217.

Berger, M., Gray, J., Roth, B.L., 2009. The expanded biology of serotonin. Annu. Rev. Med. 60, 355–366.

Burnstock, G., 2007. Purine and pyrimidine receptors. Cell. Mol. Life Sci. 64, 1471–1483.

Cazzola, M., Calzetta, L., Matera, M.G., 2011. β_2-Adrenoceptor agonists: current and future direction. Br. J. Pharmacol. 163, 4–17.

Dani, J.A., Bertrand, D., 2007. Nicotinic acetylcholine receptors and nicotinic cholinergic mechanisms of the central nervous system. Ann. Rev. Pharmacol. Toxicol. 47, 699–729.

Filip, M., Bader, M., 2009. Overview on 5-HT receptors and their role in physiology and pathology of the central nervous system. Pharmacol. Rep. 61, 761–777.

Foster, A.C., Kemp, J.A., 2006. Glutamate- and GABA-based CNS therapeutics. Curr. Opin. Pharmacol. 6, 7–17.

Gether, U., Andersen, P.H., Larsson, O.M., et al., 2006. Neurotransmitter transporters: molecular function of important drug targets. Trends Pharmacol. Sci. 27, 375–383.

Kruse, A.C., Kobilka, B.K., Gautam, D., et al., 2014. Muscarinic acetylcholine receptors: novel opportunities for drug development. Nat. Rev. Drug Discov. 13, 549–560.

Leurs, R., Vischer, H.F., Wijtmans, M., et al., 2011. En route to new blockbuster anti-histamines: surveying the offspring of the expanding histamine receptor family. Trends Pharmacol. Sci. 32, 250–257.

Ogden, K.K., Traynelis, S.F., 2011. New advances in NMDA receptor pharmacology. Trends Pharmacol. Sci. 32, 726–733.

Olsen, R.W., Sieghart, W., 2008. GABA$_A$ receptors: subtypes provide diversity of function and pharmacology. Neuropharmacology 56, 141–148.

Piletz, J.E., Aricioglu, F., Cheng, J.T., et al., 2013. Agmatine: clinical applications after 100 years in translation. Drug Discov. Today 18, 880–893.

Salio, C., Lossi, L., Ferrini, F., et al., 2006. Neuropeptides as synaptic transmitters. Cell Tissue Res. 326, 583–598.

Youdim, M.B.H., Edmondson, D., Tipton, K., 2006. The therapeutic potential of monoamine oxidase inhibitors. Nat. Rev. Neurosci. 7, 295–309.

2

The cardiovascular system

5

Ischaemic heart disease

MYOCARDIAL PERFUSION

The coronary arteries receive about 5% of the cardiac output at rest, and the myocardium extracts about 75% of the oxygen from the perfusing blood. When metabolic demand from the myocardium increases (e.g. with exercise), there is little additional oxygen available to be extracted from the perfusing blood, and coronary artery blood flow must increase to supply the necessary oxygen. Up to a three- to fourfold rise in coronary blood flow is achieved at maximum exercise. Myocardial perfusion occurs largely during diastole, when the muscle of the heart is relaxed and not compressing the intramyocardial vessels. Therefore, unlike other organs that are perfused during systole, myocardial perfusion is reliant on diastolic blood pressure.

Ischaemic heart disease arises when blood flow to the cardiac muscle is reduced by restriction of flow in the coronary circulation. Most frequently, this is due to atheromatous plaques in the large epicardial coronary arteries (Fig. 5.1). Atheromatous plaques most often form in areas where linear blood flow is disturbed, such as bends in the vessel or near branching vessels. Less commonly, myocardial ischaemia can occur in the presence of structurally normal epicardial coronary arteries. In this situation it arises either from abnormal regulation of the microvascular circulation within the myocardium, from intense vasoconstriction of an epicardial artery (coronary vasospasm) or from coronary artery embolism.

The major risk factors for atheromatous coronary artery disease (similar to atheroma in other parts of the vascular tree) are male sex, smoking, hypertension, hypercholesterolaemia and diabetes mellitus. The effects of these risk factors are additive, and when several are present, coronary atheroma occurs more extensively and at a younger age.

Atheromatous plaques initially enlarge by stretching the medial smooth muscle (vascular remodelling) and do not begin to narrow the lumen of the vessel until 40–50% of the circumference of the vessel is diseased. Even when luminal narrowing occurs, there is sufficient coronary blood flow reserve so that symptoms only arise in most people when about 75% of the cross-sectional area of the vessel lumen is occluded.

Coronary artery atheroma can diffusely involve a long segment of the vessel, but plaques are often confined to a small segment of the artery. Localised plaques frequently involve only part of the circumference of the arterial wall, leaving the rest free of significant disease and still able to respond to vasoconstrictor and vasodilator influences. At the site of an atheromatous plaque, there is turbulent blood flow. The consequent changes in shear stress at the endothelial surface impair endothelial function and reduce local generation of vasodilator substances such as nitric oxide (NO; see the discussion of organic nitrates that follows). Therefore diseased segments of a coronary artery are particularly prone to vasospasm, which produces dynamic flow limitation superimposed on the fixed atheromatous narrowing. Well-developed collateral coronary arteries are found in up to one-third of people. When these open, they

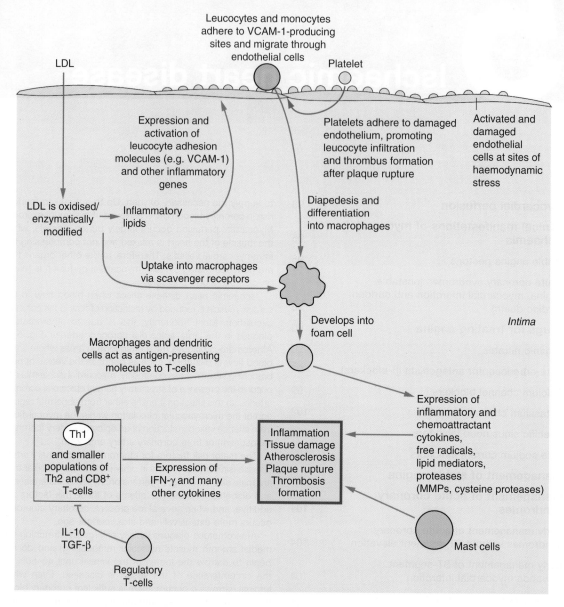

Fig. 5.1 Aspects of inflammatory processes that contribute to coronary heart disease. Many factors contribute to coronary heart disease: endothelium is damaged and activated by haemodynamic stress; platelets adhere and promote leucocyte infiltration and thrombus formation; low-density lipoprotein (LDL) is oxidised and taken up via scavenger receptors into monocyte-macrophages, subsequently forming foam cells. Dysfunctional expression of a host of cytokines, lipid mediators, free radicals and proteases exacerbates inflammation, endothelial damage, atheroma formation, plaque rupture and thrombus formation. These processes are influenced by risk factors such as smoking, heredity, hypercholesterolaemia, hypertension, obesity, diabetes, age and gender. *IFN-γ,* Interferon-γ; *IL-10,* interleukin-10; *MMPs,* matrix metalloproteases; *TGF-β,* tumour growth factor β; *Th,* T-helper cell; *VCAM-1,* vascular cell adhesion molecule 1.

can deliver blood to ischaemic tissues by bypassing the atheromatous narrowing or by retrograde filling of the distal part of the diseased vessel from another part of the coronary circulation. This improves perfusion distal to the diseased segment of the artery.

There are two morphological types of atheromatous plaque. Some have a lipid-rich core, with a substantial infiltration of inflammatory cells and a thin fibrous cap. Such plaques are relatively unstable ('vulnerable' plaques) and are more prone to plaque disruption by ulceration or rupture of the cap, leading to thrombus formation (discussed later). Other plaques have a fibrotic core with a thick fibrous cap. These plaques are more stable and resistant to erosion. Both stable and unstable plaques can coexist in the coronary circulation.

CLINICAL MANIFESTATIONS OF MYOCARDIAL ISCHAEMIA

STABLE ANGINA PECTORIS

Reversible myocardial ischaemia is the consequence of an imbalance between oxygen supply and oxygen demand in a part of the myocardium (Fig. 5.2) due to an inability to increase local coronary blood flow sufficiently to meet the metabolic demands of the heart. Angina pectoris is pain arising from heart muscle after it switches to anaerobic metabolism, and is a symptom of reversible myocardial ischaemia. Stable angina is relatively predictable ischaemic chest pain that is most frequently experienced on exertion or with emotional stress and is rapidly relieved by rest. Reversible myocardial ischaemia can also present with shortness of breath (due to diastolic stiffening of the left ventricle when a reduced cellular energy supply impairs the uptake of Ca^{2+} by the sarcoplasmic reticulum; see also heart failure with preserved ejection fraction [Chapter 7]), or it can occur without symptoms (silent ischaemia). Vasospasm at the site of an atheromatous plaque accentuates the reduction in flow produced by a fixed atheromatous obstruction, and when it is present angina occurs at a lower workload.

People with stable angina have an increased risk of subsequent myocardial infarction or sudden cardiac death, due to rupture of an unstable atheromatous plaque (discussed later). On average the annual rate of such events is about 2%.

Decreased oxygen supply

↓ **Coronary blood flow**

↓ Vessel calibre

↑ Heart rate
  (↓ diastolic filling time)

↓ Perfusion pressure

↑ Ventricular wall tension (compression of intramyocardial vessels)

Increased oxygen demand

↑ **Heart rate**

↑ **Myocardial contractility**

↑ **Ventricular wall tension**

↑ Filling pressure (preload)

↑ Resistance to ejection (afterload)

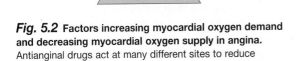

Fig. 5.2 Factors increasing myocardial oxygen demand and decreasing myocardial oxygen supply in angina. Antianginal drugs act at many different sites to reduce myocardial oxygen demand and increase oxygen supply.

ACUTE CORONARY SYNDROMES (UNSTABLE ANGINA, MYOCARDIAL INFARCTION AND SUDDEN CARDIAC DEATH)

Acute coronary syndromes have a common pathophysiological origin, arising from disruption of an unstable atheromatous plaque (vulnerable plaque) in a coronary artery. Plaque disruption can be precipitated by sudden stresses on the cap produced by pulsatile blood flow across the plaque, by elastic recoil of the vessel in diastole or by vasospasm. As a consequence of these stresses the thin cap over the unstable plaque fissures or ulcerates, leading to plaque rupture and exposure of the core of the plaque to circulating blood. Plaque rupture initiates platelet adhesion and then aggregation (see Chapter 11), followed by thrombus formation and local vasospasm. These processes lead to a sudden reduction in blood flow. Platelet–thrombin microemboli can break off from the thrombus and become lodged in small arterioles downstream from the thrombus, contributing to ischaemia.

Unstable angina

Unstable angina occurs if there is incomplete occlusion of the coronary artery following plaque rupture, but with critical reduction in blood flow so that oxygen supply is either inadequate at rest or on minimal stress. Angina may then occur at rest or with very little exertion. Unstable angina is distinguished pathologically from other acute coronary syndromes because perfusion of the ischaemic tissue remains sufficient to prevent necrosis of myocytes, so serum markers of myocardial damage do not increase. Unlike myocardial infarction, symptoms of unstable angina are usually relieved by glyceryl trinitrate (GTN) (discussed later), or resolve spontaneously within 30 minutes.

Following an episode of unstable angina, the thrombus may become incorporated into the ruptured plaque so that after healing the plaque is substantially larger, leading to greater long-term luminal narrowing.

Myocardial infarction and sudden cardiac death

Myocardial infarction most commonly arises from complete coronary artery occlusion following disruption of an unstable atheromatous plaque. Occlusion often occurs at the site of an atheromatous lesion that previously was only producing minor or moderate stenosis of the artery and in the majority of cases did not cause symptoms prior to disruption. Muscle necrosis begins if the occlusion lasts for longer than 20–30 minutes.

Myocardial infarction is usually associated with intense, prolonged chest pain and sympathetic nervous stimulation which increases cardiac work. However, about 15% of infarctions do not present with pain, and may go unrecognised (silent infarction). The diagnosis of acute myocardial infarction requires a rise in the plasma concentrations of sensitive biochemical markers, such as cardiac-specific myoglobin or troponin, which are released from necrotic myocytes. Cell death begins in the subendocardial muscle, which is furthest from the epicardial blood supply (the endocardium receives its oxygen from the ventricular cavity), and unless perfusion is restored, it progressively extends across the full thickness of the myocardium (transmurally) over the next few hours. Activation of endogenous fibrinolysis (see Chapter 11) and the presence of a good collateral circulation are factors that favour reperfusion of the ischaemic area and naturally limit the size of the infarct. If very early reperfusion occurs, the damage is usually confined to the subendocardial myocardium.

A full-thickness (or transmural) myocardial infarction usually produces characteristic changes on the electrocardiograph (ECG), with early ST-segment elevation and eventually pathological Q waves. This presentation is referred to as an ST-elevation myocardial infarction (STEMI). A subendocardial infarction often presents without diagnostic ECG changes. In these cases the ECG may show ST-segment depression or T-wave inversion, or even be normal. The resulting infarction is classified as a non-ST-elevation myocardial infarction (NSTEMI), because of the absence of the characteristic ST-segment changes usually found with more extensive myocardial damage.

Myocardial infarction principally affects the left ventricular muscle, and the amount of muscle lost and the resulting effect on left ventricular function correlate well with both early and late survival. Infarction of the anterior muscle of the left ventricle (usually resulting from an occlusion in the left coronary artery system) causes greater myocardial loss than does inferior infarction of the ventricle (usually from right coronary artery occlusion). The amount of muscle loss also determines the extent of left ventricular remodelling (a geometrical change in the left ventricle that begins with healing of the infarct), which determines the risk of subsequent heart failure.

Sudden cardiac death results when fatal ventricular arrhythmias arise from ischaemic tissue, or from ventricular rupture.

DRUGS FOR TREATING ANGINA

Drug treatment for angina is directed either:

- to reduce oxygen demand by decreasing cardiac work, and/or
- to increase oxygen supply by improving coronary blood flow.

Drugs can be taken to relieve the ischaemia rapidly during an acute attack of angina or as regular prophylaxis to reduce the risk of subsequent episodes. Several classes of drug are used to treat angina.

ORGANIC NITRATES

glyceryl trinitrate, isosorbide mononitrate

Mechanism of action and effects

The organic nitrates are vasodilators that relax vascular smooth muscle by mimicking the vasodilator effects of endogenous NO. Enzymatic degradation of the nitrate releases NO, which combines with thiol groups in vascular endothelium to form nitrosothiols. Nitrosothiols activate guanylyl cyclase and generate the intracellular second messenger cyclic guanosine monophosphate (cGMP; Fig. 5.3). Cyclic GMP activates protein kinase G, which reduces the availability of intracellular Ca^{2+} to the contractile mechanism of vascular smooth muscle, causing relaxation and vasodilation. Vasodilation is produced in three main vascular beds:

- **Venous capacitance vessels.** This leads to peripheral pooling of blood and reduced venous return to the heart. This lowers left ventricular filling pressure (preload), decreases ventricular wall tension and therefore reduces myocardial oxygen demand. Venous dilation is a major contributor to the relief of angina and is produced at moderate plasma nitrate concentrations. However, tolerance to this action occurs rapidly during continued treatment.
- **Arterial resistance vessels.** This leads to reduced resistance to left ventricular emptying (afterload). This lowers blood pressure, decreases cardiac work and contributes to a reduced myocardial oxygen demand. Arterial dilation occurs at higher plasma nitrate concentrations than venodilation, but tolerance arises less readily during long-term treatment.
- **Coronary arteries.** Nitrates have little effect on total coronary blood flow in angina; indeed, total flow may be reduced because of a decrease in perfusion pressure. However, blood flow through collateral vessels may be improved, and nitrates also relieve coronary artery vasospasm. Therefore, blood supply may be improved to ischaemic areas of the myocardium. Coronary artery dilation occurs at low plasma nitrate concentrations, and tolerance is slow to develop.

Pharmacokinetics

Glyceryl trinitrate (GTN) is the most widely used organic nitrate. It is well absorbed from the gut but undergoes extensive first-pass metabolism in the liver to inactive metabolites. To increase its bioavailability, GTN is given by one of four routes that avoid first-pass metabolism:

- **Sublingual.** When GTN is delivered under the tongue, it is absorbed rapidly across the buccal mucosa. GTN has a very short half-life (< 5 minutes), which limits the duration of action to approximately 30 minutes. GTN tablets lose their potency with prolonged storage, and a metered-dose aerosol spray is a more stable and convenient method of delivery.
- **Buccal.** A tablet containing GTN in an inert polymer matrix is held between the upper lip and gum, which permits the slow release of the drug to prolong the duration of action.
- **Transdermal.** GTN is absorbed well through the skin and can be delivered from an adhesive patch via a rate-limiting membrane or matrix. Steady release of the drug maintains a stable blood concentration for at least 24 hours after application of the patch.
- **Intravenous.** The short duration of action of GTN is an advantage for intravenous dose titration.

Isosorbide 5-mononitrate does not undergo first-pass metabolism. It has a half-life of 3–7 hours, and modified-release formulations are often used to prolong the duration of action.

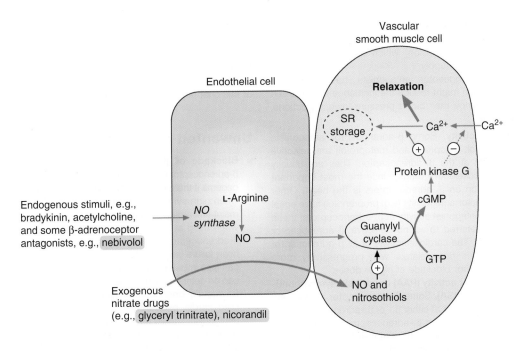

Fig. 5.3 **Actions of endogenous nitric oxide and exogenous nitrates.** Endogenous nitric oxide (NO) from endothelial cells relaxes vascular smooth muscle by activating guanylyl cyclase, with subsequent formation of cyclic guanosine monophosphate (cGMP). This activates protein kinase G, which decreases Ca^{2+} influx into the cell, increases Ca^{2+} storage in the sarcoplasmic reticulum (SR), and increases myosin light-chain dephosphorylation. Exogenous agents such as organic nitrates and nicorandil react with tissue thiols, generating NO or nitrosothiols, which then activate guanylyl cyclase and increase cGMP.

Unwanted effects

- Venodilation can produce postural hypotension, dizziness, syncope and reflex tachycardia. Tachycardia can be reduced by concurrent use of a β-adrenoceptor antagonist.
- Arterial dilation causes throbbing headaches and flushing, but tolerance to these effects is common during treatment with long-acting nitrates.
- Tolerance to the therapeutic effects of nitrates develops rapidly if there is a sustained high plasma nitrate concentration. Tolerance is therefore a particular problem with delivery of GTN via transdermal patches or with long-acting nitrates. The cause is incompletely understood, but an important mechanism may be increased degradation of NO by oxygen free radicals in the target cells. Reflex activation of the sympathetic nervous system and the renin–angiotensin system in response to hypotension may also counteract the vasodilator actions of the nitrates. Tolerance can be avoided by a 'nitrate-low' period of several hours in each 24 hours. This is preferable to a 'nitrate-free' period, which carries a risk of rebound angina. A nitrate-low period is achieved by asymmetric dosing with conventional formulations of isosorbide mononitrate (e.g. twice daily, at 8 a.m. and 1 p.m.) or by using a once-daily formulation that allows plasma nitrate concentrations to fall overnight. Transdermal GTN patches must be removed for part of each 24 hours (e.g. overnight) to prevent tolerance.
- Drug interactions are most troublesome with phosphodiesterase inhibitors, such as sildenafil, used in the treatment of erectile dysfunction. These inhibit cGMP metabolism (see Chapter 16), and co-administration can result in marked hypotension.

BETA-ADRENOCEPTOR ANTAGONISTS (β-BLOCKERS)

Examples

atenolol, bisoprolol, carvedilol, metoprolol, nebivolol, propranolol

Mechanism of action and effects in angina

All β-adrenoceptor antagonists (often referred to simply as β-blockers) act as competitive antagonists of catecholamines at β-adrenoceptors. They achieve their therapeutic effect in angina by blockade of the cardiac $β_1$-adrenoceptor with reduced generation of intracellular cAMP. As a result, they

- Decrease heart rate (by inhibition of the cardiac I_f pacemaker current in the sinoatrial node; see Chapter 8). This is most marked during exercise, when the rate of rise in heart rate is blunted;
- Reduce the force of cardiac contraction (see Chapter 7);
- Lower blood pressure by reducing cardiac output (a consequence of both the decreased heart rate and force of myocardial contraction).

The overall effect is to reduce myocardial oxygen demand. The slower heart rate also lengthens diastole and gives more time for coronary perfusion, which effectively improves myocardial oxygen supply.

Some β-adrenoceptor antagonists have additional properties, which might reduce the incidence of unwanted effects or enhance their blood pressure-lowering actions. These include:

- **Cardioselectivity.** Some β-adrenoceptor antagonists (e.g. atenolol, bisoprolol and metoprolol) are selective antagonists at the β_1-adrenoceptor. They are usually called cardioselective drugs, since the most important site of action on β_1-adrenoceptors is the heart. Other β-adrenoceptor antagonists (e.g. propranolol) have equal or greater antagonist activity at β_2-adrenoceptors; these drugs are referred to as 'nonselective' β-adrenoceptor antagonists. The cardioselectivity of all β-adrenoceptor antagonists is dose-related, with progressively more β_2-adrenoceptor blockade at higher doses.
- **Partial agonist activity (PAA) or intrinsic sympathomimetic activity (ISA).** Some β-adrenoceptor antagonists are partial agonists at either β_1- or β_2-adrenoceptors. For example, pindolol is a β_1-adrenoceptor antagonist that also has weak agonist activity at β_2-adrenoceptors, and as such it will produce vasodilation in some vascular beds (see Fig. 6.6). Drugs with PAA at the β_1-adrenoceptor have less inhibitory effect on heart rate, and force of contraction and may be less effective than full antagonists in the treatment of severe angina, but their PAA means they are less likely to cause a resting bradycardia. Beta-adrenoceptor antagonists with PAA are not widely used.
- **Vasodilator activity.** Pure β_1-adrenoceptor antagonists do not cause vasodilation. In fact reflex sympathetic nervous system stimulation of α_1-adrenoceptors in response to the fall in cardiac output produces vasoconstriction. However, some β-adrenoceptor antagonists have additional properties that override this and produce arterial vasodilation. Mechanisms of vasodilation include β_2-adrenoceptor PAA (e.g. pindolol; discussed earlier), α_1-adrenoceptor blockade (e.g. carvedilol) or an increase in endothelial NO synthesis (e.g. nebivolol; see Fig. 6.6). Vasodilation does not have any proven advantage for the treatment of angina, but may be useful when β-adrenoceptor antagonists are given for the treatment of hypertension (see Chapter 6) or heart failure (see Chapter 7).

Pharmacokinetics

Highly lipophilic β-adrenoceptor antagonists, such as propranolol and metoprolol, are well absorbed from the gut but undergo extensive first-pass metabolism in the liver, which has considerable variability among individuals. Reduction in heart rate during exercise is closely related to the plasma concentration of the drug, so dose titration of lipophilic β-adrenoceptor antagonists is usually necessary to achieve an optimal clinical response. Lipophilic β-adrenoceptor antagonists generally have short half-lives and are often available in modified-release formulations to prolong their duration of action.

Hydrophilic β-adrenoceptor antagonists, such as atenolol, are incompletely absorbed from the gut and are eliminated unchanged in the urine. The dose range to maintain effective plasma concentrations is narrower than for those drugs that undergo metabolism. The half-lives of hydrophilic β-adrenoceptor antagonists are usually longer than those of lipophilic drugs (see the drug compendium at the end of this chapter).

Unwanted effects

- **Blockade of β_1-adrenoceptors.** A large dose of a β-adrenoceptor antagonist can precipitate acute pulmonary oedema if there is preexisting poor left ventricular function, when high sympathetic nervous activity is necessary to maintain cardiac output. However, there is a paradox that when used at low doses with gradual-dose titration, a β-adrenoceptor antagonist is part of the core therapy of heart failure (see Chapter 7). A reduction in cardiac output can also impair blood supply to peripheral tissues, which can be detrimental in critical leg ischaemia or can provoke Raynaud's phenomenon (see Chapter 10). Excessive bradycardia occasionally occurs, and β-adrenoceptor antagonists should be used with caution or avoided in the presence of advanced atrioventricular conduction defect (heart block). Drugs with PAA at β_1-adrenoceptors produce less resting bradycardia.
- **Blockade of β_2-adrenoceptors.** Bronchospasm can be precipitated in people with asthma or asthma-COPD overlap syndrome due to antagonist activity at β_2-adrenoceptors in bronchial smooth muscle. Bronchospasm can arise even with cardioselective drugs. Nonselective β-adrenoceptor antagonists can prolong hypoglycaemia, which may be a problem in people with diabetes mellitus treated with insulin (see Chapter 40). Gluconeogenesis, a component of the metabolic response to hypoglycaemia, is dependent upon β_2-adrenoceptor stimulation in the liver. Beta-adrenoceptor antagonists also blunt the autonomic response that alerts the person to the onset of hypoglycaemia.
- **Central nervous system effects.** These include sleep disturbance, vivid dreams and hallucinations. All are more common with lipophilic drugs, which readily cross the blood–brain barrier. Other consequences of CNS action include fatigue and subtle psychomotor effects (e.g. lack of concentration and sexual dysfunction).
- **Effects on blood lipid levels.** Most β-adrenoceptor antagonists raise the plasma concentration of triglycerides and lower the concentration of high-density lipoprotein (HDL) cholesterol (see Chapter 48). These changes are modest but potentially atherogenic. They are most marked with nonselective β-adrenoceptor antagonists, but less so if the drug has PAA.
- **Sudden withdrawal syndrome.** Upregulation of β-adrenoceptors during long-term treatment makes the heart more sensitive to catecholamines when the drug is withdrawn. Sudden withdrawal may give rise to palpitation due to an increase in heart rate and force of cardiac contraction. Beta-adrenoceptor antagonists should be stopped gradually in people with ischaemic heart disease, to avoid precipitating unstable angina or myocardial infarction.
- **Drug interactions.** The calcium channel blocker verapamil and, to a lesser extent, diltiazem (discussed later) have

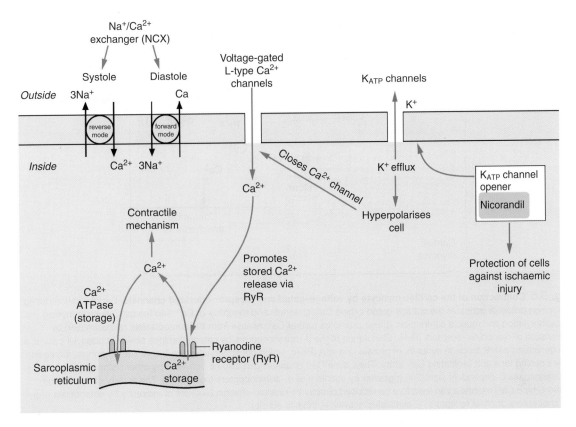

Fig. 5.4 **The control of calcium regulation and actions of potassium channel openers in cardiac myocytes and blood vessels.** Calcium concentrations in cardiac cells and in vascular smooth muscles are under the influence of a number of different mechanisms. Calcium entry through voltage-gated L-type Ca^{2+} channels stimulates ryanodine receptors (RyR) in the sarcoplasmic reticulum, releasing stored Ca^{2+} (a process known as Ca^{2+}-induced calcium release, CICR). Intracellular Ca^{2+} is also regulated by exchange with Na^+ via the Na^+/Ca^{2+} exchangers (NCX) in the cell membrane. Vascular smooth muscle cells have ATP-sensitive inward rectifier K^+ channels (K_{IR}) which combine with sulfonylurea receptors to form ATP-sensitive K^+ channels (K_{ATP}). Hyperpolarisation of the cell by drugs which open K_{ATP} channels, such as nicorandil, closes voltage-gated L-type Ca^{2+} channels and causes relaxation.

potentially hazardous additive effects with β-adrenoceptor antagonists, since both reduce the force of cardiac contraction and slow heart rate.

CALCIUM CHANNEL BLOCKERS

dihydropyridines: amlodipine, nifedipine
nondihydropyridines: diltiazem, verapamil

Mechanism of action and effects

Calcium is essential for excitation–contraction coupling in muscle cells. The following mechanisms of regulating intracellular free Ca^{2+} concentration are important pharmacologically (Figs 5.4 and 5.5):

■ In smooth muscle and cardiac muscle cells, Ca^{2+} can enter cells through transmembrane voltage-gated and ligand-gated channels (see Figs 5.4 and 5.5).

■ In striated and cardiac muscle cells, a rise in intracellular free Ca^{2+} promotes release of further Ca^{2+} from the sarcoplasmic reticulum through actions at ryanodine receptors (see Figs 5.4 and 5.5).
■ Ligand-gated channels linked to G-protein-coupled receptors promote release of Ca^{2+} from intracellular stores in the sarcoplasmic reticulum.
■ Ca^{2+} leaves striated and cardiac muscle cells in exchange for Na^+ via the Na^+/Ca^{2+} exchanger (Fig. 5.4).

Therefore, in striated muscle, free Ca^{2+} in the cytosol comes only from the sarcoplasmic reticulum, while in smooth muscle it must enter the cell through transmembrane Ca^{2+} channels. Cardiac muscle uses both mechanisms. There are at least five different types of transmembrane Ca^{2+} channels, two of which are found in myocytes and smooth muscle cells:

■ Voltage-gated L-type Ca^{2+} channels (long-acting, high-threshold-activated, slowly inactivated) are found in the cell membranes of a large number of excitable cells, including cardiac and vascular smooth muscle. Ca^{2+} enters the cell through these channels when the cell membrane

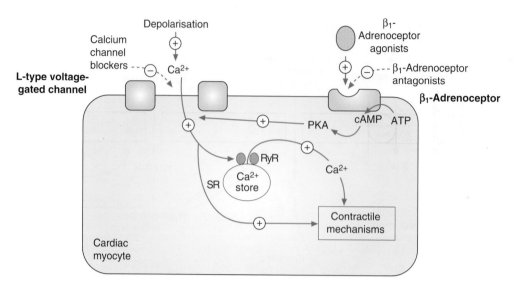

Fig. 5.5 **Contraction of the cardiac myocyte by voltage-gated and receptor-operated channels.** Depolarisation during the action potential activates the voltage-gated L-type Ca^{2+} channels and the influx of Ca^{2+} into the cell results in myosin phosphorylation and muscle contraction. It also promotes further Ca^{2+} release from the sarcoplasmic reticulum (SR) by stimulation of ryanodine receptors (RyR). Stimulation of the β_1-adrenoceptors by catecholamines activates adenylyl cyclise, and the generated cAMP binds to subunits of protein kinase A (PKA), which phosphorylates the L-type Ca^{2+} channels, increasing their opening time and facilitating Ca^{2+} entry. The L-type Ca^{2+} channels can also be activated by other pathways, such as phospholipase C-dependent signalling triggered by agonism of α_1-adrenoceptors (not shown). The activity of the voltage-gated L-type Ca^{2+} channels can therefore be reduced directly by calcium channel blockers or indirectly by antagonists of β_1-adrenoceptors or other receptors. +, stimulates activity; –, inhibits activity.

is depolarised. The cardiac and vascular smooth muscle L-type Ca^{2+} channels have different subunit structures. L-type channels are important therapeutically.

- Voltage-gated T-type Ca^{2+} channels (transient, low threshold-activated, fast inactivated) are found in pacemaker cells of the sinoatrial and atrioventricular nodes, and are also present in vascular smooth muscle.

Calcium channel blockers have different chemical structures, but their common action is to reduce Ca^{2+} influx through voltage-gated L-type Ca^{2+} channels in smooth and cardiac muscle. None of the currently available calcium channel blockers affects T-type channels to any important extent, or influences ligand-gated Ca^{2+} channels (which are involved in neurotransmitter release and respond to endogenous agonists such as noradrenaline; Fig. 5.5).

There are clinically important differences among the different types of calcium channel blockers, which bind to discrete receptors on the L-type Ca^{2+} channel. The receptor for verapamil is intracellular, while diltiazem and the dihydropyridines (e.g. nifedipine, amlodipine) have extracellular binding sites; however, the receptor domains for verapamil and diltiazem overlap. Verapamil and diltiazem exhibit frequency-dependent receptor binding and gain access to the Ca^{2+} channel when it is in the open state; in contrast, the dihydropyridines preferentially bind to the channel in its inactivated state. As more Ca^{2+} channels are in the inactive state in relaxed vascular smooth muscle than in cardiac muscle, dihydropyridines selectively bind to Ca^{2+} channels in vascular smooth muscle. These receptor binding characteristics account for the relative vascular selectivity of

the dihydropyridines and for the antiarrhythmic properties of verapamil and diltiazem (see Chapter 8).

Calcium channel blockers produce a number of effects that are important in the treatment of angina:

- **Peripheral arterial dilation.** Although all calcium channel blockers are vasodilators, dihydropyridine derivatives such as nifedipine and amlodipine are the most potent and have the greatest vascular selectivity. Arterial dilation reduces peripheral resistance and lowers blood pressure. This reduces the work of the left ventricle and therefore reduces myocardial oxygen demand. Most dihydropyridines have a rapid onset of action. A rapid reduction in blood pressure can lead to reflex sympathetic nervous system activation and tachycardia (Fig. 5.6). Amlodipine or modified-release formulations of short-acting dihydropyridines are more slowly absorbed and gradually reduce blood pressure with little reflex tachycardia.
- **Coronary artery dilation.** Prevention or relief of coronary vasospasm improves myocardial blood flow.
- **Negative chronotropic effect.** Verapamil and diltiazem (but not the dihydropyridines) slow the rate of firing of the sinoatrial node and slow the conduction of the electrical impulse through the atrioventricular node (see also Chapter 8). Reflex tachycardia does not occur with these drugs, and they also slow the rate of rise in heart rate during exercise.
- **Reduced cardiac contractility.** Most calcium channel blockers (but particularly verapamil) have some negative inotropic effect. Amlodipine does not impair myocardial contractility.

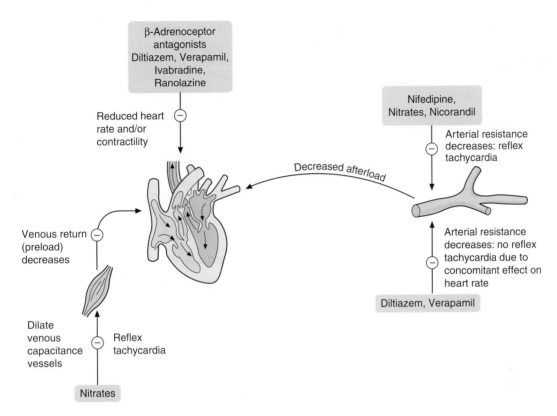

Fig. 5.6 The major sites of action of antianginal drugs. The antianginal drugs reduce cardiac work and myocardial oxygen demand either by peripheral vasodilation (which reduces afterload and preload) or by reducing heart rate and/or myocardial contractility. Myocardial oxygen supply may also be enhanced, either by coronary artery dilation or due to increased diastolic filling time. Nitrates, the dihydropyridine calcium channel blocker nifedipine, and the potassium channel opener nicorandil can cause reflex tachycardia due to a rapid fall in blood pressure. This is not a problem with the nondihydropyridines diltiazem and verapamil, which concomitantly slow the heart rate. Reflex tachycardia to nifedipine can be minimised with a modified-release formulation, or a more slowly acting dihydropyridine such as amlodipine can be used.

Pharmacokinetics

Most calcium channel blockers are lipophilic compounds with similar pharmacokinetic properties. They are almost completely absorbed from the gut lumen, but variable first-pass metabolism can limit bioavailability. Their half-lives are mostly in the range of 2–12 hours, and modified-release formulations are commonly used to prolong their duration of action. In contrast, amlodipine is slowly absorbed and does not undergo first-pass metabolism. It has a very long half-life of about 1–2 days. Verapamil can be given intravenously, usually for the treatment of supraventricular arrhythmias (see Chapter 8).

Unwanted effects

- Arterial dilation can produce headache, flushing and dizziness, although tolerance often occurs with continued use. Ankle oedema, which is frequently resistant to diuretics, probably arises from increased transcapillary hydrostatic pressure. Tolerance to oedema does not occur. Vasodilatory unwanted effects are most common with the dihydropyridines and least troublesome with verapamil.
- Reduced cardiac contractility can precipitate heart failure in people with preexisting poor left ventricular function, particularly with verapamil. Amlodipine does not depress cardiac contractility.
- Tachycardia and palpitations can arise with dihydropyridines, especially with rapid-release formulations.
- Bradycardia and heart block can occur with verapamil and diltiazem.
- Altered gut motility can occur. Constipation is most common with verapamil and less so with diltiazem. Amlodipine and other dihydropyridines can cause heartburn by relaxing the lower oesophageal sphincter.
- Gum hyperplasia.
- Several drug interactions may present: Verapamil and diltiazem can slow the heart rate excessively if they are used in combination with other drugs that have similar effects on atrioventricular nodal conduction (e.g. digoxin [see Chapter 8] or β-adrenoceptor antagonists). The metabolism of many calcium channel blockers can be inhibited or accelerated by drugs that affect the hepatic cytochrome P450 enzymes.

POTASSIUM CHANNEL OPENERS

nicorandil

Mechanism of action

There are many different K$^+$ channels in cell membranes (see Chapter 8, Table 8.1). Of these, the adenosine triphosphate (ATP)-inhibited K$_{ATP}$ channels are the target for nicorandil (see Fig. 5.4). K$_{ATP}$ channels are found in many tissues, but have a variety of tissue-specific subunit configurations, making targeted drug action on the channels possible. Nicorandil opens K$_{ATP}$ channels in vascular smooth muscle cells, so that K$^+$ leaves the cell, increasing the negative potential inside the cell (hyperpolarisation). This means that the cell becomes more difficult to depolarise and the membrane voltage-gated L-type Ca^{2+} channels are less likely to open (see the previous discussion of calcium channel blockers). As less Ca^{2+} is available to the muscle contractile mechanism, there is vasodilation in systemic and coronary arteries (see Fig. 5.4). The fall in blood pressure reduces myocardial oxygen demand, and preventing coronary vasospasm can improve myocardial perfusion. The enhanced K$_{ATP}$ channel activity may also protect myocardial cells against ischaemic injury.

Nicorandil also has a nitrate moiety, and part of its vasodilator action is via generation of NO in vascular smooth muscle (see organic nitrates, noted previously). This may account for the venodilation produced by the drug, which reduces venous return and further reduces myocardial oxygen demand.

Pharmacokinetics

Nicorandil is eliminated by hepatic metabolism and has a short half-life of 1 hour. However, the tissue effects correlate poorly with the plasma concentration and the biological effect lasts up to 12 hours.

Unwanted effects

- Arterial dilation causes headache in 25–50% of people, but tolerance usually occurs with continued use. Palpitation (caused by reflex activation of the sympathetic nervous system in response to a fall in blood pressure) and flushing are less common than headache.
- Dizziness.
- Nausea and vomiting.
- Skin, eye and mucosal ulceration, including gastrointestinal ulcers. Nicorandil should be stopped if ulceration occurs.

SPECIFIC SINUS NODE INHIBITORS

ivabradine

Mechanism of action

In cardiac pacemaker cells (especially the sinoatrial node), the pacemaker I_f current is responsible for spontaneous depolarisation (see Chapter 8). This is an inward current of positive ions through f-channels that carry both Na$^+$ and K$^+$, which are activated by the negative intracellular potential in diastole or by cyclic nucleotides. Ivabradine is a specific inhibitor of the I_f current, and its major effect is to slow the rate of firing of the sinus node. The degree of channel inhibition is use-dependent, since ivabradine binds to the open channel from the internal side of the cell membrane. As a result, the efficacy of ivabradine increases with the frequency of channel opening and is greatest at higher heart rates. Unlike β-adrenoceptor antagonists, ivabradine has no effect on myocardial contractility.

Pharmacokinetics

Ivabradine undergoes extensive first-pass metabolism in the gut wall and liver to an active metabolite. It has a short half-life of 2 hours.

Unwanted effects

- Bradycardia, first-degree heart block. It is recommended that the resting heart rate should not be allowed to fall below 50 beats/minute.
- Ventricular ectopics.
- Headache and dizziness.
- Dose-related ocular symptoms, including phosphenes (flashes of light), stroboscopic effects and blurred vision from inhibition of the I_f in the eye.

LATE SODIUM CURRENT INHIBITORS

ranolazine

Mechanism of action

Transmembrane Na$^+$ channels are activated during the initial electrical excitation of myocardial cells, and most are inactivated during the plateau phase of the action potential. However, a small proportion of the Na$^+$ channels remain open, giving rise to a late Na$^+$ current. In hypoxic tissues this current is increased and the consequent rise in intracellular Na$^+$ concentration activates the reverse mode of the Na$^+$/Ca^{2+} exchanger in the cell membrane, leading to removal of Na$^+$ from the cell. This promotes intracellular Ca^{2+} accumulation and increased diastolic myocardial tension (see Fig. 5.4). Ranolazine attenuates the late transcellular Na$^+$ current in ischaemic myocardial cells and reduces Ca^{2+} accumulation. There are two potentially beneficial consequences of this effect: the lower wall tension in the ventricles reduces myocardial oxygen demand, and it will also reduce compression of small intramyocardial coronary vessels, thus improving myocardial perfusion in diastole.

Pharmacokinetics

Ranolazine is extensively metabolised in the liver. It has a short elimination half-life of about 2 hours, and a modified-release formulation is used.

Unwanted effects

- Nausea, dyspepsia and constipation.
- Headache, dizziness and lethargy.
- Prolongation of the QT interval on the ECG (see Chapter 8), with the potential to provoke cardiac arrhythmias if used with other drugs that have the same effect.

MANAGEMENT OF STABLE ANGINA

The principal aims of treatment for stable angina are to relieve symptoms and to improve prognosis. Angina has a pronounced circadian rhythm and occurs most frequently in the hours after waking, so a drug given for prevention of symptoms should ideally be effective at this time. There is no evidence that control of symptoms will affect either survival or the risk of a subsequent myocardial infarction. Improvement in prognosis is achieved mainly by using drugs that do not directly affect symptoms.

There are several important principles of management of stable angina:

- Lifestyle changes. Stopping smoking reduces the progression of coronary atheroma and reduces the risk of developing an acute coronary syndrome by up to 50%. It also reduces coronary vasospasm and may improve symptoms. Weight loss in obese people will also reduce symptoms by reducing cardiac work. Regular exercise improves fitness and attenuates the rise in heart rate on exercise, which will increase exercise duration before the onset of angina.
- Reduction of high blood pressure and control of diabetes mellitus will reduce progression of atheroma.
- Treatment of exacerbating factors for angina, such as anaemia, arrhythmias or thyrotoxicosis.
- Sublingual GTN remains the treatment of choice for an acute anginal attack. It relieves symptoms within minutes, but gives only short-lived protection (20–30 minutes). GTN can also be taken immediately before an activity that is likely to produce angina.
- Unless anginal attacks are infrequent, a prophylactic antianginal drug should be used. A rise in heart rate is one of the main precipitating factors for angina, and a drug that lowers heart rate such as a β-adrenoceptor antagonist, or a rate-limiting calcium channel blocker like verapamil or diltiazem, is first-line treatment. Ivabradine can be used if other heart-rate-limiting drugs are not tolerated. Nitrates are less suitable as first-line prophylactic agents because of the risk of tolerance. If symptoms are not controlled by optimal doses of a single drug, then a combination of a β-adrenoceptor antagonist with a calcium channel blocker (not verapamil) can be used. Alternatively, a β-adrenoceptor antagonist or calcium channel blocker can be combined with a long-acting nitrate. Symptoms and their response to treatment are a poor guide to the severity of coronary artery disease, and quantifying the amount of ischaemic myocardium with noninvasive myocardial perfusion imaging is a more accurate predictor. A large area of ischaemic myocardium, or failure to control symptoms with two prophylactic drugs in adequate dosages, should lead to consideration of coronary angiography, with a view to revascularisation. 'Triple therapy' (e.g. β-adrenoceptor antagonist, calcium channel blocker and a long-acting nitrate) has not been shown convincingly to be better than two agents, but such combinations may give further symptomatic benefit if coronary revascularisation is not possible, not wanted or while awaiting coronary angiography. Nicorandil is generally used in combination therapy. Ranolazine may be helpful when symptomatic hypotension precludes the use of other drugs.

- Low-dose aspirin reduces the risk of myocardial infarction by about 35%. Clopidogrel is an alternative if aspirin is not tolerated, but the combination does not have any additive benefit in stable coronary artery disease (see Chapter 11).
- Lowering the total plasma cholesterol to less than 4.0 mol/L by diet and a statin (see Chapter 48) reduces the risk of nonfatal myocardial infarction, cardiac death and the need for a coronary artery revascularisation procedure by more than 30%.
- ACE inhibitors (see Chapter 6) have no antianginal action, but reduce the risk of myocardial infarction and death by about 15%.
- Percutaneous coronary intervention (PCI) consists of angioplasty and usually insertion of a stent to maintain vessel patency. PCI improves symptoms, but only reduces cardiovascular death or myocardial infarction if there is a large area of ischaemic myocardium. Insertion of a coronary artery stent is followed by combination antiplatelet therapy with aspirin and clopidogrel (see Chapter 11) to minimise stent thrombosis, which carries a high risk of myocardial infarction or death. Short-term use of a glycoprotein IIb/IIIa antagonist such as abciximab (see Chapter 11) at the time of angioplasty further improves outcome for high-risk procedures. Re-stenosis after angioplasty is due to intimal hyperplasia and smooth muscle proliferation encroaching on the lumen of the vessel, and usually occurs within 6 months of the procedure. Angioplasty without stenting is followed by a re-stenosis rate of about 40% at 6 months, which can be reduced to about 20% by the use of a bare-metal stent. Drug-eluting stents, which are coated with a polymer matrix containing an antiproliferative drug such as sirolimus or tacrolimus (see Chapter 38), reduce the risk of re-stenosis at 6 months to about 6%. The combination of aspirin and clopidogrel is used for 1 month after a bare metal stent and for a year after a drug-eluting stent, after which the clopidogrel can be stopped.
- Coronary artery bypass grafting (CABG) improves long-term prognosis compared with medical treatment in people with a left mainstem coronary artery stenosis, and in those with 'triple vessel disease' (significant stenoses of the left anterior descending, left circumflex and right coronary arteries) who have impaired left ventricular function. In less severe disease it is used for symptom relief.

MANAGEMENT OF ACUTE CORONARY SYNDROMES

EARLY MANAGEMENT OF ACUTE CORONARY SYNDROMES WITHOUT ST-SEGMENT ELEVATION

Acute coronary syndromes require urgent treatment even if there is no ECG evidence of myocardial infarction at presentation. Unstable angina, if left untreated, progresses in about 10% of cases to myocardial infarction or death. The management of an acute coronary syndrome is initially determined by the ECG. In the absence of ST-segment elevation on the ECG, management is based on the assumption that a myocardial infarction has occurred, until the result of a sensitive marker of myocardial damage such as plasma troponin I or T is obtained. A rise in one of these markers will differentiate NSTEMI from unstable angina. If there is no evidence of myocardial damage and the ECG does not show ischaemic changes, then the risk of subsequent myocardial infarction or sudden death is lower.

- Initial treatment is with sublingual or intravenous GTN, which may reduce pain by relief of coronary artery vasospasm at the site of the arterial occlusion and increase coronary blood flow. Analgesia with an intravenous opioid such as morphine (see Chapter 19), together with an antiemetic, is used to treat pain that does not settle with a nitrate. Intramuscular injection of morphine should be avoided, since a low cardiac output and poor tissue perfusion often delay absorption. Supplementary oxygen may be required if the arterial oxygen saturation is below 94% with the aim of maintaining it between 94% and 98%, unless there is a risk of type 2 respiratory failure. If there is no hypoxaemia, oxygen should be avoided, since it may increase myocardial damage.
- A loading dose of aspirin and clopidogrel (see Chapter 11) should be given. If an NSTEMI is confirmed, then dual antiplatelet therapy with clopidogrel and low-dose aspirin is continued for up to 1 year. This reduces the risk of subsequent myocardial infarction by a further 20% compared with aspirin alone. After a year, the clopidogrel is stopped, but aspirin is continued indefinitely. Low-dose aspirin is used alone after an episode of unstable angina, since dual antiplatelet therapy has no advantage.
- Full anticoagulation, usually with fondaparinux (see Chapter 11), is initially used together with dual antiplatelet therapy. Fondaparinux has largely replaced low-molecular-weight heparin (which carries a higher risk of bleeding), unless coronary angiography is planned within 24 hours of admission. The risk of further myocardial infarction or death within 14 days is reduced by about 60% using combined treatment with antiplatelet therapy and an anticoagulant. If PCI is carried out, the direct thrombin inhibitor bivalirudin (see Chapter 11) in combination with clopidogrel and aspirin will reduce the risk of ischaemic events during and after the procedure. Heparin combined with a glycoprotein IIb/IIIa antagonist such as tirofiban (see Chapter 11) can be used instead of bivalirudin, but there is a higher risk of bleeding. There is some evidence of benefit from combining an oral anticoagulant with

dual antiplatelet therapy after the acute phase, but the increased risk of bleeding means that this is not widely used.

- A β-adrenoceptor antagonist is the first-choice antianginal treatment, and can reduce ischaemic events after presentation with unstable angina. A heart rate-limiting calcium channel blocker, such as verapamil or diltiazem, can be used if a β-adrenoceptor antagonist is contraindicated or not tolerated. If further treatment is needed, then a dihydropyridine calcium channel blocker such as nifedipine, or nicorandil, or a nitrate via a buccal tablet or by intravenous infusion can be used with a β-adrenoceptor antagonist. Apart from β-adrenoceptor antagonists, antianginal drugs do not improve prognosis in unstable angina.
- In the acute phase of an NSTEMI, early angiography, followed when appropriate by CABG or PCI, will reduce the risk of reinfarction or death by about 40%. If there is no evidence of myocardial infarction, then angiography should be undertaken if symptoms do not settle with conservative treatment or there is evidence of reversible myocardial ischaemia on noninvasive stress testing.

EARLY MANAGEMENT OF ST-SEGMENT ELEVATION MYOCARDIAL INFARCTION

The presence of ST-segment elevation on the ECG usually heralds a more extensive myocardial infarction (STEMI), and early opening of the occluded artery to reperfuse the myocardium limits the extent of myocardial damage and improves long-term outcomes. Reperfusion should be considered if there is characteristic ST-segment elevation in two or more contiguous leads or left bundle branch block on the ECG and a good history of acute myocardial infarction. In the latter situation, an acute myocardial infarction cannot be easily diagnosed from the ECG, but mortality is high. The greatest reduction in mortality is achieved in people at highest risk of death (i.e. anterior infarcts rather than inferior), older people (>65 years of age) and those with a presenting systolic blood pressure below 100 mm Hg. Reperfusion therapy significantly reduces mortality if undertaken within 12 hours of the onset of pain, but the survival advantage is greater the earlier treatment is administered.

- Analgesia and oxygen may be given as described previously for unstable angina/NSTEMI. An intravenous β-adrenoceptor antagonist can be given to reduce cardiac work, especially if there is hypertension, but should be avoided if there are signs of heart failure.
- 'Primary' PCI (coronary angioplasty, usually with insertion of a stent) is the treatment of choice for reperfusion in STEMI if angiography can be started within 120 minutes of presentation. There is a greater reduction in mortality than using thrombolytic therapy. 'Rescue' PCI can be considered if thrombolysis has failed to reperfuse the infarct-related vessel. Anticoagulation with low-molecular-weight or unfractionated heparin (see Chapter 11) is given at the time of primary PCI, in addition to dual oral antiplatelet therapy. A combination of aspirin with an oral ADP receptor antagonist (either prasugrel, ticagrelor or clopidogrel; see Chapter 11) should be continued for at least 12 months after a STEMI, and is essential if a drug-eluting stent has been inserted.

Heart failure
Cardiogenic shock
Cardiac rupture
    Free wall rupture
    Ventricular septal defect
Arrhythmias
    Ventricular fibrillation
    Ventricular tachycardia
    Supraventricular tachycardias
    Sinus bradycardia and heart block
Pericarditis
    Intracardiac thrombus

■ Natural fibrinolysis can be enhanced by intravenous fibrinolytic (thrombolytic) therapy (see Chapter 11) to rapidly reperfuse the occluded artery and limit the size of the infarct. Treatment with fibrinolytic therapy is now limited mainly to people who cannot be managed by primary PCI within 2 hours of the time fibrinolysis could be given. The preferred agents are alteplase (recombinant tissue plasminogen activator, rt-PA) or a synthetic rt-PA analogue such as tenecteplase. Alteplase and related compounds are relatively short acting, and subsequent anticoagulation reduces reocclusion of the artery. Fondaparinux (see Chapter 11) for 8 days after fibrinolysis reduces mortality and reinfarction by up to 25% more than heparin. Streptokinase is rarely used now, since it has a lower success rate for opening occluded arteries and produces symptomatic hypotension during about 10% of administrations.

In addition to the management discussed previously, complications of myocardial infarction may require specific treatment (Box 5.1).

SECONDARY PROPHYLAXIS AFTER MYOCARDIAL INFARCTION

The management of unstable angina after the acute episode is similar to that of stable angina. Secondary prophylaxis after myocardial infarction to reduce late mortality requires a broad-based approach. The following interventions produce independent benefits:

■ Stopping smoking reduces mortality after a myocardial infarction by up to 50%.
■ Rehabilitation programmes which include exercise reduce mortality by up to 25% and improve psychological recovery. Weight loss should be encouraged in obese people, and a Mediterranean diet is recommended.
■ Low-dose aspirin combined with clopidogrel or ticagrelor (see Chapter 11) inhibits platelet aggregation and reduces mortality in the first few weeks when started within 24 hours of the onset of pain. Overall mortality is reduced by at least 25%. The combination is effective following both STEMI and NSTEMI.
■ Beta-adrenoceptor antagonists, started orally soon after STEMI or NSTEMI, reduce both death and reinfarction by about 25%. The mechanism is unknown. The greatest benefit is seen in those at highest risk (e.g. following anterior infarction) and in those who have had serious postinfarct arrhythmias, postinfarct angina or heart failure. Treatment should be continued for at least 12 months, or indefinitely if there is left ventricular dysfunction. Heart failure should be stabilised before a β-adrenoceptor antagonist is given (see Chapter 7).
■ An ACE inhibitor (see Chapter 6) is of greatest benefit if there is clinical or radiological evidence of heart failure after STEMI or NSTEMI, with a reduction in mortality of about 25% over the subsequent year. There is a smaller survival advantage if there is significant left ventricular dysfunction after the infarction (an ejection fraction of 40% or less) without clinical evidence of heart failure, with a 20% reduction in mortality over 3–5 years. ACE inhibitors reduce mortality when there is well-preserved left ventricular function, although the absolute risk reduction is smaller. ACE inhibitors also reduce nonfatal reinfarction by an unknown mechanism. The benefits of an ACE inhibitor are greatest with high doses. An angiotensin receptor antagonist (see Chapter 6) has similar efficacy following myocardial infarction, and should be considered if an ACE inhibitor is poorly tolerated.
■ Verapamil and diltiazem produce a small reduction in reinfarction, but do not reduce mortality. They may be detrimental if there have been symptoms or signs of heart failure. These drugs should be considered as an option only for those at high risk who cannot tolerate a β-adrenoceptor antagonist and who do not have significant left ventricular dysfunction. Dihydropyridine calcium channel blockers have no effect on prognosis after myocardial infarction.
■ Long-term anticoagulation with warfarin or rivaroxaban (see Chapter 11) reduces mortality and reinfarction to a similar extent to low-dose aspirin. In combination with aspirin, they produce an additional reduction in both fatal and nonfatal events, but with an increased risk of bleeding.
■ A Mediterranean diet reduces mortality after myocardial infarction. A further reduction in mortality may be achieved with supplementary omega-3 fatty acids. An antiarrhythmic effect may be responsible for these benefits (see Chapter 48).

SELF-ASSESSMENT

True/false questions

1. The increased oxygen demand produced by a rise in cardiac workload is met by an increase in coronary blood flow.
2. NO causes vasodilation by increasing cAMP in vascular smooth muscle cells.
3. In angina, GTN increases total coronary blood flow.
4. Topical absorption of GTN from a transdermal patch avoids first-pass metabolism.
5. GTN can be taken safely with a β-adrenoceptor antagonist.
6. All β-adrenoceptor antagonists have vasodilator activity.
7. Resting bradycardia is less likely with a β-adrenoceptor antagonist with ISA.
8. The antianginal action of amlodipine arises from its negative chronotropic and inotropic effects on the heart.

9. Enhancing the efflux of K^+ ions hyperpolarises vascular smooth muscle cells.
10. Ivabradine slows the heart rate and reduces myocardial contractility.
11. PCI reduces mortality after a STEMI more than thrombolytic therapy.
12. Drug-eluting stents reduce the risk of re-stenosis after angioplasty.

One-best-answer (OBA) questions

1. Identify the least accurate statement about angina and myocardial infarction.
   A. Isosorbide mononitrate does not undergo first-pass metabolism.
   B. Verapamil can reduce arterial blood pressure without causing reflex tachycardia.
   C. Antiplatelet drugs such as tirofiban can reduce the risk of myocardial infarction in high-risk individuals with unstable angina.
   D. Cholesterol reduction is of little benefit in reducing the risk of recurrence of myocardial infarction.
   E. Nifedipine does not improve prognosis after myocardial infarction.
2. Which change to the treatment regimen would be most likely to reduce the risk of tolerance developing to isosorbide mononitrate?
   A. Switch to its longer-acting precursor, isosorbide dinitrate.
   B. Give GTN in addition by the buccal route when necessary.
   C. Switch to a continuously applied transdermal GTN patch.
   D. Schedule doses so that there is a period of low plasma concentration of isosorbide mononitrate each day.
   E. Administer isosorbide mononitrate together with a β-adrenoceptor antagonist
3. Which drug combination is most likely to have an *adverse* effect on cardiac function in a person with angina?
   A. GTN with atenolol
   B. Verapamil with atenolol
   C. Amlodipine with atenolol
   D. GTN with nicorandil
   E. GTN with low-dose aspirin

Case-based questions

Mr T.K., a 65-year-old man who works as a landscape gardener, has been having episodes of chest pain that he likened to indigestion. They were brought on by moderately strenuous exercise and relieved by rest but not by antacids. The symptoms had been present for approximately 1 year, but recently the frequency and intensity of the pains had become worse and were now occurring several times a week. He is hypertensive, and his serum cholesterol is 6.6 mmol/L. He smokes 40 cigarettes per day and is overweight. He drinks about 10 units of alcohol a week. He had a good exercise tolerance during a diagnostic exercise test, but his ECG showed anterolateral ST-segment depression at peak

exercise. There is no evidence of heart failure. A diagnosis of angina is made and medical treatment started.

Six months later, despite continuing medication, Mr T.K. awoke with severe chest pains and dyspnoea that was not relieved by GTN. An ECG showed an acute STEMI.
A. How could his acute attacks of angina be treated?
B. The frequency of his attacks requires prophylactic treatment. What options are available to reduce the frequency of anginal attacks?
C. What other drugs could be useful to improve his prognosis?
D. Would lifestyle changes help Mr T.K.?
E. In unstable angina, which drug treatments would likely reduce the progression of the episodes to myocardial infarction or sudden death?
F. What is the likely cause of the myocardial infarction?
G. Why is it important to give reperfusion therapy as quickly as possible?
H. Mr T.K. is given the fibrinolytic agent alteplase (recombinant tissue plasminogen activator, rt-PA) because of fears that he would get an allergic response to streptokinase. Is this justified?
I. He is given 150 mg aspirin orally after an initial loading dose. What is the mechanism of action of low-dose aspirin, and would it have any added benefit if fibrinolytic therapy is also given?
J. Consideration is given to giving fondaparinux to Mr T.K., but this is considered unnecessary because he had been given rt-PA. Is this decision correct?
K. Following his myocardial infarction, long-term prophylaxis was considered. Which of the following drugs would have been likely to be of benefit: an ACE inhibitor, low-dose aspirin, a β-adrenoceptor antagonist, diltiazem, verapamil or warfarin?

ANSWERS

True/false answers

1. **True.** Increased coronary blood flow meets the increased myocardial oxygen demand, as the proportion of oxygen removed from the coronary artery blood is high (75%) even at rest.
2. **False.** NO vasodilates by increasing synthesis of cGMP, which reduces intracellular Ca^{2+}. Organic nitrates act by the same pathway.
3. **False.** Although GTN can reduce coronary vasospasm or dilate collateral blood vessels, it does not increase total coronary blood flow. Its main actions are peripheral venodilation, which reduces venous return (preload), and reduced peripheral resistance (afterload), both of which reduce cardiac work and oxygen demand.
4. **True.** GTN taken orally undergoes extensive first-pass metabolism due to delivery to the liver in the hepatic portal circulation; this is avoided by transdermal or sublingual administration, from which the drug gains direct access to the systemic circulation.
5. **True.** The main antianginal action of β-adrenoceptor antagonists is to reduce myocardial oxygen demand by reducing heart rate and contractility. They thus reduce the reflex tachycardia that may occur with GTN and other nitrates.

6. **False.** Blockade of β_1-adrenoceptors produces reflex vasoconstriction, but some β-adrenoceptor antagonists produce peripheral vasodilation by partial agonism at β_2-adrenoceptors (e.g. pindolol), by α_1-adrenoceptor blockade (e.g. carvedilol) or by activation of NO synthesis (e.g. nebivolol).

7. **True.** Drugs with intrinsic sympathomimetic (partial agonist) activity at β_1-adrenoceptors produce less bradycardia at rest, but may be less effective than full antagonists in reducing heart rate on exertion.

8. **False.** Dihydropyridine calcium channel blockers mainly reduce myocardial oxygen demand by reducing peripheral arterial resistance and venous return; they do not reduce heart rate and amlodipine does not reduce myocardial contractility.

9. **True.** Potassium channel openers such as nicorandil hyperpolarise vascular myocytes by enhancing K^+ efflux; this closes voltage-gated L-type Ca^{2+} channels, leading to smooth muscle relaxation.

10. **False.** Ivabradine slows the heart by a direct action at the sinoatrial node without effect on myocardial contractility, unlike β-adrenoceptor antagonists.

11. **True.** PCI with stent insertion within 120 minutes of a STEMI is preferred to thrombolytic therapy and can also be used when thrombolysis has failed.

12. **True.** Stents coated with polymers that elute an antiproliferative drug (e.g. tacrolimus) can reduce re-stenosis compared with bare-metal stents.

OBA answers

1. **Answer D** is the least accurate statement.
   A. Correct. Isosorbide mononitrate can therefore give a more predictable response of greater duration than the dinitrate.
   B. Correct. Unlike the dihydropyridines, verapamil also acts on the heart, and reflex tachycardia does not occur.
   C. Correct. Platelet inhibition with tirofiban, an intravenous glycoprotein IIb/IIIa antagonist, reduces the risk of MI or death in those at high risk (see also Chapter 11). These agents are most effective after an NSTEMI.
   D. **Incorrect.** Cholesterol reduction to less than 4.0 mmol/L should be attempted and statins reduce reinfarction and cardiac death by 25–30% (see Chapter 48).
   E. Correct. Dihydropyridine calcium channel blockers do not improve prognosis after myocardial infarction. Verapamil and diltiazem produce a small reduction in reinfarction, but do not reduce mortality and may be detrimental if there are signs of heart failure.

2. **Answer D** is correct. The only way to reduce tolerance is to allow daily periods with low plasma concentrations of organic nitrate. Tolerance will develop to all the organic nitrates independent of the route of administration if plasma concentrations remain high continuously; answers A–C would therefore increase the risk of tolerance. A β-adrenoceptor antagonist (answer E) will reduce reflex tachycardia but not the development of tolerance.

3. **Answer B** is correct.
   A. Incorrect. Atenolol prevents reflex tachycardia caused by the nitrate.

B. **Correct.** Verapamil and atenolol both have a negative inotropic effect, and this could be a problem, particularly if there are signs of heart failure. They also have a negative chronotropic effect, and the combination can cause severe bradycardia and heart block.
C. Incorrect, although amlodipine and atenolol might cause excessive hypotension.
D. Incorrect. Nicorandil does not have a direct effect on the heart.
E. Incorrect. Aspirin will reduce the risk of myocardial infarction.

Case-based answers

A. Sublingual GTN is the first-choice drug for rapid relief of Mr T.K.'s acute anginal attacks, although protection is only short-lived.

B. For prophylaxis, a β-adrenoceptor antagonist is often the treatment of first choice, or a calcium channel blocker if a β-adrenoceptor antagonist is contraindicated. If symptoms are not well controlled with either agent alone, a combination of both drugs, or the addition of a long-acting nitrate could be used, but the benefit of triple therapy is not convincing. Dual therapy with atenolol and diltiazem could significantly decrease the number of anginal attacks compared with either drug alone, and will also lower blood pressure and heart rate, which are precipitating factors for angina. The combination should be carefully monitored, however, because of the risk of compounding bradycardia or heart failure.

C. Additional therapy to improve prognosis includes low-dose aspirin or a statin drug to lower plasma cholesterol, both of which have been shown to reduce the risk of subsequent myocardial infarction.

D. Smoking, lack of exercise and obesity are all risk factors for coronary heart disease. T.K. is exposed to these increased risks and should address them by lifestyle changes.

E. The most consistent evidence is for combined use of aspirin with a β-adrenoceptor antagonist.

F. The most likely cause is coronary artery occlusion at the site of a ruptured atheromatous plaque, causing myocardial necrosis.

G. The benefit of reperfusion therapy is strongly dependent upon the delay between symptoms and administration. The benefit is greatest within 6 hours from the onset of pain, but there is good evidence for benefit until at least 12 hours. If angiography can be started within 2 hours of presentation, PCI (coronary angioplasty with stent) produces a greater reduction in mortality than thrombolytic therapy. PCI may also be used for rescue if fibrinolysis fails.

H. Allergic reactions to streptokinase are extremely rare. Mr T.K. had not had a previous myocardial infarction and had not previously been given streptokinase, so would be unlikely to have high titres of streptokinase-neutralising antibodies. It would, therefore, be safe to give him streptokinase unless he had severe symptomatic hypotension. However, alteplase or an rt-PA derivative is usually preferred.

I. Low doses of aspirin selectively reduce production of the platelet-aggregating agent thromboxane A_2 by platelets, while having less effect on the production of the antiaggregating agent prostacyclin (prostaglandin I_2) from endothelial cells. Aspirin (combined with clopidogrel or ticagrelor) and fibrinolytic therapy have an additive benefit for treating acute myocardial infarction, reducing subsequent reinfarction or death.

J. The decision is incorrect. Giving fondaparinux (or heparin) is necessary to prevent reocclusion of the artery, as rt-PA is short-acting.

K. ACE inhibitors (or angiotensin II receptor antagonists), low-dose aspirin, β-adrenoceptor antagonists and warfarin

all reduce mortality and the risk of reinfarction. The β-adrenoceptor antagonist will need to be given under close observation, as it carries a risk of worsening heart failure. Verapamil and diltiazem do not reduce mortality and may be detrimental in people who have signs of heart failure. Warfarin (or rivaroxaban) reduces reinfarction and mortality to a similar extent as low-dose aspirin, and additional reductions are seen in combination with low-dose aspirin, but with a greater risk of bleeding.

FURTHER READING

Stable angina

Camm, A.J., Manolis, A., Ambrosio, G., et al., 2015. Unresolved issues in the management of chronic stable angina. Int. J. Cardiol. 201, 200–207.

Husted, S.E., Ohman, E.M., 2015. Pharmacological and emerging therapies in the treatment of chronic angina. Lancet 386, 691–701.

Jones, D.A., Timmis, A., Wragg, A., 2013. Novel drugs for treating angina. Br. Med. J. 347, f4726.

Pfisterer, M.E., Zellweger, M.J., Gersh, B.J., 2010. Management of stable coronary artery disease. Lancet 375, 763–772.

Piccolo, R., Giustino, G., Mehran, R., et al., 2015. Stable coronary artery disease: revascularisation and invasive strategies. Lancet 386, 702–713.

Unstable angina and NSTEMI

Aronow, W.S., 2010. Office management of myocardial infarction. Am. J. Med. 1213, 593–595.

Timmis, A., 2015. Acute coronary syndrome. Br. Med. J. 351, h5153.

STEMI

Gershlick, A.H., Banning, A.P., Myat, A., et al., 2013. Reperfusion therapy for STEMI: is there still a role for thrombolysis in the era of primary percutaneous coronary intervention? Lancet 382, 624–632.

Keeley, E.C., Hillis, L.D., 2007. Primary PCI for myocardial infarction with ST-segment elevation. N. Engl. J. Med. 356, 47–54.

Reed, G.W., Rossi, J.E., Cannon, C.P., 2016. Acute myocardial infarction. Lancet doi:http://dx.doi.org/10.1016/S0140-6736(16)30677-8.

Compendium: drugs used to treat ischaemic heart disease

Drug	Characteristics
Nitrates	
Used for treatment of angina and in the management of heart failure.	
Glyceryl trinitrate	Given sublingually, buccally (as aerosol spray), topically (transdermal patch) or as an intravenous infusion. Half-life: 1–3 min
Isosorbide dinitrate	Precursor of isosorbide mononitrate. Given sublingually, orally (as normal or modified-release tablets), topically or by intravenous infusion. Half-life: 0.5–2 h
Isosorbide mononitrate	Given orally for prophylaxis of angina; also available in modified-release formulations. Half-life: 3–7 h
Beta-adrenoceptor antagonists	
Beta-adrenoceptor antagonists are used in a wide variety of indications in addition to ischaemic heart disease, including hypertension, chronic heart failure and arrhythmias, and also in anxiety, glaucoma, migraine prophylaxis and phaeochromocytoma. All are given orally unless otherwise indicated. For completeness, all oral or parenteral β-adrenoceptor antagonists are listed here irrespective of their licensed clinical uses.	
Acebutolol	β_1-Adrenoceptor-selective (10% partial agonism). Half-life: 7 h
Atenolol	β_1-Adrenoceptor-selective. Given orally, or by injection or intravenous infusion. Half-life: 7 h. Also available in combination with nifedipine, and with chlortalidone or other diuretics (see Chapter 14)
Betaxolol	β_1-Adrenoceptor-selective. Used topically for glaucoma (see Chapter 50). Half-life: 13–24 h
Bisoprolol	β_1-Adrenoceptor-selective (but cardioselectivity less than atenolol). Half-life: 11 h
Carvedilol	Non-selective; also vasodilates due to α_1-adrenoceptor antagonism. Half-life: 6 h
Celiprolol	β_1-Adrenoceptor-selective; also vasodilates due to partial β_2-adrenoceptor agonism. Used for hypertension. Half-life: 5 h

Compendium: drugs used to treat ischaemic heart disease (cont'd)

Drug	Characteristics
Esmolol	β_1-Adrenoceptor-selective. Given only by intravenous infusion for termination of supraventricular arrhythmias. Half-life: 9 min
Labetalol	β_1-Adrenoceptor-selective; also vasodilates due to α_1-adrenoceptor antagonism. Used for hypertension. Given orally, or by intravenous injection or infusion. Half-life: 3 h
Metoprolol	β_1-Adrenoceptor-selective (but cardioselectivity less than atenolol). Given orally, or by injection or intravenous infusion. Half-life: 3–10 h
Nadolol	Nonselective. Half-life: 17–24 h
Nebivolol	β_1-Adrenoceptor-selective; also vasodilates by generation of NO. Used in hypertension and as adjunct in chronic heart failure. Half-life: 10 h
Oxprenolol	Nonselective; 18% nonselective partial agonist activity. Half-life: 2 h
Pindolol	Nonselective; also vasodilates due to 35% partial β_2-adrenoceptor agonist activity. Also available in combination with clopamide (diuretic). Half-life: 3–4 h
Propranolol	Nonselective. Given orally or by intravenous injection. Half-life: 4 h
Sotalol	Nonselective β-adrenoceptor and K^+ channel antagonist. Used mainly in arrhythmias (as class III drug, see Chapter 8). Half-life: 7–18 h
Timolol	Nonselective; also available in combination formulations with diuretics. Also used topically for glaucoma (see Chapter 50). Half-life: 2–5 h

Calcium channel blockers

Indications include angina, hypertension, Raynaud's phenomenon, arrhythmias and subarachnoid haemorrhage (see Chapters 6, 8, 9 and 10). All are given orally unless stated otherwise.

Dihydropyridines

Dihydropyridines have less effect on the myocardium than verapamil and have little or no detrimental effect in heart failure. They have no antiarrhythmic activity. Modified-release formulations reduce fluctuations in blood pressure and reflex tachycardia and are preferred for the treatment of angina and hypertension.

Amlodipine	Similar to nifedipine, but longer duration of action and used once daily; no negative inotropic action. Half-life: 30–60 h
Felodipine	Similar to nifedipine, but longer duration of action and used once daily. Half-life: 12–25 h
Isradipine	Used only in hypertension. Half-life: 2–6 h
Lacidipine	Used only in hypertension. Half-life: 7–8 h
Lercanidipine	Used only in hypertension. Half-life: 3–5 h, but long duration of action (24 h) and used once daily
Nicardipine	Similar to nifedipine, but probably even less effect on myocardial contractility. Half-life: 1–12 h. Modified-release formulation also available
Nifedipine	Dilates peripheral and coronary arteries with little effect on myocardium and no antiarrhythmic activity. Modified-release formulations available; liquid capsule has rapid onset of action. Also available in combination with atenolol. Half-life: 2–4 h
Nimodipine	Selective for cerebral arteries. Used in ischaemic neurological deficits following subarachnoid haemorrhage. Given orally or by intravenous infusion. Half-life: 8–9 h

Nondihydropyridines

In contrast to dihydropyridines, these calcium channel blockers are also used for treatment and prevention of supraventricular arrhythmias, but are less effective for Raynaud's phenomenon. Modified-release formulations are available.

Diltiazem	Reduces heart rate and has some negative inotropic effect. Used in angina and hypertension; should be avoided in heart failure. Half-life: 2–5 h
Verapamil	Reduces heart rate with marked negative inotropic effect. Used in angina, hypertension and arrhythmia; should be avoided in heart failure. Given orally or by slow intravenous injection. Half-life: 2–5 h, but 5–12 h after chronic dosing

Compendium: drugs used to treat ischaemic heart disease (cont'd)

Drug	Characteristics
Potassium channel activators	
Nicorandil	Vasodilates by hyperpolarising vascular smooth muscle; also acts as a nitrate. Used for angina. Given orally. Half-life: 1 h
Specific sinus node inhibitor	
Ivabradine	Used for angina, and with other drugs for chronic heart failure. Given orally. Half-life: 2 h
Late sodium current inhibitor	
Ranolazine	Used as adjunctive treatment for patients inadequately controlled by, or intolerant to, other antianginal drugs. Half-life: 1.5–2 h

6 Systemic and pulmonary hypertension

SYSTEMIC HYPERTENSION

The cause of systemic hypertension in the majority of people is unknown (essential hypertension), with a complex interplay between genetic and environmental influences. Abnormal regulation of the physiological mechanisms that normally control arterial blood pressure (BP) may be an important factor. A small number of people with hypertension have an identifiable underlying cause (secondary hypertension).

CIRCULATORY REFLEXES AND THE CONTROL OF SYSTEMIC BLOOD PRESSURE

Systemic BP is determined by the cardiac output (CO) and total peripheral resistance (TPR).

$$BP = CO \times TPR$$

BP is maintained within fairly narrow limits due to modulation by a series of physiological reflexes. They are triggered by both acute and chronic changes in BP,

and function as both short-term and long-term control mechanisms. Important regulatory systems responsible for these actions include:

- the autonomic nervous system,
- the renin–angiotensin–aldosterone system,
- local chemical mediators at the vascular endothelium.

The autonomic nervous system regulates arterial BP in several ways.

- In the heart, the sympathetic nervous system acts mainly through β_1-adrenoceptors to increase myocardial contractility and heart rate, generating a greater CO and increasing BP (see Chapter 4). The parasympathetic nervous system acts through muscarinic receptors to reduce the heart rate and therefore decreases CO and BP.
- In arterial resistance vessels, sympathetic nervous stimulation produces arteriolar vasoconstriction through stimulation of postsynaptic α_1-adrenoceptors. Arteriolar vasoconstriction raises BP, but also increases the afterload on the heart. CO is maintained by an increase in cardiac contractility via β_1-adrenoceptors.
- In venous capacitance vessels, sympathetic stimulation of postsynaptic α_1-adrenoceptors produces venous constriction. This increases venous return to the heart (preload), raises CO and increases BP (see Chapter 7).

The autonomic nervous system is normally responsible for immediate modulation of BP. Change in systemic BP is detected by baroreceptors (stretch receptors) in the aorta and carotid arteries. When BP rises, stretch of the baroreceptors increases afferent nerve impulses to the nucleus tractus solitarius (NTS), a coordinating area in the medulla which controls the autonomic outflow to the cardiovascular system (Fig. 6.1). The increase in afferent impulses inhibits sympathetic nervous system activity via the rostral ventrolateral medulla (RVLM), and increases parasympathetic nervous system activity via the vagal nucleus (VN), returning the BP to normal. The opposite occurs when BP falls.

A slower compensatory mechanism for a reduction in BP is initiated by the release of renin from the juxtaglomerular apparatus of the kidney (Fig. 6.2). The major stimuli leading to renin release are reduced renal perfusion pressure, decreased Na^+ in the distal renal tubule and β_1-adrenoceptor stimulation. Renin is a protease that acts on circulating renin substrate (angiotensinogen) to release the decapeptide angiotensin I. This is further cleaved by angiotensin-converting enzyme (ACE) to the octapeptide angiotensin II. There are several additional enzymatic pathways for generating angiotensin II that do not involve ACE (see Fig. 6.8). Angiotensin II acts on various tissues via specific angiotensin AT$_1$ and AT$_2$ receptors (see Fig. 6.2). Its action at the AT$_1$ receptor produces vasoconstriction, and also enhances sympathetic nervous tone by facilitating presynaptic neuronal release of noradrenaline (NA) and through stimulation of central

sympathetic outflow. Angiotensin II has a number of additional properties which promote salt and water retention (Fig. 6.3), one of the most important being the release of aldosterone from the adrenal cortex. Aldosterone acts at the distal renal tubule to conserve salt and water at the expense of K$^+$ loss (see Chapter 14). Therefore angiotensin II and aldosterone raise BP by a combination of vasoconstriction and increasing circulating blood volume. Angiotensin II has additional actions at the AT$_2$ receptor that oppose some of those at the AT$_1$ receptor (see Fig. 6.2).

The integration of the fast-responding sympathetic nervous system and the slower-responding renin–angiotensin–aldosterone system in response to a fall in BP is shown in Fig. 6.3.

Additional mechanisms involved in controlling vascular tone and blood volume include circulating or local endothelial hormones and metabolites, such as natriuretic peptides, antidiuretic hormone, prostaglandins, bradykinin, nitric oxide (NO), endothelin and adenosine.

AETIOLOGY AND PATHOGENESIS OF SYSTEMIC HYPERTENSION

There is no absolute cut-off between normal and high BP. BP in all populations is normally distributed with a slight skew because of a small number of individuals with very high BP. The risk of cardiovascular events attributable to BP is also a continuous variable, increasing as BP rises. Defining a point at which BP is 'high' is therefore arbitrary, but it is usually set at values greater than 140/90 mm Hg. Using this definition, hypertension is a common condition found in 20–30% of the population of the developed world, with the prevalence increasing with age.

Hypertension is usually characterised by increased peripheral arterial resistance, which arises from arteriolar smooth muscle constriction and hypertrophy, leaving a smaller vessel lumen and an increase in the wall-to-lumen

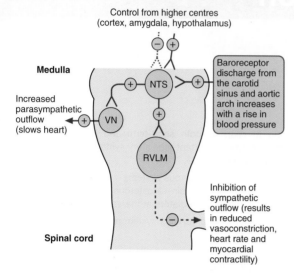

Fig. 6.1 **The role of baroreceptors in regulating blood pressure.** Increased blood pressure (BP) increases neural discharge from the baroreceptors (stretch receptors) in the carotid sinus and aortic arch, resulting in a compensatory inhibition in sympathetic outflow from the rostral ventrolateral medulla (RVLM) and an increase in the parasympathetic outflow from the cardioinhibitory vagal nucleus (VN). Both effects act to lower BP, which is also influenced by control from higher centres acting at the nucleus of the tractus solitarius (NTS). See Fig. 6.7 for sites of action of centrally acting antihypertensive drugs. +, stimulation; –, inhibition.

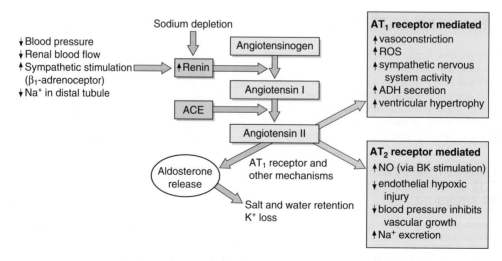

Fig. 6.2 **Formation and actions of angiotensin II.** Angiotensin II acts on angiotensin type 1 (AT$_1$) and type 2 (AT$_2$) receptors. Current therapeutic drugs act predominantly to block AT$_1$ receptors. The number of AT$_2$ receptors is low relative to that of AT$_1$ receptors but increases in pathological conditions. *ACE,* Angiotensin converting enzyme; *ADH,* antidiuretic hormone; *BK,* bradykinin; *NO,* nitric oxide; *ROS,* reactive oxygen species.

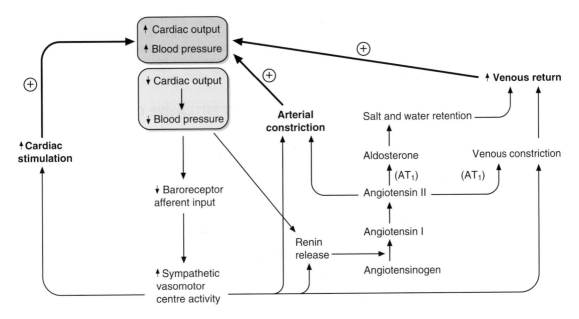

Fig. 6.3 **The control of blood pressure via the sympathetic and renin–angiotensin–aldosterone systems.** A fall in cardiac output (CO) or blood pressure (BP; *yellow box*) produces relatively rapid responses mediated by increased sympathetic activity and slower responses mediated by renin–angiotensin–aldosterone mechanisms. The outcomes are increased cardiac stimulation, increased arterial constriction and increased venous return, restoring BP. *AT₁*, Angiotensin II type 1 receptor.

ratio (vascular remodelling). CO is often normal in younger people with hypertension, but is usually reduced in the elderly.

The cause of the inappropriately raised peripheral resistance is unknown in the majority of people with hypertension, who are said to have 'essential hypertension'. Essential hypertension probably has a polygenic inheritance, leading to several clinical subtypes with different underlying pathogenic mechanisms. Environmental influences and factors such as diet, level of exercise, obesity and alcohol intake all interact with the genetic predisposition to determine the final level of BP. There is evidence that reduced renal Na^+ excretion plays a central role in the pathogenesis of essential hypertension, and the kidney requires a higher-than-normal BP to maintain a normal extracellular fluid volume. However, the disturbance in essential hypertension is much more widespread than the kidney, with cell membrane abnormalities found in many organs.

Isolated systolic hypertension (systolic BP > 160 mmHg, diastolic BP < 90 mmHg), usually found in older people, is the consequence of stiffening of large 'conductance' arteries. These vessels normally expand to accommodate the blood expelled from the heart in systole, which slows the pulse wave and increases the time taken for it to reach the peripheral resistance vessels. The pulse wave is normally reflected back from the peripheral vessels in diastole, and supports the diastolic BP and therefore coronary artery perfusion. If the compliance of the large arteries is reduced, then the pulse wave reaches the peripheral vessels early and is reflected back in systole. This increases systolic BP and reduces diastolic pressure. In isolated systolic hypertension, coronary artery perfusion can be impaired, while cardiac work is increased.

A secondary underlying cause of high BP, which often has a renal or endocrine origin, can be identified in about 5% of people with hypertension (Table 6.1).

Table 6.1 Principal causes of secondary hypertension

	Causes
Renal	Renal artery stenosis, glomerulonephritis, interstitial nephritis, arteritis, polycystic disease, chronic pyelonephritis
Endocrine	Conn's syndrome (aldosterone excess), Cushing's syndrome (glucocorticoid excess), phaeochromocytoma (catecholamine excess), acromegaly
Pregnancy	Preeclampsia and eclampsia
Drugs	Oestrogen, corticosteroids, NSAIDs, ciclosporin

NSAIDs, Nonsteroidal antiinflammatory drugs.

CONSEQUENCES OF HYPERTENSION

Hypertension does not usually cause symptoms but produces progressive structural changes in the heart and circulation. The principal complications of hypertension are ischaemic heart disease (especially in middle-aged Europeans and Americans), and cerebrovascular disease (especially in Asians and older people), which usually presents as thromboembolic stroke or, less commonly, as cerebral haemorrhage (see Chapter 9). Ischaemic complications of hypertension are more likely to occur if it is accompanied by hypercholesterolaemia, diabetes mellitus and smoking.

The underlying reasons for the complications of hypertension include accelerated formation of atheromatous plaques in many parts of the arterial circulation and development of microaneurysms on intracerebral blood vessels. Sustained hypertension predisposes to left ventricular muscle hypertrophy (LVH). LVH is an independent risk factor for the complications of hypertension, particularly ischaemic heart disease (since the muscle outgrows its blood supply), heart failure with preserved ejection fraction (see Chapter 7) and arrhythmias leading to sudden death (see Chapter 8). The cardiovascular changes and consequent clinical complications of hypertension are often referred to as 'target organ damage'. The underlying vascular lesions that occur in hypertension and their resulting complications are shown in Fig. 6.4.

Sometimes BP is raised only when the measurement is taken by a doctor or, to a lesser extent, by a nurse. This phenomenon is termed *white coat* or *office* hypertension, and appears to carry little risk of complications but can eventually lead to sustained hypertension. Hypertension should therefore be confirmed by ambulatory 24 hours BP monitoring or home BP monitoring, unless target organ damage gives a clear indication that treatment is necessary. White coat hypertension often persists despite drug treatment, which can then result in quite troublesome *hypotension* away from the surgery or clinic. There is also a phenomenon of 'masked' hypertension, when BP is normal in the clinic but high at home. This appears to carry a similar risk of complications as sustained hypertension.

Accelerated or malignant hypertension is an infrequently encountered condition produced by very high BP or a rapid rise in BP. It is characterised pathologically by arterial fibrinoid necrosis and identified clinically by the presence of flame-shaped haemorrhages, hard exudates and 'cotton wool' spots in the retina or by papilloedema, which can lead to visual disturbance. If untreated, accelerated hypertension usually leads to death from renal failure, heart failure or stroke within 5 years.

ANTIHYPERTENSIVE DRUGS

Not surprisingly, since the cause of hypertension is unclear, treatment cannot be directed precisely at the underlying mechanism(s). Most antihypertensive drugs are vasodilators, and they often modulate the natural hormonal or neuronal mechanisms responsible for BP regulation. Less commonly, a hypotensive action is partially achieved by reducing CO. The principal classes of antihypertensive drugs and their sites of action are shown in Table 6.2 and Fig. 6.5.

Drugs acting on the sympathetic nervous system

Beta-adrenoceptor antagonists (β-blockers)

atenolol, bisoprolol, nebivolol

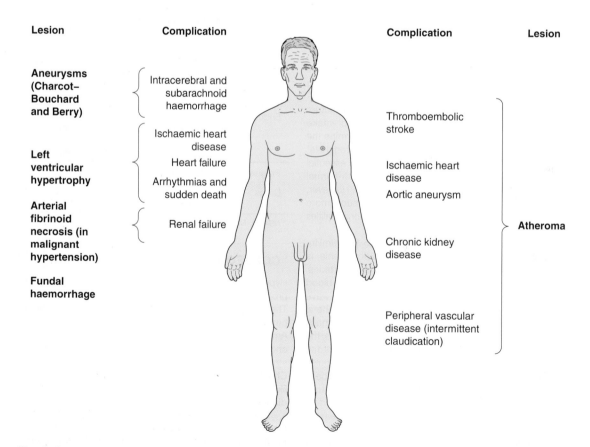

Lesion	Complication		Complication	Lesion
Aneurysms (Charcot–Bouchard and Berry)	Intracerebral and subarachnoid haemorrhage		Thromboembolic stroke	
Left ventricular hypertrophy	Ischaemic heart disease / Heart failure / Arrhythmias and sudden death		Ischaemic heart disease / Aortic aneurysm	**Atheroma**
Arterial fibrinoid necrosis (in malignant hypertension)	Renal failure		Chronic kidney disease	
Fundal haemorrhage			Peripheral vascular disease (intermittent claudication)	

Fig. 6.4 **Complications of hypertension.** Hypertension causes vascular lesions and damage throughout the body.

Table 6.2 Principal classes of antihypertensive drugs and their sites of action

Sites of action	Drugs
Sympathetic nervous system	β-Adrenoceptor antagonists
	α_1-Adrenoceptor antagonists
	Selective imidazoline I_1 receptor agonists
	Centrally acting α_2-adrenoceptor agonists
	Adrenergic neuron blockers
Hormonal control (renin–angiotensin system)	ACE inhibitors
	Angiotensin II receptor (AT_1) antagonists
	Direct renin inhibitors
Vasodilation by other mechanisms	Diuretics
	Calcium channel blockers
	Potassium channel openers
	Hydralazine and nitrovasodilators
	Endothelin ET receptor antagonists
	Prostaglandins
	PDE-5 inhibitors
	Guanylate cyclase stimulators

ACE, Angiotensin-converting enzyme; *PDE,* phosphodiesterase.

Mechanism of action in hypertension

Beta-adrenoceptor antagonists (often referred to as β-blockers) reduce BP in several ways (Fig. 6.6). Selective β_1-adrenoceptor antagonists are as effective as nonselective drugs, indicating that β_2-adrenoceptor blockade makes little contribution. The more important actions for reducing BP are likely as follows:

- Reduction of heart rate and myocardial contractility, which decreases CO.
- Antagonist action at renal juxtaglomerular β_1-adrenoceptors, which reduces renin secretion and therefore generation of angiotensin II and aldosterone. This produces arterial vasodilation and reduces plasma volume.
- Peripheral arterial vasodilation is not a direct effect of pure β-adrenoceptor antagonists, but is an additional property of some compounds that have a hybrid action (such as nebivolol; see Fig. 6.6C, and see especially Chapter 5).
- Blockade of presynaptic β-adrenoceptors in sympathetic neurons supplying arteriolar resistance vessels reduces the release of NA and thus attenuates reflex arterial vasoconstriction. The clinical importance of this effect is uncertain.

For further details about β-adrenoceptor antagonists, see Chapter 5 and Box 6.1.

Box 6.1   Clinical uses of β-adrenoceptor antagonists

Treatment of hypertension (this chapter)
Prophylaxis of angina (see Chapter 5)
Secondary prevention after myocardial infarction (see Chapter 5)
Treatment of heart failure (see Chapter 7)
Prevention and treatment of arrhythmias (see Chapter 8)
Control of symptoms in thyrotoxicosis (see Chapter 41)
Alleviation of symptoms in anxiety (see Chapter 20)
Prophylaxis of migraine (see Chapter 26)
Topical treatment of glaucoma (see Chapter 50)

Alpha-adrenoceptor antagonists (α-blockers)

Examples

α_1-adrenoceptor-selective antagonists: doxazosin, prazosin
nonselective α-adrenoceptor antagonists: phenoxybenzamine (irreversible), phentolamine (reversible)

Mechanisms of action

Alpha-adrenoceptor antagonists (often referred to as α-blockers) lower BP by blockade of postsynaptic α_1-adrenoceptors, leading to:

- dilation of arteriolar resistance vessels, which lowers peripheral resistance;
- dilation of venous capacitance vessels, which reduces venous return and therefore CO.

When BP falls as a result of using a selective α_1-adrenoceptor antagonist, this is detected by arterial baroreceptors. The baroreceptors initiate an increase in sympathetic discharge from the medulla, causing a reflex tachycardia (see Figs 6.1 and 6.3). However, NA released from cardiac sympathetic nerve terminals also stimulates inhibitory α_2-adrenoceptors on the presynaptic sympathetic neuron (see Fig. 6.6A). Selective α_1-adrenoceptor antagonists do not block the presynaptic α_2-adrenoceptors on sympathetic nerve terminals, and therefore the sympathetic stimulation of the heart is attenuated and reflex tachycardia is unusual. By contrast, nonselective α-adrenoceptor antagonists block both postsynaptic α_1-adrenoceptors and presynaptic α_2-adrenoceptors, and their use is accompanied by a marked reflex tachycardia. Nonselective α-adrenoceptor antagonists are rarely used in clinical practice except for the perioperative management of phaeochromocytoma.

Alpha-adrenoceptor antagonists produce a potentially beneficial effect on plasma lipids by increasing high-density lipoprotein (HDL) cholesterol and reducing triglycerides (see Chapter 48). Whether this has any relevance for the prevention of atheroma in individuals with hypertension is uncertain. Selective α_1-adrenoceptor antagonists are also

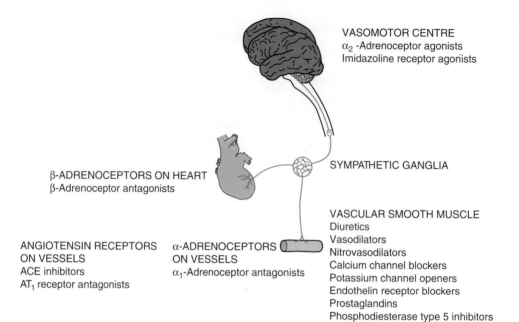

VASOMOTOR CENTRE
α_2-Adrenoceptor agonists
Imidazoline receptor agonists

SYMPATHETIC GANGLIA

β-ADRENOCEPTORS ON HEART
β-Adrenoceptor antagonists

VASCULAR SMOOTH MUSCLE
Diuretics
Vasodilators
Nitrovasodilators
Calcium channel blockers
Potassium channel openers
Endothelin receptor blockers
Prostaglandins
Phosphodiesterase type 5 inhibitors

ANGIOTENSIN RECEPTORS
ON VESSELS
ACE inhibitors
AT_1 receptor antagonists

α-ADRENOCEPTORS
ON VESSELS
α_1-Adrenoceptor antagonists

ADRENAL CORTEX
ACE inhibitors
AT_1 receptor antagonists

KIDNEY TUBULES
Diuretics
ACE inhibitors

JUXTAGLOMERULAR CELLS
THAT RELEASE RENIN
β-Adrenoceptor antagonists
Direct renin inhibitor

Fig. 6.5 The main classes of antihypertensive drugs and their sites of action. *ACE*, Angiotensin converting enzyme; AT_1, angiotensin II type 1 receptor.

used to treat the symptoms of bladder outlet obstruction (see Chapter 15).

Pharmacokinetics

Selective α_1-adrenoceptor antagonists undergo extensive first-pass hepatic metabolism. The compounds differ principally in their half-lives and, therefore, duration of action; for example, prazosin has a half-life of 3 hours, whereas doxazosin has a half-life of 9–12 hours. The nonselective drug phentolamine is given intravenously and has a short half-life (1.5 hours); phenoxybenzamine has a longer half-life (24 hours) and can be given orally.

Unwanted effects

- Postural hypotension caused by venous pooling; this can be particularly troublesome following the first dose.
- Lethargy, headache, dizziness.
- Nausea.
- Rhinitis.
- Urinary frequency or incontinence.
- Palpitation from reflex cardiac stimulation with nonselective drugs.

Centrally acting antihypertensive drugs
Selective imidazoline receptor agonists

 Example

moxonidine

Mechanism of action

Imidazoline I_1 receptors are important for the regulation of sympathetic drive (Fig. 6.7). These receptors are concentrated in the RVLM, a part of the brainstem involved in sympathetic control of BP (see Fig. 6.1). Increased neuronal activity in the RVLM, either through baroreceptor stimulation or by direct stimulation of I_1 receptors by moxonidine, will decrease sympathetic outflow, which results in a fall in BP with no reflex tachycardia. Unlike other centrally acting drugs (clonidine and methyldopa, discussed later), moxonidine has a low affinity for presynaptic α_2-adrenoceptors.

Pharmacokinetics

Moxonidine has a short half-life (2–3 hours) but a prolonged duration of action, which may reflect its high affinity for I_1 receptors.

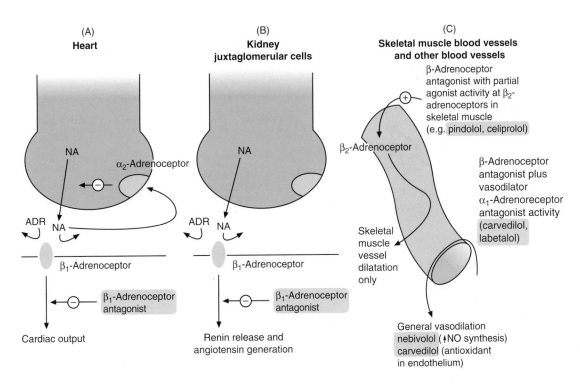

Fig. 6.6 **Sites of action of the β-adrenoceptor antagonists relevant to their use as antihypertensive agents.** (A) In the heart, the β_1-adrenoceptor antagonist drugs reduce stimulation of the β_1-adrenoceptors by noradrenaline (NA) and circulating adrenaline (ADR). Presynaptic stimulation of α_2-adrenoceptors, which inhibits noradrenaline release, still functions normally. (B) In the kidney, β_1-adrenoceptor blockade reduces the activity of the renin–angiotensin system. (C) Some selective β_1-adrenoceptor antagonists have hybrid activity: pindolol and celiprolol have intrinsic sympathomimetic activity, acting as partial agonists at β_2-adrenoceptors in skeletal muscle blood vessels, leading to vasodilation and reduced peripheral resistance. As partial agonists, these drugs reduce heart rate and cardiac output (CO) less than full antagonists. Nebivolol may dilate blood vessels more generally by releasing nitric oxide (NO). Carvedilol and labetalol also have α_1-adrenoceptor antagonist activity, reducing peripheral resistance.

Unwanted effects

- Dry mouth.
- Nausea.
- Fatigue, headache, dizziness.

Centrally acting α_2-adrenoceptor agonists

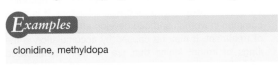

clonidine, methyldopa

Unwanted effects limit the use of centrally acting α_2-adrenoceptor agonists, although methyldopa is a drug of choice in the treatment of hypertension in pregnancy (described later).

Mechanisms of action

The α_2-adrenoceptor agonists act at presynaptic inhibitory autoreceptors in the central nervous system (CNS) to reduce sympathetic nervous outflow and increase vagal outflow from the medulla (see Fig. 6.7). This produces both peripheral arterial and venous dilation.

Methyldopa is a prodrug that is metabolised in the nerve terminal as a 'false substrate' in the biosynthetic pathway for NA to produce α-methyl NA, a potent α_2-adrenoceptor agonist. Clonidine is a direct-acting α_2-adrenoceptor agonist that is also an agonist at imidazoline I_1 receptors (discussed previously; see Fig. 6.7). Clonidine has some peripheral postsynaptic α_1-adrenoceptor agonist activity, which produces direct peripheral vasoconstriction; this initially offsets some of the central BP-lowering effect.

Pharmacokinetics

Methyldopa undergoes dose-dependent first-pass metabolism. It is eliminated by hepatic metabolism and has a half-life of 1–2 hours. Clonidine is excreted by the kidneys and has a half-life of about 24 hours.

Unwanted effects

- Sympathetic blockade: failure of ejaculation, and postural or exertional hypotension (unusual with clonidine, owing to its direct peripheral action).
- Unopposed parasympathetic action: diarrhoea.
- Dry mouth.

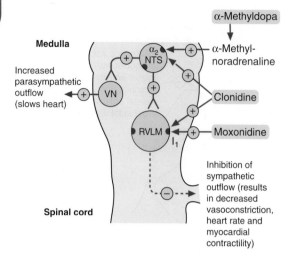

Fig. 6.7 Mechanisms of centrally acting antihypertensive drugs. These drugs act on the same medullary centres that respond to raised blood pressure (BP; see Fig. 6.1). Methylnoradrenaline and clonidine stimulate α_2-adrenoceptors in the nucleus of the tractus solitarius (NTS). Moxonidine, and possibly also clonidine, act on imidazoline I_1 receptors in the rostral ventrolateral medulla (RVLM). α_2, α_2-Adrenoceptors; I_1, I_1-imidazoline receptors; *VN,* vagal nucleus.

- CNS effects: sedation and drowsiness occur in up to 50% of people who take methyldopa; depression is occasionally seen.
- Fluid retention with peripheral oedema.
- Methyldopa induces a reversible positive Coombs's test in 20% of people, resulting from production of IgG to red cell membrane constituents; however, haemolytic anaemia is rare.
- Sudden withdrawal of clonidine can produce severe rebound hypertension with tachycardia, sweating and anxiety.

Drugs affecting the renin–angiotensin system
Angiotensin-converting enzyme inhibitors

enalapril, lisinopril, ramipril

Mechanisms of action

ACE inhibitors lower BP by several mechanisms (Figs 6.2, 6.5 and 6.8).

- Inhibition of tissue ACE in the vascular wall is central to the hypotensive effect of these drugs (see Fig. 6.8). Reduced tissue concentrations of angiotensin II lead to arterial dilation and, to a lesser extent, venous dilation. Angiotensin II production is not completely inhibited owing to alternative pathways for its generation by proteases,

including chymase and chymotrypsin-like angiotensin-II-generating enzyme (CAGE). The activity in these pathways is enhanced due to stimulation of renin release by the fall in BP after ACE inhibition.
- Competitive inhibition of plasma ACE reduces generation of circulating angiotensin II and consequently reduces the release of aldosterone (see Fig. 6.8).
- Reduction in angiotensin II-mediated potentiation of the sympathetic nervous system (see Figs 6.2 and 6.3) prevents reflex tachycardia.
- Angiotensin II is implicated in the development of arterial remodelling and LVH in hypertension. ACE inhibitors are more effective in producing regression of LVH than diuretics or β-adrenoceptor antagonists.
- ACE also degrades other peptides, including the vasodilator bradykinin (see Fig. 6.8). ACE inhibitors increase bradykinin in the vascular wall, and this may contribute to their hypotensive actions.
- There are many clinical uses of ACE inhibitors other than hypertension; these are listed in Box 6.2.

Pharmacokinetics

Many ACE inhibitors are given orally as prodrugs because the active forms are polar and poorly absorbed from the gut. The prodrugs are converted in the gut or liver to the active agent; for example, ramipril is converted to the active compound ramiprilat. In contrast, lisinopril is absorbed adequately as an active molecule. Most ACE inhibitors are excreted by the kidney with half-lives ranging from about 1–5 hours (ramiprilat) to about 30–35 hours (enalaprilat).

Unwanted effects

- Persistent dry cough that is not dose-related occurs in 10–30% of people who take ACE inhibitors. It is more common in women and can develop after many months of treatment. It may be caused by accumulation in the lungs of irritant kinins that are normally metabolised by ACE.
- Postural hypotension, which is rare unless there is salt and water depletion (e.g. as a result of therapy with diuretics). Profound hypotension can occur in such individuals, particularly after the first dose. This is rarely a problem in the treatment of hypertension, but can be in the treatment of severe heart failure (see Chapter 7).
- Renal impairment, especially in those with severe bilateral renal artery stenosis who rely on angiotensin-mediated efferent glomerular arterial vasoconstriction to maintain glomerular perfusion pressure.
- Disturbance of taste (which may be permanent), nausea, vomiting, dyspepsia or bowel disturbance.

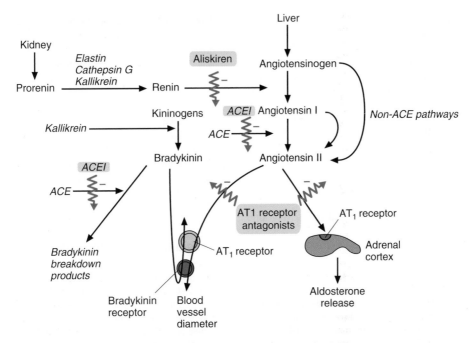

Fig. 6.8 **The biological actions of angiotensin II and bradykinin and drugs that modify these actions.** Angiotensin II causes vasoconstriction by stimulating angiotensin type 1 (AT$_1$) receptors in the blood vessels and causes Na$^+$ retention by stimulating AT$_1$ receptors in the adrenal cortex, which results in aldosterone release. Bradykinin causes vasodilation by acting on vascular smooth muscle cells and on endothelial cells. Angiotensin converting enzyme inhibitors (ACEIs) block angiotensin II formation from angiotensin I (although alternative, nonangiotensin-converting enzyme [ACE]-dependent protease pathways remain that can result in some angiotensin II formation). ACE inhibitors also reduce the breakdown of bradykinin, contributing to their vasodilator effects. Angiotensin II receptor antagonists block AT$_1$ receptors in blood vessels and the adrenal cortex. Aliskiren directly inhibits the actions of renin on angiotensinogen.

- Rashes.
- Angioedema, which is more frequent in people of Afro-Caribbean origin.

Angiotensin II receptor antagonists

candesartan, losartan, valsartan

Mechanism of action

The angiotensin II receptor antagonists are selective for the AT$_1$ receptor subtype, which is found in the heart, blood vessels, kidney, adrenal cortex, lungs and brain. They have less effect at the AT$_2$ receptor subtype (see Fig. 6.2). Actions of angiotensin II via the AT$_1$ receptor that are inhibited by these drugs include vasoconstriction, aldosterone release with salt and water retention, sympathetic nervous system stimulation, and cell growth and proliferation. Angiotensin II receptor antagonists lower BP mainly by arterial vasodilation. In contrast to ACE inhibitors, kinin degradation is unaffected by angiotensin II receptor antagonists, and inhibition of the effects of angiotensin II is more complete (see Fig. 6.8). There are many clinical uses of angiotensin II receptor antagonists other than hypertension; these are listed in Box 6.2.

Pharmacokinetics

Losartan is partially converted to an active metabolite, which is responsible for most of the pharmacological effects and has a longer half-life (6 hours) than the parent drug (2 hours). Losartan and its active metabolite are eliminated by the kidneys. Candesartan is given as a prodrug that is activated in the liver. It is eliminated by the kidneys and has a half-life of 10 hours. Valsartan is eliminated unchanged in the bile and has a half-life of 6 hours.

Unwanted effects

Drugs in this class are usually well tolerated. Their major advantages over ACE inhibitors are the low incidence of cough, and that angioedema is rare. Unwanted effects include:

- headache, dizziness;
- arthralgia or myalgia;
- fatigue.

Direct renin inhibitors

aliskiren

Mechanism of action

Aliskiren is a selective renin inhibitor with low affinity for other proteases. It binds competitively to the active site of the enzyme and inhibits the generation of angiotensin I (see Fig. 6.8). Vasodilation is achieved by reduced angiotensin II synthesis, without the compensatory increase in plasma renin activity that occurs with an ACE inhibitor or angiotensin II receptor antagonist. Aliskiren is not widely used for the treatment of hypertension because of concerns over increased vascular events when it is combined with an ACE inhibitor or an angiotensin II receptor antagonist, especially in people with type 2 diabetes mellitus.

Pharmacokinetics

Aliskiren is metabolised in the liver and has a very long half-life of 40 hours.

Unwanted effects

- Diarrhoea.
- Cough.
- Renal function may deteriorate when aliskiren is combined with an ACE inhibitor or an angiotensin II receptor antagonist, and in people with diabetes mellitus and renal impairment. These combinations also increase the risk of stroke.

Vasodilators

Diuretics

Thiazide or thiazide-type diuretics are most frequently used to lower BP, but loop and potassium-sparing diuretics are used in some situations.

Mechanism of action in hypertension

Full details of the sites and mechanisms of action of diuretics on the kidney and their unwanted effects are considered in Chapter 14. Actions involved in lowering BP include the following:

- An initial hypotensive effect is produced by intravascular salt and water depletion. However, compensatory mechanisms such as activation of the renin–angiotensin–aldosterone system largely restore plasma and extracellular fluid volumes (see Fig. 6.3), unless salt and water retention was a major component of the initial hypertension (e.g. in advanced chronic kidney disease or as a consequence of other antihypertensive treatment).
- Direct arterial dilation is responsible for the longer-term reduction in BP. The mechanism of vasodilation is not well understood. It may result from reduced Ca^{2+} entry into the smooth muscle of the arteriolar resistance vessel walls, perhaps as a consequence of intracellular Na^+ depletion.

Thiazide and thiazide-type diuretics

These drugs produce their maximum BP-lowering effect at doses lower than those required for significant diuretic activity. This is an advantage, since most unwanted effects are dose-related. They become less effective at low glomerular filtration rates.

Loop diuretics

Loop diuretics are usually less effective than thiazides in the treatment of essential hypertension. Despite having a more powerful diuretic action, their duration of action is too short. However, hypertension with advanced chronic kidney disease or hypertension resistant to multiple drug treatment is more likely to be associated with fluid retention and often responds better to a loop diuretic than to a thiazide.

Potassium-sparing diuretics

Spironolactone, a specific aldosterone antagonist, is particularly effective for hypertension caused by primary hyperaldosteronism (Conn's syndrome). It is also very effective in the treatment of resistant hypertension. Amiloride and triamterene, which directly block distal renal tubule Na^+ channels (see Chapter 14), are less effective than thiazides in essential hypertension.

Calcium channel blockers

The calcium channel blockers lower BP principally by arterial vasodilation. For clinical uses, see Box 6.3. For further details, see Chapter 5.

Potassium channel openers

Mechanism of action

Vascular smooth muscle possesses ATP-sensitive K^+ channels (K_{ATP}) that are responsible for repolarisation of the cell (see also Chapter 8). Minoxidil opens K_{ATP} channels, causing an efflux of K^+ which hyperpolarises the cell and leads to closure of voltage-gated Ca^{2+} channels and muscle relaxation

Box 6.3	Clinical uses of calcium channel blockers

Treatment of hypertension (this chapter)
Prophylaxis of angina (see Chapter 5)
Treatment of Raynaud's phenomenon (see Chapter 10)
Prevention and treatment of supraventricular arrhythmias (see Chapter 8)
Subarachnoid haemorrhage (see Chapter 9)

(see also Chapter 5). Minoxidil is one of the most powerful peripheral arterial dilators.

Pharmacokinetics

Minoxidil is mainly metabolised in the liver and has a short half-life (3–4 hours).

Unwanted effects

- Arterial vasodilation produces flushing and headache.
- The reflex sympathetic nervous system response to vasodilation causes tachycardia and palpitation (which can be blunted by concurrent use of a β-adrenoceptor antagonist, ACE inhibitor or angiotensin II receptor antagonist).
- Salt and water retention occurs through stimulation of the renin–angiotensin–aldosterone system (see Fig. 6.2). Along with increased transcapillary pressure from vasodilation, this can produce peripheral oedema, which can be reduced by the concurrent use of diuretics.
- Hirsutism; therefore rarely used for treatment of women. Topical minoxidil is used as a treatment for male pattern baldness.

Hydralazine

Hydralazine is rarely used for long-term treatment of hypertension, but is an important treatment for hypertension in late pregnancy (preeclampsia), since it maintains uterine blood flow.

Mechanism of action

The mechanism of action of hydralazine is uncertain, but it is dependent on the production of NO by vascular endothelium, particularly in arterioles, leading to activation of guanylyl cyclase and the intracellular production of cGMP. This will produce smooth muscle relaxation by mechanisms similar to those of organic nitrates (see Fig. 5.3).

Pharmacokinetics

Hydralazine undergoes extensive first-pass metabolism in the gut wall and liver, principally by N-acetylation. Genetically determined slow acetylators (see Table 2.9) are more sensitive to clinical doses of hydralazine and more susceptible to some of the unwanted effects.

Unwanted effects

- Arterial vasodilation with reflex sympathetic activation produces tachycardia, flushing, hypotension and fluid retention.
- Headache, dizziness.
- A systemic lupus erythematosus (SLE)-like syndrome, which usually occurs after several months of treatment, is dose-related and more common in slow acetylators. It resembles the naturally occurring disease but does not produce renal or cerebral damage and is slowly reversed if treatment is stopped. A positive antinuclear antibody is found in many individuals who do not develop the syndrome.

Nitrovasodilators

sodium nitroprusside

Because it must be given intravenously, the use of nitroprusside is limited to the emergency management of hypertensive crises.

Mechanism of action

Nitroprusside is a nitrovasodilator; it reacts with oxyhaemoglobin in erythrocytes to produce methaemoglobin, cyanide and NO. The NO gives the drug a mechanism of action similar to that of organic nitrates (see Chapter 5), producing dilation of arterioles and veins.

Pharmacokinetics

Nitroprusside is given by intravenous infusion, and its duration of action is less than 5 minutes. The cyanide by-product is liberated from erythrocytes and reduces aerobic metabolism in tissues by inhibiting mitochondrial cytochrome oxidase; free cyanide is converted in the liver to less toxic thiocyanate, but thiocyanate accumulates with prolonged infusion. Therefore treatment with nitroprusside is usually limited to a maximum of 3 days.

Unwanted effects

- Headache, dizziness.
- Nausea, retching, abdominal pain.
- Thiocyanate accumulation causes tachycardia, sweating, hyperventilation, arrhythmias and metabolic acidosis from inhibition of aerobic metabolism in cells.

TREATMENT OF SYSTEMIC HYPERTENSION

Morbidity and premature deaths associated with untreated hypertension are considerable (see Fig. 6.4) and increase with advancing age. Therefore treatment of older people with hypertension prevents more events in the short term than treating a similar number of younger people. However, early treatment will prevent vascular damage occurring in the younger individuals with hypertension – an important consideration since the vascular changes are not completely reversible once established.

If evidence of target organ damage is present or the person has diabetes mellitus, drug treatment reduces complications when introduced at 'office' BPs above 140/90 mm Hg. However, if there is no target organ damage, drug treatment may not alter the outcome until the 'office' systolic pressure is sustained above 160 mm Hg, or the diastolic BP is sustained above 100 mm Hg. Treating isolated systolic hypertension (systolic >160 mm Hg, diastolic <90 mm Hg) in the elderly gives similar benefits to the treatment of diastolic hypertension in this age group. In all cases, in the absence of target organ damage hypertension should be confirmed by ambulatory or home blood pressure monitoring before treatment.

The optimal target BP in uncomplicated hypertension is the subject of some controversy. It is often advocated that in people under the age of 80 years, an office systolic BP below 140 mm Hg and a diastolic pressure below 90 mm Hg (or a home BP below 135/85 mm Hg) are optimal. In those aged over 80 years, a target of 150/90 mm Hg is recommended. When there is target organ damage or diabetes mellitus, a lower target BP of 130/80 mm Hg is recommended, to minimise the risk of progressive vascular disease. Some recent evidence suggests that lower BP targets at all ages may have additional benefit. Even if the target pressures cannot be achieved, any BP reduction in severe hypertension will reduce the risk of complications. There is no recommended lower limit for BP reduction, except in people with significant coronary artery disease. In this situation, lowering the diastolic BP below 70 mm Hg may reduce coronary artery perfusion and increase the risk of myocardial infarction.

It is rarely possible to correct the underlying cause of hypertension. Lifestyle modifications such as weight loss, restriction of alcohol and salt intake, and increasing exercise may be enough to lower the BP satisfactorily in some individuals with mild hypertension. In people with more severe hypertension these measures can produce a substantial reduction in BP but rarely restore it to normal values. The decision to treat hypertension with drugs should be determined largely by an assessment of the overall risk of complications in that individual. Drug treatment is usually started if BP remains higher than the levels discussed previously, despite nonpharmacological approaches.

Drug regimens in hypertension

Lowering BP by a very modest amount with drugs (even if the target levels described previously are not achieved) produces a substantial ($\approx$40%) reduction in the risk of stroke, as well as reducing the risk of heart failure by 50% and reducing the incidence of chronic kidney disease. Drug treatment also reduces the risk of coronary artery disease in the elderly by about 25%. Evidence for a reduction in heart disease in the young is less convincing, but this may reflect the short duration of the trials (up to 5 years). In people with LVH, regression of left ventricular mass during treatment of hypertension will reduce cardiovascular events by 60% compared with those in whom left ventricular mass is unchanged.

Treatment regimens that are based on diuretics, calcium channel blockers, ACE inhibitors or angiotensin II receptor antagonists have generally shown equal efficacy in reducing vascular events. In contrast β-adrenoceptor antagonists are less effective at preventing the complications of hypertension and are no longer recommended as first-line therapy. Treatment of hypertension should follow a 'stepped care' approach (Fig. 6.9). A single drug will achieve good BP control in about one-third of people with hypertension. If the initial choice of drug fails to produce a sufficient reduction in BP, then the first drug should be continued and a second drug should be added.

The British Hypertension Society (BHS) and the National Institute of Health and Care Excellence (NICE) have endorsed a protocol for combining BP-lowering drugs, which is based on their mode of action (see Fig. 6.9). The underlying principle is that younger people (under 55 years) with hypertension are more likely to have high plasma renin concentrations, and therefore a drug that suppresses the

Choosing drugs for patients newly diagnosed with hypertension

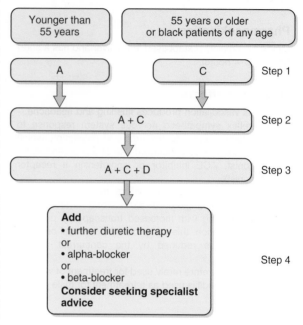

Fig. 6.9 **The British Hypertension Society recommendations for combining blood-pressure-lowering drugs.** Steps 1–4 reflect hypertension severity and risk, and initial treatment is influenced by age and ethnic origin. Black patients are those of African or Caribbean descent, and not mixed race, Asian or Chinese descent. A, ACE inhibitor (consider angiotensin II receptor antagonist if intolerant to ACE inhibitor); C, calcium channel blocker; D, thiazide-type diuretic.

renin–angiotensin–aldosterone system is most likely to be effective when used alone. An ACE inhibitor is usually the drug of choice, or an angiotensin II receptor antagonist if an ACE inhibitor is not tolerated. Conversely, older people or those of Afro-Caribbean origin at any age with hypertension are more likely to have 'low renin' hypertension, and a calcium channel blocker or thiazide diuretic is more likely to produce a substantial reduction in BP. A calcium channel blocker is generally preferred to a diuretic, as the combination with an ACE inhibitor appears to be more effective for reducing cardiovascular events. Use of a drug that suppresses the renin–angiotensin system creates the equivalent of a low-renin state, whereas calcium channel blockers and diuretics increase plasma renin. This provides the rationale for combination therapy with drugs from complementary classes at step 2. Optimal third-step therapy is the combination of an ACE inhibitor (or angiotensin II receptor blocker), calcium channel blocker, and a thiazide or thiazide-like diuretic. These recommendations are based on the probability of achieving optimal BP control and the evidence that the achieved BP, rather than the means by which it was achieved, is important for improving outcome.

Both thiazide diuretics and β-adrenoceptor antagonists increase the risk of developing new-onset diabetes mellitus, particularly when used together. This combination is not recommended for those who are at increased risk of glucose intolerance, such as people who are obese, those with a strong family history of type 2 diabetes mellitus, or people of South Asian or Afro-Caribbean origin who have a higher risk of developing diabetes mellitus. In contrast, both ACE inhibitors and angiotensin II receptor antagonists reduce the risk of developing diabetes mellitus.

Resistant and refractory hypertension

If three drugs with complementary actions, taken in adequate dosage, are insufficient to control the BP, then the person is said to have 'resistant' hypertension. There are several possible causes of apparently resistant hypertension. These include:

- poor adherence to prescribed therapy, which is the most common reason (see Chapter 55);
- 'white coat' hypertension, which responds poorly to drug treatment;
- secondary hypertension, most often caused by renal artery stenosis or Conn's syndrome;
- concurrent use of drugs that raise BP, such as a nonsteroidal antiinflammatory drug or a glucocorticoid or excessive alcohol consumption;
- obstructive sleep apnoea;
- intravascular volume expansion, due to antihypertensive drug therapy or chronic kidney disease.

A volume overload state is a common reason for resistance, and spironolactone added to a thiazide diuretic may be the optimal choice as the fourth drug unless serum potassium is raised. If expansion of the plasma volume is contributing to drug resistance, a loop diuretic rather than a thiazide may be more effective. An α-adrenoceptor antagonist or β-adrenoceptor antagonist are further options as the fourth drug for resistant hypertension. In men, minoxidil is a particularly powerful hypotensive agent, but excess hair growth limits its use for women. In a few individuals, treatment with five or more drugs may be necessary.

Failure to respond to intensive treatment with five drugs is called refractory hypertension. If poor adherence to treatment is not the cause, then increased sympathetic nervous system drive may be a major factor sustaining the BP.

Additional treatment to reduce risk of vascular complications

Control of hypertension should be seen as part of a strategy to tackle all factors that increase the risk of cardiovascular disease. Smoking cessation is important. A statin is recommended for primary prevention of cardiovascular disease in people with hypertension and a predicted risk of cardiovascular disease greater than 10% in the subsequent 10 years, or in those with diabetes mellitus who have a greatly increased risk (see Chapter 48).

Hypertension in special groups

There may be reasons for selecting particular classes of drugs rather than following the standard algorithm, particularly if there are co-morbid conditions that need treatment (Table 6.3). Although people of Afro-Caribbean origin respond less well to ACE inhibitors or angiotensin II receptor antagonists as first-line therapy than Caucasians, an ACE inhibitor is still preferred as first-line therapy if they have diabetes mellitus because of the renal protection it gives.

Accelerated or malignant hypertension

Immediate treatment is important for people with hypertension who have retinal haemorrhages and exudates or papilloedema ('hypertensive urgency'), or who have hypertensive encephalopathy, including posterior reversible encephalopathy syndrome (PRES) ('hypertensive emergency'). Rapid BP reduction is potentially dangerous, since autoregulation of cerebral blood flow is reset at a higher level than normal. A sudden fall in perfusion pressure can lead to a profound drop in cerebral blood flow and ischaemic cerebral damage.

Table 6.3 Selection of antihypertensive drugs for coexisting conditions

	Diuretic	β-Adrenoceptor antagonist	Angiotensin-converting enzyme inhibitor	Calcium channel blocker	α₁-Adrenoceptor antagonist
Angina	+/–	+	+/–	+	+/–
After myocardial infarction	+/–	+	+	–	+/–
Congestive heart failure	+	+	+	–	+/–
Diabetes mellitus (with or without nephropathy)	+/–	+/–	+	+/–	+/–
Raynaud's phenomenon	+/–	–	+	+	+
Gout	–	+/–	+/–	+/–	+/–
Prostatism	–	+/–	+/–	+/–	+
Supraventricular arrhythmias	+/–	+	+/–	+ (diltiazem or verapamil only)	+/–
Migraine	+/–	+	+/–	+/–	+/–

+, Treatment of choice; +/–, no obvious advantage/not preferred; –, usually contraindicated.

Intravenous drugs should usually be avoided unless there is encephalopathy, which necessitates very rapid BP reduction. Oral amlodipine is the most widely recommended treatment, which gradually reduces the BP over 24 hours or more.

Renal artery stenosis

If hypertension is caused by renal artery stenosis, ACE inhibitors or angiotensin II receptor antagonists usually produce an excellent reduction in BP. However, they can lead to deterioration in renal function, especially if there are bilateral stenoses. Renal artery angioplasty with insertion of a stent is recommended when the stenosis is caused by fibromuscular dysplasia. In atherosclerotic renovascular disease, angioplasty is not usually recommended for either preservation of renal function or BP control, since cholesterol embolisation to small arteries in the kidney during angioplasty may cause worsening of renal function.

Diabetic nephropathy

ACE inhibitors and angiotensin II receptor antagonists protect the kidney more than other classes of antihypertensive drug in both prevention and treatment of diabetic nephropathy. In particular, they reduce progression from microalbuminuria to overt nephropathy. The benefit from these classes of antihypertensive drugs is probably not simply due to BP reduction. They produce afferent glomerular artery vasodilation by inhibiting the generation or action of angiotensin II, and therefore reduce glomerular perfusion pressure. Other complications of hypertension in people with diabetes mellitus are prevented equally well by other antihypertensive drugs.

Phaeochromocytoma

Phaeochromocytoma is a catecholamine-secreting tumour, often arising from the adrenal gland. NA-secreting tumours most often lead to sustained hypertension, through vasoconstriction mediated by α_1-adrenoceptor stimulation. Treatment should be started with a nonselective α-adrenoceptor antagonist (usually phenoxybenzamine) to prevent excessive vasoconstriction, followed by a β-adrenoceptor antagonist to block the arrhythmogenic effects of the catecholamines on the heart. Definitive treatment, whenever possible, is by surgical removal of the tumour.

Primary hyperaldosteronism

This can be caused by bilateral adrenal hyperplasia or, less commonly, by an adrenal adenoma (Conn's syndrome). The drug treatment of choice is spironolactone, to directly block the effects of aldosterone at its renal tubular receptor. If there is an adenoma, surgical excision should be considered.

Pregnancy

There are two issues specific to pregnancy:

- **Preexisting chronic hypertension.** The risk of hypertension to mother and fetus is probably not great until the systolic BP reaches 150 mm Hg or the diastolic BP reaches 95 mm Hg. Treatment of BP at lower levels carries a risk of impairment of fetal growth. Many antihypertensive drugs should be avoided if possible in early pregnancy because they are teratogenic, or their potential for teratogenicity is not known (see Chapter 56). The drugs with the best safety record for preexisting hypertension in women who wish to become pregnant are labetalol,

methyldopa and nifedipine. In the second trimester, the risk of fetal malformations is lower, but thiazide diuretics and pure β-adrenoceptor antagonists are usually avoided because they may retard fetal growth by reducing placental blood flow. ACE inhibitors or angiotensin II receptor antagonists may cause oligohydramnios (reduced amniotic fluid production), renal failure and hypotension in the fetus, or intrauterine death, and should be avoided especially in the second and third trimesters of pregnancy.

- **Preeclampsia.** This usually occurs after 20 weeks of gestation. It presents as hypertension with oedema and proteinuria or hyperuricaemia in women whose BP had previously been normal. If this condition is untreated, there is a risk to the mother of convulsions, cerebral haemorrhage, abruptio placentae, pulmonary oedema and renal failure, and a risk to the fetus of severe growth retardation or even death. Once the diagnosis is established, bed rest is supplemented by antihypertensive drugs, as described previously for preexisting hypertension in pregnancy. Labetalol given by intravenous infusion is favoured in severe preeclampsia.

PULMONARY ARTERIAL HYPERTENSION

Pulmonary hypertension is most commonly secondary to chronic obstructive lung disease and some other lung disorders, where it arises as a result of destructive changes affecting the structure of the vascular bed. It also occurs with multiple small pulmonary emboli, which silt up the peripheral pulmonary arteries and increase vascular resistance, and a variety of less common disorders. However, some people develop increased pulmonary arterial vascular resistance for unknown reasons (primary pulmonary hypertension [PPH]), which has distinctive pathological findings of either the formation of plexiform vascular lesions or thrombotic arteriopathy. The most common presenting complaint in PPH is shortness of breath, although fatigue, chest pain, syncope, peripheral oedema and palpitation also frequently occur. The sustained increase in pulmonary vascular resistance leads to progressive right heart failure.

DRUGS FOR TREATING PULMONARY HYPERTENSION

Endothelin receptor antagonists

Examples

ambrisentan, bosentan

Mechanism of action

In PPH the expression of endothelin is increased in the pulmonary vasculature. Endothelin-1 is a powerful vasoconstrictor and smooth muscle mitogen which exerts its effects via two receptors, ET_A and ET_B. ET_A receptors on vascular smooth muscle cells primarily mediate vasoconstriction and cell proliferation, while a smaller population of ET_B receptors on endothelial cells mediates vasodilation via NO release; they are also responsible for clearance of endothelin from the circulation. Bosentan is an antagonist at both endothelin ET_A and ET_B receptors, while ambrisentan is selective for ET_A receptors.

Pharmacokinetics

Ambrisentan and bosentan are metabolised in the liver and have half-lives of 13–16 hours and 5 hours, respectively.

Unwanted effects

- Gastrointestinal disturbances, including diarrhoea and gastro-oesophageal reflux.
- Vasodilator effects, including flushing, hypotension, palpitation, oedema and syncope.
- Headache.
- Drug interactions: bosentan inhibits the metabolism of warfarin by CYP2C9, with the risk of excessive anticoagulation.

Prostaglandins

epoprostenol, iloprost

Epoprostenol is naturally occurring prostacyclin (prostaglandin I_2, PGI_2), and iloprost is a synthetic prostacyclin analogue. Prostacyclin is a vasodilator that also inhibits platelet aggregation (see Chapter 11), and both effects may be useful in the management of PPH. Iloprost is given by inhalation, but its short duration of action requires use every 2–3 hours, and it is associated with a high incidence of flushing, headache, jaw pain and cough. Epoprostenol must be given by continuous intravenous infusion, so it is only used when other treatments are ineffective.

Phosphodiesterase-5 inhibitors

sildenafil, tadalafil

Cyclic GMP production in the pulmonary vasculature may be a protective mechanism against PPH. Oral phosphodiesterase (PDE) type 5 inhibitors that inhibit breakdown of cGMP, such as sildenafil and tadalafil (see Chapter 16), reduce pulmonary artery pressure.

Guanylate cyclase stimulator

riociguat

Mechanism of action

Stimulation of soluble guanylate cyclase by riociguat mimics the action of NO by generating cGMP, which vasodilates the pulmonary arteries.

Pharmacokinetics

Riociguat is metabolised in the liver and has a half-life of about 12 hours.

Unwanted effects

- Epistaxis, haemoptysis.
- Vasodilator effects, including hypotension, oedema.
- Headache.
- Nausea, vomiting, dyspepsia, gastro-oesophageal reflux, constipation, diarrhoea.

MANAGEMENT OF PULMONARY ARTERIAL HYPERTENSION

Secondary pulmonary hypertension in chronic lung disease is most effectively managed by alleviating hypoxaemia when possible, using bronchodilators or long-term domiciliary oxygen therapy. There is no specific drug therapy. Chronic pulmonary embolic disease is treated by lifelong anticoagulation, usually with warfarin. Riociguat may improve exercise tolerance.

PPH can be treated with drugs that reduce pulmonary vascular resistance. About 25% of people with PPH maintain a vasoactive pulmonary vascular bed (defined as a 20% decrease in pulmonary vascular resistance on acute challenge with a vasodilator). In this situation, treatment with a calcium channel blocker such as nifedipine will improve both symptoms and survival. However, most people with PPH show little evidence of vascular reactivity, and in this situation calcium channel blockers usually produce excessive systemic hypotension before useful pulmonary vasodilation is achieved. For such individuals, treatment is considered with an endothelin antagonist, inhaled prostacyclin, a PDE-5 inhibitor or riociguat. All these drugs can improve symptoms and quality of life, but have not been shown to improve survival. Combination therapy using drugs from more than one class is probably more effective for reducing pulmonary artery pressure than single agents, but optimal combinations have not yet been determined. Riociguat should not be used with PDE-5 inhibitors because of the risk of excessive hypotension.

SELF-ASSESSMENT

True/false questions

1. Stretch of baroreceptors increases the afferent impulses to the vasomotor centre, resulting in a rise in BP.
2. Nifedipine lowers BP principally by arterial vasodilation.
3. Moxonidine stimulates imidazoline receptors in the medulla.
4. Propranolol lowers BP by peripheral vasodilation.
5. Thiazide diuretics reduce Na^+ and water reabsorption in the distal convoluted tubule.

6. Thiazide diuretics reduce BP in the long term at doses that do not cause diuresis.
7. Thiazide diuretics are the drugs of choice for treating pregnancy-related hypertension.
8. The potassium-sparing diuretics amiloride and spironolactone have the same mechanism of action in the renal tubule.
9. Selective blockade of α_1-adrenoceptors by prazosin increases NA release.
10. ACE inhibitors prevent the conversion of angiotensinogen to angiotensin I.
11. ACE inhibitors prevent the breakdown of bradykinin.
12. Minoxidil blocks K^+ channels in smooth muscle cell membranes.
13. Nitroprusside can be given for up to 3 months.
14. PDE type 5 inhibitors are used in PPH.
15. Ambrisentan selectively blocks pulmonary vasoconstriction mediated by endothelin ET_A receptors.

One-best-answer (OBA) question

1. Identify the *least* accurate statement about antihypertensive drugs.
   A. Thiazide diuretics increase the risk of diabetes mellitus.
   B. β-Adrenoceptor antagonists are first-line therapy for hypertension.
   C. BP is not always lowered adequately by a single drug.
   D. Angiotensin II receptor antagonists selectively block angiotensin AT_1 receptors.
   E. Nifedipine is more likely to cause reflex tachycardia than verapamil.

Extended-matching-item question

1. Choose which drug class A–D would be a *good* choice for initial treatment of the people newly diagnosed with hypertension in scenarios 1.1–1.3 provided. An answer may be used more than once.
   A. An ACE inhibitor or angiotensin II receptor antagonist
   B. A nonselective β-adrenoceptor antagonist
   C. A calcium channel blocker
   D. A thiazide diuretic
      1.1. An obese man of Afro-Caribbean origin aged 75 years with a BP of 150/100 mm Hg and no evidence of target organ damage
      1.2. A Caucasian female aged 40 years with type 1 diabetes mellitus and a BP of 150/100 mm Hg
      1.3. A woman 24 weeks pregnant with preexisting chronic hypertension and a BP of 150/100 mm Hg

Case-based question

Mr A.T., a 60-year-old man with type 2 diabetes mellitus, smokes 20 cigarettes a day. His plasma lipid levels are normal, and there is no indication of proteinuria. His ECG is normal. His height is 1.70 m, and his weight is 95.5 kg. He has no evidence of fluid retention or heart failure. Following treatment with a calcium channel blocker, his BP has reduced from 175/110 mm Hg, but he remains hypertensive (155/95 mm Hg) and he then has a non-ST elevation myocardial infarction. What changes in his therapy would you consider?

ANSWERS

True/false answers

1. **False.** Baroreceptor impulses to the vasomotor centre reduce sympathetic outflow, enhance vagal outflow and lower BP.
2. **True.** Calcium channel blockers act by opening L-type voltage-gated Ca^{2+} channels, and nifedipine, a dihydropyridine, is relatively selective for these channels in arterial smooth muscle. The nondihydropyridines verapamil and diltiazem have additional cardiodepressant properties.
3. **True.** Moxonidine selectively stimulates imidazoline I_1 receptors in the RVLM; this decreases sympathetic outflow and reduced BP.
4. **False.** Propranolol lowers BP by reducing CO and by reducing renin production, but only β_1-adrenoceptor antagonists with partial agonist activity at β_2-adrenoceptors (such as pindolol) or those drugs with other hybrid properties (such as nebivolol) produce direct peripheral vasodilation.
5. **True.** All diuretics reduce Na^+ and water reabsorption in the renal tubule; thiazides act at the Na^+/Cl^- co-transporter (NCC) in the distal convoluted tubule.
6. **True.** The initial hypotensive effect of thiazides is due to diuresis reducing blood volume, but in the longer term they cause arterial vasodilation at low doses by an unknown mechanism.
7. **False.** Thiazide diuretics cause fetal growth retardation by reducing plasma volume and placental blood flow; the centrally acting drug methyldopa, the calcium channel blocker nifedipine and the vasodilating beta-blocker labetalol are most often used in pregnancy.
8. **False.** Spironolactone competes with aldosterone for the mineralocorticoid receptor (MR), blocking its stimulation of the Na^+/K^+-ATPase pump and expression of the epithelial Na^+ channel (ENaC); this reduces uptake of Na^+ and loss of K^+ from the tubule. Amiloride, however, directly blocks ENaC (see Chapter 14).
9. **False.** Prazosin and related drugs dilate blood vessels by selective blockade of α_1-adrenoceptors; they do not block the presynaptic α_2-adrenoceptors, and stimulation of these receptors to limit further NA release can still take place.
10. **False.** Angiotensinogen is converted to angiotensin I by renin. ACE effects the subsequent conversion of angiotensin I to angiotensin II.
11. **True.** ACE inhibitors reduce the breakdown of bradykinin, a potent vasodilator, and this action may contribute to their antihypertensive effects, but also to the persistent cough that occurs in some people taking them.
12. **False.** Minoxidil is an ATP-sensitive potassium channel (K_{ATP}) opener; it causes an efflux of K^+ ions resulting in hyperpolarisation of arterial smooth muscle cells and vasodilation.
13. **False.** Nitroprusside is converted to cyanide and then to thiocyanate. The toxicity of these metabolites limits its use to 3 days for emergency management of some hypertensive states.

14. **True.** PPH is often associated with poor vascular reactivity, but vasodilation may be achieved by endothelin antagonists, PDE type 5 inhibitors, prostacyclin or riociguat.

15. **True.** Ambrisentan (and macitentan) selectively block vasoconstriction mediated by ET_A receptors; endothelial ET_B receptors which mediate vasodilation via NO are relatively unaffected.

One-best-answer (OBA) answer

1. **Answer B** is the least accurate.
   A. True. Thiazides increase the risk of new-onset diabetes, particularly when combined with β-adrenoceptor antagonists.
   B. **False.** β-Adrenoceptor antagonists are relegated in the BHS guidelines, as they are less effective in reducing the risk of myocardial infarction and stroke than other antihypertensive drugs.
   C. True. Satisfactory lowering of BP is achieved with a single drug in only 30–40% of people with hypertension.
   D. True. Angiotensin II receptor antagonists block the vasoconstrictor and aldosterone secretory actions of angiotensin II at AT_1 receptors; AT_2 receptors are involved in vascular growth and are less affected by these drugs.
   E. True. Nifedipine selectively dilates arterioles and may cause reflex tachycardia; this is unlikely with verapamil, which has negative chronotropic activity.

Extended-matching-item answers

1.1. **Answer C** (a calcium channel blocker) would be a good choice in this 75-year-old Afro-Caribbean man. The elderly and people of Afro-Caribbean origin usually have low plasma renin concentrations, so an ACE inhibitor or angiotensin II receptor antagonist would be less effective. A thiazide diuretic or a β-adrenoceptor antagonist might increase the risk of diabetes mellitus in this obese man.

1.2. **Answer A** (an ACE inhibitor or, if poorly tolerated, an angiotensin II receptor antagonist) would be a good choice in a 40-year-old white female. A thiazide diuretic or a β-adrenoceptor antagonist may exacerbate the diabetes mellitus.

1.3. **Answer C** (a calcium channel blocker) would be an appropriate first choice in a pregnant woman with preexisting hypertension. All the other drugs can cause unwanted effects on the fetus.

Case-based answer

Mr A.T.'s BP has not reached the target level (office 140/90 mm Hg or home 135/85 mm Hg). His BP may be reduced further by introducing an ACE inhibitor, which improve survival after a myocardial infarction, especially when there is left ventricular impairment. ACE inhibitors also protect the kidney in diabetic nephropathy and could be considered in this situation. The addition of a β-adrenoceptor antagonist could also be considered for additional long-term prognostic benefit, particularly if there is left ventricular impairment.

FURTHER READING

Systemic hypertension

Bramham, K., Nelson-Piercy, C., Brown, M.J., et al., 2013. Postpartum management of hypertension. Br. Med. J. 346, f894.

Brown, M.J., Cruikshank, J.K., MacDonald, T.M., 2012. Navigating the shoals in hypertension: discovery and guidance. Br. Med. J. 344, d8218.

Myat, A., Redwood, S.R., Qureshi, A.C., et al., 2012. Resistant hypertension. Br. Med. J. 345, e7473.

Poulter, N.R., Prabhakaran, D., Caulfield, M., 2015. Hypertension. Lancet 386, 801–812.

Sundström, J., Arima, H., Jackson, R., et al., 2015. Effects of blood pressure reduction in mild hypertension: a systematic review and meta-analysis. Ann. Intern. Med. 162, 184–191.

Xie, X., Atkins, E., Lv, J., et al., 2016. Effects of intensive blood pressure lowering on cardiovascular and renal outcomes: updated systematic review and meta-analysis. Lancet 387, 435–443.

Yoder, S.R., Thomberg, L.L., Bisognano, J.D., 2009. Hypertension in pregnancy and women of childbearing age. Am. J. Med. 122, 890–895.

Pulmonary hypertension

Haeck, M.L.A., Vliegen, H.W., 2015. Diagnosis and treatment of pulmonary hypertension. Heart 101, 311–319.

Kiely, D.G., Elliot, C.A., Condliffe, R., 2013. Pulmonary hypertension: diagnosis and management. Br. Med. J. 346, f2028.

Shah, S.J., 2012. Pulmonary hypertension. J. Am. Med. Assoc. 308, 1366–1374.

Compendium: drugs used to treat hypertension

Drug	Characteristics
β-Adrenoceptor antagonists	
All β-adrenoceptor antagonists except esmolol and sotalol are used for hypertension; see Chapter 5 for individual drugs.	
α-Adrenoceptor antagonists	
Selective α₁-adrenoceptor antagonists	
Doxazosin	Used for hypertension and benign prostatic hyperplasia (see Chapter 15). Given orally. Half-life: 9–12 h
Indoramin	Used for hypertension and benign prostatic hyperplasia. Given orally. Half-life: 5 h
Prazosin	Used for hypertension, congestive heart failure, Raynaud's phenomenon and benign prostatic hyperplasia. Given orally. Half-life: 2–3 h
Terazosin	Used for hypertension and benign prostatic hyperplasia. Given orally. Half-life: 12 h
Nonselective α-adrenoceptor antagonists	
Used in phaeochromocytoma only.	
Phenoxybenzamine	Used for hypertensive episodes associated with phaeochromocytoma. Given orally or by intravenous infusion. Half-life: 24 h
Phentolamine	Used for diagnosis and hypertensive episodes in phaeochromocytoma. Given by intravenous injection. Half-life: 1.5 h
Centrally acting antihypertensive drugs	
Clonidine	Selective α₂-adrenoceptor agonist. Used for hypertension, migraine and menopausal flushing. Given orally or by slow intravenous injection. Half-life: 20–25 h
Methyldopa	Selective α₂-adrenoceptor agonist. Used particularly for hypertension in pregnancy. Given orally. Half-life: 1–2 h
Moxonidine	Selective imidazoline I₁ receptor agonist. Used for resistant hypertension. Given orally. Half-life: 2–3 h
Guanethidine	Blocks release and depletes stores of noradrenaline in adrenergic nerves. Used only for hypertensive crisis, but other drugs usually preferred. Given by intramuscular injection. Half-life: 2 days
ACE inhibitors	
ACE inhibitors are used for hypertension, heart failure, prophylaxis of ischaemic heart disease and diabetic nephropathy. All are given orally; many are prodrugs activated by metabolism in liver or gut.	
Captopril	Parent drug is active. Half-life: 2 h
Enalapril maleate	Prodrug converted to enalaprilat. Half-life: 35 h
Fosinopril sodium	Prodrug converted to fosinoprilat. Half-life: 12 h
Imidapril hydrochloride	Prodrug converted to imidaprilat. Half-life: 8 h
Lisinopril	Parent drug is active. Half-life: 12 h
Moexipril hydrochloride	Prodrug converted to moexiprilat. Half-life: 10 h
Perindopril erbumine and perindopril arginine	Prodrugs converted to perindoprilat. Half-life: 17 h
Quinapril	Prodrug converted in liver to quinaprilat. Half-life: 2 h
Ramipril	Prodrug converted to ramiprilat. Half-life: 1–5 h. Also available in combination with felodipine
Trandolapril	Prodrug converted to trandolaprilat. Half-life: 16–24 h
Angiotensin II receptor (AT₁) antagonists	
Used for hypertension, heart failure, prophylaxis after myocardial infarction and diabetic nephropathy. All are given orally.	
Azilsartan	Given as prodrug (azilsartan medoxemil). Used for essential hypertension. Half-life: 11 h
Candesartan	Given as prodrug (candesartan cilexitil). Half-life: 9–12 h

Compendium: drugs used to treat hypertension (cont'd)

Drug	Characteristics
Eprosartan	Half-life: 5–7 h
Irbesartan	Half-life: 11–15 h
Losartan	Half-life: 2 h
Olmesartan	Given as prodrug (olmesartan medoxomil). Half-life: 13–16 h
Telmisartan	Half-life: 16–24 h
Valsartan	Half-life: 5–7 h
Direct renin inhibitor	
Aliskiren	Nonpeptide inhibitor of renin. Given orally. Half-life: 40 h
Diuretics	
Diuretics are commonly used to treat hypertension; see Chapter 14 for individual drugs.	
Calcium channel blockers	
All calcium channel blockers except nimodipine are used for treatment of hypertension; see Chapter 5 for individual drugs.	
Potassium channel opener	
Minoxidil	Used with a β-adrenoceptor antagonist and a diuretic for severe hypertension resistant to other drugs. Given orally. Half-life: 3–4 h
Hydralazine and nitrovasodilators	
Drugs used under special circumstances.	
Diazoxide	Given in hypertensive emergencies by intravenous bolus injection. Half-life: 28 h
Hydralazine	Used as an adjunct for moderate or severe hypertension, for heart failure and for hypertensive crisis. Given orally, by slow intravenous injection or by intravenous infusion. Half-life: 2–4 h
Sodium nitroprusside	Used for hypertensive crisis, for controlled hypotension in anaesthesia and for acute heart failure. Given intravenously. Half-life: <5 min
Endothelin receptor antagonists	
Block vasoconstrictor activity of endothelin; used for primary pulmonary hypertension	
Ambrisentan	Selective antagonist of endothelin ET_A receptors. Given orally. Half-life: 13–16 h
Bosentan	Nonselective antagonist of endothelin ET_A and ET_B receptors. Given orally. Half-life: 5 h
Macitentan	Noncompetitive ET_A/ET_B receptor antagonist, selective for ET_A subtype. Half-life: 48 h
Prostaglandins	
Vasodilator and antiplatelet drugs; used for primary pulmonary hypertension.	
Epoprostenol	Natural prostacyclin (PGI_2). Used when other drugs are ineffective. Given by continuous intravenous infusion. Half-life: <3 min. See also Chapter 11
Iloprost	Synthetic prostacyclin analogue. Given by nebuliser. Half-life: 20–30 min
PDE-5 inhibitors	
Vasodilate by reducing breakdown of cGMP by PDE5; used for primary pulmonary hypertension.	
Sildenafil	Given orally or intravenously. Half-life: 2 h. See also Chapter 16
Tadalafil	Given orally or intravenously. Half-life: 17 h. See also Chapter 16
Guanylate cyclase stimulator	
Riociguat	Vasodilates by increasing synthesis of cGMP by guanylate cyclase. Used for primary pulmonary hypertension. Given orally. Half-life: 12 h

ACE, Angiotensin-converting enzyme; *PDE,* phosphodiesterase.

7 Heart failure

There is no universally accepted definition of heart failure. The heart failure syndrome is usually said to exist when there is inadequate oxygen delivery to peripheral tissues, either at rest or during exercise, due to dysfunction of the heart or when adequate oxygen delivery can be maintained only with an elevated left ventricular filling pressure.

MAINTENANCE OF CARDIAC OUTPUT

There are four major determinants of cardiac output:

- preload: this is governed by the ventricular end-diastolic volume, which in turn is related to ventricular filling pressure and therefore to venous return of blood to the heart,
- heart rate,
- myocardial contractility,
- afterload: the systolic wall tension in the ventricle, which reflects the resistance to ventricular emptying within both the heart (during isovolumic contraction) and in the peripheral arterial bed.

The output from both the right and left sides of the heart is normally balanced. Overall cardiac output is regulated mainly by changes in heart rate and preload. Heart rate is modulated by the autonomic nervous system, with sympathetic nervous stimulation increasing the heart rate and parasympathetic stimulation via the vagus nerve slowing the rate.

The relationship between preload and stroke volume (the amount of blood ejected from the ventricle during systole with each contraction) is shown in Fig. 7.1. The degree of stretch of the ventricular muscle (preload) determines the force of cardiac contraction (the Frank–Starling phenomenon). The curve describing this relationship is governed by intrinsic myocardial contractility: thus, the curve is shifted upwards and to the left when contractility is augmented, for example, by sympathetic nervous stimulation. If myocardial contractility is normal, the left ventricular filling pressure lies on the steep part of the curve, making stroke volume very sensitive to small changes in preload.

The relationship between afterload and stroke volume is shown in Fig. 7.2. Afterload is determined largely by peripheral arterial resistance but also by the size of the ventricle. Enlargement of the left ventricular cavity (e.g. as a result of increased venous return or preload) increases wall tension, and the heart must generate greater pressure both to initiate and to maintain contraction. Preload and afterload are therefore interrelated. A rise in afterload will cause a fall in stroke volume, but the consequent sympathetic stimulation of a healthy ventricle will increase myocardial contractility and restore stroke volume.

PATHOPHYSIOLOGY OF HEART FAILURE

Heart failure is a syndrome that has several underlying causes (Box 7.1). Occasionally it arises suddenly, such as after acute myocardial infarction or acute mitral regurgitation from rupture of the chordae tendineae or from papillary muscle dysfunction. More commonly the onset is gradual and arises from progressive loss of myocardial function or a slow degenerative change in valve function.

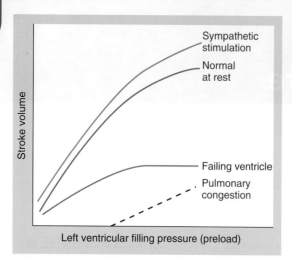

Fig. 7.1 **The Frank–Starling relationship between preload (left ventricular filling pressure) and stroke volume in healthy and failing hearts.** In the severely failing heart, increases in filling pressure and heart rate are insufficient to restore cardiac output; thus pulmonary congestion will occur.

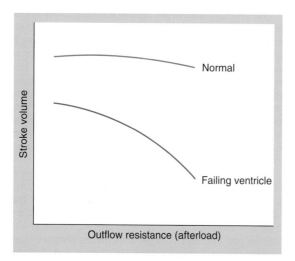

Fig. 7.2 **The relationship between afterload (outflow resistance) and stroke volume in the presence of normal and reduced myocardial contractility.** Sympathetic stimulation maintains the stroke volume of the normal heart (but not of the failing heart) against an increasing afterload.

The underlying problem in heart failure is reduced cardiac output and therefore low blood pressure, but the syndrome of heart failure arises largely from neurohumoral responses to low blood pressure and reduced renal perfusion. This is principally due to the sympathetic nervous system and the renin–angiotensin–aldosterone system (Fig. 7.3). The consequences of these compensatory mechanisms are vasoconstriction of both arteries and veins and excessive salt and water retention by the kidneys. Although these are the

Box 7.1	Causes of heart failure

Coronary artery disease
Hypertension
Myocardial disease: cardiomyopathies, myocarditis
Valvular heart disease
Constrictive pericarditis
Congenital: atrial septal defect, ventricular septal defect, aortic coarctation
Infiltrative: amyloid, sarcoid, iron
Iatrogenic: β-adrenoceptor antagonists (high doses), antiarrhythmics, calcium channel blockers, cytotoxics, alcohol, irradiation
Arrhythmias, especially incessant tachyarrhythmias

normal physiological responses to reduced blood pressure, in the setting of a failing heart they have limited benefit.

In the failing ventricle, the Frank–Starling curve is shifted downwards and to the right (failing-ventricle curve, see Fig. 7.1) and the maximum achievable stroke volume is reduced. The curve is also flatter, indicating that stroke volume has become less responsive to changes in preload. As a result of activation of the compensatory mechanisms, retention of salt and water expands plasma volume and venoconstriction enhances venous return to the heart. These factors increase the filling pressure of the left ventricle in an attempt to restore the resting stroke volume. The heart rate will also increase, which will raise cardiac output despite a lower stroke volume. However, a persistently high level of sympathetic nervous system tone results in downregulation of cardiac β₁-adrenoceptors and therefore less ability to rely on increased heart rate to maintain cardiac output. If these responses are successful in restoring a normal resting cardiac output, the heart failure is said to be *compensated*. However, the cardiac output may be unable to rise further to meet the needs of the body during exertion. *Decompensation* occurs when the combination of the increases in preload and heart rate fail to restore a normal resting cardiac output (see Fig. 7.3).

In response to the rise in atrial and ventricular filling pressures, there is release of A-type natriuretic peptide (ANP) and B-type natriuretic peptide (BNP). These peptides promote natriuresis and vasodilation but are relatively ineffective in the presence of neurohumoral activation. The natriuretic peptides are degraded by neprilysin, a neutral endopeptidase enzyme, which has several other substrates including angiotensin II, bradykinin, endothelin and vasopressin.

In most cases of heart failure, the impairment of function initially affects the left ventricle. As the central blood volume continues to increase in an attempt to raise the stroke volume, the hydrostatic pressure in the pulmonary veins will rise. When this hydrostatic pressure exceeds the plasma colloid oncotic pressure that holds fluid in the blood vessel, fluid leaves the capillaries; it moves into the interstitium of the alveoli and then into the alveolar spaces, producing pulmonary oedema (see Fig. 7.2). Eventually, the raised pulmonary vascular pressure compromises right ventricular output and leads to right heart failure (producing biventricular failure, or congestive cardiac failure), and oedema develops in the peripheral and splanchnic tissues.

Peripheral arterial resistance (afterload) will also rise as a result of the compensatory mechanisms (see Fig. 7.2). The failing ventricle cannot meet this demand with an

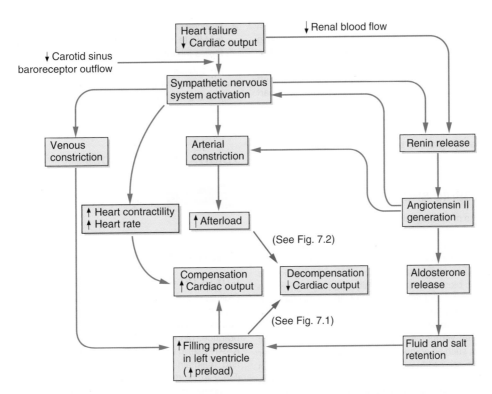

Fig. 7.3 **Neurohumoral consequences of heart failure.** In the mildly impaired heart, a fall in cardiac output results in a cascade of compensatory events *(green arrows)*, including sympathetic stimulation of heart rate and contractility, constriction of arteries and veins, and activation of the renin–angiotensin–aldosterone system; overall these compensatory mechanisms restore cardiac output. If cardiac function is significantly impaired *(red arrows)*, an increased preload cannot restore an adequate stroke volume (decompensation) (see Fig. 7.1); the increased afterload will put additional strain on the failing heart and further decrease cardiac output (see Fig. 7.2). In chronic heart failure these effects are compounded by cardiac remodelling and downregulation of cardiac β_1-adrenoceptors.

increase in myocardial contractility, so stroke volume will fall (see Fig. 7.2), with further cardiac decompensation.

Following myocyte loss, such as occurs with myocardial infarction or dilated cardiomyopathies, adaptive changes take place in the surviving myocytes and extracellular matrix – a process known as remodelling. This is driven by several factors, including the local effects of catecholamines, angiotensin II, aldosterone, and proinflammatory cytokines, eventually producing a more globular, dysfunctional left ventricle. This type of heart failure is characterised by a reduced ejection fraction (heart failure with reduced ejection fraction [HFREF] or systolic heart failure). In aortic or mitral valve regurgitation, heart failure arises because the left ventricle must dilate to accommodate the normal forward stroke volume and also the regurgitant volume (the volume leaking back into the left ventricle or left atrium, respectively). Eventually, the left ventricle dilates to the point where contractility is reduced and it is unable to maintain an effective stroke volume.

Heart failure can also arise from impaired diastolic relaxation when contractile function in systole is normal but ventricular filling is reduced. Stroke volume is reduced but ejection fraction is normal. This is known as heart failure with preserved ejection fraction (HFPEF) or diastolic heart failure. If the left ventricle fails to relax adequately, it will not accommodate the venous return, leading to pulmonary venous congestion and a low cardiac output, which activates the same compensatory neurohumoral responses found in HFREF. HFPEF characteristically occurs in older people in association with left ventricular hypertrophy, but it also contributes to heart failure in ischaemic left ventricular dysfunction (see Chapter 5) and aortic stenosis.

Symptoms in heart failure are caused by a reduced cardiac output ('forward failure') or venous congestion ('backward failure'). The most common complaints are breathlessness from increased pulmonary venous pressure and fatigue resulting from the reduced cardiac output and impaired skeletal muscle perfusion. In response to the reduced perfusion, biochemical changes also occur in skeletal muscle, making it less efficient. Other symptoms, such as the discomfort of peripheral oedema and anorexia due to bowel congestion, are attributable to a high systemic venous pressure. Increased stimulation of β-adrenoceptors in the heart can lead to life-threatening ventricular arrhythmias.

ACUTE LEFT VENTRICULAR FAILURE

Acute left ventricular failure usually results from a sudden inability of the heart to maintain an adequate cardiac output and blood pressure. It can follow acute myocardial infarction or acute mitral or aortic valvular regurgitation or arise from the onset of a brady- or tachyarrhythmia if there is preexisting poor left ventricular function. The sudden fall in cardiac output leads to reflex arterial and venous constriction (see Fig. 7.3). There is a rapid rise in filling pressure of the left ventricle as a result of increased venous return. If the heart is unable to expel the extra blood, the hydrostatic pressure in the pulmonary veins rises until it exceeds the plasma oncotic pressure and produces acute pulmonary oedema. The principal symptom is breathlessness, usually at rest, with orthopnoea or paroxysmal nocturnal dyspnoea.

CARDIOGENIC SHOCK

The syndrome of cardiogenic shock arises when the systolic function of the left ventricle is suddenly impaired to such a degree that there is insufficient blood flow to meet resting metabolic requirements of the tissues. This definition excludes shock caused by hypovolaemia. The clinical hallmarks are a low systolic blood pressure (usually <90 mm Hg), with a reduced cardiac output and an elevated left ventricular filling pressure. Cardiogenic shock can follow acute myocardial infarction and in this situation usually indicates loss of at least 40% of the left ventricular myocardium. Other mechanical disturbances, such as acute mitral regurgitation or ventricular septal rupture, can produce cardiogenic shock in association with a lesser degree of myocardial damage. Less commonly, the syndrome is associated with right ventricular infarction. The mortality of cardiogenic shock, even with intensive treatment, is in excess of 70%.

CHRONIC HEART FAILURE

Myocardial damage from ischaemic heart disease is the most common cause of chronic heart failure, but potentially correctable causes – such as valvular lesions as well as treatable exacerbating factors such as anaemia or arrhythmias – may be identified. In most people with heart failure there are signs of both right and left ventricular failure (biventricular or congestive heart failure). Chronic heart failure has a high mortality. People with left ventricular systolic dysfunction who have symptoms only on exertion have a 2-year mortality risk of about 20%, whereas the 1-year mortality is 80% if there are symptoms at rest. In HFREF the degree of left ventricular dysfunction is a guide to prognosis. Death occurs from either progressive heart failure or ventricular arrhythmias.

POSITIVE INOTROPIC DRUGS FOR THE TREATMENT OF HEART FAILURE

Myocardial contractility can be improved by increasing the availability of free intracellular Ca^{2+} to interact with contractile proteins or increasing the sensitivity of the myofibrils to Ca^{2+}. Only drugs that increase myocardial intracellular Ca^{2+} are established in clinical use; they work by one of two distinct mechanisms:

- an action on the cell membrane Na^+/K^+-ATPase pump (e.g. digitalis glycosides),

- by increasing intracellular cyclic adenosine monophosphate (cAMP) (e.g. inotropic sympathomimetics, phosphodiesterase inhibitors).

An additional advantage of the positive inotropic drugs that increase myocardial cAMP is their ability to enhance the reuptake of Ca^{2+} by the sarcoplasmic reticulum in diastole. This improves diastolic relaxation in addition to augmenting systolic contractility.

DIGITALIS GLYCOSIDES

digoxin

Mechanism of action and effects

Effect on myocardial contractility

Digitalis glycosides are compounds with a steroid nucleus that were originally isolated from a species of foxglove (*Digitalis purpura*). Digoxin, the drug most widely used in clinical practice, binds to the energy-dependent Na^+ pump (Na^+/K^+-ATPase) in the myocyte membrane. This pump establishes and maintains the Na^+ and K^+ gradients across the cell (Fig. 7.4), producing low intracellular Na^+ and high intracellular K^+ concentrations. A separate passive transmembrane exchange of Na^+ and Ca^{2+} occurs driven by the Na^+ concentration gradient, with Na^+ entering the cell while Ca^{2+} is translocated out. The rate of this exchange is dependent on the intracellular Na^+ concentration. Digoxin partially inhibits the Na^+/K^+-ATPase, which increases the intracellular Na^+ concentration. This lowers the concentration gradient for Na^+ across the cell membrane, which in turn reduces the Na^+/Ca^{2+} exchange, so that Ca^{2+} is retained in the cell. The excess intracellular Ca^{2+} is stored in the sarcoplasmic reticulum during diastole and released during cell membrane excitation, leading to enhanced myocardial contraction.

Effects on cardiac action potential and intracardiac conduction

Digoxin can be arrhythmogenic but also has actions that are useful for treating certain arrhythmias.

Direct actions of digoxin on the heart can provoke arrhythmias by increasing myocardial cell excitability (see Chapter 8) as follows:

- Reduction of the resting membrane potential. The cell membrane Na^+/K^+-ATPase pump extrudes three Na^+ ions out of the cell for every two K^+ ions that enter, which increases the negative intracellular electrical potential and hyperpolarises the cell, making it less excitable (see Chapter 8). Inhibition of this membrane pump by digoxin causes the cell membrane potential to become less negative and closer to the threshold potential for depolarisation. Action potentials, and therefore arrhythmias are therefore more readily initiated.

- Triggering of spontaneous release of Ca^{2+} from the sarcoplasmic reticulum. This leads to transient depolarisation of the cell immediately following an action potential ('delayed afterdepolarisation'), which can initiate arrhythmias (see Chapter 8).

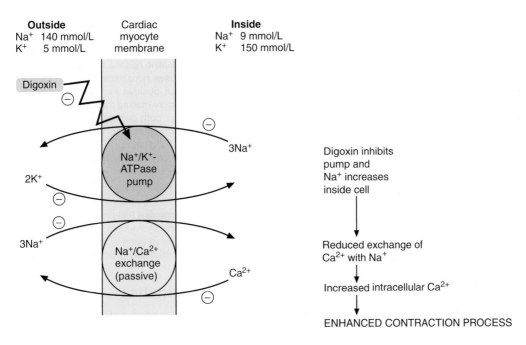

Fig. 7.4 The action of digoxin on the cardiac myocyte. Digoxin increases intracellular Na⁺ by inhibiting the Na⁺/K⁺-ATPase. This reduces the Na⁺ gradient for the passive export of Ca²⁺, resulting in increased intracellular Ca²⁺ and enhanced contractile responses.

Digoxin also has useful indirect actions on the heart that arise from stimulation of the central vagal nucleus and enable it to be used for treating arrhythmias (see Chapter 8). The vagal effects on the heart are as follows:

- decreased automaticity of the sinoatrial node which slightly slows the heart rate in sinus rhythm,
- increased refractory period of the atrioventricular node, which slows impulse transmission to the ventricles and is useful in the management of the fast ventricular rates resulting from atrial flutter and fibrillation (see Chapter 8).

Pharmacokinetics

Digoxin is eliminated by the kidneys via glomerular filtration and active tubular secretion. The half-life of digoxin is very long (about 1.5 days) and is increased if renal function is impaired; the dose must be reduced in the presence of renal impairment to avoid toxicity (see below). If an early onset of action is required, loading doses should be given over the first 24 or 36 hours (see Chapter 2). If a rapid response is essential, digoxin can be given by slow intravenous injection.

Unwanted effects

Digitalis glycosides have a narrow therapeutic index, and toxicity is mostly dose-related.

- Gastrointestinal disturbances: anorexia, nausea and vomiting (largely a central effect at the chemoreceptor trigger zone), and diarrhoea.
- Neurological disturbances: fatigue, malaise, confusion, vertigo, coloured vision (especially yellow halos around

lights, possibly from inhibition of Na⁺/K⁺-ATPase in the cones of the retina).
- Distinctive changes on the electrocardiogram (ECG): this includes nonspecific T-wave changes and sagging of the S–T segment with an upright T-wave ('reverse tick'), often referred to as the 'digoxin effect'. These ECG effects do not indicate toxicity but can be mistaken for myocardial ischaemia.
- Consequences of intracellular Ca²⁺ overload: increased excitability of the atrioventricular node and Purkinje fibres produces atrial or nodal ectopic beats, atrial or nodal tachycardia, ventricular ectopic beats, or (less commonly) ventricular tachycardia.
- Consequences of increased vagal activity: excessive atrioventricular nodal block ('heart block') can occur. When associated with increased atrial excitability, this produces atrial tachycardia with atrioventricular nodal block, a rhythm characteristic of digitalis toxicity.
- Gynaecomastia: during long-term treatment, the steroid structure allows digitalis glycosides to stimulate oestrogen receptors in breast tissue.

Exacerbating factors for digitalis glycoside toxicity

- Hypokalaemia: reduced extracellular K⁺ concentration increases the effects of digitalis glycosides on the Na⁺/K⁺-ATPase pump. Care must be taken if potassium-losing diuretics, such as furosemide (see Chapter 14), are used with digitalis glycosides.
- Renal impairment: reduces the excretion of digoxin.
- Hypoxaemia: this sensitises the heart to digitalis glycoside-induced arrhythmias.

■ Hypothyroidism: the renal elimination of digoxin is decreased because of a reduced glomerular filtration rate.

■ Drugs that displace digoxin from tissue binding sites and interfere with its renal excretion: these include verapamil (see Chapter 5) and quinidine (see Chapter 8), which can double the plasma concentration of digoxin. Amiodarone (see Chapter 8) produces a less marked effect.

Treatment of digitalis toxicity

Digitalis glycoside toxicity can be treated by:

■ withholding further doses of digitalis glycoside,

■ using K^+ supplementation (see Chapter 14) for hypokalaemia. This is usually given orally but should be given by slow intravenous infusion if there are dangerous arrhythmias,

■ using atropine (see Chapter 8) for sinus bradycardia or atrioventricular block (with temporary transvenous pacing for marked bradycardia unresponsive to atropine),

■ digoxin-specific antibody fragments for serious digoxin toxicity (see Chapter 53).

INOTROPIC SYMPATHOMIMETICS

selective β_1-adrenoceptor agonist: dobutamine
selective β_2-adrenoceptor agonist and dopamine receptor agonist: dopexamine
nonselective β-adrenoceptor, α-adrenoceptor, and dopamine receptor agonist: dopamine

Mechanisms of action and effects

The mechanisms of action of the inotropic sympathomimetic drugs are also considered in Chapter 4. Noradrenaline and adrenaline are not used for their inotropic action because they produce marked vasoconstriction through effects on α-adrenoceptors.

Isoprenaline is a nonselective β-adrenoceptor agonist that is now available in the United Kingdom only on special order. It is sometimes used to increase heart rate in the emergency treatment of bradycardias through its action on both β_1- and β_2-adrenoceptors (see Chapter 8). Dobutamine, a synthetic dopamine analogue, is a selective β_1-adrenoceptor agonist that produces a powerful inotropic response, with relatively less increase in heart rate than isoprenaline and little direct effect on vascular tone, even at high concentrations. Dopexamine has agonist activity at β_2-adrenoceptors, increasing heart rate and producing vasodilation. It has less activity at β_1-adrenoceptors, giving a weak direct positive inotropic effect. It also acts on peripheral dopamine receptors and produces some increase in renal blood flow, but, unlike dopamine, it does not cause peripheral vasoconstriction with high doses.

Dopamine has dose-related actions at several receptors.

■ At low doses, it selectively stimulates peripheral dopamine receptors, which are structurally distinct from those in the central nervous system. This produces renal arterial vasodilation and diuresis (via D_1 receptors) and peripheral arterial vasodilation (via D_2 presynaptic receptors, which inhibit noradrenaline release from sympathetic nerves).

■ At moderate doses, nonselective β-adrenoceptor stimulation produces a positive inotropic response (Fig. 7.5). Tachycardia is more marked than with dobutamine because of stimulation of both cardiac β_1- and β_2-adrenoceptors and the reflex response to β_2-adrenoceptor-mediated peripheral arterial dilation.

■ At high doses, α_1-adrenoceptor stimulation produces peripheral vasoconstriction, which also affects the renal arteries and overcomes D_1-receptor-mediated renal vasodilation.

The doses of dopamine that produce these different effects differ widely among individuals. Unfortunately there is no dose that can be relied upon to act selectively at dopamine receptors without stimulating adrenoceptors.

Pharmacokinetics

All inotropic sympathomimetics are administered by intravenous infusion because of their very short half-lives (<12 minutes). Metabolic inactivation is by the same monoamine oxidase (MAO) and catechol-O-methyltransferase (COMT) pathways as for noradrenaline (see Chapter 4). Desensitisation and downregulation of β-adrenoceptors (see Chapter 1) rapidly reduce the response to sustained infusions over 48–72 hours. Because of its unpredictable vasoconstrictor actions, dopamine is usually given in a large central vein.

Unwanted effects

■ excessive cardiac stimulation, with tachycardia, palpitations and arrhythmias,

■ nausea and vomiting,

■ chest pain, dyspnoea,

■ headache.

PHOSPHODIESTERASE INHIBITORS

enoximone, milrinone

Mechanism of action and effects

Milrinone and enoximone are specific inhibitors of the type 3 isoenzyme of phosphodiesterase found in cardiac and smooth muscle. The inotropic action of these drugs on the heart is due to an increase in intracellular cAMP with increased mobilisation of intracellular Ca^{2+} (see Fig. 7.5). Unlike β-adrenoceptor agonists, the activity of phosphodiesterase inhibitors is not limited by desensitisation of cell surface receptors because they act at a site beyond the receptor. Since they have complementary sites of action, phosphodiesterase inhibitors and β-adrenoceptor agonists will have additive effects on the heart. Phosphodiesterase type 3 inhibition

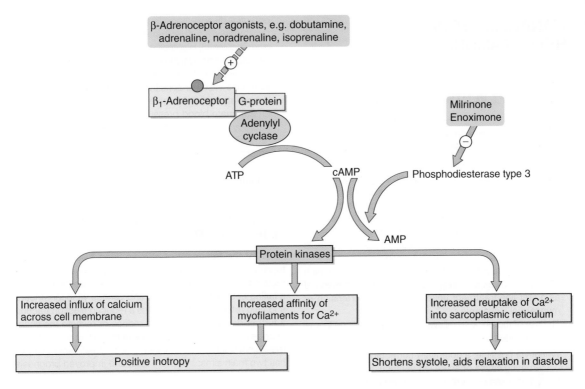

Fig. 7.5 Mechanisms by which sympathomimetics and phosphodiesterase inhibitors exert their positive inotropic effects. *AMP*, Adenosine monophosphate; *ATP*, adenosine triphosphate; *cAMP*, cyclic adenosine monophosphate.

in vascular smooth muscle produces peripheral arterial vasodilation.

Pharmacokinetics

Phosphodiesterase inhibitors are given by intravenous infusion. Milrinone is eliminated by the kidney and enoximone by hepatic metabolism. They have elimination half-lives of about 1 hour.

Unwanted effects

- These are mainly a consequence of excessive cardiac stimulation and include ectopic beats and both ventricular and supraventricular arrhythmias.
- Nausea, vomiting, diarrhoea (milrinone).
- Headache.
- Long-term oral use increases mortality in heart failure. Oral use has therefore been abandoned.

ANGIOTENSIN RECEPTOR NEPRILYSIN INHIBITORS

sacubitril valsartan

Mechanism of action and effects

Sacubitril is an inhibitor of neprilysin. Previous attempts to treat heart failure with a neprilysin inhibitor were unsuccessful, possibly because the inhibition of angiotensin II breakdown antagonises the beneficial effects on natriuretic peptides. Combining a neprilysin inhibitor with an angiotensin-converting enzyme (ACE) inhibitor increased the risk of angioedema from dual inhibition of the breakdown of bradykinin. The combination of sacubitril with an angiotensin II receptor antagonist was therefore a logical next step, as only one of the enzymes responsible for breakdown of bradykinin is inhibited. The addition of sacubitril to valsartan produces greater vasodilation and natriuresis.

Pharmacokinetics

Sacubitril valsartan is a molecular combination of the two drugs that dissociates into the individual component molecules after absorption. Sacubitril is a prodrug that is converted to sacubitrilat by esterases. Sacubitrilat is eliminated by the kidneys and has a half-life of 12 hours.

Unwanted effects

These are similar to those of an angiotensin II receptor antagonist but with a greater risk of hypotension.

MANAGEMENT OF HEART FAILURE

ACUTE LEFT VENTRICULAR FAILURE

The immediate aim of pharmacological treatment in acute left ventricular failure is to reduce excessive venous return to the heart. Treatment includes the following steps:

- Oxygen in high concentration via a facemask.
- Intravenous injection of a loop diuretic such as furosemide (see Chapter 14), which initially produces venodilation and peripheral venous pooling. Symptoms are therefore improved even before the onset of a diuresis that reduces plasma volume and further decreases preload.
- Noninvasive ventilatory support can be useful if there is severe breathlessness with acidaemia.
- Sublingual glyceryl trinitrate (GTN) (see Chapter 5), which dilates venous capacitance vessels, is not recommended as a first-line treatment unless there is hypertension or myocardial ischaemia.
- The use of morphine to relieve breathlessness is no longer recommended.

Whenever possible, a potentially correctable precipitating or exacerbating cause of acute left ventricular failure should be treated; for example, arrhythmias, anaemia, thyrotoxicosis, acute mitral regurgitation, or critical aortic stenosis. However, there is often underlying impairment of left ventricular systolic function, when management as for chronic heart failure is subsequently necessary.

CARDIOGENIC SHOCK

The immediate aim of treatment is resuscitation while looking for a remediable cause. If the underlying cause is ischaemic heart disease, then early coronary revascularisation is crucial to increase the probability of survival. Supportive measures include the following:

- Oxygen given in high concentration via a facemask.
- Correction of any acid–base imbalance (especially acidosis) and electrolyte abnormalities (particularly hypokalaemia).
- Correction of any cardiac rhythm disturbance (see Chapter 8).
- Ensuring adequate left ventricular filling pressure. This can be low after right ventricular infarction despite a high central venous pressure (right ventricular filling pressure). If intravenous volume is adequate but tissue perfusion remains impaired, dobutamine is the inotropic drug of choice. It is often given in combination with low-dose dopamine, with the intention that the dopamine will improve renal perfusion; however, there is little evidence that the addition of dopamine is beneficial.
- Phosphodiesterase inhibitors are sometimes given to improve myocardial contractility and produce peripheral vasodilation. They are usually reserved for those who fail to improve with maximum tolerated doses of dobutamine.
- When there is profound hypotension, noradrenaline (norepinephrine) (see Chapter 4) can be infused intravenously to produce α_1-adrenoceptor-mediated peripheral vasoconstriction and maintain vital organ perfusion. The

potential disadvantage is that the increase in peripheral resistance will further impair cardiac output. Vasopressin (see Chapter 43) is sometimes given to raise blood pressure, as vascular sensitivity to noradrenaline is impaired in shock. Vasopressin is a direct-acting vasoconstrictor that also increases vascular sensitivity to noradrenaline.

- Vasodilators can be given to 'offload' the heart once an adequate blood pressure has been established. This strategy is particularly helpful if there is significant mitral regurgitation, since reduced resistance to left ventricular emptying will diminish the regurgitant volume. Either glyceryl trinitrate (see Chapter 5) or nitroprusside (see Chapter 6) is used.

HEART FAILURE WITH REDUCED EJECTION FRACTION

Much of the treatment of chronic heart failure is directed towards counteracting the compensatory mechanisms for the reduced cardiac output and low blood pressure generated by a failing heart – that is, arterial and venous vasoconstriction and fluid retention. When there is a reduced ejection fraction, a further desirable action is to reduce or reverse the shape change (remodelling) that occurs in the failing ventricle and makes contraction less efficient. Overall, treatment of HFREF has two main aims: symptom relief and improved prognosis.

Nonpharmacological treatment

A number of lifestyle changes can be helpful.

- Weight reduction should be encouraged for an obese person; this improves exercise tolerance.
- Bed rest may be appropriate to rest the heart during acute episodes of fluid retention.
- Modest salt restriction is desirable (severe salt restriction is unpleasant and unnecessary).
- Fluid restriction is rarely required unless profound hyponatraemia accompanies severe oedema. In this situation, diuretics may be ineffective until the plasma Na^+ concentration is corrected.
- If possible, drugs that exacerbate heart failure by producing myocardial depression (e.g. most calcium channel blockers) or by promoting fluid retention (e.g. nonsteroidal anti-inflammatory drugs) should be withdrawn. Beta-adrenoceptor antagonists can cause myocardial depression but should not be stopped, although a high dose may have to be reduced. Alcohol intake should be moderate at most, since alcohol depresses myocardial contractility and can be arrhythmogenic.
- A graded exercise programme for people with stable heart failure can improve symptoms.

Diuretics

Diuretics remain the mainstay of treatment for chronic heart failure with fluid retention and are very effective for relief of symptoms (see Chapter 14). A loop diuretic (usually furosemide), taken once daily in the morning, is typically used. There is no evidence that the use of a loop or thiazide diuretic alters prognosis in heart failure. Hypokalaemia is unusual when loop diuretics are used in chronic heart failure, especially as an ACE inhibitor or angiotensin II receptor antagonist is usually taken concurrently (see below). Nevertheless, the use of a potassium-sparing diuretic is advisable if the plasma K^+ falls below 3.5 mmol/L, especially if digoxin or anti-arrhythmic therapy is given concurrently (because of an increased risk of generating cardiac rhythm disturbances). Spironol-actone is preferred in this situation and is also a standard treatment in severe heart failure, when it reduces mortal-ity by 25% if a low dose is added to maximal therapy with other drugs. Eplerenone has a similar benefit for heart failure following acute myocardial infarction. In more severe heart failure the fluid retention may not respond to usual doses of a loop diuretic. Strategies for the manage-ment of diuretic-resistant fluid retention are considered in Chapter 14.

Angiotensin-converting enzyme inhibitors and angiotensin II receptor antagonists

An ACE inhibitor (see Chapter 6) is now considered to be essential in the treatment of HFREF and is usually started at the same time as a diuretic. By reducing angiotensin II synthesis, ACE inhibitors produce arterial and venous dilation, which improves cardiac function by decreasing ventricular end-diastolic volume and increasing cardiac output (see Figs 7.1 and 7.2). ACE inhibitors usually improve breathlessness and fatigue, and exercise tolerance increases. Despite early haemodynamic changes, the full symptomatic response is often delayed for 4–6 weeks after the start of treatment. A further benefit of ACE inhibitors is improved survival, which may be due to a reversal of the remodelling of the left ventricle. High doses of an ACE inhibitor are more effective than low doses and reduce mortality by 20–25% in HFREF.

ACE inhibitors promote K^+ retention by the kidney; the combination of an ACE inhibitor with spironolactone is used to improve prognosis in severe heart failure but carries a small additive risk of hyperkalaemia.

If an ACE inhibitor is not tolerated, usually because of cough, an angiotensin II receptor antagonist (see Chapter 6) can be substituted. These agents have similar efficacy to ACE inhibitors.

Sacubitril valsartan

Compared with an ACE inhibitor the use of the angiotensin II receptor antagonist valsartan together with the neprilysin inhibitor sacubitril reduces hospitalisation as well as mortality by up to 20%. This combination is being increasingly used as a first-line treatment in place of an ACE inhibitor.

Beta-adrenoceptor antagonists

Beta-adrenoceptor antagonists (see Chapter 5) are highly effective for the treatment of HFREF, usually after the condition has been stabilised with an ACE inhibitor (or an angiotensin II receptor antagonist) and a diuretic. Beta-adrenoceptor antagonists were once considered to be contraindicated in heart failure because of their negative inotropic properties. However, if introduced gradually after starting with a low dose, they improve both symptoms and

Box 7.2	Possible beneficial effects of β-adrenoceptor antagonists in heart failure

Reduced workload of ischaemic myocardium
Restoration of cardiac excitation–contraction coupling and improved intracellular Ca^{2+} handling
Reduced cardiac hypertrophy and fibrosis
Reduced myocyte apoptosis
Antiarrhythmic effects

survival. The survival advantage is additive to that produced by an ACE inhibitor, with a further reduction of 30–35% in mortality at all classes of severity of heart failure. Possible explanations for the benefit of β-adrenoceptor antagonists are numerous (Box 7.2), but a reduction in cardiac remodelling is probably important. Unless there are contraindications (which does not include chronic obstructive pulmonary disease [COPD]), all people who have HFREF should be considered for treatment with a β-adrenoceptor antagonist once they are clinically stable. There remains some doubt about the value of a β-adrenoceptor antagonist in people who are in atrial fibrillation, in whom the benefit may be less than for those in sinus rhythm. The only compounds licensed for use in heart failure in the United Kingdom are bisoprolol, carvedilol and nebivolol, although there are also data to show the efficacy of a modified-release formulation of metoprolol.

Ivabradine

The sinus node inhibitor ivabradine (see Chapter 5) is advocated for those who have a heart rate above 75 beats/minute despite use of the maximum tolerated dose of a β-adrenoceptor antagonist. Ivabradine reduces hospital admissions but has no effect on mortality.

Digoxin

Digoxin is widely used to control heart rate when heart failure is associated with atrial fibrillation and a rapid ventricular rate. The use of digoxin for heart failure associated with sinus rhythm has been more controversial, but its positive inotropic effect can be useful as a supplement to standard therapy when there is severe left ventricular systolic dysfunction and symptoms persist. Digoxin improves symptoms and the need for hospitalisation; survival may be improved if the serum digoxin concentration is kept low.

Other vasodilators

Treatment with a combination of hydralazine (see Chapter 6) and isosorbide dinitrate or mononitrate (see Chapter 5) in addition to a diuretic and digoxin provides balanced arterial and venous dilation. This combination improves exercise tolerance in heart failure but produces only a modest reduction in mortality, although there may be greater benefits in people of Afro-Caribbean origin. The combination can be tried for people who cannot tolerate an ACE inhibitor or angiotensin II receptor antagonist (see Chapter 6).

Cardiac resynchronisation therapy and implantable cardioverter defibrillators

Cardiac resynchronisation therapy (CRT), or biventricular electrical pacing, is helpful in severe heart failure when the ECG shows bundle branch block and the ventricles display marked dyssynchronous contraction on echocardiography. The pacing of both ventricles simultaneously restores synchronous contraction and improves cardiac output.

About half of all people with heart failure die suddenly of ventricular arrhythmias; an implantable cardioverter defibrillator (ICD) can improve prognosis when there is severe left ventricular impairment and a propensity to ventricular arrhythmias. Combined cardiac resynchronisation–defibrillator devices (CRT-Ds) are also available.

Antiarrhythmic drugs do not improve survival in heart failure.

HEART FAILURE WITH PRESERVED EJECTION FRACTION

The optimal management of HFPEF is unclear. Most of the interventions that improve prognosis in HFREF have little impact on survival when ejection fraction is preserved; therefore treatment is mainly directed at symptom relief using the drugs discussed previously (with the exception of positive inotropic agents such as digoxin).

SELF-ASSESSMENT

True/false questions

1. When blood pressure falls, sympathetic outflow increases because of an increase in the sensory input from the baroreceptors in the carotid sinus.
2. In the healthy heart, a rise in afterload increases myocardial contractility.
3. Breathlessness and fatigue are common symptoms of heart failure.
4. Pulmonary oedema occurs when the hydrostatic pressure in the pulmonary veins is less than the plasma osmotic pressure.
5. In severe heart failure, the body's attempts to compensate for the cardiac dysfunction are detrimental.
6. Digoxin is the mainstay of the treatment of heart failure.
7. Digoxin inhibits the Na^+/K^+-ATPase pump on the cardiac myocyte membrane.
8. Hypokalaemia reduces the effect of digoxin on the Na^+/K^+-ATPase pump.
9. Digoxin inhibits the vagus nerve, thus decreasing the refractory period of the atrioventricular node.
10. Dobutamine produces peripheral vasodilation by its effect on β_2-adrenoceptors.
11. Sustained infusion of dobutamine desensitises the receptor response.
12. Milrinone is given intravenously to improve tissue perfusion in cardiogenic shock.
13. Angiotensin-converting enzyme (ACE) inhibitors should not be given together with K^+-sparing diuretics.
14. ACE inhibitors may cause cough by reducing the synthesis of bradykinin.
15. Survival in chronic heart failure is improved by β-adrenoceptor antagonists.
16. Hydralazine is a vasodilator with a predominant effect on veins.
17. Natriuretic peptides are synthesised by neprilysin.
18. Sacubitril valsartan is no more effective than an ACE inhibitor in heart failure with reduced ejection fraction.

One-best-answer (OBA) question

1. Which cardiovascular action of dopamine is mediated by D_2 receptors?
   A. Diuresis
   B. Peripheral arterial vasodilation
   C. Positive inotropy
   D. Renal arterial vasodilation
   E. Tachycardia

Case-based questions

Mr D.Y. is 78 years of age and had a large anterior myocardial infarction 3 years ago. Echocardiography revealed significant left ventricular systolic dysfunction with an ejection fraction of 30%. He presents with several symptoms, including fatigue, decreased exercise ability, shortness of breath, and peripheral oedema. Examination shows cardiomegaly, a raised jugular venous pressure, and crackles in the lungs. An ECG shows that he is in sinus rhythm.

1. What are the choices of diuretic open to you in treating Mr D.Y.?
2. Potassium loss produced by diuretics may lead to hypokalaemia. What is an effective way of reducing urinary K^+ loss?
3. Mr D.Y. was started on an ACE inhibitor. What precautionary measures should be taken in starting this new medication?
4. Could long-term oral digoxin be used as part of the treatment for Mr D.Y.?
5. Could the use of a β-adrenoceptor antagonist make Mr D.Y.'s condition worse?

ANSWERS

True/false answers

1. **False.** A falling blood pressure reduces the baroreceptor reflex input to the vasomotor centre, resulting in increased sympathetic outflow.
2. **True.** A rise in afterload decreases stroke volume initially, but the consequent sympathetic stimulation increases contractility in the healthy heart and restores the stroke volume. In the failing heart, contractility increases less readily and stroke volume falls.
3. **True.** The breathlessness is caused by increased pulmonary venous pressure, leading to pulmonary oedema; fatigue is caused by reduced cardiac output and impaired perfusion of skeletal muscle.
4. **False.** Oedema occurs when the net hydrostatic pressure, which moves fluid out of the vessel, is

greater than the plasma osmotic pressure, which moves interstitial fluid into the vessel.

5. **True.** The fall in cardiac output activates the sympathetic nervous system and the renin–angiotensin–aldosterone system; these changes are appropriate to restore blood pressure in the event of haemorrhage but are unhelpful in severe heart failure as they increase preload, afterload, and heart rate, hence increasing the workload of the failing heart.

6. **False.** Digoxin may be of benefit, but the mainstay of treatment is a diuretic such as furosemide and an ACE inhibitor (or angiotensin II receptor antagonist). If diuretics are given concurrently with digoxin, a potassium-sparing diuretic such as spironolactone may also be required to prevent hypokalaemia; hypokalaemia increases the risk of digoxin-induced rhythm disturbances.

7. **True.** By blocking the Na^+/K^+-ATPase pump, cellular export of Na^+ is reduced and intracellular Na^+ concentrations rise. The reduced Na^+ concentration gradient across the cell membrane reduces the linked export of Ca^{2+} ions. Increased intracellular Ca^{2+} concentrations enhance contractility.

8. **False.** Potassium ions and digoxin compete for the pump; therefore hypokalaemia can increase the activity and proarrhythmic risk of digoxin.

9. **False.** As well as its direct effects on the heart, digoxin increases vagal outflow from the vasomotor centre. This increases the refractory period of the atrioventricular node and is the reason why digoxin is useful in some arrhythmias, such as atrial fibrillation.

10. **False.** Dobutamine is a selective β_1-adrenoceptor agonist and does not produce peripheral vasodilation.

11. **True.** Stimulation of β_1-adrenoceptors by dobutamine results in cAMP synthesis and increased cardiac contractility. Prolonged stimulation (48–72 hours) desensitises the receptors; this does not occur with phosphodiesterase type 3 inhibitors, such as milrinone, which bypass the receptor and raise levels of cAMP by blocking its breakdown.

12. **True.** Milrinone inhibits the breakdown of intracellular cAMP by phosphodiesterase type 3 in cardiac and vascular smooth muscle, resulting in an inotropic effect and peripheral vasodilation; it is used to treat cardiogenic shock not responding to full doses of dobutamine.

13. **False.** The combination of an ACE inhibitor and spironolactone provides additive clinical benefit, but care must be taken to avoid dangerous hyperkalaemia, with regular monitoring of the plasma K^+ concentration. This is because ACE inhibitors reduce aldosterone-dependent reabsorption of Na^+ in the collecting duct. Because Na^+ reabsorption at this site occurs in exchange for K^+ efflux, ACE inhibitors may increase K^+ retention, particularly in combination with potassium-sparing diuretics.

14. **False.** ACE inhibitors reduce the breakdown of bradykinin by ACE (also known as kininase II); increased bradykinin levels in the lungs are thought to be responsible for the cough seen in some people taking ACE inhibitors. An alternative strategy is to use an angiotensin II receptor antagonist.

15. **True.** ACE inhibitors, β_1-adrenoceptor antagonists and spironolactone improve survival in chronic heart failure, possibly by reducing the cardiac remodelling effects of catecholamines, angiotensin II and aldosterone, respectively.

16. **False.** Hydralazine is predominantly an arterial vasodilator, whereas isosorbide mononitrate mainly acts as a venodilator; their combined use may be effective in chronic heart failure in people intolerant of ACE inhibitors or angiotensin II receptor antagonists.

17. **False.** Neprilysin degrades A- and B-type natriuretic peptides and also other vasoactive peptides including angiotensin II, bradykinin, endothelin and vasopressin.

18. **False.** Sacubitril valsartan is more effective in reducing morbidity and mortality than an ACE inhibitor.

One-best-answer (OBA) answer

1. **Answer B** is correct. Peripheral arterial vasodilation is produced by low concentrations of dopamine acting at presynaptic D_2 receptors, thus reducing the release of noradrenaline; however, high concentrations of dopamine acting at α_1-adrenoceptors cause peripheral arterial vasoconstriction. Diuresis (answer A) and renal arterial vasodilation (answer D) are produced by low doses of dopamine acting at D_1 receptors. Moderate doses of dopamine produce positive inotropic effects (answer C) by acting nonselectively at myocardial β-adrenoceptors and by acting at β_2-adrenoceptors to cause peripheral vasodilation, leading to reflex tachycardia (answer E).

Case-based answers

1. The treatment of first choice for fluid retention in chronic heart failure is a diuretic. For mild symptoms, a thiazide diuretic may be adequate, but in most people a loop diuretic such as furosemide is used. The loss of renal function in the elderly and renal underperfusion in heart failure means that thiazide diuretics are less effective in older people with this condition, such as Mr D.Y.

2. Hypokalaemia is arrhythmogenic and should be avoided in people with heart failure, particularly those taking digoxin. Urinary K^+ loss caused by a loop diuretic or thiazide can be reduced by combination with a K^+-sparing diuretic such as amiloride or spironolactone. Amiloride directly blocks epithelial Na^+/K^+ exchange in the collecting duct. In severe heart failure, spironolactone, which competes with aldosterone for the mineralocorticoid receptor, also improves prognosis, possibly by blocking aldosterone-dependent cardiac remodelling.

3. ACE inhibitors reduce preload and afterload by reducing the production of angiotensin II, a powerful vasoconstrictor, and reducing blood volume (via reduced aldosterone production). They also slow the progression of heart failure and improve survival. There is a small risk of severe hypotension following the first dose; omission of the diuretic immediately prior to this may be helpful.

4. The place of digoxin is well established in heart failure associated with atrial fibrillation and a rapid ventricular rate, but the benefit of a low dose of digoxin combined with a diuretic and an ACE inhibitor is now established in heart failure with severe left ventricular systolic dysfunction and sinus rhythm.

5. When used injudiciously, β-adrenoceptor antagonists may worsen heart failure by reducing cardiac output; however, low doses are beneficial (see Box 7.2) if the patient's condition has been stabilised with diuretics and an ACE inhibitor.

FURTHER READING

Bangash, M.N., Kong, M.-L., Pearse, R.M., 2011. Use of inotropes and vasopressor agents in critically ill patients. Br. J. Pharmacol. 165, 2015–2033.

Hammond, D.A., Smith, M.N., Lee, K.C., et al., 2016. Acute decompensated heart failure. J. Intensive Care Med. pii: 0885066616669494. [Epub ahead of print] PubMed PMID: 27638544.

Houston, B.A., Kalathiya, R.J., Kim, D.A., et al., 2015. Volume overload in heart failure. Mayo Clin. Proc. 90, 1247–1261.

Krum, H., Teerlink, J.R., 2011. Medical therapy for chronic heart failure. Lancet 378, 713–721.

McMurray, J.J.V., 2010. Systolic heart failure. N. Engl. J. Med. 362, 228–238.

Metra, M., Felker, G.M., Zaca, V., et al., 2010. Acute heart failure: multiple clinical profiles and mechanisms require tailored therapy. Int. J. Cardiol. 144, 175–179.

Owens, A.T., Brozena, S.C., Jessup, M., 2016. New management strategies in heart failure. Circ. Res. 118, 480–495.

Redfield, M.M., 2016. Heart failure with preserved ejection fraction. N. Engl. J. Med. 375, 1868–1877.

Thiele, H., Ohman, E.M., Desch, S., et al., 2015. Management of cardiogenic shock. Eur. Heart J. 36, 1223–1230.

Yang, E.H., Shah, S., Criley, J.M., 2012. Digoxin toxicity: a fading but crucial complication to recognize. Am. J. Med. 125, 337–343.

Compendium: drugs used to treat heart failure

Drug	Characteristics
Digitalis glycoside	
Increase intracellular Ca^{2+} by inhibiting Na^+/K^+-ATPase in myocyte membrane.	
Digoxin	Used in heart failure and for supraventricular arrhythmias (particularly atrial fibrillation, see Chapter 8). Given orally. Half-life: 20–50 h
Inotropic sympathomimetics	
β-Adrenoceptor agonists, some with additional actions; rapidly metabolised by local monoamine oxidase (MAO) and catechol-O-methyltransferase (COMT) pathways, giving very short half-lives, so all are given by intravenous infusion.	
Dobutamine	Selective $β_1$-adrenoceptor agonist; inotropic action with little effect on heart rate or vascular tone. Used after myocardial infarction, cardiac surgery, cardiomyopathies, septic shock, and cardiogenic shock. Half-life 2 min
Dopamine	Nonselective β-adrenoceptor agonist; increases cardiac contractility and heart rate; agonism of peripheral dopamine receptors increases renal perfusion, offset by $α_1$-adrenoceptor-mediated vasoconstriction at high doses. Used for cardiogenic shock in exacerbations of chronic heart failure and in heart failure associated with cardiac surgery. Half-life: 7–12 min
Dopexamine	Selective $β_2$-adrenoceptor agonist; increases cardiac contractility and rate; agonism of renal dopamine receptors increases renal perfusion. Used for inotropic effect after myocardial infarction, cardiac surgery, cardiomyopathies, septic shock, and cardiogenic shock. Half-life: 7 min
Isoprenaline	Nonselective β-adrenoceptor agonist. Used in emergency treatment of bradycardia. Available in the United Kingdom only from 'special order' manufacturers. Given intravenously. Half-life: 2 min
Phosphodiesterase inhibitors	
Inhibit phosphodiesterase (PDE) type 3 in myocytes.	
Enoximone	Used for congestive heart failure where cardiac output is reduced and filling pressure increased. Given by intravenous infusion. Half-life: 4–10 h
Milrinone	Used for short-term treatment of severe congestive heart failure and acute heart failure. Given by intravenous infusion. Half-life: 0.8–0.9 h
Angiotensin receptor neprilysin inhibitor (ARNI)	
Sacubitril valsartan	Conjugate of sacubitril with the angiotensin II receptor antagonist valsartan; sacubitril is a prodrug of sacubitrilat, which inhibits the breakdown of A- and B-type natriuretic peptides by neprilysin. Used for symptomatic chronic heart failure with reduced ejection fraction. Given orally. Half-life: (sacubitril) 1–2 h, (sacubitrilat) 12 h, (valsartan) 10 h

8

Cardiac arrhythmias

BASIC CARDIAC ELECTROPHYSIOLOGY

Action potentials in myocardial cells and the highly regulated cardiac contractions that result are a product of transmembrane ion currents generated by the movement of ions through membrane channels (see Chapter 1). A variety of specific channels exist for transmembrane Na^+, Ca^{2+} and K^+ transport in the myocardium (Figs 8.1 and 8.2). These channels cycle through three states: resting, open or closed (inactive and refractory). Whether the channels are open to allow ion flow or are closed is determined by the electrical potential across the cell membrane; therefore they are called *voltage-gated ion channels*. The direction in which ions move is dependent on the type of channel, the concentration gradient of the ions and the transmembrane electrical potential (see Figs 8.1 and 8.2). As a result of activity in some of these ion channels, the resting potential inside a cardiac cell is approximately −70 to −80 mV compared with the extracellular environment. Depolarisation of these cells generates an action potential that passes from one cell to the next.

The sinoatrial (SA) node, atrioventricular (AV) node, bundle of His and Purkinje system are part of the *specialised conducting system* of the heart; it ensures that a depolarising impulse is conducted rapidly and synchronously through the ventricular myocardium. In addition, the AV node slows impulse conduction. This allows time for the completion of mechanical events in the atrium and therefore enables ventricular filling before ventricular contraction begins. Once the impulse is passed from these specialised cells to myocytes, depolarisation initiates myocyte contraction and also triggers depolarisation in adjacent myocytes. This ensures conduction of the impulse progressively throughout the myocardium.

The action potentials in cells of the SA and AV nodes, Purkinje fibres and ventricular muscle vary substantially in their characteristics depending on the ion channels that are activated (see Figs 8.1, 8.2 and 8.5). Action potentials in cardiac cells can be divided into four phases (see Figs 8.1A and 8.2), although phases 1 and 2 are not clearly evident in the SA and AV nodes (see Fig. 8.1A).

CELLS WITH PACEMAKER ACTIVITY

The myocardial cells of the specialised conducting system (SA node, AV node, bundle of His and Purkinje system) are distinguished electrophysiologically from cardiac myocytes by their intrinsic ability to depolarise spontaneously in phase 4 and independently generate an action potential. These cells are said to possess *automaticity* and are termed *pacemaker cells*. This contrasts with cardiac myocytes, which have a stable resting potential and do not show phase 4 spontaneous depolarisation (compare Fig. 8.1A and C).

The primary pacemaker that drives normal repetitive cardiac contractions is the SA node. The cells of the SA

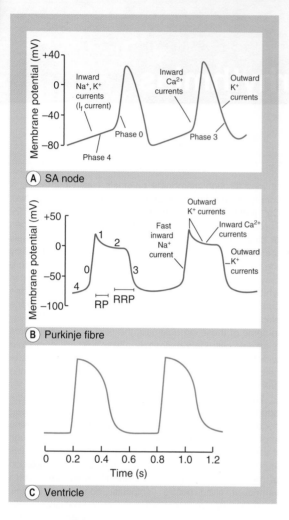

A SA node

B Purkinje fibre

C Ventricle

Fig. 8.1 Action potentials show variations in pattern among different populations of myocytes in different regions of the heart. The patterns are determined by the opening and closing of selective gates for Na^+, Ca^{2+} and K^+ ions, and this figure should be studied in conjunction with Fig. 8.2. The overall stability of the resting transmembrane ionic balance is controlled by active pumps, such as the Na^+/K^+-ATPase pump, which maintain the Na^+ concentration gradient at about 140 mM outside the cell versus 10–15 mM inside and the K^+ concentration gradient at 140 mM inside and 4 mM outside the cell. This results in an electrical potential at rest of approximately −70 to −80 mV inside the cell relative to outside the cell. Large ion fluxes at rest are prevented by specific pumps and closure of voltage-gated channels. Action potentials in the atrioventricular (AV) node, bundle of His and ventricle are controlled by the sinoatrial (SA) node when the heart is in sinus rhythm. The rate of spontaneous depolarisation of the SA node determines its primacy as a pacemaker in the healthy heart. Phase 0 (panels B and C) occurs when the membrane potential reaches a defined threshold potential and an 'all-or-none' influx of Na^+ through voltage-dependent fast Na^+ channels occurs; this is transient and the gates close after a few milliseconds. Phase 0 is much slower in the SA and AV nodes than in ventricular cells and depends mainly on Ca^{2+} influx (panel A). This causes the conduction velocity in the SA node to be considerably lower than in the Purkinje fibres, and the refractory period is longer in proportion to the total duration of the action potential. Phase 1, called the early repolarisation and notch, results from K^+ efflux (the transient outward current I_{to1}) and reduced Na^+ influx (see Fig. 8.2). The phase 2 plateau is primarily a result of Ca^{2+} influx (slow inward, or SI, current) which is balanced by K^+ efflux over a slow time course. Phase 3 repolarisation results from inactivation of Ca^{2+} influx and increasing K^+ efflux via a number of currents (see text, Table 8.1 and Fig. 8.2). Part of the overall importance of the K^+ currents lies in maintaining a stable resting membrane potential. Phase 4 (panels A and B) is termed the *diastolic* or *pacemaker depolarisation* generated on hyperpolarisation. The phase 4 inward 'funny' current (I_f) involves Na^+ and K^+ and is gated both by changes in voltage and by cAMP. The I_f current controls the rate of spontaneous beating of the heart and is regulated by the sympathetic and parasympathetic nervous systems. Ca^{2+} currents may also be involved in pacemaker activity in phase 4. *RP*, Absolute refractory period; *RRP*, relative refractory period.

node have the fastest rate of spontaneous depolarisation, producing a normal sinus rhythm of 60–100 impulses per minute at rest. The secondary pacemaker, the AV node, depolarises more slowly and can generate 40–60 impulses per minute, while the tertiary pacemakers (the bundle of His, its branches and the Purkinje fibres) can fire 20–40 times per minute. The secondary and tertiary pacemakers will be utilised only if there is a failure of pacemakers that have a faster rate of spontaneous depolarisation.

CONTROL OF DEPOLARISATION IN PACEMAKER AND NONPACEMAKER CELLS

The negative internal resting membrane potential is maintained by high K^+ permeability of resting cell membranes through inward rectifying voltage- and ligand-gated K^+ channels, which close when the cell depolarises. Progressive spontaneous depolarisation in phase 4 distinguishes pacemaker cells from other cells in the heart. This depolarisation of pacemaker cells results from influx of positive ions (Na^+ and K^+) into the cell through f-channels that generate the strangely termed cardiac pacemaker *'funny' current* (I_f) (see Figs 8.1A and 8.2). The funny current (I_f) is unusual because it is generated by

mixed-ion transport through a single channel, is activated by the negative intracellular potential in diastole, and has slow activation and deactivation rates. Nonpacemaker cells have a minimal or no I_f.

The intrinsic rate of firing of a pacemaker cell depends on four factors:

- the resting intracellular potential,
- the resting potential at which the I_f is activated,
- the rate of spontaneous depolarisation by the I_f,
- the threshold potential for initiating full depolarisation.

Activation of the I_f in the SA node is modulated by the autonomic nervous system via intracellular cyclic adenosine monophosphate (cAMP). Stimulation of β_1-adrenoceptors

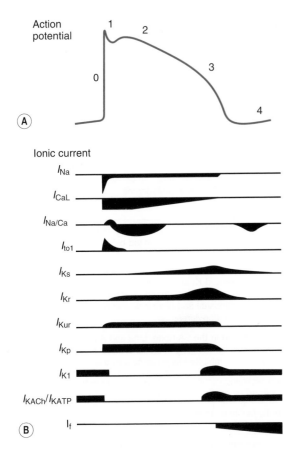

Action potential

Ionic current

I_{Na}

I_{CaL}

$I_{Na/Ca}$

I_{to1}

I_{Ks}

I_{Kr}

I_{Kur}

I_{Kp}

I_{K1}

I_{KACh}/I_{KATP}

I_f

Fig. 8.2 **A schematic representation of the influx and efflux of Na$^+$, Ca^{2+} and K$^+$ in Purkinje fibres.** This figure should be examined in conjunction with Table 8.1 and other explanations given in the text. A downward inflection represents an influx of the ion and an upward inflection an efflux. (Modified and reproduced with permission from Tamargo J, Caballero R, Gomez R, et al. Pharmacology of cardiac potassium channels. Cardiovasc Res 2004; 62:9–33.)

generates cAMP and shifts the intracellular potential for activation of the channel to a less negative voltage, while vagal stimulation via muscarinic M$_2$ receptors inhibits cAMP production so that activation of the channel requires a more negative intracellular voltage.

Full depolarisation of the SA or AV node occurs when, as a result of the I_f, the internal membrane potential reaches a threshold potential that opens voltage-gated L-type Ca^{2+} channels so that Ca^{2+} influx into the cell occurs (phase 0) (see Fig. 8.1A; I_{CaL} in Fig. 8.2). The SA node is the dominant pacemaker because activation of the I_f current in the SA node occurs at a less negative intracellular potential and has a faster intrinsic rate of depolarisation than in the AV node or Purkinje fibres. Therefore spontaneous diastolic depolarisation in the SA node is initiated earlier after repolarisation and the threshold potential for full depolarisation of the cell (phase 0) is reached sooner.

Phase 0 of the action potential in Purkinje fibres and atrial and ventricular myocytes is initiated by a rapid influx of Na$^+$ through voltage-gated Na$^+$ ion channels (fast Na$^+$ channels) (see Fig. 8.1B; I_{Na} in Fig. 8.2). In cells other than the triggering pacemaker, the depolarising current in phase 0 is initiated

by propagation of the depolarising wave between cells. At the end of phase 0, the intracellular voltage potential briefly becomes positive, at which point a voltage-triggered 'gate' closes and inactivates the depolarising Na$^+$ or Ca^{2+} channels (see Fig. 8.1A and B). The slow influx of Ca^{2+} that generates phase 0 in the AV node is the reason for slow conduction of the depolarising impulse through the AV node.

CONTROL OF CELL REPOLARISATION IN PACEMAKER AND NONPACEMAKER CELLS

Once depolarised, cardiac cells undergo repolarisation to return the membrane potential to its resting level. This creates the conditions for the next action potential to be initiated (see Figs 8.1 and 8.2). In both pacemaker and nonpacemaker cells, repolarisation (phase 3) is achieved by the opening of cell membrane K$^+$ channels known as rectifiers (see Table 8.1 for explanation). In the Purkinje system and nonpacemaker cardiac cells, initial repolarisation through the I_{to} channel (phase 1) is interrupted by influx of Ca^{2+} through L-type channels (phase 2, the plateau phase; I_{CaL} in Fig. 8.2), which balances K$^+$ efflux (see Fig. 8.1B, phase 2). This plateau is essential for excitation–contraction coupling. Eventually the K$^+$ current dominates in these cells through activation of I_{Kr}, I_{Ks} and I_{K1} channels (phase 3) and the cell returns to a negative intracellular resting potential. Repolarisation is also helped by Ca^{2+} extrusion from the cell through the Na$^+$/Ca^{2+} ion exchanger and by Ca^{2+} uptake by the sarcoplasmic reticulum.

In the resting phase between action potentials, Na$^+$ and K$^+$ transmembrane concentration gradients are restored by an energy-dependent ion exchange pump (Na$^+$/K$^+$-ATPase; see Fig. 7.4), and the low intracellular Ca^{2+} concentration is restored by the Na$^+$/Ca^{2+} ion exchanger.

During the period between phase 0 and the end of phase 2 of the action potential, the myocardial cell is refractory to any further depolarisation (the *absolute refractory period*, RP; see Fig. 8.1B). This is because the depolarising channels are held in the inactivated state until a sufficiently negative potential is restored inside the cell. During phase 3, a large depolarising stimulus can open sufficient Na$^+$ or Ca^{2+} channels (many of which will have returned to the resting state) to overcome the K$^+$ efflux and initiate a further action potential. This part of the action potential is the *relative refractory period* (RRP; see Fig. 8.1B).

The sum of the individual action potentials that pass from one cell to another through the heart can be recorded as the surface electrocardiogram (ECG) (Fig. 8.3).

MECHANISMS OF ARRHYTHMOGENESIS

Arrhythmias are disorders of rate and rhythm of the heart, which can arise as the result of either abnormal impulse generation or abnormal impulse conduction. There are three mechanisms of arrhythmogenesis:

- **Increased automaticity.** Dominant ectopic pacemakers (pacemakers other than the SA node) can arise when pacemaker cells in the specialised conducting tissue develop a more rapid phase 4 depolarisation than that of the SA node. Ectopic pacemakers can also arise when

Table 8.1 Selected examples of K⁺ channels and associated currents

Type of gating	Examples of distribution	Comment
K_V voltage-gated channel family		
K_V channels carrying delayed inward rectifying currents	Widely distributed, including brain, heart, pancreas	Multiple subtypes of K⁺ channels are involved in delayed inward rectification and are responsible for slow (I_{Ks}), rapid (I_{Kr}) and ultrarapid (I_{Kur}) K⁺ currents involved in repolarisation in phases 2 and 3 in the heart. Inhibited by some class I and class III antiarrhythmics (e.g. amiodarone and sotalol)
K_V channel carrying transient outward rectifying (I_{KTO}) current		A genetically distinct member of the K_V family of channels. Responsible for the I_{to1} transient current in phase 1. Activated by adenosine; inhibited by quinidine, amiodarone
K_{ir} family		
Inward rectifying	Heart, muscle, brain, pancreas	Inward rectifying, rapidly inactivates cardiac Na⁺ channels; sets resting membrane potential (I_{K1}, I_{Kr}). Inhibited by amiodarone
Ligand-gated channels		
ATP-sensitive channels (K_{ATP})	Heart, muscle, pancreas, mitochondria	Composed of coexpressed K_{ir} and sulfonylurea subunits with varied configurations in different tissues. Provide a weak inward rectifying current. Opened by minoxidil and nicorandil and by ischaemia; inhibited by ATP and sulfonylureas
Acetylcholine-sensitive channel (K_{ACh})	SA node, AV node and atria	This is G-protein-linked in the SA node, atria and AV node and is a member of the K_{ir} family, resulting in an inward rectifying (K_{ir}) current. Opened by adenosine; inhibited by atropine and disopyramide
Two-pore channel (K_{2P})	Heart, brain, pancreas	Weak inward rectifying current; modulates resting membrane potential. Opened by arachidonic acid
Calcium-activated (K_{Ca} family)		Members of K_{ir} family of channels
Large conductance channel (B_{Kca})	Heart, brain, pancreas	Possible roles in neuroprotection, erectile dysfunction and other disorders
Intermediate conductance channel (I_{Kca})	T-lymphocytes, smooth muscle, brain, heart	Opened by hydralazine

This table should be studied in conjunction with Fig. 8.2. Potassium channels are diverse in structure and behaviour. Each channel consists of four membrane-spanning subunits, with each subunit consisting of two to six linked membrane segments which make up the water-filled pore. This allows many different configurations of K⁺ channels, many of which have particular physiological roles. Channels with subunit variations are associated with different types of current which are involved in repolarisation at different phases of the cardiac action potential. The channels can be open or closed depending on the voltage across the cell or the presence of a selective ligand. Rectifying current: an inward rectifying current means that, under conditions of equivalent but opposing electrochemical potentials, these channels pass more current inwards than outwards. An outward rectifying current is similar but in an outward direction.

rapid spontaneous phase 4 depolarisation develops in myocytes that usually have a stable phase 4. Ischaemia or other changes in the microcellular environment can create conditions that allow a nonspecialised myocardial cell to express f-channels and become a pacemaker. Increased automaticity can produce various superventricular and ventricular arrhythmias (VAs).

- **Reentry.** This is the cause of most clinically important arrhythmias. It is initiated when a depolarising impulse, which is often a premature (ectopic) beat from elsewhere in the heart, arrives at a part of the myocardium that is still in its refractory period. A refractory part of the myocardium is usually created by a fast conducting pathway that has a slow recovery from depolarisation. If the impulse is able to access an adjacent part of the myocardium, it can bypass the refractory tissue. When this alternative pathway has a slower rate of conduction but a fast recovery rate, the impulse may subsequently arrive at the distal part of the refractory tissue when this tissue has had sufficient time to repolarise. The impulse can then be conducted retrogradely through this previously refractory tissue (Fig. 8.4C). When the retrograde conduction is complete and if there has been sufficient time for the alternative pathway to repolarise, a self-perpetuating circuit of electrical activity will be initiated (a reentry circuit). Once established, the reentry circuit acts as a pacemaker that initiates impulses which are then propagated through the heart.

Functional reentry circuits can be localised within a small area of myocardium that has been damaged by pathology such as fibrosis or ischaemia (microreentry). This underlies arrhythmias such as atrial or ventricular fibrillation (VF). The myocardium can also support large anatomical reentry circuits (macroreentry). These circuits arise over a larger area of myocardium and cause arrhythmias such as atrial or ventricular flutter or AV nodal reentry.

Macroreentry is also found when there is a congenital accessory pathway that connects the atria and ventricles, which provides an alternative pathway to the AV node for conducting electrical activity between the atria and ventricles. The reentry circuit between the atria and ventricles includes both the accessory pathway (antegrade conduction) and the AV node (retrograde conduction) (AV reentry). An example of this type of macroreentry circuit is Wolff–Parkinson–White syndrome.

■ **Triggered activity.** A cell can develop transient rapid depolarising activity during or following repolarisation ('afterdepolarisations'), which will initiate an action potential if they reach the threshold potential of the cell. Afterdepolarisations are said to be 'early' if they occur during phase 3 repolarisation (RRP in Fig. 8.1B) or 'delayed' if they occur in phase 4. Early afterdepolarisations (EADs) occur when the repolarising K^+ current through the I_{Kr} is decreased; they are due to either opening of L-type Ca^{2+} channels, increased current through the Na^+/Ca^{2+} ion exchanger, or increased late Na^+ current. Delayed afterdepolarisations (DADs) are due to intracellular Ca^{2+} overload and follow spontaneous Ca^{2+} release from the sarcoplasmic reticulum during prolonged repolarisation. This activates the cell membrane $3Na^+/Ca^{2+}$ exchange transporter and produces a net depolarising current. Triggered activity is a relatively uncommon mechanism of arrhythmogenesis but can underlie a variety of atrial arrhythmias and VAs. EADs are responsible for the proarrhythmic activity of class Ia and III antiarrhythmic agents and are also more common in pathophysiological states such as heart failure and ventricular hypertrophy. DADs are provoked by digitalis glycosides and also promoted by ischaemia, hypokalaemia and increased circulating catecholamines.

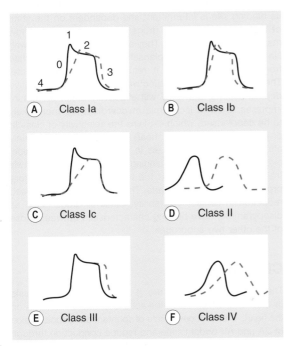

Fig. 8.3 Effects of different classes of antiarrhythmic drugs on the cardiac action potential in ventricular cells (panels A, B, C and E) and the AV node (panels D and F). (A) *Class Ia drugs* block fast Na^+ channels in phase 0 with moderate potency and some K^+ channels; repolarisation is prolonged. (B) *Class Ib drugs* weakly block fast Na^+ channels in phase 0 only in abnormal tissue, with little effect on K^+ channels. (C) *Class Ic drugs* potently block fast Na^+ channels and weakly block Ca^{2+} channels and some K^+ channels. (D) *Class II drugs* reduce phase 4 and phase 0 depolarisation in AV and SA nodes; repolarisation in the AV node is prolonged. (E) *Class III drugs* block some K^+ channels, inhibiting repolarisation and prolonging the action potential. (F) *Class IV drugs* block L-type Ca^{2+} channels, slowing phase 0 and phase 4 depolarisation particularly in the AV node, with less effect in the SA node; repolarisation is prolonged.

MECHANISMS OF ACTION AND CLASSIFICATION OF ANTIARRHYTHMIC DRUGS

A widely used classification of antiarrhythmic drugs (the Vaughan Williams classification) is based on their effects on the action potential (Fig. 8.5). This classification has many flaws and does not take account of the multiple actions possessed by some drugs or the fact that the effects of drugs on diseased myocardium may differ from those on healthy myocardium. However, there is no widely accepted alternative classification.

VAUGHAN WILLIAMS CLASSIFICATION

The Vaughan Williams classification recognises four classes of drug (Table 8.2).

Table 8.2 Principal indications for antiarrhythmic drugs

Class	Examples	Supraventricular arrhythmias	Ventricular arrhythmias
Ia	Disopyramide (procainamide)	+	+
Ib	Lidocaine	−	+ (especially after myocardial infarction)
Ic	Flecainide, propafenone	+	+
II	β-Adrenoceptor antagonists	+	+ (especially after myocardial infarction)
III	Amiodarone, sotalol	+	+
IV	Calcium channel blockers	+	−

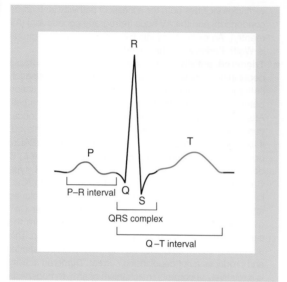

Fig. 8.4 The waveform for cardiac events seen on a surface electrocardiogram. The P wave represents the spread of depolarisation through the atria and the QRS complex is the spread through the ventricles. The T wave represents repolarisation of the ventricle. The P–R interval is the time of conductance from atrium to ventricles, and the QRS time is the time the ventricles are activated. The duration of the ventricular action potential is given by the Q–T interval.

Class I

All class I drugs inhibit fast Na$^+$ channels and slow the rate of rise of phase 0; therefore they reduce the rate of the myocardial cell's depolarisation. They are often called *membrane stabilisers*. They readily penetrate the phospholipid bilayers of the cell membrane, where they concentrate in the hydrophobic core and bind to hydrophobic amino acids in the Na$^+$ channel (see also local anaesthetics; see Chapter 18). Class I drugs are subdivided according to their effects on the duration of the action potential.

- Class Ia drugs, such as disopyramide, slow impulse conduction by producing moderate Na$^+$ channel blockade. In addition, they block some K$^+$ channels (see Table 8.1, and Figs 8.1 and 8.5A), which prolongs repolarisation and therefore extends the duration of the action potential. *They are effective for the treatment of both supraventricular arrhythmias and VAs* (see Table 8.2).
- Class Ib drugs, such as lidocaine, slow impulse conduction by producing weak Na$^+$ channel blockade in abnormal tissue (such as ischaemic myocardium) with no effect in healthy tissue. They do not block K$^+$ channels and have either no effect on repolarisation or may shorten it (see Fig. 8.5B). *They are effective only for the treatment of VAs.*
- Class Ic drugs, such as flecainide, slow impulse conduction by producing marked Na$^+$ channel blockade. They produce weak blockade of some K$^+$ channels (see Table 8.1), and

also block inward Ca^{2+} channels. There is minimal effect on repolarisation (see Fig. 8.5C). *They are effective for the treatment of both atrioventricular arrhythmias and VAs.*

The different effects of the class I subgroups result from their diverse ion-channel binding characteristics. During the time course of the action potential, access of the drug to its binding site is intermittent and dependent on the state of the channel. Class Ib drugs (such as lidocaine) show marked use-dependence. They associate more rapidly with Na$^+$ channels during depolarisation and rapidly dissociate from the channel when it returns to the resting state. Therefore they are more effective when there are repetitive depolarisations, and they will effectively block premature impulses. Cells in ischaemic myocardium are more likely to be depolarised, which explains the selectivity of class Ib drugs for VA in ischaemic heart disease (ischaemia mainly affects the ventricles). Class Ic drugs (such as flecainide) also show use-dependent binding but dissociate more slowly from their binding sites in the Na$^+$ channel and therefore produce prolonged blockade. This results in a widespread reduction in cellular excitability. Class Ia drugs (such as disopyramide) have binding characteristics between those of the other two subgroups.

Class II

The class II drugs are the β-adrenoceptor antagonists (β-blockers), which block the actions of catecholamines on the heart. They reduce the rate of spontaneous depolarisation of SA and AV nodal tissue and reduce conduction through the AV node by their action on adrenoceptor-sensitive f-channels (see Fig. 8.5D). They can also inhibit ectopic pacemakers that have developed dominant automaticity. *Beta-adrenoceptor antagonists are effective for the treatment of both supraventricular arrhythmias and VAs, particularly if these are catecholamine-dependent.*

Class III

Class III drugs such as amiodarone prolong the duration of the action potential by inhibiting some K$^+$ channels involved in repolarisation, thus increasing the absolute RP of the cell (see Table 8.1 and Fig. 8.5E). *They are effective for the treatment of both supraventricular arrhythmias and VAs.*

Class IV

There are two types of Ca^{2+} channels in the heart; the class IV drugs are calcium channel blockers that selectively block the L-type Ca^{2+} channel. They slow conduction of the action potential, particularly in the AV node. They have a lesser effect on the rate of depolarisation at the SA node (see Fig. 8.5F). *They are effective only for the treatment of supraventricular arrhythmias except in very rare situations.*

Unclassified drugs

Four drugs used in the treatment of rhythm disturbances do not fit into the Vaughan Williams classification: digitalis glycosides, adenosine, magnesium sulphate and atropine.

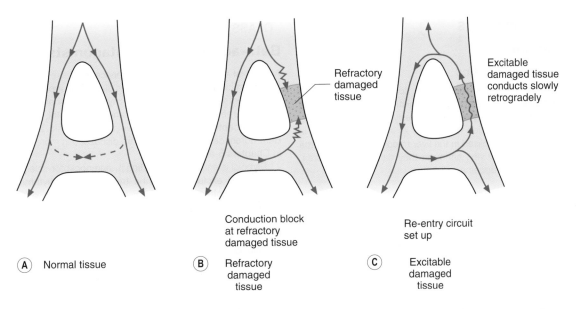

Fig. 8.5 Conduction in normal and damaged cardiac tissue. (A) In normal tissue, conduction is carefully ordered. When an action potential has been generated, the cells cannot be immediately reactivated because of refractoriness of the myocardial cells. If conducted impulses meet, they die out. (B) If an area of damage or dysfunction is present, impulses are conducted abnormally. If an action potential arrives at the area of damaged tissue and it is fully refractory, the impulse is blocked and an arrhythmia will not develop. (C) If an action potential arrives at a damaged area and is capable of being excited and conducting in a retrograde direction, a perpetuating abnormal reentry circuit may be set up.

PROARRHYTHMIC ACTIVITY OF ANTIARRHYTHMIC DRUGS

Many antiarrhythmic drugs have the potential to precipitate serious arrhythmias, such as incessant ventricular tachycardia (VT). Several of them (particularly class Ia agents and sotalol) prolong the Q–T interval on the ECG (see Fig. 8.3). This predisposes to a polymorphic VT known as torsade de pointes, which has a characteristic twisting QRS axis on the ECG and can degenerate into VF. Drug-induced ventricular rhythm disturbances are particularly refractory to treatment.

There are probably multiple mechanisms of drug-induced arrhythmogenesis. Several risk factors have been identified, including the following.

- Excessive slowing of cardiac impulse conduction, such as occurs with marked blockade of Na^+ channels.
- Excessive prolongation of the action potential, especially if this is due to blockade of the I_{Kr} repolarising current (see Table 8.1 and Fig. 8.2). Prolonged repolarisation may cause EAD (see previous discussion) or a selective effect of the drugs on some cells in the myocardium can lead to differential rates of repolarisation that predispose to reentry circuits.
- Mutations in genes coding for channels that regulate Na^+, K^+ and Ca^{2+} transmembrane ion flows exist in 5–10% of people and are probably subclinical variants of the congenital long QT syndrome. A common mutation involves the human ether-a-go-go-related gene hERG) that encodes a subunit of the I_{Kr} channel. These individuals are more susceptible to torsade de pointes when exposed to a drug that prolongs the Q–T interval.

- Structural heart disease, especially ischaemic heart disease, with greater slowing of conduction in diseased myocardium.
- Hypokalaemia.
- Increased circulating catecholamines.
- Female gender: about 70% of those who develop torsade de pointes are women.

CLASS IA DRUGS

Disopyramide

Disopyramide is no longer widely used in the United Kingdom because of its unwanted effects.

Pharmacokinetics

Disopyramide is metabolised in the liver to a compound with less antiarrhythmic activity but greater antimuscarinic activity. The half-life of disopyramide is 4–10 hours.

Unwanted effects

- Gastrointestinal disturbances.
- Powerful negative inotropic effect; disopyramide should be avoided in people with left ventricular dysfunction.
- Proarrhythmic effects (see above).
- Antimuscarinic effects (see Chapter 4), especially urinary retention, dry mouth and blurred vision.

CLASS IB DRUGS

Lidocaine

Pharmacokinetics

Extensive first-pass metabolism to a potentially toxic metabolite means that oral administration of lidocaine is not practicable. It is given intravenously, initially as a loading dose by bolus injection followed by an infusion. Lidocaine is extensively metabolised in the liver to compounds with little antiarrhythmic activity, although they can cause seizures. The half-life of lidocaine is 2 hours.

Unwanted effects

- Central nervous system (CNS) toxicity: muscle twitching, seizures, respiratory depression, dizziness, drowsiness, paraesthesia,
- Negative inotropic effect,
- Bradycardia.

CLASS IC DRUGS

Flecainide

Pharmacokinetics

Flecainide is absorbed orally, but an intravenous formulation is also available for rapid onset of action. Flecainide has a half-life of 14 hours.

Unwanted effects

- Oedema,
- Fever,
- Dyspnoea,
- CNS toxicity – dizziness, fatigue, visual disturbances,
- Negative inotropic effect,
- Proarrhythmic effects, possibly more marked after recent myocardial infarction, when flecainide may increase mortality.

Propafenone

Propafenone has weak β-adrenoceptor antagonist activity in addition to its class Ic action.

Pharmacokinetics

Propafenone undergoes extensive first-pass metabolism by cytochrome P450-mediated oxidation, which is saturable, so the half-life is dose-dependent. Elimination is much slower in subjects with CYP2D6 genetic polymorphism.

Unwanted effects

- Gastrointestinal disturbances: nausea, vomiting, diarrhoea, bitter taste,
- Cholestasis, hepatitis,
- CNS toxicity – dizziness, anxiety, confusion, ataxia, headache, insomnia, seizures,
- Negative inotropic effect, producing hypotension,
- Weak β-adrenoceptor antagonist activity – can cause bronchoconstriction in people with asthma,
- Proarrhythmic effects.

CLASS II DRUGS

Beta-adrenoceptor antagonists

Antagonist activity at cardiac β_1-adrenoceptors is responsible for the antiarrhythmic effects of this class. The most widely used agents for the treatment of rhythm disturbances are atenolol, metoprolol, bisoprolol and propranolol, but all β-adrenoceptor antagonists have antiarrhythmic activity. Beta-adrenoceptor antagonists are discussed in more detail in Chapters 5 and 6.

Esmolol is an ultra-short-acting β_1-adrenoceptor-selective agent used exclusively for the treatment of arrhythmias. It is most often used when arrhythmias arise during anaesthesia.

Pharmacokinetics

Esmolol is given by bolus intravenous injection. Its half-life is very short (about 9 minutes), as it is metabolised rapidly by esterases after uptake by erythrocytes.

CLASS III DRUGS

Amiodarone

Amiodarone is a drug with multiple antiarrhythmic actions. It has class III actions by blocking several types of K^+ channels and shows use-dependence (see above). However, amiodarone also has a class Ib-like action on Na^+ channels as well as noncompetitive β-adrenoceptor antagonist (class II) activity and calcium channel-blocking (class IV) actions. The antiarrhythmic effects produced early after intravenous infusion are believed to be due to β-adrenoceptor antagonist activity, since the class III effect is delayed.

Pharmacokinetics

Amiodarone can be given by mouth or by intravenous infusion for a more rapid onset of action. It has a large volume of distribution as a result of extensive uptake in adipose tissue. Both amiodarone and its major hepatic metabolite have extremely long half-lives (50–60 days), so a prolonged loading dose regimen is used for both routes of administration.

Unwanted effects

- Gastrointestinal disturbances – for example, constipation and nausea, occurring most often during the loading period.
- Reversible corneal microdeposits develop in almost all people and can cause dazzling by lights when driving at night.
- Amiodarone has a high iodine content and a structural relationship to thyroid hormone. In iodine-sufficient areas (such as the United Kingdom), inhibition of intracellular thyroxine (T_4) transport and 5′-deiodinase by amiodarone reduces the conversion of T_4 to active triiodothyronine (T_3) (see Chapter 41). This produces hypothyroidism in about 10% of those treated. Hypothyroidism can be treated by levothyroxine replacement without stopping amiodarone (see Chapter 41). Amiodarone can also exacerbate underlying asymptomatic autoimmune thyroid disease. By contrast, in people who are iodine-deficient, amiodarone

can produce a destructive thyroiditis with release of preformed thyroid hormone, leading to thyrotoxicosis in up to 10% of those taking it. Amiodarone-induced thyrotoxicosis is often resistant to treatment. Thyroid function should be checked every 6 months during treatment.

- Photosensitive skin rashes are common, and the use of wide-spectrum sunscreen is recommended. Slate-grey skin discoloration can also occur.
- Peripheral neuropathy or myopathy.
- Hepatitis and cirrhosis occur rarely.
- Progressive pneumonitis and lung fibrosis are rare but serious effects of long-term treatment.
- Proarrhythmic effects.
- Drug interactions: the plasma concentrations of warfarin (see Chapter 11) and digoxin (see Chapter 7) are increased by amiodarone, with consequent potentiation of their effects. Amiodarone inhibits the metabolism of warfarin. It displaces digoxin from tissue stores and inhibits its renal excretion, both of which actions increase the risk of digoxin toxicity.

Unlike most antiarrhythmic drugs, amiodarone does not have negative inotropic effects.

Sotalol

Sotalol is a nonselective β-adrenoceptor antagonist (see Chapter 5) with additional class III properties. It selectively blocks the I_{Kr} current (which is particularly involved in phase 2 and 3 repolarisation) and shows reverse use-dependence (higher receptor binding when the channel is closed), so that sotalol is most effective at slow rates of cell depolarisation (bradycardia). Sotalol is a racemic mixture; the L-isomer has both β-adrenoceptor antagonist and class III activity, whereas the D-isomer has only class III activity. The class III activity gives sotalol a greater proarrhythmic potential than other β-adrenoceptor antagonists (see above). Sotalol is reserved for the treatment of significant cardiac rhythm disturbances and is not used for the other indications for β-adrenoceptor antagonists.

Pharmacokinetics

Sotalol is excreted unchanged in the urine. Its half-life is 7–18 hours.

Unwanted effects

These are discussed in Chapter 5. Sotalol also has proarrhythmic activity (see above).

CLASS IV DRUGS

Calcium channel blockers

Verapamil and diltiazem (see Chapter 5), but not the dihydropyridine calcium channel blockers such as amlodipine, have antiarrhythmic activity. Verapamil can be given intravenously for a rapid effect but should not be given together with a β-adrenoceptor antagonist because of summation of myocardial depression and AV nodal conduction block. Details of calcium channel blockers can be found in Chapter 5.

OTHER DRUGS FOR CARDIAC RHYTHM DISTURBANCES

Those drugs used for the management of rhythm disturbances that do not fit into the Vaughan Williams classification are considered here.

Digitalis glycosides

Digitalis glycosides (such as digoxin) are not strictly antiarrhythmic, but they are useful for controlling ventricular rate in atrial flutter and atrial fibrillation (AF) by reducing conduction through the AV node. Digitalis glycosides are discussed in Chapter 7.

Adenosine

Mechanism of action and effects

Adenosine is a purine nucleoside with electrophysiological actions mediated by the A_1 subtype of specific G protein-coupled adenosine receptors. These receptors activate inward rectifier K_{ACh} channels, enhancing the flow of K^+ out of myocardial cells and hyperpolarising the resting cell (see Table 8.1). In addition, adenosine antagonises the stimulatory effects of noradrenaline on Ca^{2+} currents. These actions combine to stabilise the myocardial cell transmembrane ion fluxes. Adenosine has potent effects on the SA node, producing sinus bradycardia. It also slows impulse conduction through the AV node but has no effect on conduction in the ventricles. Consequently it is useful only for the management of supraventricular arrhythmias, particularly those caused by AV nodal reentry mechanisms.

An additional action of adenosine at A_2 adenosine receptors reduces Ca^{2+} uptake in vascular smooth muscle and produces vasodilation. In the coronary circulation, preferential dilation of healthy arteries produces coronary blood flow 'steal', which reduces flow in stenosed arteries. This receptor action enables adenosine to be used as a pharmacological stress to induce myocardial ischaemia in people with coronary artery disease, which can then be assessed by imaging the myocardium with radionuclide scanning, magnetic resonance imaging or echocardiography.

Pharmacokinetics

Adenosine is given by rapid bolus intravenous injection. The effect is terminated by uptake into erythrocytes and endothelial cells, followed by metabolism to inosine and hypoxanthine. Adenosine has a half-life of less than 10 seconds and its duration of action is less than 1 minute.

Unwanted effects

Unwanted effects are common and occur in about 25% of those given adenosine, but they last less than 1 minute. They include the following.

- Bradycardia and AV block.
- Malaise, facial flushing, headache, chest pain or tightness, bronchospasm; adenosine should be avoided in people with asthma.
- Drug interactions – dipyridamole (see Chapter 11) potentiates the effects of adenosine, while methylxanthines such as aminophylline (see Chapter 12) inhibit its action.

Atropine

Atropine (see Chapter 4) is an antimuscarinic drug given by intravenous bolus injection that reduces the inhibitory effect of the vagus nerve on the heart. Blockade of muscarinic M_2 receptors increases the rate of firing of the SA node and increases conduction through the AV node. This is due to inhibition of inward rectifying K_{ACh} channels, which prevents hyperpolarisation of the cell membrane (see Table 8.1) and enhanced activation of pacemaker f-channels by increasing the availability of cAMP. Atropine is used specifically for the treatment of sinus bradycardia and AV block. It is metabolised in the liver and has a half-life of 2–5 hours.

Magnesium sulphate

Intravenous magnesium sulphate is used to control the ventricular arrhythmia torsade de pointes and digitalis-induced VA. The mechanism is not well understood, but may involve blockade of transmembrane Ca^{2+} currents. Flushing is the main unwanted effect.

DRUG TREATMENT OF ARRHYTHMIAS

Arrhythmias can be asymptomatic or can produce a variety of consequences that range from mild symptoms to a life-threatening reduction of cardiac output. The probability of developing symptoms depends on several factors, the most important of which are the rate of an abnormal rhythm and the presence of underlying heart disease. The range of consequences of rhythm disturbances includes:

- awareness of palpitation,
- dizziness,
- syncope,
- precipitation of angina or heart failure,
- sudden death.

Treatment may not be necessary for brief self-terminating arrhythmias with minimal symptoms; reassurance may be all that is required. For some arrhythmias it may be possible to remove or treat an underlying cause, such as an electrolyte disturbance.

The choice of treatment depends on the situation. With most tachyarrhythmias, sinus rhythm should be restored if possible. Direct current (DC) cardioversion is used to achieve this in severe, life-threatening, or drug-resistant arrhythmias. Drug therapy is used if there is less need for an immediate effect or to control the ventricular rate if the abnormal rhythm cannot be terminated. Radiofrequency ablation of an arrhythmogenic focus or pathway is increasingly used to prevent arrhythmia. This is carried out after intracardiac electrophysiological studies, using a cardiac catheter. Long-term drug treatment for bradyarrhythmias is not possible; an implanted pacemaker may be necessary.

SUPRAVENTRICULAR ARRHYTHMIAS

Atrial premature beats

Atrial premature beats are very common and usually benign, but sometimes they arise as a consequence of digoxin toxicity; frequent multifocal atrial ectopics can also result from organic heart disease. Other than treatment of an underlying cause, specific drug therapy is rarely needed. Some people are disturbed by a postectopic pause followed by a more forceful beat when sinus rhythm recommences. If treatment is required, a β-adrenoceptor antagonist or a calcium channel blocker such as verapamil or diltiazem can be used to suppress the ectopics.

Atrial tachycardia

Atrial tachycardia (AT) is an infrequent rhythm disturbance usually arising from an automatic focus that produces an atrial rate of 150–250 beats/minute. There is often an associated AV conduction block with faster heart rates, since the AV node will still be in its refractory period when some of the impulses reach it. This prevents all of the atrial impulses reaching the ventricle and results in a slower ventricular rate. AT is not usually associated with significant cardiac disease but can be a manifestation of digitalis toxicity. If drug therapy is necessary, an AV nodal blocking agent such as a β-adrenoceptor antagonist or calcium channel blocker (verapamil or diltiazem) will control the ventricular rate but rarely restores sinus rhythm. Sinus rhythm can be achieved with a class Ic antiarrhythmic agent such as flecainide given with an AV nodal blocking drug (flecainide alone increases the risk of 1:1 AV nodal conduction and a paradoxical increase in the ventricular rate if the atrial rate slows sufficiently, but sinus rhythm is not restored). Sotalol or amiodarone can also be used to maintain sinus rhythm. Ablation of the initiating focus may also be considered.

A less common form of AT is multifocal AT arising from several ectopic foci, usually in people with severe pulmonary disease. If treatment is needed, calcium channel blockers are usually used for ventricular rate control.

Atrial flutter

In atrial flutter, the atrial rate is usually 250–350 beats/minute and the impulses are conducted to the ventricles with 2:1 or greater degrees of AV block. Flutter waves may be obvious on the ECG or appear if the ventricular rate is slowed by transiently increasing the degree of AV block using vagal stimulation (such as carotid sinus massage) or the administration of adenosine. Atrial flutter usually arises from a macro reentrant circuit in the right atrium. Underlying causes include recent cardiac surgery, cor pulmonale and congenital heart disease, but it can arise for no obvious reason. It may be paroxysmal and can degenerate into AF.

Drug therapy is relatively unsuccessful for restoring sinus rhythm, and DC cardioversion (synchronised to discharge on the R wave of the ECG) or rapid 'overdrive' electrical pacing to capture the ventricle followed by a gradual reduction in the paced rate may be required. Class Ic and III antiarrhythmic agents, such as sotalol or amiodarone, can prevent recurrence of paroxysmal atrial flutter. If a class Ic agent such as flecainide or propafenone is used, an AV nodal blocking drug (such as a β-adrenoceptor antagonist or a calcium channel blocker) should be given concurrently, since the atrial rate could slow with 1:1 AV conduction, causing an unacceptably high ventricular rate (see also AT, discussed earlier).

Control of the ventricular rate in atrial flutter can be achieved in a similar manner to that in AF (see below), but treatment is often less successful. For this reason, radiofrequency ablation of the reentrant pathway via a cardiac catheter is becoming increasingly popular. Anticoagulant prophylaxis against thromboembolism should be given, similar to the treatment for AF.

Atrial fibrillation

Apart from ectopic beats, AF is the most common rhythm disturbance in clinical practice. It has a variety of underlying causes (Box 8.1), some of which may be treatable. In younger people, AF often occurs without any obvious underlying cause; it is then called 'lone' AF. The arrhythmia usually arises from multiple microreentry circuits in the atria, although a rapid ectopic focus in a pulmonary vein may be responsible for triggering the reentry circuits in paroxysmal AF. The ventricular rate will depend on AV nodal function, so that when the AV node conducts well, AF produces a rapid but irregular ventricular rate. AF predisposes to left atrial thrombus formation that begins in the left atrial appendage and can lead to systemic emboli, which most commonly cause stroke. Clinically, three forms of AF are recognised: paroxysmal (intermittent self-limiting episodes), persistent (present for more than 7 days but less than 1 year) and permanent (present for more than 1 year after unsuccessful attempts to maintain sinus rhythm or if a decision has been made not to attempt this).

Management of AF has four components:

- To identify and treat an underlying cause whenever possible.
- To restore or maintain sinus rhythm in paroxysmal or persistent AF (Box 8.2). It is desirable to attempt to restore sinus rhythm in younger people or those who tolerate the rhythm disturbance poorly. In these individuals, symptoms and exercise tolerance are usually improved when they are in sinus rhythm, but the risk of stroke is not removed (see below). There is less justification for restoring sinus rhythm in older people who tolerate the rhythm well because there is no reduction in the risk of thromboembolic events (see below) and their quality of life may not improve. Restoration of sinus rhythm is usually possible in lone AF or when a precipitating factor has been treated. It can be achieved with drugs (pharmacological or chemical

cardioversion), especially if the rhythm disturbance is of recent onset (there is a 40–80% success rate if the arrhythmia is of less than 7 days' duration). QRS-synchronised DC cardioversion is usually required for a more prolonged duration. Pharmacological cardioversion is most rapidly achieved (within a few hours) by using a single oral dose of a class Ic drug such as flecainide or propafenone. These drugs should be avoided if there is underlying structural heart disease, when intravenous amiodarone is preferred, although this takes longer to restore sinus rhythm. Recurrence of AF is most frequent during the first 3–6 months after restoration of sinus rhythm. Drugs are not always recommended for prophylaxis to maintain sinus rhythm after a first cardioversion because of their proarrhythmic effects. However, if there is a high risk of recurrence, sinus rhythm can be maintained with a class Ic drug, sotalol, amiodarone, or dronedarone (see the compendium at the end of this chapter). Amiodarone is the most successful single drug for long-term prevention of recurrence; although it maintains sinus rhythm in only about 75% of people at 1 year, it is superior to the 40% maintenance of sinus rhythm with the other drugs. Digitalis glycosides are ineffective for restoring or maintaining sinus rhythm in paroxysmal AF and should be avoided. Radiofrequency isolation of a pulmonary vein trigger area via a cardiac catheter is becoming increasingly used for younger people with paroxysmal or persistent AF. Other curative procedures are infrequently used.

- To control a rapid ventricular response in persistent or permanent AF. For ventricular rate control both at rest and on exercise, a drug that slows AV nodal conduction – such as a β-adrenoceptor antagonist, verapamil, or diltiazem – should be used. Rate control at rest can be achieved with digoxin, but a rapid heart rate often still occurs during exercise (see Chapter 7), so it is only used alone for sedentary people. A β-adrenoceptor antagonist, verapamil, diltiazem, or amiodarone can be used together with digoxin if rate control is difficult to achieve. Sotalol has no additional benefit in sustained AF and should be avoided because of its greater proarrhythmic activity compared with that of other β-adrenoceptor antagonists. Dronedarone is not used for rate control due to evidence of increased mortality. If drug combinations do not provide satisfactory rate control, AV nodal ablation with insertion of a pacemaker can be considered.

- To reduce thromboembolism by long-term anticoagulation (see Chapter 11). Anticoagulation with warfarin is the treatment of choice in AF associated with rheumatic heart disease or thyrotoxicosis, which have a high risk

---

Box 8.1   **Causes of atrial fibrillation**

Structural heart disease
Hypertension
Coronary heart disease
Valvular heart disease (especially mitral)
Cardiomyopathies
Cardiac surgery
Congenital heart disease (especially atrial septal defect)

Other causes
Major infections
Thyrotoxicosis, myxoedema
Alcohol intoxication
Systemic illness (e.g. amyloid, sarcoidosis)
Pulmonary embolism

Box 8.2   **Factors predicting a high probability of successful restoration of sinus rhythm in people with atrial fibrillation**

Short duration of atrial fibrillation (<1 year)
Younger age (<50 years)
Absence of underlying heart disease
Normal left ventricular function
Little or no enlargement of the left atrium
Withdrawal or treatment of a precipitating factor (e.g. thyrotoxicosis, alcohol)

Table 8.3 CHA$_2$DS$_2$–Vasc score[a] for assessing risk of stroke in nonrheumatic atrial fibrillation

Score	Annual risk of stroke (%)	Recommended thromboprophylaxis
0	0	None
1	1.3	None if only point for being female; consider warfarin or other oral anticoagulant if male
2	2.2	Warfarin or other oral anticoagulant
3	3.2	Warfarin or other oral anticoagulant
4	4.0	Warfarin or other oral anticoagulant
5	6.7	Warfarin or other oral anticoagulant
6	9.8	Warfarin or other oral anticoagulant
7	9.6	Warfarin or other oral anticoagulant
8	6.7	Warfarin or other oral anticoagulant
9	15.2	Warfarin or other oral anticoagulant

[a]The CHA$_2$DS$_2$–Vasc score is a summation of the following component scores: **c**ongestive heart failure, 1; **h**ypertension, 1; **a**ge >75 years, 2; **d**iabetes mellitus, 1; prior **s**troke or transient ischaemic attack, 2; **a**ge 64–74 years, 1; **vasc**ular disease (prior myocardial infarction, peripheral arterial disease, aortic plaque), 1; age 64–74, 1; female gender, 1.

of embolism. In nonrheumatic AF, the risk of embolism is related to the number of associated risk factors according to the CHA$_2$DS$_2$–Vasc score (Table 8.3). Most people with AF, whether sustained or paroxysmal, should take thromboprophylaxis. Warfarin, maintaining the international normalised ratio (INR) between 2 and 3 (see Chapter 11), reduces the risk of thromboembolism by about two-thirds. Non-vitamin K-dependent oral anticoagulants (NOACs) have similar efficacy to warfarin in nonvalvular AF. These include dabigatran, apixaban, edoxaban and rivaroxaban (see Chapter 11) and are increasingly preferred to warfarin because they pose a lower risk of intracranial bleeding and there is no need for monitoring. Oral anticoagulation has little advantage in those at very low risk, when the increased risk of bleeding outweighs the benefit. Even after restoration of sinus rhythm in paroxysmal or persistent AF, people at high risk of thromboembolic events should continue to take thromboprophylaxis, since the risk of stroke does not decrease. This may reflect the high risk of recurrence (often asymptomatic) of AF. Aspirin is ineffective for thromboprophylaxis and should not be used for this purpose. For those unable to take an anticoagulant, occlusion of the left atrial appendage with a mechanical device can be considered.

Junctional (nodal) tachycardias

Junctional tachycardias usually arise from a reentry circuit and are often initiated by an ectopic beat. A macroreentry circuit can form within the AV node if there are two functional intranodal pathways with different recovery times (AV nodal reentrant tachycardia or AVNRT). Such circuits account for 60% of supraventricular tachycardias (SVTs) excluding AF/flutter and are not usually associated with structural cardiac disease. Alternatively, a macroreentry circuit may involve an accessory AV pathway connecting the atria and ventricles, as in Wolff–Parkinson–White syndrome (AV reentrant tachycardia or AVRT), which accounts for 30% of SVTs excluding AF/flutter.

Termination of an acute attack of nodal tachycardia can often be achieved with vagotonic manoeuvres such as carotid sinus massage or by a bolus injection of adenosine. For AVNRT, β-adrenoceptor antagonists, diltiazem or verapamil can be used to treat acute episodes or for prophylaxis. However, if there is an accessory AV pathway (AVRT) diltiazem, verapamil and digoxin should be avoided because selective blockade of the AV node by these drugs can predispose to rapid conduction of atrial arrhythmias through the accessory pathway. AVRTs often respond well to flecainide, sotalol or amiodarone. Radiofrequency ablation of the reentry circuit via a cardiac catheter is being employed increasingly for both AVNRTs and AVRTs.

Immediate management of narrow-complex tachycardia of uncertain origin

If the rhythm is regular, it is often not possible to determine from the ECG whether a narrow-complex tachycardia has an atrial or nodal origin. If vagotonic manoeuvres are unsuccessful and the person is haemodynamically stable, intravenous adenosine should be given. This often converts a junctional tachycardia to sinus rhythm or can slow the ventricular rate sufficiently to identify the origin of the rhythm on an ECG (e.g. revealing flutter waves). If there is a history of severe asthma, intravenous verapamil may be preferred. DC cardioversion should be considered if there is haemodynamic instability.

VENTRICULAR TACHYARRHYTHMIAS

Ventricular ectopic beats

Ventricular ectopic beats often occur in healthy individuals or in association with a variety of cardiac disorders such as ischaemic heart disease and heart failure. They are often asymptomatic. Frequent ventricular ectopic beats after myocardial infarction predict a poorer long-term outcome; however, suppressing such ectopics with class I antiarrhythmic drugs increases mortality and should be avoided. In contrast, β-adrenoceptor antagonists after myocardial infarction may suppress the ectopic beats and reduce the risk of sudden death (see Chapter 5). A β-adrenoceptor antagonist can also suppress ventricular ectopic beats induced by stress or anxiety. In the absence of ischaemic heart disease, symptomatic ventricular ectopic beats that do not respond to a β-adrenoceptor antagonist can be suppressed by a class I drug such as flecainide. Radiofrequency catheter ablation is considered for multiple ventricular ectopic beats that disturb the person's well-being and are not controlled by drugs.

Ventricular tachycardia

VT presents with broad QRS complexes on the ECG (broad-complex tachycardia). Although broad complexes can arise with SVTs (when there is bundle branch block), broad-complex tachycardia is usually treated on the assumption that it is VT. VT is often associated with serious underlying heart disease, such as ischaemic heart disease or heart failure, and is more common following myocardial infarction. It can be either sustained or nonsustained. Sustained VT can be associated with a minimal or absent cardiac output ('pulseless' VT) when it is treated in the same way as VF (see below). Polymorphic or incessant VTs can arise as a complication of antiarrhythmic drug therapy (see above) and with other drugs that prolong the Q–T interval on the ECG.

For sustained VTs, drug options include class Ib antiarrhythmic agents such as lidocaine (especially after myocardial infarction), and amiodarone. Ablation or an implantable cardioverter defibrillator (ICD) is often appropriate to avoid sudden cardiac death. A β-adrenoceptor antagonist can be used with an ICD to reduce the frequency of shocks. Sustained VT is often associated with a poor long-term outlook in ischaemic heart disease, and coronary revascularisation with or without an ICD is often used. During and after the acute phase of myocardial infarction, a β-adrenoceptor antagonist is the treatment of choice to suppress nonsustained VTs.

Polymorphic or incessant VTs do not respond well to conventional treatments. Withdrawal of a precipitant drug, correction of electrolyte imbalance and intravenous magnesium sulphate are the therapies of choice. Temporary transvenous overpacing at a rate of 90–110 beats/minute may prevent recurrence. In the congenital form of long QT syndrome a β-adrenoceptor antagonist is the mainstay of treatment.

Ventricular fibrillation

VF is a potentially lethal arrhythmia that constitutes one form of 'cardiac arrest'. An algorithm for the management of cardiac arrest is regularly updated by the Resuscitation Council (UK) and is shown in Fig. 8.6. The important principles of prolonged resuscitation are the maintenance of adequate cardiac output by external chest compression and oxygenation by artificial inflation of the lungs while attempting to restore sinus rhythm. VF is the commonest arrhythmia in cardiac arrest and it should be assumed to be present unless an ECG is available to show otherwise. It should be treated with immediate DC cardioversion. Adrenaline (epinephrine; see Chapter 4) may be given to vasoconstrict the peripheries and thus maintain pressure in the central arteries perfusing the heart and brain. For recurrent VF, an automatic ICD is usually required. Suppression by long-term use of antiarrhythmic drugs such as sotalol or amiodarone is less commonly used.

BRADYCARDIAS

Sinus bradycardia

Treatment with atropine may be necessary if sinus bradycardia is causing symptoms (e.g. after myocardial infarction or an overdose of a β-adrenoceptor antagonist). Hypotension precipitated by drugs such as streptokinase (see Chapter 11) is often associated with vagally mediated bradycardia, which will respond to atropine.

Atrioventricular block ('heart block')

AV block can be congenital or may accompany a variety of heart diseases. When it occurs after myocardial infarction, it is usually temporary if the infarct is inferior but is often permanent after anterior infarction. First-degree heart block (prolongation of the P–R interval on the ECG but with all P waves conducted to the ventricles) or Wenckebach (Mobitz type 1) second-degree heart block (progressive P–R prolongation until there is a nonconducted P wave) rarely requires treatment. Higher degrees of second-degree block (Mobitz type 2 with regular nonconducted P waves without a preceding P–R prolongation) and third-degree heart or complete heart block (when all P waves are nonconducted and there is a slow escape rhythm arising from tissues below the AV node) should be treated. If complete AV block arises suddenly, loss of consciousness (Stokes–Adams attack) or death can occur. If the onset of heart block is acute, atropine should be given intravenously to increase AV conduction. Alternatively, an intravenous infusion of the nonselective β-adrenoceptor agonist isoprenaline can be used (see Chapter 7). However, external or temporary transvenous electrical cardiac pacing is usually required in an emergency. If the AV block is permanent, the implantation of a permanent electrical cardiac pacemaker is almost always necessary.

SELF-ASSESSMENT

True/false questions

1. The SA node and the AV node have pacemaker activity.
2. Pacemaker cells in the SA node discharge at a higher frequency than those in other parts of the heart.
3. Spontaneous or pacemaker depolarisation during diastole results solely from the influx of Na^+.
4. The influx of Na^+ during phase 0 lasts for only milliseconds.
5. Cells are unable to generate further action potentials during phases 0, 1 and 2 of the action potential.
6. Reducing the gradient of the slope of phase 4 will slow the normal pacemaker rate.
7. Sympathetic and vagal stimulation reduce the slope of phase 4 depolarisation and slow the pacemaker rate.
8. Healthy nonpacemaker cells remain quiescent if not excited by an impulse arising from other regions in the heart.
9. Flecainide blocks Na^+ channels.
10. Beta-adrenoceptor antagonist drugs are useful in stress-induced tachycardias.
11. The antiarrhythmic action of amiodarone depends only on blockade of K^+ channels.
12. Amiodarone reaches steady-state concentrations after several months of treatment.
13. Adenosine is effective in the treatment of VA.
14. Verapamil affects both the plateau phase 2 and phase 4 of the action potential cycle.
15. Combining verapamil and a β-adrenoceptor antagonist may cause AV nodal conduction block.

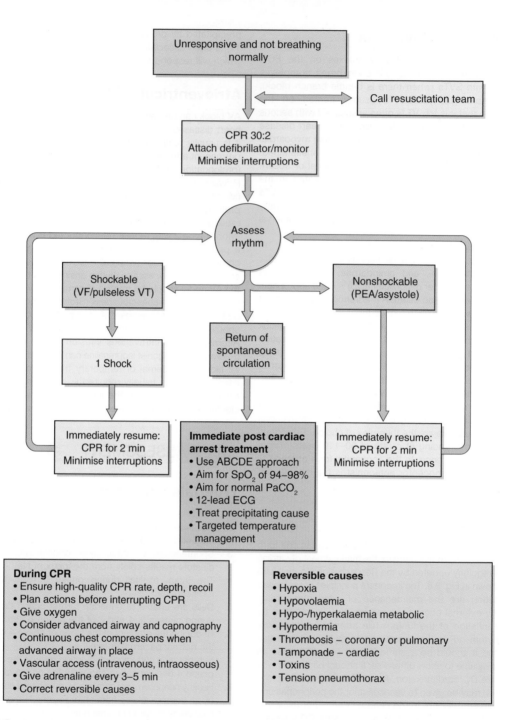

Fig. 8.6 An algorithm for the management of cardiac arrest. *CPR*, Cardiopulmonary resuscitation; *ECG*, electrocardiogram; *EMS*, emergency medical services; *PEA*, pulseless electrical activity; *VF*, ventricular fibrillation; *VT*, ventricular tachycardia. (Modified from the Resuscitation Council [UK] 2015 guidelines for advanced life support. https://www.resus.org.uk/resuscitation-guidelines/adult-advanced-life-support/#algorithm.)

One-best-answer (OBA) question

1. Which change in the flow of ions into or out of cardiac myocytes would most likely prevent arrhythmias?
   A. Increased influx of Na^+ during phase 0 of the action potential
   B. Increased influx of Ca^{2+} during phase 4 of the action potential
   C. Decreased influx of Na^+ during phase 0 of the action potential
   D. Increased influx of Ca^{2+} during phase 2 of the action potential
   E. Decreased efflux of K^+ in phase 3 of the action potential

Case-based questions

Mr G.H., aged 48 years, consulted his GP complaining of palpitations and was found to have an irregular pulse with a rate of 120 beats/minute. He had been suffering from shortness of breath and faintness for the previous 6 hours. The symptoms started after a drinking binge 36 hours earlier. Examination, blood tests (including thyroid function tests), ECG and a chest radiograph showed no coexisting heart disease, diabetes or hypertension. The ECG confirmed AF.

1. What are the options available for treating Mr G.H.?
2. Before any treatment could be instituted, Mr G.H. spontaneously reverted to sinus rhythm. He was well for a year but then returned to his GP with a 3-day history of palpitations, breathlessness, chest pain and dizziness. Examination and an ECG again showed AF. He was referred to a cardiologist and echocardiography showed no evidence of structural cardiac disease. Electrical DC cardioversion was carried out and the rhythm reverted to sinus rhythm. Over the next 5 years, episodes of AF occurred with increasing frequency, and eventually sinus rhythm could not be restored with a variety of antiarrhythmic drugs or by DC conversion. What prophylactic treatment should be considered at the time of DC cardioversion? What drug treatments may be useful after DC cardioversion?

ANSWERS

True/false answers

1. **True.** The SA and AV nodes, the bundle of His and the Purkinje system are pacemaker cells and form the specialised conducting system of the heart.
2. **True.** Pacemaker cells in the SA node therefore initiate cardiac rhythm.
3. **False.** Slow spontaneous depolarisation in pacemaker cells results from an inward flow of Na^+ and K^+ ions (the funny current, I_f).
4. **True.** The fast Na^+ channels for influx close at the end of phase 1.
5. **True.** However, during phase 3, the cells are only relatively refractory to further depolarising stimuli and a sufficient stimulus can fire an action potential during this phase.
6. **True.** The slope in phase 4 controls the normal pacemaker rate as it determines the time taken to reach the threshold potential.
7. **False.** Vagal stimulation reduces the slope of phase 4 and slows the rate of firing, but sympathetic stimulation increases the slope and hence also the firing rate.
8. **True.** However, if the intracellular Ca^{2+} concentration rises abnormally (e.g. under the influence of cardiac glycosides or catecholamines), this can exchange with Na^+ passing inwards, causing membrane depolarisations called *afterdepolarisations* or triggered activity.
9. **True.** All class I antiarrhythmics such as flecainide (class Ic) block fast Na^+ channels and slow the rate of rise of phase 0, therefore reducing myocardial excitability.
10. **True.** Beta-adrenoceptor antagonists reduce the pacemaker depolarisation rate by inhibiting the sympathetic stimulation of the cAMP-dependent funny current (I_f) in the SA and AV nodes.
11. **False.** Like other class III agents, amiodarone blocks several types of K^+ channels but also has a class Ib-like action on Na^+ channels, class II activity (noncompetitive β-adrenoceptor antagonism), and class IV activity (calcium channel blockade).
12. **True.** The accumulation of amiodarone to steady state after about 6 months is due to its lipophilicity, resulting in a high apparent volume of distribution and very long half-life (50–60 days).
13. **False.** Adenosine has no beneficial effect on VA. Its main effect involves enhancing K^+ conductance and inhibiting Ca^{2+} influx, resulting in reduced AV nodal conduction and an increase in the AV nodal refractory period. Adenosine is useful in supraventricular arrhythmias, particularly when caused by AV nodal reentry mechanisms; it has high efficacy and a very short duration of action.
14. **True.** L-type Ca^{2+} channels are involved in the phase 2 plateau, while both T- and L-type channels contribute to depolarisation in phase 0 and the funny current in phase 4. Verapamil acts both to slow the rate of pacemaker depolarisation and reduce the plateau phase, thus shortening the action potential. These effects make verapamil useful in SVTs but not in VA.
15. **True.** Verapamil is a highly negatively inotropic calcium channel blocker, reduces cardiac output, slows the heart rate and impairs AV conduction, so it may cause AV nodal block or heart failure when used with β-adrenoceptor antagonists.

One-best-answer (OBA) answer

1. **Answer C** is correct because decreased Na^+ inflow during phase 0 slows the rate of depolarisation and is one of the mechanisms by which class I antiarrhythmics exert their therapeutic actions. Answers A and B are incorrect as they would increase depolarisation rate in phase 4 and the rate of firing of the SA and AV nodes. Answers D and E are incorrect as they would shorten action potential duration, thus increasing the likelihood of arrhythmias.

Case-based answers

1. The aim at this stage is to restore and maintain sinus rhythm in Mr G.H., who appears to have no structural heart disease. Since the arrhythmia is of short duration,

pharmacological cardioversion may be successful. This could be achieved by flecainide, propafenone or amiodarone. Amiodarone is usually reserved for people with significant cardiac dysfunction or those refractory to other agents. Flecainide and propafenone should be avoided in people with significant cardiac dysfunction or concomitant ischaemic heart disease. However, they are probably suitable for this man. Digoxin, calcium channel blockers and β-adrenoceptor antagonists are ineffective for *terminating* AF. Synchronised DC cardioversion is successful in up to 90% of people with AF who have no structural heart disease or heart failure, who are below 50 years of age, and whose duration of AF is less than 1 year. It could be considered if drugs are unsuccessful. About 50% of the time, recent-onset AF (of less than 48 hours' duration) spontaneously converts to sinus rhythm. In Mr G.H., the AF could have been brought on by excessive alcohol use (the so-called holiday heart). If he moderates his alcohol intake, prophylaxis would not be necessary after a single attack.

2. Anticoagulation with warfarin is essential for at least 3–4 weeks before and 4 weeks after a DC cardioversion to minimise the risk of a systemic embolus. For prophylaxis against recurrence, antifibrillatory drugs are usually given for at least 3–6 months following DC cardioversion, since this is the period of highest risk of recurrence. Digoxin, verapamil and β-adrenoceptor antagonists are not effective for prophylaxis. After 5 years of recurrence of AF, sinus rhythm cannot be restored. Therefore the aim in Mr G.H. is to control the ventricular rate. Digoxin suppresses AV nodal conduction and can reduce the ventricular response rate. This is mediated through potentiation of vagal effects on the heart and is less effective during exercise; therefore, a β-adrenoceptor antagonist or calcium channel blocker (such as verapamil) is preferred. However, β-adrenoceptor antagonists in high doses and verapamil are negatively inotropic; if there is significant cardiac dysfunction or heart failure, they are contraindicated. The positive inotropic action of digoxin might be helpful if there is coexisting left ventricular impairment. The major long-term consequence of AF is the risk of thromboembolism, which is greatest in those over 75 years of age. For Mr G.H., no thromboprophylaxis is required as he is at a relatively low risk of stroke because of his age and lack of any coexisting hypertension, diabetes mellitus, or significant left ventricular impairment.

FURTHER READING

Dumotier, B.M., 2014. A straightforward guide to the basic science behind arrhythmogenesis. Heart 100, 1907–1915.

Freedman, B., Potpara, T.S., Lip, G.Y.H., 2016. Stroke prevention in atrial fibrillation. Lancet 388, 806–817.

Gupta, A., Lawrence, A.T., Krishnan, K., et al., 2007. Current concepts in the mechanisms and management of drug-induced QT prolongation and torsade de pointes. Am. Heart J. 153, 891–899.

Link, M.S., 2012. Evaluation and initial treatment of supraventricular tachycardia. N. Engl. J. Med. 367, 1438–1448.

Piccini, J.P., Fauchier, L., 2016. Rhythm control in atrial fibrillation. Lancet 388, 829–840.

Prystowsky, E.N., Padanilam, B.J., Joshi, S., et al., 2012. Ventricular arrhythmias in the absence of structural heart disease. J. Am. Coll. Cardiol. 59, 1733–1744.

Resuscitation Council (UK). Adult advanced life support, 2015. https://www.resus.org.uk/resuscitation-guidelines/adult-advanced-life-support. (Accessed 10 October 2016).

Roberts-Thomson, K.C., Lau, D.H., Sanders, P., 2011. The diagnosis and management of ventricular arrhythmias. Nat. Rev. Cardiol. 8, 311–321.

Van Gelder, I.C., Rienstra, M., Crijns, H.J.G.M., et al., 2016. Rate control in atrial fibrillation. Lancet 388, 818–828.

Vogler, J., Breithardt, G., Eckardt, L., 2012. Bradyarrhythmias and conduction blocks. Rev. Esp. Cardiol. 65, 656–667.

Whinnett, Z.I., Sohaib, S.M.A., Davies, D.W., 2012. Diagnosis and management of supraventricular tachycardia. BMJ 345, e7769.

Ziff, O.J., Camm, A.J., 2016. Individualized approaches to thromboprophylaxis in atrial fibrillation. Am. Heart J. 173, 143–158.

Compendium: drugs used to treat cardiac arrhythmias

Drug	Characteristics
Drugs are listed by their main effect on the cardiac action potential according to the Vaughan Williams classification, although some antiarrhythmic drugs have multiple sites and mechanisms of action. The types of arrhythmias commonly treated are AF, AT, SVT, VA, VF and VT.	
Class I drugs: sodium channel blockers ('membrane stabilisers')	
Disopyramide	Class Ia drug. Used for SVT, VF and VT but rarely in the United Kingdom. Given orally or by slow intravenous injection (over at least 5 min) or intravenous infusion. Half-life: 4–10 h
Flecainide	Class Ic drug. Used for AF, SVT. Given orally or by slow intravenous injection (over 10–30 min) or intravenous infusion (for resistant ventricular tachyarrhythmias). Half-life: 12–30 h
Lidocaine	Class Ib drug. Used for VT in haemodynamically stable patients and for VF and pulseless VT in cardiac arrest refractory to defibrillation. Given by intravenous injection or intravenous infusion. Half-life: 2 h
Mexelitine	Class 1b drug. Available in the United Kingdom only from special-order manufacturers or specialist importers; used for life-threatening VA. Given orally or intravenously. Half-life: 10–12 h

Compendium: drugs used to treat cardiac arrhythmias (cont'd)

Drug	Characteristics
Procainamide	Class Ia drug. Available in the United Kingdom only from special-order manufacturers or specialist importers; used for VA. Given by slow intravenous injection or intravenous infusion. Half-life: 6–9 h
Propafenone	Class Ic drug; also has some β-adrenoceptor antagonist (class II) activity. Used for VA and some SVTs. Given orally. Half-life: 4–17 h

Class II drugs: β-adrenoceptor antagonists

β-Adrenoceptor antagonists are used in a wide variety of indications and are listed in the drug compendium at the end of Chapter 5. The β-adrenoceptor antagonists most commonly used in arrhythmia are atenolol, bisoprolol, esmolol and propranolol. See also sotalol in class III below.

Class III drugs: potassium channel blockers

Amiodarone	Blocks potassium channels but also has class Ib, class II and class IV actions. Used for paroxysmal SVT, VT, AF and VF, with treatment usually initiated in hospital or under specialist supervision. Given orally or by intravenous injection (over 3 min) for VF. Half-life: 50–60 days
Dronedarone	Multichannel blocker; related to amiodarone but has less complicated dosing due to shorter half-life. Used for maintenance of sinus rhythm after cardioversion in those who are clinically stable with paroxysmal or persistent AF when alternative treatments are unsuitable. Given orally. Half-life: 25–30 h
Sotalol	Blocks potassium channels but is also a nonselective β-adrenoceptor antagonist (class II). Used for life-threatening VT and prophylaxis of SVT and AF. Given orally or by intravenous injection (over 10 min). Half-life: 7–18 h

Class IV drugs: calcium channel blockers

Dihydropyridine calcium channel blockers (see Chapter 5) have no antiarrhythmic activity.

Diltiazem	Nondihydropyridine calcium channel blocker. Not licensed for arrhythmia in the United Kingdom. Given orally. Half-life: 2–5 h
Verapamil	Nondihydropyridine calcium channel blocker. Used for SVT. Given orally or by intravenous injection. Half-life: 2–7 h

Other drugs

Adenosine	Purine nucleoside. Used as the treatment of choice for terminating paroxysmal SVT. Given intravenously. Half-life: 10 s
Atropine	Muscarinic receptor antagonist. Used for bradycardia, especially if complicated by hypotension. Given intravenously. Half-life: 2–5 h
Digoxin	Cardiac glycoside (see Chapter 7). Used for AF. Given orally or intravenously. Half-life: 20–50 h
Magnesium sulphate	Magnesium salt. Used for emergency treatment of *serious arrhythmias*, especially in presence of hypokalaemia, hypomagnesaemia or torsade de pointes. Given intravenously over 10–15 min

AF, Atrial fibrillation; *AT,* atrial tachycardia; *SVT,* supraventricular tachycardia; *VA,* ventricular arrhythmias; *VF,* ventricular fibrillation; *VT,* ventricular tachycardia.

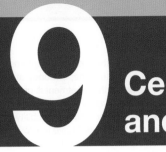

9 Cerebrovascular disease and dementia

STROKE

AETIOLOGY

Strokes are a major cause of morbidity and mortality, particularly in older people. They present as transient or permanent neurological disturbances caused by ischaemic infarction or haemorrhagic disruption of neuronal pathways in the brain.

Ischaemic strokes and transient ischaemic attacks

Ischaemic strokes and transient ischaemic attacks (TIAs) account for about 85% of cerebrovascular events. Cerebral infarction can result from intracerebral arterial thrombosis or emboli travelling to the cerebral arteries, typically from an unstable atheromatous plaque in an internal carotid artery (see also Chapter 5) or from the heart. Following occlusion of a cerebral artery, the extent and duration of the resulting functional deficit are very variable.

TIAs arise from small cerebral arterial emboli that briefly interrupt blood flow but disperse rapidly. They produce short-lived neurological signs and symptoms but leave no functional deficit 24 hours later. A completed stroke results from more prolonged cerebral ischaemia, which produces infarction. The neurological disturbance in completed stroke persists for more than 24 hours and frequently there is some permanent loss of function. Following a TIA there is a high risk of a completed stroke in the subsequent 7 days and a 30% risk of a completed stroke in the subsequent 5 years. However, the risk varies widely according to the features at presentation.

Haemorrhagic strokes

Primary intracerebral haemorrhage is responsible for up to 15% of strokes. It often arises from rupture of microaneurysms on intracerebral arteries, usually in association with hypertension. Less commonly, a haemorrhagic stroke arises from an intracerebral arteriovenous malformation or secondary to a subarachnoid haemorrhage. Haemorrhagic strokes frequently leave a permanent functional deficit.

PREVENTION AND TREATMENT

Current treatments produce only a modest limitation of the neurological deficit in acute ischaemic stroke and there are no specific treatments for haemorrhagic stroke. Most management is therefore directed to

- primary prevention of a first event,
- prevention of recurrence of stroke or of other cardiovascular events,
- rehabilitation after the stroke.

About one-third of strokes are recurrent. The recurrence rate for ischaemic stroke is about 3–7% per year for individuals who are in sinus rhythm and about 12% per year for those in atrial fibrillation.

Primary prevention of ischaemic stroke

- **Blood pressure reduction.** Hypertension is the single most powerful predictor of both ischaemic and haemorrhagic stroke. Pooled trial results indicate that a reduction in diastolic blood pressure by 5–6 mm Hg reduces the risk of stroke by about 40% (see Chapter 6). For isolated systolic hypertension, a similar reduction in risk has been shown after an average reduction of 11 mm Hg in systolic blood pressure.
- **Smoking cessation.** The risk of ischaemic stroke is reduced by up to 40% by 2–5 years after smoking cessation. This is probably due to slower progression of arterial atherothrombotic disease.
- **Inhibition of blood clotting.** Oral anticoagulation (see Chapters 8 and 11) in people with atrial fibrillation reduces

the risk of a first ischaemic stroke by 70%. Warfarin, at a dosage giving an international normalised ratio (INR) of 2–3, or one of the non-vitamin K-dependent oral anticoagulants (e.g. apixaban, dabigatran or rivaroxaban) can be used. For people in sinus rhythm, anticoagulation has no advantage over aspirin. Warfarin reduces the risk of stroke following myocardial infarction if there is intracardiac clot associated with an akinetic area of the left ventricular wall.

- Low-dose aspirin does *not* prevent a first ischaemic stroke when taken by healthy individuals who are in sinus rhythm or atrial fibrillation. For people with atrial fibrillation, treatment with aspirin and clopidogrel reduces the risk of a first ischaemic stroke less than anticoagulation but with the same bleeding risk (see Chapter 8).
- **Cholesterol reduction.** Reduction of a raised plasma cholesterol with a statin (see Chapter 48) produces a 25% reduction in the risk of a first stroke, although much of the evidence for this effect derives from trials in people who already have clinical evidence of vascular disease or diabetes mellitus.
- **Carotid endarterectomy or stenting.** This is sometimes recommended for asymptomatic carotid artery disease when the stenosis exceeds 60%, but the annual risk of an ischaemic stroke is low in this situation.

Primary prevention of haemorrhagic stroke

- Blood pressure reduction. Lowering a raised blood pressure is the only means of reducing the risk of cerebral haemorrhage.

Treatment of acute ischaemic stroke

Fibrinolytic therapy with recombinant tissue plasminogen activator (rt-PA, alteplase; see Chapter 11) can reduce the long-term neurological deficit after an ischaemic stroke. If treatment is started within 4.5 hours of the onset of symptoms, thrombolysis reduces the risk of death or dependency at 3 months, with greater benefit the earlier that treatment is given. Overall, 7% more people who are given a fibrinolytic drug after an ischaemic stroke will have no or minimal disability 3 months later and an additional one-third will have improved function. About 6% of people who are treated will have a symptomatic intracranial haemorrhage after thrombolysis, with a higher risk in those with a blood pressure above 185/110 mm Hg or when treatment is delayed, which can outweigh the benefit from neuronal salvage. Indications and usual contraindications for fibrinolytic therapy in acute stroke are shown in Box 9.1. Anticoagulants or antiplatelet drugs should not be given for 24 hours after thrombolysis.

There have been recent advances in the treatment of acute ischaemic stroke. Intra-arterial alteplase may be more effective in large ischaemic strokes than intravenous delivery. Mechanical thrombectomy devices to treat proximal artery thrombus are increasingly used alone or as an adjunctive treatment after thrombolysis and extend the time for intervention up to 6 hours. The use of sensitive brain imaging may help to identify those who have potentially recoverable neurological injury from those with irreversible infarction.

Secondary prevention of recurrent ischaemic stroke

Many treatments are similar to those used for primary prevention of ischaemic stroke (see above).

- **Blood pressure reduction.** Lowering blood pressure after a stroke will reduce the risk of recurrence by 30–40%. There is considerable reluctance to reduce blood pressure in the first few days after a stroke because of concern that cerebral perfusion pressure may fall too much if the normal cerebral arterial autoregulation has been disturbed by the stroke. However, there is some evidence that early treatment (after the first 24 hours) may be advantageous.

Box 9.1 Usual indications and contraindications for thrombolysis in acute ischaemic stroke

Indications for thrombolysis
- Clinical diagnosis of ischaemic stroke causing measurable neurological deficit for at least 30 min
- Onset of symptoms less than 4.5 h before beginning treatment
- The patient and family understand the potential risks and benefits of therapy
- Intracranial haemorrhage excluded by CT or MRI of the head

Potential contraindications to thrombolysis
- Severe stroke deficit on clinical assessment
- Head trauma or prior stroke in past 3 months
- Any previous stroke with concomitant diabetes mellitus
- Gastrointestinal or genitourinary haemorrhage in previous 21 days
- Arterial puncture in noncompressible site during previous 7 days
- Major surgery in previous 14 days
- History of previous intracranial haemorrhage
- Evidence of acute trauma or haemorrhage
- Taking an oral anticoagulant (or if so, INR greater than 1.4 when treating in under 3 h)
- Heparin within 48 h unless the activated partial thromboplastin time is normal
- Seizure at the onset of the stroke
- Systolic blood pressure above 185 mm Hg or diastolic blood pressure above 110 mm Hg
- Platelet count of less than 100×10^9 L
- Blood glucose less than 2.7 mmol/L

CT, Computed tomography; *INR,* international normalised ratio; *MR,* magnetic resonance.

- **Inhibition of platelet aggregation.** Low-dose aspirin with dipyridamole can be used following a TIA for people who are in sinus rhythm. The combination reduces the risk of a subsequent nonfatal stroke by about 35% and is more effective than aspirin alone. This combination is recommended for up to 2 years after a TIA, when the risk of recurrent stroke is highest, after which aspirin is often used alone. Clopidogrel alone (see Chapter 11) is as effective as the combination of aspirin and dipyridamole after ischaemic stroke and is now the preferred treatment. By contrast, the combination of aspirin and clopidogrel is no more effective than aspirin alone for long-term prevention (unlike the case in acute coronary syndromes; see Chapter 5) and increases the risk of serious bleeding. However, there may be some benefit from the combination for short-term treatment (7–30 days) immediately after a stroke or TIA in those at high risk for recurrence. Warfarin has no role in preventing recurrent stroke in people who are in sinus rhythm.
- **Inhibition of blood clotting.** After a first stroke in people with atrial fibrillation, oral anticoagulation reduces the risk of a further stroke by two-thirds. Antiplatelet drugs have no protective effect in this situation (see Chapter 11).
- **Cholesterol reduction.** Cholesterol reduction with a statin is effective in the secondary prevention of ischaemic stroke, reducing recurrent stroke by 20% for every 1 mmol/L reduction in low-density lipoprotein (LDL) cholesterol. However, the greatest advantage of cholesterol reduction in this situation lies in the prevention of ischaemic cardiac events, since coronary artery disease often coexists with atheromatous cerebrovascular disease.
- **Carotid endarterectomy or stenting.** This reduces the risk of recurrent stroke if there have already been transient focal neurological symptoms in the cerebral territory supplied by a diseased carotid artery. If the stenosis is ≥70% of the vessel diameter (but without near total occlusion), then endarterectomy reduces the risk of recurrent stroke by about two-thirds over the subsequent 2 years (despite a perioperative risk of stroke or death of 3–5%). There is no benefit from surgery if the occlusion is less than 50%, and only marginal benefit if the occlusion is between 50% and 69%. Surgery should be carried out within 2 weeks of the initial ischaemic event, when the risk of recurrence is highest.

Secondary prevention of recurrent haemorrhagic stroke

- **Blood pressure reduction.** Lowering blood pressure after a haemorrhagic stroke will reduce the risk of recurrence by up to 40%. The reduction in risk from treating hypertension is greater than for ischaemic stroke, and even lowering a 'normal' blood pressure may be effective. As for ischaemic stroke, unless the blood pressure exceeds 185/105 mm Hg, treatment is usually delayed to allow for the return of autoregulation of cerebral blood flow.

SUBARACHNOID HAEMORRHAGE

Most subarachnoid haemorrhages are caused by rupture of a saccular (or berry) aneurysm on an intracranial artery, usually on or close to the circle of Willis. These aneurysms are acquired during life and the cause is unknown, although there is an association with hypertension and conditions that increase cerebral blood flow, such as arteriovenous malformations. About 5% of all strokes are caused by subarachnoid haemorrhage. Sudden onset of a severe occipital headache is the most common presenting symptom, but focal neurological signs or progressive confusion and impaired consciousness can occur. Rebleeding is a significant cause of disability and death; early surgical intervention in survivors of the initial bleed reduces this risk. However, a more common cause of permanent neurological disability or later death is delayed cerebral ischaemia. This is produced by cerebral vasospasm, which develops in about 25% of cases, usually at least 3 days after the haemorrhage. The mechanism is poorly understood but involves activation of voltage-dependent L-type Ca^{2+} channels in intracranial arteries. It presents with confusion, decreased consciousness, and new focal neurological deficits.

DRUGS FOR SUBARACHNOID HAEMORRHAGE

Nimodipine

Nimodipine is a dihydropyridine L-type calcium channel blocker (for mechanism of action, see Chapter 5). It is an arterial vasodilator with some selectivity for cerebral arteries that reduces the risk of vasospasm following subarachnoid haemorrhage but probably produces most of its benefits by protecting ischaemic neurons from Ca^{2+} overload. There is a theoretical risk that cerebral arterial vasodilation may actually facilitate further bleeding, but this does not appear to be a problem in practice.

Pharmacokinetics

Nimodipine undergoes extensive first-pass metabolism in the liver and gut wall. It has a half-life of 8–9 hours and is eliminated by metabolism in the liver.

Unwanted effects

These are mainly caused by arterial dilation and include:

- hypotension, which can have a detrimental effect on cerebral perfusion,
- headache, flushing, sweating.

MANAGEMENT OF SUBARACHNOID HAEMORRHAGE

Initial treatment of subarachnoid haemorrhage aims to reduce ischaemic cerebral damage. Nimodipine is usually given orally for 5–10 days. Intravenous fluids are given to maintain euvolaemia and avoid hypotension. The optimum blood pressure in the early period after the haemorrhage is not known, but hypotension should be avoided and blood pressure lowered modestly in those who present with significant hypertension. Mannitol (see Chapter 14) may be used to reduce cerebral oedema.

The definitive management of subarachnoid haemorrhage is surgical, with endovascular coil occlusion of the aneurysm or clipping of the neck of the aneurysm that produced the bleeding. In the last 20 years, early surgical intervention combined with medical therapy has reduced mortality from 20% to about 5–10%.

DEMENTIA

Dementia usually begins with forgetfulness and is characterised by disorientation in unfamiliar surroundings, variable mood, restlessness, and poor sleep. Deterioration in social behaviour with self-neglect often follows and may be accompanied by personality change including loss of inhibition. Most dementia results from Alzheimer's disease, cerebrovascular disease (multi-infarct dementia), or a combination of the two, but there are other causes (Box 9.2). Memory impairment in dementia is associated with bilateral hippocampal damage.

ALZHEIMER'S DISEASE

Alzheimer's disease is the commonest cause of dementia in people over the age of 65 years. About 10% of people over the age of 65 and about 30% of those over the age of 85 have some signs of Alzheimer's disease. The onset of symptoms is gradual, with progressive deterioration, unlike the case with vascular dementia. It is a neurodegenerative disorder that begins pathologically 20–30 years before the clinical onset.

The cause of Alzheimer's disease is unknown, but there are several factors associated with the disease.

- **Amyloid protein.** Beta-amyloid is deposited in the medial temporal lobe and cerebral cortex of people with Alzheimer's disease as senile plaques. The initiating factor may be an imbalance between the production and clearance of β-amyloid in the brain, leading to toxic effects on neuronal synapses. Deposition of β-amyloid may be the driver for hyperphosphorylation of tau protein (found in axons, where it promotes microtubule assembly and vesicle transport), which then aggregates into the neurofibrillary tangles characteristic of Alzheimer's disease.
- **Genetic predisposition.** This accounts for about 70% of the risk. Mutations of the apolipoprotein E ε4 allele (APOE ε4, essential for amyloid β clearance) confer a higher risk of late-onset Alzheimer's disease, while mutations in genes coding for β-amyloid precursor protein and presenilin 1 and 2 explain the rare familial version of the disease.
- **Inflammatory factors.** Activated microglia and reactive astrocytes surround the senile plaques, and there is a local increase in proinflammatory mediators.

Box 9.2	Causes of dementia
Treatable causes of dementia	**Irreversible and partially treatable causes of dementia**
Hypothyroidism	Vascular dementia
Neurosyphilis	Alzheimer's disease
Vitamin B₁ deficiency	Lewy body-type dementia
Normal-pressure hydrocephalus	Parkinson's disease dementia
Frontal lobe tumours	Progressive supranuclear palsy
Cerebral vasculitis	Multiple-system atrophy
Cerebral hypoperfusion	

- **Glutamate excitotoxicity.** Amyloid deposits may promote neuronal damage by increasing the neuronal release of glutamate. This acts at *N*-methyl-D-aspartate (NMDA) receptors to generate glutamate-induced excitotoxicity of cholinergic neurons. Hyperactivity of glutamatergic neurons is a common finding in Alzheimer's disease.
- **Oxidative stress.** There is evidence of excessive free radical production in Alzheimer's disease. Increased oxidative stress may contribute to the condition by producing vascular damage, reducing β-amyloid clearance, and promoting metabolic derangement in neurons.
- **Loss of cholinergic neurotransmission.** There is a marked loss of acetylcholine neurotransmitter synthesis in the cerebral cortex and the hippocampus, particularly affecting the areas involved in cognition and in memory. There is also loss of cholinergic neurons. Depletion of other neurotransmitters is a late and inconsistent finding.
- **Vascular disease.** There is considerable overlap between Alzheimer's disease and vascular dementia, and the presence of vascular disease may influence the formation or elimination of amyloid plaques.

Drugs for Alzheimer's disease

Anticholinesterases

donepezil, galantamine, rivastigmine

Mechanisms of action and effects

The basis of the cholinergic hypothesis of Alzheimer's disease is that loss of cholinergic neurons in the basal forebrain nuclei results in abnormal function at cholinergic terminals in the hippocampus and neocortex, which are involved in memory and cognition. Anticholinesterases increase cholinergic transmission in the brain by inhibiting acetylcholinesterase in the synaptic cleft (see Chapter 4).

- Donepezil is a reversible inhibitor of acetylcholinesterase with a high degree of selectivity for the central nervous system (CNS).
- Galantamine is a reversible inhibitor of acetylcholinesterase that also has agonist activity at presynaptic nicotinic receptors by allosterically enhancing the receptor response to acetylcholine.
- Rivastigmine is a slowly reversible inhibitor of acetylcholinesterase with selectivity for the CNS, but it also inhibits pseudocholinesterase (butyrylcholinesterase), which is present in tissues and plasma.

Pharmacokinetics

Donepezil and galantamine are metabolised in the liver; galantamine has a half-life of 5–7 hours while the half-life of donepezil is very long, at 70–80 hours. Rivastigmine is rapidly inactivated by cholinesterase-mediated hydrolysis and has a short half-life of 1–2 hours.

Unwanted effects

- Anorexia, nausea and vomiting, diarrhoea, abdominal pain.

- Drowsiness, hallucination, agitation, dizziness, insomnia, headache.
- Rash, pruritus.
- Bradycardia.

N-methyl-D-aspartate receptor antagonists

memantine

Mechanism of action and effects

Memantine is a derivative of the antiviral drug amantadine (see Chapter 24) and is a noncompetitive antagonist at glutamate NMDA receptors. This may prevent glutamate-induced excitotoxicity by limiting long-lasting influx of Ca^{2+} into neurons but without interfering with the actions of glutamate, which are involved in memory and learning. Memantine is also a 5-HT$_3$ receptor antagonist and a noncompetitive nicotinic receptor antagonist, but the significance of these actions for the treatment of dementia is unknown. Memantine can be used together with an anticholinesterase.

Pharmacokinetics

Memantine is excreted unchanged by the kidneys. It has a very long half-life of 60–80 hours.

Unwanted effects

- Constipation.
- Headache, dizziness, drowsiness.
- Hypertension.
- Dyspnoea.

Treatment of Alzheimer's disease

In the United Kingdom, drug treatment for Alzheimer's disease is started only for people who have a Mini-Mental State Examination (MMSE) score of 10–20 points (moderate dementia). The diagnosis of Alzheimer's disease should first be confirmed in a specialist memory clinic. Current treatments for Alzheimer's disease do not alter progression of the underlying pathology. Since the pathological changes are apparent many years before symptoms arise, intervention before neurodegenerative disease is established might be beneficial. This will become possible only with the introduction of markers for early diagnosis.

All cholinesterase inhibitors produce a similar modest improvement in symptoms and a delay in the decline of cognitive function and memory, in up to two-thirds of those who are treated. Efficacy should be assessed by questioning the person treated or a caretaker after 2–4 months of treatment at the maximum tolerated dose. Treatment should be continued only if the 'global, functional and behavioural condition remains at a level where the drug is considered to be having a worthwhile effect'. Cholinesterase inhibitors delay the decline in mental function by about 3–6 months, but it is not arrested. Rapid progression resumes when the drugs are stopped, but there may be limited benefit from restarting treatment even if it is longer than a month after withdrawal. Anticholinesterases produce some improvement in other functional measures and behaviour, which also affect the quality of life.

Memantine produces moderate improvement in cognition and a reduction in functional decline; it is usually well tolerated. However, it may be ineffective in the early stages of Alzheimer's disease. The combination of a cholinesterase inhibitor with memantine can produce additive benefits.

Neuropsychiatric complications of Alzheimer's disease, such as depression and severe aggression, may require treatment. However, the value of antidepressant therapy is uncertain and antipsychotic drugs can produce significant unwanted effects with only modest benefit.

VASCULAR DEMENTIA

Cerebrovascular disease is a particularly common cause of dementia in people above 85 years of age; overall it is the second most frequent cause of dementia. The deterioration in mental function is produced by multiple cerebral infarcts (multi-infarct dementia), particularly if they affect the white matter. The risk of dementia is increased ninefold in people with stroke. In some of these, dementia may be produced by specific, strategically located infarcts, especially in the angular gyrus of the inferior parietal lobule. In contrast to Alzheimer's disease, the initial presentation is usually more acute and cognitive decline has a stepwise course arising from recurrent cerebrovascular events.

Treatment

- Prophylaxis against cerebral emboli with aspirin or warfarin, depending on the heart rhythm (see prevention of stroke, discussed previously), is often recommended. However, there is no evidence that aspirin is of benefit in vascular dementia in people who are in sinus rhythm.
- Control of hypertension (see Chapter 6). Calcium channel blockers reduce the risk of vascular dementia, but it is likely to be an effect related to blood pressure reduction rather than a more specific effect of this class of drug.
- Anticholinesterases or memantine may produce some improvement in function in vascular dementia.
- Immunosuppressant drugs (see Chapter 38) can be used in the rare cases caused by cerebral vasculitis.

SELF-ASSESSMENT

True/false questions

1. Aspirin reduces the risk of a first stroke in healthy individuals.
2. Aspirin cannot prevent a first stroke in people with persistent atrial fibrillation.
3. Approximately 85% of all strokes have a haemorrhagic aetiology.
4. If thrombolysis with rt-PA (alteplase) is given in acute stroke, antiplatelet and anticoagulant therapies should not be given concurrently.
5. Anticoagulation with warfarin and antiplatelet therapy with aspirin are equal first-choice drugs for the

secondary prevention of recurrent ischaemic strokes in the presence of sinus rhythm.
6. Cerebral ischaemia depolarises neurons and causes the release of large amounts of glutamate.
7. Donepezil is an acetylcholinesterase inhibitor with selectivity for the CNS.
8. Nimodipine reduces the risk of vasospasm following subarachnoid haemorrhage.
9. The NMDA receptor antagonist memantine reduces neurotoxicity caused by the excitatory transmitter glutamate.
10. Cerebral emboli arising from the heart are invariably caused by atrial fibrillation.

One-best-answer (OBA) question

1. Choose the most accurate statement about Alzheimer's disease.
   A. Alzheimer's disease is associated with reduced cholinergic and glutamatergic neurotransmission.
   B. Rivastigmine is prescribed in Alzheimer's disease irrespective of the MMSE score.
   C. Memantine is a muscarinic receptor agonist.
   D. Anticholinesterases should not be coprescribed with memantine.
   E. Unlike donepezil, rivastigmine inhibits both acetyl-cholinesterase and butyrylcholinesterase.

Case-based questions

A 70-year-old man has a blood pressure of 190/110 mm Hg despite intensive antihypertensive drug treatment. He was admitted to hospital 6 hours after the acute onset of unilateral weakness and sensory loss. At the time of admission to hospital, most of the neurological signs had resolved. He had no headache or vomiting and remained conscious and in sinus rhythm. Following clinical examination and a computed tomography (CT) brain scan, this episode was diagnosed as a TIA.
1. Should thrombolysis be given?
2. What other therapies should be instituted immediately?
3. What secondary prevention strategy should be employed?

ANSWERS

True/false answers

1. **False.** Aspirin does not reduce the risk of a first stroke in healthy individuals in sinus rhythm.
2. **False.** Aspirin reduces the risk of a first embolic stroke in atrial fibrillation by about 25% but is less effective than warfarin.
3. **False.** About 85% of strokes have an ischaemic aetiology; up to 15% are caused by intracerebral haemorrhage.
4. **True.** The immediate risk of intracranial haemorrhage with alteplase could be compounded by simultaneous administration of antiplatelet or anticoagulant agents. These should be considered later, when the effect of the thrombolytic has waned.

5. **False.** In people in sinus rhythm, aspirin alone (or together with dipyridamole) reduces the risk of stroke; warfarin is no more effective and poses a greater risk of major bleeding.
6. **True.** The excitatory transmitter glutamate can cause a substantial rise in intracellular Ca^{2+}, causing Ca^{2+} overload and cell death by the generation of free radicals.
7. **True.** Anticholinesterase drugs enhance cholinergic activity in the hippocampus and neocortex, improving memory and cognition.
8. **True.** By blocking L-type calcium channels in the CNS, nimodipine reduces vasospasm and also protects ischaemic neurons from Ca^{2+} overload.
9. **True.** Memantine blocks NMDA (glutamate) receptors and reduces the glutamate-induced excitotoxicity of cholinergic neurons.
10. **False.** Cerebral emboli arising from the heart can also be caused by infected or damaged prosthetic valves or following damage to the myocardium.

One-best-answer (OBA) answer

1. Answer E is correct.
   A. Incorrect. Alzheimer's disease is associated with reduced cholinergic transmission and increased glutamatergic transmission.
   B. Incorrect. In the UK, it is advised that the anticho-linesterases should not be prescribed if the MMSE is below 10.
   C. Incorrect. Memantine is a glutamate NMDA receptor antagonist.
   D. Incorrect. Anticholinesterases and memantine can be useful coprescribed.
   E. **Correct.** Rivastigmine inhibits both acetylcholinesterase and pseudocholinesterase (butyrylcholinesterase), but it is unclear whether its additional inhibition of the latter provides extra clinical benefit.

Case-based answers

1. Thrombolysis is inappropriate in this situation. This man's blood pressure is high and a considerable time (>4.5 hours) has passed since the onset of symptoms. The rapid resolution of signs indicates a TIA, for which thrombolysis is not given. Although thrombolysis has been shown in some trials to be useful in the treatment of stroke, safe and effective use is determined by a rigid set of criteria, as there is a significant risk of intracranial haemorrhage.
2. The patient's blood pressure must be brought under control. Reduction in blood pressure has a major effect on the prevention of a recurrent stroke. He should also be given the antiplatelet drugs aspirin and dipyridamole, or clopidogrel alone.
3. Antiplatelet therapy should be continued. Dipyridamole has additional benefit when given together with aspirin. Cholesterol reduction with a statin is effective in the secondary prevention of ischaemic stroke. It would be worth treating this man with a statin even if his cholesterol were not raised. An important reason for cholesterol reduction is the prevention of ischaemic cardiac events, since coronary artery disease often coexists with atheromatous cerebrovascular disease.

FURTHER READING

Stroke

Davis, S.M., Donnan, G.A., 2012. Secondary prevention after ischaemic stroke or transient ischaemic attack. N. Engl. J. Med. 366, 1914–1922.

Elgendy, I.Y., Mahmoud, A.N., Mansoor, H., et al., 2016. Evolution of acute ischaemic stroke therapy from lysis to thrombectomy: similar or different to acute myocardial infarction? Int. J. Cardiol. 222, 441–447.

Feher, A., Pusch, G., Koltai, K., et al., 2011. Statin therapy in the primary and secondary prevention of ischaemic cerebrovascular disease. Int. J. Cardiol. 148, 131–136.

Prabhakaran, S., Ruff, I., Bernstein, R.A., 2015. Acute stroke intervention: a systematic review. J. Am. Med. Assoc. 313, 1451–1462.

Rothwell, P.M., Algra, A., Amarenco, P., 2011. Medical treatment in acute and long-term secondary prevention after transient ischaemic attack and ischaemic stroke. Lancet 377, 1681–1692.

Salman, R.A., Labovitz, D.L., Stapf, C., 2009. Spontaneous intracerebral haemorrhage. Br. Med. J. 339, b2586.

Subarachnoid haemorrhage

D'Souza, S., 2015. Aneurysmal subarachnoid haemorrhage. J. Neurosurg. Anasthesiol. 27, 222–240.

van Gijn, J., Kerr, R.S., Rinkel, G.J., 2007. Subarachnoid haemorrhage. Lancet 369, 306–318.

Dementia

Briggs, R., Kennelly, S.P., O'Neill, D., 2016. Drug treatment in Alzheimer's disease. Clin. Med. 16, 247–253.

Mitchell, S.L., 2015. Advanced dementia. N. Engl. J. Med. 372, 2533–2540.

Robinson, L., Tang, E., Taylor, J.P., 2015. Dementia: timely diagnosis and early intervention. Br. Med. J. 350, h3029.

Scheltens, P., Blennow, J., Breteler, M.M.B., et al., 2016. Alzheimer's disease. Lancet 388, 505–517.

Compendium: drugs used to treat cerebrovascular disease and dementia

Drug	Characteristics
Anticholinesterase drugs	
Donepezil	Acetylcholinesterase inhibitor. Used for mild to moderate dementia in Alzheimer's disease. Given orally. Half-life: 70–80 h
Galantamine	Acetylcholinesterase inhibitor and nicotinic receptor agonist. Used for mild to moderate dementia in Alzheimer's disease. Given orally. Half-life: 5–7 h
Rivastigmine	Inhibitor of acetylcholinesterase and pseudocholinesterase. Used for mild to moderate dementia in Alzheimer's disease; also used in Parkinson's disease. Given orally or by transcutaneous patch. Half-life: 1–2 h
Other drugs	
Aspirin, clopidogrel, dipyridamole	Antiplatelet drugs (see Chapter 11)
Memantine	Glutamate NMDA receptor antagonist; significance of additional actions at $5-HT_3$, nicotinic and dopamine D_2 receptors is unclear. Used for moderate to severe dementia in Alzheimer's disease. Given orally. Half-life: 60–80 h
Nimodipine	Dihydropyridine calcium channel blocker (see Chapter 5) selective for cerebral arteries. Use is confined to the prevention and treatment of ischaemic neurological deficits following aneurysmal subarachnoid haemorrhage. Given orally or by intravenous infusion. Half-life: 8–9 h

Peripheral vascular disease

ATHEROMATOUS PERIPHERAL VASCULAR DISEASE

Atherothrombotic disease is by far the most important cause of peripheral vascular disease. Disease in peripheral arteries principally affects the aorta and renal and lower limb arteries. The risk factors for its development are similar to those for coronary artery and cerebrovascular disease (see Chapters 5 and 9). The strongest associations of peripheral vascular disease are with increasing age, smoking and a raised systolic blood pressure, and to a lesser extent with diabetes mellitus, a raised plasma low-density lipoprotein (LDL) cholesterol and lack of exercise. Not surprisingly, symptomatic ischaemic heart disease and cerebrovascular disease coexist in up to 50% of people with peripheral vascular disease and are responsible for about 70% of their excess mortality. Only about 50% of people with peripheral vascular disease are alive 10 years after diagnosis; this is three times the mortality of people of similar age without peripheral vascular disease.

SYMPTOMS OF PERIPHERAL VASCULAR DISEASE

Symptoms usually arise as a consequence of atherosclerotic stenosis of a lower limb artery. A stenosis of more than 50% of the diameter of an arterial lumen is usually necessary to produce symptoms. However, the severity of reduction in blood flow to the limb does not correlate well with symptoms, and an important factor is ischaemia–reperfusion injury to the muscle and altered oxidative metabolism. Hypoxia of skeletal muscle occurs when blood flow through the diseased artery fails to increase sufficiently to meet the increased metabolic demand of the muscle during exercise. This produces intermittent claudication, which is ischaemic pain in the muscles of the limb arising from metabolic changes that accompany the switch to anaerobic metabolism. Intermittent claudication is precipitated by exercise and relieved by rest. Depending on whether the vascular narrowing is distal or proximal, pain can be experienced in the calf, thigh or buttock. The presence of a collateral arterial circulation (see Chapter 5) will reduce the severity of the symptoms and influence the long-term outcome. In three-quarters of people with peripheral vascular disease, the symptoms stabilise within a few months of presentation. The remaining 25% experience steady progression, but only 1% of symptomatic individuals per year will develop critical ischaemia, which causes pain at rest and ultimately distal gangrene (described later).

DRUGS FOR PERIPHERAL VASCULAR DISEASE

Cilostazol

Mechanism of action

Cilostazol is a reversible inhibitor of the phosphodiesterase type 3 (PDE3) enzyme and therefore reduces breakdown of cAMP (see Table 1.1). PDE3 is present in vascular smooth muscle cells and platelets, and its inhibition causes vasodilation, inhibits platelet activation and aggregation, and prevents release of prothrombotic inflammatory substances. Cilostazol also inhibits cellular adenosine reuptake, which promotes vasodilation, has favourable effects on plasma lipids by increasing high-density lipoprotein (HDL) cholesterol, and inhibits cell proliferation in vascular smooth muscle.

Pharmacokinetics

Cilostazol undergoes hepatic metabolism via cytochrome P450 to two metabolites with antiplatelet activity, one of which is more active than cilostazol. Cilostazol has a half-life of about 12 hours.

Unwanted effects

- Diarrhoea.
- Headache.
- Palpitation and tachycardia.
- Other PDE3 inhibitors such as milrinone have been shown to increase mortality in people with heart failure (see

Chapter 7); cilostazol does not appear to increase the risk of life-threatening arrhythmias, but is contraindicated in people with heart failure, cardiac arrhythmias and ischaemic heart disease.

- Increased risk of bleeding when combined with aspirin and clopidogrel.
- Blood dyscrasias.
- Drug interactions: the dose of cilostazol should be reduced with concomitant use of drugs that inhibit cytochrome P450 isoenzymes 3A4 (such as clarithromycin, itraconazole) or 2C19 (erythromycin, omeprazole).

Naftidrofuryl oxalate

Mechanism of action and effects

Naftidrofuryl oxalate promotes the production of high-energy phosphates adenosine triphosphate (ATP) in ischaemic tissue by activating the mitochondrial enzyme succinic dehydrogenase. It is also a 5-hydroxytryptamine type 2 (5-HT$_2$) receptor antagonist, which leads to arterial vasodilation and reduced platelet aggregation. These actions could improve blood flow to ischaemic tissues and tissue nutrition.

Pharmacokinetics

Naftidrofuryl is metabolised in the liver. It has a half-life of 3–4 hours.

Unwanted effects

- Nausea, epigastric pain.
- Rash.
- Hepatitis is a rare but potentially serious complication.

MANAGEMENT OF INTERMITTENT CLAUDICATION

Nonpharmacological treatment

- Stopping smoking slows the progression of peripheral atherosclerosis and may improve walking distance by improving blood oxygen transport. It will also reduce the risk of coronary and cerebrovascular events, and is therefore a cornerstone of long-term management.
- Regular supervised exercise, up to the point of claudication, can improve maximum walking distance by 150% over 8–12 weeks.

Pharmacological treatment

Much of the treatment of peripheral vascular disease is aimed at reducing the risk of myocardial infarction and stroke, which are the main reasons for excess mortality.

- Low-dose aspirin inhibits platelet aggregation and reduces cardiac and cerebrovascular events (see Chapter 11).
- Intensive management of hypertension reduces progression of atheroma. Conventional antihypertensive therapy is used (see Chapter 6). Although β-adrenoceptor antagonists could theoretically exacerbate intermittent claudication by reducing cardiac output and impairing vasodilation of arteries supplying skeletal muscle (see Chapter 5), there is

little evidence of a deleterious effect, except when there is critical limb ischaemia.

- Lowering serum LDL cholesterol (see Chapter 48) can stabilise or regress atherosclerotic plaques. It is not known whether this improves limb survival or reduces the need for subsequent surgery. A greater benefit of lowering cholesterol may be reduced morbidity and mortality from coexistent ischaemic heart disease (see Chapter 5).
- Naftidrofuryl oxalate improves maximum walking distance by up to 60%, but this is often insufficient to make a difference to quality of life. A trial of treatment may be justified for those who remain restricted by the disease after 6–12 months of conservative treatment, and for whom surgical intervention is inappropriate or has failed. Withdrawal is advised after 3–6 months of treatment to assess whether spontaneous improvement has occurred.
- Cilostazol can improve maximum walking distance by up to 25% over 3–6 months of treatment, but the impact of this on quality of life is often minimal. It is not known whether cilostazol has any effect on long-term outcome or on the subsequent need for surgery.

Surgical treatment

Surgical treatment is usually considered if quality of life is significantly impaired by claudication or if tissue integrity is at risk. Percutaneous transluminal angioplasty, often with insertion of a stent, is used particularly for stenoses above the inguinal ligament, while bypass surgery is used for most other disease.

ACUTE AND CRITICAL LIMB ISCHAEMIA

An arterial embolus is the usual cause of acute limb ischaemia and can arise from an intracardiac thrombus, usually associated with atrial fibrillation (see Chapter 8) or following a myocardial infarction, or from aortic or internal iliac artery thrombus. An embolus can occlude a previously healthy artery and presents with acute onset of severe pain at rest, associated with signs of critically impaired tissue perfusion.

Critical limb ischaemia results from chronic, severe, subtotal occlusion of an artery, and may be due to partial occlusion of the vessel from thrombus on a ruptured atherosclerotic plaque. The symptoms include rest pain in the foot, often worse at night and relieved by hanging the leg out of the bed.

MANAGEMENT OF ACUTE AND CRITICAL LIMB ISCHAEMIA

Unless treatment of acute or acute-on-chronic critical limb ischaemia is rapid, the person may be left with a chronically ischaemic limb, or occasionally the limb may be lost through gangrene.

If the limb is still viable, then a peripheral arterial angiogram should be carried out. For acute embolic arterial occlusion of an otherwise healthy vessel, embolectomy is the treatment of choice. Intraarterial thrombolysis with recombinant tissue plasminogen activator (rt-PA; alteplase; see Chapter 11) is used to dissolve an acute thrombus occluding a previously diseased vessel. Alteplase can be infused via a catheter for up to 24 hours or given as repeated boluses. Reperfusion takes several hours, and in about 25% of acute vascular occlusions lysis is not achieved, especially if there is embolic occlusion. The risk of intracerebral haemorrhage is also a concern. A surgical bypass may be considered if there is no time for thrombolysis or for treatment of chronic limb ischaemia.

Secondary prevention measures to reduce other cardiovascular events (described previously) should also be started.

RAYNAUD'S PHENOMENON

Raynaud's phenomenon is a profound and exaggerated vasospastic response of blood vessels in the extremities on exposure to cold, change in environmental temperature or during emotional upset. This leads to episodes of ischaemia that most commonly affect the fingers (occasionally also the toes, ear lobes or the nipples). A typical attack initially produces pallor of the affected part, followed by one or both of cyanosis and then erythema as blood flow returns to the affected area. Each attack can last several minutes or up to a few hours. About two-thirds of cases occur in women (typically beginning under the age of 40 years), in whom the overall prevalence is about 15%. Common symptoms include discomfort, numbness and tingling, with loss of function and pain if the condition is severe. Less commonly, digital ulceration can occur.

The majority of cases of Raynaud's phenomenon are idiopathic (primary Raynaud's phenomenon; also called Raynaud's disease). The cause of the excessive vascular reactivity is unknown, although there is a genetic predisposition. Vascular function in other tissues is often abnormal in primary Raynaud's phenomenon – for example, in the cerebral arteries (giving an association with migraine), the coronary arteries (producing variant angina) or, more rarely, in the pulmonary arteries (leading to primary pulmonary hypertension).

In about 10% of cases, Raynaud's phenomenon is secondary to another disorder. This is most commonly scleroderma, but there are many other associated conditions (Box 10.1). Structural damage to arteries is common in secondary Raynaud's phenomenon, and digital ulceration is much more common than in the primary type.

Other disorders of the peripheral circulation should also be considered in the differential diagnosis of Raynaud's phenomenon:

- Acrocyanosis usually affects the hands and produces persistently cold, bluish fingers which are often sweaty or oedematous. The management of this condition is similar to that of Raynaud's phenomenon.
- Chilblains are an inflammatory disorder with erythematous lesions on the feet, or less commonly the hands or face, that are precipitated by rapid rewarming after exposure to cold and humidity. The lesions are often painful or itchy. Treatments used for Raynaud's phenomenon may help, with the addition of topical nonsteroidal antiinflammatory agents (see Chapter 29).
- Erythromelalgia is a painful, burning condition often affecting the hands and feet that, unlike Raynaud's

Box 10.1	Conditions associated with Raynaud's phenomenon

Connective tissue disorders
  Systemic sclerosis
  Systemic lupus erythematosus
  Rheumatoid arthritis
  Dermatomyositis and polymyositis
Obstructive arterial disorders
  Carpal tunnel syndrome
  Thoracic outlet syndrome
  Atherosclerosis
  Thromboangiitis obliterans
Drugs and chemicals
  Ergotamine
  Beta-adrenoceptor antagonists
  Bleomycin, vinblastine, cisplatin
  Oral contraceptives
  Vinyl chloride
Occupational
  Vibrating tools
  Cold environment
Blood disorders
  Polycythaemia
  Cold agglutinin disease
  Monoclonal gammopathies
  Thrombocytosis

phenomenon, is usually provoked by heat. It sometimes responds to treatment with a calcium channel blocker (see Chapter 5) or gabapentin (see Chapter 23).
- Vibration white finger is a patchy digital vasospasm associated with prolonged use of vibrating tools. If drug treatment is necessary, it is similar to that for Raynaud's phenomenon.

MANAGEMENT OF RAYNAUD'S PHENOMENON

Many people with Raynaud's phenomenon are only mildly inconvenienced by their symptoms and respond to simple measures. Drug treatment is usually reserved for those experiencing pain, impairment of function or trophic changes. Responses to individual treatments are unpredictable, and are less satisfactory in secondary Raynaud's phenomenon because of structural changes to the vessel wall.

Nonpharmacological treatment

- Often minimising changes in ambient temperature with insulating clothing is enough to reduce the number of attacks. Electrically heated gloves or socks may be useful for more severely affected people.
- Smoking should be strongly discouraged. Nicotine promotes vasospasm and may also reduce the threshold for other provoking factors.
- Aggravating factors should be withdrawn or corrected whenever possible (see Box 10.1). Beta-adrenoceptor antagonists (see Chapter 5) produce peripheral circulatory problems sufficient to necessitate stopping treatment in about 3–5% of people who take them.
- Surgical sympathectomy is occasionally used for advanced disease.

Pharmacological treatment

Arterial vasodilators

- Calcium channel blockers (see Chapter 5): modified-release nifedipine is the drug of first choice for Raynaud's phenomenon, and usually reduces the frequency, duration and intensity of vasospastic episodes. Several other dihydropyridines are probably equally effective, but diltiazem is less effective and verapamil ineffective in this condition.
- Naftidrofuryl oxalate may produce a modest reduction in the severity of attacks.
- Alpha$_1$-adrenoceptor antagonists (see Chapter 6): moxisylyte is typically used and does not lower blood pressure to the same degree as other α_1-adrenoceptor antagonists.
- Angiotensin II receptor antagonists (see Chapter 6)
- Sildenafil (see Chapter 16) has been used successfully in secondary Raynaud's phenomenon that is resistant to other vasodilators.
- Bosentan, an endothelin receptor antagonist (see Chapter 6), is effective in severe Raynaud's phenomenon.
- Fluoxetine (see Chapter 22), a selective serotonin reuptake inhibitor (SSRI) antidepressant, is helpful in some cases.
- Calcitonin gene-related peptide (CGRP) is effective for prolonged periods when given by short intravenous infusions over 5 or more consecutive days. It is a neurotransmitter for vasodilator cutaneous sensorimotor nerves in the fingers and toes. CGRP is usually reserved for failure to respond to epoprostenol (described later).

Drugs acting primarily on blood components

- Prostaglandins: short intravenous infusions of epoprostenol (prostacyclin, prostaglandin I$_2$, see Chapter 11) over at least 5 consecutive days produce immediate vasodilation. There is long-term improvement in symptoms and healing of ulcers over a period of 10–16 weeks. These effects are believed to be caused by reduced platelet aggregation, increased red cell deformability and reduced neutrophil adhesiveness, which together improve blood flow. Epoprostenol is rapidly inactivated in plasma by hydrolysis and has a very short half-life of about 3 minutes. Unwanted effects are due to vasodilation and include flushing, headache and hypotension.
- Inositol nicotinate (a nicotinic acid derivative) produces a gradual onset of clinical response and only modest improvement in symptoms. Its action may result more from fibrinolysis (reducing plasma viscosity) and reduction in platelet aggregation than from vasodilation.

SELF-ASSESSMENT

True/false questions

1. Diabetes mellitus, hypertension and smoking confer an additive risk of developing peripheral vascular disease.
2. People with intermittent claudication do not have an increased risk of developing coronary artery disease.
3. Statin drugs are indicated in people with symptomatic atherosclerotic peripheral vascular disease.
4. Epoprostenol mimics the actions of thromboxane A$_2$.
5. Bosentan is an endothelin receptor antagonist used in Raynaud's phenomenon.
6. Verapamil is the calcium channel blocker of choice in the treatment of Raynaud's phenomenon.

One-best-answer (OBA) question

1. What is the mechanism of action of cilostazol?
   A. Cilostazol decreases plasma HDL cholesterol.
   B. Cilostazol inhibits PDE3 in vascular tissues.
   C. Cilostazol inhibits succinic dehydrogenase in mitochondria.
   D. Cilostazol is a 5-hydroxytryptamine type 2 (5-HT$_2$) receptor antagonist.
   E. Cilostazol is an α_1-adrenoceptor antagonist.

Case-based questions

Mr T.H., aged 67 years, has type 1 diabetes mellitus and smokes 20 cigarettes a day. His plasma total cholesterol is raised at 7.2 mmol/L, and his blood pressure is 160/110 mm Hg. After walking 50 metres, he develops pain in his left calf muscle, which is relieved by rest. He occasionally has rest pain at night. On examination, both popliteal and posterior tibial pulses are absent, and femoropopliteal atherosclerotic disease is diagnosed.

1. Comment on the usefulness and drawbacks of the following drugs to treat Mr T.H.'s peripheral vascular disease.
   A. Propranolol
   B. Atenolol
   C. Nifedipine
   D. A statin
   E. Low-dose aspirin
   F. Cilostazol
2. What other therapy could be of benefit?
3. Should the use of an electric blanket be discouraged?

ANSWERS

True/false answers

1. **True.** The risk factors for peripheral vascular disease are similar to those for coronary artery and cerebrovascular disease.
2. **False.** There is a two- to fourfold increase in risk of developing coronary disease, stroke or heart failure compared with age-matched subjects who do not have intermittent claudication.
3. **True.** Lowering serum LDL cholesterol can stabilise or regress atherosclerotic plaques.
4. **False.** Epoprostenol is prostacyclin (PGI$_2$), which has actions on vessels and platelets opposite to those of thromboxane A$_2$.
5. **True.** Bosentan produces vasodilation by blocking the action of endothelin-1 at its ET-A and ET-B receptors;

it is used for Raynaud's phenomenon in people with systemic sclerosis.

6. **False**. Verapamil is ineffective in the treatment of Raynaud's phenomenon, and the agent of choice is nifedipine.

One-best-answer (OBA) answer

1. **Answer B** is correct; cilostazol increases cAMP levels in vascular smooth muscle cells and platelets by inhibiting phosphodiesterase (PDE) type 3. Answer A is incorrect, as cilostazol decreases plasma HDL cholesterol. Answers C and D are mechanisms that contribute to the activity of naftidrofuryl oxalate. Moxisylate is a prodrug converted to metabolites that block α_1-adrenoceptors (answer E).

Case-based answers

1. The usefulness and drawbacks of drugs A–F in treating Mr T.H. are as follows:

   A. Beta-adrenoceptor antagonists should probably be avoided in this man. They would not be the drug of choice in the initial treatment of his high blood pressure (see Chapter 6), and by reducing cardiac output and inhibiting vasodilation, they could further reduce blood flow in critical limb ischaemia.

   B. Cardioselective β-adrenoceptor antagonists such as atenolol do not cause deterioration in walking distance when used without a vasodilator.

   C. Vasodilators will lower blood pressure but do not improve walking distance. In some people, they may redirect blood from the maximally dilated ischaemic tissues to healthy tissues (vascular steal). This can be particularly troublesome in critical limb ischaemia, or when the cardiac output is also reduced by concurrent use of a β-adrenoceptor antagonist.

   D. Lowering LDL cholesterol can stabilise atherosclerotic plaques, perhaps reducing the consequences of coexistent heart disease; it is not known whether walking distance or limb survival are improved.

   E. Low-dose aspirin inhibits platelet aggregation and reduces future cardiac events, which are common in people with peripheral vascular disease.

   F. Cilostazol can increase walking distance by up to 25%.

2. Intensive management of blood pressure, control of diabetes and antiplatelet therapy will reduce the risk of cardiac events. An exercise programme can improve walking distance. Smoking is a major contributory factor to impaired walking distance and cardiac events.

3. An electric blanket should be discouraged, as excessive warming of limbs may dilate normal arteries, 'stealing' blood from diseased arteries.

FURTHER READING

Foley, T.R., Armstrong, E.J., Waldo, S.W., 2016. Contemporary evaluation and management of lower extremity peripheral artery disease. Heart 102, 1436–1441.

Goundry, B., Bell, L., Langtree, M., et al., 2012. Diagnosis and management of Raynaud's phenomenon. Br. Med. J. 344, e289.

Kullo, I.J., Rooke, T.W., 2016. Peripheral artery disease. N. Engl. J. Med. 374, 861–871.

Wigley, F.M., Flavahan, N.A., 2016. Raynaud's phenomenon. N. Engl. J. Med. 375, 556–565.

Compendium: drugs used to treat peripheral vascular disease

Drug	Characteristics
Cilostazol	Reversibly inhibits phosphodiesterase (PDE) type 3 and blocks adenosine reuptake in vascular smooth muscle cells, causing vasodilation; also has antiplatelet activity and increases plasma HDL cholesterol. Given orally. Half-life: 12 h
Epoprostenol	Prostaglandin I_2 (prostacyclin); vasodilator and antiplatelet activity. Freshly reconstituted from dry powder before intravenous infusion. Half-life: <3 min
Inositol nicotinate	Hydrolysed to nicotinic acid (niacin), a vasodilator, but not recommended; also used for hyperlipidaemias. Given orally
Moxisylyte	Formerly known as thymoxamine in the United Kingdom. Prodrug converted to desacetylmoxisylyte, which blocks α_1-adrenoceptors. Used for the short-term treatment of primary Raynaud's phenomenon. Given orally. Half-life: 1–2 h
Naftidrofuryl oxalate	Activates mitochondrial succinic dehydrogenase and is a $5\text{-}HT_2$ receptor antagonist. Given orally. Half-life: 3–4 h
Pentoxifylline	PDE inhibitor; increases erythrocyte flexibility and decreases blood viscosity, possibly by increasing erythrocyte cAMP, but not recommended. Given orally. Half-life: 1 h

Haemostasis is a complex process involving vasoconstriction, platelet aggregation, blood coagulation and the interactions among them. The descriptions of the processes of platelet aggregation and coagulation pathways in this chapter are restricted to essential knowledge required for understanding the actions of pharmacological agents.

PLATELETS AND PLATELET AGGREGATION

Platelets are critical components of the blood for initiating thrombus formation and have a lifespan in the circulation of 8–10 days, with about 10–12% being replaced each day. Platelets adhere to an injured blood vessel, following which they are activated and then aggregate. Intact endothelium produces substances such as prostacyclin and nitric oxide that inhibit platelet activation. When the integrity of vascular endothelium is breached, subendothelial proteins such as von Willebrand factor (vWF) and collagen come into contact with blood. These proteins interact with a family of platelet-surface glycoprotein (GP) receptors (integrin receptors), particularly GPIb (vWF receptor) and GPVI (collagen receptor), resulting in platelets adhering to the site of injury. This forms a platelet plug that seals the breached endothelial surface (Fig. 11.1).

Platelet adhesion initiates a process known as platelet activation, which is a prerequisite for platelet aggregation and the extension of the platelet plug. Platelet activation is initiated by exposure to soluble agonists, such as exposed collagen and thrombin generated by local coagulation. These activators lead to an increase in intracellular Ca^{2+} and the activation of myosin light-chain kinase (MLCK). MLCK phosphorylates myosin light chains in the platelet which interact with actin, disrupting the platelet cytoskeleton and changing the shape of the platelet. Platelet shape change initiates a release reaction that expels several mediators, such as platelet factor 4, adrenaline, adenosine diphosphate (ADP) and serotonin from the platelet. The increase in platelet intracellular Ca^{2+} also activates phospholipase A_2, which liberates arachidonic acid (AA) from membrane phospholipids. AA is converted by cyclo-oxygenase type 1 (COX-1) in the platelet to thromboxane A_2, the most potent naturally occurring proaggregating agent, which diffuses from the platelet.

Outside the platelet ADP, thrombin, collagen and thromboxane A_2 interact with specific platelet surface receptors and trigger intracellular pathways that express and activate GPIIb/IIIa collagen receptors on the surface of the platelets (see Figs 11.1 and 11.2). ADP amplifies platelet activation by other agonists. The GPIIb/IIIa receptors on the surface of the platelets are crosslinked by fibrinogen in the plasma, producing irreversible platelet aggregation.

The substances released from platelets during activation also facilitate haemostasis by:

- Reducing prostacyclin (prostaglandin I_2, PGI_2) synthesis by vascular endothelium. Prostacyclin is a vasodilator and a potent inhibitor of platelet aggregation.
- Inhibiting the action of heparin sulfate produced by vascular endothelium. This enhances activity of the coagulation cascade.

The expression of platelet GPIIb/IIIa surface receptors can be inhibited by an increase in the concentration of cyclic nucleotides (cyclic adenosine monophosphate [cAMP] and cyclic guanosine monophosphate [cGMP]) in the platelet. This is the mechanism by which prostacyclin (PGI_2) inhibits platelet aggregation (see Figs 11.1 and 11.2).

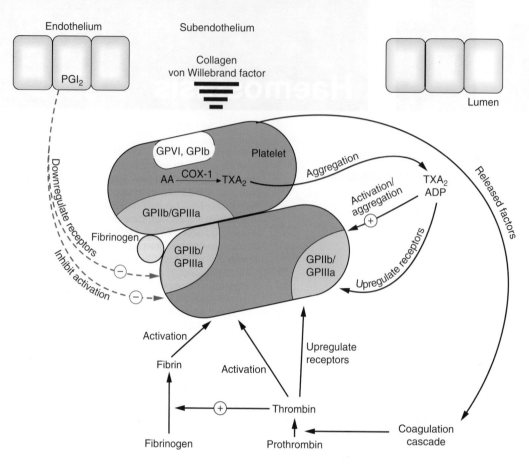

Fig. 11.1 **Platelets and platelet aggregation.** Subendothelial macromolecules such as von Willebrand factor and collagen interact with glycoprotein receptors (GPVI and GPIb) on platelets, causing activation of platelets and upregulation of GPIIb/IIIa receptors, which are crosslinked by fibrinogen, resulting in aggregation. During the initial processes of aggregation, stimulation of the synthesis and release of a number of platelet-derived substances, such as adenosine diphosphate (ADP), thromboxane A_2 (TXA_2), which is synthesised from arachidonic acid (AA) by cyclo-oxygenase-1 (COX-1), and other factors (described previously) further promote aggregation by upregulation of GPIIb/IIIa receptors. Conversely, prostacyclin (PGI_2) from endothelial cells inhibits the activation and upregulation of GPIIb/IIIa receptors. The mechanisms of action of antiplatelet drugs that act on these pathways are shown in Fig. 11.2. Platelet activation is also stimulated by thrombin generated from prothrombin by the coagulation cascade (see Fig. 11.3).

Polyunsaturated (omega-3) fatty acids in fish oils are precursors for thromboxane A_3, which causes less platelet aggregation than thromboxane A_2; they also increase production of a modified form of prostacyclin (PGI_3) by vascular endothelium, which has equal antiaggregatory activity to PGI_2. Therefore a high intake of fish oils creates a state in which platelets are less able to aggregate.

BLOOD COAGULATION AND THE COAGULATION CASCADE

Both procoagulant and anticoagulant factors regulate haemostasis. Activation of the coagulation cascade is divided into extrinsic and intrinsic pathways (Fig. 11.3). The factors involved in these cascades amplify the coagulation response and work together to produce a thrombus. The extrinsic pathway accounts for most of the coagulation in vivo, but both coagulation pathways respond to breaches in endothelial integrity much more slowly than platelet aggregation. The following description of the pathways is simplified to identify the key steps at which drugs can modulate coagulation.

The extrinsic coagulation pathway is initiated by exposure of blood to tissue factor (TF) on the surface of subendothelial cells after vascular injury, and is activated rapidly within minutes of endothelial disruption. Formation of complexes of TF with factor VIIa in the presence of phospholipids and Ca^{2+}, results in the conversion of inactive factor X to active Xa.

The intrinsic coagulation pathway is triggered by contact of blood with a negatively charged surface such as subendothelial collagen, and its activation is delayed by more than 10 minutes after tissue disruption. The intrinsic coagulation pathway comprises a series of enzyme-mediated

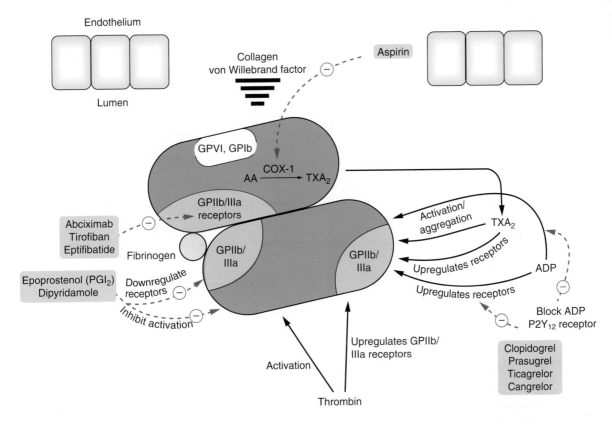

Fig. 11.2 Sites of action of major antiplatelet drugs. Drugs act directly or indirectly to block activation of platelets and inhibit upregulation of the glycoprotein GPIIb/IIIa receptors (integrin receptor family), which are necessary for platelet aggregation. Abciximab is an antibody, tirofiban a nonpeptide inhibitor and eptifibatide a peptide inhibitor of these glycoprotein receptors. Epoprostenol and dipyridamole inhibit activation of platelets and downregulate the glycoprotein receptors by increasing cAMP. Clopidogrel and related drugs inhibit ADP ($P2Y_{12}$) receptors and prevent ADP-induced upregulation of the glycoprotein GPIIb/IIIa receptors. Aspirin inhibits the generation of thromboxane A_2 (TXA_2) by cyclo-oxygenase-1 (COX-1), which otherwise causes platelet activation and upregulation of GPIIb/IIIa receptors. *AA*, Arachidonic acid; *ADP*, adenosine diphosphate. For the sites of action of anticoagulant drugs that directly or indirectly inhibit thrombin, see Fig. 11.3.

reactions involving serial activation of several clotting factors and eventually activation of factor X.

The two coagulation pathways converge with activation of factor X, which mediates the hydrolysis of prothrombin to thrombin (factor IIa; see Fig. 11.3). Thrombin converts the soluble protein fibrinogen to an insoluble fibrin gel. Thrombin also activates factor XIII, which crosslinks the fibrin polymers and forms a fibrin mesh that traps circulating platelets, leucocytes and red blood cells.

The actions of thrombin and several other activated coagulation factors (see Fig. 11.3) are inhibited by circulating antithrombin. Antithrombin inhibits coagulation factors after forming complexes with heparin-like molecules that are produced by intact endothelial cells, and with heparin released from mast cells. Once sufficient thrombin has been produced to overcome the effect of circulating antithrombin, it is able to initiate coagulation.

Each activated clotting factor is inactivated extremely rapidly so that the coagulation process remains localised at the site of the initiating event. However, aggregates of platelets combined with fibrin thrombi can embolise and occlude more distal parts of the circulation.

ARTERIAL AND VENOUS THROMBOSIS

There are differences in the composition of an arterial or venous thrombus. Arterial thrombosis occurs in the setting of high flow and high shear stress, and platelets play a prominent role in the initiation and growth of the thrombus. In contrast, venous thrombi form in a low-flow, low-shear stress environment. Venous thrombus usually forms initially as a result of stasis in the valve pockets of deep veins, and consists mainly of fibrin and red cells with few platelets.

ANTIPLATELET DRUGS

CYCLO-OXYGENASE INHIBITORS

Example

aspirin

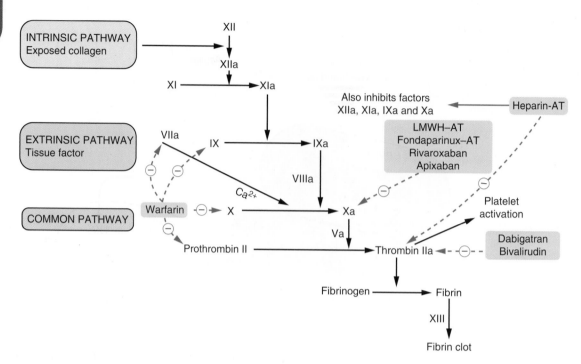

Fig. 11.3 The coagulation cascade and action of anticoagulants. Roman numerals indicate the individual clotting factors in the cascade. Coagulation is initiated by vascular tissue damage, causing exposure of subendothelial collagen (which activates clotting factor XII) and tissue factor (a receptor for clotting factor VII). Sequential activation of clotting factors in the intrinsic and extrinsic pathways results in the generation of thrombin (factor IIa), which generates fibrin from fibrinogen. Platelet products, phospholipids from damaged cells, Ca^{2+} ions and many other factors are involved at numerous sites in the coagulation cascade, and thrombin from the coagulation cascade also enhances activation of platelets. Unfractionated heparin forms complexes with the anticlotting factor antithrombin III (AT); the heparin–AT complex inhibits thrombin and the other activated clotting factors listed. Low-molecular-weight heparins (LMWH) and fondaparinux also form complexes with AT but in a different manner that inhibits factor Xa selectively. The xaban drugs (such as rivaroxaban, apixaban) are direct inhibitors of factor Xa, while dabigatran and bivalirudin directly inhibit thrombin (factor IIa). Warfarin and other coumarin anticoagulants inhibit vitamin K-dependent synthesis of the clotting factors VII, IX, X and II (prothrombin) in the liver.

Mechanism of action on platelets

The highly potent platelet-aggregating agent thromboxane A_2 is formed in platelets from AA by the enzyme COX-1. After release from the platelet, thromboxane A_2 acts via thromboxane (TP) receptors on the surface of the platelet to generate the intracellular second messengers inositol triphosphate (IP_3) and diacylglycerol (DAG). These lead to Ca^{2+} release in the cell and expression and activation of GPIIb/IIIa receptors (described earlier).

Inhibition of COX-1 by aspirin reduces platelet thromboxane A_2 synthesis and inhibits platelet aggregation, but does not eliminate it completely, because other pathways for platelet activation still function (see Figs 11.1 and 11.2). Aspirin (acetylsalicylic acid) irreversibly inhibits COX-1 by acetylation (see Chapter 29), and since platelets lack a nucleus and cannot synthesise new enzyme, their ability to aggregate will be reduced throughout the lifespan of the platelet. The antiplatelet action of aspirin occurs at very low doses that have little analgesic or anti-inflammatory actions. At higher doses, aspirin also inhibits the production of prostacyclin by vascular endothelium, which may offset some of the beneficial effects on platelets. Details of the pharmacology of aspirin can be found in Chapter 29.

PHOSPHODIESTERASE INHIBITORS

dipyridamole

Mechanism of action

Dipyridamole inhibits the cellular reuptake of adenosine. The increased plasma concentration of adenosine inhibits platelet aggregation by activating cell surface adenosine A_2 receptors and stimulating intracellular adenylyl cyclase and production of the intracellular cyclic nucleotides cGMP and cAMP, which inhibit expression of cell surface GPIIb/IIIa receptors (see Fig. 11.2). Adenosine also produces vasodilation. Dipyridamole also inhibits phosphodiesterase (PDE) types 3 and 5. Since PDE degrades intracellular cyclic nucleotides, this also contributes to reduced platelet activation.

Pharmacokinetics

Dipyridamole is metabolised in the liver and has a half-life of 12 hours. A modified-release formulation is better tolerated than the standard formulation.

Unwanted effects

- Diarrhoea, nausea, vomiting.
- Myalgia.
- Dizziness, headache.
- Flushing, hypotension, tachycardia.
- Hypersensitivity reactions, including rash, urticaria, bronchospasm and angioedema.

ADENOSINE DIPHOSPHATE RECEPTOR ANTAGONISTS

Examples

clopidogrel, prasugrel, ticagrelor

Mechanism of action

ADP receptor antagonists inhibit platelet aggregation by binding selectively to purinergic $P2Y_{12}$ receptors (see Fig. 11.2). ADP activates platelets via two surface receptors, $P2Y_1$ and $P2Y_{12}$. Stimulation of $P2Y_1$ receptors increases intracellular Ca^{2+}, and initiates platelet shape change and reversible aggregation. Stimulation of $P2Y_{12}$ receptors inhibits adenylyl cyclase, and reduces generation of the intracellular cyclic nucleotides that inhibit activation of GPIIb/IIIa receptors.

Clopidogrel and prasugrel are irreversible $P2Y_{12}$ receptor inhibitors, while ticagrelor binds to a different site on the receptor and produces reversible inhibition. There is considerable interindividual variability in the degree of platelet inhibition by clopidogrel, and it has a slow onset of action (about 5 days for full effect) without a loading dose. Both prasugrel and ticagrelor are more predictable inhibitors of platelet activation than clopidogrel, and have a more rapid onset of action.

Pharmacokinetics

Clopidogrel is a prodrug. It is activated by metabolism in the liver to a derivative that has a half-life of 7 hours. Prasugrel is also a prodrug that is metabolised in the liver to an active metabolite which has a very long half-life of 8 days. Ticagrelor is active as the parent drug, and also has an active metabolite. The offset of action of ticagrelor over 3 days is much slower than would be predicted from its short half-life.

Unwanted effects

- Bleeding; a greater risk with prasugrel and ticagrelor than clopidogrel.
- Gastrointestinal upset, especially dyspepsia, abdominal pain and diarrhoea with clopidogrel.
- Dyspnoea with ticagrelor.

GLYCOPROTEIN IIB/IIIA RECEPTOR ANTAGONISTS

Examples

abciximab, eptifibatide, tirofiban

Mechanism of action

Abciximab is a murine/human chimaeric monoclonal antibody to the GPIIb/IIIa receptors with the Fc fragment removed to prevent clearance of antibody-bound platelets from the circulation. Abciximab binds irreversibly to the GPIIb/IIIa receptors and blocks the binding of fibrinogen (see Fig. 11.2). Abciximab can reduce platelet aggregation by more than 90%.

Eptifibatide is a synthetic peptide that binds reversibly to and blocks the GPIIb/IIIa receptor. Tirofiban is a nonpeptide reversible antagonist of the GPIIb/IIIa receptor.

Pharmacokinetics

All GPIIb/IIIa antagonists are given intravenously, usually as an initial bolus to achieve rapid inhibition of platelets, followed by continuous infusion. The duration of action of abciximab is longer than predicted from its very short half-life of 30 minutes, due to its slow dissociation from the receptor over several hours. After stopping abciximab, platelet aggregation largely recovers by 48 hours as new platelets are synthesised.

Eptifibatide is partially metabolised and partly excreted by the kidneys and has a half-life of about 2.5 hours. Tirofiban is eliminated by the kidneys and has a half-life of 2 hours. Platelet aggregation recovers more rapidly after treatment with eptifibatide or tirofiban than with abciximab due to rapid dissociation of the drug from the receptor.

Unwanted effects

- Bleeding, especially in the elderly and those of low body weight; the risk is reduced if the dose is adjusted for body weight.
- Thrombocytopenia.
- Abciximab can cause nausea, vomiting, hypotension, bradycardia, headache and, occasionally, hypersensitivity reactions.

Epoprostenol

Mechanism of action

Epoprostenol (prostacyclin, prostaglandin I_2) acts at prostacyclin IP receptors to increase platelet cAMP, which at low concentrations inhibits platelet aggregation and at higher concentrations reduces platelet adhesion. Epoprostenol is also a peripheral arterial vasodilator.

Pharmacokinetics

Epoprostenol is given by intravenous infusion. Unlike most other prostaglandins it is not significantly metabolised in the lung, as it is rapidly metabolised by hydrolysis in plasma and peripheral tissues, giving a very short half-life of about 3 minutes.

Unwanted effects

These can be reduced by starting the infusion with a low dose and include:

- facial flushing;
- headache;
- hypotension;
- jaw pain, arthralgia;
- gastrointestinal disturbances.

CLINICAL USES OF ANTIPLATELET DRUGS

Aspirin has often been used as the sole antiplatelet drug in a variety of ischaemic vascular conditions. However, there are some situations where clopidogrel is more effective, or where combinations of aspirin and another antiplatelet agent give better outcomes than aspirin alone. A combination of antiplatelet drugs inevitably carries a greater risk of bleeding than a single agent. Main uses of antiplatelet drugs are listed here.

- Secondary prevention of embolic stroke and transient ischaemic attacks (aspirin, clopidogrel, dipyridamole). Clopidogrel alone is more effective than aspirin alone for the secondary prevention of stroke. Dipyridamole combined with aspirin is better than aspirin alone for prevention of recurrent transient ischaemic attacks, and is equally effective as clopidogrel after stroke. The combination of aspirin and clopidogrel is no more effective than clopidogrel alone yet has a higher risk of bleeding (see Chapter 9).
- Secondary prevention after acute coronary syndrome (aspirin, clopidogrel, prasugrel, ticagrelor). The combination of aspirin and clopidogrel is better than aspirin alone for reducing further vascular events after myocardial infarction.
- Reduction of ischaemic complications produced by stent thrombosis following percutaneous coronary intervention (PCI) with stent insertion (aspirin, clopidogrel, prasugrel, ticagrelor, eptifibitide, tirofiban). These complications include nonfatal myocardial infarction, death and the need for emergency surgical revascularisation. Aspirin with clopidogrel, prasugrel or ticagrelor are given for up to a year (longer for a drug-eluting stent than a bare metal stent). Abciximab, tirofiban or eptifibatide can be used at the time of the procedure in people at high risk of complications.
- Secondary prevention of myocardial infarction in stable angina or peripheral vascular disease (aspirin, clopidogrel). Either aspirin or clopidogrel alone is effective, and there is no evidence to support combination therapy (see Chapters 5 and 10).
- Primary prevention of ischaemic heart disease (aspirin). This is a controversial area, with the potential for serious haemorrhage offsetting much of the potential benefit. Use of aspirin should be confined to people at very high risk of developing cardiovascular disease.
- Anticoagulation in extracorporeal circulations e.g. cardiopulmonary bypass and renal haemodialysis (epoprostenol).
- Symptom relief in Raynaud's phenomenon (epoprostenol; see Chapter 10).
- Dipyridamole is used as a pharmacological stress for the coronary circulation to detect myocardial ischaemia in people who are unable to exercise. This is related to its ability to block the cellular uptake of adenosine. In the heart, adenosine acts on specific receptors in the small resistance coronary arteries to produce vasodilation. Dipyridamole can divert blood away from myocardium supplied by stenosed coronary arteries by preferentially dilating healthy vascular beds (vascular steal).

ANTICOAGULANT DRUGS

Anticoagulation can be achieved with either injectable or oral drug therapy. Increasingly, oral anticoagulant therapy with direct-acting (nonvitamin K-dependent) anticoagulants is likely to supersede the long-established use of heparin followed by warfarin to initiate long-term anticoagulation.

INJECTABLE ANTICOAGULANTS

Heparins

Examples

Unfractionated heparin
Low molecular weight heparins: enoxaparin, tinzaparin
fondaparinux

Heparins are a family of highly sulphated acidic mucopolysaccharides (glycosaminoglycans) that are found in mast cells, basophils and vascular endothelium. Heparins have a variable molecular weight of between 3000 and 30 000 Da according to the numbers of polysaccharide subunits.

Mechanism of action and effects

Heparin is available as an unfractionated preparation, or as low-molecular-weight heparins (LMWHs), which consist of the heparin subfractions that have molecular weights of less than 7000 Da.

Unfractionated heparin forms a complex with and alters the conformation of antithrombin III; this complex can then inactivate thrombin and factors IXa, Xa, XIa and XIIa (see Fig. 11.3). LMWH interacts with antithrombin III in a different manner to unfractionated heparin, and the LMWH–antithrombin complexes have a more selective anticoagulant action, mainly inhibiting factor Xa (see Fig. 11.3).

Additional actions of heparins are as follows:

- promotion of tissue factor pathway inhibitor (TFPI) release from the vascular wall, which contributes to the antithrombotic effects of heparin. TFPI inhibits the formation of factor Xa.
- inhibition of platelet aggregation through binding to platelet factor 4 (mainly unfractionated heparin).
- activation of lipoprotein lipase, which in addition to promoting lipolysis also reduces platelet adhesiveness.

Pharmacokinetics

Heparins are inactive orally and are given intravenously or by subcutaneous injection. They have a rapid onset of action. Heparins do not cross the placenta or enter breast milk. The two principal forms of heparin have different pharmacokinetic properties.

Unfractionated heparin

This is extracted from porcine intestinal mucosa or bovine lung and consists of an average of 45 polysaccharide units. It has dose-dependent (saturable) pharmacokinetics, giving a very short half-life of about 30 minutes at low doses, increasing to 2–3 hours at higher doses. Variable binding to plasma proteins contributes to interindividual variation in the dose required to achieve target levels of anticoagulation. Most heparin is metabolised in endothelial cells after binding to cell surface receptors. Unfractionated heparin is usually given by continuous intravenous infusion for full anticoagulation. Low doses are used by subcutaneous injection for prophylaxis against venous thrombosis, although bioavailability by this route is only about 30%.

Low-molecular-weight heparins (LMWHs)

LMWHs have an average of 15 polysaccharide units. They are almost completely absorbed after subcutaneous administration and only need to be given once or twice daily by subcutaneous injection for full anticoagulation. LMWHs have a low affinity for plasma protein binding sites and for endothelial cell heparin receptors. They have two routes of elimination: a rapid, saturable liver uptake and slower renal excretion. The different LMWHs have half-lives in the range of 2–6 hours. When the dose of an LMWH is based on body weight, it produces a more predictable anticoagulant effect compared with unfractionated heparin.

Control of heparin therapy

The therapeutic index for heparin is low. The degree of anticoagulation with unfractionated heparin is usually monitored with the activated partial thromboplastin time (APTT; a global test of the activity of the intrinsic coagulation pathway), which should be prolonged by 1.5–2.0 times the control value for full anticoagulation. Monitoring is not required when low-dose unfractionated heparin is used subcutaneously for prophylaxis. The anticoagulant effect of LMWHs can be monitored by the extent of inhibition of factor Xa, but this is not carried out routinely since their effect is much more predictable than that of unfractionated heparin.

Unwanted effects

- Haemorrhage is the most common complication. The risk is greater in the elderly, especially if there is a history of heavy alcohol intake. The effect of unfractionated heparin can be rapidly reversed by intravenous injection of protamine sulphate, a basic peptide which binds strongly to the acidic heparin components. Protamine binds poorly to LMWHs and only partially reverses their action.
- Osteoporosis is a rare complication which can occur when heparin is given for several weeks; heparin binds to osteoblasts and inhibits their activity. The risk is less with LMWHs.
- Heparin-induced thrombocytopenia (HIT) usually occurs 5–15 days after starting intravenous heparin. It affects about 2% of those treated, and arises from the development of antibodies to the heparin–platelet factor 4 complex. This causes platelet activation, aggregation and thrombosis. LMWHs are much less likely to cause HIT, since they have much less affinity for platelet factor 4. Danaparoid (see the drug compendium at the end of this chapter) can be used if continued parenteral anticoagulation is necessary.
- Hyperkalaemia by inhibition of aldosterone secretion. This is most likely to occur after at least 7 days of treatment.
- Hypersensitivity reactions.

Fondaparinux

Mechanism of action

Fondaparinux is a synthetic pentasaccharide almost identical to the natural pentasaccharide sequence of heparin that binds to antithrombin III. It selectively enhances the innate ability of antithrombin III to inhibit factor Xa, but does not inactivate thrombin. Fondaparinux has no effect on platelets.

Pharmacokinetics

Fondaparinux is given by subcutaneous injection. It is predictably absorbed from the injection site and has a long half-life (18 hours).

Unwanted effects

- Haemorrhage.
- Anaemia, thrombocytopenia.
- Oedema.
- Gastrointestinal upset.

ORAL ANTICOAGULANTS

Vitamin K antagonists

Examples

warfarin, acenocoumarol (especially in Europe)

Mechanism of action

Hepatic synthesis of clotting factors II (prothrombin), VII, IX and X requires gamma-carboxylation of glutamate residues within the clotting factor by gamma-glutamyl carboxylase. An essential cofactor for gamma-carboxylation is vitamin K, which is generated by the intestinal flora. During the carboxylation reaction the reduced form of vitamin K (hydroquinone) is oxidised by gamma-glutamyl carboxylase to vitamin K epoxide, which is then restored to the hydroquinone form by vitamin K epoxide reductase (VKOR). The so-called vitamin K antagonists inhibit VKOR, preventing the regeneration of active vitamin K hydroquinone and inhibiting gamma-carboxylation of the vitamin K idependent clotting factors (see Fig. 11.3). There is a delay in the onset of the anticoagulant effect due to the presence of previously synthesised clotting factors in the circulation; these must be cleared and replaced by the noncarboxylated forms, which cannot be activated in the coagulation cascade.

Pharmacokinetics

Warfarin is eliminated by cytochrome P450-mediated hepatic metabolism (CYP2C9) and has a long half-life of 1–2 days. Functional CYP2C9 polymorphisms contribute to considerable interindividual variability in warfarin sensitivity. However, the plasma concentration of warfarin does not correlate directly with the clinical effect of the drug, which is determined by the balance between the rates of synthesis and degradation of clotting factors. The maximum effect of an individual dose of warfarin is reflected in the blood coagulation time some 24–48 hours later. On stopping treatment, the duration of anticoagulant action is determined largely by the time required to synthesise new clotting factors, which is approximately 2–4 days.

Monitoring of oral vitamin K antagonist therapy

Factor VII is the clotting factor that is most sensitive to vitamin K deficiency, since it has the shortest half-life of the vitamin K-sensitive clotting factors. Therefore a test of the extrinsic coagulation pathway – the prothrombin time – is used as a measure of effectiveness. The degree of prolongation of the prothrombin time is standardised by comparison with control plasma from a single source, with the result referred to as the international normalised ratio (INR). Therapeutic INR ranges differ according to the condition being treated:

- An INR of 2–2.5 is used for prophylaxis of deep vein thrombosis (thromboprophylaxis).
- An INR of 2–3 is used for thromboprophylaxis in hip surgery and fractured femur operations, for treatment of deep vein thrombosis and pulmonary embolism, and for prevention of thromboembolism in atrial fibrillation.
- An INR of 3–4.5 is used for prevention of recurrent deep vein thrombosis and for preventing thrombosis on mechanical prosthetic heart valves.

The percentage of time in therapeutic range (TTR) for the INR is often used to determine the effectiveness of long-term anticoagulation with vitamin K antagonists. A TTR greater than 65% is considered acceptable. Persistently lower values despite counselling on adherence and correction of interfering factors suggest that alternative anticoagulants should be considered where appropriate.

Unwanted effects

Warfarin is an important example of a drug with a narrow therapeutic index and a significant risk of unwanted effects, as well as drug interactions.

- Haemorrhage. The most effective antidote to warfarin is phytomenadione (vitamin K_1). For major bleeding, this is given intravenously and controls bleeding within 6 hours. An immediate coagulant effect is achieved by giving an intravenous injection of prothrombin complex concentrate (containing vitamin K-dependent clotting factors) or an infusion of fresh frozen plasma. After giving a large dose of phytomenadione, it can be difficult to restore therapeutic anticoagulation with warfarin for up to 3 weeks. If the INR is >8.0 but there is no bleeding or only minor bleeding, then a smaller dose of phytomenadione can be given intravenously or orally with less disturbance of subsequent anticoagulation.
- Alopecia, skin necrosis and hypersensitivity reactions occur rarely.
- Warfarin crosses the placenta and can have undesirable effects on the fetus. It is teratogenic and should be avoided in the first trimester of pregnancy, except when essential; furthermore, it should not be used in the last trimester, as it increases the risk of intracranial haemorrhage in the baby during delivery.
- Drug interactions are particularly important. The anticoagulant effect of warfarin can be increased by broad-spectrum antibacterial agents that suppress the production of vitamin K by gut bacteria. Drugs such as amiodarone (see Chapter 8) and cimetidine (see Chapter 33) inhibit CYP2C9-mediated metabolism of warfarin and enhance its effects. Drugs that induce CYP2C9 – for example, phenytoin (see Chapter 23) and alcohol (see Chapter 54) – reduce the effect of warfarin by increasing its elimination. Foods rich in vitamin K, such as some green vegetables, also reduce the effect of warfarin.

Nonvitamin K-dependent oral anticoagulants

Direct factor Xa inhibitors

apixaban, edoxaban, rivaroxaban

Mechanism of action

Apixaban, edoxaban and rivaroxaban are orally active factor Xa inhibitors that bind reversibly to the active site of factor Xa. They inhibit both free factor Xa and factor Xa that is bound to the prothrombinase complex. Unlike warfarin, they produce a rapid onset of predictable anticoagulation.

Pharmacokinetics

Apixaban, epixaban and rivaroxaban are partially metabolised in the liver and partially excreted by the kidneys. Their half-lives are around 10 hours.

Unwanted effects

- Nausea, and less often other gastrointestinal upset.
- Haemorrhage. The risk of bleeding is less than with warfarin, especially intracerebral haemorrhage, but there is a higher risk of gastrointestinal bleeding. If bleeding occurs, the short half-life means that stopping treatment may be all that is required. There is no direct antidote (although adexanet alpha, a decoy receptor for factor Xa inhibitors, is under development as a specific reversal agent), but serious bleeding can be reduced with intravenous prothrombin complex concentrates or activated factor X.
- Drug interactions: rivaroxaban is a substrate for P-glycoprotein (P-gp), and its excretion is reduced by drugs that inhibit P-gp, such as ketoconazole.

Direct thrombin inhibitors

dabigatran etexilate

Mechanism of action

Dabigatran is a selective direct competitive thrombin inhibitor that binds to and inhibits both circulating and thrombus-bound thrombin (factor IIa). It produces a rapid onset of predictable anticoagulation.

Pharmacokinetics

Dabigatran etexilate is a prodrug that undergoes first-pass metabolism to its active derivative dabigatran. The active metabolite has a short half-life of about 40 minutes.

Unwanted effects

- Nausea, dyspepsia, diarrhoea, abdominal pain.
- Haemorrhage, but with a lower risk than warfarin at equally effective doses. Idarucizumab is a monoclonal antibody fragment that is a specific antidote for dabigatran and rapidly reverses its anticoagulant effect. It is reserved for serious haemorrhage caused by dabigatran.

CLINICAL USES OF ANTICOAGULANTS

Rapid anticoagulation can be achieved with LMWH or unfractionated heparin, and warfarin started simultaneously for long-term anticoagulation. The heparin is stopped when the INR reaches the desired therapeutic range. The nonvitamin K-dependent oral anticoagulants (NOACs) have a rapid onset of action, and in the case of rivaroxaban there is trial evidence that initial anticoagulation with heparin is not needed. Compared with warfarin, they have fewer drug interactions and do not need monitoring of their anticoagulant effect, which is predictable from standard doses. It is important to remember that the INR is unreliable as a guide to the extent of anticoagulation when NOACs are taken. In most situations where warfarin is used, NOACs have similar or greater efficacy compared to warfarin, with a lower risk of intracranial bleeding. Therefore there is increasing use of drugs such as apixaban, edoxaban, rivaroxaban and dabigatran in place of warfarin.

VENOUS THROMBOEMBOLISM

Deep vein thrombosis usually arises following stasis of blood in the deep venous circulation, although some episodes arise from excessive coagulability of blood. The most common sites are leg and pelvic veins, sometimes extending into the inferior vena cava. Less commonly, thrombus forms in veins in the arm, usually due to compression of venous outflow. Many episodes of deep vein thrombosis occur in hospital, particularly in people over 40 years of age following major illness, trauma or surgery. Factors predisposing to venous thromboembolism in a hospital setting (Table 11.1) include prolonged immobility and a variety of coexisting medical conditions such as cancer. Spontaneous thromboembolism can occur after long journeys, such as by road or air, and in various inherited or acquired disorders of the coagulation system. Use of the combined oral hormonal contraceptive, especially in older women who smoke (see Chapter 45), is also a factor.

After an initial spontaneous deep vein thrombosis, the risk of recurrence is about 25% after 4 years, but is much lower after postoperative thrombosis. Following a deep vein thrombosis, chronic postphlebitic syndrome can develop, with pain, swelling and ulceration of the affected leg.

Pulmonary embolism is a major cause of morbidity and death. Most serious pulmonary emboli arise from deep vein thrombosis in the lower limb, particularly if the thrombus extends to the larger veins above the calf. Acute pulmonary embolism can present with a variety of symptoms. Massive pulmonary emboli produce shock or sustained hypotension, while smaller emboli can present with chest pain, dyspnoea or haemoptysis. Massive pulmonary emboli causing

Table 11.1 Risk of thromboembolism in people admitted to hospital

Risk	Procedure
Low	Minor surgery, no other risk factor Major surgery, age <40 years, no other risk factors Minor trauma or illness
Moderate	Major surgery, age ≥40 years or other risk factor Heart failure, recent myocardial infarction, malignancy, inflammatory bowel disease Major trauma or burns Minor surgery, trauma or illness in patient with previous deep vein thrombosis or pulmonary embolism
High	Fracture or major orthopaedic surgery of pelvis, hips or lower limb Major pelvic or abdominal surgery for cancer Major surgery, trauma or illness in patient with previous deep vein thrombosis or pulmonary embolism Lower limb paralysis Major lower limb amputation

haemodynamic instability are fatal in about 60% of cases if untreated. Pulmonary embolism has been estimated to be responsible for up to 10% of all deaths in hospital. Mortality is much lower if the person is haemodynamically stable. Chronic pulmonary embolic disease can lead to pulmonary arterial hypertension with progressive dyspnoea (see Chapter 6).

Prevention of deep vein thrombosis

In people who are relatively immobile in hospital, the most appropriate method to prevent deep vein thrombosis will depend on the degree of risk.

Mechanical methods

These are used for people who are at moderate risk of thromboembolism and include graduated elastic compression stockings and intermittent pneumatic compression devices to improve venous flow and limit stasis in venous valve pockets. They can also be used to supplement pharmacological prophylaxis in people at high risk.

Low-dose subcutaneous heparin

This is the treatment of choice for many people in a hospital setting who are at high or moderate risk of thromboembolism. Low-dose heparin reduces both initiation and extension of fibrin-rich thrombi at doses that have little effect on measurements of blood coagulation; therefore laboratory monitoring is unnecessary. Low-dose unfractionated heparin reduces deep venous thrombosis and fatal pulmonary emboli by about two-thirds, with minimal risk of serious bleeding, although minor bleeding is increased. LMWHs or fondaparinux are more effective than unfractionated heparin for those at highest risk.

Oral anticoagulants

Low-dose dabigatran, apixaban and rivaroxaban are at least as effective as LMWHs for thromboprophylaxis in people undergoing hip and knee orthopaedic surgery. Bleeding rates are similar to LMWH. Prophylaxis should be started before surgery. Although a meta-analysis of several studies suggests that low-dose aspirin reduces the development of deep venous thrombosis, it is less effective than heparin.

Treatment of established venous thromboembolism

The goals of treatment for deep vein thrombosis are to prevent pulmonary emboli and to restore patency of the occluded vessel, with preservation of the function of venous valves. In about 50% of people with deep venous thrombosis, the vein will recanalise within 3 months if appropriately treated. The use of compression stockings in the first few weeks after a deep venous thrombosis of the leg reduces the incidence of postphlebitic syndrome.

Therapeutic anticoagulation

This is the treatment of choice for deep vein thrombosis and for most pulmonary emboli. LMWH or fondaparinux given subcutaneously are still the most widely used initial treatment. They have a rapid onset of effect and are preferred to unfractionated heparin because of their more predictable action. Unfractionated heparin is used for people with significant renal impairment. Heparin is usually given for 3–5 days, with concurrent initiation of treatment with warfarin. Heparin can be stopped once warfarin has produced adequate anticoagulation (i.e. the INR is within the therapeutic range, as described previously). When deep vein thrombosis occurs in someone with cancer, there is a high risk of both bleeding and recurrence during treatment with warfarin. In this situation, prolonged treatment with LMWH (6 months, or lifelong if remission is not achieved) is usually advocated. The optimal duration of anticoagulant therapy is not well defined, but suggested periods are shown in Table 11.2.

Rivaroxaban can be used alone instead of sequential heparin and warfarin, has equal efficacy and is more convenient. It is increasingly used as a convenient alternative strategy. At present there is only evidence for the efficacy of apixaban, edoxaban and dabigatran in venous thromboembolism after initial treatment with LMWH.

Surgical venous thrombectomy

This may be required for massive iliofemoral thrombosis if it threatens the viability of the limb. Pulmonary embolectomy is occasionally carried out for large pulmonary emboli.

Thrombolysis and percutaneous thrombectomy

Pharmacological thrombolysis (discussed later) has no advantage over warfarin in uncomplicated deep venous thrombosis. However, it is used to disintegrate massive pulmonary emboli (either intravenously or by infusion directly into the pulmonary artery), and reduces mortality in haemodynamically unstable patients. Percutaneous mechanical thrombectomy (fragmentation and removal of the thrombus) and surgical embolectomy are occasionally used if there are contraindications to thrombolysis.

Other treatments

When pulmonary emboli recur despite adequate anticoagulation, or when anticoagulation is contraindicated, inferior vena caval plication or insertion of a 'filter' device to trap emboli in the inferior vena cava can be considered.

ANTICOAGULATION FOR ARTERIAL THROMBOEMBOLISM

Warfarin is used long term for the prevention of thrombosis on prosthetic heart valves. Nonvitamin K-dependent oral anticoagulants are ineffective for preventing thrombus on mechanical heart valves, and should never be used.

Atrial fibrillation and mural thrombus in the left ventricle following a myocardial infarction predispose to arterial embolism and are indications for anticoagulation. Dabigatran, apixaban, edoxaban and rivaroxaban are at least as effective as warfarin for prevention of thromboembolism in non-valvular atrial fibrillation and have a lower risk of serious intracranial haemorrhage (see Chapter 8). When combined with dual antiplatelet therapy, apixaban reduces the composite endpoint of mortality, reinfarction and ischaemic stroke after an acute coronary syndrome, but with the risk of more bleeding (see Chapter 5).

THE FIBRINOLYTIC SYSTEM

Fibrinolysis is the physiological mechanism for dissolving the fibrin meshwork in a thrombus. The process is initiated by activation of plasminogen, a circulating α_2-globulin, to generate the fibrinolytic enzyme plasmin (Fig. 11.4). Tissue plasminogen activator (t-PA) released from damaged vessels cleaves plasminogen to plasmin. Plasminogen activator inhibitors 1 and 2 rapidly inactivate circulating t-PA. However, t-PA binds to fibrin locally at the site of release and converts fibrin-bound plasminogen to plasmin. Plasmin splits both fibrinogen and fibrin into degradation products, and if this occurs at the site of a thrombus, it produces lysis of the clot matrix. Fibrinolytic therapy

Table 11.2 Suggested duration of anticoagulant therapy for venous thromboembolism

Risk of recurrence	Clinical setting	Duration
Low	Temporary risk factors for thromboembolism Unprovoked distal deep vein thrombosis	3 months
Intermediate	Continuing medical risk factors for thromboembolism First unprovoked proximal deep vein thrombosis	Indefinite with annual review
High	Recurrent thromboembolism Inherited thrombophilic tendency Cancer-associated venous thromboembolism	Indefinite

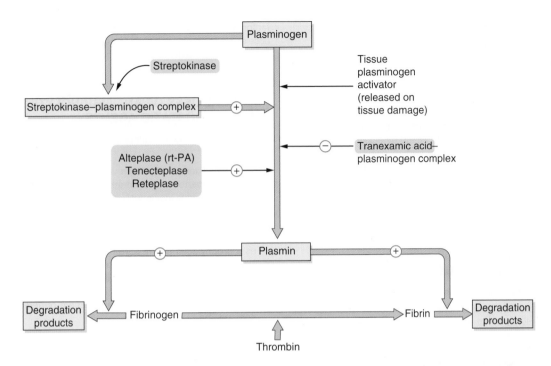

Fig. 11.4 The fibrinolytic system. The fibrinolytic system is linked closely to platelet function and the coagulation cascade. When a clot is formed via the prothrombotic system, activation of plasminogen to the fibrinolytic enzyme plasmin is initiated by several tissue plasminogen activators, thus lysing the clot. The drugs promoting fibrinolysis act as plasminogen activators (alteplase and analogues) or bind to plasminogen (streptokinase), promoting plasmin activity. The antifibrinolytic drug tranexamic acid inhibits plasminogen activation. *rt-PA*, Recombinant tissue-type plasminogen activator.

(thrombolysis) is achieved by using a plasminogen activator in such large quantities that the inhibitory controls are overwhelmed.

FIBRINOLYTIC (THROMBOLYTIC) AGENTS

alteplase (recombinant tissue-type plasminogen activator, rt-PA), streptokinase, tenecteplase

Mechanism of action

Fibrinolytic drugs enhance fibrinolysis by substituting for the naturally occurring t-PA. They bind to and activate plasminogen to plasmin, which degrades fibrin thrombi. Alteplase is a genetically engineered copy of the naturally occurring t-PA that binds directly to fibrinogen and fibrin. It has a wide range of clinical uses. Tenecteplase is a genetically engineered modified form of t-PA with increased fibrin specificity, less sensitivity to plasminogen activator inhibitors and a longer duration of action than alteplase. Tenecteplase is only licensed for treatment of myocardial infarction.

Streptokinase is obtained from haemolytic streptococci and is inactive until it forms a complex with circulating plasminogen; the resultant streptokinase–plasminogen activator complex substitutes for t-PA in the fibrinolytic cascade, causing plasminogen activation. Streptokinase is used much less frequently than other fibrinolytic drugs.

The effectiveness of any fibrinolytic agent is greatest with fresh thrombus and if a large surface area of thrombus is exposed to the drug.

Pharmacokinetics

All fibrinolytic agents are given intravenously or intraarterially. Alteplase and related compounds are metabolised in the liver. They have a more rapid onset of action than streptokinase, and consequently the reperfusion of occluded vessels is faster. Infusions of alteplase are given over 1–3 hours, depending on the condition being treated. Tenecteplase is given as a single bolus. Because of a short duration of action, when alteplase or its derivatives have been used to lyse coronary artery thrombus, subsequent anticoagulation with heparin for 48 hours is necessary to reduce the risk of reocclusion.

The streptokinase–plasminogen activator complex is degraded enzymatically in the circulation. After the use of streptokinase, or following a streptococcal infection, neutralising antibodies can form and persist for several years. These antibodies combine with streptokinase and clear it from the plasma before it forms an active complex, and substantially reduce the effectiveness of streptokinase. For this reason, repeat use of streptokinase is not recommended. Streptokinase is usually given as a short (1 hour) infusion for the treatment of coronary artery occlusion, although longer infusions are usual for peripheral arterial occlusions or pulmonary embolism. The long duration of action means that anticoagulation is not necessary after streptokinase has been given.

Unwanted effects

- Nausea and vomiting.
- Haemorrhage is usually minor, but serious bleeding (e.g. intracerebral haemorrhage) occurs in about 1% of those treated. Bleeding can be stopped by antifibrinolytic drugs (discussed later) or by transfusion of fresh frozen plasma.
- Hypotension. This is dose-related and more common with streptokinase. It may be caused by enzymatic release of the vasodilator bradykinin from its circulating precursor. If the infusion of the fibrinolytic is stopped for a brief period, the blood pressure usually recovers rapidly and treatment can be continued.
- Allergic reactions. These are rare but can occur with streptokinase as a consequence of its bacterial origin.

CLINICAL USES OF FIBRINOLYTIC AGENTS

Fibrinolytic agents are used to treat the following:

- acute myocardial infarction (although this use has declined with the greater availability of primary coronary angioplasty; see Chapter 5);
- ischaemic stroke (alteplase only; see Chapter 9);
- pulmonary embolism or deep venous thrombosis, in a minority of cases (described previously);
- peripheral arterial thromboembolism with acute limb ischaemia (see Chapter 10);
- central venous catheters occluded by thrombus (alteplase, which is particularly useful to restore patency of 'long lines' inserted for intravenous nutrition or administration of cytotoxic drugs).

ANTIFIBRINOLYTIC AND HAEMOSTATIC AGENTS

Antifibrinolytic agents

tranexamic acid

Mechanisms of action

Tranexamic acid competitively inhibits the activation of plasminogen, so fibrinolysis is inhibited. The theoretical risk of creating a thrombotic tendency does not appear to be a clinical problem.

Pharmacokinetics

Tranexamic acid is a synthetic amino acid that can be given orally or intravenously. It has a short half-life (1–2 hours).

Unwanted effects

- Nausea, vomiting, diarrhoea.

Desmopressin

Desmopressin (see Chapter 43) briefly increases the plasma concentrations of clotting factor VIII and von Willebrand factor, an adhesion protein in blood vessel walls. Factor VIII accelerates the process of fibrin formation, and von Willebrand factor enhances platelet adhesion to subendothelial tissue.

CLINICAL USES OF ANTIFIBRINOLYTIC AND HAEMOSTATIC AGENTS

The use of haemostatic agents is limited, but includes the following:

- Tranexamic acid is used to prevent bleeding after surgery (e.g. prostatectomy or bladder surgery) or after dental extraction in individuals with haemophilia.
- Desmopressin is used in mild congenital bleeding disorders such as haemophilia A or von Willebrand's disease; it is given to reduce spontaneous or traumatic bleeding, or as a prophylactic before surgery.
- Tranexamic acid is used for the treatment of menorrhagia and epistaxis, or for bleeding following an overdose of a fibrinolytic drug.
- Tranexamic acid is used for the treatment of hereditary angioedema.

SELF-ASSESSMENT

True/false questions

1. Unfractionated heparin and low-molecular-weight heparins (LMWH) directly inhibit thrombin in the coagulation cascade.
2. Heparin can be used to prevent clotting of blood collected in laboratory test tubes.
3. Once administered, the action of heparin cannot be reversed.
4. Fondaparinux is a pentapeptide activator of antithrombin III.
5. Warfarin readily crosses the placenta.
6. Warfarin prevents the synthesis of vitamin K-dependent clotting factors.
7. The activity of warfarin is inhibited by broad-spectrum antibacterial agents.
8. Clopidogrel has its antithrombotic action by enhancing the action of ADP on platelets.
9. Abciximab is an antibody directed against the glycoprotein GPIIb/IIIa receptor on platelets.
10. Aspirin is a reversible inhibitor of cyclo-oxygenase type 1 (COX-1).
11. Aspirin inhibits platelet aggregation at doses below those needed for an anti-inflammatory effect.
12. Fibrinolytic infusions of recombinant tissue-type plasminogen activator (rt-PA; alteplase) for myocardial infarction are usually given over the course of 1 hour, whereas streptokinase is given for 3–24 hours.
13. Tenecteplase is a modified form of t-PA with a longer half-life than alteplase.
14. Apixaban is a direct inhibitor of factor Xa.
15. Dabigatran inhibits thrombin in the plasma and within the thrombus.
16. Tranexamic acid enhances plasminogen activation.

One-best-answer (OBA) question

1. Identify the most accurate statement about anticoagulant drugs.
   A. INR needs to be regularly monitored in people treated with heparin.
   B. Heparin is the drug of choice if an oral anticoagulant is required for rapid anticoagulant activity before surgery.
   C. Dosage adjustment of warfarin is required if a person is prescribed concomitant treatment with the H_2 receptor antagonist cimetidine.
   D. In overdose, the effects of warfarin cannot be reversed.
   E. During treatment with a broad-spectrum antibacterial, the anticoagulant effects of enoxaparin may be inhibited.

Case-based questions

A 51-year-old obese female is treated with oestrogen replacement therapy for 18 months because of perimenopausal symptoms. She is scheduled for a hip replacement.
1. Is prophylactic pre-operative anticoagulant therapy necessary for this woman?
2. Should thromboprophylaxis be started before surgery?
3. Should a heparin or warfarin be chosen for prophylaxis, and what routes of administration are appropriate?
4. The hip replacement was carried out successfully and the woman was discharged from hospital after 5 days, although heparin therapy was continued for a further 5 days. Why is therapy continued for this extended period, and what out-of-hospital therapeutic prophylaxis could be considered?

ANSWERS

True/false answers

1. **False.** Heparins first form a complex with antithrombin III; the complex then inactivates thrombin and other clotting factors, including factors IXa, Xa and XIa. Complexes of LMWH with antithrombin have a more selective action on factor Xa.
2. **True.** The complexing of heparin with antithrombin III in plasma means it can anticoagulate blood in vitro.
3. **False.** The action of unfractionated heparin (but not LMWH) can be reversed by the strongly basic protein protamine, which rapidly binds to it, forming an inactive complex.
4. **False.** All heparins are mucopolysaccharides, not polypeptides. Fondaparinux is similar in structure to the pentasaccharide sequence within heparin that binds to antithrombin.
5. **True.** Warfarin can cause fetal abnormalities and, unless essential, should not be given in early or late pregnancy.
6. **True.** Warfarin inhibits vitamin K epoxide reductase (VKOR); this reduces the regeneration of the active (hydroquinone) form of vitamin K required for gamma-carboxylation of clotting factors II (prothrombin), VII, IX and X in the liver.
7. **False.** Vitamin K is produced by gut bacteria, and their elimination by broad-spectrum antibacterials reduces vitamin K formation. This further impairs the synthesis of vitamin K-dependent clotting factors and *enhances* the anticoagulant activity of warfarin.
8. **False.** Clopidogrel and related drugs prevent the platelet aggregatory action of ADP by blocking its purinergic (P2Y$_{12}$) receptors.
9. **True.** The increased expression of GPIIb/IIIa receptors on activated platelets is essential for aggregation as fibrinogen links adjacent platelets by binding to these glycoproteins; abciximab is an antibody inhibitor of GPIIb/IIIa receptors.
10. **False.** Aspirin (acetylsalicylic acid) irreversibly inhibits COX-1 by acetylating its active site. At low doses this produces a selective antiplatelet action, as the platelet is nonnucleated and unable to replace the COX-1 enzyme by gene transcription and protein synthesis.
11. **True.** Thromboxane A2 (TXA2) required for platelet aggregation is synthesised by COX-1, whereas prostaglandins are synthesised during inflammation predominantly by induced cyclo-oxygenase type 2 (COX-2). Aspirin is 160 times more active at inhibiting COX-1 than COX-2, so it has no anti-inflammatory effect at the low doses required to inhibit TXA2 synthesis.
12. **False.** Streptokinase is usually infused for 1 hour and alteplase for 3 hours. Streptokinase has a longer half-life (1 hour, alteplase 0.5 hour), permitting a shorter infusion time.
13. **True.** Alteplase is identical to the naturally occurring t-PA, while tenecteplase has been modified for greater fibrin specificity and a longer duration of action.
14. **True.** Apixaban, edoxaban and rivaroxaban are orally active direct inhibitors of factor Xa.
15. **True.** Unlike heparin, which only inhibits plasma thrombin (via antithrombin III), dabigatran directly inhibits both free thrombin and thrombus-bound thrombin.
16. **False.** Tranexamic acid is an antifibrinolytic agent that inhibits plasminogen activation, reducing fibrin degradation and the risk of bleeding.

One-best-answer (OBA) answer

1. **Answer C** is the accurate statement.
   A. Incorrect. Regular INR monitoring is required in people taking warfarin but not heparin, when the activated partial thromboplastin time (APTT) is used. Monitoring is not required when LMWHs are used subcutaneously.
   B. Incorrect. Heparin is inactive orally and must be given by intravenous or subcutaneous routes.
   C. Correct. Warfarin is metabolised by the liver cytochrome P450 CYP2C9, and cimetidine inhibits this isoenzyme. A reduction in warfarin dose may be required, or the replacement of cimetidine with another H_2 antihistamine or a proton pump inhibitor without an interaction with warfarin.
   D. Incorrect. The effects of warfarin can be reversed with vitamin K_1.
   E. Incorrect. Broad-spectrum antibacterials can suppress the production of vitamin K by gut bacteria and increase the activity of warfarin, but would not affect the actions of heparin.

Case-based answers

1. Anticoagulant therapy is necessary. Postoperative venous thromboembolism occurs in 40–50% of people who

undergo hip replacement, and fatal pulmonary embolism in 1–5%, if prophylactic anticoagulant therapy is not given. This woman is also at increased risk because of obesity.

2. This is controversial. Initiating prophylaxis postoperatively allows more effective haemostatic control during and immediately after surgery, and does not reduce the effectiveness of treatment.

3. Heparins are active given intravenously or subcutaneously, and their onset of action is rapid, whereas warfarin takes several days for full effectiveness but can be given orally.

Heparin would therefore be chosen if started pre- or postoperatively.

4. The woman is obese, a risk factor for postoperative venous thrombosis. Daily self-administered subcutaneous prophylaxis with an LMWH or fondaparinux could be used. These drugs have more predictable anticoagulant activity, longer durations of action and a lower risk of producing thrombocytopenia than unfractionated heparin. Low doses of dabigatran, apixaban or rivaroxaban started before surgery are as effective as LMWHs for thromboprophylaxis in people undergoing hip and knee orthopaedic surgery.

FURTHER READING

Antiplatelet agents

Antiplatelet Trialist's Collaboration, 2002. Collaborative meta-analysis of randomised trials of antiplatelet therapy for prevention of death, myocardial infarction and stroke in high risk patients. Br. Med. J. 324, 71–86.

Floyd, C.N., Ferro, A., 2013. Mechanisms of aspirin resistance. Pharmacol. Ther. 141, 69–78.

Mega, J.L., Simon, T., 2015. Pharmacology of antithrombotic drugs: an assessment of oral antiplatelet and anticoagulant treatments. Lancet 386, 281–291.

Sambu, N., Curzen, N., 2011. Monitoring the effectiveness of antiplatelet therapy: opportunities and limitations. Br. J. Clin. Pharmacol. 72, 83–696.

Schneider, D.J., 2011. Antiplatelet therapy: glycoprotein IIb–IIIa antagonists. Br. J. Clin. Pharmacol. 72, 672–682.

Wells, P.S., Forgie, M.A., Rodger, M.A., 2014. Treatment of venous thromboembolism. JAMA 311, 2545.

Wiviott, S.D., Steg, P.G., 2015. Clinical evidence for oral antiplatelet therapy in acute coronary syndrome. Lancet 386, 292–302.

Anticoagulants

Arbit, B., Nishimura, M., Hsu, J.C., 2016. Reversal agents for direct oral anticoagulants: a focused review. Int. J. Cardiol. 223, 244–250.

Blann, A.D., Lip, G.Y.H., 2016. Non-vitamin K antagonist oral anticoagulants (NOACs) for the management of venous thromboembolism. Heart 102, 975–983.

Cayley, W.E., 2007. Preventing deep vein thrombosis in hospital inpatients. Br. Med. J. 335, 147–151.

Lapner, S.T., Kearon, C., 2013. Diagnosis and management of pulmonary embolism. Br. Med. J. 346, f757.

Verheught, F.W.A., Granger, C.B., 2015. Oral anticoagulants for stroke prevention in atrial fibrillation: current status, special situations and unmet needs. Lancet 386, 303–310.

Welsh, R.C., Roe, M.T., Steg, P.G., et al., 2016. A critical reappraisal of aspirin for secondary prevention in patients with ischemic heart disease. Am. Heart J. 181, 92–100.

Fibrinolytic drugs

Bivard, A., Lin, L., Parsons, M.W., 2013. Review of stroke thrombolytics. J. Stroke 15, 90–98.

Nordt, T.K., Bode, C., 2003. Thrombolysis: newer thrombolytic agents and their role in clinical medicine. Heart 89, 1358–1362.

Haemostatic drugs

Mannucci, P.M., Levi, M., 2007. Prevention and treatment of major blood loss. N. Engl. J. Med. 356, 2301–2311.

Compendium: drugs used to affect haemostasis

Drug	Characteristics
Antiplatelet drugs	
Inhibit platelet activation and aggregation by a range of mechanisms.	
Abciximab	Antibody; produces long-lasting blockade of platelet glycoprotein IIb/IIIa receptors. Specialist use only, as adjunct to heparin and aspirin in high-risk PCI. Given intravenously. Half-life: 0.5 h
Aspirin	Cyclo-oxygenase inhibitor; deacetylated to salicylic acid. Low dose used for the secondary prevention of thrombotic cerebrovascular or cardiovascular disease. Given orally. Half-life: 0.3h (aspirin), 3–20 h (salicylic acid)
Cangrelor	Reversible antagonist of platelet adenosine diphosphate (ADP; $P2Y_{12}$) receptors. Used with aspirin to prevent thrombotic cardiovascular during percutaneous coronary intervention (PCI) when other oral ADP antagonists are not suitable (specialist use). Given intravenously. Half-life: 2–4 min
Clopidogrel	Prodrug of irreversible ADP ($P2Y_{12}$) receptor antagonist. Used for the prevention of ischaemic events in people with a history of symptomatic ischaemic disease. Given orally. Half-life: 6–8 h
Dipyridamole	Phosphodiesterase inhibitor; also enhances antiplatelet and vasodilator activity of adenosine. Used as an adjunct to oral anticoagulants in people with prosthetic heart valves and for the secondary prevention of ischaemic stroke. Given orally, or by intravenous injection (for diagnostic purposes). Half-life: 12 h

Compendium: drugs used to affect haemostasis (cont'd)

Drug	Characteristics
Epoprostenol	Prostacyclin (prostaglandin I_2); antiaggregatory action and potent vasodilator. Used in combination with heparin during renal dialysis; also used with oral anticoagulants for resistant primary pulmonary hypertension. Given intravenously. Half-life: 3 min
Eptifibatide	Cyclic hexapeptide; inhibits glycoprotein IIb/IIIa receptor. Used as an adjunct to heparin and aspirin in high-risk people with unstable angina (specialist use only). Given intravenously. Half-life: 1.5–2 h
Prasugrel	Prodrug of irreversible antagonist of platelet ADP (P2Y$_{12}$) receptors. Uses similar to clopidogrel, but more rapid onset and greater inhibition of platelet aggregation. Given orally. Half-life: 2–15 h (active metabolite)
Ticagrelor	Reversible antagonist of platelet ADP (P2Y$_{12}$) receptors. Used in combination with low-dose aspirin for the prevention of atherothrombotic events in people with acute coronary syndrome. Given orally. Half-life: 7 h
Tirofiban	Nonpeptide inhibitor of glycoprotein IIb/IIIa receptor. Used as an adjunct to heparin and aspirin in high-risk people with unstable angina (specialist use only). Given intravenously. Half-life: 2 h

Anticoagulants

Heparin-like anticoagulants

Heparin-like anticoagulants are polysaccharides that enhance the inhibitory action of antithrombin on thrombin and/or factor Xa; they are given by injection. Low-molecular-weight heparins (LMWHs) and the pentasaccharide fondaparinux have more predictable anticoagulant activity, longer durations of action and fewer unwanted effects than unfractionated heparin; they do not usually require monitoring of clotting time and are commonly given by subcutaneous injection, or intravenously. The half-lives provided are based on duration of anticoagulant activity, not on plasma drug concentrations.

Dalteparin sodium	LMWH. Used for treatment and prevention of venous thromboembolism; also used in myocardial infarction, unstable angina and to prevent clotting in extracorporeal circuits. Half-life: 2–4 h
Danaparoid sodium	Heparinoid substance. Used in prophylaxis of deep vein thrombosis on a named-patient basis only. Half-life: 17–28 h
Enoxaparin	LMWH. Used similar to dalteparin. Half-life: 3–6 h
Fondaparinux	Synthetic pentasaccharide; antithrombin-dependent anticoagulant action is selective for factor Xa. Used for prophylaxis of thromboembolism in people undergoing major orthopaedic surgery of the legs. Half-life: 18 h
Heparin (unfractionated)	Antithrombin-dependent inhibitor of factor Xa and thrombin. LMWHs are preferred for routine use, but unfractionated heparin can be used in patients at high risk of bleeding. Given as an intravenous loading dose followed by an intravenous infusion or intermittent subcutaneous injection for initial treatment of deep vein thrombosis and pulmonary embolism; also used for prophylaxis of venous thromboembolism in people with renal failure. Half-life (0.4–2.5 h) is dose-dependent due to saturable metabolism in tissues
Tinzaparin	LMWH. Uses similar to dalteparin. Half-life: 3–4 h

Vitamin K antagonists

Inhibit vitamin K epoxide reductase required for hepatic synthesis of clotting factors II (prothrombin), VII, IX and X. Warfarin is the drug of choice, and the others are seldom required. Slow onset of action (48–72 h) necessitates combination with heparins if immediate action is required.

Acenocoumarol	Coumarin anticoagulant. Uses as for warfarin. Given orally. Half-life: 8–11 h
Phenindione	Synthetic anticoagulant. Uses as for warfarin. Given orally. Half-life: 5–6 h
Warfarin	Coumarin anticoagulant. Used for treatment of deep vein thrombosis and pulmonary embolism, and for prophylaxis of embolism in rheumatic heart disease, atrial fibrillation and after insertion of prosthetic heart valves. Given orally. Half-life: 20–50 h

Direct factor Xa inhibitors

Apixaban	Used for treatment and prevention of thromboembolism, particularly after hip and knee replacement surgery. Given orally. Half-life: 9–12 h
Edoxaban	Used for treatment and prevention of recurrent venous thromboembolism. Given orally. Half-life: 10–14 h
Rivaroxaban	Used for treatment and prevention of thromboembolism, particularly after hip and knee replacement surgery. Given orally. Half-life: 9–12 h

Compendium: drugs used to affect haemostasis (cont'd)

Drug	Characteristics
Direct thrombin inhibitors	
Argatroban monohydrate	Nonpeptide inhibitor of thrombin. Used for anticoagulation in people with heparin-induced thrombocytopenia type II. Given intravenously. Half-life: 52 min
Bivalirudin	Peptide related to hirudin (found in saliva of medicinal leeches). Used with aspirin and clopidogrel for people undergoing percutaneous coronary intervention, and in unstable angina and acute myocardial infarction. Given intravenously. Half-life: 0.5 h
Dabigatran etexilate	Prodrug of dabigatran, a nonpeptide inhibitor acting on both free and clot-bound thrombin (factor IIa). Used for treatment and prophylaxis of thromboembolic events, particularly in orthopaedic surgery. Half-life: 40 min
Fibrinolytic (thrombolytic) agents	
Activate plasminogen to plasmin. Used in the treatment of myocardial infarction; all are macromolecules given intravenously.	
Alteplase (recombinant tissue-type plasminogen activator)	Tissue-type plasminogen activator. Given by intravenous injection or infusion. Half-life: 0.5 h
Reteplase	Recombinant plasminogen activator. Given by intravenous injection over not more than 2 min. Half-life: 0.3–0.5 h
Streptokinase	Streptococcal plasminogen activator. Also used for life-threatening venous thrombosis and pulmonary embolism. Given by intravenous infusion. Half-life: 2 h
Tenecteplase	Modified tissue-type plasminogen activator; higher selectivity than alteplase for fibrin. Given by intravenous injection over 10 s. Half-life: 1.5–2 h
Urokinase	Human urokinase purified from urine. Used for deep vein thrombosis and pulmonary embolism; also used for clearing occluded catheters and cannulas. Half-life: <20 min
Antifibrinolytic drugs and haemostatic agents	
Etamsylate	Reduces capillary bleeding, probably by affecting platelet adhesion. Given orally
Tranexamic acid	Used in hereditary angioedema, epistaxis and after excessive thrombolytic dosage. Given orally or by slow intravenous injection. Half-life: 1.4 h

3

The respiratory system

12 Asthma and chronic obstructive pulmonary disease

Asthma and chronic obstructive pulmonary disease (COPD) show several similarities in their clinical features but have some distinct pathophysiological – including immunological – differences. Both are inflammatory disorders of the bronchi. Clinically, they present with airflow obstruction (a forced expiratory volume in 1 second [FEV_1] below 80% of predicted and a ratio of FEV_1 to forced vital capacity of less than 70%). The differentiation is further complicated by the recognition of an asthma-COPD overlap syndrome (ACOS).

- Asthma is a heterogeneous disease, usually characterised by chronic airway inflammation. It is defined by the history of respiratory symptoms such as wheezing, shortness of breath, chest tightness and cough that vary over time and in intensity, together with variable expiratory airflow limitation.
- COPD is characterised by persistent airflow limitation that is usually progressive and associated with enhanced chronic inflammatory responses in the airways and the lungs to noxious particles and gases. Exacerbations and comorbidities contribute to the overall severity of COPD in individual people.
- ACOS is characterised by persistent airflow limitation with several features usually associated with asthma, and several features usually associated with COPD. ACOS is therefore identified by the features that it shares with both asthma and COPD.

ASTHMA

The characteristic feature of asthma is reversible airflow obstruction. Asthma is often associated with an atopic disposition, and exposure to allergens or other environmental air pollutants may then result in expression of the condition. However, more severe and adult-onset asthma is often nonallergic and accounts for 10–30% of cases.

The most common symptoms of asthma are chest tightness, wheezing, breathlessness and cough, although cough may be the only symptom in younger people, often at night. Airflow obstruction in asthma typically shows marked variability over time and greater than 15% improvement in response to any inhaled bronchodilator (discussed later). The symptoms are due to a combination of smooth muscle constriction in the airway and bronchial inflammation.

The pathogenesis of asthma is complex, and our knowledge is incomplete (Figs 12.1 and 12.2). Immune dysfunction leads to airway inflammation in asthma and may result from impaired regulation and imbalance between different T-lymphocyte subsets and also epithelial and airway dendritic cells. Inflammation of the bronchial mucosa is prominent, with infiltration of activated T-helper 2 lymphocytes, eosinophils and mast cells. These inflammatory cells release several powerful chemical mediators that promote hyperplasia of bronchial smooth muscle, increased smooth muscle reactivity, oedema of the bronchial wall, deposition of subepithelial collagen and increased airway secretions. Dysregulation of numerous inflammatory mediators appears to be involved in asthma, including cysteinyl-leukotrienes, histamine, proteases and a variety of cytokines and chemokines, but unlike COPD, there is little evidence of an increase in reactive oxygen species.

Fig. 12.1 shows how exposure of atopic individuals to a relevant allergen (such as pollen or the faeces of house-dust mite) crosslinks immunoglobulin E (IgE) bound to mast cell membrane receptors and causes mast cell degranulation. Degranulation and the subsequent pathological processes can also occur in hypersensitive nonatopic asthmatics with

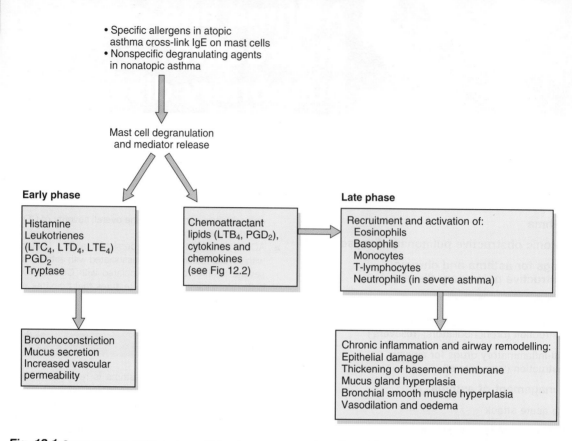

Fig. 12.1 **Some aspects of the early- and late-phase responses in asthma.** Allergen crosslinking of the IgE overexpressed on mast cells of atopic individuals, and nonimmunogenic stimuli in more severe nonatopic asthma, can degranulate mast cells, resulting in the release of preformed mediators such as histamine from mast cell granules, and de novo synthesis of lipid mediators such as leukotrienes (LT) and prostaglandin (PG) D_2, which directly produce early-phase bronchoconstriction and initiate the acute inflammatory response. These mediators, together with inflammatory cytokines and chemokines, attract and activate cells including eosinophils, monocytes and T lymphocytes that are responsible for further inflammatory mediator production and persistent chronic inflammation. *IgE,* Immunoglobulin E.

normal levels of IgE, triggered by other factors such as upper respiratory tract infections, particularly with human rhinovirus. Degranulation of mast cells produces immediate bronchoconstriction (early phase) due to the synthesis and release of a number of spasmogens, of which the most potent are the cysteinyl-leukotrienes LTC_4 and LTD_4 (see Fig. 12.1). Chemotactic mediators are also synthesised and released, including prostaglandin (PG)D_2, leukotriene E_4, interleukins (IL-3, IL-5, IL-6, IL-8), and chemokines such as eotaxin, monocyte chemoattractant proteins (MCP) and RANTES (regulated on activation, normal T-cell expressed and secreted). These promote an influx of inflammatory cells which 4–6 hours later results in a delayed bronchoconstrictor response (late phase) and the commencement of a cascade of other pathological events in the airways. The persistent release of spasmogens and inflammatory mediators by these infiltrating cells can leave the bronchi hyperreactive to various irritants for several weeks. The inflammatory mediators produce mucosal oedema, which narrows the airways, and also stimulate smooth muscle contraction leading to bronchoconstriction. Excessive production of mucus can cause further airways obstruction by plugging the bronchiolar lumen.

In *mild to moderate* asthma, both large and small airways are involved in the inflammatory process, but the degree of submucosal fibrosis and mucus secretion is modest, with no parenchymal destruction.

In *severe* asthma there is evidence of additional, greater infiltration of neutrophils, tissue destruction and airways remodelling, with progressive thickening and loss of elastic recoil, especially in the small airways.

CHRONIC OBSTRUCTIVE PULMONARY DISEASE

About 95% of people with COPD in the developed world are, or have been, cigarette smokers. There is wide variability in the rate of decline in pulmonary function in persistent smokers, with about 10–20% showing an accelerated decline that may reflect a genetic susceptibility. Less common causes of COPD are exposure to air pollution (including biomass fuels, which are a common cause of COPD in the developing world) and inherited α_1-antiprotease (α_1-antitrypsin) deficiency.

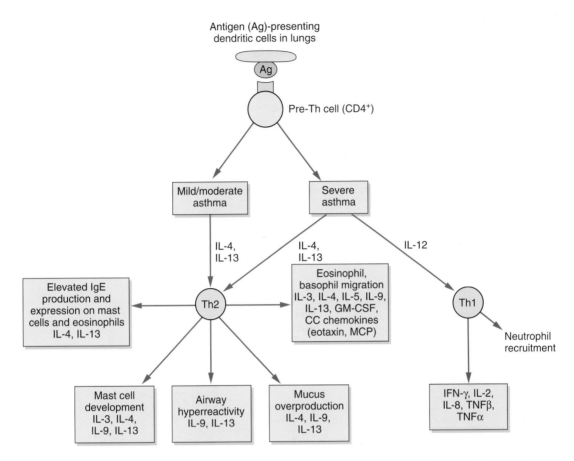

Fig. 12.2 **T-cells and asthma.** In allergic asthma there are complex and still poorly understood imbalances in the immune system. These include alterations in the functioning of several T-cell subsets and additional dysregulation in epithelial cells, fibroblasts and airway dendritic cells. In mild to moderate allergic asthma, the T-helper cell type 2 (Th2) response is amplified, and Th2 cytokines contribute to many of the pathophysiological features of asthma. In severe asthma there is an additional pathological role for T-helper type 1 (Th1) cytokines and neutrophils. *GM-CSF*, Granulocyte–macrophage colony stimulating factor; *IFN*, interferon; *IgE*, immunoglobulin E; *IL*, interleukin; *MCP*, monocyte chemoattractant proteins; *TNF*, tumour necrosis factor.

COPD is a symptom complex that is characterised by persistent airflow obstruction, with most people showing limited reversibility in response to a bronchodilator; however, up to 60% of people with COPD do show bronchial hyper-responsiveness and considerable bronchodilator-induced reversibility of the airflow obstruction. They have a mixed inflammatory pattern in the airways, which is now recognised as the ACOS.

The airflow obstruction in COPD is usually slowly progressive and results from a combination of decreased bronchial luminal diameter affecting small airways, produced by wall thickening, intraluminal mucus and changes in the fluid lining together with dynamic airways collapse due to emphysema (discussed later). It is often accompanied by chronic bronchitis (production of mucoid sputum for all or part of the year).

The most frequent symptoms of COPD are gradually progressive breathlessness and cough. The cough is often productive and usually worse in the morning, but its severity is unrelated to the degree of airflow obstruction. Repeated respiratory infections are common, and are often associated with exacerbations of the airflow obstruction and symptomatic deterioration.

In COPD there is an inflammatory process that particularly affects the peripheral airways. The predominant infiltrating cells are neutrophils and macrophages, but ongoing damage to the lung even after the trigger is removed is probably due to $CD8^+$ T-lymphocyte-mediated inflammation (Fig. 12.3). There is increased oxidative stress due to reactive oxygen species derived from cigarette smoke and other pollutants and released from neutrophils and inflammatory macrophages. The inflammation produces a marked fibrotic reaction with parenchymal destruction and excessive bronchial mucus secretion. Corresponding histological changes include an increase in goblet cells in the bronchial mucosa and an increase in muscle mass in the bronchial wall, accompanied by interstitial fibrosis. Apoptosis of endothelial and alveolar cells reduces the ability of the lung to repair itself in response to sustained injury from the inhaled pollutants.

Emphysema is a pathological description, and is defined as enlargement of airways distal to the terminal bronchioles owing to destructive changes that may involve the entire acinus

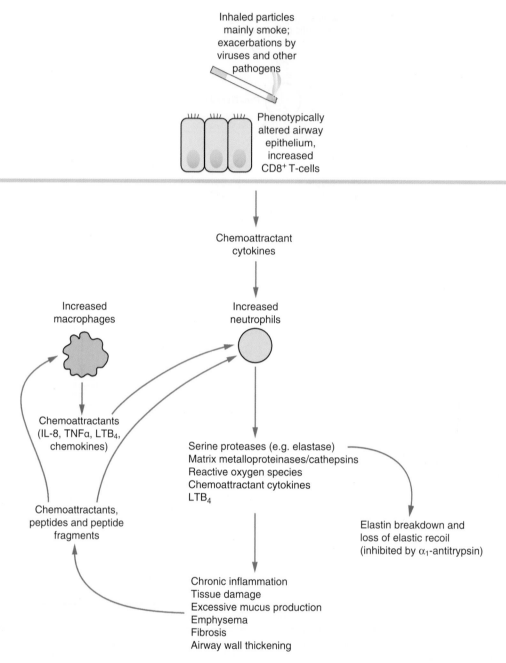

Fig. 12.3 **Pathophysiological factors in chronic obstructive pulmonary disease.** Irritants and particles in cigarette smoke trigger mucus production and activation of macrophages, which release chemoattractants that recruit neutrophil leucocytes to the airways. Neutrophils release elastase, which breaks down elastin, and other factors that cause tissue damage and promote chronic inflammation. A small percentage of people are particularly susceptible to the development of COPD due to variability in inflammatory or protective gene products, including α_1-antitrypsin, which normally inhibits neutrophil elastase. Chronic alterations in the function of neutrophils, macrophages and subsets of T-cells result in parenchymal damage, loss of elastic recoil and episodes of infection. *COPD,* Chronic obstructive pulmonary disease; *IL-8,* interleukin-8; *LTB$_4$,* leukotriene B$_4$; *TNFα,* tumour necrosis factor alpha.

(panacinar) or the central part of the acinus (centriacinar). Lung parenchymal destruction is largely mediated by tissue proteases and cathepsins that are released by neutrophils and macrophages. Generation of excessive amounts of reactive oxygen species inhibits the antiproteases that normally protect the lung against such attack. This explains the susceptibility of people with inherited α_1-antiprotease deficiency to emphysema. Tissue destruction leads to a loss of lung recoil on expiration, which is a major factor in reduced expiratory flow. Emphysema is probably the dominant factor in severe COPD.

DRUGS FOR ASTHMA AND CHRONIC OBSTRUCTIVE PULMONARY DISEASE

DRUG DELIVERY TO THE LUNG

For the treatment of airways disease, direct delivery of drug to the lung by inhalation allows the use of smaller doses than with systemic use, and therefore reduces the incidence of unwanted systemic effects (see Table 12.1). It also allows rapid onset of action of 'rescue' medication. The drug is usually delivered directly to the airways in an aerosol form or a dry powder. The size of the inhaled particle is an important factor that determines whether or not it will reach the airways and where in the airways it will be deposited. The optimal particle size is 2–5 μm. Particles larger than 10 μm impact on the upper airways and will be swallowed. Particles smaller than 1 μm are not deposited in the lower respiratory tract and will reach the alveoli and be absorbed into the blood, or are exhaled. Other factors that influence particle deposition include the pattern of inhalation, the properties of the carrier and the type and severity of the lung disease. There are several methods for the delivery of the inhaled drug.

Pressurised metered-dose inhaler

This is the most common device for delivery of bronchodilator and anti-inflammatory drugs used in the treatment of asthma and COPD. The propellant in the device is a pressurised hydrofluoroalkane (HFA), and activation delivers a measured dose of aerosol via an atomisation nozzle. One variant of this type of inhaler (soft-mist inhaler) generates two fine jets of liquid that converge and release a soft mist when they collide with 60–80% of the particles at optimal size. A pressurised metered-dose inhaler (pMDI) should be shaken before use. Optimal delivery of the drug requires:

- adequate inspiratory flow rate;
- gentle, slow, long inspiration preceded by full expiration;
- breath hold of at least 5 seconds.

Manually activated pMDIs depend on coordination of timing of dose release and inspiration. About one-third of users find coordination difficult, and even if it is optimal, up to 70–90% of the aerosol may be deposited in the oropharynx and swallowed. This is avoided if a breath-actuated pMDI is used. However, breath actuation requires air to be drawn through the mouthpiece at a flow rate of at least 30 L/

Table 12.1 Comparison of aerosol and oral therapy for asthma

	Aerosol	Oral
Ideal pharmacokinetics	Slow absorption from the lung surface and rapid systemic clearance	Good oral absorption and slow systemic clearance
Dose	Low dose delivered rapidly to target, with low systemic drug concentrations	High systemic dose necessary, which achieves appropriate concentration in the lung more slowly than by inhaled route
Incidence of unwanted effects	Usually low	High (but depends on drug)
Distribution in the lung	Rapid, but may be reduced in severe disease	Slow, but unaffected by airway disease
Adherence	Good with bronchodilators, but may be poor with prophylactic use of anti-inflammatory drugs	Good
Ease of administration	May be difficult for small children and infirm people[a]	Good
Effectiveness	Good in mild to moderate disease	Good even in severe disease

[a]May be improved by spacer devices. Nebulisers can be used for severe exacerbations.

minute, and people who have severe airflow obstruction cannot achieve this.

Pressurised metered-dose inhaler with a spacer

A spacer device (a plastic reservoir) can be attached to the pMDI to act as a chamber from which the suspended aerosol particles can be inhaled. The use of a spacer removes the need to coordinate aerosol activation and inspiration. A spacer can be large volume, which retains more of the aerosol, or small volume, which is more convenient but in which the aerosol impacts to a greater extent on the wall of the spacer. The spacer can be designed as a holding chamber by incorporating a one-way valve that retains the aerosol in the chamber for longer. A spacer is essential for young children, and for very young children a holding chamber can be attached to a facemask. The inhaler is activated into the spacer, and tidal breathing through the mouthpiece delivers the drug. Inhalation of the contents should be completed within 10 seconds of inhaler activation. The spacer allows evaporation of propellant and may create more droplets of the correct size to deposit in the airways. It also reduces drug deposition in the oropharynx, due to reduced particle velocity. Electrostatic charge on the plastic wall can attract particles and reduce drug delivery, so nonelectrostatic materials are preferred. The device should be washed in mild detergent once a month and air-dried to minimise the electrostatic charge. The addition of a spacer makes a metered-dose inhaler system less portable and may reduce adherence with treatment. Breath-actuated metered-dose inhaler devices cannot be used with a spacer.

Dry-powder inhaler

Dry-powder inhalers contain particles of drug of optimal size for deposition. Inspiration through the device generates turbulence, which disperses the particles in the inspired air. Some devices use a single-dose capsule that is loaded in the device and pierced, while in others the source is a bulk powder with the device metering the dose and a counter showing how many doses remain. Some devices produce an audible click to indicate successful activation. Optimal drug delivery requires:

- a deep, forceful, long inhalation over at least 5 seconds;
- breath hold for at least 10 seconds.

Nebulisers

Nebulisers are devices used with a facemask or mouthpiece to deliver the drug from a reservoir solution. There are two types:

- Jet nebulisers use compressed air or oxygen passing through a narrow orifice at 6–8 L/minute to suck drug solution from a reservoir into a feed tube. There are fine ligaments in this tube, and the impact of the solution on these ligaments generates droplets (Venturi principle). Baffles trap the larger droplets.
- Ultrasonic nebulisers use a piezoelectric crystal vibrating at high frequency to create the aerosol, and do not require gas flow. The vibrations are transmitted through a buffer to the drug solution and form a fountain of liquid in the nebulisation chamber. Ultrasonic nebulisers produce a more uniform particle size than jet nebulisers, but are less widely used due to cost.

Up to 10 times the amount of drug is required in a nebuliser to produce the same degree of bronchodilation achieved by a metered-dose inhaler. Drug delivery is more efficient via a mouthpiece than via a mask from which drug can be deposited in the nasal passages.

SYMPTOM-RELIEVING DRUGS FOR AIRFLOW OBSTRUCTION (BRONCHODILATORS; 'RELIEVERS')

β_2-Adrenoceptor agonists

Examples

short-acting: salbutamol, terbutaline
long-acting: formoterol, salmeterol
ultra-long-acting: indacaterol

Mechanism of action and effects

β_2-Adrenoceptors are widely distributed in the lung, and the receptor density is higher in bronchial smooth muscle than in other cell types such as epithelial and endothelial cells and mast cells. Stimulation of these receptors by an agonist stabilises the receptor in its active rather than inactive configuration. This results in increased generation of cyclic adenosine monophosphate (cAMP) by adenylyl cyclase, and activation of protein kinase A (PKA), which phosphorylates myosin light chain proteins that are central to the regulation of smooth muscle tone. β_2-Adrenoceptor agonists also reduce Ca^{2+} entry into muscle cells and activate K^+ channels that hyperpolarise the smooth muscle cell. Major beneficial actions of a β_2-adrenoceptor agonist are:

- bronchodilation due to relaxation of bronchial smooth muscle cells;
- inhibition of mediator release from mast cells and infiltrating leucocytes;
- enhanced mucociliary clearance.

However, in addition to their beneficial effects on the airway, frequent use of a β_2-adrenoceptor agonist in asthma can enhance Th2 inflammatory pathways and also downregulate β_2-adrenoceptors. Regular use of a β_2-adrenoceptor agonist without an inhaled corticosteroid is therefore not advised. There is evidence of synergy between inhaled corticosteroids and inhaled β_2-adrenoceptor agonists, with the latter enhancing the gene-transcription effects of corticosteroids, and corticosteroids increasing β_2-adrenoceptor gene transcription and enhancing coupling of the receptor to adenylyl cyclase.

Some β_2-adrenoceptor agonists, such as salbutamol, terbutaline and salmeterol, have about 60% partial agonist activity at the receptor (low-efficacy agonists) compared with formoterol and indacaterol, which have full agonist activity (high-efficacy agonists). The relevance of these differences to treatment outcomes and unwanted effects is unclear.

Pharmacokinetics

The selectivity of β_2-adrenoceptor agonists for the β_2-adrenoceptor subtype is dose-dependent. Inhalation of drug aids selectivity, since it delivers small doses to the airways and minimises systemic exposure of β-adrenoceptors outside the lungs (see Table 12.1). The dose–response relationship for bronchodilation is log-linear, and a 10-fold increase in dose is required to double the bronchodilator response.

Short-acting β_2-adrenoceptor agonists, such as salbutamol, have a rapid onset of action, often within 5 minutes, and produce bronchodilation for up to about 6 hours. Their duration of action is far longer than the natural adrenoceptor agonists such as adrenaline, because they are not substrates for the norepinephrine uptake transporter (NET) on the presynaptic neuron or for catechol-O-methyltransferase, the enzyme that metabolises catecholamines outside adrenergic neurons.

Salmeterol and formoterol have a longer duration of action (up to 12 hours) because they are more lipophilic than short-acting agents and bind to the lipid of the cell membrane. Salmeterol has a slower onset of action than short-acting agents, but the onset with formoterol is rapid. Indacaterol is a lipophilic β_2-adrenoceptor agonist with a rapid onset and ultralong duration of action (up to 24 hours).

Salbutamol and terbutaline can also be given orally (as conventional or modified-release formulations), by subcutaneous or intramuscular injection, or by intravenous infusion. Much larger doses are required to deliver an adequate amount of drug to the lungs by any of these routes, compared with inhaled doses. This reduces the selectivity for β_2-adrenoceptors, and systemic unwanted effects can be troublesome.

Unwanted effects

- Fine skeletal muscle tremor from stimulation of β_2-adrenoceptors.
- Tachycardia and arrhythmias result from both β_1- and β_2-adrenoceptor stimulation in the heart when high doses of inhaled drug are used, or after oral or parenteral administration.
- Hypokalaemia with high doses, due to promotion of cellular uptake of K^+ by a cAMP-dependent action of β_2-adrenoceptor agonists on the Na^+/K^+ pump. Nebulised salbutamol is used as a treatment for hyperkalaemia. Hypomagnesaemia and hyperglycaemia can also occur. These effects do not persist during long-term use.
- Paradoxical bronchospasm has been reported with inhalation, usually when given for the first time or with a new canister.
- Headache.
- Nervous tension.
- Tolerance to the bronchodilator effects with prolonged use of β_2-adrenoceptor agonists is modest, but desensitisation and downregulation of the β_2-adrenoceptor do occur. The process of receptor desensitisation appears to be more rapid for mast cells than for bronchial smooth muscle, and the prevention of exercise-induced bronchoconstriction is more affected than the symptom relief that these drugs produce.
- Regular use of high doses of short-acting or inhaled long-acting β_2-adrenoceptor agonists has been linked with increased mortality in people with asthma, although a causal relationship remains controversial. One possibility is that they precipitate serious cardiac arrhythmias when combined with hypoxaemia during severe asthma exacerbations. It is also possible that their use might allow people to tolerate initial exposure to larger doses of allergens or irritants, which then produce an enhanced late asthmatic response.

Antimuscarinics

ipratropium, tiotropium

Mechanism of action and effects

The main type of muscarinic receptor in the airways is the M_3 receptor, which is involved in direct bronchoconstriction, glandular mucus secretion and mucociliary clearance from the bronchi. M_3 receptor stimulation activates phospholipase C with subsequent formation of inositol triphosphate (IP_3) and diacylglycerol (DAG), which are key events in the signalling pathway that increase intracellular Ca^{2+} (see Chapter 1 and Fig. 1.5).

Ipratropium binds nonselectively to all five subtypes of muscarinic receptor (M_1 to M_5). The recommended dose

is determined by unwanted effects and is well below the dose that produces maximal bronchodilation. By contrast, tiotropium and other long-acting antimuscarinics are functionally selective for the M_3 receptor due to a higher affinity for binding to the receptor or due to lower reversibility of binding at M_3 than at other muscarinic receptors.

The main benefit of muscarinic antagonists is in COPD. They are of less value for bronchodilation in acute mild to moderate asthma, but ipratropium has a place when added to a β_2-adrenoceptor agonist in severe exacerbations of asthma.

Pharmacokinetics

The antimuscarinic drugs are derived from atropine but are N-quaternary cations that are poorly absorbed orally and do not cross the blood–brain barrier. They are given exclusively by inhalation as a powder or aerosol or via a nebuliser. They have a slower onset of action (30–60 minutes) than salbutamol (5–10 minutes), probably due to slow absorption from the surface of the airways. The duration of action of antimuscarinics is related to the rate of removal locally from the airways, and not the half-life of elimination from the circulation. Long-acting antimuscarinics such as tiotropium are active for 24 hours or more, allowing once-daily dosing.

Unwanted effects

Direct delivery of antimuscarinic drugs to the lung is the main reason for the relative lack of unwanted systemic effects.

- Dry mouth is the most common unwanted effect.
- Nausea, constipation.
- Headache.
- Cough.
- Tiotropium can cause urinary retention in men with prostatism.
- Exacerbation of angle-closure glaucoma (see Chapter 50).

Methylxanthines

aminophylline, theophylline

Mechanism of action and effects

Methylxanthines are a group of naturally occurring substances found in coffee, tea, chocolate and related foodstuffs. Naturally occurring theophylline (1,3-dimethylxanthine), and its ester derivative aminophylline, are the only compounds in clinical use. They are chemically similar to caffeine. Methylxanthines have vasodilatory, anti-inflammatory and immunomodulatory actions. The potential effects of methylxanthines are numerous, controversial and of uncertain importance.

- Inhibition of the enzyme phosphodiesterase (PDE), which degrades cyclic nucleotide second messengers, may partly explain the actions of methylxanthines. Theophylline preferentially inhibits the isoenzymes PDE3 (which degrades cAMP and cyclic guanosine monophosphate [cGMP]) and PDE4 (which degrades cAMP). PDE3 is found in bronchial smooth muscle and PDE4 in several inflammatory cell types, including mast cells. The rise in intracellular cAMP in bronchial smooth muscle stimulates large-conductance voltage-gated Ca^{2+}-activated K^+ channels (BK_{Ca}) in the cell membrane, leading to cell hyperpolarisation and muscle relaxation. However, theophylline only produces bronchodilation at relatively high plasma concentrations, and drugs that are more effective PDE inhibitors (such as dipyridamole) do not bronchodilate. Prolonging the duration of action of cyclic nucleotides may potentiate the action of β_2-adrenoceptor agonists and produce a synergistic dilator effect on bronchial smooth muscle. PDE inhibition also stimulates ciliary beat frequency in the airways and enhances water transport across the airway epithelium, which increases mucociliary clearance. In contrast, theophylline increases the force and rate of contraction of cardiac muscle through its effect on cAMP (see Chapter 7), but also causes arterial vasodilation by inhibiting the breakdown of cGMP.

- Adenosine receptor antagonism may be relevant to some of the clinical effects of methylxanthines (see also the section on adenosine in Chapter 8). Adenosine releases histamine and leukotrienes from mast cells, which results in the constriction of hyperresponsive airways in individuals with asthma. Theophylline is a potent antagonist at adenosine A_1, A_2 and A_3 receptors (see Chapter 1) and may reduce bronchoconstriction by this mechanism. Adenosine receptor antagonism is responsible for central nervous system (CNS) stimulation, which improves mental performance and alertness, has positive inotropic and chronotropic effects on the heart, and in the kidney reduces tubular Na^+ reabsorption, which leads to natriuresis and diuresis.

- Activation of histone deacetylases (HDACs; see the section on corticosteroids later in this chapter): acetylation of core histones, which form part of the structure of chromatin, activates gene transcription, while their deacetylation suppresses gene transcription, including transcription of proinflammatory genes. Theophylline at low concentrations activates HDAC in nuclear extracts, indicating an action independent of adenosine and other surface receptors, and also increases HDAC activity in bronchial biopsies from people with asthma. Anti-inflammatory effects of theophylline occur at drug plasma concentrations similar to those that produce clinical benefit. The action of theophylline on HDAC may potentiate the anti-inflammatory effects of corticosteroids (see Chapter 44).

- Increased diaphragmatic contractility and reduced fatigue have been reported at lower plasma theophylline concentrations than those required for bronchodilation. This may improve lung ventilation.

Pharmacokinetics

The extent of absorption of theophylline from the gut is unpredictable, with considerable interindividual variation. This, and the short but highly variable plasma half-life, has resulted in the widespread use of modified-release formulations. Theophylline has a narrow therapeutic index, and since different formulations vary in their release characteristics, they are not readily interchangeable. Theophylline is metabolised in the liver by cytochrome P450 (mainly CYP1A2), giving the potential for drug interactions. Aminophylline is a more water-soluble ester prodrug, which is hydrolysed rapidly after absorption from the gut to theophylline and ethylenediamine.

Aminophylline can also be given by intravenous infusion. Measurement of blood theophylline concentrations is valuable as a guide to effective dosing.

Unwanted effects

Most are dose-related and can arise within the accepted therapeutic plasma concentration range.

- Gastrointestinal upset, including nausea, vomiting (PDE4 inhibition in the vomiting centre) and diarrhoea.
- CNS stimulation, including insomnia, irritability, dizziness, headache (PDE3 inhibition) and occasionally seizures at high plasma concentrations (adenosine receptor antagonism).
- Hypotension from peripheral vasodilation (PDE3 inhibition). In contrast, cerebral arteries are constricted by methylxanthines (adenosine receptor antagonism).
- Cardiac stimulation produces various arrhythmias.
- Hypokalaemia can occur acutely, especially after intravenous injection, which also promotes cardiac arrhythmias.
- Tolerance to the beneficial effects of methylxanthines can occur.
- Drug interactions can be troublesome, due to the narrow therapeutic index of theophylline. Hepatic CYP1A2 enzyme inhibitors such as ciprofloxacin, erythromycin, clarithromycin, fluconazole and ketoconazole (see Chapter 51 and Table 2.7) can precipitate theophylline toxicity.

ANTI-INFLAMMATORY DRUGS FOR AIRWAYS OBSTRUCTION ('PREVENTERS')

Corticosteroids

Examples

beclometasone dipropionate, budesonide, fluticasone propionate, hydrocortisone, prednisolone

Mechanism of action and effects

Corticosteroids with powerful glucocorticoid activity (but without significant mineralocorticoid activity) are the most effective class of drug in the treatment of chronic asthma, but are relatively ineffective in COPD. They suppress inflammation and the immune response but are not bronchodilators and are therefore of no benefit in the initial stages of an acute attack of asthma.

Intracellular events involved in the anti-inflammatory action of corticosteroids are described in Chapters 38 and 44. The inhibition of transcription of genes coding for the cytokines involved in inflammation is particularly important in asthma. Higher glucocorticoid concentrations also activate anti-inflammatory genes and genes linked to glucocorticoid unwanted effects. Following a delay of 6–12 hours, corticosteroids reduce airway responsiveness to several bronchoconstrictor mediators and, with chronic therapy, inhibit both the early and late reactions to allergen.

Anti-inflammatory effects of corticosteroids in asthma include:

- Reduced airway oedema and leucocyte recruitment by induction of tight junctions in vascular endothelial cells.

- Reduced inflammatory cell activation (including macrophages, T-lymphocytes, eosinophils and airway epithelial cells) with reduced inflammatory cytokine, chemokine, adhesion molecule and inflammatory enzyme expression (see Chapter 38). In allergic disease, suppression of Th2 cells and their cytokines is particularly important.
- Reduced inflammatory cell recruitment to the airways (particularly eosinophils, but also T-lymphocytes, mast cells and others) through reduction in chemotactic mediators and adhesion molecules, and reduced cell survival (enhanced apoptosis).
- Decreased local generation of inflammatory prostaglandins and leukotrienes due to inhibition of phospholipase A_2 by annexin 1 (lipocortin), which reduces mucosal oedema (see also Chapter 29).
- β_2-Adrenoceptor upregulation and better coupling to adenylyl cyclase, which restores responsiveness to β_2-adrenoceptor agonists.
- Enhanced activity of the M_2 autoreceptors on acetylcholine nerve endings inhibits acetylcholine release and relieves vagally mediated bronchoconstriction.
- Suppression of the excess epithelial cell shedding and goblet cell hyperplasia found in the bronchial epithelium in asthma.

Inhaled corticosteroids produce some improvement in asthmatic symptoms after 24 hours and a maximum response after 1–2 weeks. Reduction in airway responsiveness to allergens and irritants occurs gradually over several months, but many of the chronic structural changes in the airways in asthma are not affected by corticosteroids.

Pharmacokinetics

Whenever possible, corticosteroids are given by inhalation of an aerosol or dry powder in order to minimise systemic unwanted effects, but they can be used intravenously or orally in severe asthma. Desirable properties of an inhaled corticosteroid include a low rate of absorption across mucosal surfaces (such as the lung, but also the gut for the swallowed fraction of the drug) and rapid inactivation once absorbed. Beclometasone dipropionate fulfils the former criterion, but it is only slowly inactivated once it reaches the systemic circulation. Inhaled budesonide (which is inactivated by extensive first-pass metabolism in the liver following oral absorption) or fluticasone (which is very poorly absorbed from the gut) may be preferred if high doses of inhaled drug are needed, or for the treatment of children in whom the systemic effects can be more problematic.

Unwanted effects

The unwanted effects of oral and parenteral corticosteroids are described in Chapter 44. Inhaled corticosteroids only have systemic actions when given in high doses. The amount of the drug that is swallowed can be minimised by using a large-volume spacer (described previously); large aerosol particles, which would otherwise be deposited on the oropharyngeal mucosa, are trapped in the spacer, and only the smaller particles are inhaled.

There are some specific problems with inhaled corticosteroids:

- Dysphonia (hoarseness), caused by drug deposition on vocal cords and myopathy of laryngeal muscles, occurs in

up to one-third of those using inhaled corticosteroids. This may be less troublesome with breath-actuated delivery, since the method of inspiration leads to protection of the vocal cords by the false cords.
- Oral candidiasis can occur but can be prevented by using a spacer device or by gargling with water after use of the inhaler.
- Prolonged use of high doses of inhaled corticosteroid has been associated with systemic unwanted effects. These include adrenal suppression, osteoporosis and reduced growth velocity in children. In older people with COPD there is an increased risk of pneumonia.

Cromones

Examples

sodium cromoglicate, nedocromil sodium

The cromones are used to prevent asthma attacks, but they are usually less effective than inhaled corticosteroids, and only about one-third of people benefit from treatment. Cromones have no bronchodilator activity and are of no use in acute attacks of asthma. The major use of cromones is as prophylactic agents in the treatment of mild to moderate antigen-, pollutant- and exercise-induced asthma. They are also used as nasal inhalants to treat seasonal allergic rhinitis (see Chapter 39) and in ophthalmic solutions to treat allergic conjunctivitis (see Chapter 50).

Mechanisms of action and effects

- Mast cell stabilisation. Sodium cromoglicate was originally introduced as a mast cell stabiliser. It enhances the phosphorylation of a protein that normally forms a substrate for intracellular protein kinase C, and interferes with the signal transduction for inflammatory mediator release. This action may protect against immediate bronchoconstriction induced by allergens, exercise or cold air.
- Inhibition of sensory C-fibre neurons by antagonism of the effects of the tachykinins, substance P and neurokinin B, which are involved in generation of sensory stimuli. This is probably responsible for protection against bronchoconstriction produced by irritants such as sulphur dioxide.
- Inhibition of accumulation of eosinophils in the lungs, and reduced activation of eosinophils, neutrophils and macrophages in inflamed lung tissue. These actions may be important in preventing the late-phase response to allergen and the development of bronchial hyperreactivity.
- Inhibition of B-cell switching to IgE production probably also contributes to the long-term effects.

A single dose of either nedocromil sodium or sodium cromoglicate will prevent the early-phase bronchoconstrictor response to allergen, but treatment for 1–2 months may be necessary to block the late-phase reaction.

Pharmacokinetics

Both sodium cromoglicate and nedocromil sodium are highly ionised and poorly absorbed across biological membranes.

They are therefore largely retained at the site of action on bronchial mucosa after inhalation as a powder or from a metered-dose aerosol inhaler. Swallowed drug is voided in the faeces.

Unwanted effects

- Cough, wheeze and throat irritation may be provoked transiently following inhalation.
- Headache.
- Nausea, vomiting, dyspepsia and abdominal pain with nedocromil sodium.

Leukotriene receptor antagonists

montelukast, zafirlukast

Mechanisms of action and effects

The leukotriene receptor antagonists (LTRAs) are taken orally and inhibit the bronchoconstriction induced by the cysteinyl-leukotrienes (LTC$_4$, LTD$_4$ and LTE$_4$; see Figure 29.1) by blocking the CysLT$_1$ receptor on bronchial smooth muscle. Cysteinyl-leukotrienes are released from various cells, including activated mast cells and eosinophils, in response to several airway insults, and their synthesis is increased by many mediators, such as cytokines. Cysteinyl-leukotrienes also contribute to airway oedema, enhanced secretion of mucus and airway eosinophilia (see Fig. 12.1).

LTRAs reduce both the early and late bronchoconstrictor responses to inhaled allergen, and may be most useful in mild and moderate asthma, exercise-induced bronchoconstriction and hypersensitivity reactions provoked by nonsteroidal anti-inflammatory drugs (NSAIDs; see Chapter 29). The effects are additive to those of inhaled corticosteroid.

Pharmacokinetics

Montelukast and zafirlukast are well absorbed from the gut and metabolised in the liver. The half-life of montelukast is 3–5 hours and that of zafirlukast 10 hours.

Unwanted effects

- Headache.
- Gastrointestinal upset.

Phosphodiesterase type 4 inhibitor

roflumilast

Mechanism of action and effects

Phosphodiesterase type 4 (PDE4) is the main isoenzyme present in cells involved in the inflammatory process in COPD. PDE4 degrades the intracellular second messenger cAMP, and inhibition of this enzyme with roflumilast has several anti-inflammatory actions:

- Decreased cytokine and chemokine release from neutrophils, eosinophils, macrophages and T-lymphocytes.
- Decreased expression of adhesion molecules on T-lymphocytes and other inflammatory cells. Along

with the reduced chemokine release, this results in less accumulation of these cells in the airway.
- Decreased apoptosis of airway cells, which may assist in sputum clearance.

Roflumilast is highly selective for PDE4 (splice variants PDE4A, PDE4B and particularly PDE4D), and therefore has little action in tissues that express other PDE isoenzymes. It is effective in patients with COPD with chronic bronchitis (prominent cough and sputum production), who have frequent exacerbations. In these individuals, roflumilast improves lung function and reduces exacerbation frequency.

Pharmacokinetics

Roflumilast is well absorbed from the gut, and is metabolised by the liver. It has a long but variable half-life, with an average of about 17 hours.

Unwanted effects

PDE4 has several isoforms that are found in the gut, adipose tissue and neurons, and inhibition of these is responsible for most unwanted effects with roflumilast, which often resolve with continued use:

- nausea, anorexia, abdominal pain, diarrhoea;
- weight loss;
- headache, insomnia.

Magnesium sulfate

Mechanism of action and effects

Intravenous magnesium sulfate can be given for the treatment of severe asthma in adults if life-threatening features are present. Magnesium bronchodilates by blocking Ca^{2+} channels in smooth muscle cell membranes, therefore reducing Ca^{2+} influx into the cell.

Pharmacokinetics

Magnesium sulfate is given by slow intravenous infusion, and it is widely distributed. The Mg^{2+} is excreted by the kidney with a half-life of 4 hours.

Unwanted effects

- Atrioventricular block.
- Enhancement of neuromuscular blockade by neuromuscular blocking agents.
- Diarrhoea.
- Potentiates the hypotensive effects of calcium channel blockers.

Antibody to immunoglobulin E

omalizumab

Mechanism of action

Omalizumab is a recombinant humanised IgG1k monoclonal antibody that binds selectively to IgE to form complexes which are removed from the circulation by the reticuloendothelial system and endothelial cells. This leads to a reduction in IgE receptor expression and in mediator release from mast cells and basophils. Treatment with omalizumab gradually reduces airway inflammation in asthma, with a peak response after 12–16 weeks. Omalizumab is used for the treatment of persistent severe allergic asthma in adults and children over 12 years that cannot be controlled with high-dose inhaled corticosteroids with a long-acting β_2-adrenoceptor agonist and other standard therapies for asthma.

Pharmacokinetics

Omalizumab is given subcutaneously every 2–4 weeks in a dose that is determined by the recipient's plasma IgE concentration and body weight. Omalizumab has a very long half-life of about 26 days.

Unwanted effects

- Anaphylaxis occurs in 1–2 of every 1000 people given omalizumab.
- Headache.
- Injection-site reactions.

MANAGEMENT OF ASTHMA

Treatment of asthma has two aims:

- relief of symptoms;
- reduction of airways inflammation.

THE ACUTE ATTACK

Mild infrequent attacks of asthma can often be controlled by occasional use of a short-acting inhaled β_2-adrenoceptor agonist. Antimuscarinic agents are less effective unless asthma coexists with COPD. More severe attacks of asthma require intensive treatment with bronchodilators and systemic corticosteroids. The signs of severe and life-threatening acute asthma are shown in Table 12.2.

Treatment of severe acute asthma should include:

- ensuring adequate hydration;
- high-flow oxygen via a facemask to achieve an arterial oxygen saturation of above 90%;
- inhaled short-acting β_2-adrenoceptor agonist such as salbutamol, preferably via an oxygen-driven nebuliser, or via a metered-dose inhaler with a large-volume spacer if a nebuliser is not available;
- high-dose oral prednisolone or initial intravenous hydrocortisone followed by oral prednisolone.

If response to treatment is poor after 15–30 minutes, or if there are life-threatening features, additional treatment should be given:

- inhaled ipratropium via an oxygen-driven nebuliser.

If response is poor after a further 15–30 minutes, then consider:

- intravenous aminophylline,
- intravenous magnesium sulfate,
- assisted ventilation if there is not rapid clinical improvement.

After recovery from a severe asthma attack, prednisolone should be continued for at least 5 days or until there are no residual symptoms, especially at night, and the peak

Table 12.2 Signs of severe and life-threatening acute asthma

Severe acute asthma[a]	Life-threatening acute asthma
Any one of the following:	Any one of the following in a patient with severe acute asthma:
PEF 33–50% of predicted or previous best	PEF <33% of predicted or previous best
Pulse ≥110 beats/min	Arterial oxygen saturation (SpO_2) <92%
Respiratory rate ≥25/min	Partial arterial pressure of oxygen (PaO_2) <8 kPa
Inability to complete a sentence in one breath	Normal[b] partial arterial pressure of carbon dioxide ($PaCO_2$) 4.6–6.0 kPa
	Arrhythmia or hypotension
	Exhaustion, altered consciousness level, poor respiratory effort
	Silent chest
	Cyanosis

[a]Moderate acute asthma is defined as worsening symptoms with PEF 50–75% of predicted or previous best, but no features of severe acute asthma. [b]Raised $PaCO_2$, or a requirement for mechanical ventilation with raised inflation pressures, or both, is a sign of near-fatal acute asthma.
PEF, Peak expiratory flow.

expiratory flow is at least 80% of the person's previous best. High doses of prednisolone can be stopped abruptly if used for 3 weeks or less, but should be reduced gradually if they have been used for a longer period (see Chapter 44).

PROPHYLAXIS OF CHRONIC ASTHMA

An initial attempt should be made to identify and exclude precipitating factors – for example, allergens, occupational precipitants, NSAIDs (described later) and β-adrenoceptor antagonists (including eye drops; see Chapter 5). Long-term treatment is guided by a stepwise treatment plan. Inhaled medication is the mainstay of treatment, and it is central to successful management that an appropriate inhaler device is selected after careful assessment of the person's preferences and abilities.

Step 1. Occasional relief bronchodilator. An inhaled short-acting β_2-adrenoceptor agonist, such as salbutamol, taken as required. For those who are intolerant to this treatment, inhaled ipratropium and oral theophylline are alternative options, but there is a higher risk of unwanted effects with the latter. Step 2 treatment should be considered if more than two doses of short-acting β_2-adrenoceptor agonist are required in a week, there are night-time symptoms at least once a week or if there has been an exacerbation of asthma in the previous 2 years.

Step 2. Regular inhaled preventer therapy. For adults, a regular standard-dose inhaled corticosteroid such as beclometasone is used in addition to step 1 therapy. A LTRA, theophyline or an inhaled cromone could be tried, but are generally less effective than inhaled corticosteroids.

Step 3. Initial add-on therapy. If symptoms in an adult are not controlled by standard doses of inhaled corticosteroid, a long-acting β_2-adrenoceptor agonist such as salmeterol is usually more effective than increasing the dose of corticosteroid. An inhaled short-acting β_2-adrenoceptor agonist can still be used as required. If there is no response to the long-acting β_2-adrenoceptor agonist, it should be stopped and the corticosteroid dose increased. The corticosteroid dose can also be increased if there was some response to a long-acting β_2-adrenoceptor agonist but the symptoms are still not controlled. For persistent poor control, sequential add-on therapy with an LTRA, a modified-release theophylline formulation or a modified-release oral β_2-adrenoceptor agonist should be tried. For children under 5 years, an LTRA is added to a regular inhaled corticosteroid with an inhaled short-acting β_2-adrenoceptor agonist as required.

Step 4. Persistent poor control. High-dose inhaled corticosteroid with an inhaled long-acting β_2-adrenoceptor agonist plus a short-acting β_2-adrenoceptor agonist as required, and a 6-week sequential trial of one of the following:

- LTRA,
- oral modified-release theophylline formulation,
- modified-release oral β_2-adrenoceptor agonist.

Step 5. Continuous or frequent use of oral corticosteroids. Oral prednisolone is taken in addition to high-dose inhaled corticosteroids, with an inhaled long-acting β_2-adrenoceptor agonist plus a short-acting β_2-adrenoceptor agonist as required.

ASPIRIN-INTOLERANT ASTHMA

About 5–20% of people with asthma experience acute exacerbations when they take aspirin or other NSAIDs in a laboratory setting (see Chapter 29), and the syndrome may be underrecognised clinically. Individuals with the full clinical syndrome of aspirin-intolerant asthma (or aspirin-exacerbated respiratory disease; AERD) usually have an eosinophilic rhinosinusitis and nasal polyposis in addition to asthma. The condition may be initiated by priming of the respiratory mucosa by an immune reaction to a viral infection or other insult, which chronically upregulates the cysteinyl-leukotriene biosynthetic pathway. The production of bronchoconstrictor leukotrienes nevertheless remains under partial inhibitory control of prostaglandin (PG)E$_2$.

Aspirin is an irreversible cyclooxygenase type 1 (COX-1) and COX-2 inhibitor with selective action on COX-1. COX inhibition reduces PGE$_2$ synthesis, which removes its inhibition of leukotriene synthesis, provoking acute bronchospasm (see Fig. 29.1). Other NSAIDs that inhibit COX-1 also induce bronchoconstriction, but the selective COX-2 inhibitors very rarely provoke asthma. In sensitive individuals, asthma symptoms begin within 3 hours of ingesting aspirin, accompanied by profuse rhinorrhoea, conjunctival injection and, sometimes, flushing or urticaria. Airway inflammation can persist for many weeks after an aspirin challenge.

LTRAs produce symptom relief in some people with aspirin-intolerant asthma. Treatment of acute aspirin-intolerant asthma is the same as for any other episode. Sometimes long-term use of an oral corticosteroid is the only way to control persistent symptoms; in such cases, desensitisation to aspirin should be attempted. Nasal polypectomy may be necessary to control rhinosinusitis.

MANAGEMENT OF CHRONIC OBSTRUCTIVE PULMONARY DISEASE

There are two goals in the treatment of COPD: to minimise symptoms (including a reduction in acute exacerbations) and to preserve lung function.

- Cessation of smoking (see Chapter 54) is the only effective way to alter the natural history of COPD. Smoking cessation slows the rate of decline in lung function to that naturally seen with ageing, although any loss of lung function due to smoking cannot be restored. Occupational exposure to inhaled pollutants should also be minimised.
- **Pneumococcal and influenza vaccination.** These can reduce infective exacerbations in people with COPD.
- **Inhaled bronchodilators.** The principles are similar to those for asthma, although the limited reversibility of the airway obstruction means that the benefit is less marked, except during an acute exacerbation of symptoms. Some improvement in symptoms and functional capacity can occur without changes in standard lung function tests, and the main benefit is improved lung emptying during expiration, with reduced hyperinflation at rest. Inhaled bronchodilators reduce the frequency of exacerbations of COPD. Short-acting β_2-adrenoceptor agonists and antimuscarinic agents are equally effective for mild symptoms. For continuing breathlessness, either a long-acting β_2-adrenoceptor agonist (with a short-acting bronchodilator as required) or a long-acting antimuscarinic drug such as tiotropium (with a short-acting β_2-adrenoceptor agonist as required) may give better symptom relief and reduce the risk of exacerbations. Long-acting antimuscarinics are also available in combined formulations, with a long-acting β_2-adrenoceptor agonist for maintenance therapy of COPD (see the drug compendium at the end of the chapter). Theophylline or roflumilast are usually reserved for advanced COPD when symptoms persist or there are frequent exacerbations despite use of inhaled long-acting bronchodilators and corticosteroids. Nebulised bronchodilators can be useful for severe exacerbations.
- **Corticosteroids.** The chronic airway inflammatory changes in most people with COPD do not respond to corticosteroids; nevertheless, an oral corticosteroid should be used for 7–14 days when treating an acute exacerbation of symptoms. Long-term use of an inhaled corticosteroid can reduce the number and severity of exacerbations, and should be considered if there are two or more exacerbations in a 12-month period. An inhaled corticosteroid can also produce some symptomatic benefit for people who remain breathless despite the use of a long-acting bronchodilator, or those with an FEV$_1$ of less than 50% of predicted. About 10% of people with COPD will have an improvement in their forced expiratory volume with an inhaled corticosteroid. However, there is an increased risk of pneumonia with inhaled corticosteroid, especially in the elderly with COPD.

- **Antibacterial drugs.** One-third of infective exacerbations are due to viral infection, but antibacterial drugs (see Chapter 51) produce earlier symptomatic improvement if there is moderate-to-severe acute exacerbation of symptoms with purulent sputum.
- **Mucolytic agents.** Mecysteine hydrochloride, erdosteine or carbocisteine (see Chapter 13) may reduce the frequency of exacerbations of COPD. An initial 1-month trial should be considered if COPD is accompanied by a chronic productive cough or if there are prolonged severe exacerbations. Treatment should only be continued if there is a perceived benefit.
- **Oxygen therapy.** This is extremely important to treat hypoxaemia during acute exacerbations. Care must be taken to raise the arterial oxygen saturation (if possible to ≥90%) without increasing the arterial carbon dioxide tension. To avoid suppressing hypoxic drive in type 2 respiratory failure (hypoxaemia with a raised arterial carbon dioxide concentration), low-dose supplementary oxygen may be necessary (e.g. 24% via a Venturi mask or 1–2 L/minute via a nasal cannulae). Long-term domiciliary oxygen treatment, usually from an oxygen concentrator which removes nitrogen from air and delivers via nasal cannulae, improves symptoms and survival in COPD with respiratory failure (with an arterial oxygen tension less than 7.3 kPa). This should only be considered if respiratory failure persists for 3–4 weeks despite optimal drug therapy and without a clinical exacerbation. Those in the household must be warned of the risk of fire if people smoke when receiving oxygen therapy. To improve survival in COPD with respiratory failure, oxygen must be used for at least 15 hours per day.
- **Ventilatory support.** This may be required during exacerbations. Intubation and mechanical ventilation may be necessary, but noninvasive assisted ventilation is preferable. Nasal intermittent positive-pressure ventilation (NIPPV) is increasingly being used during exacerbations for people who fail to respond to maximal medical therapy, especially if there is carbon dioxide retention.
- **Pulmonary rehabilitation.** This improves exercise capacity and reduces the sensation of breathlessness, and can substantially improve morale.

SELF-ASSESSMENT

True/false questions

1. Asthma is defined as irreversible airflow obstruction resulting from chronic airway inflammation.
2. An influx of Th2 lymphocytes occurs in the late airway response to inhaled allergen challenge of people with asthma and atopy.
3. The β_2-adrenoceptor agonists are effective in preventing exercise-induced asthma.
4. The β_2-adrenoceptor agonists have no effect on mucus clearance.
5. Tolerance to β_2-adrenoceptor agonists can occur.
6. The mechanisms of action of theophylline are unclear.
7. The plasma concentration of theophylline is increased by simultaneous administration of erythromycin or ciprofloxacin.

8. Methylxanthines cause drowsiness.
9. An unwanted effect of theophylline is stimulation of the heart.
10. Ipratropium is more effective than salbutamol for preventing bronchospasm following a challenge with an allergen.
11. Tiotropium is a selective antagonist of muscarinic M_2 receptors.
12. Ipratropium causes bradycardia.
13. Ipratropium is poorly absorbed from the bronchi into the systemic circulation.
14. Leukotriene C_4 is an important bronchodilator released from eosinophils.
15. Cysteinyl-leukotrienes are important in the precipitation of asthma in people who are intolerant to NSAIDs.
16. Montelukast inhibits 5-lipoxygenase that converts arachidonic acid to leukotrienes.
17. The LTRA are only given prophylactically.
18. Glucocorticoids reduce eosinophil recruitment to the bronchial mucosa.
19. Roflumilast is a nonselective inhibitor of PDE isoenzymes.
20. Omalizumab binds to IgE receptors on mast cell membranes, preventing binding of allergen.

One-best-answer (OBA) questions

1. What is the most likely unwanted effect of high-dose salbutamol?
   A. Bradycardia
   B. Hypokalaemia
   C. Hypoglycaemia
   D. Mydriasis
   E. Hypermagnesaemia
2. What is the mechanism of action of corticosteroids in asthma therapy?
   A. They reduce airway inflammation by inhibiting eosinophil apoptosis
   B. They reduce airway narrowing by relaxing bronchial smooth muscle
   C. They reduce release of mast cell mediators by blocking allergen–IgE interaction
   D. They downregulate β_2-adrenoceptors on bronchial smooth muscle
   E. They reduce oedema by inducing endothelial tight junctions

Extended-matching-item question

Match each statement to the most appropriate option (A–G).
   A. Theophylline
   B. Celecoxib
   C. Prostaglandin D_2
   D. Salbutamol
   E. Montelukast
   F. Indometacin
   G. Leukotriene B_4
1. It increases the synthesis of cAMP.
2. It decreases the breakdown of cAMP.
3. It results in an increase in leukotriene synthesis in susceptible people with asthma.
4. It inhibits NSAID-induced bronchoconstriction.
5. It causes bronchoconstriction.

Case-based question

Which option (A–H) is the most appropriate for add-on treatment to the current medication prescribed in each case scenario (1–5)?

- A. Tiotropium
- B. Ciprofloxacin
- C. Salmeterol
- D. A spacer device
- E. Modified-release theophylline
- F. Intravenous magnesium sulfate
- G. Oral prednisolone
- H. Modified-release theophylline.

Case 1. A 25-year-old woman was admitted to the emergency department with an acute exacerbation of her asthma. Her peak expiratory flow was 150 L/minute. Her pulse rate was 145 beats/minute, her respiratory rate was 30/minute, her respiration was shallow and she was confused. She was treated with 60% oxygen, nebulised salbutamol, nebulised ipratropium, intravenous aminophylline and intravenous hydrocortisone. Arterial blood gases on admission, breathing air, showed PaO_2 8.4 kPa, $PaCO_2$ 7.2 kPa and pH 7.29. There was little clinical improvement, and she was transferred to the intensive care unit.

Case 2. A 64-year-old man had mild asthma that was well controlled, taking salbutamol two to three times a week and inhaled beclometasone twice daily. He complained of soreness of the mouth and hoarseness and was advised about oral hygiene.

Case 3. A 67-year-old man had COPD with a chronic cough producing clear sputum. The cough and sputum production had not recently changed. He had stopped smoking 3 months previously because of his dyspnoea. Prior to that time, he had smoked 20 cigarettes a day for 50 years. He denied alcohol use. He had no other significant medical illnesses. His FEV_1 was 1.34 L (about 45% of that predicted). He was taking salbutamol four times daily. A trial of inhaled beclometasone 3 months previously had provided no benefit and had been stopped.

Case 4. A 60-year-old woman attended the emergency department with increasing shortness of breath and production of green–yellow sputum and fever over the previous 4 days. She was known to have COPD. She was taking daily salbutamol and ipratropium by breath-actuated inhalers.

Case 5. A 30-year-old man had mild asthma and allergic rhinitis. He was taking inhaled salbutamol and beclometasone, both twice daily. Recently he had been waking most nights with a persistent cough. He was a nonsmoker and had no other medical history.

ANSWERS

True/false answers

1. **False.** Airflow obstruction in asthma is mostly reversible, either spontaneously or as a result of treatment.
2. **True.** Th2 lymphocyte infiltration generates cytokines and chemokines that promote activation, recruitment and survival of eosinophils and other leucocytes, and increase the expression of IgE receptors on mast cells and eosinophils.
3. **True.** Salbutamol is effective if taken before exercise, but the longer-acting β_2-adrenoceptor agonists are slower in onset. Cromoglicate taken prophylactically may also be effective.
4. **False.** β_2-Adrenoceptor agonists increase ciliary action and mucus clearance.
5. **True.** Tolerance to β_2-adrenoceptor agonists may occur due to downregulation of their target receptor, an effect counteracted by use of corticosteroids.
6. **True.** Methylxanthines probably bronchodilate by inhibiting PDE, but also block adenosine receptors on airway smooth muscle, while inhibition of HDAC may account for reported anti-inflammatory effects at low doses.
7. **True.** Erythromycin and ciprofloxacin inhibit liver cytochrome P450 enzymes, resulting in slower metabolism of theophylline.
8. **False.** Methylxanthines present in coffee increase alertness and can cause irritability and headache.
9. **True.** All methylxanthines have positive inotropic and chronotropic activity, and a narrow therapeutic index.
10. **False.** Ipratropium is less effective against allergen challenge but can be useful as an adjunct and in the management of COPD.
11. **False.** Tiotropium is a selective antagonist of M_3 receptors on airway smooth muscle, with less antagonism of inhibitory M_2 autoreceptors on parasympathetic nerves than ipratropium.
12. **False.** Ipratropium can cause a modest tachycardia owing to blockade of muscarinic receptors in the heart.
13. **True.** Ipratropium and tiotropium have quaternary structures and are therefore only poorly absorbed, minimising unwanted systemic effects.
14. **False.** Leukotriene C_4 (and its extracellular metabolite LTD_4) are potent bronchoconstrictors, and also increase mucus secretion, oedema and eosinophilia in the airway.
15. **True.** In susceptible individuals, NSAIDs that inhibit COX-1 may cause acute bronchospasm either by shunting arachidonic acid from the COX pathway to the leukotriene pathway or, more probably, by liberating the leukotriene pathway from partial inhibition by COX-1-derived prostaglandin E_2.
16. **False.** Montelukast and zafirlukast are antagonists of the cysteinyl-leukotriene receptor type 1 ($CysLT_1$), not inhibitors of 5-lipoxygenase.
17. **True.** The LTRA are oral drugs taken once or twice daily for prophylaxis of asthma; they may also benefit comorbid conditions such as allergic rhinitis.
18. **True.** Glucocorticoids act at the transcriptional level to inhibit numerous steps in the inflammatory pathways involved in the pathogenesis of asthma, including the proliferation, recruitment, activation and survival of eosinophils and other leucocytes.
19. **False.** Roflumilast is a highly selective inhibitor of PDE4, which is found in inflammatory cells.
20. **False.** Omalizumab binds to circulating and tissue IgE, leading to its clearance by endothelial cells. This results in a reduction in the numbers of IgE receptors on mast cells and other cells.

One-best-answer (OBA) answers

1. **Answer B** is correct. Salbutamol is a β_2-adrenoceptor agonist that can produce hypokalaemia by increasing cellular uptake of K^+. At high doses it may cause tachycardia not bradycardia (answer A), hyperglycaemia not hypoglycaemia (answer C) and hypomagnesaemia not hypermagnesaemia (answer E), while mydriasis (answer D) is not likely with a β-adrenoceptor agonist, as adrenergic control of pupil diameter is mediated by α-adrenoceptors.

2. **Answer E** is correct. Corticosteroids induce endothelial tight junctions, which reduces vascular permeability and leucocyte migration into tissue. They reduce airway inflammation by *promoting* eosinophil apoptosis (answer A). They are *not* bronchodilators (answer B) and do not block allergen–IgE interaction (answer C). They may also *upregulate* β_2-adrenoceptors on bronchial smooth muscle (answer D).

Extended-matching-item answers

1. **Answer D** is correct. Salbutamol acts selectively on the β_2-adrenoceptors in airways, activating adenylyl cyclase and increasing cAMP.

2. **Answer A** is correct. Theophylline inhibits the breakdown of cAMP by PDE.

3. **Answer F** is correct. Indometacin (and other NSAIDs that inhibit COX-1) can induce bronchoconstriction in aspirin-sensitive people with asthma. Celecoxib, a selective COX-2 inhibitor, is unlikely to cause this reaction, but should still be used with care.

4. **Answer E** is correct. Montelukast is a selective antagonist of $CysLT_1$ receptors for the bronchoconstrictor cysteinyl-leukotrienes ($LTC_4/D_4/E_4$), synthesis of which is triggered by nonselective NSAIDs.

5. **Answer C** is correct. Prostaglandin D_2 is a broncho-constrictor released by mast cells.

Case-based answers

Case 1. **Answer F** is correct. This woman is being treated according to the British Thoracic Society guidelines; an appropriate add-on medication for use in this life-threatening situation is intravenous magnesium sulfate.

Case 2. **Answer D** is correct. This man should be advised to use a spacer with all inhaled drugs. This improves the effectiveness of the medication and will reduce deposition of corticosteroid in the mouth and oropharynx, reducing the occurrence of fungal growth and hoarseness.

Case 3. **Answer A** is correct. A long-acting antimuscarinic provides equal or greater benefit to β_2-adrenoceptor agonists in COPD and will reduce the volume of sputum produced. Corticosteroids are of modest benefit in only a small percentage of people with COPD.

Case 4. **Answer B** is correct. This woman has an infection-related exacerbation of her COPD and should be treated with an appropriate antibacterial drug. Nebulised salbutamol and ipratropium should also be started.

Case 5. **Answer C** is correct. Approximately 80% of severe asthmatic attacks occur between midnight and 8 a.m. Salbutamol is a short-acting β_2-adrenoceptor agonist, providing relief for 2–6 hours. A trial of salmeterol or formoterol, which provide bronchodilation for 12 hours or longer, should be considered. The long-acting drugs should not be used for relief of acute asthma episodes.

FURTHER READING

General

Barnes, P.J., 2011. Glucocorticoids: current and future direction. Br. J. Pharmacol. 163, 29–43.

Cazzola, M., Calzetta, L., Matera, M.G., 2011. β_2-Adrenoceptor agonists: current and future direction. Br. J. Pharmacol. 163, 4–17.

Dolovich, M.B., Dhand, R., 2011. Aerosol drug delivery: developments in device design and clinical use. Lancet 377, 1032–1045.

Moulton, B.C., Fryer, A.D., 2011. Muscarinic receptor antagonists, from folklore to pharmacology; finding drugs that actually work in asthma and COPD. Br. J. Pharmacol. 163, 44–52.

Asthma

Bradding, P., Arthur, G., 2016. Mast cells in asthma—state of the art. Clin. Exp. Allergy 46, 194–263.

Bush, A., Saglani, S., 2010. Management of severe asthma in children. Lancet 376, 814–825.

Laidlaw, T.M., Boyce, J.A., 2016. Aspirin-exacerbated respiratory disease—new prime suspects. N. Engl. J. Med. 374, 484–488.

Lazarus, S.C., 2010. Emergency treatment of asthma. N. Engl. J. Med. 363, 755–764.

Lin, C.H., Cheng, S.L., 2016. A review of omalizumab for the management of severe asthma. Drug Des. Devel. Ther. 10, 2369–2378.

Martinez, F.D., Vercelli, D., 2013. Asthma. Lancet 382, 1360–1372.

Olin, J.T., Wechsler, M.E., 2014. Asthma: pathogenesis and novel drugs for treatment. BMJ 349, g5517.

Reddel, H.K., Bateman, E.D., Becker, A., 2015. A summary of the new GINA strategy: a roadmap to asthma control. Eur. Respir. J. 46, 622–639.

Wechsler, M.E., 2014. Getting control of uncontrolled asthma. Am. J. Med. 127, 1049–1059.

Chronic obstructive pulmonary disease

Aaron, S.D., 2014. Management and prevention of exacerbations of COPD. BMJ 349, g5237.

Brusselle, G.G., Joos, G.F., Bracke, K.R., 2012. New insights into the immunology of chronic obstructive pulmonary disease. Lancet 378, 1015–1026.

Decramer, M., Janssens, W., Miravitelles, M., 2012. Chronic obstructive pulmonary disease. Lancet 379, 1341–1351.

Park, H.Y., Man, S.F.P., Sin, D.D., 2012. Inhaled corticosteroids for chronic obstructive pulmonary disease. BMJ 345, e6843.

Postma, D.S., Rabe, K.F., 2015. The asthma-COPD overlap syndrome. N. Engl. J. Med. 373, 1241–1249.

Wedzicha, J.A., Calverley, P.M., Rabe, K.F., 2016. Roflumilast: a review of its use in the treatment of COPD. Int. J. Chron. Obstruct. Pulmon. Dis. 11, 81–90.

Woodruff, P.G., Agusti, A., Roche, N., et al., 2015. Current concepts in targeting chronic obstructive pulmonary disease pharmacotherapy: making progress towards personalized management. Lancet 385, 1789–1798.

Compendium: drugs used to treat asthma or chronic obstructive pulmonary disease

Drug	Characteristics
β₂-Adrenoceptor agonists	
Bronchodilators; most commonly given by inhalation. Short-acting drugs are used for acute exacerbations and long-acting drugs for chronic management of asthma and COPD.	
Bambuterol	Prodrug slowly converted to terbutaline in plasma. Used rarely for asthma; not recommended for children or in pregnancy. Given orally. Half-life: 8–22 h
Ephedrine	Direct- and indirect-acting nonselective sympathomimetic; converted to norephedrine. Not recommended. Given orally. Half-life: 6 h
Formoterol	Long-acting. Given by inhalation for management of chronic asthma in people using an inhaled corticosteroid. Also available combined with fluticasone or budesonide. Half-life: 2–3 h
Indacaterol	Ultra-long-acting. Used for maintenance treatment of COPD. Given by inhalation. Also available combined with glycopyrronium. Half-life: 40–52 h
Olodaterol	Ultra-long-acting. Used for maintenance treatment of COPD. Also available combined with tiotropium. Half-life: 7.5 h
Salbutamol	Short-acting. Given by inhalation, orally, intravenously or subcutaneously. Also available combined with ipratropium. Half-life: 4–6 h
Salmeterol	Long-acting. Given by inhalation for management of chronic asthma in people using an inhaled corticosteroid. Also available in combination with fluticasone. Half-life: 3–5 h
Terbutaline	Short-acting. Given by inhalation, orally, intravenously or subcutaneously. Half-life: 14–18 h
Vilanterol	Ultra-long-acting. Given by inhalation combined with fluticasone or umeclidinium. Half-life: 19 h
Antimuscarinics	
Given by inhaler; little drug is absorbed from the airway. Muscarinic antagonists selective for M₃ receptors allow higher doses and have longer duration of action.	
Aclidinium bromide	Long-acting. Used for maintenance treatment of patients with COPD. Also available combined with formoterol. Half-life: 5 h
Glycopyrronium	Long-acting. Used for maintenance treatment of patients with COPD. Also available combined with indacaterol. Half-life: 33–57 h (after inhalation)
Ipratropium bromide	Short-acting, nonselective antimuscarinic. Used for short-term relief in asthma and for COPD. Also available combined with salbutamol. Half-life: 4 h
Tiotropium	Long-acting. Used for COPD in adults, and with inhaled corticosteroids and long-acting β₂-agonist bronchodilators in poorly controlled asthma. Also available combined with olodaterol. Half-life: 5–6 days
Umeclidinium	Long-acting. Used for maintenance treatment of people with COPD. Also available in combination with vilanterol. Half-life: 19 h
Methylxanthines	
Nonselective PDE inhibitors.	
Aminophylline	Mixture of theophylline and ethylenediamine improves solubility. Given orally, or by injection for acute severe asthma
Theophylline	Given orally, usually as a modified-release preparation, for asthma prophylaxis. Half-life: 1–13 h
Corticosteroids	
Given by inhalation for chronic asthma and COPD. See Chapter 44 for corticosteroids (such as prednisolone and hydrocortisone) given orally or intravenously in the treatment of acute asthma.	
Beclometasone dipropionate	Converted to highly active monopropionate. Inhaled using aerosol or powder formulation; also given in combination with formoterol. Half-life: 15 h
Budesonide	Inhaled using aerosol or powder formulation. Also given in combination with formoterol. Half-life: 2 h
Ciclesonide	Prodrug converted to active metabolite. Inhaled using powder formulation. Half-life: 7 h

Compendium: drugs used to treat asthma or chronic obstructive pulmonary disease (cont'd)

Drug	Characteristics
Fluticasone propionate	Inhaled using aerosol or powder formulation; any swallowed dose undergoes 100% first-pass hepatic metabolism. Also available combined with salmeterol, vilanterol or formoterol
Mometasone furoate	Inhaled using powder formulation; not recommended for children. Half-life: 5 h
Cromones	
Mast cell stabilisers. Given by inhaler; minimal absorption from lung.	
Nedocromil sodium	Used for asthma prophylaxis. Half-life: 23 h
Sodium cromoglicate	Used for asthma prophylaxis. Half-life: 1.3 h
Leukotriene receptor antagonists	
Bronchodilator and anti-inflammatory drugs used prophylactically in chronic asthma.	
Montelukast	Leukotriene D_4 receptor (CysLT$_1$) antagonist. Given orally at bedtime. Half-life: 3–5 h
Zafirlukast	Leukotriene D_4 receptor (CysLT$_1$) antagonist. Given orally twice daily; not recommended for children under 12 years. Half-life: 10 h
Phosphodiesterase type 4 inhibitor	
Roflumilast	Selective PDE4 inhibitor used in bronchitic exacerbations of severe COPD. Given orally. Half-life: 17 h
Magnesium sulfate	
Magnesium sulfate	Smooth muscle relaxant. Given intravenously in life-threatening acute asthma in adults. Half-life: 4 h
Antibody to immunoglobulin E	
Omalizumab	Recombinant monoclonal antibody; binds to human IgE and prevents activation of IgE receptors on mast cells and other cells. Given by subcutaneous injection every 2–4 weeks in severe, uncontrolled allergic asthma. Half-life: 22–28 days

COPD, Chronic obstructive pulmonary disease; *IgE*, immunoglobulin E; *PDE*, phosphodiesterase.
The half-life refers to the systemic elimination half-life from the general circulation, which may not correlate with the duration of action following inhalation when this is dependent on very slow uptake from the airways.

Respiratory disorders: cough, respiratory stimulants, cystic fibrosis, idiopathic pulmonary fibrosis and neonatal respiratory distress syndrome

COUGH

Cough is a protective mechanism that removes excessive mucus, abnormal substances such as fluid or pus, or inhaled foreign material from the upper airways. Epithelial ciliary action and bronchial peristalsis initially move foreign material from smaller airways to the main bronchi and the bifurcation of the trachea, from where it can be more easily expelled. A cough is initiated by a short inspiration, followed by brief closure of the glottis. Forced expiration against the closed glottis raises intrathoracic pressure, and sudden opening of the glottis expels air at a rate up to 85% of the speed of sound, which is sufficient to dislodge secretions and debris from the airway surface. The high flow rates produce vibration of upper airway structures and the typical sound of coughing. Coughing is under both voluntary and involuntary control.

The cough reflex is initiated by irritant receptors located at the epithelial surface of the airway mucosa, which can be activated by either chemical or mechanical stimuli. Rapidly adapting pulmonary stretch receptors that respond mainly to mechanical stimuli may be of primary importance in eliciting the cough reflex. These cough receptors are mainly found on the pharynx, trachea and where the trachea branches into the main bronchi, although they are also present in lesser numbers in other parts of the upper airway and external ear. Peptides such as bradykinin produced following viral infection or allergen challenge likely sensitise the sensory arm of the cough reflex.

Afferent fibres from the cough receptors travel via the vagus and superior laryngeal nerves to a loose medullary 'cough network'. Neuronal pathways connect this network to the respiratory pattern generator, from where efferent fibres travel in the vagus nerve to the glottis and pharynx and various somatic nerves to respiratory muscles to initiate the cough. Projections from the cerebral cortex to the medulla can also initiate cough in response to a sensation of airway irritation (voluntary cough) or modulate the cough reflex.

Numerous mediators are involved in the cough reflex pathways in the medulla. Opioid receptors have an inhibitory action on the cough reflex, but do not appear to be involved in voluntary cough. The complexity of these pathways is illustrated by the number of mediators and antagonists that can experimentally initiate or inhibit cough.

Coughing has several diverse causes (Box 13.1). A cough is considered useful if it aids clearing excess secretions or inhaled foreign matter from the airway. By contrast, an unproductive cough has no useful function. An effective cough that can clear the airway depends on the ability to generate high airflow. An ineffective cough may result from respiratory muscle weakness, or when the mucus on the airway wall is thick and adhesive.

There are three clinical categories of cough:

- acute cough, lasting less than 3 weeks;
- subacute cough, lasting 3–8 weeks;
- chronic cough, lasting more than 8 weeks.

Acute cough is most often caused by acute viral upper respiratory tract infection (the common cold), and most subacute cough also results from an initial viral infection. Chronic productive cough is usually related to smoking or bronchiectasis. The most common causes of a chronic nonproductive cough in nonsmokers are upper airway cough syndrome (also called postnasal drip syndrome), asthma and gastro-oesophageal reflux disease. There is also an entity called unexplained cough, predominantly affecting middle-aged women and associated with cough reflex hypersensitivity, for which investigations fail to identify a cause.

DRUGS FOR TREATMENT OF COUGH

Antitussives (cough suppressants)

Cough suppressants fall into three classes.

Acute respiratory infection
  Upper respiratory tract infection
  Pneumonia, including aspiration
Chronic respiratory infection
  Cystic fibrosis
  Bronchiectasis
  Postnasal drip (upper airway cough syndrome)
Airway disease
  Asthma
  Chronic obstructive pulmonary disease
Parenchymal lung disease
  Interstitial fibrosis
Irritants
  Cigarette smoke
  Inhaled foreign body
Bronchopulmonary malignancy
Drug-induced
  Angiotensin-converting enzyme (ACE) inhibitors
  Inhaled drugs

Centrally acting drugs (opioids)

Opioids increase the threshold for stimulation of neurons in the medullary cough network, and probably modulate a gating mechanism in the brain analogous to that identified for pain reception. They are most effective for cough arising from the lower airways. Weak opioid analgesics (see Chapter 19) are most commonly used, especially codeine and pholcodine. Morphine is used for cough in terminal conditions. Dextromethorphan is an antitussive that is structurally related to opioids, but is a glutamate NMDA receptor antagonist with no analgesic or sedative action.

Peripherally acting drugs

Local anaesthetics such as lidocaine (see Chapter 18) are used as an oropharyngeal spray to reduce cough during bronchoscopy. Antihistamines (see Chapter 39) reduce postnasal drip from allergic rhinitis, which can stimulate cough, but they have no direct antitussive activity. Nevertheless, sedative antihistamines, such as diphenhydramine, are commonly used in compound cough preparations on sale direct to the public.

Locally acting drugs

Demulcents line the surface of the upper airway above the larynx, reducing local irritation. Many cough lozenges and the syrup in simple linctus act by this mechanism.

Expectorants

Expectorants such as guaifenesin and squill are often included in compound cough preparations (sometimes with a cough suppressant!), with the intention of making cough more effective by increasing the volume of mucus secretion. There is no evidence that they have any clinical value.

Mucolytics

Mucolytics such as erdosteine and carbocisteine reduce the viscosity of bronchial secretions by breaking disulphide crosslinks between mucin monomers. Carbocisteine also reduces goblet cell hyperplasia. However, there is no evidence that they improve the ability to expectorate sputum. Taken orally, mucolytics can reduce the frequency of exacerbations in chronic obstructive pulmonary disease and bronchiectasis, but this is probably more related to their antioxidant properties.

Dornase alfa (recombinant human deoxyribonuclease I, or rhDNase I) is an enzyme that digests extracellular DNA. In cystic fibrosis, there is almost no mucin in the airway secretions, which largely comprises a polymer network of DNA from degraded inflammatory cells and F-actin. Dornase alfa is given to people with cystic fibrosis by inhalation using a jet nebuliser, and reduces sputum viscosity and adhesiveness. Unwanted effects such as transient pharyngitis and hoarseness can occur.

MANAGEMENT OF COUGH

An acute cough should be treated only if it is unproductive or excessive. A self-limiting nonproductive acute cough, such as that caused by a viral illness, can be suppressed by simple linctus or a weak opioid given for a maximum of 5 days. Sedative antihistamines in compound cough preparations should not be given to children under the age of 6 years. Codeine should be avoided in children under the age of 12 years, since it is variably metabolised to morphine and rapid metabolisers may develop unpredictable excessive respiratory depression.

In chronic cough, treatment should be directed at the underlying cause. Specific treatment for cough-variant asthma, postnasal drip and gastro-oesophageal reflux will often resolve cough associated with these conditions. Cough is a common unwanted effect of angiotensin-converting enzyme (ACE) inhibitors (see Chapter 6) and occurs in up to 15% of people who take them. It sometimes appears only a few hours after starting treatment, but can first arise after several months of treatment. Changing to another class of drug is usually necessary to eliminate the cough.

Chronic nonproductive cough in terminal lung cancer can be treated with a powerful opioid such as morphine. If an underlying cause for a chronic cough is not found, symptomatic therapy is frequently ineffective.

RESPIRATORY STIMULANTS (ANALEPTIC DRUGS)

Doxapram stimulates the medullary respiratory centre both by a direct action and by peripheral stimulation of the carotid body. It increases respiratory drive and arousal, and improves both rate and depth of ventilation. Given by intravenous injection, its action is very brief, owing to rapid metabolism by the liver, and a continuous infusion is needed for a more prolonged effect. Restlessness, muscle twitching and vomiting are common unwanted effects. Seizures can occur due to generalised stimulation of the central nervous system. Doxapram has a limited place in the short-term treatment of ventilatory failure, such as in hypercapnoeic respiratory failure due to chronic obstructive pulmonary disease which is causing drowsiness. When combined with physiotherapy, doxapram can encourage coughing and clearance of excessive secretions. However, its use has largely been superseded by noninvasive ventilatory support, such as with nasal intermittent positive pressure ventilation. There is also a minor role for doxapram to reverse postoperative respiratory depression.

Acetazolamide is an inhibitor of carbonic anhydrase that stimulates the respiratory centre by creating a mild metabolic acidosis. It is used in the prevention and management of acute altitude sickness (see Chapter 14).

CYSTIC FIBROSIS

Cystic fibrosis is an autosomal recessive disorder caused by a single gene mutation on the long arm of chromosome 7. This gene encodes the cystic fibrosis transmembrane conductance regulator (CFTR), a cAMP regulated Cl^- and HCO_3^- channel in the apical membranes of many epithelial cells. The channel requires ATP to open it, and then permits passive movement of ions out of the cell along electrochemical gradients. In the airway epithelium, CFTR also inhibits nearby Na^+ channels. If the *CFTR* gene is faulty, then the function of the transporter is impaired or absent, and Cl^- transport is defective in epithelial cells in many organs, including the respiratory, hepatobiliary, gastrointestinal and reproductive tracts, and the pancreas. As a result of the defective ion flows, secretions become thicker. This causes obstruction in (and destruction of) exocrine glandular ducts, and in the lungs, it clogs respiratory cilia with mucus. There are six classes of *CFTR* gene mutations, grouped according to their known or putative effects on the CFTR protein, and around 2000 individual gene mutations have been found. The various classes of mutation confer different severities of disease. Other genes also modify the effects of the CFTR gene and contribute to the phenotypic variability of the condition.

The major cause of morbidity and mortality in cystic fibrosis is lung disease. The airway epithelium normally protects against infection and toxins by providing a mechanical barrier, participating in the innate immune system and initiating the adaptive immune response. The mucus secreted onto the respiratory epithelium in healthy lungs has an inner, low viscosity layer to permit free ciliary motion and a thicker outer layer that traps pathogens and particles. In cystic fibrosis, the periciliary liquid layer of the mucus is defective, which makes it more viscous and renders the cilia ineffective. The resulting stasis permits accumulation of mucus, debris and pathogens, and creates an environment for bacterial colonisation. The consequence is persistent endobronchial bacterial infection and a chronic inflammatory response in the airway, punctuated by recurrent episodes of acute infection. Together, these lead to progressive bronchiectasis and chronic airflow obstruction.

The other most common and disabling clinical consequence of cystic fibrosis, affecting about 90% of those with the condition, is pancreatic exocrine insufficiency. Viscous secretions obstruct the pancreatic ductules and prevent pancreatic enzymes from reaching the gut, leading to fat malabsorption. About 30% also develop pancreatic fibrosis and replacement of pancreatic tissue with fat that produces endocrine insufficiency and type 1 diabetes mellitus. Less commonly, people with cystic fibrosis develop meconium ileus in infancy or obstructive biliary tract disease in adult life.

Death in 90% of people with cystic fibrosis is due to progressive lung disease, but median life expectancy has risen steadily to about 41 years due to improved treatment.

DRUG TREATMENT OF CYSTIC FIBROSIS

Treatment of cystic fibrosis in early years would ideally be directed at improving the function of the CFTR channel. Ivacaftor is a small molecule that potentiates the action of the CFTR in class III gene mutations (about 5% of those with cystic fibrosis). It improves lung function, reduces respiratory exacerbations and promotes weight gain. There are no specific treatments that affect CFTR channel function in the other classes of mutation.

Treatment of lung disease

Much of the treatment for cystic fibrosis remains supportive, including physiotherapy. Nebulised hypertonic saline improves mucociliary clearance, and reduces the frequency of infective exacerbations. It can sometimes produce bronchospasm, which can be prevented by prior use of an inhaled β_2-adrenoceptor agonist such as salbutamol (see Chapter 12). Airway obstruction is treated in the same way as chronic obstructive airway disease (see Chapter 12).

DNA released from dying neutrophils in the airways contributes to the increased sputum viscosity in cystic fibrosis. Inhaled dornase alfa improves lung function in the short- to medium-term (although long-term benefits are much less certain) and results in fewer exacerbations of lung disease. Improved lung function should be measurable after 2 weeks in responders.

Prevention of infection and cross-infection (especially from other people with cystic fibrosis and during hospital admission) is a key element in the management of cystic fibrosis. Rapid and intensive treatment of clinical infection slows the decline in lung function and is the main reason for the prolongation of life expectancy in recent years. The most common lung pathogens in the very young person with cystic fibrosis are *Staphylococcus aureus* (50%), *Haemophilus influenzae* (30%) and *Pseudomonas aeruginosa* (20%). In the first 3 years of life, prophylactic antistaphylococcal therapy with flucloxacillin is usually given to reduce exacerbations of lung disease (see Chapter 51). By adolescence, *P. aeruginosa* becomes the predominant pathogen. Colonisation with *P. aeruginosa* can be prevented or reduced by regular treatment with inhaled nebulised tobramycin or nebulised colistimethate sodium combined with oral ciprofloxacin. Exacerbations of infection require oral or intravenous antimicrobials (see Chapter 51).

Since inflammation is a major component of the airway disease, several antiinflammatory therapies have been studied. Oral corticosteroids reduce the rate of decline in lung function and reduce the frequency of infections, but unwanted effects preclude their long-term use. Inhaled corticosteroids do not improve lung function unless there is associated airway hyperreactivity.

Treatment of malabsorption

Nutritional supplements are important because of the frequency of fat malabsorption and impaired absorption of fat-soluble vitamins. Pancreatic enzyme supplements (Pancreatin) are used from the diagnosis of pancreatic insufficiency. Pancreatin contains protease, lipase and amylase, enzymes which are inactivated by gastric acid and by heat. Supplements should be taken with food (but not mixed with very hot food) and either with gastric acid suppression therapy (e.g. given 1 hour after a histamine H₂ receptor antagonist such as ranitidine; see Chapter 33) or as enteric-coated formulations to protect them from gastric acid. Pancreatin preparations in clinical use are all of porcine origin. Dosage is adjusted according to the size, number and consistency of stools. Unwanted effects include irritation of the mouth and perianal skin, nausea, vomiting and abdominal discomfort. Some higher-strength formulations of pancreatin should be avoided in children under 15 years of age with cystic fibrosis, since they have been associated with the formation of large bowel strictures.

Pancreatin is also used for pancreatic exocrine insufficiency following pancreatectomy, gastrectomy or chronic pancreatitis.

IDIOPATHIC PULMONARY FIBROSIS

Pulmonary fibrosis is a form of interstitial lung disease. It has a characteristic histological finding of usual interstitial pneumonia (fibrotic foci surrounded by normal lung tissue), which may result from aberrant wound healing following repetitive alveolar cell epithelial injury. Median survival after diagnosis varies from 2 to 3.5 years, with a slow progressive decline in respiratory function.

There are no curative therapies. Pirfenidone has antiinflammatory and antifibrotic actions, and when used in mild to moderate disease slows progression of the fibrosis. It may act by inhibition of transforming growth factor-β and altering collagen synthesis. Gastrointestinal unwanted effects and photosensitive rash are the most common problems encountered with treatment. Acute exacerbations of symptoms are treated with a corticosteroid. When there is hypoxaemia at rest or desaturation with physical activity, supplemental oxygen therapy can improve symptoms and quality of life. Lung transplantation may be considered.

NEONATAL RESPIRATORY DISTRESS SYNDROME

Pulmonary surfactant is responsible for reducing surface tension at the air–liquid interface in the alveoli, preventing lung collapse at resting lung pressures. Surfactant is a macromolecular complex largely composed of phospholipids (80–85%), mainly phosphatidylcholine of which dipalmitoylphosphatidylcholine is the major surface-active component; neutral lipids (5–10%); and surfactant-specific proteins A–D (5–10%). The phospholipid forms a monolayer at the air–liquid interface which displaces water and reduces the force of attraction between the water molecules that promotes collapse of alveoli at end-expiration. This stabilises the alveoli by reducing the deflating force during expiration. Surfactant proteins B and C are hydrophobic and involved in

spreading of the surfactant layer at the air–liquid interface. The hydrophilic surfactant proteins A and D are involved in surfactant metabolism and in host defence by enhancing phagocytosis of pathogens.

Surfactant is synthesised by type II alveolar epithelial cells and is normally present in substantial amounts at full-term delivery. However, preterm infants (especially those born at or before 28 weeks gestation) have immature lungs which may produce too little surfactant. These infants develop difficulty breathing within minutes or hours of delivery, a condition called neonatal respiratory distress syndrome.

Mortality is high in neonatal respiratory distress syndrome. In women at risk of preterm delivery, a corticosteroid such as betamethasone (see Chapter 44) given to the mother at least 12 hours, and preferably 48 hours, before delivery can enhance pulmonary maturity in the neonate which may prevent neonatal respiratory distress syndrome.

Surfactant is given as soon as possible after delivery to infants with neonatal respiratory distress syndrome, or to those considered to be at high risk of developing it. Surfactant combined with noninvasive ventilation reduces the risk of death by 40%. Treatment also reduces the risk of pneumothorax and of subsequent chronic lung disease. Delivery of surfactant was originally via an endotracheal tube, but techniques that avoid intubation such as aerosols or delivery via a thin plastic catheter are being studied.

There are two natural therapeutic surfactants: beractant (bovine lung extract) and poractant alfa (porcine lung phospholipid fraction). Synthetic compounds have been developed with peptides that mimic the natural surfactant proteins, but these appear to be less effective. Therapeutic use of pulmonary surfactants has been associated with intrapulmonary haemorrhage in neonates.

Pulmonary surfactant is also useful in neonates with meconium aspiration syndrome and in acute neonatal respiratory distress due to group B streptococcal sepsis. There is some evidence of improved outcomes when pulmonary surfactant is given to children with acute respiratory distress syndrome due to acute lung injury.

SELF-ASSESSMENT

True/false questions

1. Postviral cough can last for 3–6 weeks.
2. Angiotensin II receptor antagonists frequently cause cough.
3. Many compound cough preparations sold over-the-counter contain sedating antihistamines.
4. Dextromethorphan is a synthetic opioid with cough suppressant, sedative and analgesic activity.
5. There is little evidence that any preparation can specifically facilitate expectoration.
6. Pulmonary surfactant increases surface tension in the alveoli.
7. Therapeutic surfactant is identical to natural human surfactant.
8. Doxapram should not be used in postoperative respiratory failure.
9. The mucolytic carbocisteine acts by inhibiting the production of mucus.

10. Dornase alfa breaks down extracellular DNA in sputum.
11. Ivacaftor improves CFTR function in over 90% of people with cystic fibrosis.
12. Pirfenidone is used in idiopathic pulmonary fibrosis.

ANSWERS

True/false answers

1. **True.** Treatment of postviral cough should include increased humidity of inspired air and cough suppressants; other drugs are of little value.
2. **False.** Angiotensin II receptor antagonists do not cause cough. However, inhibitors of ACE, which reduce the formation of angiotensin II, also prevent the breakdown of bradykinin and this causes cough in 15% of people.
3. **True.** Diphenhydramine and chlorphenamine are common constituents of over-the-counter cough mixtures.
4. **False.** Dextromethorphan has the same cough-suppressant potency as codeine but does not share its sedative or analgesic effects; dextromethorphan may act by blocking *N*-methyl-D-aspartate (NMDA) receptors.
5. **True.** Expectorants may nevertheless serve a useful placebo function.
6. **False.** Surfactant has a detergent-like action to lower surface tension, enabling the alveoli to expand and retain an expanded shape.
7. **False.** Therapeutic surfactants such as beractant and poractant alfa are animal products lacking the two hydrophilic surfactant proteins, SP-A and SP-D.
8. **False.** Doxapram is sometimes used in hospitals for postoperative respiratory failure. It stimulates the respiratory centre and the carotid chemoreceptors, but its precise mode of action is unknown.
9. **True.** Mucolytics reduce mucus viscosity by breaking the disulphide cross-bridges that maintain the polymeric gel-like structure of mucus, but carbocisteine also inhibits mucus secretion by reducing goblet cell hyperplasia.
10. **True.** Dornase alpha is a recombinant deoxribonuclease that digests DNA released by dying neutrophils in sputum; it is given by nebuliser to reduce viscosity of lung secretions in cystic fibrosis.
11. **False.** Ivacaftor improves CFTR function only in the 4–5% of people with CF and only those with the G551D mutation.
12. **True.** Pirfenidone has antiinflammatory and antifibrotic activity in IPF.

FURTHER READING

Cough

Davies, L., Calverley, P.M.A., 2010. The evidence for the use of oral mucolytic agents in chronic obstructive pulmonary disease (COPD). Br. Med. Bull. 93, 217–227.

Dicpinigaitis, P.V., Morice, A.H., Birring, S.S., et al., 2014. Antitussive drugs—past, present, and future. Pharmacol. Rev. 66, 468–512.

Smith, J.A., Woodcock, A., 2016. Chronic cough. N. Engl. J. Med. 375, 1544–1551.

Rubin, B.K., 2007. Mucolytics, expectorants and mucokinetic medications. Respir. Care. 52, 859–865.

Cystic fibrosis

Cuthbert, A.W., 2011. New horizons in the treatment of cystic fibrosis. Br. J. Pharmacol. 163, 141–172.

Elborn, J.S. 2016. Cystic fibrosis. Lancet. 388, 2519–2531.

Mogayzel, P.J., Naureckas, E.T., Robinson, K.A., et al., 2013. Cystic fibrosis pulmonary guidelines. Chronic medications for maintenance of lung health. Am. J. Respir. Crit. Care Med. 187, 680–689.

Plant, B.J., Goss, C.H., Plant, W.D., et al., 2013. Management of comorbidities in older patients with cystic fibrosis. Lancet Respir. Med. 1, 164–174.

Idiopathic pulmonary fibrosis

Rafii, R., Juarez, M.M., Albertson, T.E., et al., 2013. A review of current and novel therapies for idiopathic pulmonary fibrosis. J. Thorac. Dis. 5, 48–73.

Neonatal respiratory distress syndrome

Duffett, M., Choong, K., Ng, V., et al., 2007. Surfactant therapy for acute respiratory failure in children: a systematic review and meta-analysis. Crit. Care 11, R66. doi:1186/cc5944.

Ramanthan, R., Kamholz, K., Fujii, A.M., 2013. Is there a difference in surfactant treatment of respiratory distress syndrome in premature neonates? A review. J. Pulmon. Resp. Med. S13, 004. doi:10.4172/2161-105X.S13-004.

Compendium: drugs used to treat respiratory disorders

Drug	Characteristics
Cough suppressants	
Cough suppressants listed here are opioid derivatives (see Chapter 19), usually given orally as a linctus. Sedating antihistamines (see Chapter 39) are also sometimes given for cough suppression.	
Codeine	Use is associated with constipation. Half-life: 3–4 h
Dextromethorphan	Fewer unwanted effects than codeine. Half-life: 3 h
Methadone	Used mainly in palliative care for the distressing cough of terminal lung cancer (but less than other opioids). Half-life: 6–8 h
Morphine	Used in palliative care for the distressing cough of terminal lung cancer. Half-life: 1–5 h
Pholcodine	Fewer unwanted effects than codeine. Mild sedative activity. Long half-life (32–43 h)
Mucolytics	
Carbocisteine	Reduces mucus viscosity and inhibits goblet cell hyperplasia; used in chronic obstructive pulmonary disease (COPD) and bronchiectasis, given orally. Half-life: 2 h
Dornase alfa	Recombinant human deoxyribonuclease preparation used for cystic fibrosis, given by nebuliser. Not detectable in blood, but activity in sputum is measurable for at least 6 h
Erdosteine	Reduces mucus viscosity by breaking cross-links in mucus glycoproteins. Used in COPD and bronchiectasis, given orally as a prodrug. Half-life: 1.5 h
Ivacaftor	Potentiates CFTR function in cystic fibrosis patients with the G551D mutation, given orally. Half-life: 12 h
Pulmonary surfactants	
Used for respiratory distress in preterm infants.	
Beractant	Given by endotracheal tube; alveoli are stabilised against collapse by reduction of surface tension, without systemic absorption of the surfactant
Poractant alfa	See beractant
Respiratory stimulant	
Doxapram	Stimulates carotid chemoreceptors; used only under expert supervision for short-term treatment of ventilatory failure, given by intravenous injection (over 30 s) or by continuous intravenous infusion. Half-life: 2–4 h
Antifibrotic	
Pirfenidone	Antiinflammatory and antifibrotic drug, given orally for mild-to-moderate idiopathic pulmonary fibrosis in adults. Half-life: 2–3 h

4

The renal system

14 Diuretics

Almost all diuretics act on the kidney to increase the tubular concentration and elimination of Na^+ ions (natriuresis), with a concurrent excretion of water. Loss of water with the Na^+ ions depletes intravascular volume.

FUNCTIONS OF THE KIDNEY

The kidney has several important functions:

- regulation of plasma fluid volume, electrolyte concentrations and osmolarity;
- regulation of acid–base balance;
- elimination of waste products (mainly nitrogen-containing compounds);
- conservation of essential nutrients, such as glucose and amino acids;
- production and secretion of hormones;
- gluconeogenesis.

Of these, a basic knowledge of the mechanisms of electrolyte and fluid handling by the kidney is essential for understanding the uses and unwanted effects of diuretics. The following account is simplified to emphasise the functions relevant to the actions of diuretics.

THE KIDNEY AND MAINTENANCE OF SALT AND WATER BALANCE

Each day the renal glomeruli of a healthy adult filter about 140–170 L of fluid from plasma, along with ions and small molecules. This is about 20% of the volume of plasma that enters the glomerular capillaries. Since the urine output is only 2–3 L/day, it is clear that most of the filtered fluid and solutes are reabsorbed from the tubule into the blood. Different regions of the tubule and collecting duct vary in their capacity to reabsorb water and solutes (Figs 14.1 and 14.2).

The proximal convoluted tubule

In the proximal convoluted tubule, up to 65% of the filtered Na^+ is reabsorbed together with an equivalent (iso-osmotic) amount of water. Therefore, on leaving the proximal tubule, the tubular fluid still has the same osmolality as plasma. Reabsorption of ions from the proximal tubule into the renal tubular cells is passive (see Fig. 14.1, site 1). The activity of the Na^+/K^+-ATPase pump on the basolateral surface of the tubular cell (transporting three Na^+ out of the tubular cell in exchange for two K^+) helps establish the electrochemical gradient for passive Na^+ reabsorption from the tubular lumen into the tubule cell. Water reabsorption occurs via transmembrane aquaporin (AQP) channels. The passage of water through these channels from the lumen of the proximal renal tubule is driven by the osmotic gradient across the tubular cells, which is created by the active transport of Na^+ out of the cell across the basolateral membrane. The extent of the proximal tubular reabsorption of Na^+ and water is also influenced by various neural and hormonal influences, such as the sympathetic nervous system, angiotensin II, endothelin and dopamine. Most of the filtered K^+ and Cl^- are also reabsorbed by the proximal tubule.

The proximal tubule has organic anion transporters (OATs) that secrete organic anions into the tubular lumen (see Fig. 14.1, site 1; see also Table 2.1) and other transporters that reabsorb water-soluble essential nutrients, such as water-soluble vitamins, glucose and amino acids, from the lumen. The OATs are important for the transport of many drugs and their metabolites from the blood into the tubule. Bicarbonate is also reabsorbed from the proximal tubule

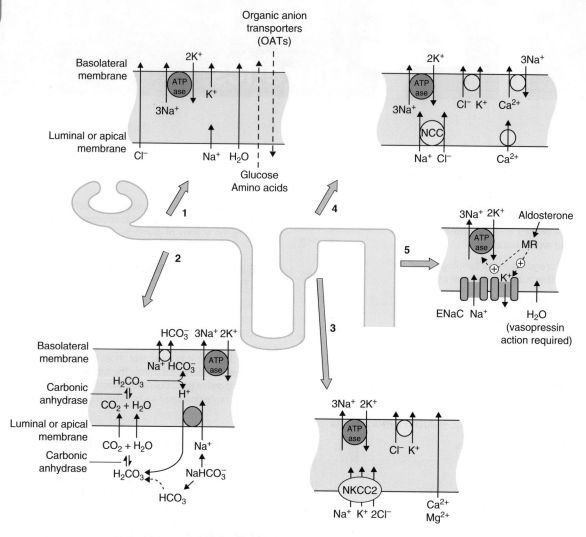

Fig. 14.1 Transport mechanisms for solutes in the kidney. In all segments of the renal tubule, there is active transport of Na^+ out of and K^+ into the cell across the basolateral membrane using Na^+/K^+-ATPase proton pumps. This sets up electrochemical gradients for the transport of other ions. In the proximal tubule (sites 1 and 2), considerable amounts of Na^+, glucose and amino acids are taken up from the lumen, along with water which crosses via aquaporin (AQP) channels. The principal function of the organic anion transporters (OATs) at site 1 is the elimination of metabolites of ingested xenobiotics (see Chapter 2). Transport by OATs also enables diuretic drugs such as furosemide and bendroflumethiazide to gain access to their sites of action on apical membranes in the tubule. Hydrogen ions are excreted in exchange for Na^+ uptake and this, in part, depends upon the activity of carbonic anhydrase (site 2). In the ascending limb of the loop of Henle (site 3), the luminal membrane has a $Na^+/K^+/2Cl^-$ co-transporter (NKCC2) but is impermeable to water. In the proximal part of the distal tubule (cortical diluting segment; site 4) Na^+ and Cl^- ions are reabsorbed by the Na^+/Cl^- co-transporter (NCC), but water is not reabsorbed. Ca^{2+} also exchanges with three Na^+ at the basolateral border at this site. In the distal part of the distal tubule and collecting duct (site 5), Na^+ is reabsorbed from the lumen via an epithelial Na^+ channel (ENaC), in exchange for loss of K^+ into the lumen. The expression and activity of ENaC and the basolateral Na^+/K^+-ATPase pump are regulated by aldosterone acting via mineralocorticoid receptors (MR). Water is reabsorbed in the collecting duct under the influence of antidiuretic hormone (ADH, vasopressin), acting through vasopressin receptors in the basolateral membrane.

by a mechanism dependent on the enzymatic activity of carbonic anhydrase (see Fig. 14.1, site 2).

The loop of Henle

The descending limb of the loop of Henle has AQP channels and is permeable to water, but is impermeable to Na^+. The

interstitial fluid is hypertonic as a result of ion transport in the thick portion of the ascending limb of the loop of Henle (discussed later). Therefore water passes from the tubule into the interstitium of the renal medulla along a concentration gradient. Approximately 10–15% of the total filtered water is absorbed at this site. As a result, tubular fluid reaching the ascending limb of the loop of Henle is hypertonic.

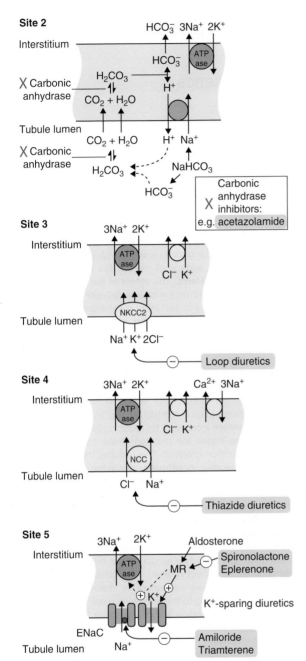

Fig. 14.2 Sites of action of diuretics. For location of these sites in the tubule, see Fig. 14.1. Osmotic diuretics increase osmotic pressure through the tubule, reducing electrolyte reabsorption across the luminal membrane. Other drugs gain access to their sites of action after secretion into the tubule by the organic anion transporters (OATs) in the proximal tubule. Acetazolamide inhibits carbonic anhydrase (site 2) and is a weak self-limiting diuretic, now largely used for other conditions such as glaucoma. Loop diuretics such as furosemide block the luminal $Na^+/K^+/2Cl^-$ co-transporter (NKCC2) and inhibit up to 20–25% of filtered Na^+ reabsorption (site 3). The thiazide diuretics inhibit the luminal Na^+/Cl^- co-transporter (NCC; site 4) and reduce reabsorption of 3–5% of filtered Na^+. The aldosterone antagonists spironolactone and eplerenone compete with aldosterone for the mineralocorticoid receptor (MR), blocking the induction by aldosterone of the expression and activity of the epithelial Na^+ channel (ENaC) and the basolateral Na^+/K^+-ATPase pump (site 5). Amiloride and triamterene act directly on ENaC to block Na^+ reabsorption. Potassium-sparing diuretics inhibit the reuptake of less than 2% of filtered Na^+.

co-transporter is recycled back into the tubular lumen, which ensures that there is always enough tubular K^+ to continue to favour Na^+ reabsorption. K^+ recycling creates a lumen-positive transepithelial voltage gradient, which drives a paracellular ionic current that is responsible for Ca^{2+} and Mg^{2+} reabsorption. Fluid leaving the thick portion of the ascending limb of the loop of Henle and entering the distal tubule is hypotonic with respect to plasma.

The reabsorption of Na^+, but not water, by the thick portion of the ascending limb of the loop of Henle establishes the hypertonicity of the medullary interstitium, which is maintained in part because the medulla has a very low blood flow. This hypertonicity generates the corticomedullary concentration gradient that drives water reabsorption from the descending limb of the loop of Henle. The interstitial hypertonicity in the renal medulla is also responsible for an osmotic gradient across the collecting ducts, which permits the formation of hypertonic urine (discussed later).

The distal convoluted tubule

The hypotonic filtrate leaving the loop of Henle passes into the distal convoluted tubule which is impermeable to water but has a luminal thiazide-sensitive Na^+/Cl^- co-transporter (NCC; see Fig. 14.1, site 4). The driving force for this co-transporter is again generated by the Na^+/K^+-ATPase pump in the basolateral membrane. About 10–15% of the filtered Na^+ load can be reabsorbed at this site. The rich blood supply to this region allows rapid diffusion of the reabsorbed ions into the plasma and prevents the interstitium from becoming hypertonic. Reabsorption of Ca^{2+} is also regulated at this site, under the influence of parathyroid hormone and calcitriol (see Chapter 42). The rate of Ca^{2+} transport is inversely related to that of Na^+ transport.

The thick portion of the ascending limb of the loop of Henle is relatively impermeable to water but has an active $Na^+/K^+/2Cl^-$ co-transporter complex (NKCC2) in the luminal (apical) membrane (see Fig. 14.1, site 3). Na^+ is transported from the tubular cells to the interstitium by the Na^+/K^+-ATPase pump in the basolateral membrane. This creates a low intracellular Na^+ concentration in the tubular cells and generates the Na^+ ion gradient that drives the luminal NKCC2 co-transporter. The thick portion of the ascending limb of the loop of Henle can reabsorb up to 25% of the Na^+ filtered at the glomerulus. K^+ that is carried from the tubule into the cells by the NKCC2

The connecting tubule and the collecting ducts

The tubular fluid that has become yet more hypo-osmolar with respect to plasma while in the distal convoluted tubule is delivered to the connecting tubule and then to the collecting ducts. The connecting tubule has properties intermediate between the distal convoluted tubule and the collecting ducts. There are two main cell types in this region, the principal cells and the intercalated cells.

The principal cells predominate in the cortical portion of the collecting duct. They reabsorb Na^+ through a highly specific amiloride-sensitive epithelial Na^+ channel (ENaC) accompanied by obligatory K^+ loss into the urine (see Fig. 14.1, site 5). Aldosterone acts in the principal cells at cytosolic mineralocorticoid receptors (MRs), inducing transcription of gene-encoding components of ENaC and the basolateral Na^+/K^+-ATPase pump. Therefore the consequence of the action of aldosterone is increased reabsorption of Na^+ from the tubule and the concomitant loss of K^+ into the lumen. The natriuretic peptides, atrial natriuretic peptide (ANP) and brain natriuretic peptide (BNP), decrease Na^+ reabsorption at this site by receptor-mediated phosphorylation of ENaC. Overall, only about 3–5% of filtered Na^+ is reabsorbed at the distal part of the distal tubule. The distal renal tubule is the primary site in the kidney responsible for maintenance of K^+ homeostasis.

The principal cell is also the site of action of vasopressin (antidiuretic hormone [ADH]; see Chapter 43). Vasopressin is secreted by the posterior pituitary gland, binds to receptors on principal cells, and increases the expression of luminal aquaporin (AQP2) channels. This increases the permeability of the cell to water. In the absence of vasopressin, the collecting duct is impermeable to water and the tubular fluid remains hypo-osmolar with respect to plasma. In the presence of vasopressin, water reabsorption is increased down the osmotic gradient established by the thick ascending limb of the loop of Henle into the hypertonic medullary interstitium. This concentrates the tubular fluid as it passes through the collecting duct.

Intercalated cells are more prominent in the medullary collecting duct (not illustrated in Figs 14.1 and 14.2). They express H^+-ATPases that help regulate acid–base balance by secreting or reabsorbing H^+ and HCO_3.

AUTOREGULATION BY TUBULOGLOMERULAR FEEDBACK AND HORMONAL CONTROL

There are additional regulatory mechanisms that control overall function of the nephrons. The first is autoregulation of glomerular perfusion pressure in response to changes in blood pressure through a myogenic reflex that constricts the afferent arteriole when blood pressure increases. The second is tubulo-glomerular feedback, in which the macula densa senses the concentration of Cl^- in the loop of Henle. When the Cl^- concentration rises due to a rise in glomerular filtration rate, the macula densa secretes either adenosine or possibly ATP, which vasoconstricts the afferent arteriole. Tubulo-glomerular feedback is also linked to secretion of renin from the juxtaglomerular apparatus. This enhances the release of aldosterone from the adrenal cortex and increases Na^+ reabsorption at the connecting tubule and cortical segment of the collecting duct.

DIURETIC DRUGS

LOOP DIURETICS

bumetanide, furosemide

Mechanism of action and effects

Loop diuretics are powerful natriuretic drugs which can inhibit reabsorption of up to 20–25% of the Na^+ that appears in the glomerular filtrate. They are secreted into the proximal kidney tubule by the tubular organic anion transporters (OATs) and act at the luminal surface of cells in the thick ascending limb of the loop of Henle. The extent of the natriuresis and diuresis is dependent on the rate of delivery of the drug to the renal tubule via this secretory mechanism. Once these transporters have been saturated, increasing the dose of the diuretic will not enhance its effect. Loop diuretics bind to the Na^+/K^+/$2Cl^-$ co-transporter complex (NKCC2) at the luminal border of the thick ascending limb of the loop of Henle, and inhibit Cl^- reabsorption. This diminishes the electrochemical gradient across the cell and reduces Na^+ reabsorption from the tubular fluid (see Fig. 14.2, site 3). The Na^+ concentration in the tubular fluid leaving the loop of Henle is therefore increased. By reducing Na^+ reabsorption, loop diuretics impair the creation of the corticomedullary ionic concentration gradient. This reduces the ability of the kidney to generate concentrated urine in the collecting duct and enhances water loss in urine.

The dose–response curves of loop diuretics are steep, but the oral doses required for maximal inhibition of Na^+ reabsorption show wide interindividual variation. Because they have a short duration of action, there is partial compensation for the natriuresis by subsequent rebound Na^+ uptake from the tubular fluid after their tubular action has finished. Loop diuretics remain effective even in advanced renal failure, but larger doses are necessary to deliver an effective concentration of drug to the remaining renal tubules, as the reduced tubular secretion allows more time for metabolism of the drug in the liver.

When injected intravenously, furosemide releases vasodilator prostaglandins, such as prostacyclin, into the circulation and produces a short-lived venodilation. Pooling of blood in these capacitance vessels reduces central blood volume, which can be useful in the treatment of acute left ventricular failure (see Chapter 7). Loop diuretics also produce arterial vasodilation, but because of their short duration of action, they are not widely used to treat hypertension, except in renal failure or when there is plasma volume expansion (such as in drug-resistant hypertension), where their diuretic action can be useful.

Pharmacokinetics

Furosemide is incompletely and erratically absorbed from the gut, with considerable interindividual variation. Bumetanide is more completely and reliably absorbed. Furosemide and bumetanide can also be given intravenously. Natriuresis and diuresis begin about 30 minutes after an oral dose and last up to 6 hours; intravenous injection produces a more rapid effect, with an onset of diuresis within minutes. Loop diuretics are partially metabolised in the liver. They are highly protein bound in plasma, and little drug is filtered at the glomerulus. In renal failure there is reduced delivery of drug to the tubular fluid, since other substrates compete with the diuretic for the remaining organic anionic transporters.

Unwanted effects

- Excessive Na^+ and water loss can cause intravascular volume depletion, hypotension and renal impairment.
- Dilutional hyponatraemia can arise from excessive Na^+ loss that exceeds water loss. This is because the drugs are primarily natriuretic and stimulation of ADH secretion in response to plasma volume contraction also promotes reabsorption of water from the collecting duct. Hyponatraemia can present with lethargy, impaired consciousness, and eventually coma and seizures. Hyponatraemia is less common with loop diuretics than with thiazide diuretics.
- Hypokalaemia is dose-related, but is usually less marked than with thiazide diuretics, which have a longer duration of action. The reasons for hypokalaemia include:
  - Increased delivery of Na^+ to the distal convoluted tubule, where Na^+ reabsorption is then enhanced. This creates a negative ionic gradient from tubular cells to the tubular lumen that promotes K^+ diffusion into the tubular lumen.
  - Diuretic-induced hypovolaemia and increased tubular Cl^- concentration stimulate release of renin and therefore aldosterone. Aldosterone further enhances Na^+ reabsorption in the distal tubule at the expense of increased K^+ excretion.
  - Obligatory urinary loss of Cl^- with the increased K^+ loss creates a mild metabolic alkalosis in the plasma. To counteract the alkalosis, H^+ is shifted out of cells in exchange for intracellular accumulation of K^+, which exacerbates the hypokalaemia.
  - The consequences and treatment of hypokalaemia produced by loop diuretics are considered below.
- Hypomagnesaemia. Paracellular diffusion of filtered Mg^{2+} in the thick ascending limb of the loop of Henle is impaired by loop diuretics, which inhibit the electrical gradient necessary for Mg^{2+} reabsorption. Hypomagnesaemia predisposes to cardiac arrhythmias. Hypokalaemia often cannot be corrected unless co-existent hypomagnesaemia has been treated.
- Increased urinary Ca^{2+} excretion from inhibition of paracellular reabsorption of Ca^{2+} at the thick ascending limb of the loop of Henle. It does not produce hypocalcaemia, but this action can be helpful in the management of hypercalcaemia (see Chapter 42).
- Hyperuricaemia arises from reduced glomerular filtration of uric acid following the reduction of plasma volume. There may be an additional reduction of proximal tubular uric acid secretion as a result of competition between uric acid and the diuretic for organic anion transporters. Clinical gout is unusual and less common with loop diuretics than with thiazide diuretics.

- Incontinence can result from the rapid increase in urine volume. In older males with prostatic hypertrophy, retention of urine can occur.
- Ototoxicity. Deafness can result from cochlear toxicity, or tinnitus and vertigo from vestibular toxicity, especially when renal failure reduces the rate of drug excretion or when very large doses of a loop diuretic are used. Ototoxicity is more common with furosemide than bumetanide and is usually reversible.

THIAZIDE AND RELATED DIURETICS

Examples

bendroflumethiazide, chlortalidone, hydrochlorothiazide, indapamide

Mechanisms of action and effects

Thiazides and related diuretics have a lower efficacy than loop diuretics, achieving a maximum natriuresis of about 3–5% of the filtered Na^+ load, and have shallow dose–response curves. Thiazides (such as bendroflumethiazide and hydrochlorothiazide) are structurally related to sulphonamides. Several structurally unrelated thiazide-type drugs, such as chlortalidone and indapamide, share the same site of action and are considered to be thiazides in the following discussion. All these drugs are highly protein-bound, and therefore little drug is filtered at the glomerulus and they are secreted by OATs into the proximal tubule. All these drugs act at the luminal surface of the distal convoluted tubule and inhibit the NCC (see Fig. 14.2, site 4); this inhibits transport of Na^+ and Cl^- into the tubular cell. The concentration of Na^+ in fluid leaving the distal convoluted tubule is therefore increased.

Thiazides produce arterial vasodilation during long-term use, which appears to be the basis of their hypotensive effect (see Chapter 6), but the mechanism of vasodilation is unclear. It may involve an action on the arterial wall, since the vasodilator action occurs at lower dosages than required for significant diuresis. However, an indirect vasodilator effect arising from salt depletion may be important, since thiazides do not lower blood pressure in end-stage renal disease.

Pharmacokinetics

Thiazide and related diuretics are fairly well absorbed from the gut, and most are metabolised in the liver. The onset of diuresis is slow, but they have a longer duration of action than loop diuretics, which varies among the drugs; for example, bendroflumethiazide produces a natriuresis for up to 6–12 hours and chlortalidone for 48–72 hours. Thiazide and related diuretics are less effective when the glomerular filtration rate is below 20 mL/minute.

Unwanted effects

- Hypokalaemia. This is due to greater delivery of Cl^- to the connecting tubule, eliciting a release of renin and therefore aldosterone. A reduced intracellular Ca^{2+} concentration (discussed later) also activates ENaCs in the distal convoluted tubule, which promotes K⁺ secretion into the tubule. Hypokalaemia is more frequent with thiazides than with loop diuretics, partly due to their longer duration of action. The greatest reduction in plasma K⁺ usually occurs within 2 weeks of starting treatment. The management of thiazide-related hypokalaemia is considered below.

- Hyponatraemia. This is due to impaired urine-diluting ability, but without the impaired concentrating ability created by loop diuretics. Prolonged block of Na⁺/Cl⁻ co-transport in the distal convoluted tubule (a cortical diluting site where water cannot be reabsorbed) and vasopressin release in response to reduced plasma volume impairs free water clearance. The combination of a thiazide with amiloride (discussed later) is particularly associated with dilutional hyponatraemia (see loop diuretics). Hyponatraemia usually occurs within 2 weeks of starting treatment. Rapid recurrence of hyponatraemia with re-exposure to thiazides suggests a genetic predisposition in some individuals.
- Hyperuricaemia (see the section on loop diuretics). Gout occurs infrequently and is less common in women.
- Decreased urinary Ca²⁺ excretion, in contrast to increased excretion with loop diuretics. Reduced Na⁺ concentration in the tubular cell activates the Na⁺/Ca²⁺ ATPase antiporter in the basolateral membrane of the distal convoluted tubule. This exchanger uses the electrochemical gradient for Na⁺ across the cell membrane to transport Ca²⁺ from the cell into the interstitium, which then promotes Ca²⁺ reabsorption from the tubular lumen. Hypercalcaemia does not usually occur, unless there is another underlying disturbance of Ca²⁺ metabolism, such as hyperparathyroidism. The reduction in urinary Ca²⁺ loss is useful for the prevention of renal stones resulting from hypercalciuria.
- Glucose intolerance. This is dose-related, with a progressive increase in plasma glucose over several months. The major cause is prolonged hypokalaemia and the consequent reduced intracellular K⁺ concentration which inhibits insulin release and impairs tissue uptake of glucose in response to insulin. A direct action of thiazides producing hyperpolarisation of islet cell membranes and inhibiting insulin release may also contribute. The glucose intolerance usually reverses over several months if the thiazide is stopped.
- Hyperlipidaemia. There is a dose-related increase in low-density lipoprotein cholesterol and triglycerides. The long-term effects (>1 year) are small unless high doses of thiazides are used.
- Impotence. This is reported by up to 10% of middle-aged hypertensive men treated with high doses of thiazides (see Chapter 16).
- Nocturia and urinary frequency can result from prolonged diuresis.

POTASSIUM-SPARING DIURETICS

 Examples

amiloride, eplerenone, spironolactone, triamterene

Mechanism of action and effects

Drugs in this class produce a diuresis while preventing urinary K⁺ loss. The maximum natriuresis achieved by potassium-sparing diuretics is small (usually 1–2% of filtered Na⁺). All potassium-sparing diuretics act at the late distal convoluted tubule and cortical collecting duct. Spironolactone, its active metabolite canrenone, and eplerenone are the only diuretics that do not act at the luminal membrane of the tubular cells. They compete with aldosterone for the cytoplasmic MR in the distal convoluted tubular cells and block transcriptional upregulation of the ENaC and the basolateral Na⁺/K⁺-ATPase pump. They therefore antagonise the effects of aldosterone on Na⁺ reabsorption and K⁺ excretion (see Fig. 14.2, site 5). Spironolactone and eplerenone only work in the presence of aldosterone, so their natriuretic effect is enhanced in primary and secondary hyperaldosteronism.

Amiloride and triamterene have a different mechanism of action: they directly block the ENaC at the luminal surface of the renal tubule (see Fig. 14.2). Their action is independent of the presence of aldosterone.

With potassium-sparing diuretics, Na⁺ and water loss is accompanied by preservation of plasma K⁺, because the reduced Na⁺ reabsorption limits ATP-dependent Na⁺ exchange with K⁺ at the basolateral membrane (see Fig. 14.2, site 5). When used together with a thiazide or a loop diuretic, potassium-sparing diuretics reduce or eliminate the excess urinary K⁺ loss.

Pharmacokinetics

All potassium-sparing diuretics are taken orally. Spironolactone is metabolised in the wall of the gut and the liver to canrenone, which has a much longer half-life and is probably responsible for most of the diuretic effect. The onset of action of spironolactone and eplerenone is slow, starting after 1 day and becoming maximal by 3–4 days, largely a consequence of their transcriptional mechanism of action.

Triamterene is extensively metabolised in the liver, and tubular secretion of the sulfate ester metabolite is responsible for the diuretic action. Amiloride is secreted unchanged into the proximal renal tubule. The onset of action of both drugs is rapid.

Unwanted effects

- Hyperkalaemia. This is more common in the presence of preexisting renal disease, in the elderly and during combination treatment with angiotensin-converting enzyme (ACE) inhibitors or angiotensin II receptor antagonists (see Chapter 6). Retention of Mg²⁺ also occurs, in contrast to the loss of Mg²⁺ with thiazides and loop diuretics.
- Hyponatraemia. This is more common with thiazide/amiloride combinations.
- Spironolactone has an antiandrogenic effect, a consequence of its ability to bind to androgen receptors and prevent their interaction with dihydrotestosterone. This can cause gynaecomastia and impotence in males, and menstrual irregularities in women. The antiandrogenic effect is sometimes used in women to treat hirsutism (such as in polycystic ovary syndrome), male-pattern hair loss and acne. Eplerenone has greater aldosterone receptor selectivity and does not have antiandrogenic actions.
- Gastrointestinal disturbances.

CARBONIC ANHYDRASE INHIBITORS

acetazolamide

Mechanism of action and uses

Acetazolamide inhibits carbonic anhydrase, an enzyme which is responsible for the small amount of active Na^+ reabsorption in the proximal tubule in exchange for H^+ secretion into the tubule (see Fig. 14.2, site 2). Acetazolamide increases HCO_3^-, Na^+ and K^+ loss into tubular fluid, producing alkaline urine. H^+ is retained in plasma, producing a mild acidosis. However, the fall in plasma HCO_3^- concentration stimulates carbonic anhydrase activity, which rapidly leads to tolerance to the diuretic action of acetazolamide. The diuretic action of acetazolamide is therefore weak and not clinically useful. Acetazolamide has a role in prevention and treatment of altitude sickness (discussed later) and in glaucoma (see Chapter 50).

Pharmacokinetics

Acetazolamide is secreted into the proximal renal tubule by organic acid transporters (OATs) and works at the luminal surface of the proximal tubule. It is eliminated unchanged in the urine.

Unwanted effects

- Nausea, vomiting, anorexia, taste disturbance.
- Paraesthesia, dizziness, fatigue, irritability, ataxia, depression.
- Hypokalaemia (see the discussion on loop diuretics for mechanisms).

OSMOTIC DIURETICS

mannitol

Mechanism of action and uses

Mannitol is a polyol (sugar alcohol) with a low molecular weight that is filtered at the glomerulus but not reabsorbed from the renal tubule. It exerts osmotic activity within the proximal convoluted tubule and the descending limb of the loop of Henle, which limits passive tubular reabsorption of water. Water loss produced by mannitol is accompanied by a variable natriuresis.

Unlike other diuretics, the osmotic action of mannitol produces an initial expansion of plasma and extracellular fluid volume, and it has little value as a diuretic. Mannitol does not readily cross the blood–brain barrier and has a role in the management of acute brain injury.

Pharmacokinetics

Mannitol is given by intravenous infusion and is excreted unchanged at the glomerulus. It has a half-life of 2 hours, which is substantially increased in renal impairment.

Unwanted effects

- Expansion of plasma volume can precipitate heart failure, and subsequently hypovolaemia and hypotension result from diuresis.
- Urinary K^+ loss can lead to hypokalaemia (see the discussion on loop diuretics).
- Hypernatraemia with repeated dosing.

MANAGEMENT OF DIURETIC-INDUCED HYPOKALAEMIA

A modest reduction in plasma K^+ concentration is common during treatment with loop or thiazide diuretics. Marked hypokalaemia (below 3.0 mmol/L) predisposes to cardiac rhythm disturbances (including ventricular arrhythmias), particularly in the presence of acute myocardial ischaemia, during treatment with digitalis glycosides (see Chapter 7), or with antiarrhythmic agents that prolong the Q–T interval on the electrocardiogram (see Chapter 8). It may also precipitate encephalopathy in people with liver failure. The risk of hypokalaemia is greatest with:

- thiazide diuretics, because of their longer duration of action, rather than loop diuretics;
- low oral intake of K^+;
- high doses of diuretic;
- hyperaldosteronism, for example in hepatic cirrhosis or nephrotic syndrome.

The addition of a potassium-sparing diuretic will prevent and treat diuretic-induced hypokalaemia, but it is unnecessary to routinely prescribe a potassium-sparing diuretic with a thiazide or loop diuretic. A pragmatic approach is to use combination treatment for those at high risk for hypokalaemia, or those who develop significant hypokalaemia during regular diuretic treatment.

Oral K^+ supplements should not be given to prevent hypokalaemia, but can be used to correct hypokalaemia. They are less effective than a potassium-sparing diuretic unless used in large quantities (>30 mmol daily), which often cause gastric irritation. Modified-release tablets and effervescent formulations of K^+ are available to improve tolerability. Oral K^+ supplements should not be used together with potassium-sparing diuretics.

Intravenous K^+ replacement is rarely needed unless there is severe K^+ depletion. Rapid intravenous injection of K^+ can produce potentially lethal hyperkalaemia (provoking asystole), and a maximum infusion rate of 20 mmol/hour (and usually much lower) is recommended. Continuous ECG monitoring and hourly measurement of the plasma K^+ concentration is advisable if a high infusion rate is necessary. Hypomagnaesaemia often coexists with diuretic-induced hypokalaemia, and it is usually impossible to correct the hypokalaemia unless the serum Mg^{2+} is corrected first with either intravenous magnesium sulfate or an oral preparation such as magnesium-L-aspartate.

MAJOR USES OF DIURETICS

Diuretics can be used to treat a number of conditions.

Diuretics for treatment of oedema in heart failure, nephrotic syndrome and hepatic cirrhosis

Oedema in heart failure is discussed in Chapter 7. Spironolactone and eplerenone play an important role in heart failure, as they are the only diuretics that improve prognosis.

For nephrotic syndrome, a loop diuretic is usually used. Modest doses of a loop diuretic provide a near-maximal response if renal function is normal, but large doses are sometimes necessary if there is renal impairment. Once the glomerular filtration rate (GFR) falls below 10 mL/minute, then the effect of a loop diuretic is minimal.

Spironolactone is the diuretic of choice in ascites associated with liver disease, due to the marked secondary hyperaldosteronism. It is also important to avoid hypokalaemia, which can precipitate hepatic encephalopathy. A loop diuretic can be added to a high dose of spironolactone if the loss of fluid is inadequate (see Chapter 36).

Management of oedema resistant to diuretics

Resistance to loop diuretics can result from several mechanisms:

- reduced GFR due to low perfusion or abnormal glomerular haemodynamics;
- postdiuretic effect with avid proximal tubular reabsorption of Na^+ after the effect of the diuretic has worn off;
- 'braking phenomenon' due to upregulation of the $Na^+/K^+/2Cl^-$ co-transporters in the loop of Henle;
- rebound Na^+ retention in the distal renal tubule due to renin-aldosterone system activation;
- tolerance with long-term diuretic use due to hypertrophy of epithelial cells of the cortical collecting duct, which increases Na^+ reabsorption at this site.

There are various strategies that can be considered if fluid retention is resistant to oral furosemide:

- Salt restriction and avoidance of salt-retaining drugs, such as nonsteroidal anti-inflammatory drugs (NSAIDS; see Chapter 29). Water restriction may be necessary if there is dilutional hyponatraemia, since raising the serum Na^+ concentration improves diuretic responsiveness.
- Divided oral doses of a loop diuretic can be used to give more prolonged drug delivery to the kidney. This also reduces postdiuretic rebound Na^+ retention.
- Oral bumetanide can be used rather than furosemide, because of its more consistent oral absorption.
- A loop diuretic can be given by intravenous infusion (often over 24 hours) to prolong the duration of action and give a more sustained natriuresis and diuresis. Slow intravenous infusion of higher drug doses will also help avoid ototoxicity.
- The addition of a thiazide or related diuretic to a loop diuretic. Sequential inhibition of tubular Na^+ reabsorption

can produce a dramatic diuresis and natriuresis. However, hyponatraemia, hypokalaemia, hypovolaemia and renal impairment are all more frequent with such combinations.
- Secondary hyperaldosteronism can develop with high doses of a loop diuretic, and the addition of spironolactone can be particularly useful.

Diuretics for treatment of hypertension

Low doses of a thiazide or related diuretic are usually used for treatment of hypertension for their vasodilator action, rather than the diuretic effect. Spironolactone can be added for treatment of resistant hypertension. A loop diuretic is used instead of a thiazide diuretic for drug-resistant hypertension, since there is often expansion of plasma volume. Loop diuretics are also more effective when there is renal impairment (especially a GFR below 20 mL/minute). See also Chapter 6.

Diuretic use in hypercalciuria with renal stone formation

Thiazides reduce urinary Ca^{2+} excretion, and this can be exploited to prevent recurrence of Ca^{2+}-containing kidney stones (usually calcium oxalate). Increased urinary Ca^{2+} excretion often occurs when the serum Ca^{2+} is normal (idiopathic hypercalciuria) and reflects abnormally high Ca^{2+} absorption from the gut. Thiazide diuretics are effective in conjunction with a low-Na^+ and low-protein diet for preventing further stone formation. High dietary Na^+ enhances Ca^{2+} excretion in urine because less Ca^{2+} is reabsorbed in the proximal convoluted tubule.

Carbonic anhydrase inhibitors for glaucoma

Acetazolamide and other topical carbonic anhydrase inhibitors are used to reduce intraocular pressure in glaucoma (see Chapter 50). Tolerance does not occur to this effect, unlike the diuretic action.

Acetazolamide for altitude sickness

An unlicensed use for acetazolamide is the prevention and treatment of the symptoms of altitude sickness. This occurs when a person rapidly ascends to altitude before the body has acclimatised to the low inspired oxygen concentration. It produces headache, nausea, dizziness and fatigue. Symptoms are initially worse at night, with periodic breathing leading to disturbed sleep. Slow ascent to altitude is the most important way to prevent acute mountain sickness, and symptoms generally subside within 2–4 days. Acetazolamide works by inducing a mild metabolic acidosis that drives ventilation and should be taken for 2 days before ascending to altitude. It is continued for 3 days once the highest altitude is reached.

Acetazolamide for hypoventilation in chronic obstructive pulmonary disease

Acetazolamide creates a mild metabolic acidosis in plasma. This can stimulate respiration in the short term, and reduce carbon dioxide retention (see Chapter 12).

Mannitol for acute brain injury

Mannitol is sometimes used to reduce ischaemic cerebral damage (e.g. after neurosurgery or in acute traumatic brain injury). This is achieved by a reduction in plasma viscosity and increase in cardiac output that improves blood flow to areas of the brain where autoregulation is disturbed. The osmotic action of mannitol may be beneficial during more prolonged administration, but this requires an intact blood–brain barrier. Fluid loss via the kidney should be replaced with intravenous crystalloid to avoid dehydration.

SELF-ASSESSMENT

True/false questions

1. A fall in plasma K^+ concentration can affect cardiac muscle function.
2. The main renal site of K^+ loss in the urine is from the proximal convoluted tubule.
3. The Na^+/K^+-ATPase pump is only found on the basolateral membrane of the loop of Henle.
4. The thick ascending limb of the loop of Henle is impermeable to water.
5. Osmotic diuretics are poorly reabsorbed from the renal tubule.
6. Osmotic diuretics should not be given in heart failure.
7. The carbonic anhydrase inhibitor acetazolamide is used in the treatment of glaucoma.
8. All thiazide diuretics are shorter acting than loop diuretics.
9. Thiazide diuretics act by inhibiting Na^+/Cl^- co-transport in the basolateral membrane.
10. Thiazide diuretics increase urinary Ca^{2+} excretion.
11. Thiazide diuretics may exacerbate diabetes mellitus.
12. Spironolactone and amiloride act by the same mechanism to reduce K^+ loss.
13. Potassium-sparing diuretics and ACE inhibitors can cause a harmful interaction.
14. Thiazide or loop diuretics should not be given together with potassium-sparing diuretics.
15. NSAIDs reduce the response to diuretics.

One-best-answer (OBA) questions

1. What is the mechanism of action of triamterene?
   A. Antagonism of a cytosolic receptor
   B. Blockade of a $Na^+/K^+/2Cl^-$ co-transporter
   C. Blockade of a selective Na^+ channel
   D. Blockade of a Na^+/Cl^- symporter
   E. Reduction in HCO_3^- reabsorption

2. Which is the *most accurate* statement about loop diuretics?
   A. They are useful in the treatment of acute pulmonary oedema.
   B. They should not be taken together with thiazides.
   C. They do not produce hypokalaemia.
   D. They increase the hypertonicity of the interstitium in the medullary region.
   E. They reduce the risk of ototoxicity with aminoglycoside antibacterial drugs.

Extended-matching-item question

Choose the *most likely* option (A–F) related to the case scenarios 1–3 provided.
A. Raised serum K^+ concentration
B. Lowered serum K^+ concentration
C. Increased natriuresis
D. Reduced natriuresis
E. Raised plasma glucose
F. Lowered plasma glucose

Case 1. A 58-year-old woman was taken to the emergency department with dyspnoea and bradycardia (40 beats/minute). She previously had a myocardial infarction and coronary stenting. She was taking the diuretics bendroflumethiazide and eplerenone, and recently had her dose of the ACE inhibitor lisinopril increased.

Case 2. A 48-year-old man has been treated for 4 years with the thiazide-related diuretic chlortalidone for his hypertension and was seeking medical advice about his increased tiredness and lethargy.

Case 3. A 55-year-old man with congestive heart failure was treated with digoxin and lisinopril. Furosemide was added because of oedema, and he subsequently complained of palpitations. He was admitted to hospital, and the electrocardiogram showed atrial tachycardia.

ANSWERS

True/false answers

1. **True.** Hypokalaemia can also affect brain and skeletal muscle function.
2. **False.** Much of the filtered K^+ is reabsorbed in the proximal tubule and loop of Henle, and its loss into the urine occurs mainly in the collecting ducts.
3. **False.** The basolateral Na^+/K^+-ATPase pump is present throughout the renal tubule.
4. **True.** Impermeability to water and the NKCC2 transporter that co-transports Na^+, K^+ and Cl^- ions from the lumen into the tubular cell in the thick ascending limb together generate the hyperosmotic interstitium important in concentrating urine in the collecting duct.
5. **True.** Osmotic diuretics are retained within the tubule where their osmotic activity reduces passive reabsorption of water in the proximal tubule and descending limb of the loop of Henle.
6. **True.** By extracting water from intracellular compartments and expanding extracellular and intravascular fluid volumes, osmotic diuretics can precipitate pulmonary oedema.

7. **True.** Acetazolamide reduces the formation of aqueous humour.

8. **False.** Some thiazide diuretics such as chlortalidone can produce a diuresis for 48–72 hours, while the action of most loop diuretics is relatively short-lived.

9. **False.** Thiazide diuretics act from within the renal tubular lumen on the thiazide-sensitive NCC on the luminal (apical) membrane.

10. **False.** Thiazide diuretics do not increase urinary Ca^{2+} excretion, unlike the loop diuretics.

11. **True.** Thiazide diuretics may exacerbate diabetes mellitus, probably through hypokalaemia reducing insulin release from pancreatic β-cells.

12. **False.** Amiloride blocks the ENaC directly, whereas spironolactone competes with aldosterone at MRs, thus reducing the transcriptional expression of ENaC. The reduced Na^+ reabsorption produced by both drugs in the collecting duct reduces the loss of K^+ into the urine.

13. **True.** ACE inhibitors, by reducing angiotensin-induced aldosterone secretion, will reduce K^+ excretion and hence increase plasma K^+ concentration, particularly when combined with potassium-sparing diuretics.

14. **False.** Thiazides and loop diuretics increase Na^+ concentrations in the tubular fluid reaching the collecting duct; the excessive loss of K^+ that results can be reduced by combining the thiazide or loop diuretic with a potassium-sparing diuretic.

15. **True.** NSAIDs inhibit prostaglandin synthesis in the kidney and this reduces renal blood flow, leading to reduced natriuretic responses to thiazide and loop diuretics.

One-best-answer (OBA) answers

1. **Answer C** is correct. Triamterene is a potassium-sparing diuretic that directly blocks a selective Na^+ channel (ENaC) on the luminal membrane of tubule cells in the collecting duct. Answer A is the mechanism of action of aldosterone (mineralocorticoid) receptor antagonists such as spironolactone. Answers B, D and E are the mechanisms of action of loop diuretics, thiazides and carbonic anhydrase inhibitors, respectively.

2. **Answer A** is correct.
   A. **Correct.** Loop diuretics are widely used in the control of oedema in heart failure for the elimination of excessive salt and water load. The direct venodilator activity of furosemide after intravenous injection reduces central blood volume.
   B. Incorrect. A thiazide diuretic can be added to a loop diuretic to act sequentially at different sites in the nephron, thus producing a marked natriuresis and diuresis.
   C. Incorrect. Delivery of greater concentrations of Na^+ to the collecting ducts increases the exchange for K^+ at that site, thus increasing K^+ loss.
   D. Incorrect. By inhibiting the $Na^+/K^+/2Cl^-$ co-transporter (NKCC2), the medullary interstitial hypertonicity falls and this reduces the reabsorption of water in the collecting ducts (in the presence of ADH).
   E. Incorrect. Loop diuretics alone can cause ototoxicity (especially at high doses or in renal impairment) and also when taken with other ototoxic drugs such as aminoglycosides.

Extended-matching-item answers

Case 1. **Answer A.** The combination of a potassium-sparing diuretic (eplerenone) and an ACE inhibitor (lisinopril) may have raised the plasma K^+ concentration, and this may have been the cause of the profound bradycardia.

Case 2. **Answer E.** Thiazide-like diuretics can worsen insulin resistance, resulting in an increased plasma glucose concentration within weeks. In the longer term there is a small increase in the risk of diabetes mellitus.

Case 3. **Answer B.** The loop diuretic may cause hypokalaemia. This enhances the toxicity of digoxin, resulting in arrhythmias.

FURTHER READING

Asmar, A., Mohandas, R., Wingo, C.S., 2012. A physiologic-based approach to the treatment of a patient with hypokalaemia. Am. J. Kidney Dis. 60, 492–497.

Cox, Z.L., Lenihan, D.J., 2014. Loop diuretic resistance in heart failure: resistance-etiology-based strategies to restoring diuretic efficacy. J. Card. Fail. 20, 611–622.

Duarte, J.D., Cooper-DeHoff, R.M., 2010. Mechanisms for blood pressure lowering and metabolic effects of thiazide and thiazide-like diuretics. Expert Rev. Cardiovasc. Ther. 8, 793–802.

Jentzer, J.C., DeWald, T.A., Hernandez, A.F., 2010. Combination of loop diuretics with thiazide-type diuretics in heart failure. J. Am. Coll. Cardiol. 56, 1527–1534.

Roush, G.C., Kaur, R., Ernst, M.E., 2014. Diuretics: a review and update. J. Cardiovasc. Pharmacol. Ther. 19, 5–13.

Sica, D.A., 2012. Diuretic use in renal disease. Nat. Rev. Nephrol. 8, 100–109.

ter Maaten, J.M., Valente, M.A.E., Damman, K., et al., 2015. Diuretic response in acute heart failure—pathophysiology, evaluation and therapy. Nat. Rev. Cardiol. 12, 184–192.

Wile, D., 2012. Diuretics: a review. Ann. Clin. Biochem. 49, 419–431.

Compendium: diuretic drugs

Drug	Characteristics
Carbonic anhydrase inhibitors	
Acetazolamide	Little clinical value as a diuretic due to rapid tolerance; used orally in glaucoma (see Chapter 50) and in altitude sickness. Half-life: 6–9 h
Osmotic diuretics	
Mannitol	Given by rapid intravenous infusion in cerebral oedema; not used in heart failure due to expansion of plasma volume. Half-life: 2 h, but very prolonged (36 h) in renal failure
Loop diuretics	
Used for heart failure and oedema, and oliguria due to renal failure.	
Bumetanide	Given orally or by intravenous or intramuscular injection. Half-life: 1–2 h
Furosemide	Given orally or by intravenous or intramuscular injection. Half-life: 1 h
Torasemide	Given orally. Known as torsemide in the United States; little used in the United Kingdom. Half-life: 2–4 h
Thiazide and related diuretics	
Given orally; used for heart failure, oedema and, in lower doses, hypertension.	
Bendroflumethiazide	Complete absorption from gut; 30% excreted in urine unchanged (3–9 h)
Chlortalidone	Thiazide-related diuretic with long half-life (50–90 h)
Cyclopenthiazide	No advantages over other thiazides and now little used in the United Kingdom
Hydrochlorothiazide	Now used in the United Kingdom only in antihypertensive combined formulations, but available as a single formulation in continental Europe. Half-life: 8–12 h
Indapamide	Thiazide-related diuretic. Half-life: 10–22 h
Metolazone	Thiazide-related diuretic; effective even in advanced renal failure. Half-life: 4–5 h
Xipamide	Thiazide-related diuretic. Half-life: 5 h
Potassium-sparing diuretics	
Given orally; used for prevention of diuretic-induced hypokalaemia, hyperaldosteronism and ascites associated with liver cirrhosis.	
Amiloride	Potassium-sparing diuretic used in combination with thiazides and loop diuretics to conserve K^+. Half-life: 6–9 h
Eplerenone	Aldosterone antagonist with greater selectivity than spironolactone for mineralocorticoid receptor; reduced antiandrogenic effects; used in heart failure. Half-life: 4–6 h
Spironolactone	Aldosterone antagonist used in primary hyperaldosteronism (Conn's syndrome), liver cirrhosis (ascites), acne, female hirsutism. Active metabolite (canrenone). Half-life: 17–22 h
Triamterene	Potassium-sparing diuretic used in combination with thiazides and loop diuretics to conserve K^+. Half-life: 2 h

15 Disorders of micturition

PATHOPHYSIOLOGY OF MICTURITION

The urinary bladder is surrounded by a smooth muscle called the detrusor muscle, which relaxes to allow bladder filling up to 500–600 mL. The detrusor contracts in response to stimulation by the parasympathetic nervous system (via muscarinic M_3 receptors), which empties the urine contained in the bladder into the urethra. Sympathetic nervous system tone inhibits contraction of the detrusor (via β_2- and β_3-adrenoceptors). There is a smaller muscle, the trigone, between the ureteric orifices and bladder neck. The trigone is particularly sensitive to stretch and has an important role in the reflex that initiates bladder emptying.

The urethra has several mechanisms that aid continence and prevent the involuntary leakage of urine. The submucosal layer of the urethra is a highly vascular tissue that creates a 'washer' effect when compressed. The urethra is surrounded by an external urethral sphincter of skeletal muscle innervated by the pudendal nerve and is under voluntary control. Additional smooth muscle bundles pass either side of the urethra to form the internal urethral sphincter, which is constricted by sympathetic nervous stimulation (via α_{1A}- and

to a lesser extent α_{1B}-adrenoceptor subtypes). Pelvic floor muscles also support the urethra when abdominal pressure increases, particularly in women. The internal and external urethral sphincters combine with the pelvic floor muscles to constrict the urethra, which prevents bladder emptying and maintains continence by keeping the urethral closure pressure above the pressure in the bladder (Fig. 15.1). The coordination of bladder filling, maintaining continence and bladder emptying is a complex process.

During bladder filling (storage phase), sympathetic nervous system stimulation relaxes the detrusor muscle and contracts the smooth muscle of the internal urethral sphincter. Voluntary stimulation of the striated muscle of the external urethral sphincter, aided by pelvic muscle control, contributes to maintenance of continence. The urge to micturate occurs in adults at a bladder volume of 200–300 mL, when the signals from stretch receptors in the bladder reach a frequency to initiate reflex bladder contraction. Higher centres can then inhibit the micturition reflex.

Bladder emptying (voiding phase) is initiated by myogenic stretch receptor activity produced by distention of the trigone, and by sensory signals from the urothelium (the epithelial cell lining of the bladder). Release of ATP from the urothelium stimulates P2X purinoceptors which, along with other modulators of bladder receptor activity, initiate sensory impulses in the afferent nerves. Conscious sensations of bladder fullness are processed by the cerebral cortex, which then sends signals to the micturition centre when it is appropriate to empty the bladder. The pontine micturition centre initiates activity in efferent motor pathways to the detrusor muscle, producing bladder contraction and voiding. At the same time, stimulation of muscarinic M_2 receptors on presynaptic nerve terminals opposes the effects of sympathetic activity on the bladder. Noncholinergic-mediated efferent impulses (ATP neurotransmission acting via P2X purinoceptors) also contribute to bladder contraction, and this component becomes more prominent in overactive bladders. Contraction of the detrusor is coordinated with inhibition of the tonic control of the urethral sphincters, thus relaxing the bladder outflow tract. Bladder emptying may be augmented by contraction of the diaphragm and abdominal muscles.

DISORDERS OF MICTURITION

Disorders of micturition can arise from a disturbance of bladder function or from abnormalities affecting the bladder outflow tract and urethra. They produce a constellation of symptoms known as lower urinary tract symptoms (LUTS; see Fig. 15.1). When someone presents with LUTS, it is

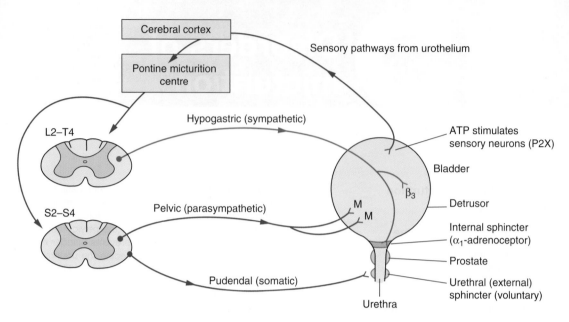

Fig. 15.1 **Aspects of the bladder/prostate structures and the innervation involved in the micturition reflex.** Bladder filling provides neuronal signals to the micturition centre via sensory input from purinoceptors on neurons in the urothelium. To accommodate filling and continence, sympathetic stimulation both relaxes the smooth muscle of the bladder via β_2- and β_3-adrenoceptors and stimulates sphincter mechanisms through α_1-adrenoceptor subtypes. Somatic control of the external sphincter also aids continence. Voluntary urination involves parasympathetic stimulation of bladder smooth muscle through M_3 and M_2 muscarinic receptor subtypes (M), and inhibition of the sympathetic and somatic outflow. Aspects of bladder control may involve other less understood transmitter substances. For example, γ-aminobutyric acid (GABA) interneurons inhibit bladder contraction. *P2X,* Purinergic receptors.

important to consider reversible contributory factors such as urinary tract infection, use of diuretics (which increase urinary flow rates), use of α_1-adrenoceptor antagonists for treatment of hypertension (which affect bladder neck function), and stool impaction (which inhibits sacral parasympathetic neurotransmission).

Urinary incontinence is the involuntary leakage of urine. This affects up to 50% of women older than 20 years, and becomes more common with increasing age in both women and men. There are four main types of urinary incontinence:

- Urgency urinary incontinence associated with overactive bladder syndrome.
- Stress urinary incontinence due to urethral sphincter incompetence.
- Mixed urinary incontinence (both stress and urgency urinary incontinence).
- Overflow incontinence with continuous urine leakage. This results from hypotonic bladder or bladder outlet obstruction, which produce urinary retention.

OVERACTIVE BLADDER SYNDROME

Detrusor instability produces uncontrolled bladder contractions during normal filling. Symptoms include urinary urgency, nocturia and frequency (overactive bladder syndrome), often accompanied by urgency incontinence (a sudden compelling desire to urinate). Most cases in women are idiopathic but probably have a neurogenic component, while in men, bladder outflow obstruction is the most common initiating factor (discussed later). Upper motor neuron lesions, such as those produced by stroke, spinal cord injuries or multiple sclerosis, can also produce an overactive bladder.

DRUGS FOR TREATMENT OF OVERACTIVE BLADDER SYNDROME

Increased understanding of the neural pathways involved in initiating micturition is opening up new avenues for drug therapy to augment the relatively ineffective treatments currently available.

Muscarinic receptor antagonists

darifenacin, fesoterodine, oxybutynin, solifenacin, tolterodine, trospium

Oxybutynin is a selective antagonist of M_1 and M_3 receptors and has additional weak muscle-relaxant properties through calcium channel blockade and local anaesthetic activity. It is rapidly absorbed from the gut and metabolised in the liver to an active metabolite. Oxybutynin has a short half-life (1–3 hours), and use of standard formulations can result in large fluctuations in plasma drug concentrations and increase the severity of unwanted effects. Modified-release and transdermal formulations prolong the duration of action. Oxybutynin is lipophilic and crosses the blood–brain barrier, where it can produce sedation, insomnia, confusion and cognitive problems by M_1 receptor blockade. M_3 receptor blockade in salivary glands causes dry mouth.

Tolterodine, fesoterodine and trospium are nonselective muscarinic receptor antagonists with no additional properties. They are less lipophilic than oxybutynin and do not readily cross the blood–brain barrier, producing fewer cognitive unwanted effects. Both tolterodine and trospium have short half-lives. Tolterodine is better tolerated in a modified-release formulation.

Darifenacin and solifenacin are more selective antagonists of M_3 receptors and also have fewer central nervous system actions than oxybutynin.

β_3-adrenoceptor agonist

mirabegron

Stimulation of β_3-adrenoceptors in the bladder trigone by mirabegron flattens and lengthens the bladder base, which facilitates urine storage. Mirabegron reduces symptoms of urinary frequency and urgency with efficacy similar to that of muscarinic receptor antagonists. The main adverse effects are an increase in blood pressure and heart rate, and mirabegron is contraindicated in people with severe hypertension.

Management of overactive bladder syndrome

First-line approaches to management include reduction in excessive fluid intake, weight loss, smoking cessation and behavioural training that includes pelvic floor muscle rehabilitation and suppression of urge. If this is not sufficient, then a muscarinic receptor antagonist is usually used. Transdermal delivery should be considered if oral treatment is poorly tolerated. Oxybutynin should not be given to frail older people with cognitive impairment. The need for continued use of muscarinic receptor antagonists should be reviewed after 6 months. Mirabegron is an option for those who fail to respond to muscarinic receptor antagonists, or who cannot tolerate them.

Oral desmopressin, a synthetic vasopressin (ADH) analogue (see Chapter 43), is sometimes helpful to reduce nocturia in overactive bladder syndrome. The nasal spray formulation is no longer licensed for this indication, because of the risk of water intoxication.

Intravesical botulinum toxin type A (see Chapter 27) can be considered if conservative treatment is ineffective, but intermittent bladder catheterisation may be needed for urinary retention. Options for intractable symptoms include percutaneous sacral nerve stimulation or surgery.

HYPOTONIC BLADDER

Hypotonic bladder is often a result of lower motor neuron lesions, or can arise from bladder distension following chronic urinary retention. Hypotonic bladder leads to incomplete bladder emptying, with urinary retention and overflow incontinence. Muscarinic receptor antagonists discussed previously and drugs with antimuscarinic properties (such as tricyclic antidepressants; see Chapter 22) make the symptoms worse.

Treatment depends on the cause.

- Chronic urinary retention is often caused by bladder outlet obstruction. If renal function is impaired, it should initially be managed by bladder catheterisation. Correction of the underlying cause is the mainstay of treatment if a long-term urinary catheter is to be avoided.
- Neurogenic problems usually require long-term bladder catheterisation.

URETHRAL SPHINCTER INCOMPETENCE

Urethral sphincter incompetence produces stress incontinence in women (urine leakage with effort, exertion, sneezing or coughing) or sphincter weakness incontinence in men. Urethral hypermobility is the usual pathology, and the most common cause in women is loss of collagenous support in the pelvic floor or perineum resulting from trauma or hormonal changes. Internal urethral sphincter dysfunction is less common, arising from pelvic trauma, childbirth, radiation or following prostatectomy in males. Drugs such as α_1-adrenoceptor antagonists can make stress incontinence worse.

Pelvic floor muscle training for at least 8–12 weeks is the recommended treatment. Minimal access surgical sling procedures or colposuspension to provide urethral support are among the surgical options.

Drug therapy is limited and only recommended if surgical treatment is not suitable. In postmenopausal women, topical oestrogen (see Chapter 45) may be helpful. Oestrogen stimulates urethral mucosal proliferation and enhances the internal urethral sphincter response to neural stimulation. Duloxetine is a serotonin and noradrenaline reuptake inhibitor (SNRI; see Chapter 22) that augments sympathetic nervous system activity. It relaxes the detrusor and enhances external urethral sphincter activity by increasing efferent impulses in the motor neurons of the pudendal nerve when the bladder is placed under stress. Duloxetine significantly reduces the frequency of incontinence episodes in about half of those treated. It is recommended for people who are averse to surgery or who are poor candidates for surgery.

LOWER URINARY TRACT SYMPTOMS IN MEN AND BENIGN PROSTATIC HYPERTROPHY

Most LUTS in men are caused by prostatic hypertrophy; there are a large number of other possible causes including urethral

Voiding symptoms	Postmicturition symptoms	Storage symptoms
Hesitancy	Feeling of incomplete bladder emptying	Urgency
Slow stream	Urinary retention	Frequency
Intermittent stream	Post-micturition dribble	Nocturia
Straining to pass urine		Urgency incontinence
Splitting or spraying of stream		
Terminal dribbling		

stricture, prostate cancer and overactive bladder syndrome. Benign prostatic hypertrophy (BPH) usually produces mixed storage symptoms, voiding symptoms and postmicturition symptoms (Box 15.1). The storage symptoms result from functional changes in the detrusor. Isolated storage symptoms in men are usually due to overactive bladder.

Symptoms of BPH are present in more than 25% of men older than 60 years, and up to 70% of men older than 70 years. Left untreated, spontaneous improvement occurs or symptoms remain stable in up to half of those affected. Acute urinary retention occurs at a rate of 1–2% per year. Scoring systems can reliably quantify the extent to which symptoms affect the quality of life and therefore guide treatment.

DRUGS FOR BENIGN PROSTATIC HYPERTROPHY

Alpha$_1$-adrenoceptor antagonists

doxazosin, tamsulosin

Selective α_1-adrenoceptor antagonists inhibit contraction of hypertrophied smooth muscle in prostatic tissue and also the internal urethral sphincter without affecting the detrusor. Relaxation of these muscles improves urine flow rate and symptoms of BPH. Tamsulosin has modest selectivity for the α_{1A}-adrenoceptor subtype in the smooth muscle of the prostate, but it can still cause postural hypotension by an effect on arterial smooth muscle. More information about α_1-adrenoceptor antagonists is found in Chapter 6.

5α-Reductase inhibitors

dutasteride, finasteride

Inhibition of 5α-reductase reduces the enzymatic conversion of testosterone to dihydrotestosterone (DHT) in prostatic cells, but does not affect circulating testosterone levels. DHT is involved in prostate growth, and inhibition of

its production can reduce prostate volume by up to 30%. There are two isoenzymes of 5α-reductase, both found in the prostate. Finasteride only inhibits the type 2 isoenzyme, while dutasteride inhibits both the types 1 and 2 isoenzymes. Despite the different patterns of isoenzyme inhibition, the efficacy of these drugs is similar.

Pharmacokinetics

Both finasteride and dutasteride are well absorbed after oral administration and eliminated by hepatic metabolism. Finasteride has a half-life of about 6 hours, whereas the half-life of dutasteride is extremely long, at about 4 weeks.

Unwanted effects

- Reduced libido.
- Erectile impotence or decreased ejaculation.
- Breast tenderness or enlargement.
- Reduction of the plasma concentration of prostate-specific antigen by an average of 50%, which should be considered when screening for prostate cancer.

Plant extracts

saw palmetto plant extracts, β-sitosterol plant extract

Plant extracts are available over the counter, but their composition is not standardised. There is little convincing evidence that they are effective for symptoms of LUTS in BPH. It is uncertain how they might work, but they may reduce the synthesis of DHT or inhibit expression of prostatic growth factors. Plant extracts are well tolerated, with unwanted effects mainly confined to gastrointestinal upset.

TREATMENT OF LOWER URINARY TRACT SYMPTOMS WITH BENIGN PROSTATIC HYPERTROPHY

Many symptomatic individuals do not require or want treatment, and a policy of 'watchful waiting' will be appropriate. There is no evidence that medical treatment avoids the need for surgery in the long term.

Selective α_1-adrenoceptor antagonists are the first-choice drugs for improving symptoms and urinary flow rates. Symptoms improve within a few days, but maximum benefit may take several weeks. About two-thirds of those treated will respond, but selective α_1-adrenoceptor antagonists do not reduce the risk of urinary retention or the subsequent need for surgery for BPH.

5α-Reductase inhibitors usually take 6 months to improve LUTS, but the improvements are maintained. These drugs may be more effective with larger-volume prostates, as they reduce prostatic volume by about 25%. Unlike α_1-adrenoceptor antagonists, 5α-reductase inhibitors reduce both the risk of urinary retention and the need for surgery for BPH.

Additional symptomatic benefit can be obtained from combining an α_1-adrenoceptor antagonist with finasteride or dutasteride. If storage symptoms persist despite use of an α_1-adrenoceptor antagonist, then a muscarinic receptor antagonist can be added. Tadalafil, a phosphodiesterase

> **Box 15.2   Indications for surgery in patients with benign prostatic hypertrophy**
>
> Acute retention of urine
> Chronic retention of urine
> Recurrent urinary tract infection
> Bladder stones
> Renal impairment owing to benign prostatic hypertrophy
> Large bladder diverticula
> Severe symptoms

inhibitor used for erectile dysfunction (see Chapter 16), also improves symptoms of LUTS and increases urinary flow rate in men with BPH. Its place in management is not clear.

Surgical treatment is usually required for severe LUTS or for complications of BPH (Box 15.2). Transurethral resection of the prostate improves symptoms in 70–90% of those treated. Long-term sequelae of this procedure include impotence (5–10%), retrograde ejaculation (80–90%) and incontinence (<5%). Several less invasive procedures are now available, but they may be less successful for relieving symptoms and do not reduce the risk of long-term consequences, although they produce fewer immediate postoperative complications.

SELF-ASSESSMENT

True/false questions

1. Urinary bladder function is controlled by both voluntary and involuntary nervous pathways.
2. The antimuscarinic drug darifenacin causes urinary frequency and urge incontinence.
3. The antidepressant drug duloxetine can be used to treat stress incontinence.
4. Blockade of α_1-adrenoceptors in the bladder neck smooth muscle improves urine flow rates.
5. Finasteride reduces prostate volume by blocking testosterone receptors.

Extended-matching-item questions

Choose the *most appropriate* pharmacological option A–E for each case scenario (1–3) provided.
A. Tamsulosin
B. Finasteride
C. Duloxetine
D. Amitriptyline
E. Oxybutynin

1. A 50-year-old man with a 2-year history of difficulty in urinating and hesitancy was found to have BPH with a significantly enlarged prostate. He was given a 1-month trial of treatment with an α_1-adrenoceptor antagonist, which did not improve his symptoms. He did not at this stage want to undergo surgery. What pharmacological treatment might be of benefit?

2. A 30-year-old woman with normal bladder function complained of difficulty in urination after being prescribed new medication for neuropathic pain. She was found to have urinary retention. What class of medicine could cause this effect?
3. A 60-year-old woman had severe urge incontinence. She urinated 16–20 times a day and had leakage two to three times a day and at night. What treatment could she be given?

Case-based question

A 65-year-old man developed progressive urinary problems over a 5-year period. He had difficulty passing urine and was getting up three times in the night to pass urine. A rectal examination by his general practitioner (GP) showed an enlarged prostate. Ultrasound, flow tests and a normal prostate-specific antigen measurement suggested BPH.

1. What pharmacological approaches to the treatment of BPH could be considered?
2. What are the unwanted effects of these treatments?
3. What are the possible outcomes of not giving treatment?

ANSWERS

True/false answers

1. **True.** Bladder function is controlled by involuntary parasympathetic and sympathetic innervation of the detrusor and sphincter muscles, and by voluntary control via the somatic nervous system.
2. **False.** Darifenacin blocks muscarinic receptors with some selectivity for the M_3 subtype, inhibiting the parasympathetic effects on the detrusor muscle. It is used for treatment of overactive bladder.
3. **True.** Duloxetine inhibits the reuptake of serotonin and noradrenaline and increases the contractility of the urethral sphincters.
4. **True.** Selective antagonism of the α_{1A}-adrenoceptor subtype in bladder smooth muscle may reduce unwanted vasodilator effects.
5. **False.** Finasteride and dutasteride block the conversion of testosterone to DHT by inhibiting 5α-reductase in the prostate.

Extended-matching-item answers

1. Answer **B**. Finasteride inhibits the conversion of testosterone to DHT, which is a promoter of prostatic cell growth. A reduction of up to 30% in prostate size can be obtained. Symptomatic benefit may be increased if finasteride and an α_1-adrenoceptor antagonist are given together.
2. Answer **D**. The tricyclic antidepressant amitriptyline is also an antagonist at muscarinic receptors and may inhibit the micturition reflex.
3. Answer **C**. Duloxetine could be tried if the condition were caused by sphincter incompetence. Duloxetine increases the levels of noradrenaline and serotonin in the synapse and the activity of the motor neurons in the pudendal nerve. Pelvic floor exercises should also be suggested, as drug therapy is of limited benefit.

Case-based answers

1. Drugs may be used in mild disease and while awaiting a transurethral resection of the prostate. Selective α_1-adrenoceptor antagonists increase urine flow to a limited extent but also decrease urgency, frequency and hesitancy. The 5α-reductase inhibitor finasteride slowly reduces prostate size.

2. α_1-Adrenoceptor antagonists can cause postural hypotension, especially with the first dose. They cause dizziness and can interact with other drugs to lower blood pressure. Finasteride can reduce libido and cause impotence.

3. The outcome is variable; symptoms may not worsen appreciably for many years, but moderate symptoms can lead to a poor quality of life. Complications include urinary retention, incontinence and renal insufficiency owing to hydronephrosis.

FURTHER READING

Marinkovic, S.P., Rovner, E.S., Moldwin, R.M., et al., 2012. The management of overactive bladder syndrome. Br. Med. J. 344, e2365.

Myers, D.L., 2014. Female mixed urinary incontinence: a clinical review. J. Am. Med. Assoc. 311, 2007–2014.

Nygaard, I., 2010. Idiopathic urgency urinary incontinence. N. Engl. J. Med. 363, 1156–1162.

Rees, J., Bultitude, M., Challacombe, B., 2014. The management of lower urinary tract symptoms in men. Br. Med. J. 348, g3861.

Robinson, D., Cardozo, L., 2012. Antimuscarinic drugs to treat overactive bladder. Br. Med. J. 344, e2130.

Sanna, A.V., Wei, J.T., 2012. Benign prostatic hyperplasia and lower urinary tract symptoms. N. Engl. J. Med. 367, 248–257.

Wood, L.N., Anger, J.T., 2014. Urinary incontinence in women. Br. Med. J. 367, g4531.

Compendium: drugs used to treat disorders of micturition

Drug	Characteristics
Drugs for urinary retention	
All drugs taken orally.	
α_1-Adrenoceptor antagonists	
Relax internal sphincter smooth muscle to improve urinary flow; may cause hypotension.	
Alfuzosin	Similar to doxazosin but selectivity for α_{1A}-adrenoceptors in the urinary tract; may reduce vasodilator effects at α_{1B}- and α_{1D}-adrenoceptors. Half-life: 4–10 h
Doxazosin	May cause postural hypotension especially with first dose. Half-life: 10–20 h
Indoramin	See doxazosin. Half-life: 2–10 h
Prazosin	See doxazosin. Half-life: 2–4h
Tamsulosin	Relatively selective for α_{1A}-adrenoceptors in the urinary tract. Half-life: 15 h
Terazosin	See doxazosin. Half-life: 10–12 h
Parasympathomimetic	
Bethanechol	Muscarinic agonist increases bladder detrusor activity; largely superseded by bladder catheterisation
5α-Reductase inhibitors	
Used as alternative to α_1-adrenoceptor antagonists, particularly in men with significantly enlarged prostates.	
Dutasteride	Similar profile to finasteride, but blocks 5α-reductase types 1 and 2. Very long half-life (4–5 weeks), requiring about 6 months to reach steady state
Finasteride	Reduces prostate growth by blocking synthesis of dihydrotestosterone by 5α-reductase type 2. Half-life: 3–16 h

Compendium: drugs used to treat disorders of micturition (cont'd)

Drug	Characteristics
Drugs for urinary frequency, enuresis and incontinence	
All drugs taken orally.	
Muscarinic receptor antagonists	
Nonselective drugs given as extended-release or transdermal formulations may have fewer antimuscarinic effects. Newer drugs are selective for muscarinic receptor subtypes.	
Darifenacin	Selective M_3 receptor antagonist used for urinary frequency, urgency and incontinence. Half-life: 13–19 h
Flavoxate	Nonselective muscarinic antagonist; fewer unwanted effects than oxybutynin, but also weaker clinical action
Fesoterodine	Nonselective muscarinic antagonist used for urinary frequency, urgency and incontinence; prodrug converted to an active metabolite of tolterodine. Half-life: 4–20 h
Oxybutynin	Nonselective muscarinic antagonist used for urinary frequency, urgency and incontinence, and for nocturnal enuresis in children. Antimuscarinic side-effects at M_1 receptors in central nervous system limit the use of higher doses. Half-life: 1–3 h
Propantheline	Quaternary amino compound; rarely used. Half-life: 1–2 h
Propiverine	Nonselective muscarinic antagonist used for urinary frequency, urgency and incontinence. Half-life: 4 h
Solifenacin	Selective M_3 receptor antagonist used for urinary frequency, urgency and incontinence. Half-life: 55 h
Tolterodine	Selective M_2/M_3 muscarinic antagonist used for urinary frequency, urgency and incontinence, and for nocturnal enuresis in children. Half-life: 2–10 h
Trospium	Nonselective muscarinic antagonist used for urinary frequency, urgency and incontinence. Half-life: 1–2 h
Serotonin and noradrenaline reuptake inhibitor	
Duloxetine	Used for moderate to severe stress incontinence in women. Half-life: 9–19 h
β_3-Adrenoceptor agonist	
Mirabegron	Used for overactive bladder syndrome in adults. Half-life: 50 h

16 Erectile dysfunction

PHYSIOLOGY OF ERECTION

Achieving and maintaining an erection is a spinal reflex that involves a complex series of interactions among the central nervous system (CNS), the autonomic nervous system and local mediators. Mechanical stimulation produces erection with little input from the CNS. The CNS can initiate erection in the absence of direct mechanical stimulation, when psychological, visual, olfactory, auditory and tactile stimuli are all important. The primary innervation that initiates penile erection is the parasympathetic nervous system through the sacral plexus. There are several components involved in achieving full penile erection:

- Parasympathetic stimulation (via release of acetylcholine) relaxes smooth muscle in the trabecular arteries supplying the vascular erectile tissues of the penis, the corpora cavernosa and to a lesser extent the corpus spongiosum. These tissues run the length of the penis and contain sinusoids that fill with blood (Fig. 16.1).
- Pressure rises within the corpora cavernosa as they become engorged and the sinusoids expand. The penis elongates and widens.
- The rise in pressure in the sinusoids compresses the venous plexus and reduces venous outflow, thus enhancing the erection (the corporeal veno-occlusive mechanism).

- The pudendal nerve (carrying parasympathetic innervation) stimulates the ischiocavernosus and bulbospongiosus muscles at the base of the penis. This further compresses the veins of the corpora cavernosa against the tunica albuginea, reduces venous outflow from the penis and maintains full erection. Muscle fatigue eventually permits venous outflow and detumescence. Basal tone in the sympathetic nervous system produces vasoconstriction in the penile arteries and inhibits erection.

Many locally produced mediators are involved in achieving and maintaining an erection. Nitric oxide (NO) is crucial for the smooth muscle relaxation in penile arteries. It is synthesised by blood vessel endothelial cells and released in response to parasympathetic stimulation and also nonadrenergic noncholinergic (NANC) nerves in the corpora cavernosa. Nitric oxide generates intracellular cyclic guanosine monophosphate (cGMP), which activates protein kinase G. cGMP is degraded to GMP in the vascular smooth muscle by phosphodiesterase type 5 (PDE5; see Table 1.1), which terminates its effects. Inhibition of PDE5 is a primary target for the pharmacological treatment of erectile dysfunction (discussed later).

Other vasodilators are involved in penile vascular smooth muscle relaxation, including vasoactive intestinal peptide (VIP), calcitonin gene-related peptide (CGRP) and prostaglandin E_1, but their precise roles are less understood. Numerous CNS facilitatory mediators have been identified, including dopamine, acetylcholine and a variety of peptides. These are involved in the psychological preparedness that is essential for an erection to occur.

ERECTILE DYSFUNCTION

Erectile dysfunction is defined as the consistent inability to achieve or sustain an erection of sufficient rigidity for sexual intercourse. It is a common problem, affecting up to 50% of adult men, with up to 10% over the age of 40 years having complete erectile dysfunction. Any disease process that affects penile neural supply, arterial inflow or venous outflow can produce erectile dysfunction. There is a physical cause in about 80% of cases (Box 16.1), but a psychological component often coexists. Psychogenic erectile dysfunction is more common in younger men. Drugs are an important cause of erectile dysfunction, particularly many antihypertensive, psychotropic and 'recreational' drugs (including alcohol), which account for up to 25% of cases. Drugs can also affect libido and therefore arousal, or inhibit ejaculation in those who achieve an erection (Table 16.1).

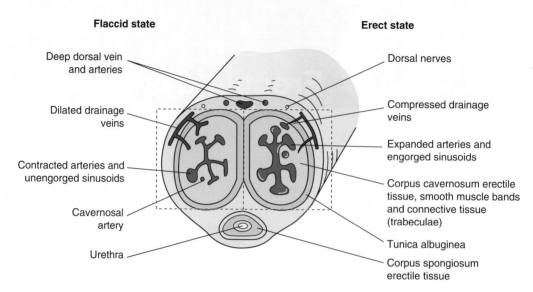

Flaccid state

Deep dorsal vein and arteries

Dilated drainage veins

Contracted arteries and unengorged sinusoids

Cavernosal artery

Urethra

Erect state

Dorsal nerves

Compressed drainage veins

Expanded arteries and engorged sinusoids

Corpus cavernosum erectile tissue, smooth muscle bands and connective tissue (trabeculae)

Tunica albuginea

Corpus spongiosum erectile tissue

Fig. 16.1 **Cross-section of the penis, showing structures involved in erection.** This diagram shows only part of the rich nervous and vascular filling and drainage system in the penis. The left-hand area shows the situation in the flaccid penis, and the right-hand area shows the erect penis. The rising pressure during erection limits the venous outflow, thus maintaining the erection. The penis contains three cylinders of erectile tissue: two corpora cavernosa and the corpus spongiosum. The corpus spongiosum contains the urethra. The cylinders of erectile tissue are divided into spaces known as sinusoids or lacunae, which are lined by vascular epithelium. The walls of these spaces are made up of thick bundles of smooth muscle cells within a framework of fibroblasts, collagen and elastin (trabeculae). The erectile tissues are supplied with blood from the cavernosal and helicine arteries, which drain into the sinusoidal spaces. Blood is drained from the sinusoidal spaces through emissary veins. The venules join together to form larger veins that drain into the deep dorsal vein or other veins at different parts of the penis. Arterial and sinusoid dilation is important for erection, while swelling is limited by the inelastic tunica albuginea.

| Box 16.1 | Common causes of erectile dysfunction |

Diabetes
Vascular disease
Prostate surgery
Drugs and substance abuse (see Table 16.1)
Testosterone deficiency (e.g. hyper- or hypothyroidism)
Neurological disease (e.g. multiple sclerosis, Alzheimer's disease, epilepsy)
Spinal cord injury
Psychological factors (20% as a primary cause; more commonly secondary to physical problems)

DRUGS FOR ERECTILE DYSFUNCTION

ORAL PHOSPHODIESTERASE INHIBITORS

Examples

sildenafil, tadalafil, vardenafil

Mechanism of action and uses

Sildenafil, tadalafil and vardenafil are orally active analogues of cGMP that selectively inhibit PDE5 and inhibit degradation of cGMP generated by nitric oxide release in penile tissue. PDE5 is also found in lower concentrations in other vascular and visceral smooth muscles, and in skeletal muscle and platelets.

Sexual stimulation to initiate release of nitric oxide is essential for these drugs to produce an erection, and the drug will then prolong the vasodilator effect of nitric oxide on penile arterial smooth muscle. If an appropriate dose of the drug is used, about 60% of men with erectile dysfunction will achieve erections sufficient to permit intercourse. The response is often better if precipitating factors are also treated, such as depression or excess alcohol consumption.

Sildenafil and tadalafil are also used to treat pulmonary hypertension (see Chapter 6).

Pharmacokinetics

The median time to onset of action is about 30 minutes. The absorption of sildenafil and vardenafil is delayed by a fatty meal, whereas the absorption of tadalafil is rapid and unaffected by food. All are eliminated by hepatic metabolism, mediated primarily by CYP3A4. Sildenafil and vardenafil have

Table 16.1 Drugs that commonly cause male sexual dysfunction

	Ejaculatory dysfunction	Erectile dysfunction	Loss of libido
Antihypertensives			
Beta-adrenoceptor antagonists		+	
Alpha-adrenoceptor antagonists	+		
Methyldopa	+	+	+
Thiazide diuretics		+	
Psychotropic drugs			
Phenothiazines	+	+	+
Benzodiazepines	+	+	+
Tricyclic antidepressants		+	+
Selective serotonin reuptake inhibitors		+	+
Other prescription drugs			
Spironolactone			+
Digoxin		+	
Cimetidine/ranitidine		+	
Metoclopramide		+	+
Carbamazepine		+	+
Recreational drugs			
Alcohol	+	+	
Marijuana		+	
Cocaine		+	+
Amphetamines	+	+	+
Anabolic steroids		+	+

half-lives of less than 6 hours. The half-life of tadalafil is longer (17 hours), and its duration of action is up to about 24–36 hours; therefore the timing of sexual activity in relation to drug intake is less relevant with this drug.

Unwanted effects

- Dyspepsia, nausea, vomiting.
- Hypotension, dizziness, flushing, headache and nasal congestion from systemic vasodilation.
- Myalgia, back pain.
- PDE6 (involved in phototransduction in the eye) is inhibited by high doses of sildenafil, but less so by tadalafil or vardenafil. PDE6 inhibition can cause visual disturbance (enhanced perception of bright lights, or a 'blue halo' effect) and raised intraocular pressure. Ischaemic optic neuropathy can cause sudden visual impairment.
- Priapism, a painful and sustained erection, is a rare consequence of PDE5 inhibitor use.
- Drug interactions: Oral PDE5 inhibitors should not be used together with nitrates or nicorandil (see Chapter 5), because of a synergistic effect on vascular nitric oxide with exaggerated vasodilator effects. Several antiviral drugs, such as saquinavir (see Table 2.7 and Chapter

51), inhibit the CYP3A4 isoenzyme that metabolises oral PDE5 inhibitors, and can potentiate their effects.

ALPROSTADIL

Alprostadil is a synthetic prostaglandin E_1 analogue. It vasodilates by acting on smooth muscle cell surface receptors to increase intracellular cyclic adenosine monophosphate (cAMP), which in turn reduces the intracellular Ca^{2+} concentration. Intracavernosal injection of alprostadil can enhance erections if penile arterial flow is normal, such as occurs with neurogenic and psychogenic impotence. It should not be used if the person has bleeding tendencies, and may be problematic if there is poor manual dexterity or morbid obesity. The injection is made into the side of the penis, directly into the corpus cavernosum. Local pain after injection is a common unwanted effect, reported by one-third of users, and can be reduced by the addition of a local anaesthetic such as procaine (see Chapter 18) to the injected fluid. Rapid local metabolism of alprostadil minimises unwanted systemic effects, but headache and dizziness can occur. Priapism is the most worrying complication, and may require aspiration and lavage of the corpora cavernosa.

Alprostadil is also available as a cream for application to the tip of the penis (formulated to enhance dermal penetration) or for intraurethral application using a small pellet. These formulations are less effective than the injection. In responders, an erection develops within 30 minutes and lasts for 1–2 hours. Alprostadil has uterine-stimulant activity, and when the cream or pellet is used, a condom is recommended if the partner is pregnant.

MANAGEMENT OF ERECTILE DYSFUNCTION

Initial management of erectile dysfunction involves assessment and treatment of any underlying psychological cause or physical disease or, if possible, withdrawal of a causative drug. A psychogenic cause is most common in younger men and should be suspected if nocturnal and early morning erections are maintained, or an erection is achieved through masturbation. Causes and treatment options for persistent organic erectile dysfunction include:

- Lifestyle changes such as exercise, stopping smoking and weight loss can be effective for mild dysfunction.
- Testosterone-replacement therapy for hypogonadism (see Chapter 46), an uncommon cause of impotence.
- Hyperprolactinaemia impairs erection and is most commonly caused by drug therapy (e.g. with phenothiazines); it can be improved by oral dopamine agonists (see Chapter 43) if the cause cannot be treated.
- Herbal remedies are widely promoted but lack good-quality evidence to support their use. They include Panax ginseng (stimulates nitric oxide release), Butea superba (action unknown) and yohimbine (CNS presynaptic α2-adrenoceptor agonist).
- An oral PDE5 inhibitor. Alprostadil is used as a second-line treatment if a PDE5 inhibitor is contraindicated or poorly tolerated.
- Mechanical aids, such as the vacuum constriction device, are usually advised for older people who do not respond to pharmacological treatment and do not wish to have surgery.
- Penile implants using a malleable or inflatable prosthesis.

PREMATURE EJACULATION

Premature ejaculation is orgasm with expulsion of semen following minimal penile stimulation. It usually is defined as ejaculation that occurs less than 1 minute after the onset of stimulation or vaginal penetration, and can produce significant psychological distress.

Ejaculation begins with emission of fluid from the ampullary vas deferens, seminal vesicles and prostate into the urethra under control of the sympathetic nervous system. Expulsion of the resulting semen from the urethra is due to a spinal reflex that produces rhythmic urethral contractions through pudendal nerve stimulation of the bulbospongiosus muscle.

Dapoxetine is a short-acting selective serotonin reuptake inhibitor (SSRI) that prolongs intravaginal latency time from

less than a minute to an average of over 3 minutes. The mechanism of action is unclear but may involve increased serotonin in the brain stem, modulating pudendal nerve activity via descending pathways. Dapoxetine is taken 'on demand' 1–3 hours before sexual activity. The most common adverse effects are dizziness, headache and nausea.

SELF-ASSESSMENT

True/false questions

1. Sildenafil should not be taken by men already taking nitrates.
2. Sexual stimulation is a prerequisite for sildenafil to cause an erection.
3. PDE5 is only found in the vasculature in the penis.
4. Increased parasympathetic outflow to the penis causes a failure of erection.
5. Erections caused by injected drugs such as alprostadil are not easy to control.
6. Dapoxetine is a PDE5 inhibitor used for erectile dysfunction.
7. Diabetes can cause impotence.
8. The durations of action of sildenafil and tadalafil are similar.
9. Sildenafil inhibits the breakdown of cAMP.
10. Alprostadil reduces prostaglandin synthesis by inhibiting cyclo-oxygenase-1.

One-best-answer (OBA) question

Which statement concerning drug action and erectile dysfunction is the *least accurate*?
A. Alcohol can cause erectile difficulties.
B. Cimetidine can exacerbate the potential for sildenafil to cause headache.
C. Nicorandil is safe when taken together with tadalafil.
D. Amitriptyline can cause impotence.
E. Sildenafil prevents the breakdown of cGMP.

Case-based questions

Mr J.A., aged 56 years, presented with erectile dysfunction of gradual onset over the last 2–3 years. He was hypertensive, with a blood pressure of 160/96 mm Hg, and was being treated with atenolol and bendroflumethiazide. Mr J.A. also reported chest pain on strenuous exertion that was relieved by rest. He has a family history of coronary artery disease, smokes 30 cigarettes a day and drinks 4 pints of beer a night. Investigation showed that he had hypercholesterolaemia, and there were signs of peripheral arterial disease. Tests for liver function and testosterone were normal, and no organic reason for the dysfunction was found. Mr J.A. also has recurrent heartburn, for which he is taking cimetidine on most days. It was decided not to prescribe a pharmacological agent for his erectile dysfunction at this stage, but a number of suggestions and recommendations were made. After 3 months, during which time Mr J.A. followed the advice he was given, his blood pressure was within normal limits and his cholesterol was lower. He was regularly taking cimetidine. However, his erectile dysfunction persisted. Following discussions, it was decided that Mr J.A. should try sildenafil.

1. Which of these factors could contribute to his erectile dysfunction, and what recommendations would you suggest?
2. From his history, what precautions should be taken in prescribing sildenafil, and what advice should Mr J.A. be given?

ANSWERS

True/false answers

1. **True.** Nitrates result in increased nitric oxide production, and this elevates cGMP. Sildenafil elevates cGMP by blocking its breakdown, and the combination with nitrates can lead to additive unwanted effects – particularly hypotension.
2. **True.** Sildenafil and other PDE5 inhibitors prolong the vasodilator action of NO produced as a result of sexual stimulation.
3. **False.** PDE5 is found in some other blood vessels and tissues, which can result in unwanted effects when sildenafil is given.
4. **False.** Parasympathetic stimulation enhances erection, and drugs known to inhibit the parasympathetic outflow (e.g. tricyclic antidepressants) can cause erectile failure.
5. **True.** Painful priapism with erections lasting many hours can occur with intracavernosal drugs.
6. **False.** Dapoxetine is an SSRI, used for premature ejaculation.
7. **True.** Diabetes mellitus probably causes erectile problems through vascular dysfunction.
8. **False.** Tadalafil has a much longer biological half-life than sildenafil, allowing it to be taken up to 12 hours before sexual activity.
9. **False.** Sildenafil inhibits the breakdown of cGMP, not cAMP.
10. **False.** Alprostadil is a synthetic prostaglandin E_1 analogue, which vasodilates by increasing cAMP.

One-best-answer (OBA) answer

Answer C is the least accurate.
A. True. Alcohol use is a recognised cause of erectile dysfunction.
B. True. Cimetidine inhibits the isoenzyme CYP3A4 that metabolises sildenafil, enhancing its vasodilator effects, including headache.
C. **False.** Nicorandil is a K^+ channel opener (see Chapter 5) that also has a nitrate structure; this increases cGMP formation and would add to the effects of tadalafil, with the potential for increased unwanted effects.
D. True. Amitriptyline has antimuscarinic actions that could decrease blood vessel dilation in the penis, thereby inhibiting erection.
E. True. Blocking the breakdown of cGMP is the main mechanism of action of sildenafil, leading to vasodilation.

Case-based answers

1. The contribution of psychological factors to Mr J.A.'s erectile dysfunction needs to be assessed and dealt with if they are present. Vascular disease, smoking and alcohol consumption may also contribute, and Mr J.A. should be helped to manage these. Because of the evidence of peripheral vascular disease and coronary artery disease, which are known to be associated with erectile dysfunction, it would be advisable to be more intensive in treating his high blood pressure and reducing his cholesterol levels. Although this is unlikely to restore erectile function, it may improve his well-being and have a psychological benefit. Beta-adrenoceptor antagonists (atenolol) and thiazide diuretics (bendroflumethiazide) can contribute to erectile problems; Mr J.A. could be treated with an ACE inhibitor, such as enalapril, which has not been shown to contribute to impotence.
2. Cimetidine is an inhibitor of hepatic CYP3A4 (see Table 2.7) that metabolises sildenafil, so the initial dose of sildenafil should be reduced. Alternatively, Mr J.A. could use ranitidine, which does not inhibit CYP3A4. Studies of sildenafil in patients with a history of cardiovascular disease have shown that the simultaneous use of nitrates is an absolute contraindication. Mr J.A. should be told about the dangers of drug interactions and possible unwanted effects.

FURTHER READING

Gur, S., Kadowitz, P.J., Sikka, S.C., 2016. Current therapies for premature ejaculation. Drug Discov. Today 21, 1147–1154.

Muneer, A., Kalsi, J., Nazareth, I., et al., 2014. Erectile dysfunction. Br. Med. J. 348, g129.

Shamloul, R., Ghanem, H., 2013. Erectile dysfunction. Lancet 381, 153–165.

Compendium: drugs used to treat erectile dysfunction and premature ejaculation

Drug	Characteristics
Drugs used for erectile dysfunction	
All drugs for erectile dysfunction should be used with caution in people with cardiovascular disease.	
Phosphodiesterase type 5 inhibitors	
All PDE5 inhibitors are given orally.	
Avanafil	Rapid onset of action (15–30 min). Half-life: 6–17 h
Sildenafil	Taken between 30 min and 4 h before sexual activity; also used for primary pulmonary hypertension. Half-life: 2 h
Tadalafil	Long duration of action means tadalafil can be taken up to 12 h before sexual activity. Half-life: 17 h
Vardenafil	Usually taken about 1 h before sexual activity. Half-life: 4–5 h
Other drugs used for erectile dysfunction	
Alprostadil	Prostaglandin E_1 analogue. Care needed if partner is pregnant; can cause priapism. Given by intracavernosal injection, dermal cream or urethral application. Very short half-life (30 s)
Papaverine	Smooth muscle relaxant. Given by intracavernosal injection; not licensed for this indication in the United Kingdom. Half-life: 2 h
Phentolamine	An α_1-adrenoceptor antagonist. Given with papaverine by intracavernosal injection (unlicensed indication). Half-life: 1.5 h
Drug for premature ejaculation	
Dapoxetine	Selective serotonin reuptake inhibitor; may cause postural hypotension. Given orally 1–3 h before sexual activity. Half-life: 1.5 h

5

The nervous system

17

General anaesthetics

General anaesthetics act in the brain to induce reversible unconsciousness with amnesia, immobility and varying degrees of analgesia. This allows surgical or other painful procedures to be undertaken without the person being aware. General anaesthesia was introduced into clinical practice in the 19th century, with the inhalation of vapours such as diethyl ether and chloroform. Major drawbacks with such compounds included the time taken to cause loss of consciousness, slow recovery, unpleasant taste, irritant properties and their potential to explode. Cardiac and hepatic toxicity also limited the usefulness of chloroform.

The ideal general anaesthetic would possess the properties shown in Box 17.1, but no single anaesthetic agent has all of these. Therefore, to produce general anaesthesia, it is usual to administer a combination of several drugs which contribute in different degrees to sedation, analgesia and muscle relaxation, an approach known as 'balanced anaesthesia' (Table 17.1). Full general anaesthesia not only produces loss of consciousness, but also depresses brainstem reflexes with loss of spontaneous respiration and depression of heart rate and blood pressure, a state that is comparable to coma.

General anaesthesia for surgical procedures involves several steps, although not all are essential for successful anaesthesia:

■ premedication,
■ induction,
■ muscle relaxation and intubation,
■ maintenance of anaesthesia,
■ analgesia,
■ reversal.

Premedication is given to adults to reduce anxiety and produce amnesia, usually with a benzodiazepine such as diazepam (see Chapter 20). In addition, an antiemetic such as metoclopramide (see Chapter 32) may be used.

Induction and maintenance of general anaesthesia can be achieved solely by inhalation of a volatile anaesthetic agent. With this approach in adults, several stages of general anaesthesia are observed during induction (Table 17.2). The stage of excitation with struggling is overcome by using a bolus of intravenous anaesthetic for rapid induction, followed by an inhalational anaesthetic for maintenance. For short surgical procedures in adults, both induction and maintenance can be achieved with an intravenous anaesthetic alone (total intravenous anaesthesia). In children, excitation is less of a problem, and anaesthesia is often induced and maintained with an inhalational anaesthetic agent.

Full general anaesthesia produces depression of spontaneous respiration and blood pressure, requiring mechanical ventilation and perhaps circulatory support. Some short procedures do not need full general anaesthesia and can be carried out under sedation produced by an anaesthetic, with preserved respiratory and cardiovascular function.

The adequacy of general anaesthesia is assessed by monitoring the heart rate, blood pressure and other physiological functions. For example, it can be inferred that the level of anaesthesia is inadequate and that pain is being experienced if the heart rate rises, or the person develops perspiration, tears, return of muscle tone, movement or change in pupil size.

For abdominal and thoracic surgery, and for long operations, full skeletal muscle paralysis is produced by giving neuromuscular blocking drugs (see Chapter 27), in which case endotracheal intubation and mechanical ventilation are essential.

Analgesia can be provided by an intravenous opioid for systemic analgesia, or by a local anaesthetic (see Chapter 18) to provide regional analgesia, such as administration into the epidural space (epidural analgesia) or infiltration around peripheral nerves.

At the end of an operation, resumption of consciousness (reversal of anaesthesia) occurs when intravenous anaesthetics are redistributed or metabolised, or when inhalational anaesthetics are redistributed or exhaled. Residual neuromuscular blockade by competitive blocking agents may need reversal with an anticholinesterase such as neostigmine (see Chapter 27). Attentiveness, and therefore the ability to drive safely, may be impaired for up to 24 hours after general anaesthesia.

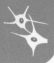

Table 17.1 The concept of 'balanced anaesthesia'

	Sedation	Analgesia	Muscle relaxation
Drugs exerting a major effect	Intravenous anaesthetics Inhalational anaesthetics Premedicant benzodiazepines	Opioids Local anaesthetics	Neuromuscular blocking drugs (see Chapter 27)
Drugs exerting a minor effect	Opioids Nitrous oxide	Nitrous oxide	Inhalational anaesthetics

Drugs are used in combination to produce the appropriate balance of sedation, analgesia and muscle relaxation while minimising unwanted effects; at particular doses and concentrations, each contributes minor or major effects to achieve this balance. Excessive or inadequate doses of any one agent could disturb the balance.

Table 17.2 The stages of anaesthesia

Stage	Description	Effects produced
I	Analgesia	Analgesia without amnesia or loss of touch sensation; disorientation, but consciousness retained
II	Excitation	Excitation and delirium with struggling; coughing and vomiting may occur; respiration rapid and irregular; frequent eye movements with increased pupil diameter; amnesia
III	Surgical anaesthesia	Loss of consciousness; subdivided into four levels or planes of increasing depth: Plane I: Decrease in eye movements and some pupillary constriction Plane II: Loss of corneal reflex; increased tear secretion Plane III: Increasing loss of laryngeal reflex; pupils dilated and light reflex lost Plane IV: Progressive decrease in thoracic breathing and general muscle tone
IV	Medullary depression	Loss of spontaneous respiration and progressive depression of cardiovascular reflexes; requires respiratory and circulatory support

Box 17.1 Properties of an ideal inhalational anaesthetic

Inherent stability at room temperature in contact with soda lime (used in anaesthesia to absorb CO_2), metals and plastic.
Nonflammable and nonexplosive when mixed with air, oxygen or nitrous oxide.
Minimal interactions with other drugs.
Lack of unwanted effects on respiratory, cardiovascular and other systems.
High lipid solubility, providing potency and allowing use of high inspired oxygen concentration.
Low blood solubility, allowing rapid induction and rapid emergence from anaesthesia, and rapid adjustment of the depth of anaesthesia.
No hangover effects.
Nontoxic, nonirritant to the airways, and no unpleasant taste or odour.
Analgesic activity.
Inexpensive; long shelf life; safe for operating theatre staff.

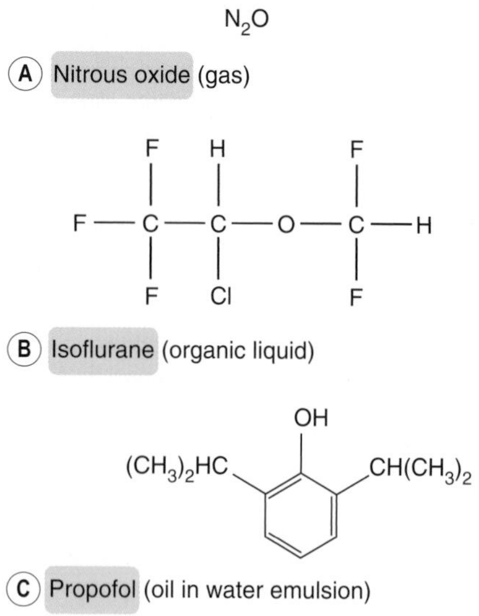

N_2O

(A) Nitrous oxide (gas)

(B) Isoflurane (organic liquid)

(C) Propofol (oil in water emulsion)

Fig. 17.1 Examples of general anaesthetics of different chemical natures.

MECHANISMS OF ACTION OF GENERAL ANAESTHETICS

General anaesthesia can be produced by compounds of widely differing chemical structure: simple gases such as nitrous oxide, volatile liquids such as isoflurane and nonvolatile solids such as propofol (Fig. 17.1).

General anaesthetics act at cell membranes, and the relationship between lipid solubility and potency led to the Meyer–Overton hypothesis that their incorporation into lipids altered the properties and function of neuronal cell membranes. However, this does not account for many of the properties of general anaesthetics. For example, the differing anaesthetic potencies of the stereoisomers of some anaesthetic agents suggest stereospecific interaction with target receptors. The general relationship between lipid solubility and anaesthetic potency is probably more important for determining the pharmacokinetic properties of the drug than for explaining its mode of action.

Although it is not known precisely how general anaesthetics work, there is increasing evidence for interactions with specific binding sites on cellular protein channels (particularly ligand-gated ion channels) to control synaptic transmission (Table 17.3). The main effects are to *inhibit* excitatory receptors, particularly *N*-methyl-D-aspartate (NMDA) receptors for glutamate and glycine, and to *enhance* the activities of inhibitory receptors, particularly GABA_A receptors for γ-aminobutyric acid (GABA) and nicotinic receptors for acetylcholine (ACh). These receptors are found in the cortex, thalamus, striatum and the brainstem. The initial effect of a general anaesthetic is to decrease spontaneous neuronal firing in the cerebral cortex, which slows cortical oscillatory activity (rhythmic, coordinated spontaneous firing). Anaesthetics reduce thalamic activity due to decreased excitatory cortico-thalamic feedback to the thalamus, which in turn may trigger a 'thalamic consciousness switch'. Effects on connections between the basal ganglia and cortex also appear to be important in the mechanism of general anaesthesia. Numerous other complex neuronal pathways are involved in the maintenance of unconsciousness, and the effect of anaesthetics on functional integration among neuronal circuits is the subject of intensive research. The many types of intravenous and inhalational anaesthetic agents differ in their interactions with specific receptors, and they target different regions of the brain, which probably explains the differences in their capacities to produce unconsciousness, amnesia, analgesia and muscle relaxation.

The various stages of anaesthesia (see Table 17.2) probably arise as a result of the progressive effects of anaesthetic agents on different neurons. A rapid action on small neurons in the dorsal horn of the spinal cord (nociceptive impulses; see Chapter 19) and inhibitory cells in the brain (see the discussion on the effects of alcohol in Chapter 54) explains the early analgesic and excitation phases. By contrast, neurons of the medullary integration centres are less sensitive.

DRUGS USED IN ANAESTHESIA

General anaesthetics are usually grouped according to their route of administration, which is either intravenous or inhalational.

INTRAVENOUS ANAESTHETICS

Examples

etomidate, ketamine, propofol, thiopental

Intravenous anaesthetics can be given by slow intravenous injection for rapid induction of anaesthesia and then replaced by inhalational anaesthetics for longer-term maintenance of anaesthesia. Both propofol and ketamine, but not etomidate or thiopental, can also be given by continuous infusion without inhalational anaesthesia for short operations (total intravenous anaesthesia) or for prolonged sedation. Ketamine has analgesic actions, unlike other intravenous anaesthetics, but it does not reliably suppress laryngeal reflexes, which can make endotracheal intubation more difficult. It is now rarely used, except for paediatric anaesthesia. Some properties of commonly used intravenous anaesthetics are shown in Table 17.4.

Pharmacokinetics

Thiopental is a thiobarbiturate that has a very rapid onset of action (within 30 seconds), owing to its high lipid solubility and ease of passage across the blood–brain barrier. The duration of action after a bolus dose is very short (about 2–5 minutes) and blood concentrations fall rapidly, initially because of distribution into lean muscle tissue (because of its high blood flow). With continuous infusion, distribution occurs more slowly into adipose tissue, which has poor blood flow (Fig. 17.2). With thiopental, total intravenous anaesthesia is not practicable, as during a lengthy procedure the brain and blood and slowly equilibrating tissues would reach equilibrium. Recovery from anaesthesia on cessation of anaesthetic administration would then depend on the elimination half-life of thiopental (3–8 hours due to hepatic metabolism), not the distribution half-life (about 3 minutes). Therefore, following induction of anaesthesia with thiopental, an inhalational agent is used for maintenance of anaesthesia.

Propofol is a lipophilic agent that is insoluble in water. It is formulated as an oil-in-water emulsion which can cause pain during injection. It has a slightly slower onset of action (about 30 seconds) compared with thiopental, and its duration of action is also limited by redistribution (distribution half-life 2–8 minutes) after a bolus dose. It can be given as an infusion

Table 17.3 Possible sites of action of inhalation and intravenous general anaesthetics

Drug group	Properties of group	Receptor and channel targets
Etomidate, propofol, thiopental	Potent amnesics Potent sedatives Weak muscle relaxants	Enhance activity at GABA_A receptors
Nitrous oxide, ketamine	Potent analgesics Weak sedatives Weak muscle relaxants	Inhibit glutamate NMDA receptors Inhibit ACh nicotinic receptors Open two-pore K$^+$ channels
Sevoflurane, isoflurane, desflurane	Potent amnesics Potent sedatives Potent muscle relaxants	Enhance activity at GABA_A receptors Enhance activity at glycine receptors Inhibit glutamate NMDA receptors Inhibit ACh nicotinic receptors Open two-pore K$^+$ channels

ACh, Acetylcholine; *GABA*, γ-aminobutyric acid; *NMDA*, N-methyl-D-aspartate.
Information in this table is mainly from Solt K, Forman SA., 2007. Correlating the clinical actions and molecular mechanisms of general anesthetics. Curr. Opin. Anaesthesiol. 20, 300–306, and is based on data from in vitro studies and in vivo studies in transgenic animals.

Table 17.4 Properties of some common intravenous anaesthetics

Drug	Type	Speed of induction	Recovery	Hangover effect	Analgesic	Comment
Thiopental	Barbiturate	Rapid	Slow	Yes	No	Causes tissue necrosis if extravasation at the site of injection; cannot be given by continuous infusion due to accumulation
Propofol	Phenol	Rapid	Rapid	Low	No	Does not accumulate; continuous infusion can be used for total intravenous anaesthesia or for sedation of adults in intensive care
Etomidate	Imidazole	Rapid	Fairly rapid	Low	No	Not infused continuously, because repeated doses suppress adrenocortical function
Ketamine	Cyclohexanone	Slower	Slower	No	Yes	Can be given by continuous infusion; produces analgesia that outlasts anaesthesia; usually used for children

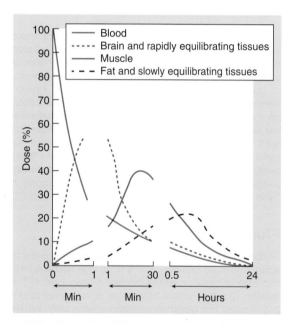

Fig. 17.2 The amounts of thiopental in blood, brain (and other rapidly equilibrating tissues), muscle and adipose tissue (and other slowly equilibrating tissues) after an intravenous infusion over 10 seconds. Note: The time axis is not linear. The continued uptake into muscle between 1 and 30 minutes lowers the concentrations in the blood and in all rapidly equilibrating tissues, including the brain, hence terminating its anaesthetic action by distribution within minutes.

for total intravenous anaesthesia or for sedation in intensive care, when its duration of action is determined by hepatic clearance (half-life 4–7 hours). If infused for less than 8 hours, propofol returns to the circulation from fatty tissue at a sufficiently slow rate that blood concentrations do not increase dramatically (giving it a context-specific half-life of <40 minutes). Therefore propofol is particularly useful for day surgery, because of the absence of hangover effects.

Ketamine can be given by intramuscular injection or intravenously by bolus injection or infusion. When used for induction or for total intravenous anaesthesia, the anaesthetic action is terminated largely by distribution (half-life about 15 minutes). With prolonged infusion the duration of action becomes dependent on hepatic metabolism (half-life 2–4 hours). Ketamine produces dissociative anaesthesia in which the person appears conscious, with eye opening, swallowing and muscle contraction, but unresponsive to pain.

Etomidate is highly lipid-soluble and has a rapid onset of action after intravenous injection. Its action is terminated by rapid hydrolysis by plasma esterases and hepatic microsomal enzymes, so that the duration of action is about 6–10 minutes with minimal hangover. It is not used to maintain anaesthesia, because prolonged infusion can suppress adrenocortical function.

Unwanted effects

- On the central nervous system (CNS): General depression of the CNS can produce respiratory and cardiovascular depression. Slow release of thiopental distributed into tissues may result in some sedation for up to 24 hours after use. Ketamine has minimal effects on ventilatory drive. Hallucinations and vivid dreams are common during recovery from ketamine in adults (emergence reactions, that can be minimised by co-administration of a benzodiazepine), but are less frequent in children.
- On muscles: Extraneous muscle movement is common with etomidate, and to a lesser degree with propofol. They can be reduced by a benzodiazepine or opioid analgesic given before induction. Ketamine increases muscle tone and can cause laryngospasm.
- On the heart: Thiopental and propofol depress the heart, producing bradycardia and reducing blood pressure. Etomidate has no effect on the heart or systemic vascular resistance. By contrast, ketamine more often produces

tachycardia and an increase in blood pressure through sympathetic nervous system stimulation.

- Nausea and vomiting during recovery are experienced by up to 40% of people but rarely persist for more than 24 hours. Propofol has an antiemetic action.
- Convulsions have been reported after propofol. These can be delayed, indicating the need for particular caution after day surgery.
- Pain on injection with etomidate and propofol. This can be reduced by injecting into a large vein, by giving an opioid analgesic just before induction, or giving intravenous lignocaine with propofol. Thiopental is an alkaline solution that is irritant; if it extravasates outside the vein, it can cause tissue necrosis.
- Propofol is not used for prolonged sedation at high doses because of the risk of 'propofol infusion syndrome', which includes metabolic acidosis, heart failure and rhabdomyolysis.

INTRAVENOUS OPIOIDS

fentanyl, remifentanil

Intravenous opioids are usually given at induction for intraoperative analgesia, which reduces the dose requirement for anaesthetic agents. They can also be used for sedation and respiratory depression during assisted ventilation in intensive care. In high doses, opioids stimulate the vagus nerve and produce bradycardia; this can be helpful to reduce the tachycardia and hypertension produced by sympathetic nervous system activation during surgery. Details of the mechanism of action of opioids can be found in Chapter 19.

Pharmacokinetics

After intravenous injection, fentanyl has a rapid onset of action within 1–2 minutes. After a single dose, the drug is distributed rapidly into skeletal muscle and then into adipose tissue (half-life about 15 minutes), and its duration of action is about 30–60 minutes. The effect can be maintained by repeated injections or infusion, but with prolonged use, tissue stores are saturated and fentanyl then has a long duration of action determined by its hepatic metabolism (half-life about 4 hours). After repeated injections, respiratory depression may become apparent during recovery from an anaesthetic.

Remifentanil is an opioid ester that has a similar rapid onset to fentanyl but a very short half-life of about 5 minutes, due to metabolism by tissue and plasma esterases. After an initial bolus dose of remifentanil, continuous intravenous infusion is used to maintain its effects.

Unwanted effects

- Muscle rigidity. This particularly affects the chest wall and jaw, and can be prevented during surgery with neuromuscular junction blocking drugs (see Chapter 27). Myoclonus and rigidity can persist after recovery, and

can be reversed with the opioid antagonist naloxone (see Chapter 19).
- Respiratory depression. This may be profound and means that assisted ventilation is usually necessary during surgery when large doses have been used.
- Nausea and vomiting.

INHALATIONAL ANAESTHETICS

desflurane, halothane, isoflurane, sevoflurane, nitrous oxide

Inhalational anaesthetics are either volatile liquids, which must be vaporised before administration, or gases. All inhalational anaesthetics must be given with adequate oxygen (usually a minimum 25% of the inspired gas mixture) to avoid hypoxia during anaesthesia.

Sevoflurane is a volatile liquid anaesthetic that can be used for both induction and maintenance of anaesthesia in children, as it has a pleasant smell. It is used in adults for maintenance of anaesthesia following induction with an intravenous anaesthetic. Recovery is rapid after sevoflurane, and therefore early postoperative analgesia may be necessary. Other volatile liquid anaesthetics such as desflurane and isoflurane irritate mucous membranes, which makes them less suitable for induction. These agents also give a slower recovery at the end of a procedure.

Nitrous oxide is a gaseous anaesthetic that is not sufficiently potent to be used alone (Table 17.5), but it has the advantage of producing analgesia (unlike the other inhalational anaesthetics). It is often used in combination with other inhalational anaesthetics, and reduces the required dose of the other agent. Nitrous oxide can only be used as the sole inhalational agent when combined with an intravenous opioid and a neuromuscular blocking drug (see Chapter 27), but there is a risk of awareness during surgery. Nitrous oxide is also used alone as an analgesic, in subanaesthetic doses.

Pharmacokinetics

The amount and duration of administration of inhaled anaesthetic required to give a sufficient concentration of the drug in the CNS for general anaesthesia will depend on the relationships shown in Fig. 17.3 and Table 17.5. The crucial factors are the alveolar concentration of the drug and its uptake from the lungs. Alveolar concentration is affected by three factors:

- The inspired concentration of the drug, which affects the rate of increase of alveolar concentration towards the inspired concentration and contributes to the speed of onset of anaesthesia.
- Alveolar ventilation (rate and depth of inspiration), which directly determines replacement of the drug in the alveoli after removal by the pulmonary circulation. This is most important if an inhaled agent is used for induction, but less significant once equilibrium has been established between the inhaled concentration and that in the brain.

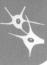

Table 17.5 Inhalational anaesthetics

Compound	Blood:gas partition coefficient	Induction time	Oil:gas partition coefficient	MAC (%)	Metabolism (%)
Nitrous oxide	0.5	Fast	1.4	>100	0
Isoflurane	1.4	Medium	91	1.12	0.2
Enflurane	1.9	Medium	96	1.7	2–10
Sevoflurane	0.6	Fast	53	2.1	≈5

The blood:gas partition coefficient correlates closely with the time to induction when the drug is used as the sole anaesthetic. The oil:gas partition correlates with the potency of the anaesthetic, which correlates inversely with the minimum alveolar concentration (MAC) necessary for surgical anaesthesia. Nitrous oxide cannot produce anaesthesia alone, so it has a theoretical MAC of >100%. Metabolism is the percentage of drug eliminated as urinary metabolites, with the remainder mainly eliminated unchanged by exhalation.

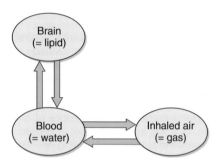

Fig. 17.3 Equilibration of inhalational general anaesthetics between air, blood and brain. The concentration ratio between blood and air at equilibrium is estimated from in vivo studies of the blood:gas partition coefficient and correlates with the induction time of the drug (see Table 17.5). The concentrations in brain and blood at equilibrium reflect the different affinities of the two body compartments for general anaesthetics. The brain:blood ratio is 1–3:1 for all commonly used anaesthetics. The concentration in the inspired air required to give the necessary concentration in brain membranes (minimum alveolar concentration [MAC]) correlates inversely with the blood:gas partition coefficient, which is an indication of the potency of the compound.

- Functional residual capacity of the lungs. If this is large, then the alveolar concentration of the drug will be diluted and the onset of action will be slower.

The rate of induction of anaesthesia with an inhaled drug is more rapid in children, as they have higher alveolar ventilation relative to functional residual capacity. Therefore alveolar drug concentration increases more rapidly to equilibration. Drug uptake from the lungs is determined by three factors:

- The blood-gas partition coefficient, which indicates the relative solubilities of the drug in blood and air. A high solubility in blood, and therefore in all rapidly equilibrating body tissues, means that a greater amount of the agent will need to be administered before its partial pressure in the blood is the same as that in the inspired air. The blood-gas partition coefficient therefore correlates with the time to induction of anaesthesia (see Table 17.5). This conforms to the basic pharmacokinetic principle that compounds with a large apparent volume of distribution take longer to reach steady state during a constant rate of drug administration (see Chapter 2).
- The cardiac output, which will determine pulmonary alveolar blood flow. A high cardiac output will remove anaesthetic more quickly from the alveoli and speed equilibrium with tissues. However, because the alveolar concentration of the drug falls more rapidly, induction does not occur faster.
- Alveolar-venous partial pressure gradient and tissue uptake. Tissue uptake will depend on blood flow, the difference in partial pressure of the drug in the blood and tissue, and the blood tissue solubility coefficient of the drug (which determines the affinity of the tissue for the drug). Although the brain has a lower affinity for inhaled anaesthetics than adipose tissue, its high perfusion allows rapid equilibration.

Anaesthetic potency of the inhaled anaesthetics is measured as the minimum alveolar concentration (MAC) of an agent necessary to prevent a withdrawal reaction in 50% of people exposed to a noxious stimulus (a midline surgical skin incision). Therefore MAC is the equivalent of the ED_{50} (the 50% effective dose) for other drugs (see Chapter 1). The MAC for inhaled anaesthetics correlates *inversely* with the oil-gas partition coefficient, which reflects the ratio between the concentration in the lipid membranes of brain cells (oil) and the inhaled concentration (gas). A potent inhalational anaesthetic agent such as enflurane has a high oil-gas partition coefficient, and this high lipid solubility means it has a low MAC (see Table 17.5).

The major route of elimination of inhalational anaesthetics is via the airways in expired air. Factors that influence the duration of the induction phase, such as ventilation rate and the blood-gas partition coefficient, will also affect the time taken to eliminate the anaesthetic. Sevoflurane has a short recovery time, due to its low blood-gas partition coefficient (see Table 17.5). The recovery time may also depend on the duration of inhalation, which determines the extent to which the drug has entered slowly equilibrating tissues. Removal of the drug from these tissues is also slow, which can maintain the plasma concentration of the drug and delay recovery. During recovery, the depth of anaesthesia reverses through the stages discussed previously (see Table 17.2) to consciousness; a rapid recovery which minimises stage II of anaesthesia (see Table 17.2) is beneficial.

Inhalational anaesthetics are also partly eliminated by metabolism, the extent of which depends on the time that the agent is retained in the body and is therefore available for metabolism. Exhalation and metabolism can be regarded as alternative pathways of elimination, the proportions of which are determined largely by the blood-gas partition coefficient of the agent (see Table 17.5).

Unwanted effects

A number of unwanted effects are common to most inhalational anaesthetics; however, each agent also has a unique profile of additional unwanted effects.

- **Cardiovascular system.** Isoflurane, isoflurane and sevoflurane reduce blood pressure mainly by arterial vasodilation. They also depress myocardial contractility and predispose to bradycardia by interfering with transmembrane Ca^{2+} flux, with a resultant decrease in cardiac output. Nitrous oxide has less depressant effect on the heart and circulation, and its use in combination with other agents that depress the heart may permit reduction in their dosage. Inhalational anaesthetics often increase cerebral blood flow, which can exacerbate an elevated intracranial pressure. Arrhythmias occasionally occur with volatile liquid anaesthetics.
- **Respiratory system.** All anaesthetic agents depress the response of the respiratory centre in the medulla to carbon dioxide and hypoxia. They also decrease tidal volume and increase respiratory rate. Desflurane and isoflurane irritate mucous membranes and can cause coughing, apnoea and laryngospasm if used for induction. Isoflurane and sevoflurane have a bronchodilator action.
- **Liver.** All inhaled anaesthetics decrease liver blood flow. Halothane commonly causes mild hepatic dysfunction, due to T-cell-mediated immune toxicity from a metabolite. About 1 in 10,000 people will develop severe hepatic necrosis following the use of halothane, especially after repeat exposure within a short time interval. Halothane is now only available in the United Kingdom on special order. Hepatotoxicity is rare with other halogenated anaesthetics.
- **Uterus.** Relaxation of the uterus may increase the risk of haemorrhage when anaesthesia is used in labour. Nitrous oxide has less effect on uterine muscle than the volatile liquid anaesthetics.
- **Skeletal muscle.** Most agents produce some muscle relaxation, which enhances the activity of neuromuscular blocking drugs (see Chapter 27). With sevoflurane this may be sufficient to enable tracheal intubation without the use of a neuromuscular blocker.
- **Chemoreceptor trigger zone.** Inhalational anaesthetics trigger postoperative nausea and vomiting. This is most pronounced with nitrous oxide.
- **Postoperative shivering.** This occurs in up to 65% of those recovering from general anaesthesia. The aetiology is unclear.
- **Malignant hyperthermia.** This is a rare but potentially fatal complication of volatile liquid anaesthetics. It is genetically determined, and results from a defect in the ryanodine receptor (RyR1) that regulates release of Ca^{2+} from the sarcoplasmic reticulum in skeletal muscle cells (see Chapter 5, Fig. 5.4). A sudden increase in intracellular Ca^{2+} provoked by an anaesthetic produces tachycardia, unstable blood pressure, hypercapnoea, fever and hyperventilation, followed by hyperkalaemia and metabolic acidosis. Muscle rigidity may occur. Treatment is with dantrolene, an RyR1 receptor antagonist (see Chapter 24).

SELF-ASSESSMENT

True/false questions

1. Inhalational anaesthetics may have their effects by interacting with specific receptors.
2. Inhalational anaesthetics are all gases.
3. Most inhalational anaesthetics are sulfur-containing compounds.
4. Halothane closely approaches the properties of an ideal inhalational anaesthetic.
5. The risk of hangover effects with inhalational anaesthetics increases if the operation is long.
6. The MAC of an inhalational anaesthetic required to produce surgical anaesthesia correlates inversely with the oil:gas partition coefficient of the drug.
7. Nitrous oxide administered alone at a concentration of 50% in inspired air reaches the MAC necessary for surgical anaesthesia.
8. Nitrous oxide is frequently given with oxygen and a halogenated anaesthetic agent to produce effective surgical anaesthesia.
9. Isoflurane is metabolised as extensively as halothane.
10. The short duration of action of thiopental is due to its distribution into richly perfused tissues such as muscles.
11. The elimination half-life of thiopental is similar to its distribution half-life.
12. Propofol can be given alone by continuous intravenous infusion to maintain anaesthesia.
13. Accidental injection of thiopental into an artery can have serious consequences.
14. Ketamine is a sedative but is without analgesic action.
15. Fentanyl should not be administered concurrently with inhalational anaesthetics.
16. With modern anaesthetics, the classical stages of anaesthesia induction are rarely seen.
17. When administering an inhalational anaesthetic, the excitement stage of anaesthesia may be prolonged if an intravenous anaesthetic is not given beforehand.
18. Most inhalational anaesthetics have a depressant effect on the cardiovascular system.
19. Inhalational anaesthetics increase the sensitivity of the respiratory centre to carbon dioxide and hypoxia.
20. Sevoflurane has the advantage of a fast onset of action and rapid elimination.

One-best-answer (OBA) questions

1. Identify the *most accurate* statement concerning the pharmacology of agents used in anaesthesia.
   A. The respiratory centre in the medulla is particularly sensitive to the depressant action of general anaesthetics.
   B. The major route of elimination of most inhalational anaesthetics is via the liver.
   C. Metoclopramide is often given as a premedication before general anaesthesia.
   D. The intravenous opioid fentanyl should not be administered together with sevoflurane.
   E. Atropine is a commonly administered preoperative agent.

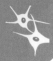

2. What are ideal properties of an inhalational anaesthetic?
   A. Stability
   B. Nonflammability
   C. Potency
   D. Analgesic action
   E. High blood:gas partition coefficient.

Case-based question

A 40-year-old woman is scheduled for a laparotomy because of abdominal swelling. She has not had a previous operation and is otherwise healthy, with normal cardiovascular and respiratory function. She was given premedication with atropine. The operation lasted 40 minutes. (Refer to Chapter 27 for information on neuromuscular junction blockers.)

A. Why is atropine little used nowadays as preanaesthetic medication in adults?

B. Do the muscarinic receptor antagonists atropine and hyoscine have the same properties?
   The woman was intubated after the administration of thiopental, fentanyl and suxamethonium (succinylcholine).

C. Why has the routine use of suxamethonium to facilitate endotracheal intubation been reduced?
   Following intubation, pancuronium and fentanyl were given and she was ventilated with nitrous oxide, enflurane and oxygen. An ovarian cyst was removed and the operation took 40 minutes.

D. Is pancuronium the most suitable choice of muscle relaxant? What alternatives are available?
   After the operation, she did not breathe spontaneously, despite the administration of neostigmine and glycopyrronium.

E. What are the possible reasons for the apnoea, and how could they be treated?

F. Would mivacurium (a short-duration muscle relaxant) have been a preferable muscle relaxant to use in this patient?

G. What is the reason for administering glycopyrronium with neostigmine at the end of the operation?

ANSWERS

True/false answers

1. **True.** It is increasingly thought that general anaesthetics act at a number of excitatory and inhibitory receptors (see Table 17.3).
2. **False.** Many inhalational anaesthetics are volatile liquids.
3. **False.** The main inhalational anaesthetics are halogenated compounds.
4. **False.** Halothane is potent but can cause hepatotoxicity, hypotension and sensitisation of the heart to catecholamines producing cardiac arrhythmias; it is now available in the United Kingdom only on special order.
5. **True.** In prolonged anaesthesia, lipid-soluble agents may accumulate in body fat stores and be slowly released after the operation.
6. **True.** The higher the oil:gas ratio, the lower the inhaled concentration of anaesthetic required to produce anaesthesia.

7. **False.** Even at concentrations higher than 50%, nitrous oxide is not potent enough to produce effective surgical anaesthesia on its own.
8. **True.** Nitrous oxide provides additional analgesic activity in combination with a fluorinated anaesthetic and oxygen.
9. **False.** Halothane undergoes substantial metabolism, but the other halogenated anaesthetics do not.
10. **True.** Rapid redistribution of thiopental from the CNS terminates its anaesthetic action.
11. **False.** The half-life of thiopental redistribution is about 3 minutes, but its elimination from the body is much slower (half-life 3–8 hours), partially accounting for the hangover effect seen with this drug.
12. **True.** Propofol is useful for short operations, but its rapid elimination and little hangover effect mean that it can also be given by continuous infusion for maintenance anaesthesia, such as in intensive care units.
13. **True.** Extravascular or intra-arterial injection of thiopental can be damaging due its high pH (approximately 9–10).
14. **False.** Ketamine does have analgesic action, unlike other available intravenous anaesthetics.
15. **False.** Fentanyl is short-acting with a rapid recovery and is increasingly used for intraoperative analgesia with inhalation anaesthetics.
16. **True.** The classical stages of anaesthetic induction were originally described following the use of slower-acting anaesthetics than those used today.
17. **True.** The intravenous agent is used to provide rapid induction of anaesthesia.
18. **True.** Most are negatively inotropic, and they depress myocardial function by interfering with Ca^{2+} fluxes. Halothane also sensitises the heart to catecholamines and can lead to arrhythmias.
19. **False.** Inhalational anaesthetics *reduce* the ventilatory response to carbon dioxide and hypoxia, and increase the arterial partial pressure of carbon dioxide.
20. **True.** Sevoflurane has a rapid onset of action and is more rapidly eliminated than halothane or isoflurane.

One-best-answer (OBA) answers

1. **Answer C** is correct, as an antiemetic such as metoclopramide is often used to reduce the risk of vomiting caused by general anaesthetics and opioid analgesics. Medullary neurons are relatively *in*sensitive to anaesthetics (answer A). Inhalation anaesthetics are eliminated mainly by exhalation, not hepatic metabolism (answer B). Fentanyl is often used as an analgesic together with inhalational anaesthetics (answer D). With modern anaesthetic practice, atropine is seldom needed to reduce bronchial and salivary secretions (answer E).
2. **Answers A–D** are desirable properties of an ideal anaesthetic. A high blood:gas ratio (answer E) is associated with a long induction time, so it is *not* an ideal property of an inhalational anaesthetic.

Case-based answers

A. Atropine (and hyoscine) block muscarinic receptors, reducing bronchial and salivary secretions, but modern anaesthetics have less irritant effect, thus reducing this problem. Muscarinic antagonists can reduce the bradycardia caused by some inhalation anaesthetics and by suxamethonium.

B. No. Atropine can cause CNS excitation, whereas hyoscine causes sedation and has antiemetic properties.

C. Relatively minor but frequent complications occur with suxamethonium, including bradycardia, postoperative myalgia, transient hyperkalaemia, and raised intraocular, intracranial and intragastric pressures. A rare but potentially fatal complication is malignant hyperthermia. The competitive blocking drug rocuronium has a short duration of action and does not cause these problems.

D. Pancuronium is probably not the ideal muscle relaxant to use, as it can cause tachycardia and hypertension and is long-acting (see Chapter 27). An alternative would be vecuronium, which has an intermediate duration of action and lacks cardiovascular effects. Rocuronium is more expensive but has a rapid onset and short duration of action and a low risk of cardiovascular effects.

E. There are at least three possible reasons for the postoperative apnoea: (1) The person could be experiencing opioid-induced respiratory depression, which could be reversed by the opioid antagonist naloxone. (2) The dose of neostigmine given may have been insufficient to reverse the competitive blockade induced by long-acting pancuronium. (3) The person could have a genetically determined deficiency of pseudocholinesterase (plasma cholinesterase, butyrylcholinesterase), found in about 1 in 3000 individuals, which would normally metabolise suxamethonium. Administration of neostigmine would exacerbate the respiratory suppression. Fresh frozen plasma (containing pseudocholinesterase) could be given.

F. Although mivacurium is a short-acting muscle relaxant, it is metabolised by pseudocholinesterase and its effect would be greatly prolonged if the person has the genetic deficiency of this enzyme.

G. Neostigmine inhibits acetylcholinesterase, increasing ACh concentrations at cholinergic synapses. It partially or fully reverses the actions of competitive blockers of N_2 receptors at the neuromuscular junction, but also enhances the activity of ACh at muscarinic receptors, causing bradycardia and bronchoconstriction. Glycopyrronium is a selective muscarinic receptor antagonist used to prevent these muscarinic effects.

FURTHER READING

Brown, E.N., Lydic, R., Schiff, N.D., 2010. General anesthesia, sleep, and coma. N. Engl. J. Med. 363, 2638–2650.

Chau, P.L., 2010. New insights into the molecular mechanisms of action of general anaesthetics. Br. J. Pharmacol. 161, 288–307.

Khan, K.S., Hayes, I., Buggy, D.J., 2013. Pharmacology of anaesthetic agents I: intravenous anaesthetic agents. Contin. Educ. Anaesth. Crit. Care. Pain. doi:10.1093/bjaceaccp/mkt039.

Khan, K.S., Hayes, I., Buggy, D.J., 2013. Pharmacology of anaesthetic agents II: inhalational anaesthetic agents. Contin. Educ. Anaesth. Crit. Care. Pain. doi:10.1093/bjaceaccp/mkt038.

Litman, R.S., Rosenberg, H., 2005. Malignant hyperthermia. Update on susceptibility testing. J. Am. Med. Assoc. 293, 2918–2924.

Solt, K., Forman, S.A., 2007. Correlating the clinical actions and molecular mechanisms of general anesthetics. Curr. Opin. Anaesthesiol. 20, 300–306.

Uhrig, L., Dehaene, S., Jarraya, B., 2014. Cerebral mechanisms of general anaesthesia. Ann. Fr. Anesth. Reanim. 33, 72–82.

Compendium: general anaesthetics

Drug	Characteristics
Intravenous anaesthetics	
Following a bolus dose, the duration of action depends on the rate of distribution and not the elimination half-life given here.	
Etomidate	Used for rapid induction (<30 s) without hangover. Suppresses adrenocortical function on continuous dosage and should not be used for maintenance anaesthesia. May cause involuntary movements. Action is terminated by rapid distribution; metabolism faster than thiopental. Half-life: 1–2 h
Ketamine	Used for paediatric anaesthesia. Analgesic activity at subanaesthetic doses. Transient psychotic effects (hallucinations, nightmares) may occur. Slower onset than other induction agents (2–5 min); action is terminated by rapid distribution. Elimination half-life: 2–4 h
Propofol	Most widely used intravenous anaesthetic; can be used for rapid induction (<30 s) or for maintenance. Rapid recovery with little hangover. Duration of action partly determined by distribution and partly by rapid glucuronidation in liver and other tissues; in prolonged use, drug has long half-life (3–12 h)
Thiopental	Rapid induction (<30 s) and recovery, but may cause sedation up to 24 h due to slow metabolism. Action is terminated by rapid distribution; on repeated dosing slow hepatic metabolism (3–8 h) can cause accumulation in poorly perfused tissues. Reconstituted solution is highly alkaline; may cause tissue necrosis with extravascular injection

Compendium: general anaesthetics (cont'd)

Drug	Characteristics
Intravenous opioids	
Provide analgesia and enhance anaesthesia.	
Alfentanil	Used especially during short procedures and for outpatient surgery; respiratory depression may persist after the end of the procedure if repeated doses are given. Half-life: 0.7–2 h
Fentanyl	Respiratory depression may persist after the end of the procedure if repeated doses are given. Half-life: 1–6 h
Remifentanil	Given intraoperatively as an intravenous infusion. Very rapid clearance by blood and tissue esterases (half-life: 0.1 h) minimises postoperative respiratory depression
Inhalational anaesthetics	
Desflurane	Not recommended for induction in children. Irritant, causing cough, laryngospasm and increased secretions. Eliminated by exhalation; very rapid recovery (minutes)
Enflurane	Powerful cardiorespiratory depressant; largely superseded by isoflurane. Eliminated mainly by exhalation
Halothane	Potent and nonirritant but largely superseded due to risk of severe hepatotoxicity on repeated exposure; now available in the United Kingdom on special order only. Eliminated by exhalation with significant hepatic metabolism (15%)
Isoflurane	An isomer of enflurane. May decrease peripheral vascular resistance. Potentiates effects of muscle-relaxant drugs. Eliminated mainly by exhalation
Nitrous oxide	Low potency compared with other inhaled agents precludes use as sole anaesthetic agent. Has analgesic activity. Rapid recovery owing to low potency and low tissue affinity. Eliminated rapidly by exhalation
Sevoflurane	Potent maintenance anaesthetic with rapid recovery; nonirritant so can also be used for inhalational induction. Eliminated rapidly by exhalation, with some metabolism (≈5%)

Various other drugs, such as analgesics (see Chapters 19 and 29), anxiolytics (see Chapter 20) and antiemetics (see Chapter 32) are used in the perioperative period.

18 Local anaesthetics

Local anaesthetics are drugs that reversibly block the transmission of pain stimuli locally at their site of administration.

Examples

bupivacaine, cocaine, lidocaine, ropivacaine

PHARMACOLOGY

MECHANISM OF ACTION

Local anaesthetics produce a reversible blockade of nerve conduction by inhibiting the influx of Na^+ across neuronal cell membranes, which prevents depolarisation of the cell. At rest, the neuronal cell membrane has only limited permeability to Na^+, but about 50–70 times greater permeability to K^+ because of the large number of channels that are open for passive transport of K^+ out of the cell. The maintenance of a negative internal resting membrane electrical potential is largely determined by the K^+ gradient across the cell membrane. Conduction of a nerve action potential results from the opening of voltage-dependent Na^+ channels and rapid influx of Na^+ to depolarise the cell (see Fig. 18.2). Na^+ channels cycle between three states:

- Resting, when the channel is closed but able to open in response to a change in transmembrane potential.
- Open, when the channel opens in response to an action potential and allows the rapid influx of Na^+ ions through to the cytoplasm and a rapid change in membrane voltage.
- Inactivated, due to a conformational change at the cytoplasmic end of the channel that occurs very soon after the action potential has passed. During this stage the channel is resistant to depolarising influences, but sensitivity returns when the membrane potential is restored to the resting level by return of Na^+ ions to the exterior of the cell.

There is considerable redundancy in membrane Na^+ channels; as a consequence, nerve conduction can continue even when 90% of the channels are inactivated.

Local anaesthetics block the voltage-dependent Na^+ channels that depolarise the cell. They bind to the Na^+ channel at a site on the inner surface of the membrane and hold them in their inactivated state. They progressively interrupt Na^+ channel-mediated depolarisation until impulse conduction fails. The probability that propagation of a nerve impulse will fail at a particular segment of the nerve is related to:

- the local concentration of the anaesthetic drug,
- the size of the nerve fibre,
- whether the nerve is myelinated,
- the length of the nerve exposed to the drug.

Nerve transmission is blocked in smaller-diameter rapid-firing fibres before that in larger fibres (Table 18.1). The myelinated Aδ and small nonmyelinated C fibres that transmit pain (nociceptive fibres) are blocked first, followed by larger sensory fibres (carrying pressure and proprioception) and finally somatic motor fibres. Therefore pain pathways are most rapidly and intensely blocked by local anaesthetics (see Table 18.1), and also show the longest duration of local anaesthetic effect. In myelinated nerves, the drug penetrates at the nodes of Ranvier and must block at least three consecutive nodes to produce a conduction block. Unmyelinated nerves must be blocked over a sufficient length and around the full circumference of the nerve.

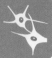

Table 18.1 Nerve fibres and their responsiveness to local anaesthetics

Fibre type	Site or function	Myelination	Diameter (μm)	Sensitivity to local anaesthesia
A fibres				
Alpha	Motor Muscle sense	Yes	12–20	+
Beta	Motor (muscle spindle) Touch, proprioception	Yes	5–12	+
Gamma	Motor (muscle spindle)	Yes	3–6	++
Delta	Pain, temperature, crude touch, pressure	Yes	2–5	+++
B fibres				
	Preganglionic autonomic	Yes	1–3	+++
C fibres				
	Pain, temperature, touch, pressure, itch	No	0.4–1.2	+++
	Postganglionic autonomic	No	0.3–1.3	+++

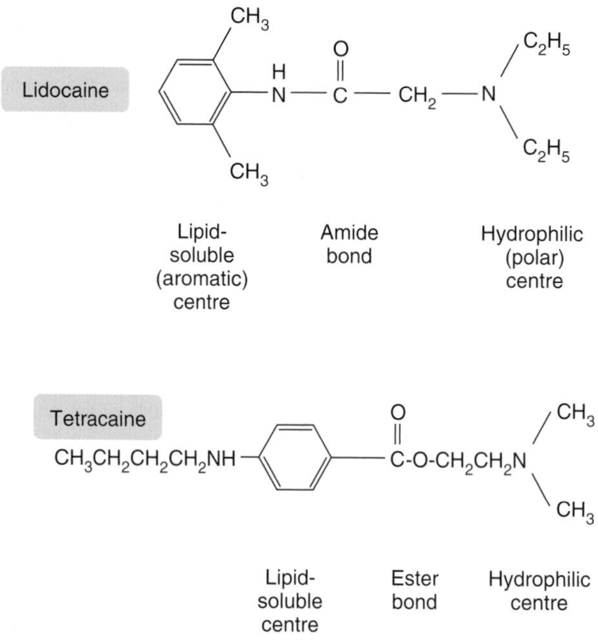

Lidocaine

Lipid-soluble (aromatic) centre | Amide bond | Hydrophilic (polar) centre

Tetracaine

CH₃CH₂CH₂CH₂NH–

Lipid-soluble centre | Ester bond | Hydrophilic centre

Fig. 18.1 **General structure of local anaesthetics.** All local anaesthetic structures contain a lipophilic (aromatic) centre and a hydrophilic (polar) centre linked by an amide (peptide) or ester bond. Local anaesthetics with an ester bond are susceptible to rapid hydrolysis at the injection site and in the plasma. The length of the intermediate bonding chain is optimal between three and seven atoms for local anaesthetic activity.

Structural requirements of local anaesthetics

All local anaesthetics have a lipid-soluble hydrophobic aromatic ring structure that is connected to a hydrophilic amine group by a short ester or amide intermediate linkage (Fig. 18.1). The length of the intermediate bonding chain is critical for local anaesthetic activity, and is optimal between three and seven atoms. The action of local anaesthetics results mainly from binding of the ionised form of the drug to

a site on the inside (cytoplasmic opening) of the Na⁺ channel. The drug must therefore diffuse through the cell membrane to access the site of action, which is made possible by the lipophilic aromatic group. The potency of a local anaesthetic is directly related to its lipid solubility.

Time to onset of action

The pK_a of the drug determines the extent of ionisation at physiological pH and the speed of onset of the conduction block. All local anaesthetics are weak bases and will be relatively more ionised (as quaternary amines) at a pH below their ionisation constant (pK_a), which for most local anaesthetics is between 7.7 and 9.1. Local anaesthetics are most water-soluble in their ionised form, and to ensure they are stable in solution, injectable preparations are formulated as hydrochloride salts with a pH of 5.0–6.0. The ionised form of the drug is unable to cross lipid membranes, and must be converted to the base (nonionised) form (a tertiary amine), which is more lipid-soluble. The time of onset of local anaesthesia is closely related to the amount of drug converted to the lipid-soluble form at physiological pH (7.4), which is in turn related to the pK_a of the drug. A drug with a high pK_a is more ionised at physiological pH, and the speed of onset of anaesthesia is slower. Alkalinisation of the injected solution by adding bicarbonate immediately before injection increases the proportion of the drug in its nonionised lipid-soluble form and increases the rate of absorption of the anaesthetic into the nerve, which will accelerate the onset of action. Care must be taken not to give too much alkali, which will cause the local anaesthetic to precipitate. The addition of alkali is most useful for infiltration anaesthesia (discussed later) and for the blocking of small nerves.

Receptor binding

A local anaesthetic must be in its ionised form to bind to its receptor within the Na^+ channel. Therefore, after passing across the cell membrane in the nonionised form, the anaesthetic must be converted to the ionised form in the cytosol. Drugs with a higher pK_a will re-ionise to a greater extent within the cell (pH 7.4) and produce more effective blockade. Local anaesthetics bind to the receptor preferentially when the channel is in either its open (activated) state or when it is inactivated (Fig. 18.2). For this reason, the effectiveness of most local anaesthetics is dependent on the frequency of firing of the neuron (use dependency), and a faster onset of local anaesthesia occurs in rapidly firing neurons. Once the local anaesthetic has bound to the channel, the influx of Na^+ is blocked and the channel remains in the *inactivated* state and resistant to further depolarisation. The local anaesthetic dissociates from the binding site when the membrane potential returns to its resting level and the channel is in the *resting* state.

Duration of action

Compounds with high protein-binding affinity stay at the site of action for longer and have a long duration of action. Thus procaine, which has a low binding affinity (6% protein bound), has a very short duration of action, whereas bupivacaine has a high binding affinity (95% protein bound) and a long duration of action.

The duration of action of any local anaesthetic can be extended considerably by co-administration with a vasoconstrictor to reduce the rate of diffusion away from the site of action. Local anaesthetics are available in formulations combined with vasoconstrictors such as adrenaline (epinephrine), phenylephrine or felypressin (a vasopressin analogue).

Binding to other receptors

Local anaesthetics bind to other ion channels and cell receptors. Binding to presynaptic Ca^{2+} channels, K^+ channels,

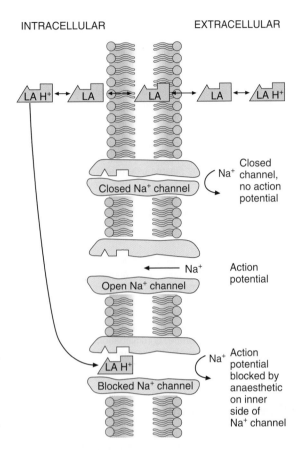

Fig. 18.2 Site and mechanism of action of local anaesthetics. Local anaesthetics are weak bases and exist in an equilibrium between ionised ($LA + H^+$) and nonionised (LA) forms. The nonionised form is lipid-soluble and crosses the axonal membrane, allowing the ionised form to bind to the intracellular end of the open Na^+ channel, holding it in an inactivated state and preventing further action potentials.

tachykinin type 1 receptors, glutamate, bradykinin B_2 and acetylcholine receptors may be involved in reducing nociceptive neurotransmission, the production of spinal anaesthesia and possibly some of the toxic effects of these drugs.

PHARMACOKINETICS

As seen previously, the speed of onset of local anaesthetic action is largely determined by the physicochemical properties of the drug molecule. The duration of action of local anaesthetics is dependent on the degree of receptor binding and on their rate of removal from the site of administration, rather than their systemic elimination by metabolism. Most local anaesthetics produce vasodilation at the site of injection, which will enhance their removal. However, cocaine, a local anaesthetic that also blocks noradrenaline reuptake by noradrenergic neurons (see Chapter 4), produces intense vasoconstriction. Because of the risk to local tissue integrity associated with the vasoconstriction, cocaine is never given by injection, and its medical use is restricted to topical anaesthesia in otolaryngology.

Once the local anaesthetic has diffused away from the site of administration, it enters the general circulation and undergoes metabolism. Most local anaesthetics have an intermediate amide bond, and are eliminated at least in part by hydrolysis of this bond by liver enzymes. The half-life of amide local anaesthetics within the circulation is generally between 1 and 3 hours. However, the plasma half-lives of anaesthetics such as procaine and tetracaine, which have an ester bond, are 3 minutes or less, since they are very rapidly hydrolysed by plasma esterases.

UNWANTED EFFECTS

Local effects

These occur at the site of administration and include irritation and inflammation. Local anaesthetics should not be injected into inflamed or infected tissues. Local ischaemia can occur if local anaesthetics are co-administered with a vasoconstrictor; therefore this should be avoided in the extremities, including the digits. Tissue damage with necrosis can follow inappropriate administration (e.g. accidental intra-arterial administration or spinal administration of an epidural dose).

Systemic effects

These are related to the anaesthetic action, and usually result from excessive plasma concentrations that affect other excitable membranes such as the heart (see the discussion on the antiarrhythmic action of lidocaine in Chapter 8). After regional anaesthesia, the maximum plasma drug concentration occurs within 30 minutes, requiring close observation for toxic effects during this period. Toxic plasma concentrations of drugs are more likely after accidental intravenous injection, or rapid absorption from highly vascular sites or from inflamed tissues. Severe toxicity can be treated with intravenous lipid emulsions, which partition the drug away from receptors within tissues, as an adjunct to resuscitation. Care should be taken to avoid inadvertent intravenous administration of a preparation containing adrenaline.

- **Central nervous system (CNS) effects.** High concentrations of local anaesthetics can produce light-headedness, paraesthesia, dizziness, nausea and vomiting, progressing to sedation and loss of consciousness. Severe toxicity produces convulsions and respiratory arrest. CNS toxicity tends to occur before cardiovascular toxicity, but this is not invariable.
- **Cardiovascular effects.** High plasma concentrations of local anaesthetic can cause tachycardia and arrhythmias. Serious arrhythmia is a particular problem with bupivacaine, particularly the $R(+)$-isomer, and is caused by its avid tissue binding in the heart. As a result of its high lipid solubility, high protein binding, and greater affinity for resting and inactive Na^+ channels, bupivacaine blocks the normal cardiac conducting system and predisposes to ventricular re-entrant pathways and intractable ventricular arrhythmias. Severe toxicity from bupivacaine is also associated with cardiovascular collapse from systemic vasodilation

and a negative inotropic effect. Levobupivacaine and ropivacaine have about the same local anaesthetic potency as bupivacaine, but less potential to produce cardiac effects, having less effect on cardiac Na^+ channels. In individuals with severe hypertension or unstable cardiac rhythm, the use of adrenaline with a local anaesthetic may be hazardous.

- **Allergy.** True allergy is rare, but can occur with ester agents due to their metabolism to p-aminobenzoic acid (PABA). For this reason, amide bond local anaesthetics are more commonly used.

TECHNIQUES OF ADMINISTRATION

The extent of local anaesthesia depends largely on the technique of administration.

SURFACE ADMINISTRATION

High concentrations (up to 10%) of drugs in an oily vehicle can slowly penetrate the skin or mucous membranes to give a localised area of anaesthesia. Lidocaine can be applied as a cream to an area before a minor skin procedure or venepuncture. Benzocaine is a relatively weak local anaesthetic that is included in some throat pastilles to produce anaesthesia of mucous membranes. Cocaine is restricted to topical use in otolaryngeal procedures, to produce vasoconstriction and reduce mucosal bleeding.

INFILTRATION ANAESTHESIA

A localised injection of an aqueous solution of local anaesthetic, sometimes with a vasoconstrictor, produces a local field of anaesthesia. The anaesthetic effect produced is more efficient than surface anaesthesia, but requires a relatively large dose. Smaller volumes can be used for field-block anaesthesia, involving subcutaneous injection close to nerves around the area to be anaesthetised. This technique is used extensively in dentistry.

PERIPHERAL NERVE BLOCK ANAESTHESIA

Injection of an aqueous solution around a nerve trunk produces a field of anaesthesia distal to the site of injection (regional anaesthesia). It can be used as the sole anaesthesia for selected surgical procedures or to reduce postoperative pain after general anaesthesia. The use of ultrasound-guided techniques has improved the placement of the anaesthetic and expanded the use of peripheral nerve blocks. Examples are axillary, supraclavicular, scalene, subclavian and sciatic and femoral nerve blocks. Concurrent infiltration of an opioid such as buprenorphine can almost double the duration of analgesia, but also increases the risk of postprocedural nausea and vomiting. Peripheral nerve block can also be used to produce temporary sympathetic nerve block, such as at the stellate ganglion (cervicothoracic sympathetic block) or lumbar sympathectomy.

EPIDURAL ANAESTHESIA

Injection or slow infusion of an aqueous solution of local anaesthetic via a catheter adjacent to the spinal column, but outside the dura mater, produces anaesthesia both above and below the site of injection after 15–30 minutes. The extent of anaesthesia depends on the volume of the drug administered and the rate of delivery. It is unaffected by the position of the person receiving the injection. Epidural anaesthesia is used extensively in childbirth for pain relief (using a local anaesthetic together with an opioid) and for surgical anaesthesia, either alone or in combination with a general anaesthetic. The catheter can also be used for postoperative analgesia using a local anaesthetic alone or combined with an opioid. The concentration of local anaesthetic used for epidural anaesthesia is the same as that for spinal anaesthesia, but the volume (10–20 mL), and therefore the dose, is greater to ensure homogeneous spread to nerve roots. For this reason, systemic unwanted effects are more frequent with epidural than with spinal anaesthesia. Sympathetic fibres are particularly sensitive to local anaesthetics (see Table 18.1), which can lead to hypotension. Hypotension is particularly a problem during pregnancy, probably related to the concurrent effects of high progesterone concentrations. Backache is a frequent postprocedural complication with both epidural and spinal anaesthesia.

SPINAL ANAESTHESIA

Spinal anaesthesia involves injection of an aqueous solution (1.5–2.5 mL) of local anaesthetic alone (often bupivacaine) or together with an opioid into the lumbar subarachnoid space, usually between the third and fourth lumbar vertebrae. The spread of anaesthetic within the subarachnoid space depends on the density of the solution (a solution in 10% glucose is more dense than cerebrospinal fluid) and the posture of the person during the first 10–15 minutes while the solution flows up or down the subarachnoid space. Anaesthesia is produced after about 5 minutes and can be used for surgical procedures below the umbilicus lasting for up to 2 hours. Spinal and epidural anaesthesia can be used together.

INTRAVENOUS REGIONAL ANAESTHESIA

This involves injection of a dilute solution of local anaesthetic into a limb after application of a tourniquet (Bier's block). It is used for manipulation of fractures and minor surgical procedures. Arterial blood flow must not be occluded for more than 20 minutes.

SELF-ASSESSMENT

True/false questions

1. The block produced by local anaesthetics is more rapid and complete when the nerve is actively firing.
2. Local anaesthetics have no systemic unwanted effects.
3. Local anaesthetics block smaller myelinated axons more effectively than larger myelinated axons.
4. The α_1-adrenoceptor antagonist prazosin is added to local anaesthetics to extend their duration of activity.
5. Local anaesthetics in their nonionised form penetrate the axon more readily than in their ionised form.
6. Ropivacaine is a long-acting local anaesthetic.
7. Bupivacaine has a high potential to produce cardiac arrhythmia.
8. The risk of systemic effects is greater with spinal anaesthesia than with epidural anaesthesia.

One-best-answer (OBA) question

Which of the following is the *most accurate* statement about local anaesthetics?
A. Raising the pH of a local anaesthetic solution will increase the speed of onset of anaesthesia.
B. Liver metabolism is the primary mechanism in terminating local anaesthetic action.
C. The effectiveness of a local anaesthetic is not altered by local tissue pH.
D. Direct effects on the blood vessel diameter of most commonly used local anaesthetics prolong their duration of action.
E. Adrenaline (epinephrine) is given with a local anaesthetic injection in digits and appendages to increase the duration of anaesthesia.

Extended-matching-item question

Choose the *most appropriate* drug from options A–F for each situation provided (1–4).
A. Cocaine
B. Adrenaline (epinephrine)
C. Salbutamol
D. Tetracaine
E. Lidocaine
F. Benzocaine
1. A child needs a minor surgical procedure on her nasopharynx, and you choose to use a single agent that could be administered topically to reduce mucous membrane bleeding.
2. An agent that would extend the duration and potency of a local anaesthetic.
3. An agent that could be applied topically to produce anaesthesia of the conjunctiva and would not cause vasoconstriction.
4. An agent that could be administered intravenously in the treatment of ventricular arrhythmias.

ANSWERS

True/false answers

1. **True.** This is because most local anaesthetics gain better access to binding sites in Na$^+$ channels that are in the open state.
2. **False.** If absorbed, systemic high doses of local anaesthetics can produce cardiovascular collapse and CNS depression.
3. **True.** For example, Aδ axons (2–5 μm diameter) are blocked more readily than motor fibres (12–20 μm diameter).

4. **False.** Prazosin is a vasodilator and would increase removal of the local anaesthetic from its injection site; a vasoconstrictor like adrenaline (epinephrine) is necessary.
5. **True.** The nonionised form is lipophilic and better able to cross the axon membrane.
6. **True.** Ropivacaine is a long-acting local anaesthetic (2–4 hours) similar to bupivacaine but is less arrhythmogenic.
7. **True.** The arrhythmogenic potential of bupivacaine is a result of its high lipid solubility, high protein binding, and greater affinity for resting and inactive Na⁺ channels.
8. **False.** The greater dose of local anaesthetic required for epidural anaesthesia carries a greater risk of unwanted systemic effects.

One-best-answer (OBA) answers

Answer A is correct.

A. Most local anaesthetics are weak bases (pK_a 7–9). Raising the pH increases the amount of the nonionised form, and therefore enhances lipid solubility and membrane penetration.
B. Local anaesthetic action is terminated mainly by uptake from tissues into the systemic circulation, not by hepatic metabolism.

C. Altered local pH could change the ratio of the ionised and nonionised forms of the local anaesthetic, affecting its potential to penetrate membranes (when nonionised) and block Na⁺ channels (as the ionised form).
D. With the exception of cocaine, local anaesthetics dilate blood vessels, hastening their removal from the site of injection and shortening their duration of action.
E. Adrenaline (epinephrine) should not be given with a local anaesthetic for injection in digits and appendages because of the risk of ischaemic necrosis.

Extended-matching-item answers

1. **Answer A**. Cocaine can be administered topically and, unlike other local anaesthetics, inhibits the neuronal uptake of released noradrenaline, resulting in vasoconstriction.
2. **Answer B**. Adrenaline (epinephrine) causes vasoconstriction and the administered local anaesthetic resides at its site of injection for a longer period.
3. **Answer D**. Tetracaine is poorly absorbed and, unlike cocaine, does not cause vasoconstriction; it is used topically for conjunctival anaesthesia.
4. **Answer E**. Lidocaine can be given intravenously for the treatment of ventricular arrhythmias (see Chapter 8).

FURTHER READING

Becker, D.E., Reed, K.L., 2012. Local anaesthetics: review of pharmacological considerations. Anaesth. Prog. 59, 90–102.

Kessler, J., Marhofer, P., Hopkins, P.M., et al., 2015. Peripheral regional anaesthesia and outcome: lessons learned from the last 10 years. Br. J. Anaesth. 114, 728–745.

Kirksey, M.A., Haskins, S.C., Cheng, J., et al., 2015. Local anaesthetic peripheral nerve block adjuvants for the prolongation of analgesia: a systematic qualitative review. PLoS ONE 10 (9), e0137312.

Scholz, A., 2002. Mechanisms of (local) anaesthetics on voltage-gated sodium and other ion channels. Br. J. Anaesth. 89, 52–61.

Compendium: local anaesthetics

Drug	Characteristics
Articaine	Used in dentistry. Half-life: 1 h
Benzocaine	Used in throat lozenges; minimal oral absorption
Bupivacaine	Used for local infiltration anaesthesia, peripheral nerve block, epidural block and sympathetic block. More cardiotoxic than lidocaine. Slow onset (1–10 min) and long duration of action (3–9 h). Half-life: 2–4 h
Cocaine	Used topically on mucosal surfaces (the only legal route). Very rapid onset of action. Profound CNS effects limit clinical usefulness. Half-life: 1–2 h
Levobupivacaine	An isomer of bupivacaine. Similar to bupivacaine but less cardiotoxic. Half-life: 1–3 h
Lidocaine	Used for local infiltration anaesthesia, intravenous regional anaesthesia, nerve blocks and dental anaesthesia; also used topically. Half-life: 1–2 h. For use in ventricular dysrhythmia, see Chapter 8
Mepivacaine	Used in dentistry. Available with or without adrenaline. Half-life: 2–3 h
Prilocaine	Used for local infiltration anaesthesia, intravenous anaesthesia, nerve blocks and dental anaesthesia; may cause methaemoglobinaemia (especially in infants). Half-life: 1–2 h
Procaine	Local infiltration anaesthesia, but rarely used now. Very rapid ester hydrolysis at site of injection and in plasma (minutes)
Ropivacaine	Similar to bupivacaine but less cardiotoxic. Used for epidural, major nerve block and field block anaesthesia. Half-life: 2–4 h
Tetracaine	Mostly used topically. Poorly absorbed and rapidly hydrolysed by pseudocholinesterase (3 min)

PAIN AND PAIN PERCEPTION

Pain is a complex phenomenon that involves the person's awareness of, and response to, a noxious stimulus. Pain is highly subjective to the individual, and psychological factors will determine the extent to which a person experiences suffering or distress (Fig. 19.1). Pain can be acute, lasting only until the initiating stimulus resolves; this is also called *nociceptive pain*. Pain can also become protracted and chronic. Ongoing tissue damage can produce chronic nociceptive pain. However, chronic pain may outlast the original trigger and become intractable as a result of persistent pathological change in the way that the nociceptive (pain-carrying) neuronal pathways function. This is called *neuropathic pain*.

Nociceptive pain is a defensive response to a variety of stimuli (e.g. mechanical, thermal or chemical) that activate nociceptor sensory units responsive to high-threshold noxious stimuli, on nerve endings. It is defensive, as it induces behaviour that avoids exacerbation of the pain and allows us to protect a damaged part of the body while it heals. Painful stimuli are transmitted to the central nervous system (CNS) by two types of peripheral nerve fibre. Fast nerve fibres connect through the neospinothalamic pathways, respond to mechanical and thermal stimuli and carry pain that is appreciated as sharp and localised. Slow nerve fibres connect through the paleospinothalamic pathways, respond to chemical stimuli and produce poorly localised aching, throbbing or burning sensations (Fig. 19.2).

Neuropathic pain results from neuronal activity that persists beyond the time expected for healing of the injury. Examples include phantom limb pain following amputation, and shingles causing pain well beyond the healing of the vesicles. Neuropathic pain can be spontaneous (stimulus-independent), where it is usually described by the sufferer as shooting or lancinating sensations, electric shock-like pain or an abnormal unpleasant sensation (dysaesthesia). Alternatively, it can be an exaggerated response to a painful stimulus (hyperalgesia) or a painful response to a trivial stimulus (allodynia). Some pain states have mixed nociceptive and neuropathic elements – for example, mechanical spinal pain with local nerve damage such as radiculopathy or myelopathy.

The pathophysiological and molecular explanations for nociceptive and neuropathic pain and the endogenous responses that modulate pain are complex. In brief, the genesis of nociceptive pain results from initial stimulation of nociceptors on afferent sensory neurons by thermal, mechanical or chemical stimuli (Fig. 19.3). Nociceptors carry many surface receptors that modulate neuronal sensitivity to stimulation, such as those for γ-aminobutyric acid (GABA), opioids, bradykinin, histamine, serotonin (5-hydroxytryptamine, 5-HT) and capsaicin, as well as mechano-sensitive ion channels (responsive to touch, pressure, etc.). The particular type of painful stimulus may determine which receptors or ion channels are activated. Activation of the ion channels or receptors results in an influx of Na^+/Ca^{2+} sufficient to generate action potentials in the nerve (see Fig. 19.3). Pain-conducting neurones are generally electrically silent and transmit impulses only when activated. In response to tissue damage or a sufficient mechanical stimulus, nociceptors are activated locally and sensitise the area to painful stimuli.

Pain is conducted by two types of axon, Aδ fibre axons (rapidly conducting) and C fibre axons (slowly conducting), that enter both the dorsal and ventral horns of the spinal cord and link to ascending pathways. The afferent impulse is transmitted across synapses in the spinal cord and in the projections of the ascending pathways to the thalamus, and from there to the reticular formation and the cortex. Neurotransmitters in these central pathways include excitatory substances such as glutamate, tachykinins (neurokinins and substance P) and calcitonin gene-related peptide (CGRP). Synaptic transmission responsible for nociceptive pain can be reduced by local inhibitory neurons, mediated by GABA. There are also important descending modulatory pathways arising from the locus coeruleus (LC), periaqueductal grey matter (PAG) and nucleus raphe magnus (NRM) that inhibit ascending

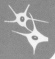

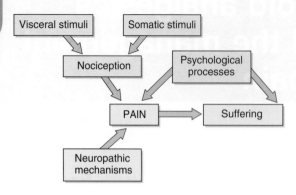

Fig. 19.1 The origin of pain and suffering.

pain pathways, with a further host of neurotransmitters including endogenous opioids, noradrenaline (acting on α_2-adrenoceptors) and serotonin. Activation of these systems inhibits neuronal Na^+/Ca^{2+} influx and enhances K^+ efflux, which produces hyperpolarisation of neurons in the pain pathways. This prevents the generation of nociceptive action potentials (Figs 19.4 and 19.5). The endogenous cannabinoids (anandamide and 2-arachidonyl glycerol) may also have modulatory functions in the descending pathways.

Persistent activation of pain pathways generates intracellular protein synthesis through stimulation of the proto-oncogene c-Fos and various inducible transcription factors in CNS neurons. These factors are responsible for the many changes in neuronal structure and the neuronal proliferation that occur in pain-transmitting pathways with chronic pain.

In neuropathic and other chronic pain states, the following mechanisms may be important:

■ Sensitisation of afferent inputs: This may include recruitment and activation of silent nociceptors and a lower threshold for generation of action potentials in the spinal cord (see Figs 19.3 and 19.5). Central sensitisation is also important with excessive neurotransmitter release. Abnormal voltage-gated Na^+ channel expression may also be important in both peripheral and central sensitisation.

■ Dysfunctional descending pain-modulatory and pain-facilitatory pathways: The functioning of the descending modulatory pathway (see Fig. 19.4) may be impaired by persistent nociceptive pain. Overactivity of endogenous pain facilitatory pathways that run in tracts from the medulla to the spinal dorsal horn then maintain neuropathic pain.

■ Loss of inhibitory neurons and generation of new synapses that act as nociceptive neurons (neuronal plasticity): In neuropathic pain, Aβ nerve fibres that normally transmit tactile stimuli can undergo phenotypic change and take on the properties of a nociceptive neuron.

ANALGESIC DRUGS

Nonsteroidal antiinflammatory drugs (NSAIDs) and opioids are the major classes of pain-relieving (analgesic) drugs. They act at different points in the pain-transmitting pathways to influence the production and recognition of pain (see Figs 19.3 and 19.4).

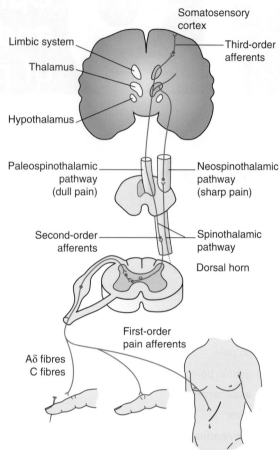

Fig. 19.2 **Ascending pathways of pain perception.** Ascending pathways are activated following stimulation of afferent sensory nociceptive nerve terminals. Thermal and mechanical influences and the release of mediators (bradykinin, serotonin, prostaglandins) can stimulate and sensitise the sensory nerve terminals of pain fibres, resulting in increased cation influx, depolarisation and generation of action potentials (see Fig. 19.3). Onward afferent transmission of ascending nerve impulses at the synapses in the dorsal horn involves transmitters such as substance P, glutamate and calcitonin gene-related peptide (CGRP; see Fig. 19.5). Hyperexcitability of pain fibres can also be promoted by other mediators. Prolonged activation of the nociceptive pathways can produce pathophysiological and phenotypic changes, resulting in neuropathic pain that persists when the original pathological cause of the pain has resolved, and generation of nociceptive signals can occur at low levels of axonal stimulation.

Nonsteroidal antiinflammatory drugs

NSAIDs block the peripheral generation of nociceptive impulses. Prostaglandins increase Na^+/Ca^{2+} influx into nociceptors and sensitise them to thermal, mechanical or chemical stimuli. NSAIDs inhibit the production of prostaglandins by the cyclo-oxygenase type 1 and type 2 (COX-1, COX-2) isoenzymes and thereby reduce the sensitivity

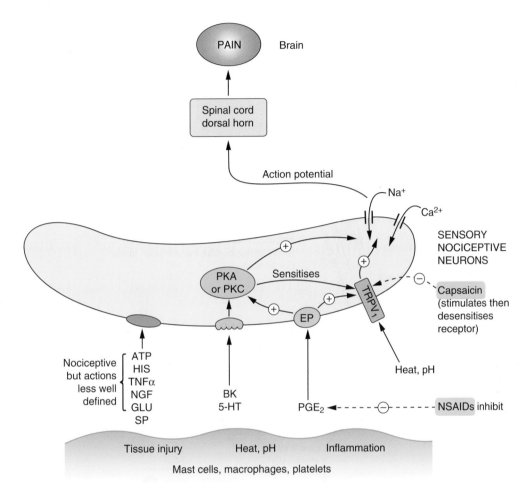

Fig. 19.3 **Mediators involved in the genesis and modulation of pain.** Numerous mediators are able to stimulate or sensitise primary sensory neurons (nociceptors), leading to activation of nociceptive fibres. Tissue injury and other noxious stimuli such as heat or extremes of pH can stimulate the release of substances that act to promote pain, such as bradykinin (BK) and serotonin (5-hydroxytryptamine, 5-HT). Prostaglandin E_2 (PGE$_2$) acting at prostaglandin E receptors (EP) sensitises the nerve endings to the actions of nociceptive mediators, including BK and 5-HT. Adenosine triphosphate (ATP) and histamine (HIS) also have nociceptive actions, acting in poorly defined ways. Heat and H^+ ions stimulate the transient receptor potential vanilloid 1 (TRPV$_1$) receptor, producing pain. The TRPV$_1$ receptor is also sensitised by many other mediators. Capsaicin and other TRPV$_1$ receptor stimulants desensitise the receptor on persistent stimulation, resulting in an analgesic effect. Nonsteroidal antiinflammatory drugs (NSAIDs) inhibit the production of PGE$_2$. Overall the effect of nociceptive stimuli is to depolarise the neuron, setting up action potentials in the fibres to the dorsal horn and pain-perceiving areas of the brain. Substance P (SP) and calcitonin gene-related peptide (CGRP) may also be involved in nociception. *GLU,* Glutamate; *NGF,* nerve growth factor; *PKA,* protein kinase A; *PKC,* protein kinase C; *TNFα,* tumour necrosis factor α.

of sensory nociceptive nerve endings to agents released by injured tissue that initiate pain, such as bradykinin and substance P. NSAIDs may also inhibit pain pathways in the CNS. Paracetamol, although not usually considered to be an NSAID, may inhibit prostaglandins in the spinal cord. These drugs are considered fully in Chapter 29.

Opioids

Opioids produce their effects via specific receptors that are closely associated with the neuronal pathways that

transmit pain from the periphery to the CNS. They act on the spinal cord and limbic system and stimulate the long descending inhibitory pathways from the midbrain to the dorsal horn.

Nonopioid, non-NSAID analgesics

A variety of drugs that were developed for other purposes are being used increasingly for their analgesic actions when NSAIDs and opioids are less effective – for example, in neuropathic pain (see Table 19.1).

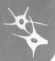

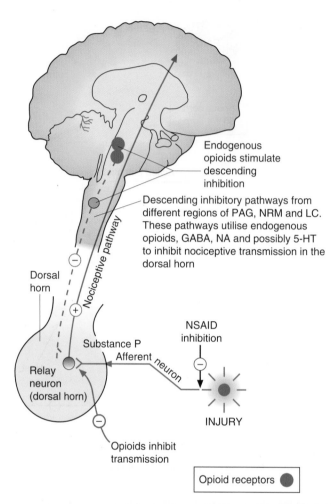

Fig. 19.4 **Transmitters and receptors for pain perception and control.** The afferent nociceptive pathways are subject to inhibitory control. Opioids act at opioid receptor-rich sites in the periaqueductal grey matter (PAG), the nucleus raphe magnus (NRM) and other midbrain sites to stimulate descending inhibitory fibres that reduce nociceptive transmission in the dorsal horn. Descending noradrenergic pathways from the locus coeruleus (LC) are also involved. Opioids also act at a local level in the dorsal horn (see Fig. 19.5). Inhibitory modulation of nociceptive transmission via local nerve networks also results from actions of other agents (see Fig. 19.5). *5-HT*, 5-Hydroxytryptamine (serotonin); *GABA*, γ-aminobutyric acid; *NA*, noradrenaline; *NSAID*, nonsteroidal anti-inflammatory drug.

OPIOID ANALGESICS

buprenorphine, codeine, diamorphine (heroin), dihydrocodeine, fentanyl, methadone, morphine, oxycodone, tramadol

Opioid is a term used for both naturally occurring and synthetic molecules that produce their effects by an agonist action at opioid receptors. The terms *opiate analgesic* (specifically, a drug derived from the juice of the opium poppy, *Papaver somniferum*) and *narcotic analgesic* (which literally means a 'stupor-inducing pain killer') are no longer preferred.

Mechanism of action

The brain produces several endogenous opioid peptide neurotransmitters, most of which contain the amino acid sequence Tyr-Gly-Gly-Phe as the message domain and act via specific opioid receptors. Among these are:

- enkephalins, two pentapeptides containing the core amino acid sequence linked to either leucine (leu-enkephalin) or methionine (met-enkephalin);
- dynorphins A and B;
- β-endorphin, a 31-amino-acid peptide with met-enkephalin at its carboxyl end;
- endomorphins 1 and 2 that have Tyr-Pro-Phe and Tyr-Pro-Trp message domain sequences.

All opioid peptides are derived by selective cleavage of larger precursor molecules. Three major classes of opioid

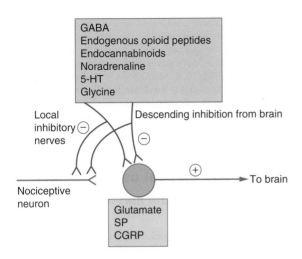

GABA
Endogenous opioid peptides
Endocannabinoids
Noradrenaline
5-HT
Glycine

Local inhibitory nerves

Descending inhibition from brain

Nociceptive neuron

To brain

Glutamate
SP
CGRP

***Fig. 19.5* Neurotransmitter substances involved in the genesis and modulation of pain.** Inhibitory modulation of nociception can occur via activation of the descending regulatory pathways and also by actions of local interneurons. *5-HT*, 5-Hydroxytryptamine (serotonin); *CGRP*, calcitonin gene-related peptide; *GABA*, γ-aminobutyric acid; *SP*, substance P.

Box 19.1 Effects of opioid receptors

Mu (μ) or MOP receptors
   Analgesia (supraspinal μ_1, spinal μ_2)
   Respiratory (μ_2)
   Euphoria
   Miosis
   Physical dependence
   Reward
   Sedation
   Inhibition of gastrointestinal motility
Kappa (κ) or KOP receptors
   Analgesia (spinal, peripheral)
   Sedation
   Miosis
   Dysphoria
Delta (δ) or DOP receptors
   Analgesia (spinal)
   Respiratory depression
   Inhibition of gastrointestinal motility
   Mood and emotional responses
Nociceptin (NOP) receptors
   Modulation of analgesic activity?

---

receptors have been identified, which mediate distinct effects (Box 19.1):

- μ (mu) receptor (MOP receptor),
- κ (kappa) receptor (KOP receptor),
- δ (delta) receptor (DOP receptor).

β-Endorphin and endomorphins act at μ receptors, met-enkephalin acts at μ and δ receptors, leu-enkephalin acts at δ receptors, and dynorphins act at κ receptors. There is a distinctive regional distribution of opioid peptides and their receptors in the CNS, with high concentrations in the limbic system and spinal cord. These regions also contain high

Table 19.1 Mechanisms of some nonopioid, non-NSAID drugs used as adjuncts in the control of pain

Drug	Mechanism
The mechanisms of pain control by these classes of drugs (listed by chapter number) are imperfectly understood, and some are selective in their areas of analgesic activity. GABA, γ-Aminobutyric acid; NMDA, N-methyl-D-aspartate; TRPV₁, transient receptor potential vanilloid 1 receptor.	
Clonidine	α_2-Adrenoceptor agonism. See Chapter 6
Ketamine, dextromethorphan	Glutamate (NMDA) receptor antagonism. See Chapter 17
Local anaesthetics	Neuronal Na^+ channel blockade. See Chapter 18
Tricyclic antidepressants (imipramine, amitriptyline)	Increased monoamine neurotransmitter availability. See Chapter 22
Gabapentin, pregabalin	Increased GABA concentrations. See Chapter 23
Carbamazepine, lamotrigine	Membrane stabilisation by Na^+ channel blockade; attenuation of glutamate-related synaptic transmission. See Chapter 23
Baclofen	$GABA_B$ receptor agonism; attenuation of glutamate-related synaptic transmission. See Chapter 24
Cannabinoids	Stimulation of cannabinoid (CB) receptors. See Chapter 32
Bisphosphonates	Inhibition of bone resorption. See Chapter 42
Glucocorticoids	Antiinflammatory activity. See Chapter 44
Capsaicin	Substance P depletion; stimulation of vanilloid (TRPV₁) receptor followed by desensitisation

concentrations of various enkephalinases, enzymes which rapidly hydrolyse endogenous opioids. The physiological effects produced by the different opioid receptors are due to their specific neuronal distributions.

A fourth member of the opioid receptor family has been identified, named the nociceptin receptor (NOP) after its specific endogenous agonist, which does not bind the major opioid peptides. It is widely distributed in the brain and has antianalgesic activity that may modulate the activity of other opioid receptors.

Opioid receptors are found on the presynaptic and postsynaptic membranes of neurons in CNS pain pathways, and also in the peripheral nervous system. The postsynaptic actions inhibit neuronal depolarisation, and the presynaptic actions inhibit neurotransmitter release. All opioid receptors are coupled to inhibitory G-proteins (G_i/G_0), and receptor activation has many intracellular consequences:

- inhibition of adenylyl cyclase with reduced intracellular generation of cyclic adenosine monophosphate, which reduces neurotransmitter release;
- inhibition of voltage-gated N-type Ca^{2+} channels in target neurons, which reduces neurotransmitter release;
- activation of voltage-gated inwardly rectifying K^+ channels, which hyperpolarises the target cells, making them less responsive to depolarising impulses;
- phosphorylation of extracellular signal-regulated kinase (ERK) and other mitogen-activated protein (MAP) kinases, which may have actions on neural cell growth and proliferation;
- phosphorylation, desensitisation and internalisation of the opioid receptors, the extent of which varies among receptor ligands and may underlie the development of opioid drug tolerance.

Morphine and synthetic opioid analgesics produce their analgesic effects by acting as agonists at opioid receptors in the CNS. The analgesic action of opioids is the result of a complex series of neuronal interactions:

- In the nucleus raphe magnus of the brain, μ-receptor stimulation decreases activity in inhibitory GABA-ergic neurons that project to descending inhibitory serotonergic neurons in the brainstem. These neurons in turn connect presynaptically with afferent nociceptive fibres in the dorsal horn of the spinal cord. Inhibition of the GABA-ergic neurons permits increased firing of the descending inhibitory serotonergic neurons. Analgesia is produced by inhibition of the release of the pain pathway mediators, substance P, glutamate and calcitonin gene-related peptide from the afferent nociceptive neurons (see Fig. 19.5).
- Activation of κ-receptors antagonises the analgesia produced by μ-receptor stimulation, but there is a direct spinal analgesic effect from unopposed κ-receptor activation.
- Opioid receptors are also present on peripheral nociceptive neurons, and a κ-receptor agonist reduces their sensitivity to pain stimuli, particularly in inflamed tissues.
- Nonneuronal κ-receptors suppress the inflammatory response, and are found on endothelial cells, T-lymphocytes and macrophages.

Opioid drugs show receptor selectivity and can have agonist, partial agonist or antagonist properties at various opioid receptor types (see the compendium at the end of the chapter). Opioid analgesics can be classified by their activity at opioid receptors:

- Full agonists: These act principally at μ-receptors and include morphine, diamorphine, fentanyl, pethidine, codeine and dihydrocodeine. They also have weak agonist activity at δ- and κ-receptors.
- Mixed agonist–antagonist: Pentazocine has agonist effects at the κ-receptor (and, to a lesser extent, the δ-receptor) and is a weak μ-receptor antagonist.
- Mixed partial agonist–antagonist: Buprenorphine is a potent partial agonist at the μ-receptor and has antagonist activity at κ-receptors. The latter action will enhance the analgesic action produced via the μ-receptors.

Some opioids have additional actions at nonopioid receptors or other cellular targets: meptazinol is a μ-receptor agonist with muscarinic receptor agonist activity, and tramadol and methadone are μ-receptor agonists that also inhibit neuronal noradrenaline and serotonin uptake. The supplementary actions of tramadol and methadone contribute to their analgesic actions, since amine-mediated neurotransmission potentiates descending inhibitory pain pathways (see Fig. 19.4). Methadone is also an antagonist at glutamate N-methyl-D-aspartate (NMDA) receptors, an action which can also inhibit pain transmission (see Fig. 19.5).

Opioid receptor antagonists such as naloxone have no analgesic actions and are used in the treatment of opioid overdose (see Chapter 53).

Effects and clinical uses

Effects on the central nervous system

Analgesia

The analgesia produced by opioids is most effective for acute or chronic nociceptive pain, but can be helpful for some types of neuropathic pain. In addition to the antinociceptive effect, opioids alter the perception of pain, making it less unpleasant. This supraspinal effect, possibly at the limbic system, is less marked with some opioids such as pentazocine. Opioid analgesics have no antiinflammatory effect. In fact, morphine can cause release of the inflammatory mediator histamine, which produces peripheral vasodilation and hypotension.

Full μ-receptor agonists are the most powerful opioid analgesics (see above and the compendium for details of full and partial agonists). However, some full μ-receptor agonists (e.g. codeine) have a low affinity for μ-receptors and have a limited analgesic effect. There is growing evidence that the antagonist action of methadone at NMDA receptors can produce effective analgesia in people who have become tolerant to high doses of morphine (discussed later). Short-acting opioids such as fentanyl and remifentanil are used intravenously to provide analgesia during general anaesthesia (see Chapter 17).

The ceiling analgesic effect of a μ-receptor partial agonist is lower than that of a full agonist. If a person receiving high doses of a potent full μ-receptor agonist is given a μ-receptor partial agonist (e.g. buprenorphine) or a μ-receptor antagonist (e.g. pentazocine), then some of the full agonist molecules will be displaced from receptor sites by the less effective partial agonist or antagonist molecules. The degree of analgesia may then be reduced, and in dependent individuals withdrawal symptoms can be produced (discussed later).

Euphoria and dysphoria

The use of morphine is often associated with an elevated sense of well-being (euphoria, mediated by μ-receptors), an action that contributes considerably to its analgesic efficacy. Agonist activity at κ-receptors produces the opposite effect (dysphoria); therefore the degree of euphoria produced will depend on the receptor-binding characteristics of the drug.

Respiratory depression

Opioids reduce the sensitivity of the respiratory centre to stimulation by carbon dioxide at doses that produce analgesia. Respiratory depression is a common cause of death in opioid overdose. Occasionally, the effect on respiratory rate can be of clinical benefit; for example, intravenous morphine relieves the dyspnoea associated with acute pulmonary oedema, and morphine is used orally or by subcutaneous infusion for the treatment of breathlessness in palliative care. Meptazinol and tramadol are claimed to cause less respiratory depression than other opioids.

Suppression of the cough centre

Opioids possess an antitussive action. Compounds such as codeine and dextromethorphan are effective for cough suppression (see Chapter 13), despite having relatively weak, or no, analgesic effects.

Vomiting

Opioids stimulate the chemoreceptor trigger zone, and morphine causes vomiting in up to 30% of people. Tolerance to the nausea and vomiting can occur with repeated doses. Powerful opioids such as morphine are usually given with an antiemetic (see Chapter 32), particularly when used for acute pain.

Miosis

Opioids stimulate the third cranial nerve nucleus, producing pupillary constriction. Pinpoint pupils, together with coma and slow respiration, are signs of opioid overdose (see Chapter 53).

Endocrine effects

Opioids inhibit the hypothalamic–pituitary–adrenal axis, leading to a progressive decline in plasma cortisol levels (see Chapter 44). They also increase prolactin release and decrease luteinising hormone release, which leads to testosterone deficiency in men and a reduction in oestrogen synthesis in women (see Chapter 45). Therefore long-term opioid treatment is associated with osteoporosis and an increased risk of fractures. Men can benefit from testosterone replacement during long-term opioid use (see Chapter 46).

Peripheral effects
Gastrointestinal tract

Opioids produce a general increase in resting tone of the gut wall and sphincters. These effects arise from stimulation of both μ- and κ-receptors on neuronal plexuses in the gut wall. An increase in biliary pressure caused by opioid-induced spasm at the sphincter of Oddi can exacerbate biliary colic. In the stomach, a decrease in motility and pyloric tone contributes to anorexia, nausea and vomiting. In the small and large intestines there is increased segmenting activity and decreased propulsive activity, which is associated with constipation. Up to 80% of people who take regular opioids will need a laxative. Methylnaltrexone, a specific antagonist of peripheral opioid receptors, is used to treat opioid-induced constipation during palliative care when conventional laxatives are inadequate. The effects of opioids on gastrointestinal motility make them useful in the treatment of diarrhoea (see Chapter 35). Pethidine and tramadol have less effect on the gastrointestinal tract than equi-analgesic doses of morphine.

Cardiovascular system

Opioids have little effect on the heart or circulation, except at high doses that can depress the medullary vasomotor centre.

Hypotension can occur with parenteral use of morphine, probably because of histamine release.

Other systems

Opioids have minor effects on other systems. For example, there is an increase in the tone of the bladder wall and sphincter, which can lead to urinary retention. There is increasing evidence that the long-term use of opioids suppresses immune function by inhibiting the development and differentiation of many types of immune cells. The clinical relevance of this is not known.

Tolerance and dependence

Tolerance and dependence during continuous opioid administration result from changes in the functioning of opioid receptors. Adaptive changes mean that more of the drug is necessary to produce the same effect (tolerance), and withdrawal of the drug produces adverse physiological effects until the compensatory changes are reset (dependence).

Tolerance to opioids occurs in two ways. Associative (learned) tolerance has a major psychological component. Nonassociative (adaptive) tolerance involves downregulation of opioid receptor signalling due to desensitisation, including uncoupling of the receptors from G-proteins, or receptor internalisation within endocytotic vesicles. These processes are induced to varying extents by different opioid receptor agonists. Other mechanisms of tolerance include increased firing of neurons in the noradrenergic pathways of the locus coeruleus (an area of the brain involved in the physiological response to stress, which is rich in inhibitory opioid receptors), activation of the reward pathway in the brain (see Chapter 54) and increased activity at NMDA receptors for excitatory glutamate-mediated neurotransmission in spinal and supraspinal circuits. Tolerance to the analgesic, euphoric and emetic actions and to respiratory depression develops rapidly during regular opioid administration, but there is less tolerance to constipation or miosis. A high degree of cross-tolerance is shown by many opioids; consequently, individuals who develop tolerance to one opioid are often (but not invariably) tolerant to another. Opioid-induced NMDA receptor activation can also produce abnormal pain sensitivity at spinal cord dorsal horn cells. This sensitisation process can be confused with tolerance and lead to opioid dose escalation. Methadone may be useful in this situation (discussed previously).

Dependence manifests itself as a withdrawal syndrome, which can be precipitated when individuals who have taken the drug for a long period of time have their intake stopped or are given an opioid antagonist or partial agonist (see Chapter 54). This is most often a problem for people who abuse the drug, but can occur from long-term intake of a prescribed opioid.

During the first 12 hours after opioid withdrawal, effects such as nervousness, sweating and craving are largely psychological, because they can be alleviated by the administration of a placebo. Following this period the effects of physiological dependence manifest themselves; for example, dilated pupils, anorexia, weakness, depression, insomnia, gastrointestinal and skeletal muscle cramps, increased respiratory rate, pyrexia, piloerection with goose pimples, and diarrhoea. The time course for the development and resolution of these symptoms varies among the opioids.

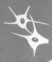

In the case of morphine, the maximum severity of withdrawal effects occurs quickly (after about 1–2 days) and subsides rapidly (about 5–10 days), and the intensity of the symptoms is often intolerable.

In contrast to morphine, withdrawal from methadone produces delayed and far less intense withdrawal effects (peak severity at almost 1 week and symptoms persist for about 3 weeks), because it has a very long half-life. Therefore morphine- or heroin-dependent individuals are often transferred from their drug of abuse to methadone prior to withdrawal (opioid-substitution therapy). Methadone also produces less euphoria than morphine or heroin. After a period of treatment with methadone, the methadone dosage is gradually reduced and the person undergoes a more tolerable withdrawal. Buprenorphine is used as an alternative to methadone, and also gives a low intensity of withdrawal symptoms. It can be taken for 6 days in a rapid detoxification programme, or as long-term maintenance for reducing relapse in people who are addicted to opioids, since its partial agonist activity blocks the 'high' from illicit opioid use.

Rapid in-hospital tapering of opioids over 2 weeks has an early 80% withdrawal success rate. On an outpatient basis, slow tapering over 6 months is more successful than rapid withdrawal, but there is only a 40% success rate. Long-term buprenorphine therapy, combined with high-intensity psychosocial group therapy, has achieved up to 75% withdrawal rates after 1 year. Detoxification from opioids can be helped by the presynaptic α_2-adrenoceptor agonists clonidine or lofexidine (a clonidine analogue with fewer unwanted effects). These inhibit the excessive sympathetic nervous system activity associated with opioid withdrawal, such as lacrimation, rhinorrhoea, muscle pain, joint pain and gastrointestinal symptoms. However, lethargy, insomnia and restlessness persist.

Naltrexone is a μ- and κ-receptor antagonist and a weak agonist at the δ-receptor. It blocks the effects of opioid agonists, and is used for prevention of relapse in people who were dependent on opioids, and who have withdrawn for at least 7–10 days.

Pharmacokinetics

Most opioids are available for oral use. Buprenorphine is formulated for sublingual absorption, and fentanyl as a sublingual or buccal tablet or as a nasal spray for rapid pain relief. Some opioids, such as morphine, buprenorphine, meptazinol, methadone, oxycodone and tramadol, can be given by intravenous or intramuscular injection. Morphine and oxycodone can also be given by subcutaneous infusion in palliative care. Diamorphine is more potent than morphine, and delivery of effective doses by subcutaneous infusion requires smaller fluid volumes, which can be useful for emaciated people. Morphine and pentazocine are available as suppositories. Fentanyl and buprenorphine can be delivered transdermally via self-adhesive patches for prolonged analgesia.

Some opioids, such as morphine, have a low and variable absorption across the gut wall, and the dose should be much smaller when given parenterally to achieve equivalent analgesia and minimise unwanted effects. Opioids are eliminated by hepatic metabolism. A metabolite of morphine, morphine 6-glucuronide, has two- to fourfold greater analgesic activity than the parent compound and is excreted by the

kidney. The dose of morphine must therefore be reduced in renal failure. Diamorphine is an acetylated morphine derivative that is converted to morphine by hydrolysis in plasma and in most tissues, including the brain. Codeine is a prodrug that is metabolised by CYP2D6 to several active metabolites. Codeine 6-glucuronide is responsible for most of the analgesic activity, while about 5% is converted to morphine. CYP2D6 shows genetic polymorphism, and about 10% of people have low CYP2D6 activity and a reduced analgesic response to codeine.

Most opioid analgesics have short half-lives in the range of 1–6 hours. For long-term pain control, morphine and some other powerful opioids are often given as a modified-release formulation to prolong the duration of action. Fentanyl has a short half-life, but when given via a transdermal delivery patch, pain relief lasts 12–24 hours due to slow drug delivery. In addition, the effect persists for several hours after removing the patch, owing to build-up of a subcutaneous drug reservoir at the site of application. Care is necessary both to maintain analgesia and to avoid unwanted opioid effects if the dose of fentanyl is increased or fentanyl patches are replaced by another opioid.

Unwanted effects

The unwanted effects of opioids are caused by their actions on those opioid receptors that are not the primary site for therapeutic benefit. For example, respiratory depression and constipation are unwanted effects when an opioid is used as an analgesic, but the same effects are therapeutically beneficial in the treatment of breathlessness or diarrhoea. Tolerance and dependence can also be regarded as unwanted problems associated with long-term use.

NONOPIOID, NON-NSAID AGENTS USED FOR ANALGESIA

A diverse group of drugs that are not conventional analgesics are used for pain control in circumstances where opioids and NSAIDs are ineffective (see Table 19.1). These are dealt with individually in the next section, and the detailed pharmacology of the drugs is given in the chapters describing their main clinical uses.

PAIN MANAGEMENT

THE ANALGESIC LADDER

Appropriate management of pain depends on its origin and severity. The analgesic ladder developed by the World Health Organization (WHO) is useful for choosing drug therapy appropriate to the level of pain (Box 19.2). An adjuvant drug (see Table 19.1) may be given concurrently at any step.

Step 1 drugs

Paracetamol (see Chapter 29) is often suitable for mild pain, such as postoperative dental pain and headache, but may be ineffective for back, hip and knee pain. An NSAID (see Chapter

Step 1. Nonopioid analgesics (e.g. paracetamol, nonsteroidal antiinflammatory drugs)
Step 2. Opioid suitable for moderate pain ± nonopioid analgesics
Step 3. Opioid suitable for severe pain ± nonopioid analgesics
   Adjuvant (nonopioid, non-NSAID) analgesics may be required at any step (see text and Table 19.1).

29) may be more appropriate if there is local inflammation, but the choice will be determined by the balance of benefits and risks of NSAIDs. Examples of pain that respond better to an NSAID are soft-tissue injury, tissue compression, visceral pain caused by pleural or peritoneal irritation, and bone pain caused by metastatic deposits. Bone metastases promote local secretion of prostaglandins, and NSAIDs can be particularly effective. Individual responses to an NSAID vary; about 60% of people will respond to an alternative drug even if the first was ineffective.

Step 2 drugs

A weak opioid should be added to a step 1 drug for moderate pain, or when the response to a step 1 drug is inadequate. Opioids suitable for moderate pain include codeine and dihydrocodeine. These are often used in combination with paracetamol, such as the compound formulation co-codamol (codeine and paracetamol), although the dose of opioid in some combinations is too low to produce useful additional analgesia. Tramadol has been advocated at this stage, but it is no more effective than co-codamol, and claims that it has less effect on respiration and gastrointestinal motility are of uncertain clinical importance. Consideration should be given to the risk of dependence if long-term use of an opioid is proposed.

Step 3 drugs

The drug of choice for moderate to severe pain is morphine. It is usually effective orally, using a rapid-onset formulation for initial pain control. Doctors are often unwilling to give adequate doses of strong opioid because of concern about dependence. In severe chronic pain this is not an issue, and it should not be used as a reason for avoiding the use of morphine in noncancer pain. Opioid dependence is not a problem when opioids are given appropriately for the relief of pain.

ACUTE PAIN

Acute pain usually has an obvious cause and is often accompanied by anxiety. For rapid pain relief in a self-limiting condition (e.g. migraine), a readily absorbed, short-acting drug will be appropriate. For more protracted conditions (e.g. sprains), a long-acting drug may be helpful to improve adherence by reducing the frequency of administration.

   The principles of the WHO analgesic ladder should be followed. Very severe acute pain (e.g. with myocardial infarction) will require a powerful opioid such as morphine given intravenously for rapid effect. Intramuscular injection should be avoided if possible, since severe pain is often accompanied by sympathetic nervous system stimulation, which produces peripheral vasoconstriction and thereby delays drug absorption. Some acute severe pain, such as that arising postoperatively or from trauma, renal colic, cholecystitis, pancreatitis or sickle cell crisis, should be treated initially with a powerful opioid and then less powerful analgesics as the condition resolves. This involves applying the steps of the WHO analgesic ladder in reverse.

POSTOPERATIVE PAIN

Postoperative pain has many components, including hyperalgesia in the area of the incision, local ischaemia in the wound and central neuronal sensitisation in addition to the inflammatory response to surgery. Many surveys show that the treatment of postoperative pain is often inadequate. There is some evidence that intraoperative and postoperative opioid use can increase the risk of hyperalgesia (acute opioid-induced hyperalgesia), an effect that can be modulated by the use of α_2-adrenoceptor agonists (such as clonidine), cyclo-oxygenase (COX)-2 inhibitors (see Chapter 29) or glutamate NMDA receptor antagonists (such as ketamine or methadone).

   Persistent postsurgical pain is common, and is usually considered to be present if symptoms continue for more than 2 months after the procedure. There are many surgical, psychosocial, genetic and environmental factors that predict the development of this condition. Postoperative regional anaesthesia and combination analgesic regimens can reduce the risk of developing the syndrome. Although the principles of the WHO pain ladder are still important for the management of postoperative pain, combinations of regional anaesthetic techniques (see Chapter 18) and analgesics (including those more commonly used for neuropathic pain) after surgery may be important to ensure optimal outcomes.

CHRONIC PAIN

Chronic pain is usually defined as pain lasting for at least 3 months, or at least until acute tissue pathology that initiated the pain would have been expected to heal. It can be a result of persistent nociceptive stimulation or can have a neuropathic origin. There are numerous psychosocial contributors to the development of chronic pain as well as physical pathology, and therefore management of much chronic pain is more effective if facilitated by multidisciplinary pain teams. Drug therapy is not the only solution for chronic pain, and depending on the cause, nonpharmacological or local treatments are often appropriate. Examples include:

- surgery for neoplastic, structural or ischaemic disorders;
- physical methods such as acupuncture, or transcutaneous electrical nerve stimulation (TENS), which activates spinal inhibitory neurons by acting as a counterirritant and local anaesthetic nerve block (see Chapter 18);
- behavioural modification (e.g. biofeedback, relaxation techniques, hypnosis);
- a corticosteroid (see Chapter 44) for raised intracranial pressure or spinal cord compression, or to reduce local inflammation which can be associated with cancer.

Many forms of chronic noncancer pain, such as fibromyalgia, osteoarthritis or low-back pain, respond better to adjuvant analgesics such as tricyclic antidepressants or anticonvulsant drugs (see the section on neuropathic pain later in the chapter) than to conventional analgesics. Combinations of both adjuvant and conventional analgesics are often used. If conventional analgesia is needed (especially for nociceptive pain and several types of cancer-related pain), then the principles of escalation of analgesia described by the WHO analgesic ladder should be followed.

For severe chronic nociceptive pain, morphine is usually used. However, the evidence for efficacy of powerful opioids in noncancer pain is limited, and the risk of unwanted effects and dependence are considerable. When an opioid is appropriate, a low initial dosage of morphine should be commenced and the daily dosage increased by 50–100% every 24 hours until the pain is moderate in intensity. Subsequently, increments of 25–50% daily are usually sufficient to achieve control without excessive unwanted effects. A modified-release formulation of morphine can be substituted once a stable dosage has been determined, although a rapid-acting formulation may still be required to treat breakthrough pain. Oral administration of morphine may not be possible if there is vomiting, dysphagia or intestinal obstruction. In these circumstances, rectal administration or subcutaneous infusion using a syringe driver should be considered. Diamorphine can also be given by epidural or intrathecal injection for intractable pain. Transdermal delivery of an opioid such as fentanyl from an adhesive patch is an alternative to modified-release oral morphine. There is substantial evidence that if a person is unable to tolerate a particular opioid, then it is worth trying an alternative opioid, which may be better tolerated. The factors that predict intolerance to a particular opioid are poorly understood, although it is now recognised that intolerance to morphine may be associated with a mutation in the multidrug resistance 1 transporter protein (see Table 2.1). Oxycodone can be effective as an alternative to morphine, and there is also evidence that the response to methadone can persist when other μ-receptor agonists are ineffective. If possible, long-term opioid use should be avoided for noncancer pain. After long-term use, the dose of opioid should be gradually tapered to avoid withdrawal effects.

NEUROPATHIC PAIN

Neuropathic pain, such as trigeminal neuralgia, postherpetic neuralgia and phantom limb pain after an amputation, often responds less well to conventional analgesia than nociceptive pain. Although the mechanisms of neuropathic pain are now better understood, there is still little agreement on how to use this knowledge to direct treatment. As with all forms of chronic pain, a multidisciplinary approach that considers the psychosocial contributors to pain and promotes appropriate physical activity is often necessary.

First-line treatment is usually with an anticonvulsant that binds to voltage-gated Ca^{2+} channels (such as gabapentin or pregabalin; see Chapter 23). Pregabalin is the first-choice treatment for postherpetic neuralgia. Tricyclic antidepressants (see Chapter 22) that increase synaptic noradrenaline and serotonin concentrations in the descending spinal inhibitory pathways are an alternative first-line approach, but the evidence of efficacy is limited (see Figs 19.4 and 19.5).

Selective serotonin and noradrenaline reuptake inhibitors (SSRIs and SNRIs, respectively), such as duloxetine (see Chapter 22), have fewer unwanted effects than tricyclic antidepressants, and duloxetine is the first choice for painful diabetic neuropathy. SSRI antidepressants have no benefit in neuropathic pain.

Stimulus-independent neuropathic pain (such as dysaesthesia) may have underlying central potentiating mechanisms and can respond to an opioid. However, although opioids may be helpful for acute management of neuropathic pain, there is little evidence for efficacy when used for more than 3 months. In this situation, the risk of dependence usually outweigh the benefits. Other pharmacological treatments that are sometimes considered include baclofen (see Chapter 24) and the NMDA receptor antagonist ketamine (see Chapter 17), which modulate spinal transmission of the pain signal.

Stimulus-evoked neuropathic pain (such as allodynia and hyperalgesia) may respond to topical treatment if it is localised. Lidocaine cream or topical patches can be effective for conditions such as mechanical allodynia in postherpetic neuralgia through its local anaesthetic actions (see Chapter 18). Alternatively, capsaicin, a derivative of red chilli peppers that stimulates C fibres in the afferent nociceptive pathway, can be applied topically as a counterirritant. This releases substance P, which stimulates the transient receptor potential vanilloid 1 ($TRPV_1$) receptor and initially provokes hyperalgesia by promoting depolarisation and action potential generation. Subsequent depletion of substance P then blocks nerve function (see Fig. 19.3). The use of cannabinoids (the active components of cannabis; see Chapter 54) is sometimes advocated for relief of hyperalgesia in conditions such as multiple sclerosis. Stimulation of cannabinoid receptors produces an antinociceptive action and inhibits pain transmission in the spinal cord.

Trigeminal neuralgia is distinct from other forms of neuropathic pain. It responds well to carbamazepine or oxcarbazepine (see Chapter 23), which can reduce the frequency and intensity of attacks. There is less evidence for the efficacy of other drugs, and surgical decompression of the nerve may be required.

SELF-ASSESSMENT

True/false questions

1. Opioids inhibit pain transmission in the dorsal horn of the spinal cord.
2. Opioids can cause euphoria or dysphoria.
3. Tolerance develops consistently to all of the biological effects of the opioids.
4. Morphine can cause vasodilation at injection sites.
5. Methadone has a rapid onset of action and a short half-life.
6. The main indication for remifentanil is for treatment of chronic intractable pain.
7. Naloxone is a short-acting opioid agonist.
8. Drugs that inhibit the reuptake of noradrenaline can be effective analgesics in neuropathic pain.
9. Anticonvulsants should not be used in the treatment of neuropathic pain.
10. Buprenorphine is a partial agonist at μ-opioid receptors.

11. Pentazocine can precipitate withdrawal symptoms in morphine addicts.
12. Pethidine (meperidine) is used in childbirth because of its short half-life.

One-best-answer (OBA) questions

1. Which is the *most appropriate* statement about opioid analgesics?
   A. In the elderly, tolerance rapidly develops to the constipating effects of morphine.
   B. An opioid analgesic is the drug of choice for phantom limb pain following a below-knee amputation after a road traffic accident.
   C. The analgesic potencies of codeine and dihydrocodeine are similar to that of morphine.
   D. Tolerance does not develop to the miotic effect of opioids.
   E. Fentanyl can be used for opioid withdrawal and maintenance of the chronically relapsing heroin addict.
2. Choose the *most accurate* statement about opioid drugs.
   A. Heroin (diamorphine) is too toxic for clinical use.
   B. Morphine suppresses pain by reducing histamine release in inflamed tissues.
   C. Fentanyl can be administered transdermally.
   D. Naloxone is used to treat opioid addiction.
   E. Morphine is acid-labile and must be given parenterally.

Case-based questions

Mr. J.H., aged 60 years, was admitted to a hospice. He had previously had a left nephrectomy for renal cell carcinoma and now has intense metastatic bone pain in his ankles, right iliac crest and left upper arm. He was also having periods of dyspnoea. Prior to admission, his medication was co-codamol three times daily and diclofenac (150 mg) at night. He was also taking cimetidine (400 mg) twice daily. His pain was not well controlled on admission. After a week of assessment and optimisation of drug therapy, Mr. J.H.'s treatment comprised the following drugs.

Morphine, modified-release	260 mg	Once or twice daily
Morphine, oral solution	50 mg	When required
Diclofenac, slow release	150 mg	At night
Dexamethasone	2 mg	Three times daily
Metoclopramide	10 mg	Three times daily
Lansoprazole	30 mg	Once daily
Docusate sodium	100 mg	Three times daily
Temazepam	20 mg	At night

1. Was Mr. J.H. taking an opioid analgesic before admission to the hospice?
2. How does morphine exert its pharmacological action as an analgesic?
3. Why was oral morphine solution (an immediate-release form) made available in addition to the modified-release formulation?
4. Was the dependence potential of morphine likely to present a problem in this man?
5. What alternative opioids might you consider as an immediate replacement for morphine?
6. How does diclofenac control inflammation, and why was it useful in this man?
7. What was the rationale for the use of dexamethasone?
8. Metoclopramide is an antiemetic. Why do you think that this man was likely to suffer from nausea and possibly vomiting?
9. How does metoclopramide act to alleviate nausea, and what other antiemetic drugs could be used?
10. Why might gastric or duodenal ulceration be a problem in this man?
11. Why was cimetidine given before admission, and why was it replaced with lansoprazole?
12. Why was constipation likely to be a problem in this man?
13. What is the mechanism of action of docusate sodium, and what alternative laxative agents could have been used?
14. Why was temazepam given?

ANSWERS

True/false answers

1. **True.** Opioids act at opioid receptors to block transmitter release and postsynaptic transmission in the dorsal horn. They also act at opioid receptors at multiple sites in the brain.
2. **True.** In people who have pain, opioid analgesia is often associated with well-being (mediated by μ-receptors), whereas in pain-free people, dysphoria can occur (κ-receptors).
3. **False.** Much less tolerance to miosis and constipation develops than to the other effects of opioids, such as analgesia and respiratory depression.
4. **True.** Morphine is an alkaloid which in parenteral doses may release histamine from mast cells, leading to itch, vasodilation and hypotension.
5. **False.** Methadone has good oral absorption and less potential to cause euphoria, so it is used in controlled withdrawal in people with opioid dependence. Its *long* half-life means that withdrawal symptoms are more gradual and less intense than with morphine or heroin.
6. **False.** Remifentanil (and alfentanil) are used parenterally as adjuncts for anaesthesia.
7. **False.** Naloxone is a short-acting opioid *antagonist*, blocking μ-, κ- and δ-receptors. It is used in opioid overdose, although severe withdrawal symptoms can occur in people addicted to opioids following naloxone administration.
8. **True.** Tricyclic antidepressants can be effective for the treatment of neuropathic pain. They may act by enhancing monoamine levels in the descending inhibitory pathways that control the pain gate mechanism. Some analgesics such as tramadol have dual activity as opioids and monoamine reuptake inhibitors.
9. **False.** Anticonvulsants such as carbamazepine and lamotrigine can be of use in the treatment of neuropathic pain, probably by stabilising neuronal membranes and inhibiting release of excitatory neurotransmitters, while gabapentin and pregabalin increase levels of the inhibitory transmitter γ-aminobutyric acid (GABA).

10. **True.** The partial agonism of buprenorphine at μ-opioid receptors is associated with lower abuse potential than morphine.
11. **True.** A partial agonist (such as pentazocine) can reduce the effects of a full agonist (such as morphine) at the same receptor.
12. **True.** The short half-life of pethidine reduces respiratory depression in the neonate and allows rapid adjustment of dosage. Pethidine also has less suppressive effect on the uterine muscles than morphine.

One-best-answer (OBA) answers

1. **Answer D** is correct.
   A. Incorrect. Constipation is a problem with long-term morphine treatment, particularly in the elderly and bed-bound, and laxatives are often required.
   B. Incorrect. Chronic pain is usually less responsive to opioids, and nonopioid treatments (e.g. anticonvulsants) may be required for neuropathic pain.
   C. Incorrect. Codeine and dihydrocodeine are *less* potent analgesics than morphine.
   D. **Correct**. Miosis is one of the signs of opioid abuse.
   E. Incorrect. Fentanyl is not suitable. Methadone can be used as a substitute in the detoxification process.
2. **Answer C** is correct
   A. Incorrect. Heroin for medical use is pure, not contaminated, as often occurs with illicitly obtained heroin. Although its potency and dependence potential can limit its clinical use, it can be effective for severe pain in terminal cancer and in acute myocardial infarction.
   B. Incorrect. Analgesia by morphine and other opioids occurs by central actions on opioid receptors and not by effects on histamine release in inflamed tissues. Unlike most opioids, however, morphine can trigger histamine release from mast cells, leading to peripheral vasodilation.
   C. **Correct**. Fentanyl can be administered by a transdermal patch due to its high potency and lipid solubility.
   D. Incorrect. The rapid-acting opioid antagonist naloxone can be used in opioid overdose but triggers severe withdrawal effects in opioid-addicted individuals. However, former opioid-dependent persons can be treated with a longer-acting opioid antagonist, naltrexone, to reduce relapse.
   E. Incorrect. Morphine can be administered by parenteral routes, but can also be given orally, although its oral bioavailability is relatively low and inconsistent.

Case-based answers

1. The simple analgesic paracetamol was given in a compound formulation with the opioid analgesic codeine (co-codamol) before Mr. J.H.'s admission to the hospice. A nonsteroidal antiinflammatory drug (NSAID) analgesic (diclofenac) was also given. Although this regimen conformed to the WHO analgesic ladder principle of combining opioid and nonopioid analgesics, codeine lacks the efficacy of morphine and failed to provide adequate pain control before admission.

2. Morphine acts mainly at opioid μ-receptors at spinal and supraspinal sites to produce analgesia. Morphine is a strong μ-receptor agonist that produces analgesia, euphoria, sedation, respiratory depression, dependence and inhibition of gastrointestinal motility.
3. Oral morphine solution is used to control breakthrough exacerbations of pain on a patient-initiated basis. Repeated use of oral morphine solution should signal a reassessment of the dose of the long-acting morphine. When the person is unable to take oral medication because of weakness or vomiting, rectal or continuous subcutaneous infusion may be required. Normally, 80% of people require less than 200 mg morphine per day to control severe pain. With terminally ill people having persistent severe pain, the dose is gradually increased over a period of 1–2 weeks until appropriate control is achieved. The maximum dose may be as high as 2–3 g per day. Unwanted effects can occur, so close monitoring is needed when an opioid is initiated or its dosage is altered.
4. For reasons that are not easily explained, opioid dependence seldom occurs in people with a high degree of pain. Possible reasons include high levels of endogenous opioids or catecholamines.
5. Diamorphine can be used instead of morphine. It is more potent but no more efficacious. Its major advantage is its high solubility, which reduces the volume of intramuscular injections or continuous subcutaneous infusion, if these are required. Infrequently, an unusual response to morphine may require its replacement by other opioids. Fentanyl delivered via a transdermal patch has fewer unwanted effects, and fentanyl nasal spray can be used for breakthrough pain.
6. Diclofenac is an aspirin-like NSAID often used in the treatment of arthritic conditions (see Chapter 29). Unlike opioids, it has both analgesic and antiinflammatory actions, due to its inhibition of the synthesis of prostaglandins by cyclo-oxygenase. The pain from bone metastases is compounded by local inflammation. Prostaglandins sensitise nociceptors to pain stimuli, and inflammatory swelling triggers pain due to increased pressure. Inflammation is reduced by diclofenac, thereby reducing the requirement for morphine.
7. Dexamethasone is a potent glucocorticoid (see Chapter 44), reducing inflammation and swelling at metastatic sites.
8. Nausea is an unwanted effect of morphine and other opioids, occurring particularly during the first week of use, but tolerance to the nausea induced by morphine occurs. Nausea may also be a consequence of the cancer itself, of related complications such as hypercalcaemia, or of cytotoxic chemotherapy or radiotherapy.
9. Metoclopramide is a dopamine antagonist that acts in the chemoreceptor trigger zone (CTZ) to reduce nausea caused by opioid analgesics, chemotherapy and radiotherapy. It also has prokinetic activity on the gut that reduces the risk of nausea and vomiting. Other dopamine antagonists such as prochloperazine can also be used (see Chapter 32).
10. Gastric and/or duodenal inflammation (which may cause considerable discomfort) or even ulceration may occur with prolonged use of diclofenac and a

corticosteroid, due to inhibition of the synthesis of protective prostaglandins in the gut wall.

11. Cimetidine is a histamine H_2 receptor antagonist that reduces histamine-mediated gastric acid secretion by the parietal cells (see Chapter 33), and was used twice-daily to reduce the risk of NSAID-induced gastric or duodenal ulceration. Cimetidine inhibits the enzymes that convert codeine into morphine and may reduce its analgesic effect. After admission, cimetidine was replaced with the proton pump inhibitor lansoprazole, which is more effective in blocking acid secretion and can be given once daily (see Chapter 33).

12. Constipation is a feature of opioid therapy. Tolerance does not develop to opioid-induced constipation. Peristalsis is reduced, while the tone of the intestinal muscle is increased.

13. Docusate sodium has some faecal-softening properties and is a stimulant of intestinal smooth muscle, which restores peristalsis. In practice, terminally ill people are often given danthron, in combination with either docusate sodium (co-danthrusate) or poloxamer (co-danthramer). Danthron is a stimulant drug and stool softener and is particularly useful when 'bowel movements must be by strain'. The irritant properties of danthron and its carcinogenic potential restrict its general use. The alternatives in use include senna preparations (stimulants) and magnesium sulfate (a bulk purgative).

14. Temazepam is a short-acting benzodiazepine anxiolytic sedative used to aid sleeping (see Chapter 20).

Note. Pain control must also take note of the psychological and social condition of the person. At all times, if pain control is inadequate, adjuvant treatments such as other drug classes (see Table 19.1), radiotherapy or transcutaneous electrical nerve stimulation (TENS) should be considered.

FURTHER READING

Freynhagen, R., Bennett, M.I., 2009. Diagnosis and management of neuropathic pain. Br. Med. J. 339, 391–395.

Freynhagen, R., Geisslinger, G., Schug, S.A., 2013. Opioids for chronic non-cancer pain. Br. Med. J. 346, f2937.

Kalso, E., Aldington, D.J., Moore, R.A., 2013. Drugs for neuropathic pain. Br. Med. J. 347, f7339.

Lobmaier, P., Gossop, M., Waal, H., et al., 2010. The pharmacological treatment of opioid addiction: a clinical perspective. Eur. J. Clin. Pharmacol. 66, 537–545.

Portenoy, R.K., 2011. Treatment of cancer pain. Lancet 377, 2236–2247.

Reid, M.C., Eccleston, C., Pillemer, K., 2015. Management of chronic pain in older adults. Br. Med. J. 350, h532.

Turk, D.C., Wilson, H.D., Cahana, A., 2011. Treatment of chronic non-cancer pain. Lancet 377, 2226–2235.

Wu, C.L., Raja, S.N., 2011. Treatment of acute postoperative pain. Lancet 377, 2215–2225.

Zakrzewska, J.M., Linskey, M.E., 2015. Trigeminal neuralgia. Br. Med. J. 350, h1238.

Compendium: opioids and related drugs

Drug	Characteristics
Opioids used primarily for analgesia	
Alfentanil	Highly potent, selective μ-receptor agonist. Used by injection for intraoperative analgesia (see Chapter 17); respiratory depression may persist after the end of the procedure if repeated doses are given. Half-life: 1–2 h
Buprenorphine	Partial μ-receptor agonist and κ-receptor antagonist. Highly potent analgesic but moderate dependence potential. Can precipitate withdrawal in individuals dependent on other opioids, and action only partly reversed by naloxone (opioid antagonist). Used as an alternative to morphine for analgesia, but nausea may limit its tolerability. Given sublingually, by slow intravenous or intramuscular injection, or as transdermal patches. Half-life: 1–7 h
Codeine	Selective μ-receptor agonist. Low potency and low dependence potential. Produces little respiratory depression. Given orally for mild to moderate pain or by intramuscular injection; also used when antitussive and antidiarrhoeal actions required. Increased response and toxicity risk in ultra-rapid CYP2D6 metabolisers. Available in combination with paracetamol. Half-life: 3–4 h
Dextropropoxyphene	Selective μ-receptor agonist; given in combination with paracetamol (co-proxamol), but licence withdrawn in United Kingdom in 2005 due to toxicity in overdose. Co-proxamol tablets (unlicensed) may still be prescribed for patients who find it difficult to change, or because alternatives are not effective or suitable
Diamorphine (heroin)	Highly potent μ-receptor agonist; the acetylated prodrug readily crosses the blood–brain barrier. Clinical uses restricted because of high tolerance and abuse potential. Given orally or by infusion for the pain of terminal cancer, and for acute severe pain (e.g. myocardial infarction); also given by intramuscular or subcutaneous injection. Rapidly hydrolysed to morphine. Half-life: 2–5 min
Dihydrocodeine	Potency and profile similar to codeine. Given orally or by intramuscular or subcutaneous injection for moderate pain. Half-life: 3–5 h

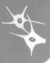

Compendium: opioids and related drugs (cont'd)

Drug	Characteristics
Dipipanone	Moderately potent analgesic; less sedating than morphine. The only available formulation in the United Kingdom contains cyclizine (an antiemetic), which makes it unsuitable for long-term use. Half-life: 3–4 h
Fentanyl	Selective μ-receptor agonist; more potent than morphine. Used orally or as transdermal patch or buccal film for chronic intractable pain, and by nasal spray for breakthrough pain. Also used as intravenous adjunct in anaesthesia (see Chapter 17); respiratory depression may persist after the end of the procedure if repeated doses are given. Half-life: 1–6 h
Hydromorphone	Selective μ-receptor agonist; similar to morphine in most properties. Given orally. Half-life: 2–3 h
Meptazinol	Selective agonist for μ₁-receptors. Less potent than morphine; low dependence potential and possibly a reduced risk of respiratory depression. Given orally or by intramuscular or slow intravenous injection. Short duration of action. Half-life: 1–3 h
Methadone	Selective μ-receptor agonist; also a monoamine reuptake inhibitor and glutamate NMDA receptor antagonist. Potency similar to morphine, but less sedating. Slow onset and long duration of action support major use for withdrawal from morphine/heroin dependence. Given orally or by subcutaneous or intramuscular injection. Half-life: 25 h
Morphine	Strong μ-receptor agonist, weak κ- and δ-receptor agonist. The standard potent opioid against which other opioids are compared. Given orally, rectally, or by subcutaneous, intramuscular or slow intravenous injection. Half-life: 1–5 h
Oxycodone	Agonist of μ- and κ-receptors; similar pharmacological profile to morphine. Used largely in palliative care as an alternative in people who cannot tolerate morphine. Given orally or by subcutaneous or slow intravenous injection. Also available in oral combination with naloxone, which is not active orally but antagonises opioid effects of oxycodone if the tablet is crushed and injected intravenously. Half-life: 3–5 h
Papaveretum	Rarely used combined formulation of morphine, papaverine and codeine; not to be confused with papaverine alone. Given by subcutaneous, intramuscular or intravenous injection
Pentazocine	κ-Receptor agonist and weak or partial antagonist at μ- and δ-receptors; will provoke a withdrawal syndrome in a morphine-dependent person. May cause hallucinations. Given orally, rectally or by slow intravenous injection; may cause irritation given subcutaneously. Half-life: 2–3 h
Pethidine (meperidine)	Selective μ-receptor agonist; less potent than morphine. Produces rapid but short-lasting analgesia; not useful for antitussive or antidiarrhoeal effects. Frequently used in labour as less respiratory depression and less suppression of uterine contractility than other opioids; antimuscarinic activity may cause tachycardia. Given orally or by subcutaneous or slow intravenous injection. Half-life: 3–8 h, but converted to long-lived active metabolite (norpethidine)
Remifentanil	Potent, selective μ-receptor agonist. Used by IV infusion for intraoperative analgesia; not used for management of chronic pain. Very rapid local metabolism. Half-life: 0.1 h
Tapentadol	Selective μ-receptor agonist and noradrenaline reuptake inhibitor. Moderate analgesic potency. Given orally for moderate to severe pain. Half-life: 4 h
Tramadol	Weak μ-receptor agonist and inhibitor of monoamine reuptake; opioid analgesia is enhanced by increased serotonergic and noradrenergic pathway activity. WHO-classified step 2 agent; low potential for respiratory depression or dependence. Given orally or by intramuscular or intravenous injection. Also available in combination with paracetamol. Half-life: 5–6 h, with active metabolite
Opioid antagonists	
Methylnaltrexone	Peripheral μ-receptor antagonist; does not cross the blood–brain barrier. Reduces opioid-induced constipation without affecting central actions (including analgesia) or inducing withdrawal; used in combination with laxatives in palliative care when laxatives alone have failed, and also to reduce postoperative paralytic ileus. Given by subcutaneous injection. Half-life: 2–3 h
Naloxone	Opioid receptor antagonist used to treat opioid overdose (see Chapters 53 and 54); also used to reverse opioid-induced respiratory depression in anaesthesia. Administered by intravenous bolus injection or infusion, with rapid onset of action (1–2 min). Half-life: 1–1.5 h
Naltrexone	Opioid receptor antagonist. Given orally to prevent relapse in formerly opioid-dependent patients. Also used for treatment of alcohol dependence (see Chapter 54). Longer duration of action than naloxone. Half-life: 4 h

Compendium: opioids and related drugs (cont'd)

Drug	Characteristics
Opioids used primarily for nonanalgesic effects	
Dextromethorphan	Only opioid activity is antitussive action; also antagonist to NMDA receptors. Given orally. Half-life: 11 h
Diphenoxylate	Opioid agonist used in acute diarrhoea (see Chapter 35); may exert its effects locally on smooth muscle rather than via opioid receptors. Given orally. Half-life: 2–3 h
Loperamide	Only opioid characteristic is an antidiarrhoeal action (see Chapter 35); tolerance does not develop. Given orally. Half-life: 9–14 h
Related drugs or actions	
Lofexidine	α_2-Adrenoceptor antagonist. Used as an adjunct in opioid withdrawal. Given orally. Half-life: 11 h

20 Anxiety, obsessive-compulsive disorder and insomnia

• •

There is considerable overlap in the pharmacology of drugs that have anxiolytic (anxiety-relieving), sedative (moderating excitement and calming) and hypnotic (sleep-inducing) properties. Compounds with sedative properties at low doses often have hypnotic effects at higher doses, while sedative drugs may have anxiolytic properties when used at doses that are too low to produce sedation. Buspirone is one compound that has anxiolytic properties but does not sedate.

ANXIETY DISORDERS

BIOLOGICAL BASIS OF ANXIETY DISORDERS

Anxiety disorders are among the most common psychiatric syndromes and affect 15% of the general population at some time during their life. The clinical manifestations of anxiety are both psychological and physical. Anxiety is only pathological when it is inappropriate to the degree of stress to which the individual is exposed. There are several anxiety syndromes, of which the most common are generalised anxiety disorder, panic disorder and phobic disorder. Generalised anxiety disorder is often misdiagnosed as depression, but the two may co-exist as mixed anxiety and depression. Many anxiety syndromes present early in life, and tend to become chronic if untreated. They are often associated with substance abuse.

Symptoms vary among the anxiety disorders, but usually include apprehension, worry, fear and nervousness. Increased sympathetic nervous system activity frequently accompanies these feelings, causing trembling, sweating, palpitation, dizziness and epigastric discomfort. Sleep is often disturbed, with difficulty getting to sleep being a common feature. Physical symptoms can be prominent (somatisation) and disabling, and are sometimes difficult to interpret because anxiety can coexist with an underlying chronic physical condition.

It is now thought that generalised anxiety disorder and major depression may share a genetic basis, and that expression of anxiety as the predominant feature is determined by environmental factors such as low socioeconomic status, childhood maltreatment and internalising problems. Dysfunction of neurotransmission in the limbic region of the brain underlies the genesis of anxiety. The amygdala is a central part of the system that processes a fear stimulus and selects a response based on previous experience. Responses are then implemented through the locus coeruleus (autonomic and neuroendocrine responses), the nucleus paragigantocellularis in the brainstem (autonomic responses) and through the hypothalamus. Structural changes in the neural pathways from the amygdala to the cortex have been identified in anxiety disorders, which may underlie hyperactive sensory processing of threat stimuli. In addition, the cognitive control mechanisms that terminate the emotional response to the sensory cues are deficient.

Many abnormalities of neurotransmission have been implicated in anxiety syndromes, but it is unclear whether these are causative or secondary changes. They include:

- Increased noradrenergic neurotransmission
- Deficient inhibition by γ-aminobutyric acid (GABA) interneurons
- Increased excitatory glutamatergic neurotransmission at N-methyl-D-aspartate (NMDA) receptors
- Supersensitivity of receptors for peptide neurotransmitters such as cholecystokinin and neuropeptide Y
- Increased serotonergic (5-hydroxytryptamine [5-HT]) neurotransmission.

There is increasing evidence for the central role of brain-derived neurotrophic factor (BDNF) in modulating neural plasticity in anxiety states (see Fig. 22.2). BDNF is regulated by most of the neurotransmitters implicated in the genesis of anxiety states, and down regulation of BDNF is found in anxiety states.

In some anxiety syndromes there is excess secretion of corticotropin-releasing hormone (CRH), but a low plasma cortisol concentration and upregulation of glucocorticoid receptors. CRH is a neurotransmitter in the limbic system, and upregulation may occur from early adverse experiences, leading to conditioning of those with a genetic predisposition to anxiety disorder in later life.

ANXIOLYTIC DRUGS

This section considers drugs primarily developed to treat anxiety (anxiolytics), although management of anxiety disorders involves many other drug classes such as antidepressants.

Benzodiazepines

chlordiazepoxide, diazepam, lorazepam, midazolam, temazepam

In addition to their anxiolytic effect, benzodiazepines have several other properties that are clinically useful. This section also considers benzodiazepines that are not used primarily for treatment of anxiety.

Mechanism of action and effects

Benzodiazepines act by potentiating the actions of GABA, the primary inhibitory neurotransmitter in the central nervous system. They act at an allosteric regulatory site closely linked to the GABA$_A$ receptor, which mediates fast inhibitory synaptic neurotransmission (Fig. 20.1). Activation of GABA receptors increases the influx of Cl$^-$ into the neuron, hyperpolarises the cell membrane and decreases cell excitability. Binding of a benzodiazepine to subunits of the receptor induces a conformational change in the GABA receptor that enhances its affinity for the neurotransmitter. Benzodiazepines have no direct action on ion flow and only enhance GABA-mediated opening of the ion channel.

The increase in inhibitory neurotransmission produced by benzodiazepines has the following potentially useful effects:

- Sedation from reduced sensory input to the reticular activating system
- Onset of sleep at high drug concentrations
- Anterograde amnesia
- Anxiolysis from actions on the limbic system and hypothalamus
- Anticonvulsant activity (see Chapter 23)
- Reduction of skeletal muscle tone (see Chapter 24).

The GABA$_A$ receptor has α, β and γ subunits, arranged in a group of five (usually two α, two β and one γ, although only α and β are essential) around a central pore (see Fig. 20.1). There are many subtypes of each subunit, and therefore many receptor configurations that have different regional distributions in the brain. Benzodiazepines bind at the interface between an α and γ subunit. GABA$_A$ receptors

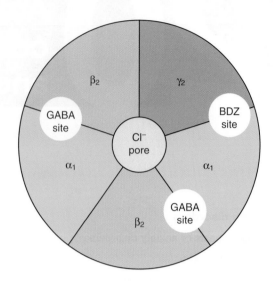

Fig. 20.1 **The GABA$_A$ receptor.** The GABA$_A$ receptor is a ligand-gated chloride ion channel and consists of five transmembrane subunits configured from the 19 possible subunits that have been identified; thus many configurations of the GABA receptor exist, which vary in their sensitivity to benzodiazepines. A common configuration comprises two α_1, two β_2, and one γ_2 subunit. Binding of GABA to the receptor at the interfaces of the α_1 and β_2 subunits mediates opening of the Cl$^-$ channel and an influx of Cl$^-$ ions, resulting in hyperpolarisation of the cell. This action is enhanced by drugs stimulating allosteric regulatory sites on the GABA receptor, distinct from the GABA-binding site. Diazepam, lorazepam and other 'classic' benzodiazepines (BDZ) bind at the interface of the α_1 and γ_2 subunits. Compounds such as zolpidem bind with high affinity for the α_1-subunits and also enhance Cl$^-$ ion influx. The intravenous anaesthetics propofol and etomidate bind to β_2- and β_3-subunits (see Chapter 17).

that have an α_1 or α_5 subunit are responsible for the sedative and amnesic properties of benzodiazepines, while both α_2 and α_3 subunits appear to be involved in the anxiolytic and muscle-relaxant effects. Anticonvulsant activity is conferred by several α subunits. The minority of GABA receptors with only α_4 or α_6 subunits do not bind benzodiazepines. The potential for selective action of benzodiazepines through preferential binding to specific subunits has not yet been realised.

Pharmacokinetics

The pharmacokinetics of individual benzodiazepines determines their major clinical uses.

Benzodiazepines that are used as hypnotics for inducing sleep (e.g. temazepam) are rapidly absorbed from the gut. This produces a fast onset of sedation, followed by sleep. A short duration of action is also desirable to minimise 'hangover' sedation in the morning. This is achieved by using drugs that are metabolised to inactive derivatives.

The anxiolytic properties of benzodiazepines are best exploited by using a compound with a long duration of action. Smaller doses can then be used to minimise sedation, and the rebound in anxiety symptoms that can occur between doses of a short-acting drug is avoided. Diazepam and other long-acting benzodiazepines are metabolised in the liver to active compounds (see Fig. 2.12) that are relatively slowly eliminated from the body. Regular dosing with long-acting benzodiazepines results in accumulation of the active metabolites with prolonged action. Long-acting benzodiazepines, such as clobazam, clonazepam, diazepam and lorazepam, are used in the prophylaxis of epilepsy (see Chapter 23). Diazepam, oxazepam or chlordiazepoxide are used to reduce symptoms during withdrawal from alcohol dependence (see Chapter 54).

Diazepam, lorazepam and midazolam can be given by intravenous injection. They are used to provide rapid conscious sedation preoperatively or before procedures such as endoscopy or for emergency treatment of generalised seizures and status epilepticus (see Chapter 23). Buccal midazolam or rectal diazepam is also used for control of seizures if the intravenous route is not available.

Unwanted effects

- Drowsiness, which may cause problems with driving or operating machinery.
- Lightheadedness.
- Confusion, especially in the elderly.
- Paradoxical increase in aggression.
- Amnesia.
- Ataxia.
- Muscle weakness.
- Potentiation of the sedative effects of other central nervous system (CNS)-depressant drugs, such as alcohol. In overdose, such combinations can lead to severe respiratory depression. Flumazenil is a competitive antagonist of benzodiazepines and can be used in acute overdose to reverse respiratory depression (see Chapter 53).
- Tolerance to the therapeutic effects of benzodiazepines is common. Rebound insomnia on withdrawal can perpetuate benzodiazepine use.
- Dependence with physical and psychological withdrawal symptoms occurs during long-term treatment. The risk is highest in people with personality disorders, or a previous history of dependence on alcohol or drugs, and is more likely to occur if high doses of benzodiazepines are used. Restricting use to a maximum of 4 weeks will minimise the risk of dependence. Withdrawal symptoms on stopping long-acting benzodiazepines may be delayed by up to 3 weeks. Anxiety is the most frequent symptom, while insomnia, depression and abnormalities of perception, such as altered sensitivity to noise, light or touch, also occur. More severe reactions such as psychosis or convulsions are rare. Some withdrawal symptoms may resemble those for which the drug was originally prescribed, encouraging continued use. Gradual withdrawal of a benzodiazepine over 4–8 weeks is desirable after long-term use, although complete withdrawal may take up to a year. Lorazepam is a potent benzodiazepine with a relatively short duration of action that proves particularly difficult to stop because of the intensity of withdrawal symptoms that begin a few hours after cessation of treatment. Substitution with the longer-acting drug diazepam may be helpful before withdrawal is attempted. There are no proven treatments for reducing symptoms associated with benzodiazepine withdrawal. β-Adrenoceptor antagonists (see Chapter 5) are sometimes helpful, or an antidepressant (see Chapter 22) if there are depressive symptoms.

Azapirones

Example

buspirone

Mechanism of action and effects

The mechanism of anxiolytic action of buspirone is unclear. Buspirone is a partial agonist at presynaptic 5-HT$_{1A}$ receptors, producing negative feedback to inhibit serotonin release. It is also a partial agonist at α_1-adrenoceptors and an antagonist at dopamine D$_2$, D$_3$ and D$_4$ receptors. It has no effect on GABA receptors. Initial exacerbation of anxiety may occur with buspirone, and the onset of the anxiolytic action is slow, beginning after 2 weeks and reaching a maximum effect at approximately 4 weeks. The mechanism of action may involve gradual changes in neural plasticity (enhancement of neural performance or changes in neural connections; see Chapter 22). Buspirone has no sedative action, and is ineffective for panic attacks.

Pharmacokinetics

Buspirone undergoes extensive first-pass metabolism in the liver. The half-life is short (2–4 hours).

Unwanted effects

- Nausea.
- Dizziness, lightheadedness and headache.
- Nervousness.

Neither tolerance nor dependence has been reported.

MANAGEMENT OF ANXIETY DISORDERS

If substance misuse is identified, it should be treated first and may improve symptoms, while comorbid depression may require an antidepressant. Mild symptoms of anxiety often respond to counselling or psychotherapy, such as relaxation response training, cognitive behavioural therapy or mindfulness, without drug therapy.

Generalised anxiety disorder with symptoms that cause marked functional impairment often requires long-term drug treatment, and there is now considerable evidence that antidepressants (see Chapter 22) are useful in this situation. Selective serotonin reuptake inhibitors (SSRIs) such as sertraline are the treatment of choice, or a serotonin and noradrenaline reuptake inhibitor (SNRI) such as venlafaxine if an SSRI is ineffective. Antidepressants can initially exacerbate anxiety, and a benzodiazepine may be necessary for the first 2–3 weeks of treatment to prevent this. The optimal duration of antidepressant treatment in generalised anxiety disorder is usually 1 year. Pregabalin, which increases inhibitory neurotransmission, is an effective alternative to antidepressants and has a rapid onset of action (see Chapter 23). Buspirone may be as effective as an antidepressant, but 2–4 weeks of treatment are necessary to see a response.

Benzodiazepines can be considered as a short-term measure for anxiety to treat crises, since they have a rapid onset of action over 15–60 minutes. However, the potential for dependence should limit their use to a maximum of 4 weeks,

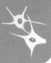

and the dose should be gradually reduced after the first 2 weeks. Buspirone has similar efficacy to benzodiazepines, but the slow onset of action makes it less versatile for managing short-term anxiety. In addition, anxiety that responds well to benzodiazepines often responds less well to buspirone, possibly due to a relative lack of effect of buspirone on somatic symptoms. Somatic symptoms of anxiety (e.g. tremor, palpitations) that are produced by overactivity in the sympathetic nervous system are often helped by a nonselective β-adrenoceptor antagonist such as propranolol (see Chapter 5).

Social anxiety disorder responds to monoamine oxidase inhibitors (MAOIs; see Chapter 22) better than to most other agents. Moclobemide is the treatment of choice, but phenelzine is also used. Phobic disorders usually need a different approach, and cognitive behavioural therapy is often more effective than drugs. Panic disorder is usually treated with tricyclic antidepressants or SSRIs, with MAOIs reserved for patients who do not respond.

OBSESSIVE-COMPULSIVE DISORDER

Obsessive-compulsive disorder (OCD) is a common condition that presents with repetitive, time-consuming obsessions and compulsions. Obsessions are unwanted intrusive thoughts, doubts or urges that are inconsistent with the person's values. Compulsions are repetitive behaviours that the person feels must be performed in response to the obsession. The neurobiology of OCD is not well understood, and it appears to be different from anxiety disorders. There is a genetic predisposition to OCD which interacts with psychological stressors to trigger the condition.

The neurobiology of OCD involves abnormalities in the frontal cortico-striatal-thalamic-cortical circuit. OCD results from a failure of the striatal portion of the basal ganglia to 'filter' excessive cortical impulses, which permits excitatory activity in the thalamus to reach the frontal cortex. This presents a barrier to removal of irrelevant worries from becoming the centre of attention. Within this circuit, reduced inhibitory neurotransmission in GABA-ergic neurons may allow unopposed excitatory glutamatergic neurotransmission.

MANAGEMENT OF OBSESSIVE-COMPULSIVE DISORDER

Psychological therapies are important, with cognitive behavioural therapy, to enable the person to tolerate anxiety. Treatment can be augmented by the use of an SSRI (see Chapter 22), but higher doses than those used for depression are often required. Clomipramine is used as a second-line option (see Chapter 22).

INSOMNIA

Defining insomnia is complicated by the considerable variability in the normal pattern of sleep. Most healthy adults sleep between 7 and 9 hours per night, but much shorter or

Table 20.1 Types of insomnia

Type of insomnia	Duration	Likely causes
Transient	2–3 days	Acute situational or environmental stress (e.g. jet lag, shift work)
Short-term	<3 weeks	Ongoing personal stress
Long-term	>3 weeks	Psychiatric illness, behavioural reasons, medical reasons

even longer periods can be normal. Insomnia is considered to be present if there is repeated inability to initiate or maintain sleep, despite adequate opportunity and time for sleep. There are three major categories of insomnia, defined by duration of symptoms (Table 20.1).

Insomnia symptom patterns include sleep-onset insomnia (difficulty falling asleep, more common in younger people), frequent nocturnal awakening (difficulty maintaining sleep, more common in older people), early morning awakening (with difficulty getting back to sleep) and difficulty functioning in the daytime due to perceived poor sleep. Obstructive sleep apnoea is a common cause of nocturnal awakening (as well as daytime sleepiness), affecting up to 10% of people who report insomnia.

The reticular formation in the midbrain, medulla and pons is responsible for maintaining wakefulness. Activity in the reticular formation is dependent on sensory input through collateral connections from the main sensory pathways. Neurotransmitter systems involved in the regulation of sleep are complex. Cortical arousal is regulated by noradrenergic pathways from the locus coeruleus, cholinergic ascending tracts from brainstem nuclei, histaminergic neurons from the tuberomammillary nucleus and serotonergic neurons from the raphe nuclei. Hypocretins are important neuropeptide transmitters in the lateral hypothalamus that promote wakefulness (see also the discussion of narcolepsy in Chapter 22). Sleep is induced by release of GABA, melatonin and galanin (a predominantly inhibitory neuropeptide) from the anterior hypothalamus, which together inhibit the arousal neurons.

SLEEP PATTERNS

The two main types of sleep pattern are rapid-eye-movement (REM) sleep and nonrapid-eye-movement (non-REM) sleep, which occur in cycles (Fig. 20.2). Non-REM sleep includes light sleep (stages 1 and 2) and deep sleep (stages 3 and 4), with two-thirds of sleep usually spent in stages 2–4. The deeper stages of sleep are the recuperative phase, while most dreaming occurs during the REM sleep periods. Increasing age is associated with more nocturnal awakening and longer periods of REM sleep.

HYPNOTIC DRUGS

Benzodiazepines

Benzodiazepines have dose-related hypnotic effects. See the previous discussion for details.

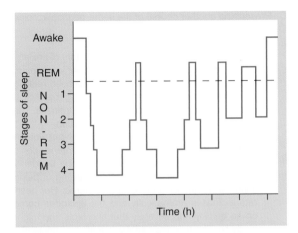

Fig. 20.2 Typical sleep pattern in a young adult. Phases of rapid-eye-movement (REM) sleep, associated with dreaming, alternate with recuperative phases of deeper, non-REM sleep.

Nonbenzodiazepine hypnotics that modulate the GABA$_A$ receptor

zaleplon, zolpidem, zopiclone

Mechanism of action and effects

Zaleplon, zolpidem and zopiclone (the so-called Z drugs) belong to different chemical classes but interact in a similar manner with the postsynaptic GABA$_A$ receptor on neuronal membranes. They bind to regulatory binding sites on the receptor that are close to, but distinct from, the benzodiazepine-binding site (see Fig. 20.1). Like benzodiazepines, they increase GABA-mediated Cl$^-$ influx into the cell, which inhibits neurotransmission. Zaleplon, zolpidem and zopiclone bind to the α_1-subunit in the GABA$_A$ receptor, and zopiclone also binds to the α_2-subunit. Although zopiclone also possesses anxiolytic and anticonvulsant activity, its short duration of action makes it unsuitable for these indications.

Pharmacokinetics

The 'Z drugs' are rapidly absorbed from the gut and metabolised in the liver. They have short half-lives (1–6 hours), which makes them well suited to their use as hypnotics.

Unwanted effects

- Bitter metallic taste (zopiclone).
- Gastrointestinal disturbances, including nausea and vomiting.
- Incoordination.
- Drowsiness, dizziness, headache and fatigue.
- Depression, confusion, amnesia.
- There is only anecdotal evidence for tolerance.
- Dependence with withdrawal symptoms has been reported.

MANAGEMENT OF INSOMNIA

Drugs play only a small part in the treatment of insomnia. Explanation of the normal variations in sleep patterns and avoidance of diuretics, drinks containing caffeine, cigarettes or alcohol in the hours before retiring can improve sleep. Eliminating excessive noise or heat in the bedroom, encouraging regular exercise in the day and minimising daytime napping may also be useful. Cognitive behavioural therapy is helpful for persistent insomnia.

Hypnotic drugs are reserved for times when abnormal sleep markedly affects quality of life. The ideal hypnotic would induce good-quality prolonged sleep without disturbance of the normal sleep pattern. It should have a rapid onset of action, with no 'hangover' sedation in the morning, and should not produce tolerance or dependence. Few drugs come close to this ideal profile. Benzodiazepines reduce sleep latency (the time between settling down and falling asleep) and prolong sleep duration. However, they reduce the time spent in REM sleep, with more time spent in stage 2 sleep. The 'Z drugs' produce less disturbance of sleep 'architecture' than benzodiazepines, having less effect on the amount of REM sleep while increasing the duration of deeper (stages 3–4) sleep. Short-acting hypnotics (such as zolpidem) are preferred if there is delayed onset of sleep, and medium-acting drugs (such as temazepam or zopiclone) for those who wake in the middle of the night. Long-acting drugs can also suppress daytime anxiety, but carry the risk of hangover sedation the following day.

Hypnotic drugs should be used only for short periods and intermittently if possible, since tolerance to hypnotics is common after 2 weeks of continuous use. If a benzodiazepine or a 'Z drug' is used every night for 4–6 weeks, then rebound insomnia, caused by mild dependence, frequently occurs when the drug is stopped. Despite this, hypnotic drugs are still widely used.

Of the other hypnotics, chloral derivatives and clomethiazole (see the compendium at the end of this chapter) should usually be avoided. Compounds with sedative actions as a part of their therapeutic profile are sometimes used as hypnotics. For example, a sedative antihistamine such as promethazine (see Chapter 39) can be helpful for children with somnambulism (sleepwalking) or night terrors, but daytime sedation and weight gain can be a problem. Sedative tricyclic antidepressants (see Chapter 22), such as amitriptyline, should be considered if there is an underlying depressive illness. If less-sedating antidepressants are used, then short-term concurrent use of a benzodiazepine may be necessary while awaiting the onset of the antidepressant effect.

Melatonin is a natural pineal hormone that regulates circadian rhythms. It can be used to treat insomnia caused by jet lag or shift work and has short-term benefit for primary insomnia with delayed onset of sleep.

SELF-ASSESSMENT

True/false questions

1. Benzodiazepines with a medium to long duration of action are useful for treating anxiety states.

2. Long-term use of benzodiazepines is recommended in anxiety states.
3. Potentiation of the CNS effects of benzodiazepines occurs with concurrent use of alcohol.
4. The CNS-depressant effects of benzodiazepines can be reversed with flumazenil.
5. Lower doses of benzodiazepines should be used in the elderly.
6. Buspirone is more sedative than temazepam.
7. Benzodiazepines used to treat anxiety should be taken for as short a time as possible.
8. Benzodiazepines have no effect on sleep patterns as measured by the duration of REM sleep.

One-best-answer (OBA) question

Choose the *most correct* statement from the following:
A. Benzodiazepines inhibit the action of GABA at the $GABA_A$ receptor.
B. Withdrawal effects may take more than 3 weeks to appear after stopping diazepam.
C. Zolpidem acts at the benzodiazepine site on the $GABA_A$ receptor.
D. Buspirone decreases anxiety within 3 days of starting the drug.
E. If there is no response to one hypnotic, it is advisable to switch to another.

Case-based questions

Mrs. F.L. is a 46-year-old mother of three who is finding it very hard to cope following the sudden death of her husband 3 months ago. She has returned to work but does not sleep properly, experiences episodes of intense anxiety during the day, and feels that she is at risk of losing her job because tiredness and anxiety about her financial difficulties prevent her from concentrating on her work.
1. What drug might you prescribe to help Mrs. F.L.'s insomnia, and what factors determine your choice of this drug?
2. How does your chosen drug work to reduce insomnia and anxiety?
3. What potential unwanted effects and drug interactions should you warn Mrs. F.L. about?
4. Mrs. F.L. returns 2 weeks later, saying that she regularly wakes at 4 am and cannot get back to sleep; consider the advantages and disadvantages of changing her drug.
5. What are the problems associated with long-term use of benzodiazepines?
6. What other options should be considered to help to manage Mrs. F.L.'s problems in the long term?

Extended-matching-item questions

Keeping in mind the equally important roles of psychological and psychiatric help, choose the *most appropriate* option from A–E for the next pharmacological course of action in the case scenarios 1 and 2 described here.
A. Gradual tapering of the medication over many months
B. Gradual tapering of the medication over several days

C. Prescribing another course of the same benzodiazepine
D. Considering giving an antidepressant
E. Immediate withdrawal of all medications

Scenario 1. A 54-year-old woman has a history of anxiety. Seven years earlier she had taken regular lorazepam, and for the last 3 years her doctor had been refilling prescription requests without reassessing the clinical need. There is no indication of depressive illness. The woman now wishes to stop her medication.

Scenario 2. You have been treating a 25-year-old woman for 1 year. She has been having up to 10 intense panic attacks a month. At any time of day, she suddenly develops a peculiar and very strong feeling of being lightheaded, jumpy and being smothered. Her heart rate increases dramatically and the episodes come on so quickly and severely that she feels she might be dying. She then feels shaky, sweaty and unsteady. Each attack quickly reaches such intensity that she is often unable to continue work and needs to go home. She has been treated with intermittent courses of diazepam for 1 year without improvement.

ANSWERS

True/false answers

1. **True.** Benzodiazepines used in anxiety, such as diazepam, have long-acting metabolites that contribute to the duration of action.
2. **False.** Dependence, tolerance and withdrawal symptoms occur with long-term continuous use of benzodiazepines.
3. **True.** Alcohol, older antihistamines and barbiturates can potentiate CNS depression by benzodiazepines.
4. **True.** Flumazenil is a competitive benzodiazepine antagonist used in acute benzodiazepine overdose.
5. **True.** Hepatic metabolism of benzodiazepines is reduced in the elderly, who are also more sensitive to their effects.
6. **False.** Buspirone has less sedative action than benzodiazepines such as temazepam.
7. **True.** Using the lowest possible dose of benzodiazepine for the shortest duration reduces the risk of tolerance and withdrawal effects.
8. **False.** Benzodiazepines affect sleep structure, with relative reduction in REM sleep. 'Z drugs' have less effect than benzodiazepines.

One-best-answer (OBA) answers

Answer B is correct.
A. Incorrect. Benzodiazepines *potentiate* the entry of Cl^- through the $GABA_A$ channel induced by GABA.
B. **Correct.** Diazepam has long-lived, active metabolites that accumulate on prolonged use and sustain its activity after stopping the drug.
C. Incorrect. 'Z drugs' act at different allosteric regulatory sites on the $GABA_A$ receptor to benzodiazepines; zolpidem binds to the α_1-subunit.
D. Incorrect. Buspirone may exacerbate anxiety initially, and its anxiolytic action requires at least 2 weeks of treatment, probably due to gradual effects on neuronal plasticity.

E. Incorrect. An alternative hypnotic is unlikely to work, and switching between hypnotics is not good practice.

Case-based answers

1. Mrs. F.L.'s insomnia and anxiety are a response to bereavement and might present fewer long-term problems than chronic 'endogenous' anxiety. The central concept in hypnotic therapy is to use the minimal effective dose for the shortest possible period. A short-acting hypnotic (e.g. temazepam or a 'Z drug') taken at night should help restore her sleep pattern and may improve her daytime tiredness. Their relatively short duration of action should minimise the risk of unwanted effects during the working day. However, if the daytime anxiety also warrants treatment, a long-acting benzodiazepine (e.g. diazepam) given at night may be the drug of choice. Only short or intermittent courses of treatment should be given. The anxiolytic buspirone is not sedative, but it is ineffective against panic attacks.

2. Benzodiazepines and 'Z drugs' are $GABA_A$ agonists that enhance $GABA_A$-mediated inhibition of neuronal activity in the brain and spinal cord. They bind to distinct allosteric sites on the $GABA_A$ receptor to enhance Cl^- entry and hyperpolarise the neurone.

3. Benzodiazepines are relatively free of serious unwanted effects if used correctly and are safe in overdose, but Mrs. F.L. should be advised that they cause sedation and may interfere markedly with driving and operating machinery (worsened by interaction with alcohol, barbiturates and sedative antihistamines). Other unwanted effects include headache, dry mouth, hypotension, anterograde amnesia, skin rashes and blood dyscrasias. 'Z drugs' may cause gastrointestinal disturbances, dizziness, sedation and other unwanted effects.

4. Rebound wakefulness may indicate a need for a long-acting benzodiazepine such as nitrazepam or diazepam, which may also help reduce Mrs. F.L.'s daytime anxiety and panic attacks. Conversely, daytime sedation may interfere with driving and work, exacerbated by long-acting metabolites of these drugs. An alternative would be to prescribe buspirone; however, this may require 2 weeks for a response.

5. Long-term use of a benzodiazepine is associated with dependence, manifested mainly as a withdrawal reaction, which may include rebound anxiety, tremor, nausea, irritability, anorexia and dysphoria. Together with rapid development of tolerance (especially to hypnotic action), these contraindicate benzodiazepine treatment for more than 2–4 weeks.

6. In the longer term a course of antidepressants may be indicated. Mrs. F.L.'s recovery from bereavement may be aided by psychological counselling and support from her family and employer.

Extended-matching-item answers

Scenario 1: Answer **A** is correct. Withdrawal from long courses of benzodiazepines is difficult. She is liable to show withdrawal symptoms or return of the original complaints that determined the original prescription. Psychological and other forms of counselling may be advisable. Withdrawal should include gradual dosage reduction and anxiety management. Long-term psychological support is equally important for successful outcome, particularly for reducing the incidence and severity of postwithdrawal syndromes.

Scenario 2: Answer **D** is correct. Continuing with a benzodiazepine is unlikely to improve matters after a year of treatment. The use of anxiolytics may be masking depression. An option might be to assess for depression and use an SSRI licensed for the treatment of anxiety and panic disorders. General assessment is also recommended to rule out other disorders, and nonpharmacological treatments should be considered.

FURTHER READING

Baldwin, D., Woods, R., Lawson, R., et al., 2011. Efficacy of drug treatment for generalized anxiety disorder: systematic review and meta-analysis. Br. Med. J. 342, d1199.

Falloon, K., Arroll, B., Elley, C.R., et al., 2011. The assessment and management of insomnia in primary care. Br. Med. J. 342, d2899.

Hoge, E.A., Ivkovic, A., Fricchione, G.L., 2012. Generalized anxiety disorder. Br. Med. J. 345, e7500.

Morin, C.M., Benca, R., 2012. Chronic insomnia. Lancet 379, 1129–1141.

Roy-Byrne, P.P., Craske, M.G., Stein, M.B., 2006. Panic disorder. Lancet 368, 1023–1032.

Schneier, F.R., 2006. Social anxiety disorder. N. Engl. J. Med. 355, 1029–1036.

Stein, M.B., Sareen, J., 2014. Generalised anxiety disorder. N. Engl. J. Med. 373, 2059–2068.

Veale, D., Roberts, A., 2014. Obsessive-compulsive disorder. Br. Med. J. 348, g2183.

Winkelman, J.W., 2015. Insomnia disorder. N. Engl. J. Med. 373, 1437–1444.

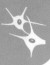

Compendium: anxiolytics, sedatives and hypnotics

Drug	Characteristics
Anxiolytics	
Short-term use; given orally unless other otherwise indicated.	
Alprazolam	Benzodiazepine; an allosteric GABA$_A$ receptor agonist. Half-life: 6–16 h
Buspirone	Partial agonist at presynaptic 5-HT$_{1A}$ receptors, which reduces 5-HT release. No effect on GABA$_A$ receptors and no sedative action; anxiolytic onset after 2 weeks. Half-life: 2–4 h
Chlordiazepoxide	Long-acting benzodiazepine anxiolytic. Also used as an adjunct in alcohol withdrawal. Half-life: 15–100 h
Diazepam	Long-acting benzodiazepine anxiolytic. May be given orally, rectally or by intramuscular or slow intravenous injection. Also used for insomnia, status epilepticus and muscle spasm and in surgical premedication. Half-life: 20–100 h
Lorazepam	Benzodiazepine anxiolytic; shorter-acting than diazepam. Also used as anticonvulsant and for surgical premedication. Half-life: 4–25 h
Oxazepam	Benzodiazepine anxiolytic; shorter-acting than diazepam. Half-life: 4–25 h
Sedatives and hypnotics	
All given orally and recommended for short-term use only (unless otherwise indicated).	
Chloral hydrate	Chlorinated derivative of ethanol; acts at GABA$_A$ receptor. Formerly used as a hypnotic in children and the elderly; now rarely used. Half-life: 8–12 h
Clomethiazole	Derivative of chloral hydrate; acts at barbiturate site on GABA$_A$ receptor. Used only for severe insomnia in the elderly (with little hangover) and for acute alcohol withdrawal (not preferred, as addictive). Half-life: 4–6 h
Flurazepam	Benzodiazepine hypnotic. Half-life: 2–4 h, with a long-lived active metabolite (30–100 h)
Loprazolam	Benzodiazepine hypnotic. Half-life: 7 h
Lormetazepam	Benzodiazepine hypnotic. Half-life: 8–10 h
Melatonin	Pineal hormone. Used for short-term insomnia in adults over 55 years. Half-life: 3–4 h
Midazolam	Benzodiazepine used primarily in surgical premedication; given by slow intravenous or intramuscular injection. Half-life: 1–5 h
Nitrazepam	Benzodiazepine hypnotic. Half-life: 20–48 h
Promethazine	H$_1$ antihistamine with prolonged sedative and hypnotic effects. Half-life: 7–14 h
Temazepam	Benzodiazepine hypnotic; also used in surgical premedication. Half-life: 5–12 h
Zaleplon	Z-drug hypnotic; binds to α_1-subunit of the GABA$_A$ receptor. Used for up to 2 weeks. Half-life: 1 h
Zolpidem	Z-drug hypnotic; binds to α_1-subunit of the GABA$_A$ receptor. Used for up to 4 weeks. Half-life: 2–3 h
Zopiclone	Z-drug hypnotic; binds to α_1- and α_2-subunits of the GABA$_A$ receptor. Used for up to 4 weeks. Half-life: 4–6 h
Drugs that reverse sedative effects of benzodiazepines	
Flumazenil	Competitive antagonist of benzodiazepine binding site; given by intravenous injection or infusion in acute benzodiazepine overdose. Half-life: 1 h

21

Schizophrenia and bipolar disorder

SCHIZOPHRENIA

The term *psychosis* indicates a mental state in which the person affected has lost contact with reality. This is usually experienced as hallucinations, delusions, or disruptions in thought processes, often with lack of insight. The most profound primary psychotic condition is schizophrenia, but the diagnosis covers a continuum that embraces the so-called schizoaffective disorders. Organic disease such as metabolic disturbance, toxic substances, or psychoactive drugs can cause psychosis (Box 21.1).

Clinical features of schizophrenia are categorised as positive or negative (Table 21.1), although none are pathognomonic of the disorder. The positive features are disordered thinking, perception, formation of ideas, or sense of self. They include hallucinations (false sensory perceptions) and delusions (false beliefs held with absolute certainty and unexplained by the person's socioeconomic background).

The negative features, deficits in normal behaviours, are often the most debilitating in the long term. Cognitive decline is an early finding in schizophrenia and precedes the psychotic symptoms. Memory deficits are accompanied by abnormalities of declarative memory, a type of memory related to the conscious recall of facts and events. This generates false memories with psychotic content.

Schizophrenia presents relatively early in life. The onset is usually gradual but can be abrupt. Once established, it has either a relapsing or persistent course.

BIOLOGICAL BASIS OF SCHIZOPHRENIA

There is a strong genetic component to schizophrenia involving several risk genes that affect early brain development and predispose an individual to developing the condition. Triggers that have a further impact on neurodevelopment – such as prenatal exposure to viral infections or obstetric complications – probably lead to the disease in only those with a genetic predisposition. Many neurobiological abnormalities have been described in schizophrenia, including disturbances in neuronal numbers and synaptic connections in the cortical, thalamic and hippocampal areas. These structural changes become more marked as the illness progresses, but the heterogeneous nature of the disease makes it difficult to determine the precise underlying neuropathology.

Dopamine–glutamate interactions and their possible involvement in schizophrenia

Schizophrenia is believed to involve interconnected abnormalities of glutamatergic and dopaminergic neurotransmission in the brain. The limbic region (amygdala, hippocampus and nucleus accumbens) and prefrontal cortex are involved in cognition, emotional memory and the initiation of behaviour. They are regulated by a complex interplay among their neuronal connections, with dopamine and glutamate as important neurotransmitters.

Most dopaminergic pathways in the central nervous system (CNS) arise from the substantia nigra (among the basal ganglia) and the ventral tegmental area in the midbrain (Fig. 21.1). One major dopaminergic pathway has its origin in the substantia nigra and projects to γ-aminobutyric acid (GABA)-ergic inhibitory interneurons in the corpus striatum through the nigrostriatal pathway (see Chapter 24). This pathway modulates motor and behavioural function through ongoing projections to the thalamus and cortex. Other major

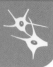

Table 21.1 Clinical features of schizophrenia

Features	Characteristics
Positive features	
Hallucinations	Third-person auditory hallucinations (voices talking about the person as 'he' or 'she')
	Second-person commands
	Olfactory, tactile, or visual hallucinations
Delusions	Thought withdrawal (thoughts being taken from the person's mind)
	Thought insertion (alien thoughts inserted in the person's mind)
	Thought broadcast (thoughts are known to others)
	Actions are caused or controlled from outside
	Bodily sensations are imposed from outside
	Delusional perception (a sudden fully formed delusion in the wake of a normal perception)
Negative features	
Loss of interest in others, initiative or sense of enjoyment	
Blunted emotions	
Limited speech	

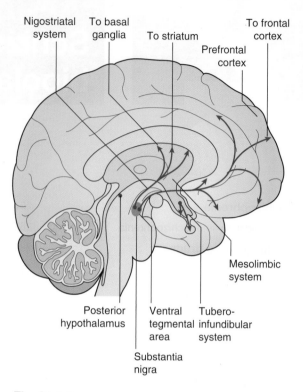

Fig. 21.1 Dopamine pathways. Major dopaminergic pathways in the central nervous system.

dopaminergic pathways connect the ventral tegmental area via the mesolimbic projections to the limbic region (especially the hippocampus). There is growing evidence that increased presynaptic dopamine synthesis and release in the corpus striatum may be the final common pathway for the positive psychotic symptoms. The involvement of dopaminergic abnormalities in cognitive decline is less clear.

Dopamine receptors in the brain belong to two families: D_1-like (coupled to a stimulatory G protein) and D_2-like (coupled to an inhibitory G protein). Postsynaptic D_1- and D_2-like receptor subtypes are found in the dopaminergic pathways in the corpus striatum, limbic system, thalamus and hypothalamus. Schizophrenia is characterised by overactivity at D_2-like receptors.

Excitatory glutamatergic neurons are involved in the regulation of dopaminergic activity in the midbrain. Glutamate *N*-methyl-D-aspartate (NMDA) receptors are also involved in brain maturation by influencing synaptic plasticity, which is achieved by changes in the receptor subunits during brain development. Failure of NMDA subunit "switching" at crucial times of "risk windows" for schizophrenia (such as birth

stress, infection, inflammation, or drug abuse) may result in the loss of important neuronal connections, particularly in the hippocampus. Hypofunction of NMDA receptors may contribute to negative symptoms and cognitive decline.

Several strands of evidence support the involvement of defective glutamatergic and overactive dopaminergic neurotransmission in the genesis of schizophrenia:

- Amfetamine-induced dopamine release is greater in people with schizophrenia.
- The dopamine concentration in the corpus striatum is higher in people with schizophrenia.
- Blockade of D_2-like receptors produces antipsychotic effects.
- Increased stimulation of D_2-like receptors worsens positive symptoms.
- Glutamate NMDA receptor antagonists (ketamine, phencyclidine) produce positive and negative symptoms and cognitive dysfunction similar to those of schizophrenia.
- Autoimmune encephalitis with antibodies to glutamate NMDA receptors produces a clinical picture indistinguishable from schizophrenia.

A third mechanism that appears to contribute to the development of schizophrenia is low-grade chronic inflammation with activation of microglial cells, the main immunocompetent cells in the brain. This may adversely affect brain development and contribute to the cognitive impairment and negative symptoms of schizophrenia.

It is likely that by the time psychotic symptoms arise, the brain is already "hard-wired" with irreversible changes in brain maturation and synaptic plasticity. Treatment at this stage may therefore control but not cure the condition.

ANTIPSYCHOTIC DRUGS

CLASSIFICATION

Antipsychotic drugs (also known as neuroleptics or major tranquillisers) have a common mechanism for their beneficial clinical effects via actions at the dopamine D_2 receptor. However, they belong to various chemical classes that differ in their propensity to cause sedation and antimuscarinic or extrapyramidal effects (Table 21.2). Antipsychotics are commonly considered in two groups: the conventional and atypical antipsychotics.

CONVENTIONAL (FIRST-GENERATION) ANTIPSYCHOTIC DRUGS

 Examples

chlorpromazine, flupentixol, haloperidol, sulpiride

Mechanism of action and effects

The antipsychotic action of all conventional antipsychotic drugs arises primarily from dopamine D_2 receptor antagonist activity in the mesolimbic pathway of the brain. High affinity for D_2 receptors and slow dissociation from these receptors is a common feature of all conventional antipsychotics. The affinity of the drug for these receptors correlates well with its effective dose. At least 65% of D_2-receptor occupancy in the mesolimbic system is required for clinical benefit during long-term treatment of psychotic disorders. However, these drugs also have D_2-receptor antagonist activity in other CNS pathways, and 80% or more D_2-receptor occupancy in the striatum will produce unwanted extrapyramidal effects (see later).

Many conventional antipsychotics also block serotonin 5-HT_{2A} and 5-HT_{2C} receptors, actions that may contribute to the suppression of negative symptoms in schizophrenia. Antagonist activity at other receptors, including α_1-adrenoceptors and histamine H_1 receptors, does not influence their efficacy in psychotic illness but can produce unwanted effects (in which respect they resemble tricyclic antidepressants; see Chapter 22). The severity of these unwanted effects varies considerably among the different drugs.

Clinical improvement with antipsychotic drugs develops slowly, despite an immediate antagonist action at dopamine receptors. There is increasing evidence that they modulate complex intracellular pathways that affect neuroplasticity in areas of the brain known to be involved in psychotic illness.

Clinically useful effects produced by antipsychotic drugs include the following:

- A depressant action on conditioned responses and emotional responsiveness. In psychoses, this is particularly helpful for the management of thought disorders, abnormalities of perception, and delusional beliefs.
- A sedative action, which is useful for the treatment of restlessness and confusion. Sensory input into the reticular activating system is reduced by the inhibition of collateral fibres from the lemniscal pathways. Spontaneous activity is preserved but arousal stimuli produce less response.
- An antiemetic effect through the activity of dopamine receptor antagonists at the chemoreceptor trigger zone (CTZ). This is useful in treating vomiting, such as that associated with drugs (e.g. cytotoxics, opioid analgesics)

Table 21.2 Unwanted effects of selected antipsychotic drugs

Example	Sedative	Antimuscarinic	Extrapyramidal	Hypotension
Conventional antipsychotics				
Chlorpromazine	+++	++	++	+++
Flupentixol	+	+	+++	+
Fluphenazine	++	+	+++	+
Haloperidol	+	+	+++	++
Pimozide	0	+	+++	+
Sulpiride	+	+	+	0
Atypical antipsychotics				
Aripiprazole	+	0	+	+
Clozapine	++	+	0	+
Lurasidone	+	0	++	0
Olanzapine	++	+	0	+
Quetiapine	++	0	0	+
Risperidone	+	0	+	+

+++, High; *++*, moderate; *+*, low; *0*, minimal.

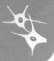
and uraemia. Some antipsychotic drugs are also effective in treating motion sickness through muscarinic receptor antagonism (see Chapter 32).

- The antihistamine effect from histamine H_1-receptor antagonism can be used for the treatment of allergic reactions (see Chapter 39).

Pharmacokinetics

Most conventional antipsychotics undergo extensive first-pass metabolism. Elimination is by metabolism in the liver. Several antipsychotic drugs – such as chlorpromazine, haloperidol, perphenazine, and zuclopenthixol – are metabolised predominantly by the polymorphic enzyme CYP2D6 (see Chapter 2). There is a relationship between the steady-state plasma concentrations of these drugs and the CYP2D6 genotype. The plasma concentrations of active drug (including metabolites) can vary up to 10-fold among individuals. However, there is a poor relationship between plasma drug concentration and clinical response, although unwanted effects may be greater at higher plasma concentrations. Sulpiride does not undergo first-pass metabolism and is largely eliminated unchanged by the kidney. The half-lives of the antipsychotics vary widely.

Since adherence to treatment is often poor in patients with psychotic disorders, depot formulations of many antipsychotics have been developed. They are given by intramuscular injection as prodrugs, where the active compound is esterified to a long-chain fatty acid and dissolved in a vegetable oil. The antipsychotic is then slowly released for between 1 and 12 weeks (depending on the formulation). When given as a depot preparation or as a short-acting formulation by deep intramuscular injection, the doses used are smaller than those for oral treatment owing to the absence of first-pass metabolism. Examples of depot preparations are flupentixol decanoate and zuclopenthixol decanoate.

Unwanted effects

The conventional antipsychotic drugs have different spectrums of unwanted effects (see Table 21.2).

- Extrapyramidal effects are most common with piperazine phenothiazines (such as prochlorperazine), the butyrophenones (such as haloperidol), and depot preparations. Most arise from D_2-receptor blockade in the nigrostriatal pathways. Clinical manifestations vary. Acute dystonias (tongue protrusion, torticollis, oculogyric crisis) are most common after the first dose or first few doses in children and young adults, akathisia (restlessness) usually follows large initial doses, and parkinsonism has a gradual onset over several weeks, usually in adults or the elderly. Extrapyramidal effects occur in more than half of those treated with conventional antipsychotics but are usually reversible if the drug is stopped. With prolonged use (several months to years) and especially in the elderly, tardive dyskinesias or tardive dystonias can develop. These consist of choreoathetoid and repetitive orofacial movements that often persist when the drug is withdrawn. Their aetiology is uncertain: upregulation of D_2 receptors may contribute, but damage to inhibitory GABAergic neurons and/or dysfunction in other neurotransmitter pathways is probably involved.

- Drowsiness and cognitive impairment can occur as a result of histamine and dopamine receptor antagonism.
- Galactorrhoea, with gynaecomastia and amenorrhoea in women, due to hyperprolactinaemia and reduced gonadotrophin secretion. The risk of osteoporosis is increased. Hyperprolactinaemia results from more than 70% D_2-receptor occupancy in the hypothalamus. Erectile dysfunction can occur from α_1-adrenoceptor antagonism and impaired arousal from antimuscarinic actions. Sexual dysfunction is a major cause of nonadherence.
- Antimuscarinic effects: peripheral antimuscarinic actions include dry mouth, constipation, micturition difficulties, blurred vision, and reduced sexual arousal (see Chapter 4); CNS muscarinic receptor blockade predisposes to acute confusional states.
- Postural hypotension, nasal stuffiness, and impaired erection and ejaculation in men due to α_1-adrenoceptor antagonism.
- Hypothermia as a consequence of depressed hypothalamic function.
- Reduced seizure threshold.
- Hypersensitivity reactions including cholestatic jaundice, skin reactions and bone marrow depression.
- Weight gain, with an increased risk of insulin resistance and glucose intolerance.
- Gastrointestinal disturbances.
- Prolongation of the Q–T interval on the electrocardiogram (ECG), a particular problem with pimozide, predisposes to ventricular arrhythmias (see Chapter 8).
- Neuroleptic malignant syndrome is a rare genetically determined disorder caused by a polymorphism in the D_2 receptor and consequent abnormal dopamine receptor antagonist activity in the corpus striatum and hypothalamus. In the presence of this polymorphism, antipsychotic drugs produce high fever, muscle rigidity, autonomic instability with hypertension, urinary incontinence and sweating, and altered consciousness. Immediate withdrawal of the antipsychotic and treatment with dantrolene or a dopamine receptor agonist (see Chapter 24) may be lifesaving. Symptoms can take up to 1 week to subside or longer after a depot preparation. Cautious reintroduction of an antipsychotic may be possible without recurrence, but at least 2 weeks should be allowed after symptoms of the syndrome have resolved.
- Sudden withdrawal after long-term use can produce nausea, vomiting, anorexia, diarrhoea, sweating, myalgia, paraesthesia, insomnia and agitation. These symptoms usually subside within 2 weeks.

ATYPICAL (SECOND-GENERATION) ANTIPSYCHOTIC DRUGS

aripiprazole, clozapine, olanzapine, risperidone

Mechanism of action and effects

The antipsychotic action of atypical antipsychotic drugs, like that of conventional antipsychotics, arises primarily from blockade of CNS dopamine D_2 receptors in mesolimbic pathways. However, the atypical antipsychotic drugs have a lower affinity for D_2 receptors and transient receptor occupancy. Therefore they are less likely than conventional antipsychotics to produce extrapyramidal movement disorders at usual doses. Antagonist activity at serotonin 5-HT$_2$ receptors may contribute to their antipsychotic action, particularly in improving negative features such as apathy and blunted emotions.

Atypical antipsychotic drugs have different patterns of activity at a variety of receptors:

- Aripiprazole has partial agonist activity at D_2 receptors, which limits the degree of receptor antagonism. It also has weak partial agonist activity at 5-HT$_{1A}$ receptors but is an antagonist at 5-HT$_{2A}$ receptors.
- Clozapine is a relatively weak D_2-receptor antagonist with selective cortical receptor occupancy and shows greater antagonist activity at D_1 receptors. It has greater antagonist activity at serotonin 5-HT$_{2A}$ receptors, α_1-adrenoceptors and muscarinic receptors.
- Olanzapine has a similar profile to clozapine, with additional antagonist activity at histamine H_1 receptors.
- Quetiapine has moderate affinity for D_1 and D_2 receptors, and is an antagonist at 5-HT$_{2A}$ and 5-HT$_{2C}$ receptors, α_1-adrenoceptors and histamine H_1 receptors.
- Risperidone has relatively high affinity for D_2 receptors. It also has antagonist activity at several 5-HT$_2$ receptor subtypes, α_1-adrenoceptors and histamine H_1 receptors.

Adherence to treatment with atypical antipsychotics is greater than for conventional antipsychotics, probably as a result of less marked unwanted effects, which may explain their apparently greater efficacy. Clozapine, however, is uniquely superior to all other drugs for the treatment of refractory schizophrenia.

Pharmacokinetics

Atypical antipsychotics undergo extensive first-pass metabolism to inactive metabolites. The half-lives of the atypical antipsychotics vary widely. Some atypical antipsychotics can be given intramuscularly in a depot formulation, such as olanzapine embonate.

Unwanted effects

The atypical antipsychotic drugs show some differences from conventional antipsychotics in their unwanted effects (see Table 21.2).

- Extrapyramidal effects are less frequent with atypical antipsychotics except at high dosages, when the risk is similar to that of conventional antipsychotics.
- Drowsiness and cognitive impairment are less marked than with conventional antipsychotics. Risperidone can cause insomnia and agitation.
- Galactorrhoea and sexual dysfunction are less common with most atypical antipsychotics except risperidone.
- Antimuscarinic effects are uncommon with atypical antipsychotics.
- Postural hypotension, especially during initial dose titration with clozapine and quetiapine.
- Reduced seizure threshold with clozapine.

- Agranulocytosis is a particular problem with clozapine (1–2% risk); regular blood tests are mandatory during treatment with this drug.
- Increased appetite with weight gain.
- Hyperglycaemia is more common than with conventional antipsychotics.
- Hyperlipidaemia.
- Neuroleptic malignant syndrome is rare.
- Sudden withdrawal syndrome.

MANAGEMENT OF SCHIZOPHRENIA

Acute psychotic symptoms such as hallucinations and delusions can be controlled relatively rapidly with an antipsychotic drug. However, reductions in thought disturbance, withdrawal, and apathy are delayed and clinical improvement is gradual over several weeks of treatment. Atypical antipsychotics should be considered in preference to conventional antipsychotics under the following circumstances:

- when choosing first-line treatment for newly diagnosed schizophrenia,
- if there are unacceptable unwanted effects with a conventional antipsychotic,
- during an acute schizophrenic episode when discussion with the affected person is not possible.

Treatment for schizophrenia is not curative and long-term maintenance therapy is usually required to prevent relapse. The optimal duration of this treatment is determined by the number of acute episodes and is usually at least 2–5 years. Intermittent treatment that is given only for relapses is associated with a higher overall relapse rate of 50–80%, compared with 25–40% in those taking prophylactic therapy. The relapse rate is lower and relief of negative symptoms better with atypical antipsychotics compared with conventional antipsychotics, possibly owing to better adherence. Adherence to maintenance treatment is often poor in schizophrenia and can be improved by use of depot injections that are given every 2–4 weeks. Continuous antipsychotic treatment provides relief of symptoms for more than 70% of people with schizophrenia, but resistance to conventional antipsychotics is particularly common if negative symptoms predominate.

There is limited evidence to support the concurrent use of a selective serotonin reuptake inhibitor (SSRI; see Chapter 22) together with an atypical antipsychotic drug for those whose negative symptoms do not respond to the antipsychotic drug alone. Clozapine is the only antipsychotic drug that is effective in treatment resistance (incomplete recovery), but close monitoring is required because of the risk of agranulocytosis. Clozapine should always be tried if symptoms have failed to respond to two antipsychotic drugs, at least one of which should be an atypical drug, each given for 6–8 weeks. Between 30% and 50% of those who are resistant to other treatments will respond to clozapine.

Various psychological treatments to improve social skills are important as an adjunct to drug treatment and should be provided, along with social support.

MANIA AND BIPOLAR DISORDER

Mania is a disorder of elevated mood that can occur alone (unipolar mania) or more usually interspersed with episodes of depression (bipolar affective disorder). Mild mania is termed hypomania. Sometimes the fluctuations of mood are less marked, in which case the disorder is termed cyclothymia.

The onset of mania can be gradual or sudden, most often between the ages of 15 and 25 years, and varies in severity from mild elation, increased drive and sociability, to grandiose ideas, marked overactivity, overspending and socially embarrassing behaviour. Mania and bipolar disorder have (and share) a stronger genetic component than any other grouping of major psychiatric disorders.

BIOLOGICAL BASIS OF BIPOLAR DISORDER

The biological basis of bipolar disorder is less well understood than that for unipolar depression. Susceptibility genes have been identified that are shared with those for schizophrenia, but the environmental stressors resulting in the expression of bipolar disorder are poorly understood. The dysregulation of neuronal function is probably triggered by altered expression of critical neuronal proteins, determined by the genetic predisposition. In bipolar disorder there is increased CNS monoamine neurotransmitter activity (particularly serotonin and dopamine) and reduced acetylcholine and GABA neurotransmission. These may all be important in orchestrating changes in neuronal number and function within the prefrontal cortex, visual association cortex and limbic circuitry.

The changes in neurotransmitter regulation produce functional disruptions in target neurons. Reduced neuronal levels of brain-derived neurotrophic factor (BDNF) may be important in the genesis of bipolar disorder (see also depression, Chapter 22). BDNF regulates several intracellular signal transduction pathways, and dysregulation of these pathways may produce the neuroplastic changes (especially synaptic plasticity) and neuronal cell loss that are features of bipolar disorder.

MOOD-STABILISING DRUGS FOR BIPOLAR DISORDER

LITHIUM

Mechanism of action

The mechanism of action of lithium is not well understood, but it has multiple effects in the CNS:

- Complex effects on the generation of intracellular second messengers in cortical neuronal pathways. Lithium attenuates the function of G_s proteins coupled to adenylyl cyclase but increases basal adenylyl cyclase activity, with consequent effects on cAMP synthesis. Lithium also inhibits intracellular inositol monophosphatase and therefore interferes with substrate generation for second messengers involved in phosphoinositide pathway signalling. These actions affect several monoaminergic and cholinergic systems in the CNS. The overall action of lithium may be to stabilise intracellular signalling by enhancing basal activity but decreasing maximum activity.
- Suppression of proapoptotic genes and increased expression of antiapoptotic genes, with consequent

neuroprotection. Lithium inhibits the multifunctional enzyme glucose synthase kinase-3 (GSK-3), a regulator of many signal transduction pathways involved in neuronal apoptosis. Inhibition of the activity of the proapoptotic enzyme caspase-3 by lithium also confers neuroprotection.
- Increased neurogenesis in the hippocampus; this may be one consequence of the complex changes in intracellular signalling, perhaps through enhanced BDNF synthesis.

Pharmacokinetics

Lithium is given as a salt (e.g. carbonate, citrate), which is rapidly absorbed from the gut. To avoid high peak plasma concentrations (which are associated with unwanted effects), modified-release formulations are normally used. Lithium is widely distributed in the body but enters the brain slowly. It is selectively concentrated in bone and the thyroid gland. Excretion is by glomerular filtration, with 80% reabsorbed in the proximal tubule by the same mechanism as Na^+; unlike Na^+, however, lithium is not reabsorbed from more distal parts of the kidney. When the body is depleted of salt and water, for example by vomiting or diarrhoea, then enhanced reabsorption of Na^+ in the proximal tubule is accompanied by enhanced lithium reabsorption, which can produce acute toxicity. Lithium has a long half-life of about 1 day. It has a narrow therapeutic index, and regular monitoring of serum concentrations is mandatory at least every 3 months during long-term treatment. The serum concentration should be measured 12 hours after dosing so that the absorption and distribution phases are completed, with the aim of maintaining a therapeutic plasma lithium concentration between 0.4 and 1.0 mmol/L.

Unwanted effects

- Nausea and diarrhoea can occur even at low plasma concentrations.
- CNS effects, including tremor, giddiness, ataxia, dysarthria, and mild cognitive and memory impairment.
- Hypothyroidism can be caused by interference with thyroxine synthesis during long-term treatment. Thyroid function should be monitored every 6 months.
- Reduced responsiveness of the distal renal tubule to antidiuretic hormone (ADH) can produce a reversible nephrogenic diabetes insipidus with polyuria and consequent polydipsia.
- Overdosage usually produces symptoms when the serum lithium concentration rises above 1.5 mmol/L. Severe toxicity (serum lithium concentration above 2.0 mmol/L) can lead to coma, convulsions, and profound hypotension with oliguria.

Drug interactions

Diuretics can reduce lithium excretion by producing intravascular volume depletion (see pharmacokinetics, discussed previously). This is most marked with thiazides (see Chapter 14) because of their prolonged action. Angiotensin-converting enzyme inhibitors, angiotensin II receptor antagonists (see Chapter 6), and some nonsteroidal anti-inflammatory drugs (see Chapter 29) also reduce the renal excretion of lithium. The risk of extrapyramidal effects may be increased when lithium is prescribed concurrently with antipsychotic drugs.

ANTICONVULSANTS

 Examples

carbamazepine, lamotrigine, sodium valproate

Mechanism of action in bipolar disorder

The mode of action of the anticonvulsants carbamazepine, lamotrigine and sodium valproate in mania may be related to the facilitation of GABAergic inhibitory neurotransmission and consequent modulation of excitatory glutamatergic neurons. Like lithium, anticonvulsants affect cAMP-mediated intracellular events and inhibit the phosphoinositide signalling pathway. They also inhibit histone deacetylase, which modulates gene expression, activates neuroprotective antiapoptotic genes, and stimulates hippocampal neurogenesis. Anticonvulsant (antiepileptic) drugs are discussed in Chapter 23.

MANAGEMENT OF BIPOLAR DISORDER

Mild to moderate symptoms of acute mania can usually be controlled by lithium, although the therapeutic effect may be delayed for at least a week. For this reason, a benzodiazepine (see Chapter 20) is usually given concurrently for the first 7 days. The anticonvulsant sodium valproate is an effective alternative to lithium for the acute phase; its sedative action produces a response in 1–4 days when used alone. Carbamazepine is an alternative option, but like lithium has a delayed onset of action and is given initially with a benzodiazepine.

If manic symptoms are more severe, it is usually necessary to give an antipsychotic drug in combination with lithium, carbamazepine or sodium valproate and perhaps initially a benzodiazepine. An atypical antipsychotic such as olanzapine, quetiapine or risperidone is usually preferred.

Depression in bipolar disorder is often treated with quetiapine or a combination of lithium and an antidepressant. The response to antidepressant therapy is less satisfactory than with unipolar depression and there is a risk of provoking a switch to mania, although this is less likely with an SSRI than a tricyclic antidepressant (see Chapter 22). Alternative treatments for bipolar depression include a combination of olanzapine with the SSRI fluoxetine or the mood-stabilising anticonvulsant lamotrigine.

Optimal duration of treatment after a first episode of mania is unclear. However, if a person with bipolar disorder has had at least two episodes of either mania or depression in 5 years, prophylactic therapy is recommended for at least 5 years. Lithium is the conventional treatment of choice for prophylaxis of both mania and depression (although the full prophylactic effect may not be apparent for 6–12 months), with quetiapine an alternative monotherapy. Antipsychotics other than quetiapine are more effective at preventing mania, whereas lamotrigine is more effective at preventing depression. Combination treatment may be required for maintenance, using lithium with valproate or an antipsychotic with valproate. If a decision is made to discontinue treatment, gradual withdrawal is recommended to reduce the risk of relapse, especially of mania.

Electroconvulsive therapy is used for refractory episodes of both mania and depression and has a much more rapid action than drug therapy. Psychological treatments are an important adjunct to drug therapy in bipolar disorder, as in the case for schizophrenia.

SELF-ASSESSMENT

True/false questions

1. It may take several weeks for the full beneficial effects of antipsychotics to be seen.
2. The positive symptoms of schizophrenia are more readily controlled than negative symptoms.
3. There is a close correlation between plasma levels of chlorpromazine and its antipsychotic effect.
4. Antipsychotics are effective in treating about 70% of people with schizophrenia.
5. Some antipsychotic drugs can be given as a depot preparation injected at 6-monthly intervals.
6. The atypical antipsychotic drugs have relatively low affinity for dopamine D_2 receptors.
7. The atypical antipsychotic clozapine has greater antimuscarinic activity than chlorpromazine.
8. Clozapine causes agranulocytosis.
9. The atypical antipsychotic drugs have relatively few effects on the extrapyramidal system.
10. Atypical antipsychotic drugs typically cause anorexia and weight loss.
11. Lithium interferes with thyroxine synthesis.
12. Lithium is reabsorbed through the distal convoluted tubule in the kidney.

One-best-answer (OBA) question

Choose the *most accurate* statement about antipsychotic drugs.
A. Adherence to atypical antipsychotic drugs is generally worse than to conventional antipsychotics.
B. Depot antipsychotic injections reduce the risk of extrapyramidal effects.
C. Dopamine receptor agonists may be lifesaving in neuroleptic malignant syndrome.
D. Haloperidol causes nausea.
E. Clozapine causes little sedation.

Extended-matching-item questions

Choose one mechanism from A to E below most likely to underlie each of the drug effects from 1 to 5:
A. Antagonism of dopamine receptors in the substantia nigra
B. Antagonism of muscarinic receptors
C. Antagonism of α_1-adrenoceptors

D. Antagonism of serotonin 5-HT$_2$ receptors
E. Antagonism of histamine receptors
   1. Antipsychotic activity
   2. Postural hypotension
   3. Sedation
   4. Constipation
   5. Extrapyramidal movement disorders

Case-based questions

Jake Smith, 20 years of age, lives with his parents. He has a diagnosis of schizophrenia, initially characterised by delusions of reference that he was being written about on social media and that the government was using Facebook to monitor his thoughts. He also experienced "running commentary" auditory hallucinations that only served to confirm his beliefs. He was suspicious of others and felt highly anxious, which affected his sleep. He was first prescribed olanzapine, which was effective in treating his delusions and anxiety. However, he became sedated and put on over 15 kg in weight. Jake again became a little more concerned about being monitored by the government, which prompted his parents to tell his nurse that they thought he was not taking his medication. In response to this, Jake's psychiatrist changed his medication to aripiprazole. Jake was pleased that he was more alert and lost 2 kg quickly. Unfortunately his mental health deteriorated and he became reclusive in his room and self-neglecting, which led to an admission to hospital. He was suspicious of everyone and nonadherent with oral medication. After a few days he was given intramuscular haloperidol for rapid tranquillisation, which was the beginning of his recovery.

1. What neural pathways are affected in schizophrenia?
2. Why are atypical antipsychotic drugs so called?
3. Discuss the use of olanzapine in Jake's treatment.
4. What is unusual about the pharmacology of aripiprazole?
5. What type of antipsychotic is haloperidol and why does it cause movement disorders?
6. What measures could be taken to improve Jake's adherence with treatment?

ANSWERS

True/false answers

1. **True.** Acute psychotic symptoms may respond relatively rapidly but further gradual improvement is seen over several weeks.
2. **True.** Negative symptoms are more difficult to treat but may respond better to atypical antipsychotics, at least in part owing to better adherence with treatment.
3. **False.** The plasma concentrations of chlorpromazine and some other antipsychotics are variable and do not correlate with their clinical effects, although unwanted effects are more apparent at higher plasma concentrations.
4. **True.** Schizophrenia is well controlled in about 70% of people taking continuous antipsychotic drug therapy.
5. **False.** Depot injections are usually given at 2- to 4-week intervals, depending on the drug dose and formulation.
6. **True.** The atypical antipsychotics have lower affinity for D$_2$ receptors and more transient D$_2$-receptor occupancy than conventional antipsychotics.

7. **False.** The atypical antipsychotics such as clozapine have less antimuscarinic activity than conventional antipsychotics.
8. **True.** The 1–2% risk of agranulocytosis with clozapine necessitates regular blood monitoring.
9. **True.** The atypical antipsychotics produce fewer unwanted extrapyramidal effects at normal doses than the conventional drugs, probably because of their lower occupancy of dopamine D$_2$ receptors in the nigrostriatal pathway.
10. **False.** Weight gain due to increased appetite is often seen with atypical antipsychotics such as clozapine and olanzapine.
11. **True.** Hypothyroidism can occur with the use of lithium; thyroid function should be monitored.
12. **False.** Lithium is reabsorbed through the proximal convoluted tubule, at the same site where Na$^+$ is absorbed.

One-best-answer (OBA) answers

Answer C is correct.
A. Incorrect. Adherence is higher with atypical drugs, probably as a result of fewer unwanted effects.
B. Incorrect. The risk of extrapyramidal effects is increased with depot injections.
C. **Correct.** Dopamine receptor agonists reverse D$_2$ receptor blockade in neuroleptic malignant syndrome.
D. Incorrect. Antipsychotics do not cause nausea and some are used in the treatment of nausea and vomiting.
E. Incorrect. Clozapine has a sedative action.

Extended-matching-item answers

1. Answer **D** is correct. Serotonin 5-HT$_2$ receptor antagonism is most likely to contribute to antipsychotic activity, particularly the negative symptoms such as social withdrawal.
2. Answer **C** is correct. Blockade of α_1-adrenoceptors on blood vessels can cause postural hypotension.
3. Answer **E** is correct. Blockade of histamine H$_1$ receptors in the CNS causes sedation.
4. Answer **B** is correct. Antimuscarinic effects include constipation, dry mouth, blurred vision and problems with micturition.
5. Answer **A** is correct. Antagonism of nigrostriatal pathway dopamine D$_2$ receptors produces extrapyramidal disorders of movement.

Case-based answers

1. Schizophrenia is associated with overactivity of dopaminergic pathways in the corpus striatum and limbic system, associated with defective glutamatergic activity. Florid schizoid symptoms may be mimicked by dopamine agonists (e.g. amphetamines) and are improved by dopamine antagonists. Antipsychotic activity correlates most closely with antagonism at dopamine D$_2$ receptors, which improves positive symptoms (e.g. delusions), and with antagonism at serotonin receptors (such as 5-HT$_{2A}$ receptors), which is associated with improvement in negative symptoms (e.g. low mood, apathy, social withdrawal).

2. Atypical antipsychotics are so-called because they produce few extrapyramidal movement disorders compared with the conventional antipsychotics. This may be because they produce lower dopamine D_2-receptor occupancy in the nigrostriatal pathway. Atypical drugs also tend to be more effective in treating negative symptoms of schizophrenia, possibly by antagonism of 5-HT_2 receptors.

3. Olanzapine is a commonly used atypical antipsychotic that is thought to act principally as a 5-HT_{2A} antagonist. There is good evidence that olanzapine and the other atypical drugs clozapine and risperidone are more effective than conventional antipsychotics, but olanzapine is noted for causing weight gain, as seen in Jake. It also blocks histamine H_1 receptors, and this may explain Jake's sedation.

4. Aripiprazole is another atypical antipsychotic used in schizophrenia, but it is also effective in bipolar disorder and as an adjunct in unipolar depression. Apart from blocking 5-HT_2 receptors, aripiprazole is a partial agonist at dopamine D_2 receptors; this may limit unwanted effects on movement and also reduce the risk of hyperprolactinaemia compared with other antipsychotics that are dopamine D_2 antagonists.

5. Haloperidol is a first-generation antipsychotic (a butyrophenone) and a highly selective dopamine D_2 receptor antagonist; it thus carries a high risk of movement disorders, but it was effective in treating Jake's acute deterioration. It is now more common to use an atypical antipsychotic for rapid relief of symptoms.

6. Jake's poor adherence with his antipsychotic medication could be addressed with a long-acting depot preparation. Support from the person's family and physician is also important in maintaining adherence. A principal cause of poor adherence is the unwanted effects of antipsychotic drugs, which vary widely from drug to drug and from person to person, so adherence may be improved by changing the antipsychotic drug.

FURTHER READING

Schizophrenia

Kahn, R.S., Sommer, I.E., 2015. The neurobiology and treatment of first-episode schizophrenia. Mol. Psychiatry 20, 84–97.

Leucht, S., Cipriani, A., Spindi, L., et al., 2013. Comparative efficacy and tolerability of 15 antipsychotic drugs in schizophrenia: a multiple-treatments meta-analysis. Lancet 382, 953–962.

Leucht, S., Tandy, M., Komossa, K., et al., 2012. Antipsychotic drugs versus placebo for relapse prevention in schizophrenia: a systematic review and meta-analysis. Lancet 379, 2063–2071.

Owen, M.J., Sawa, A., Mortensen, P.B., 2016. Schizophrenia. Lancet 388, 86–97.

Bipolar disorder

Anderson, I.M., Haddad, P.M., Scott, J., 2012. Bipolar disorder. Br. Med. J. 345, e8508.

Cipriani, A., Barbui, C., Salanti, G., et al., 2011. Comparative efficacy and acceptability of anti-manic drugs in acute mania: a multiple-treatments meta-analysis. Lancet 378, 1306–1315.

Grande, I., Berk, M., Birmaher, B., et al., 2016. Bipolar disorder. Lancet 387, 1561–11572.

Compendium: antipsychotic drugs

Drug	Characteristics
Conventional antipsychotics	
Benperidol	Butyrophenone antipsychotic. Main indication is control of deviant antisocial sexual behaviour (but efficacy uncertain). Given orally. Half-life 5–7 h
Chlorpromazine	Phenothiazine. Marked sedative effect. Oral, suppository and injection formulations available. Also used as an antiemetic in palliative care. Half-life 8–35 h
Flupentixol	Thioxanthene. Given orally (half-life 35 h) or as a depot formulation (as the decanoate ester)
Fluphenazine	Phenothiazine. Given by depot injection (as the decanoate ester)
Haloperidol	Butyrophenone. Pronounced extrapyramidal effects. Given orally and by injection (half-life 9–67 h) or as a depot formulation (as the decanoate ester)
Levomepromazine	Phenothiazine. Given orally or by intramuscular or intravenous injection. Also used for pain relief and as an antiemetic in palliative care. Half-life 15–70 h
Pericyazine	Phenothiazine. Given orally
Perphenazine	Phenothiazine. Given orally. Also used as an antiemetic. Half-life 9 h
Pimozide	Diphenylbutylpiperadine. ECG monitoring for Q–T prolongation mandatory before first use. Given orally. Half-life 55 h
Prochlorperazine	Phenothiazine. Given orally, rectally or by deep intramuscular injection. Also used as an antiemetic. Half-life 6–7 h
Promazine	Phenothiazine. Metabolite of chlorpromazine with little antipsychotic activity; used as a sedative. Given orally. Half-life >24 h
Sulpiride	Substituted benzamide. Given orally. Half-life 6–8 h

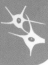

Compendium: antipsychotic drugs (cont'd)

Drug	Characteristics
Trifluoperazine	Phenothiazine. Also used as an antiemetic. Given orally. Half-life 7–18 h
Zuclopenthixol	Thioxanthene. Given orally (half-life 13–23 h) or as deep intramuscular depot formulation (as the decanoate)

Atypical antipsychotics

Drug	Characteristics
Amisulpride	D_2 and D_3 antagonist. Associated with prolongation of the Q–T interval. Given orally. Half-life 12 h
Aripiprazole	Partial agonist at D_2 and 5-HT_{1A} receptors and antagonist at 5-HT_{2A} receptors. Given orally (half-life 60 h) or as a depot formulation
Clozapine	Antagonist of D_1, D_2 (weak), D_4, 5-HT_{2A}, 5-HT_{2C}, α_1-adrenoceptors and muscarinic receptors. Highly effective antipsychotic but can cause weight gain, sedation and risk of agranulocytosis. Regular white cell count monitoring mandatory. Given orally. Half-life 6-33 h
Lurasidone hydrochloride	Antagonist of D_2, 5-HT_{2A}, 5-HT_7 and α_2-adrenoceptors, and partial agonist of 5-HT_{1A} receptors. Lowest risk of Q–T interval prolongation in class. Given orally. Half-life 20–40 h
Olanzapine	Antagonist at D_1, D_2, D_4, 5-HT_2, 5-HT_3 and histamine H_1 receptors. May cause weight gain. Given orally (half-life 21–54 h) or as a depot formulation (as the embonate)
Paliperidone	Metabolite of risperidone. Antagonist at D_2 and 5-HT_2 receptors. Given orally (half-life 23 h) or as a depot formulation
Quetiapine	Antagonist at D_2, 5-HT_{2A}, 5-HT_{2C}, α_1-adrenergic and histamine H_1 receptors. Given orally. Half-life 6 h
Risperidone	Antagonist at D_2, D_4, 5-HT_1, 5-HT_2, α_1-adrenergic and histamine H_1 receptors. Given orally or by deep intramuscular depot injection. Half-life 2–4 h and 17–22 h in rapid and slow metabolisers, respectively

Mood-stabilising drugs

Drug	Characteristics
Lithium	Given orally. Half-life 24 h

22 Depression, attention deficit hyperactivity disorder and narcolepsy

DEPRESSION

Clinical depression is characterised by diverse psychological and physical symptoms. Major depressive disorder is considered to be present if the person has had at least five of the following symptoms for at least 2 months or the symptoms have produced marked functional impairment for at least 2 weeks: depressed mood, loss of interest and enjoyment of activities, loss of energy, loss of appetite or weight disturbance (significant weight loss or gain), sleep disturbance, psychomotor changes, a sense of guilt and worthlessness, concentration difficulties or indecisiveness, or thoughts of death or suicide. Depressed mood or diminished interest or pleasure in all activities must be present to make the diagnosis, but depression can present with mainly physical rather than psychological symptoms. The existence of mixed anxiety-depression disorder is now also well recognised.

Major depressive disorder is an episodic illness that has a lifetime prevalence in about 15% of the population and recurs in almost three-quarters of people who experience an episode. In about 25% of people with depression, the condition may become chronic, with symptoms lasting for more than 2 years, whereas up to 40% of people report reduced psychosocial functioning even after recovering from a depressive episode. As the number of depressive episodes increases, the threshold for precipitation of a further episode by life stresses appears to decrease, a process referred to as "kindling". Both a genetic predisposition and the effects of adverse events in early life may determine whether a person is susceptible to depressive illness in later life.

BIOLOGICAL BASIS OF DEPRESSION

The cause of depression is unknown and there may not be a single mechanism. The neurotrophic hypothesis postulates that there are changes of connectivity between key structures in the brain that are involved in the regulation of mood and the stress response, including limbic structures (amygdala, hippocampus, and nucleus accumbens) and the prefrontal cortex. It has been suggested that the disruption of limbic connections with the prefrontal cortex impairs the normal feedback from the cortex that regulates limbic activity. Depression involves a negative emotional bias that may lead the person to preferentially recall negative events. This negative information is processed in the amygdala, which is hyperactive in people with depression.

In people who are genetically predisposed to depression, stress can initiate remodelling of the hippocampal circuits involved in regulating mood, cognition and behaviour. High plasma concentrations of the stress peptide corticotropin-releasing hormone (CRH, also known as corticotropin-releasing factor) and the stress hormone cortisol are found in more severe depressive disorders, which can lead to impaired neuroplasticity.

The monoamine theory, which has underpinned the treatment of depression for many years, is complementary to the neurotrophic hypothesis. Depression is associated with reduced central nervous system (CNS) monoaminergic neurotransmission, possibly as a result of high monoamine oxidase (MAO) A activity. This affects both serotonergic and noradrenergic pathways, which are closely involved in the regulation of mood. However, the central importance accorded to monoamines in the genesis of depression has been questioned.

Corticotropin-releasing hormone in depression

In many people with depression, there is hypersecretion of the "stressor" peptide CRH (see Chapter 43), which has detrimental effects on neural synaptic plasticity and neurogenesis and promotes neuronal excitotoxicity. CRH depresses serotonergic neurotransmission and is also a neurotransmitter that orchestrates CNS control of many behavioural, endocrine, autonomic and immunological responses. Many of these circuits involve glutamatergic neurotransmission via the excitatory N-methyl-D-aspartate (NMDA) receptor. Depressed neurotransmission in these pathways provides a potential target for the treatment of depression. CRH also increases cortisol secretion, which contributes to the loss of neuroplasticity.

Serotonergic and noradrenergic pathways in depression

Most serotonergic neurons are found in the raphe nuclei of the midbrain, from where they project to the hippocampus in the limbic system and to the cerebral cortex. Presynaptic α_2-adrenoceptors and serotonin 5-HT$_1$ autoreceptors (not shown in Fig. 22.1) inhibit serotonin release. Somatodendritic α_1- and β-adrenoceptor autoreceptors on the neuronal cell bodies of the raphe nuclei also regulate firing in serotonergic neurons. Postsynaptic 5-HT$_2$ receptors mediate the effects of serotonin; they are widely distributed in the cerebral cortex, especially the prefrontal cortex. A schematic diagram of these mechanisms is shown in Fig. 22.1.

In contrast, most noradrenergic neurons arise in the locus coeruleus and the lateral tegmental areas of the brain stem. The locus coeruleus and the raphe nuclei have many reciprocal neural projections; therefore their pathways are interdependent. For example, noradrenergic neurotransmission stimulates serotonergic neurons by activating somatodendritic α_1-adrenoceptors, but it also inhibits serotonin synthesis and release through presynaptic α_2-adrenoceptors (see Fig. 22.1).

Serotonergic pathways in the CNS are believed to be mainly involved in regulating mood, whereas noradrenergic pathways are involved in stress systems, drive and energy status. These monoaminergic circuits in the brain are closely integrated. Simplistically, it has been hypothesised that the following biological changes in the monoamine system are important in depression:

- low levels of monoamine neurotransmitters,
- upregulation of postsynaptic monoamine receptors,
- upregulation of the inhibitory presynaptic and somatodendritic autoreceptors that control monoamine release.

Overall, evidence for the monoamine theory as a molecular basis for depression is limited, but the response to drugs that increase monoamine neurotransmission supports the concept.

Regulation of brain-derived neurotrophic factor in depression

Most antidepressant drugs increase the CNS's monoamine concentrations rapidly, but the clinical benefit of antidepressant therapy is delayed. This suggests that more gradual adaptive changes occur as a result of increased monoaminergic neurotransmission.

There is evidence for a central role of brain-derived neurotrophic factor (BDNF) in the genesis of depression. Regulation of BDNF by monoamines is shown in Fig. 22.2. BDNF expression is reduced when monoamine neurotransmission is impaired, but it is also reduced in conditions of stress with elevated serum cortisol. Decreased expression of BDNF has adverse effects on neuronal plasticity and may be a major factor in the loss of neuronal circuitry and hippocampal atrophy. There is some evidence that successful antidepressant treatment is associated with increased BDNF expression and a restoration of hippocampal function and neuroendocrine regulation.

ANTIDEPRESSANT DRUG ACTION

Most of the antidepressant drugs currently used clinically target the mechanisms involved in the control of monoamine neurotransmitter turnover or monoamine receptor function. There seems to be little difference in efficacy between drugs that act predominantly on serotonergic or noradrenergic pathways, although they differ in their unwanted effect profiles. The ways in which major antidepressants work to modify monoamine turnover and function are shown in Fig. 22.1.

Long-term treatment with antidepressants promotes both the structural and functional integrity of the neural circuits that regulate mood. The postulated mechanisms by which they achieve this are complex:

- Enhanced CNS monoamine levels. The initial action of most drugs used in the treatment of depression is to enhance neurotransmission by CNS monoamines, particularly serotonin but also noradrenaline and dopamine. Increased noradrenergic activity further enhances serotonergic neurotransmission by stimulating somatodendritic α_1-adrenoceptors on serotonergic neurons. However, although antidepressants rapidly increase synaptic monoamine levels, clinical improvement is delayed. In part this may be because of a slow reduction in the number of upregulated somatodendritic and presynaptic 5-HT$_1$ inhibitory autoreceptors in depressed people (see earlier), which is necessary before activity increases in serotonergic pathways.

- Effects on postsynaptic monoamine receptor expression and intracellular signal transduction. During treatment with antidepressants there is a gradual increase in responsiveness to serotonin in the prefrontal cortex. There is considerable evidence that antidepressants reverse the changes in intracellular signalling that are found in depression (see Fig. 22.2). Antidepressants enhance the response to monoamine receptor stimulation, which increases the expression of BDNF and its receptor. This stimulates differentiation of progenitor cells into neurons and increases neuronal survival.

- Regulation of CRH production. During long-term treatment with antidepressants there is normalisation of overexpressed CRH secretion. This may be related to upregulation of CNS glucocorticoid receptors, with feedback inhibition of CRH.

- Antagonism of NMDA receptor action. Antidepressant drugs bind to a site in NMDA receptor-associated ion channels in the hippocampus and cerebral cortex and

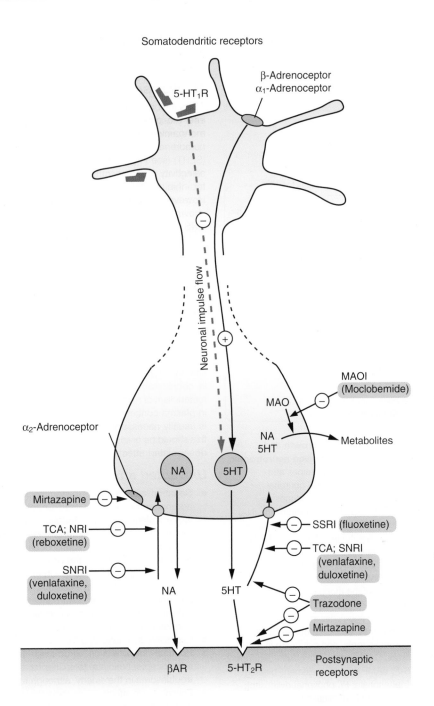

Fig. 22.1 **The actions of antidepressant drugs on CNS serotonergic and adrenergic functioning.** The primary action of many antidepressants in current clinical use (SSRI, SNRI, TCA, NRI) is to enhance the availability of serotonin (5-HT, 5-hydroxytryptamine) and/or noradrenaline (NA) in the synaptic cleft. The majority of released serotonin and noradrenaline is rapidly removed from the synapse by reuptake transporters *(yellow circles)*. Antidepressants vary in their abilities to inhibit the reuptake of serotonin or noradrenaline, thus they enhance the synaptic concentrations of these transmitters. Stimulation of presynaptic α_2-adrenoceptors reduces monoamine release; mirtazapine, by blocking these presynaptic autoreceptors, increases noradrenaline and serotonin release and transmission. Antidepressants may also block postsynaptic serotonin 5-HT$_2$ receptors, which are upregulated in depression. Monoamine oxidase (MAO) inhibitors (MAOIs) reduce the breakdown of monoamine transmitters within the presynaptic cell. *βAR,* β-adrenoceptor; *NRI,* noradrenaline reuptake inhibitor; *SNRI,* serotonin and noradrenaline reuptake inhibitor; *SSRI,* selective serotonin reuptake inhibitor; *TCA,* tricyclic antidepressant.

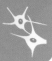

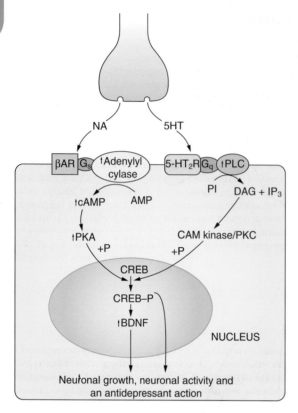

Fig. 22.2 **The regulation of neuronal growth and plasticity by monoamines and brain-derived neurotrophic factor (BDNF).** Adequate levels of monoamines and BDNF are considered necessary for normal neuronal growth and plasticity. An increase in cyclic adenosine monophosphate (cAMP) can result from noradrenaline (NA) acting on β-adrenoceptor (βAR) subtypes and an increase in diacylglycerol (DAG) from serotonin acting on 5-HT$_2$ type receptors. Other serotonin receptor subtypes (5-HT$_4$, 5-HT$_7$) and α$_1$-adrenoceptors may also contribute (not shown). This cascade may be dysfunctional in depressed individuals, including reduced synthesis of the monoamine transmitters, genetic polymorphism affecting the function or expression of monoamine receptors, and anomalies in the intracellular signalling pathways. These may result in reduced BDNF activity, leading to neuronal atrophy and cell death in the hippocampus and cortex. *CAM kinase,* calmodulin-dependent protein kinase; *CREB-P,* cAMP response element-binding protein; *IP$_3$,* inositol triphosphate; *PI,* phosphatidylinositol; *PKC,* protein kinase C; *PLC,* phospholipase C.

may protect cells against stress-induced "glutamate excitotoxicity".

ANTIDEPRESSANT DRUGS

Tricyclic antidepressant drugs

amitriptyline, imipramine, lofepramine

Tricyclic antidepressants (TCAs), once the mainstay in the treatment of depression, are now largely superseded by selective serotonin reuptake inhibitors (SSRIs).

Mechanism of action

TCAs inhibit the reuptake of monoamine neurotransmitters into the presynaptic neuron by competitive inhibition of monoamine transporter (MAT) proteins, particularly the noradrenaline transporter (NET) and the serotonin transporter (SERT) (see Fig. 22.1). Some drugs show little monoamine selectivity whereas other compounds are more selective for inhibiting the reuptake of one monoamine (Table 22.1). However, the degree of monoamine selectivity has not been shown to influence efficacy. The subsequent effects on the CNS are described in the preceding text.

Many of the unwanted effects of TCAs arise from an antagonist action at several postsynaptic receptors (e.g. muscarinic and histamine H$_1$ receptors and α$_1$-adrenoceptors) (see Table 22.1), which does not contribute to their antidepressant action.

Pharmacokinetics

All TCAs undergo extensive first-pass metabolism in the liver, forming active metabolites that are partially responsible for the variable effective half-lives of these drugs (8–90 hours; see the compendium at the end of this chapter). There is considerable interindividual variability in the first-pass metabolism of most TCAs, leading to up to 40-fold differences in plasma concentrations of the parent drug. Dose titration is usually necessary to optimise the therapeutic response; this should be gradual over 1–2 weeks to minimise unwanted dose-related effects.

Unwanted effects

- Sedation as a result of histamine H$_1$ receptor and α$_1$-adrenoceptor blockade (see Chapter 39). Amitriptyline is particularly sedative. Sedation can be useful to help restore sleep patterns in depression (using a larger dose of the sedative drug at night) but can be troublesome or even dangerous during the day.
- Antimuscarinic effects (see Chapter 4): dry mouth is a frequent occurrence; constipation, urinary retention, impotence and visual disturbances are less common. Tolerance to these effects can occur and gradual increases in dose may reduce their incidence.
- Excessive sweating and tremor.
- Postural hypotension produced by peripheral α$_1$-adrenoceptor blockade (see Chapter 4) can be particularly troublesome in the elderly, although tolerance can occur.
- Epileptogenic effects: TCAs lower the convulsive threshold, and seizures can be provoked even when there is no previous clinical history.
- Cardiotoxicity in overdose: most tricyclic drugs depress myocardial contractility. They can produce tachycardia and severe arrhythmias when taken in overdose, owing to both antimuscarinic effects and excessive noradrenergic stimulation. Lofepramine is less cardiotoxic than other drugs in this class.
- Weight gain: appetite stimulation is common, probably due to histamine H$_1$ receptor blockade.
- Hyponatraemia from inappropriate antidiuretic hormone (ADH; vasopressin) secretion, leading to drowsiness, confusion and convulsions.

Table 22.1 Comparative properties of some commonly used antidepressant drugs

	Uptake inhibition	Muscarinic receptor blockade	α₁-Adrenoceptor blockade	Histamine H₁ receptor blockade	P450-related metabolism	Sedation
Tricyclic antidepressants (TCAs)						
Amitriptyline	Serotonin = NA	+++	+++	+++	Inhibition	+++
Imipramine	Serotonin = NA	++	++	+++	Inhibition	++
Lofepramine	NA ≫ serotonin	+	+	+	?	+/−
Selective serotonin reuptake inhibitors (SSRIs)						
Citalopram	Serotonin ≫ NA	0	+	+	Weak inhibition	0
Escitalopram	Serotonin ≫ NA	0	+	+	Weak inhibition	0
Fluoxetine	Serotonin ≫ NA	0	0	0	Inhibition	0
Paroxetine	Serotonin > NA	++	+	+	Inhibition	0
Sertraline	Serotonin ≫ NA	0	++	0	Weak inhibition	0
Serotonin and noradrenaline reuptake inhibitors (SNRIs)						
Duloxetine	Serotonin ≥ NA	Low	Low	Low	Low	Low
Venlafaxine	Serotonin > NA	0	0	0	Weak inhibition	0
Noradrenaline reuptake inhibitor (NRI)						
Reboxetine	NA ≫ serotonin	Low	Low	Low	Weak inhibition	0
α₂-Adrenoceptor blocker						
Mirtazapine	0	+	+	++++	Weak inhibition	+
Serotonin 5-HT₂ receptor blocker						
Trazodone	Weak serotonin	Low	+	+	Weak inhibition	+

Drugs are listed under their conventional groupings but many have mixed or uncertain mechanisms of action; comparisons between drugs are approximate only. Other antidepressant drugs including MAO inhibitors are listed in the drug compendium. The side-effect profiles of antidepressant drugs partly reflect differential blockade of muscarinic receptors (e.g. dry mouth, tachycardia, urinary retention), α₁-adrenoceptors (e.g. postural hypotension), and histamine H₁ receptors (e.g. sedation). NA, noradrenaline.

- Sexual dysfunction with reduced interest in sex, erectile dysfunction in men and diminished arousal in women, and difficulty attaining orgasm.
- Sudden withdrawal syndrome: during long-term treatment, doses should be gradually reduced over 4 weeks to avoid agitation, headache, malaise, sweating and gastrointestinal upset, which can accompany sudden withdrawal.

Drug interactions

Several important drug interactions are recognised. TCAs potentiate the central depressant activity of many drugs, including alcohol. A dangerous interaction can result from giving an MAO inhibitor (see later) and a TCA together because of prolonged action of the increased serotonin released from the neuron. The interaction can lead to hyperpyrexia, convulsions and coma and can occur up to 2 weeks after stopping an MAO inhibitor because of the long duration of MAO inhibition.

The risk of serious arrhythmias is increased when TCAs are taken with drugs that prolong the Q–T interval on the electrocardiogram (see Chapter 8). Such drugs include the class III antiarrhythmic sotalol and all class I antiarrhythmics.

Selective serotonin reuptake inhibitors and related antidepressants

 Examples

citalopram, fluoxetine, paroxetine, sertraline

Mechanism of action

Unlike the TCAs, the SSRIs reduce the neuronal reuptake of serotonin by its presynaptic transporter protein (SERT) but have little or no effect on noradrenaline reuptake (see Table 22.1). They have a more favourable profile of unwanted effects than TCAs because of their low affinity for postsynaptic muscarinic and histamine receptors and α₁-adrenoceptors. Paroxetine is unusual among SSRIs in binding to muscarinic M₃ receptors, found in the brain, salivary glands and smooth muscle.

The proposed mechanism of action of SSRIs is as follows:

- increased synaptic serotonin concentration as a result of reduced neuronal uptake,

- downregulation of the 5-HT$_1$ somatodendritic and axon terminal presynaptic inhibitory autoreceptors on serotonergic neurons,
- increased serotonin release at the axon terminal,
- downregulation of postsynaptic 5-HT$_2$ receptors resulting from the prolonged increase in synaptic serotonin concentration.

The other cellular consequences of SSRI regulation of neurotransmitters are discussed in the preceding text.

Pharmacokinetics

SSRIs are metabolised in the liver. Paroxetine has a long half-life (10–20 hours), which is greatest in poor metabolisers of CYP2D6 substrates (30–50 hours). Citalopram, fluoxetine and sertraline have very long half-lives (23–75 hours). The active metabolite of fluoxetine has a half-life of 6 days, and the resulting very long duration of action can be a disadvantage if an MAO inhibitor is used subsequently (see later).

Unwanted effects

In contrast to the TCAs, SSRIs have few antimuscarinic effects (apart from paroxetine); they cause little sedation or weight gain and are not cardiotoxic in overdose. However, they have a range of unwanted effects.

- Nausea (frequent), dyspepsia, abdominal pain, or diarrhoea (less frequent).
- Insomnia, anxiety, and agitation.
- Anorexia with weight loss.
- Rashes.
- Hyponatraemia due to inappropriate secretion of ADH – leading to drowsiness, confusion and convulsions – is more frequent than with TCAs.
- Dry mouth and constipation with paroxetine.
- Sexual dysfunction with reduced interest in sex, erectile dysfunction in men and diminished arousal in women, and difficulty attaining orgasm. This affects up to three-quarters of people taking SSRIs.
- Increased risk of gastrointestinal bleeding due to platelet dysfunction.
- SSRIs lower the convulsive threshold; seizures can be provoked even when there is no previous clinical history.
- Sudden withdrawal syndrome after long-term use, which may be most troublesome with paroxetine. It presents with gastrointestinal symptoms; headache; anxiety; dizziness; paraesthesias;, electric shock sensations in the head, neck and spine; sleep disturbance; and sweating. This usually begins 24–72 hours after stopping treatment. To minimise these effects the dose should be reduced gradually over at least 4 weeks,
- Increase in suicidal thoughts and self-harm in people below 25 years of age in the early stages of treatment. SSRIs should be used with care in children and adolescents.
- Serotonin syndrome is the rapid onset of neuromuscular hyperactivity, autonomic dysfunction and altered mental state due to excessive serotonin levels peripherally and in the CNS. It is rare but can be life-threatening. Symptoms usually arise after an increase in the dose of an SSRI or when two drugs with serotonergic activity are used together.

Drug interactions

The most serious interaction of SSRIs is with MAO inhibitors. An interval of 5 weeks is recommended after stopping fluoxetine, or 2 weeks after paroxetine or sertraline, before an MAO inhibitor (including selegiline, see Chapter 24) is taken. Fluoxetine and paroxetine inhibit hepatic CYP2D6, which can increase the plasma concentration of drugs metabolised by this enzyme.

Serotonin and noradrenaline reuptake inhibitors

duloxetine, venlafaxine

Mechanism of action and uses

Venlafaxine and duloxetine are classified as serotonin and noradrenaline reuptake inhibitors (SNRIs), although at lower doses they have a greater effect on serotonin reuptake (see Table 22.1). Like the TCAs, they inhibit neuronal reuptake of both serotonin and noradrenaline but share with SSRIs a low affinity for muscarinic and histamine H$_1$ receptors and α_1-adrenoceptors. Their unwanted effect profiles are therefore closer to those of the SSRIs than those of the TCAs. There is some evidence that clinical improvement with venlafaxine may begin earlier than with other antidepressant drugs.

Duloxetine is also used as an adjunctive treatment for smoking cessation (see Chapter 54) and in urinary stress incontinence (see Chapter 15).

Pharmacokinetics

Venlafaxine and duloxetine undergo extensive first-pass metabolism in the liver. The main active metabolite of venlaxafine has a long half-life (11 hours), and the half-life of duloxetine is 9–19 hours.

Unwanted effects

- Nausea, vomiting, anorexia, dyspepsia, constipation.
- Hypertension, palpitation.
- Dry mouth.
- Drowsiness, insomnia, dizziness, confusion, headache, tremor.
- Sexual dysfunction.
- QT-segment prolongation on the electroencephalogram (ECG) with venlafaxine, which predisposes to ventricular arrhythmias (see Chapter 8); venlafaxine should be avoided in people at high risk for arrhythmias.
- Sudden withdrawal symptoms are more frequent than with other antidepressants, with gastrointestinal symptoms, headache, anxiety, dizziness, paraesthesia, tremor, sleep disturbance and sweating.

Selective noradrenaline reuptake inhibitors

reboxetine

Mechanism of action

Reboxetine is related to fluoxetine but is a selective noradrenaline reuptake inhibitor (NRI). Increased noradrenergic activity at somatodendritic α_1-adrenoceptors enhances serotonergic neurotransmission. Reboxetine, in common with the SSRIs, has little activity at muscarinic and histamine receptors and α_1-adrenoceptors. It therefore has fewer unwanted effects than TCAs.

Pharmacokinetics

Reboxetine is eliminated by hepatic metabolism and has a long half-life (15 hours).

Unwanted effects

- Nausea, anorexia, constipation,
- Palpitation, postural hypotension,
- Dry mouth, urinary retention, blurred vision,
- Sweating,
- Headache, insomnia, dizziness, paraesthesia.

Presynaptic α_2-adrenoceptor antagonists

mirtazapine

Mechanism of action

Mirtazapine is a tetracyclic drug unrelated structurally to the TCAs. In addition to potent postsynaptic 5-HT$_{2C}$ receptor antagonist activity in the cortex (see serotonin receptor antagonists, below), mirtazapine is an antagonist at presynaptic α_2-adrenoceptors (see Fig. 22.1). This reduces negative feedback inhibition of serotonin release from raphe nucleus neurons in their terminal projections to regions such as the cortex and hippocampus. Mirtazapine is an antagonist at histamine H$_1$ receptors but has low affinity for muscarinic receptors and postsynaptic α_1-adrenoceptors. It has minimal effects on monoamine reuptake.

Pharmacokinetics

Mirtazapine is metabolised in the liver and has a very long half-life (20–40 hours).

Unwanted effects

- Drowsiness, especially at lower doses, due to histamine H$_1$ receptor blockade. At higher doses, increased noradrenergic neurotransmission offsets some of the sedative effects.
- Increased appetite and weight gain.
- Fatigue, tremor, dizziness.
- Oedema.

Serotonin receptor antagonists

trazodone

Mechanism of action

Trazodone is a tetracyclic compound. Its most significant antidepressant action is through antagonism of postsynaptic 5-HT$_2$ receptor subtypes, which increases the activity of dopamine and noradrenaline in the frontal cortex. It also produces weak inhibition of presynaptic serotonin reuptake but does not inhibit noradrenaline reuptake. Trazodone is an α_1-adrenoceptor antagonist and a weak antagonist at histamine H$_1$ receptors.

Pharmacokinetics

Trazodone is well absorbed orally and metabolised in the liver. The half-life is 7–13 hours.

Unwanted effects

- These are similar to those of TCAs, but with fewer antimuscarinic and cardiovascular effects.
- Priapism (rare).

Irreversible monoamine oxidase A and B inhibitors

phenelzine, tranylcypromine

Mechanism of action

The primary mechanism of action of nonselective monoamine oxidase inhibitors (MAOIs) is irreversible inhibition of intracellular MAO, which is the enzyme responsible for degrading free monoamines in the presynaptic nerve terminal. This leads to the accumulation of monoamine neurotransmitters in the presynaptic neuron and increased release when the nerve is stimulated (see Fig. 22.1). There are two MAO isoenzymes (Fig. 22.3). MAO-B is the predominant enzyme in many parts of the brain, but MAO-A is present in noradrenergic and serotonergic neurons, especially in the locus coeruleus and other cells of the brain stem, as well as being the main enzyme in peripheral tissues. Inhibition of MAO-A in the brain produces the therapeutic effects of these drugs, but nonselective MAOIs target both isoenzymes. Inhibition of MAO in the gut wall and liver has important consequences (see below). MAOIs also inhibit various drug-metabolising enzymes in the liver, which predisposes to drug interactions but does not contribute to clinical efficacy.

Pharmacokinetics

All drugs in this class are irreversible enzyme inhibitors, so their prolonged duration of action is unrelated to their half-lives. Drug withdrawal is followed by gradual restoration of normal MAO activity over about 2 weeks, as new enzyme is synthesised.

Unwanted effects

- Dose-related postural hypotension can occur. Unlike the case with the TCAs, tolerance does not develop. The mechanism may involve conversion of tyramine (normally degraded by MAO) to octopamine, a false neurotransmitter

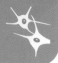

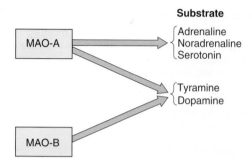

Fig. 22.3 **Monoamine oxidase (MAO) isoenzymes and MAO inhibitors (MAOI).** The relative selectivity of substrates for MAO is shown. MAO-A is the target for drugs useful in treating depression. Irreversible (nonselective) inhibitors of MAO-A and MAO-B prevent the metabolism of tyramine, which is responsible for the adverse food reaction that occurs with these drugs. Reversible inhibitors of MAO-A (RIMAs) allow tyramine still to be metabolised by MAO-B, so that the food reaction is reduced. Selective inhibitors of MAO-B enhance CNS dopamine levels and are used in treating Parkinson's disease (see Chapter 24).

that competes with noradrenaline at sympathetic nerve terminals.

- Because of its structural similarity to amphetamine (see Chapter 54), tranylcypromine causes CNS stimulation, leading to irritability and insomnia. Doses should be given early in the day to avoid disturbing sleep.

- Hepatitis is a rare idiosyncratic reaction to the hydrazine derivative phenelzine.

- Acute overdose produces delayed toxic effects after some 12 hours. Excessive adrenergic stimulation leads to chest pain, headache and hyperactivity, progressing to confusion and severe hypertension, with eventually profound hypotension and seizures.

- Food interactions can occur because MAO in the gut wall and liver usually prevents the absorption of natural amines, particularly tyramine, which is an indirect-acting sympathomimetic (see Chapter 4). If food containing tyramine – for example cheese, yeast extracts (such as Bovril, Oxo, or Marmite), pickled herrings, chianti, caviar, or broad bean pods (which contain L-3,4-dihydroxyphenylalanine [L-Dopa]) – is eaten, the increased absorption of tyramine and consequently greater release of noradrenaline result in vasoconstriction and severe hypertension. The first indication of this is a throbbing headache. A warning card should be supplied to people who take MAOIs.

Drug interactions

A number of drug interactions can occur. Indirect-acting sympathomimetics (see Chapter 4) in cold remedies (e.g. ephedrine, phenylpropanolamine), and levodopa (treatment of Parkinson's disease, see Chapter 24) will be more active, with a risk of hypertensive crisis. The toxicity of the triptans (5-HT$_1$ receptor agonists used for the treatment of migraine, see Chapter 26) will be potentiated. All these drugs should be avoided for 2 weeks after stopping an MAOI. The combination of MAOIs with TCAs or SSRIs (see earlier) can be dangerous. Other important interactions occur because MAOIs can impair

the hepatic metabolism of certain drugs, especially opioid analgesics.

Reversible inhibitors of monoamine oxidase A

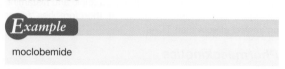

*E*xample

moclobemide

Mechanism of action and effects

Moclobemide is a reversible inhibitor of MAO-A, the same isoenzyme target for the antidepressant action of nonselective MAOIs. However, moclobemide does not inhibit MAO-B, so tyramine absorbed from the gut can still be degraded and the food reaction described previously for nonselective MAOIs is very unlikely to occur. Since the action of moclobemide on MAO-A is reversible, high concentrations of tyramine will displace the drug from the enzyme, further facilitating the degradation of tyramine. Therefore if moclobemide is taken after meals, the inhibition of MAO-A in the gut during absorption of tyramine will be minimised, providing further protection. MAO-A inhibition by moclobemide lasts less than 24 hours after a single dose.

Pharmacokinetics

Oral absorption of moclobemide is subject to substantial first-pass metabolism, partially to an active metabolite. Moclobemide undergoes hepatic metabolism and has a short half-life (1–2 hours).

Unwanted effects

- Sleep disturbance, agitation, confusion,
- Gastrointestinal upset,
- Dizziness, headache, paraesthesia,
- Dry mouth, visual disturbances,
- Oedema.

Drug interactions

Inhibition of cytochrome P450 activity in the liver by cimetidine (see Chapter 33) substantially reduces the metabolism of moclobemide; smaller starting doses are recommended in this situation. Moclobemide should not be given with other antidepressants, and the recommendations for stopping these drugs before prescribing moclobemide are the same as for nonselective MAOIs.

Melatonin receptor agonist and serotonin receptor antagonist

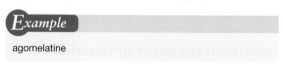

*E*xample

agomelatine

Mechanism of action and effects

Agomelatine is a synthetic agonist of melatonin, a naturally occurring substance, which is secreted by the pineal gland

and is involved in the regulation of circadian rhythms and, therefore, sleep patterns. Agomelatine is an agonist at both melatonin MT_1 receptors (attenuating alerting signals to the cortex) and MT_2 receptors (producing a phase-shifting action on the circadian rhythm of sleep). Agomelatine significantly improves sleep quality when taken at night to mimic the natural rhythm of melatonin release. It is a weak antagonist at $5\text{-}HT_{2C}$ receptors (see the previous discussion of serotonin receptor blockers) and increases noradrenaline and dopamine release in the frontal cortex. The antidepressant efficacy of agomelatine is similar to that of SSRIs.

Pharmacokinetics

Agomelatine is metabolised in the liver and has a short half-life of 1–2 hours.

Unwanted effects

- Nausea, diarrhoea, constipation, abdominal pain,
- Headache, dizziness, drowsiness, insomnia, fatigue, anxiety,
- Back pain,
- Sweating.

MANAGEMENT OF DEPRESSION

In mild to moderate depression, psychological therapies such as improving social contact and cognitive behavioural therapy are as effective as drug treatment and should be tried first. The herbal remedy *Hypericum perforatum* (St. John's wort) has no convincing efficacy compared with placebo in mild depression. St. John's wort is usually well tolerated, but it can induce cytochrome P450 and should not be taken with a prescribed antidepressant.

Drugs are usually necessary to treat moderate, severe or protracted symptoms, preferably in combination with psychological therapies. SSRIs are first-line drug treatments for depression. They are no more effective than TCAs and do not work any faster, but they are better tolerated and safer than TCAs when there is a high risk of attempted suicide.

The TCAs are now infrequently prescribed for depression. They have serious cardiotoxic effects when taken in overdose and should usually be avoided in treating people who are at high risk of attempting suicide. Encouraging adherence to treatment with TCAs may initially be difficult, since unwanted antimuscarinic effects can be troublesome before any benefit is perceived. Starting with a small dose of TCA followed by gradual dose titration can minimise unwanted effects. There is now evidence that large doses of a TCA do not necessarily enhance the treatment response but do increase unwanted effects; therefore low dosages are preferred.

All antidepressant drugs have a delayed onset of action; hence initial treatment should be continued for 3–4 weeks. If there is no response after this time and adherence to treatment is not a problem, the dose should be increased. If unwanted effects are troublesome, an alternative drug should be substituted. SNRIs should be considered if SSRIs are poorly tolerated. There is little evidence to guide therapy when there is failure to respond to an SSRI. Options include changing to another class of antidepressant, combining antidepressants (such as an SSRI with mirtazapine), or augmenting with the addition of lithium (see Chapter 21).

Up to 70% of depressed people will respond to drug therapy if the dosage is adequate, compared with about 30% taking placebo. However, only 50% will respond to an individual drug, and up to a further 20% of people with depression will respond if the drug is changed after failure of the initial treatment. Responders show an initial improvement in sleep pattern within a few days. Psychomotor retardation responds more gradually over several days, leading to greater involvement with everyday activities and enjoyment of life. Improvement in the depressed mood is delayed, beginning up to 2 or more weeks after commencing treatment with an adequate drug dosage. The response of most symptoms tends to be erratic, with good and bad days.

If there is a good response to treatment, the dosage of antidepressant can usually be reduced, but maintenance treatment should be continued for at least 4–6 months after the first episode of depression to minimise the risk of relapse. A longer period of maintenance treatment to prevent recurrence (at least a year and often longer) is often recommended for the elderly, for others who are at high risk of recurrence, and for people who have experienced two or more depressive episodes. About half of all people who experience depression only have a single episode. In individuals with recurrent illness, relapse occurs within a year in up to 65% of those who stop treatment but in only in 15% of people who continue treatment. Risk factors for relapse in major depression include

- presence of residual symptoms,
- number of previous episodes,
- severity of most recent episode,
- duration of most recent episode,
- degree of treatment resistance in previous episode.

Nonselective MAOIs are usually reserved for atypical depression with hypochondriacal and phobic symptoms or when SSRIs have failed. Small doses of the phenothiazine antipsychotic drug flupentixol (see Chapter 21) are sometimes used to treat depressed elderly people. The evidence for a true antidepressant effect of flupentixol is slight, but some symptoms undoubtedly do improve.

Treatment is most difficult in severe depression, especially if there are psychotic features or where depression forms part of a bipolar affective disorder (see Chapter 21). Electroconvulsive therapy (ECT) is used for treatment-resistant depression as well as in the elderly, who are particularly likely to show a response. Overall, ECT is probably more effective than drug therapy but does produce some lasting cognitive impairment, especially if given bilaterally rather than unilaterally or given frequently or with high currents. ECT should be combined with prolonged antidepressant drug treatment. Lithium (see Chapter 21) is used for people with severe recurrent depressive episodes and for the prophylaxis of bipolar affective disorder. The effect of lithium can take several months to become fully established. The treatment of depression in bipolar disorder is discussed in Chapter 21.

ATTENTION DEFICIT HYPERACTIVITY DISORDER AND NARCOLEPSY

Several drugs with mechanisms of action similar to those of antidepressants as well as central stimulant drugs have limited

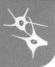

uses in the management of attention deficit hyperactivity disorder (ADHD) and narcolepsy.

ATTENTION DEFICIT HYPERACTIVITY DISORDER

ADHD is the most common behavioural and cognitive disorder in children of school age, but it often remains a problem in adult life. The core symptoms are inattention, hyperactivity and impulsivity. The cause of ADHD is poorly understood but may involve dopamine deficiency in the prefrontal cortex. There are three subtypes:

- predominantly inattentive subtype: failing to pay attention to details, difficulty with sustained attention, disorganisation and forgetfulness,
- predominantly hyperactive-impulsive subtype: excessive fidgeting and squirming, restlessness, frequently interrupting and intruding on others,
- predominantly inattentive/hyperactive-impulsive subtype: features of both subtypes in two areas of life and causing dysfunction in at least one area.

Adults with ADHD often present with poor occupational performance, marital instability, poor self-discipline or self-organisation, and restlessness. Sleep disturbances may also be prominent.

NARCOLEPSY

Narcolepsy usually begins in adolescence and is characterised by overwhelming daytime sleepiness, even if nighttime sleep has been adequate. Sudden daytime naps are frequent and there may be prolonged periods of drowsiness. Hallucinations may be troublesome on falling asleep or awaking. The condition may coexist with cataplexy, characterised by sudden loss of muscle function, ranging from weakness to collapse, that is often precipitated by laughter. People with narcolepsy have an abnormal sleep pattern, with rapid-eye-movement (REM) sleep at the onset of sleep rather than after a period of non-REM sleep (see Chapter 20). Narcolepsy has a genetic predisposition and there may be an autoimmune component. There is loss of hypocretin-secreting neurons in the hypothalamus, possibly as a result of autoimmune-mediated cell destruction. Hypocretins are neurotransmitters that regulate wakefulness by releasing dopamine and noradrenaline in the hypothalamus. The dopamine excites histaminergic tuberomammillary neurons, which are involved in control of arousal, sleep and circadian rhythms.

DRUGS FOR ATTENTION DEFICIT HYPERACTIVITY DISORDER AND NARCOLEPSY

Atomoxetine

Mechanism of action

Atomoxetine is a selective inhibitor of the presynaptic neuronal uptake of noradrenaline. There is a secondary increase in dopaminergic activity in the prefrontal cortex. Atomoxetine has antidepressant activity, but the mechanism of action in ADHD is not known.

Pharmacokinetics

Atomoxetine is metabolised in the liver; it has a half-life of 6 hours in most individuals (extensive metabolisers) but 19 hours in poor metabolisers of CYP2D6 substrates.

Unwanted effects

- Anorexia, dry mouth, nausea, vomiting, abdominal pain, constipation,
- Palpitation, hypertension, postural hypotension,
- Sleep disturbance, dizziness, headache, fatigue, irritability, depression, tremor,
- Urinary retention, sexual dysfunction.

Methylphenidate

Mechanism of action

Methylphenidate is an amphetamine derivative that activates the arousal system of the brain stem's reticular formation. Its mechanism of action is not well understood, but there is evidence that the drug blocks the presynaptic reuptake of noradrenaline and dopamine and increases dopaminergic neurotransmission in the prefrontal cortex.

Pharmacokinetics

Methylphenidate is metabolised in the liver and has a short half-life of 3 hours.

Unwanted effects

- Dry mouth, nausea, vomiting, abdominal pain,
- Palpitation, hypertension, postural hypotension,
- Sleep disturbance, dizziness, headache, fatigue, irritability, depression,
- Fever, arthralgia, rash.

Dexamfetamine

Mechanism of action

Dexamfetamine selectively releases monoamines such as noradrenaline (norepinephrine), serotonin and dopamine from CNS neurons in the mesolimbic pathway and also from the reticular formation that regulates alertness and sleep (see Chapter 54).

Pharmacokinetics

Dexamfetamine is partially metabolised in the liver and partially excreted unchanged. It has a half-life of 10–12 hours.

Unwanted effects

- Sleep disturbance, dizziness, headache, fatigue, irritability, depression, tremor, seizures, psychosis,
- Anorexia, dry mouth, gastrointestinal upset,
- Palpitations, hypertension,
- Tolerance and dependence.

Modafinil

Mechanism of action

Modafinil blocks the presynaptic reuptake of noradrenaline and dopamine, thus increasing dopaminergic neurotransmission in the prefrontal cortex. It may also reduce inhibitory neurotransmission mediated by γ-aminobutyric acid (GABA) and activate hypocretin-releasing neurons in the hypothalamus.

Pharmacokinetics

Modafinil is metabolised in the liver and has a long half-life of 15 hours.

Unwanted effects

- Anorexia, dry mouth, nausea, dyspepsia, abdominal pain, diarrhea,
- Palpitations, chest pain,
- Sleep disturbance, dizziness, confusion, agitation, depression.

MANAGEMENT OF ATTENTION DEFICIT HYPERACTIVITY DISORDER

Behavioural management, family strategies and psychotherapy have an important role. Drug treatment is considered for severe ADHD in children who are 6 years of age and older and can improve the three core symptoms. Methylphenidate is usually the first choice; dexamfetamine can be tried if there is no improvement with methylphenidate. Atomoxetine is used when stimulant drugs are ineffective. There is some concern that the benefits of the currently available compounds may be short-lived, with loss of efficacy after about 3 years. Treatment is usually continued until the child or parents want to try getting along without drugs.

MANAGEMENT OF NARCOLEPSY

Planned short naps may avoid the need for drug treatment, but drowsiness may require use of a CNS stimulant. Dexamfetamine or modafinil are usually chosen, but methylphenidate may be helpful. Cataplexy can respond to an SSRI or a TCA.

SELF-ASSESSMENT

True/false questions

1. The aetiology of depression is explained by the monoamine hypothesis.
2. Downregulation of serotonin $5-HT_2$ receptors occurs during antidepressant treatment.
3. Most TCAs inhibit the reuptake of noradrenaline and serotonin equally.
4. SSRIs should be used with caution in children and adolescents.
5. Different types of antidepressant differ little in their clinical efficacy.
6. TCAs potentiate the central depressant effects of alcohol.
7. Lofepramine is more cardiotoxic than amitriptyline.
8. Coadministration of an SSRI and a MAOI can cause cardiovascular collapse.
9. The antidepressant activity of mirtazapine is related to the blockade of serotonin receptors.
10. Trazodone is a potent inhibitor of monoamine reuptake.
11. Venlafaxine has marked sedative and antimuscarinic actions.
12. Venlafaxine has a low incidence of cardiovascular toxicity.
13. Only 30–40% of people with depression improve as a direct result of antidepressant drug treatment.
14. Lithium is used only for the treatment of bipolar affective disorder.
15. Methylphenidate is an amphetamine derivative used in the management of ADHD.
16. Narcolepsy is associated with loss of neurons that secrete hypocretins.

One-best-answer question

Which statement concerning antidepressant drugs is the *most accurate*?
A. A TCA would be more suitable than an SSRI for a patient with urinary outflow problems due to benign prostate hypertrophy.
B. The antidepressant action of trazodone is due mainly to inhibition of monoamine reuptake.
C. Moclobemide carries a high risk of unwanted interactions with food and drink.
D. An SSRI would be more suitable than a TCA to treat a person with suicidal tendencies.
E. Increases in levels of brain monoamine occur only after 2–3 weeks of treatment with an SSRIs.

Case-based questions

Darcey Ward is a 30-year-old accountant working in the City of London. She recently split from her husband and there was some uncertainty about her job, with a possible takeover and reorganisation of the company and her role. She was aware of feeling very stressed, being off her food, and sleeping poorly with vivid dreams, waking frequently, and not being able to get back to sleep after about 4 a.m. She started to feel that everything was "on top" of her and that she was no good at her job; she found herself crying every day. She didn't enjoy her social life and was becoming short-tempered with her friends, but she thought she should force herself to "put on a brave face". She visited her general practitioner (GP) who prescribed fluoxetine. After 3 months, there was little improvement in Darcey's mental health and she requested a change of medication. Her GP switched her from fluoxetine to venlafaxine and asked her to come back for a checkup in 2 weeks. As Darcey got to know her GP a little better, she said that she had not been taking her medication every day because of the effect on her sex life. Her GP took a detailed alcohol history – Darcey said that she was drinking most nights, either entertaining clients or socially after work, and they estimated a total of over 50 units per week.

1. What neurochemical and receptor changes are associated with depression?
2. What factors in Darcey's history may have contributed to her depression?
3. What type of antidepressant is fluoxetine? How does it act and what are the most common side effects of this group of antidepressants?
4. What type of antidepressant is venlafaxine and how does it act?
5. What is the evidence for the efficacy of antidepressants and what other types of therapy could Darcey try?

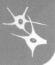

ANSWERS

True/false answers

1. **False.** The monoamine hypothesis alone cannot explain the causation of depression, in which neurotrophic factors, stress hormones and other factors play a role.
2. **True.** Downregulation of postsynaptic 5-HT$_2$ receptors (and also presynaptic autoreceptors) is thought to parallel the time course of clinical improvement, following changes in monoamine transmitter availability.
3. **False.** TCAs vary in their ability to inhibit noradrenaline and serotonin reuptake, with lofepramine being relatively more effective on NET and clomipramine on SERT.
4. **True.** Among the SSRIs (and venlaxafine and mirtazapine), only fluoxetine has shown efficacy for depression in clinical trials in people under 18 years of age; all SSRIs may be associated with a small risk of self-harm and suicidal behaviour in children and adolescents and should be used with caution.
5. **True.** Antidepressant drug groups differ more in their profiles of unwanted effects than in their clinical efficacy.
6. **True.** Alcohol should not be consumed by people taking TCAs.
7. **False.** Lofepramine is among the least cardiotoxic of the TCAs; it also causes little sedation.
8. **True.** An MAOI and an SSRI should not be combined. The combination can cause CNS excitation, tremor and hyperthermia. An MAOI should not be started until 2–5 weeks after stopping the SSRI, depending on which SSRI has been taken.
9. **True.** The main action of mirtazapine is blockade of postsynaptic 5-HT$_2$ receptors and central presynaptic α_2-adrenoceptors.
10. **False.** Trazodone is only a weak inhibitor of serotonin reuptake and does not block noradrenaline reuptake; its main action is blockade of postsynaptic 5-HT$_2$ receptors.
11. **False.** Like the TCAs, the SNRI venlafaxine inhibits both noradrenaline and serotonin reuptake, but it lacks the sedative and antimuscarinic effects of TCAs.
12. **False.** Venlafaxine causes QT-segment prolongation and predisposes to ventricular arrhythmia in high-risk depressed people, such as those with uncontrolled blood pressure.
13. **True.** Depression improves in up to 70% of people taking antidepressants compared with 30% of those on placebo.
14. **False.** Although most commonly used in bipolar affective disorder, lithium is also used in people with severe recurrent depressive episodes who do not respond to other treatment.
15. **True.** The amphetamine derivative methylphenidate is a first-line drug treatment in ADHD. In refractory ADHD, dexamfetamine or its prodrug lisdexamfetamine may be required.
16. **True.** Hypocretins promote wakefulness by releasing noradrenaline and dopamine. Increased production of hypocretins may contribute to the action of modafinil in narcolepsy.

One-best-answer (OBA) answers

Answer D is correct.
A. Incorrect. Many TCAs have antimuscarinic activity, which could exacerbate urinary retention.
B. Incorrect. Trazodone acts mainly by blockade of postsynaptic 5-HT$_2$ receptors.
C. Incorrect. Moclobemide is a reversible inhibitor of MAO-A (RIMA), so MAO-B activity remains available to metabolise dietary tyramine. The "tyramine reaction" with food and drink is much less likely to occur with moclobemide than with nonselective MAO inhibitors.
D. **Correct.** SSRIs are first-line drugs in depression; they are no more effective than TCAs but are less dangerous should a suicidal person take an overdose.
E. Incorrect. Increases in CNS monoamines occur rapidly following antidepressant treatment, but effects on mood and behaviour may depend on changes in receptor expression and neuronal growth; they may take several weeks to become apparent.

Case-based answers

1. There is a biological association of depression with reduced CNS monoamines (notably noradrenaline and serotonin). Monoamine depletion may upregulate monoamine receptors, especially postsynaptic 5-HT$_2$ receptors. It is unclear if these changes are causative, but most current antidepressant drugs act to enhance monoamine availability, possibly returning receptor expression to normal levels. Chronic depletion of monoamines may also reduce the levels of neurotrophic factors that promote neuronal health and growth. Treatment with antidepressants rapidly increases monoamine levels but takes longer to benefit depression, possibly by increasing the levels of BDNF, which promotes neurogenesis.
2. Risk factors for Darcey include female sex and a stressful home and work life, including a marital separation and what appears to be impending demotion at work. A family history of depression may be relevant. Depression is a syndrome (or cluster of symptoms), several of which Darcey exhibited over a significant period. A definitive diagnosis needs careful clinical consideration, but this patient has stress, low mood, sleep disturbance, alcohol abuse and dietary changes. It is not stated whether she has had suicidal thoughts.
3. Fluoxetine is an SSRI; others include sertraline, citalopram and escitalopram. National Institute for Health and Care Excellence (NICE) guidelines advise that an SSRI is the drug of first choice in mild/moderate depression seen in primary care. If this is unsuccessful, then another antidepressant drug type (discussed later) should be tried. SSRIs block the reuptake of serotonin (5-HT) by the serotonin transporter SERT in presynaptic neurons. SSRIs have fewer unwanted effects than most other antidepressants but can cause nausea, insomnia, agitation and decreased libido in a significant proportion of people.
4. Venlafaxine is a serotonin and noradrenaline reuptake inhibitor (SNRI). Venlafaxine blocks reuptake of serotonin by SERT and of noradrenaline (by the norepinephrine transporter NET). SNRIs do not diminish libido but are not quite as well tolerated as SSRIs. Venlaxafine may cause cardiac arrhythmia and a sudden withdrawal syndrome.

5. There is good evidence for the effectiveness of anti-depressants in moderate and severe depression, including reducing relapses. In people with mild depression, antidepressant therapy is difficult to distinguish from placebo, suggesting that these drugs may be overprescribed. Other antidepressant drug groups include (a) TCAs, which inhibit NET and SERT but are dangerous in overdose because of unwanted effects at histamine, adrenergic and muscarinic receptors; (b) noradrenaline reuptake inhibitors (NRI) such as reboxetine; (c) antagonists of presynaptic autoreceptors and/or postsynaptic 5-HT$_2$ receptors such as mirtazapine and trazodone; and (d) MAOIs, which are rarely used. Other approaches to managing depression include cognitive behavioural therapy (CBT), family therapy, and regular exercise. In addition, this woman's chronic alcohol abuse should be addressed.

FURTHER READING

Depression

Belmaker, R.H., Agam, G., 2008. Major depressive disorder. N. Engl. J. Med. 358, 55–68.

Grant, J.E., 2014. Obsessive-compulsive disorder. N. Engl. J. Med. 371, 646–653.

Hatcher, S., Arroll, B., 2012. Newer antidepressants for the treatment of depression in adults. Br. Med. J. 344, d8300.

Reid, S., Barbui, C., 2010. Long term treatment of depression with selective serotonin reuptake inhibitors and newer antidepressants. Br. Med. J. 340, 752–756.

Rodda, J., Walker, Z., Carter, J., 2011. Depression in older adults. Br. Med. J. 343, d5219.

Tanti, A., Belzung, C., 2010. Open questions in current models of antidepressant action. Br. J. Pharmacol. 159, 1187–1200.

Timonen, M., LiuKonen, T., 2008. Management of depression in adults. Br. Med. J. 336, 435–439.

Veale, D., Roberts, A., 2014. Obsessive compulsive disorder. Br. Med. J. 348, g2183.

Narcolepsy and ADHD

Scammell, T.E., 2015. Narcolepsy. N. Engl. J. Med. 373, 2654–2662.

Thapar, A., Cooper, M., 2016. Attention deficit hyperactivity disorder. Lancet 387, 1240–1250.

Verkuijl, N., Perkins, M., Fazel, M., 2015. Childhood attention-deficit/hyperactivity disorder. Br. Med. J. 350, h2168.

Young, T.J., Silber, M.H., 2006. Hypersomnias of central origin. Chest 130, 913–920.

Compendium: drugs used to treat depression, ADHD and narcolepsy.

Drug	Characteristics
Depression	
Tricyclic antidepressants (TCAs) and related compounds	
Given orally.	
Amitriptyline	TCA with sedative effect. Hazardous in overdose. Also used for nocturnal enuresis in children, for neuropathic pain, and for prophylaxis of migraine. Half-life 10–28 h
Clomipramine	TCA; relatively selective inhibitor of serotonin uptake. Sedative effect. Also used for phobic and obsessive states. Half-life 12–36 h
Dosulepin	TCA with sedative effect. Hazardous in overdose; specialist use only. Half-life 11–40 h
Doxepin	TCA with sedative effect. Half-life 30–50 h
Imipramine	TCA. Little sedative effect. Also used for nocturnal enuresis in children. Half-life 8–20 h
Lofepramine	TCA; relatively selective inhibitor of noradrenaline uptake. Little sedative effect. Low risk of fatality in overdose. Half-life 4–5 h
Mianserin	Tetracyclic antidepressant; noradrenaline reuptake inhibitor and postsynaptic 5-HT$_2$ receptor antagonist. Particularly useful when sedation is required. Risk of neutropenia and aplastic anaemia in elderly. Half-life 10–20 h
Nortriptyline	TCA. Little sedative effect. Also used for nocturnal enuresis in children and for neuropathic pain. Half-life 18–90 h
Trazodone	Tetracyclic antidepressant; antagonist of postsynaptic 5-HT$_2$ receptor subtypes and weak inhibitor of serotonin reuptake. Half-life 7–13 h
Trimipramine	TCA, with sedative effect. Half-life 20–26 h
Selective serotonin reuptake inhibitors (SSRIs)	
Given orally.	
Citalopram	Also used for panic disorder. Half-life 23–75 h
Escitalopram	Active isomer of citalopram; also used for panic disorder, generalised anxiety disorder and obsessive-compulsive disorder. Half-life 27–32 h

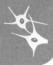

Compendium: drugs used to treat depression, ADHD, and narcolepsy (cont'd)

Drug	Characteristics
Fluoxetine	Used for major depression, bulimia nervosa and obsessive compulsive disorder. Inhibits CYP2D6. Long duration of action; half-life 48–72 h
Fluvoxamine	Also used for obsessive compulsive disorder. Half-life 7–70 h
Paroxetine	Also used for obsessive compulsive disorder, panic disorder, social phobia, posttraumatic stress and generalised anxiety disorder. Some antimuscarinic effects; risk of sudden withdrawal syndrome. Inhibits CYP450. Half-life 10–50 h
Sertraline	Also used for obsessive compulsive disorder, posttraumatic stress disorder, panic disorder and social anxiety disorder. Half-life 26 h

Serotonin and noradrenaline reuptake inhibitors (SNRIs)

Given orally.

Drug	Characteristics
Duloxetine	Also used in generalised anxiety disorder, diabetic neuropathy and stress urinary incontinence (see Chapter 15). Half-life 9–19 h
Venlafaxine	Risk of ventricular arrhythmia; risk of withdrawal effects. Also used for generalised anxiety disorder. Half-life 5 h

Irreversible monoamine oxidase A and B inhibitors (MAOIs)

Given orally.

Drug	Characteristics
Isocarboxazid	Used in refractory depression; risk of tyramine reaction. Slow onset of clinical action (weeks). Half-life 2–3 h but prolonged inhibition of MAO (days)
Phenelzine	Used in refractory depression; risk of tyramine reaction; risk of hepatitis. Slow onset of clinical action (weeks). Half-life 1 h but prolonged inhibition of MAO (weeks)
Tranylcypromine	Used in refractory depression; risk of tyramine reaction. Faster onset of action than other MAOIs but more hazardous because of stimulant action. Half-life 2–3 h but prolonged inhibition of MAO

Reversible inhibitors of monoamine oxidase A (RIMAs)

Given orally.

Drug	Characteristics
Moclobemide	Lower risk of tyramine reaction than with irreversible (nonselective) inhibitors of monoamine oxidase types A and B. Used for refractory depression and also for social phobia. Half-life 1–4 h

Other antidepressant drugs

Given orally.

Drug	Characteristics
Agomelatine	Agonist at melatonin MT1 and MT2 receptors and a weak 5-HT$_{2C}$ receptor antagonist; also has anxiolytic properties. Risk of hepatotoxicity. Half-life 1–2 h
Flupentixol	Phenothiazine antipsychotic (see Chapter 21); useful for depression with associated psychosis. Half-life 35 h
Lithium	Mechanism unknown. Used for severe recurrent depressive episodes and prophylaxis of bipolar affective disorder (see Chapter 21). Half-life 24 h
Mirtazapine	Antagonist at central presynaptic α_2-adrenoceptors and postsynaptic 5-HT$_2$ receptors. Half-life 20-40 h
Reboxetine	Noradrenaline uptake inhibitor (NRI). Half-life 15 h
Tryptophan	Amino acid. Very restricted hospital use as an adjunct to conventional treatments. Half-life 2 h

Drugs used to treat attention deficit hyperactivity disorder (ADHD) and narcolepsy

Given orally.

Drug	Characteristics
Atomoxetine	Noradrenaline reuptake blocker. Used for ADHD. Half-life 6–19 h
Dexamfetamine	Blocks monoamine reuptake. Used for refractory ADHD and narcolepsy. Half-life 11 h
Lisdexamfetamine	Prodrug of dexamfetamine. Used for refractory ADHD and narcolepsy. Half-life <1 h
Methylphenidate	Amfetamine derivative; blocks presynaptic reuptake of noradrenaline and dopamine. Used for ADHD and narcolepsy. Half-life 3 h
Modafinil	Atypical inhibitor of dopamine and noradrenaline reuptake. Used for daytime sleepiness associated with narcolepsy or sleep apnoea. Half-life 10–15 h
Sodium oxybate	Central stimulant; the sodium salt of γ-hydroxybutyric acid (GHB). Used for narcolepsy with cataplexy. Half-life <6 h

23 Epilepsy

PATHOLOGICAL BASIS OF EPILEPSY

Epileptic seizures are sudden, transient, and usually unpredictable episodes of motor, sensory, autonomic or psychic disturbances triggered by abnormal neuronal discharges in the brain. Epilepsy affects up to 0.6% of the population and is characterised by recurrent epileptic seizures without any immediate provoking cause. The clinical manifestations of epilepsy depend on the site of the discharge in the brain:

- In *partial or focal seizures* the discharge starts in a localised area of the brain and may remain localised or may secondarily spread to affect the whole brain.
- In *generalised seizures* the abnormal discharge affects the whole of the brain from the onset.

Identification of the type of seizure is important in the selection of the most appropriate therapy (Table 23.1).

The origin of epilepsy is complex. For most people with epilepsy, the initial focus of abnormal neuronal activity arises in an area of the brain with structural damage resulting from conditions such as trauma, tumours, cerebrovascular disease or haemorrhage. In about 30% of cases of epilepsy where there is no identifiable structural or metabolic disorder (idiopathic epilepsy), there is an important genetic component. Isolated seizures can also be caused by metabolic disturbances, such as hypoglycaemia or alcohol abuse.

NEUROTRANSMITTERS AND EPILEPSY

Normal coordinated activity among neurons depends on a controlled balance between excitatory and inhibitory influences on electrical activity across neuronal cell membranes. Neuronal networks cooperate by oscillatory electrical activity between different parts of the brain. Generalised epilepsy involves a change from these oscillations to excessive neuronal firing and abnormally synchronised neuronal activity across large-scale networks, in particular involving both the cortex and subcortical structures such as the thalamus (thalamocortical system). Structural changes in neuronal networks may provide a basis for the generation of abnormal discharges, with focal lesions in the neocortex and limbic structures (especially hippocampus and amygdala) promoting the formation of abnormal regional hyperexcitable circuits.

In healthy neuronal circuits, depolarising ionic currents are mainly activated by excitatory glutamate *N*-methyl-D-aspartate (NMDA) receptors. Repolarisation is initiated by γ-aminobutyric acid receptors (GABA$_B$ receptors), which act as a feedback inhibitory circuit in response to excitation. The activation of GABA$_A$ receptors hyperpolarises the cell and inhibits further impulse generation. Neuropeptide Y is coreleased with GABA and potentiates the inhibition. The balance between excitatory and inhibitory neuronal activity is important for suppressing excessive synchronisation.

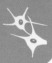

Table 23.1 Simplified classification of epileptic seizures

Seizure type	Characteristics
Partial (focal) seizures	
Simple partial seizures	Motor, somatosensory or psychic symptoms; consciousness is not impaired
Complex partial seizures	Temporal lobe, psychomotor; consciousness is impaired
Secondary generalised seizures	These begin as partial seizures
Generalised seizures	
Affect whole brain with loss of consciousness	
Clonic, tonic or tonic-clonic	Initial rigid extensor spasm, respiration stops, defaecation, micturition and salivation occur (tonic phase, ≈1 min); violent synchronous jerks (clonic phase, 2–4 min)
Myoclonic	Seizures of a muscle or group of muscles
Absence	Abrupt loss of awareness of surroundings, little motor disturbance (occur in children)
Atonic	Loss of muscle tone/strength
Unclassified seizures	—

An epileptic seizure probably begins with a localised imbalance between excitatory and inhibitory neurotransmission, which leads to a focus of neuronal instability. In some forms of epilepsy there may be a defect in neuronal transmembrane currents resulting in incomplete repolarisation of the cell. This will leave the neuron closer to its threshold potential for firing and create a hyperexcitable state. Such instability could initiate the burst of firing that produces epileptiform activity. Once an electrical discharge is triggered, spontaneous repetitive firing of the focus is maintained by a feedback mechanism known as posttetanic potentiation. The synchronisation of the electrical charge necessary to generate a seizure and subsequent generalisation of the impulse may also be enhanced by neural plasticity and the remodelling of neural connections.

Several inherited epilepsy syndromes have now been characterised at a cellular level; they arise from mutations of proteins involved in the function of ion channels. Reduction in the activity of membrane-bound ATPases linked to neuronal transmembrane ion pumps has also been found in the brains of people with primary generalised epilepsy. Ion channel dysfunction may therefore provide the basis for the genesis of many types of generalised seizures, but defective GABA-mediated inhibitory neurotransmission also appears to be a key factor.

The genesis of partial seizures does not involve large neural circuits. However, there is similar underlying excessive neuronal firing and synchronisation of firing that is localised to the cortex or limbic structures such as the hippocampus or amygdala. These circuits are generated by the abnormal functional organisation of excitatory neurons in the region associated with increased synaptic connectivity. Changes in the function of voltage-gated ion channels in these neurons may also play a role.

ANTIEPILEPTIC DRUGS

Most antiepileptic drugs produce their therapeutic effects either by blockade of depolarising ion channels, by an antagonist action at glutamate receptors, or by enhancing the inhibitory actions of GABA. Many drugs have multiple sites of action, so the drugs discussed here are grouped by their principal mode of action.

SODIUM CHANNEL BLOCKERS

Carbamazepine, oxcarbazepine, eslicarbazepine acetate

Mechanism of action and uses

The mechanisms of action of these drugs are incompletely understood, but the main action is use-dependent blockade of Na^+ channels to stabilise them in the inactive state, which inhibits repetitive neuronal firing.

Carbamazepine, oxcarbazepine and eslicarbazepine are effective in most types of epilepsy except for myoclonic epilepsy and absences, which they can exacerbate. They are also used in the management of trigeminal neuralgia (see Chapter 19), and carbamazepine is used in the management of diabetic neuropathy (see Chapter 19) and bipolar disorder (see Chapter 21).

Pharmacokinetics

Carbamazepine is metabolised in the liver to an active epoxide metabolite. The half-life of carbamazepine is initially very long, at about 1.5 days, but decreases by about a half over the first 2–3 weeks of treatment because of "autoinduction" of its own metabolism in the liver. Seizure control may then require an increase in dose. Transient unwanted neurological effects occurring in association with peak plasma drug concentrations can be minimised by the use of a modified-release formulation. The nonlinear relationship of the oral dose of carbamazepine to the plasma concentration of carbamazepine and its epoxide derivative makes the monitoring of drug plasma concentration useful to guide dose adjustment.

Oxcarbazepine is rapidly converted in the liver to active metabolites, including *S*-licarbazepine. Eslicarbazepine acetate is a prodrug converted rapidly on first-pass through the liver to *S*-licarbazepine after oral administration.

Unwanted effects

The unwanted effects of oxcarbazepine and eslicarbazepine are less frequent than those of carbamazepine.

- Nausea and vomiting (dose-related, and especially early in treatment), dry mouth.
- Oedema.
- Rashes, especially transient generalised erythema, but more severe reactions also occur. If a rash is produced by carbamazepine, oxcarbazepine can often be given without recurrence. Stevens-Johnson syndrome occasionally

occurs with carbamazepine and is more frequent in people with HLA-B*1502, who are most often of Han Chinese or Thai origin. Testing for this allele is recommended before using carbamazepine in people of these ethnic origins.

- Central nervous system (CNS) effects: headache, dizziness, drowsiness, ataxia. These are most common early in treatment and are dose-related.
- Transient leukopenia is common, especially early in treatment; also thrombocytopenia.
- Hyponatraemia, caused by potentiation of the action of antidiuretic hormone on the kidney, can lead to confusion and decreased control of seizures.
- Teratogenicity in the form of neural tube defects is common (see below).
- Induction of hepatic CYP3A4 (see Table 2.7) by carbamazepine can lead to drug interactions. The most common interaction is with the oral combined contraceptive (see Chapter 45); here the dose of oestrogen should be increased to avoid failure of contraception. The metabolism of warfarin (see Chapter 11) and ciclosporin (see Chapter 38) is also accelerated. Inhibition of CYP3A4 by erythromycin, clarithromycin or diltiazem can increase the plasma concentration of carbamazepine. Interactions of carbamazepine with other antiepileptic drugs are discussed below. Oxcarbazepine and eslicarbazepine have little effect on cytochrome P450 and therefore have few drug interactions.

Phenytoin and fosphenytoin

Mechanism of action and uses

Phenytoin and its prodrug fosphenytoin have a broad spectrum of activity and are effective against all forms of epilepsy except absences. The major mechanism of action is use-dependent blockade of Na⁺ channels, which reduces cell excitability.

Pharmacokinetics

Phenytoin is given orally for seizure prophylaxis. Slow intravenous injection is effective for rapid control of seizures. Intramuscular injection of phenytoin should be avoided, since absorption by this route is erratic and muscle damage can occur. Phenytoin is eliminated by hepatic metabolism, which is readily saturated, so the elimination changes from first-order (linear) kinetics to zero-order (nonlinear) kinetics (Fig. 23.1). A small change in dose then produces a large change in the plasma concentration and the elimination half-life is increased from about 12 hours to almost 2 days. This change in elimination kinetics occurs in some individuals at plasma drug concentrations below or near the lower end of the therapeutic range. Plasma phenytoin concentrations are closely correlated to the clinical effect, and their measurement is useful as a guide to dosing. When the plasma concentration is close to or within the therapeutic range, any further increase in dose should be small.

Phenytoin is highly protein-bound (about 90%), and changes in plasma protein concentration will affect the total plasma concentration but not the active free component. The concentration of phenytoin in saliva reflects the concentration of free drug in plasma. Measurement of the salivary concentration can be useful to guide dose adjustment when the plasma protein concentration is changing, as in

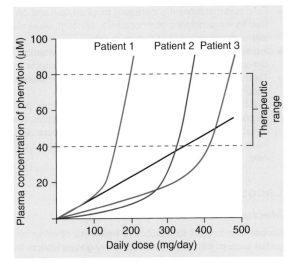

Fig. 23.1 Variation in the plasma concentration of phenytoin in relation to the daily dose. Hepatic metabolism of phenytoin becomes saturated at higher steady-state plasma concentrations, leading to "zero-order" (nonlinear) kinetics; the plasma concentration at which saturation occurs also varies markedly between individuals. The figure illustrates the relationship between daily dose and plasma concentrations in three individuals (Patients 1, 2 and 3). The straight black line illustrates the increase in plasma phenytoin concentration in Patient 1, which would occur if the metabolism followed first-order kinetics (i.e. not saturated). Small increases in phenytoin dose above those that saturate hepatic metabolism in each patient may result in plasma concentrations that exceed the desired therapeutic range. This nonlinearity can lead to difficulties in dosage adjustment.

pregnancy or nephrotic syndrome, or to avoid blood sampling in children.

Fosphenytoin is a prodrug of phenytoin for parenteral use. It can be given by intramuscular injection (absorption from this route is good, unlike that of phenytoin) or by intravenous infusion; it is completely metabolised to phenytoin.

Unwanted effects

Most unwanted effects of phenytoin and fosphenytoin are dose-related.

- Nausea, vomiting, constipation, anorexia.
- CNS effects: transient nervousness, dizziness, drowsiness, tremor and insomnia. Nystagmus, blurred vision, ataxia and dysarthria are signs of overdosage.
- Chronic connective tissue effects: gum hypertrophy, coarsening of facial features, hirsutism and acne. It is therefore usual to avoid phenytoin in young women or adolescents.
- Rashes. Stevens-Johnson syndrome occasionally occurs with phenytoin and is more frequent in people with HLA-B*1502, who are most often of Han Chinese or Thai origin. Testing for this allele is recommended before using phenytoin in people of these ethnic origins.

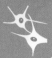

- Folic acid metabolism is increased by phenytoin and can lead to megaloblastic haemopoiesis, although anaemia with a macrocytic blood picture is rare.
- Increased vitamin D metabolism can produce vitamin D deficiency; in rare cases this results in osteomalacia.
- Teratogenicity, including facial and digital malformations, occurs in up to 10% of pregnancies.
- Induction of hepatic cytochrome P450 enzymes predisposes to several drug interactions. In particular, the metabolism of warfarin and ciclosporin are increased; interactions with other antiepileptic drugs are discussed next.

Lacosamide

Mechanism of action and uses

Lacosamide is used for adjunctive treatment of refractory partial seizures with or without secondary generalisation. Its major mechanism of action is enhancing the slow inactivation of neuronal Na^+ channels, which stabilises cell membranes.

Pharmacokinetics

Lacosamide is eliminated by metabolism and also by the kidneys. It has a half-life of about 13 hours.

Unwanted effects

- CNS effects: drowsiness, fatigue, dizziness, ataxia, nystagmus, tremor, depression, impaired concentration,
- Nausea, vomiting, flatulence, constipation,
- Pruritus.

Lamotrigine

Mechanism of action and uses

Lamotrigine has a wide spectrum of activity against partial and generalised seizures. It produces use-dependent inhibition of neuronal voltage-gated Na^+ channels. Unlike carbamazepine and phenytoin, it selectively targets dendrites of pyramidal neurons that synthesise glutamate and aspartate; lamotrigine reduces the release of glutamate.

Lamotrigine is also used for prophylaxis of depression in bipolar disorder (see Chapter 21).

Pharmacokinetics

Lamotrigine is metabolised in the liver and has a long half-life (15–60 hours).

Unwanted effects

- Nausea, vomiting, diarrhoea, dry mouth.
- CNS effects: aggression, agitation, drowsiness, headache, fatigue, insomnia, dizziness, double vision and ataxia; tremor can be troublesome at high dosages.
- Arthralgia, back pain.
- Hypersensitivity syndrome with fever, rash, lymphadenopathy and hepatic dysfunction. This is more common if lamotrigine is used together with sodium valproate.
- Rashes: some disappear despite continued treatment, but severe skin reactions, including Stevens-Johnson syndrome and toxic epidermal necrolysis, occasionally occur, particularly in children and following rapid dose escalation or with concurrent use of sodium valproate.

Zonisamide

Mechanism of action and uses

Zonisamide is used for adjunctive treatment of refractory partial seizures with or without secondary generalisation. Its main mechanism of action is use-dependent blockade of neuronal Na^+ channels, which stabilises cell membranes. It also blocks voltage-dependent T-type Ca^{2+} channels, which contributes to cell membrane stabilisation and inhibits glutamate release.

Pharmacokinetics

Zonisamide is eliminated by metabolism. It has a very long half-life in blood (about 60 hours) because of its selective binding to red blood cells.

Unwanted effects

- CNS effects: agitation, drowsiness, lethargy, dizziness, confusion, ataxia, diplopia, tremor, insomnia, emotional lability, psychosis, impaired concentration,
- Anorexia, weight loss, nausea, abdominal pain, diarrhoea, constipation,
- Rash, pruritus, peripheral oedema, alopecia.

Rufinamide

Mechanism of action and uses

Rufinamide prolongs inactivation of neuronal voltage-gated Na^+ channels, but it is unclear whether this is the only mechanism of action.

It is specifically used as adjunctive treatment of seizures in Lennox-Gastaut syndrome but is also used for refractory tonic or atonic seizures.

Pharmacokinetics

Rufinamide is metabolised in the liver and has a half-life of 6–10 hours.

Unwanted effects

- CNS effects: aggression, anxiety, dizziness, ataxia, tremor, blurred vision, nystagmus, drowsiness, gait disturbance, insomnia,
- Gastrointestinal upset: nausea, abdominal pain, constipation, diarrhoea, weight loss,
- Influenza-like symptoms.

GAMMA-AMINOBUTYRIC ACID RECEPTOR AGONISTS

Benzodiazepines

clobazam, clonazepam, diazepam, lorazepam

Mechanism of action and uses

Benzodiazepines enhance the action of the inhibitory neurotransmitter GABA on $GABA_A$ receptors. Their actions are discussed in Chapter 20. Clonazepam and clobazam are used orally for prophylaxis, usually as an adjunct to other drugs. Lorazepam, diazepam or clonazepam can be given intravenously to suppress individual seizures. If intravenous access is not available, rectal or buccal midazolam can be used. Intravenous diazepam is formulated as an emulsion to reduce the incidence of thrombophlebitis.

Pharmacokinetics

These are long-acting benzodiazepines; they are discussed in detail in Chapter 20.

Unwanted effects

These effects are discussed in Chapter 20. Partial or complete tolerance to the antiepileptic action of benzodiazepines often occurs after about 4–6 months of continuous treatment.

Phenobarbital and primidone

Mechanism of action and effects

Phenobarbital is a barbiturate whose major mechanism of action is activation of inhibitory postsynaptic neuronal GABA$_A$ receptors (see also Chapter 20). This increases the duration of opening of the transmembrane Cl⁻ channel associated with the receptor; the neuronal membrane is therefore hyperpolarised and less likely to fire. In contrast to benzodiazepines, the receptors are directly activated by phenobarbital and do not require the presence of GABA, but phenobarbital will also potentiate the effect of GABA (see Chapter 20). The action of primidone is due in part to its conversion to phenobarbital. Primidone has no advantage over phenobarbital and is generally less well tolerated. People with epilepsy who do not respond to phenobarbital or tolerate it poorly are unlikely to benefit from primidone.

Both drugs have a wide spectrum of activity and are effective in most forms of epilepsy, but the high incidence of unwanted effects means that they are infrequently used.

Pharmacokinetics

Phenobarbital is eliminated by hepatic metabolism and renal excretion. The half-life is very long, about 4 days, but with considerable interindividual variation. Primidone is converted in the liver to two active metabolites, one of which is phenobarbital.

The plasma concentrations of phenobarbital and primidone do not correlate with control of seizures; they are useful only as a guide to adherence to treatment. Control of seizures or unwanted effects should be used to determine dosages.

Unwanted effects

- CNS effects: sedation, fatigue and memory impairment are common in adults; paradoxical excitement, confusion and restlessness can occur in the elderly, and hyperactivity can occur in children.
- Cholestasis.
- Rashes.
- Folic acid metabolism is increased by phenobarbital, producing megaloblastic haemopoiesis, although anaemia with a macrocytic blood picture is rare.
- Increased vitamin D metabolism can produce vitamin D deficiency; in rare cases this results in osteomalacia.

- Tolerance to both unwanted and therapeutic effects occurs during long-term treatment.
- Dependence with a physical withdrawal reaction is seen after long-term treatment.
- Teratogenicity (see below).
- Induction of hepatic cytochrome P450 enzymes (see Chapter 2) leads to increased metabolism of phenobarbital itself and warfarin, cyclosporine and oestrogen (reducing the effectiveness of oral contraception). Interactions with other antiepileptic drugs are considered below.

GAMMA-AMINOBUTYRIC ACID REUPTAKE INHIBITOR

Tiagabine

Mechanism of action and uses

Tiagabine is a potent inhibitor of GABA transporter 1 (GAT-1) and decreases glial and presynaptic neuronal uptake of the inhibitory amino acid GABA. This prolongs the duration of action of GABA at its receptor. GAT-1 is the predominant transporter in the neocortex and hippocampus. Tiagabine is used as an adjunctive therapy for partial seizures with or without secondary generalisation.

Pharmacokinetics

Tiagabine is metabolised in the liver and has a half-life of 5–8 hours.

Unwanted effects

- CNS effects: dizziness, lethargy, nervousness, tremor, impaired concentration, speech impairment, emotional lability, tremor,
- Diarrhoea.

GAMMA-AMINOBUTYRIC ACID TRANSAMINASE INHIBITOR

Vigabatrin

Mechanism of action and uses

Vigabatrin is a structural analogue of GABA and produces irreversible inhibition of GABA transaminase (GABA-T), the enzyme that inactivates GABA. The generalised increase in CNS concentrations of GABA inhibits the spread of epileptic discharges.

Vigabatrin is used only in combination with other drugs to treat epilepsy that is resistant to other drug combinations, or when they are poorly tolerated. It is effective in partial epilepsy with or without secondary generalisation but may worsen absence, myoclonic, tonic and atonic seizures. Its use is restricted because of the unacceptably high risk of visual field defects (see below).

Pharmacokinetics

Vigabatrin is excreted unchanged by the kidney. Irreversible drug binding to its target enzyme GABA-T means that its duration of action is determined by the time required for GABA-T synthesis rather than the half-life of elimination of the drug. GABA-T activity recovers to about 60% of baseline after 5 days. Therefore the efficacy of vigabatrin is unrelated to the plasma drug concentration and the monitoring of blood concentration is of no value.

Unwanted effects

- CNS effects: sedation and fatigue, aggression, dizziness, nervousness, irritability, depression, impaired concentration, headache, blurred vision, diplopia, nystagmus and tremor.
- Nausea, vomiting, abdominal pain.
- Severe peripheral visual field defects during prolonged use. These can arise from 1 month to several years after starting treatment and are usually irreversible. Monitoring of visual fields at 6-month intervals is recommended.
- Weight gain, oedema.

DRUGS WITH MULTIPLE ACTIONS

Sodium valproate

Mechanism of action and uses

The mechanisms of action of sodium valproate are probably complex. One important action appears to be enhanced activity of glutamic acid decarboxylase (GAD), which increases the synthesis of GABA. The contribution of effects on ion channels is controversial, and there are other actions that are not yet well understood. Inhibition of histone deacetylase (HDAC) by valproate modulates the transcription of multiple genes encoding signalling proteins and ion channels. This may explain why the full benefit of treatment may not be apparent for several weeks.

Sodium valproate has a wide spectrum of antiepileptic activity and suppresses the initial seizure discharge as well as the spread of seizure activity. It is effective for all forms of epilepsy. Valproate is also used for the management of neuropathic pain (see Chapter 19) and bipolar disorder (see Chapter 21) as well as the prophylaxis of migraine (see Chapter 26).

Pharmacokinetics

Sodium valproate is metabolised in the liver and has a half-life of 9–21 hours. It is highly ionised at physiological pH but is rapidly transported across the blood–brain barrier via an anion exchange transporter. Subsequent diffusion into and out of neurons is slow, partly explaining why the drug concentration in plasma does not correlate well with its therapeutic effect. Monitoring of blood concentrations is useful only to assess compliance.

Unwanted effects

- Gastrointestinal upset: nausea, abdominal pain and diarrhoea. These can be minimised by gradual dosage titration.
- Weight gain caused by appetite stimulation.
- Transient hair loss, with regrown hair being curly.
- CNS effects: aggression, tremor, confusion, headache, memory impairment, sedation. These can be minimised by slow dosage titration.
- Thrombocytopenia or impaired platelet activity.
- Severe hepatotoxicity can develop but is rare and usually occurs in the first 6 months of therapy. This is most frequent in children under 3 years of age or in people with organic brain disorders who are receiving multiple

drug therapy for seizures. Transiently raised liver enzymes are common but usually do not progress to more serious liver dysfunction.
- Teratogenicity in the form of neural tube defects (see below).
- Inhibition of hepatic drug-metabolising enzymes – including CYP2C9, glucuronyl transferase and epoxide hydrolase – leading to interactions with other antiepileptic drugs (see below).

Topiramate

Mechanism of action and uses

Various mechanisms of action have been proposed for topiramate; the overall effects are probably due to a combination of actions on multiple targets. Potentially relevant actions include use-dependent blockade of neuronal Na^+ channels and enhanced action of GABA at a subset of $GABA_A$ receptors. It is less certain whether antagonist activity at the AMPA/kainite subtype of receptor for the excitatory amino acid glutamate or inhibition of carbonic anhydrase II and IV isoenzymes contribute to the antiepileptic effects.

Topiramate is used alone or as an add-on treatment for drug-resistant partial or generalised seizures. It is also effective for prophylaxis of migraine (see Chapter 26).

Pharmacokinetics

Topiramate is eliminated unchanged by the kidney and by hepatic metabolism. It has a long half-life (21 hours).

Unwanted effects

- CNS effects, including impaired concentration, cognitive impairment, confusion, dizziness, ataxia, paraesthesia, sleep disturbance, tinnitus, agitation, emotional lability and depression,
- Gastrointestinal upset, with nausea, vomiting, dyspepsia, taste disturbance, abdominal pain, anorexia, dry mouth and weight loss,
- Nephrolithiasis,
- Myalgia, muscle weakness,
- Rash, pruritus, alopecia,
- Teratogenicity, with increased risk of cleft palate.

NEURONAL CALCIUM CHANNEL BLOCKERS

Ethosuximide

Mechanism of action and uses

Ethosuximide is a drug of choice in absence seizures and may be effective for myoclonic seizures and tonic or atonic seizures. It is ineffective in other types of epilepsy. In absence seizures, T-type Ca^{2+} channels are believed to be responsible for generating excessive activity in thalamocortical relay neurons. Ethosuximide blocks these channels and prevents synchronised neuronal firing.

Pharmacokinetics

Absorption of ethosuximide from the gut is almost complete. Metabolism in the liver is extensive and the half-life is very long, at 40–60 hours, although it is shorter in children (30 hours). Plasma and salivary drug concentrations correlate well with control of seizures and can be used to monitor treatment.

Unwanted effects

- Gastrointestinal upset with nausea, vomiting, anorexia, abdominal pain, weight loss and diarrhoea.
- CNS effects: drowsiness, dizziness, ataxia, ataxia, headache and depression.

Gabapentin and pregabalin

Mechanism of action and uses

Although designed as a structural analogue of GABA, gabapentin does not appear to work by affecting GABA-mediated inhibition in the brain. The mechanisms of action of gabapentin and pregabalin are unclear, but both bind to the $\alpha2\delta$ subunit of P/Q-type voltage-gated Ca^{2+} channels in the neocortex and hippocampus and reduce Ca^{2+} entry into neurons. This may inhibit release of excitatory neurotransmitters such as glutamate.

Gabapentin and pregabalin are also used in the management of neuropathic pain (see Chapter 19) and pregabalin for generalised anxiety disorder (see Chapter 20).

Pharmacokinetics

Gabapentin is incompletely absorbed from the gut via a saturable transport mechanism, while pregabalin is better absorbed. Both drugs are excreted largely unchanged by the kidney, with half-lives of about 6 hours.

Unwanted effects

- Nausea, vomiting, dry mouth, dyspepsia, diarrhoea, constipation, abdominal pain.
- CNS effects, including drowsiness, dizziness, ataxia, fatigue, headache, tremor, diplopia, dysarthria, confusion and emotional lability.
- Weight gain from stimulation of appetite.
- Rhinitis, cough, dyspnoea.
- Myalgia, arthralgia.
- Rashes.

NEURONAL POTASSIUM CHANNEL OPENER

Retigabine

Mechanism of action and uses

Retigabine is used as an adjunctive (add-on) therapy for partial seizures with or without secondary generalisation. It activates voltage-gated K^+ channels (KCNQ2 and KCNQ3), which hyperpolarises neurons. It may also enhance GABA-mediated neurotransmission and reduce the release of the excitatory neurotransmitter glutamate.

Pharmacokinetics

Absorption of retigabine from the gut is almost complete. It is metabolised in the liver and the half-life is 6–10 hours.

Unwanted effects

- Increased appetite with weight gain, nausea, constipation, dyspepsia, dry mouth.
- CNS effects: anxiety, drowsiness, dizziness, vertigo, amnesia, paraesthesia, tremor, impaired concentration, confusion, diplopia, myoclonus.
- Haematuria.
- Blue-grey discolouration of nails, skin and ocular tissue. Ophthalmic examination is recommended every 6 months, and treatment should be reassessed if there are changes to vision or retinal pigmentation.
- Peripheral oedema.

SYNAPTIC VESICLE PROTEIN 2A INHIBITOR

Levetiracetam

Mechanism of action and uses

The mechanisms of action of levatiracetam remain uncertain. It blocks presynaptic Ca^{2+} channels and also binds to a protein (synaptic vesicle protein 2A [SV2A]) on the presynaptic neuronal plasma membrane. The exact function of this transmembrane transporter remains unclear, but it is involved in the regulation of neurotransmitter release. Levetiracetam produces selective inhibition of synchronised epileptiform burst firing and propagation of seizure activity in the hippocampus without affecting neuronal excitability.

Levetiracetam is used for adjunctive treatment of partial seizures with or without secondary generalisation.

Pharmacokinetics

Levetiracetam is largely eliminated unchanged by the kidney. Its half-life is 7 hours.

Unwanted effects

- CNS effects: drowsiness, lethargy, dizziness, ataxia, headache, tremor, insomnia, emotional lability, impaired concentration,
- Anorexia, nausea, vomiting, dyspepsia, diarrhoea, weight changes,
- Cough, nasopharyngitis,
- Myalgia,
- Rash.

AMPA GLUTAMATE RECEPTOR ANTAGONIST

Perampanel

Mechanism of action and uses

Perampanel is a noncompetitive antagonist at AMPA-type glutamate receptors on postsynaptic neurons. These receptors are the main mediators of fast synaptic excitation.

Perampanel is used for adjunctive treatment of partial seizures with or without secondary generalisation.

Pharmacokinetics

Perampanel is metabolised by CYP3A isoenzymes in the liver and has a very long half-life of 105 hours; when given in combination with strong inducers of CYP3A, such as carbamazepine, the half-life of perampanel is shortened to 25 hours.

Unwanted effects

- CNS effects: aggression, anxiety, dizziness, ataxia, blurred vision, drowsiness, dysarthria, gait disturbance, suicidal ideation,
- Nausea, changes in appetite, weight changes,
- Malaise.

INTERACTIONS AMONG ANTIEPILEPTIC DRUGS

Many antiepileptics affect the activity of hepatic drug-metabolising enzymes, especially cytochrome P450 isoenzymes (see Chapter 2, Table 2.7); drug interactions are therefore frequent. Interactions when two or more antiepileptics are used together can have major clinical implications for seizure control and/or toxicity. However, the extent of the interaction is variable and unpredictable.

Carbamazepine, phenobarbital, primidone and phenytoin induce various isoenzymes of CYP450 and lower the plasma concentrations of several other antiepileptic drugs. By contrast, valproate inhibits hepatic metabolism, which increases the plasma concentrations of some antiepileptic drugs.

MANAGEMENT OF EPILEPSY

TREATMENT OF INDIVIDUAL SEIZURES

The initial management of a seizure involves positioning the person to avoid injury. Particular attention must also be given to maintaining the airway and ensuring adequate oxygenation. A correctable cause of seizures such as hypoglycaemia should be sought and treated; intravenous thiamine should be given if alcohol abuse is suspected.

Prolonged or repetitive seizures lasting more than 5 minutes (convulsive status epilepticus) usually require urgent parenteral drug treatment. Intravenous lorazepam is the drug of choice. Diazepam can be used, but it can cause thrombophlebitis and has a shorter duration of action owing to more rapid tissue distribution. If necessary, a second dose of benzodiazepine can be given after 10 minutes. If intravenous access is not available, midazolam can be given by the buccal route. Diazepam rectal solution may be particularly useful for children or for initial treatment out of hospital. Close observation for signs of drug-induced respiratory depression and hypotension should be maintained after a benzodiazepine is given.

If there is no response to a benzodiazepine after 25 minutes or seizures recur, a slow intravenous injection of phenytoin or a more rapid injection of fosphenytoin or phenobarbital should be given. If seizures are still not controlled with these measures, full anaesthesia using thiopental or propofol (see Chapter 17) with assisted respiration in an intensive care unit will be necessary.

Nonconvulsive status epilepticus does not usually require urgent treatment unless there is complete loss of awareness or failure to respond to oral therapy.

PROPHYLAXIS FOR SEIZURES

A diagnosis of epilepsy requires two or more spontaneous seizures. After a single event, up to 80% of people will have a second seizure within 3 years. If a predisposing cause cannot be identified and avoided (e.g. alcohol withdrawal, photosensitive epilepsy precipitated by viewing a television screen from too close a distance), drug treatment will usually be recommended after a second seizure unless the seizures were separated by very long intervals or were mild. Occasionally treatment will be recommended after a first seizure, as when there is structural brain damage. Treatment should begin with a single drug, the choice depending on the type of epilepsy and relative toxicity of the drugs (Table 23.2).

For generalised tonic-clonic seizures or unclassifiable seizures and in the absence of factors that would lead to an alternative choice, sodium valproate is the first-line treatment because it has a wide spectrum of activity. Lamotrigine is the usual second-line choice. Carbamazepine or oxcarbazepine can also be considered. Adjunctive therapy is added for failure to control seizures with the initial drug, and at this stage several other drugs can be considered.

Absence seizures are usually treated with ethosuximide or sodium valproate, with lamotrigine as an alternative choice. Myoclonic seizures show a variable response to treatment. Sodium valproate is usually the first choice, with topiramate or levetiracetam as alternatives. Atonic seizures are usually

Table 23.2 Drug choice in the treatment of epilepsy

Type of seizure	First-line drugs	Second-line and specialist drugs
Partial seizures		
	Carbamazepine Lamotrigine Oxcarbazepine Sodium valproate Levetiracetam	Clobazam Eslicarbazepine Gabapentin Lacosamide Oxcarbazepine Phenytoin Pregabalin Tiagabine Topiramate Vigabatrin Zonisamide
Generalised seizures		
Tonic-clonic	Sodium valproate Carbamazepine Oxcarbazepine Lamotrigine	Clobazam Levetiracetam Topiramate
Myoclonic	Sodium valproate Topiramate Levetiracetam	Clobazam Clonazepam Lamotrigine Piracetam Zonisamide
Absence	Ethosuximide Sodium valproate Lamotrigine	Clobazam Clonazepam Levetiracetam Topiramate Zonisamide
Atonic	Sodium valproate Lamotrigine	Rufinamide Topiramate

seen in childhood and associated with cerebral damage. Treatment is with sodium valproate or lamotrigine.

Carbamazepine and lamotrigine are the drugs of first choice for partial seizures. Alternative options are oxcarbazepine, sodium valproate and levetiracetam. If monotherapy fails to control the seizures, then two of these drugs are usually given together. Adjunctive treatment with one of a number of other drugs is then considered if seizures are still not controlled.

When initiating treatment with any antiepileptic drug, the starting dose should be low, with gradual titration, so as to minimise unwanted effects. If seizures continue, the maximum tolerated dose should be taken. If seizures are not controlled with the first-choice drug, it becomes more important to accurately identify the type of seizure. A second drug should then be introduced and titrated to an adequate dose before the first drug is gradually withdrawn (see Table 23.2). A single drug will usually control seizures in up to 90% of people with epilepsy, although this may not be achieved with the first drug chosen. However, if the first drug does not control the seizures, the chance of a second single drug being successful is 13%; with a third it is only 4%.

Refractory epilepsy

Refractory epilepsy can indicate poor adherence to treatment, inappropriate drug choice or dosage, or that the seizures are "pseudoseizures" (nonepileptic attack disorder) rather than true epilepsy. However, seizures can be refractory to standard treatments. Multiple drug treatment (initially with two first-line drugs or a first- and a second-line drug) should be reserved for seizures that have not been controlled by treatment with two or three first- or second-line drugs given alone.

Combination therapy at maximally tolerated doses does not control the seizures in some people with epilepsy, even when there is good adherence to treatment recommendations. Lack of seizure control is more frequent if the onset was at an early age; if there are generalised, atonic, or absence seizures; or if there is underlying structural brain damage. Some data suggest that resistance can arise from overexpression of proteins that transport drugs out of the CNS neurons, such as P-glycoprotein, but the evidence for this is conflicting. Alternatively, resistance may arise from genetic variation affecting targets for drug action. For temporal lobe epilepsy there is now good evidence that surgical treatment should be considered if more than two consecutive antiepileptic drugs fail to control the seizures. Surgery for other forms of epilepsy may provide some amelioration of seizure frequency.

Therapeutic drug monitoring

It is not usually necessary to monitor concentrations of antiepileptic drug in plasma unless seizure control is poor or if poor adherence or drug toxicity is suspected. Good seizure control will often be achieved at plasma drug concentrations that are below the accepted therapeutic range; under such circumstances an increase in dosage is not necessary. By contrast, people who continue to have seizures may need plasma drug concentrations above the standard therapeutic range to achieve seizure control provided that the drug is well tolerated. The only drug for which monitoring is of proven benefit for dosage adjustment is phenytoin, primarily because metabolism may be saturated at therapeutic doses

and the pharmacokinetics become nonlinear (see Fig. 23.1). Adjustment of the dosages of carbamazepine, lamotrigine and ethosuximide may be easier if the plasma concentration is known; however, for other drug monitoring is of value only to confirm that the drug is being taken.

Duration of treatment

In the United Kingdom, a driving licence is revoked until the person has been seizure-free for 1 year or has suffered only nocturnal seizures for 3 years. A person should be advised not to drive during withdrawal of antiepileptic drugs or for 6 months afterwards. For this reason, drivers may wish to continue treatment indefinitely.

Once started, treatment should usually be continued for at least 2–3 years after the last seizure. Treatment should probably be lifelong if there is a continuing predisposing condition. If a decision is made to withdraw treatment, withdrawal should be gradual over at least 2–3 months to minimise the risk of rebound seizures. When several drugs are used, only one should be withdrawn at a time.

Following neurosurgical procedures or head injury, prophylaxis against seizures is often given for up to 3 months, particularly if there was a depressed skull fracture or an associated intracranial haematoma. However, evidence that routine use is beneficial is not strong.

Childhood febrile convulsions

Febrile convulsions occur commonly in infancy and usually do not lead to epilepsy or produce CNS damage. About 4% of children have them, and they recur in about one third. It is important to reduce pyrexia during subsequent febrile episodes, as by the removal of clothes and use of paracetamol (see Chapter 29). Routine prophylaxis with antiepileptic drugs is not recommended, but rectal diazepam is sometimes given when a child who has previously had a febrile convulsion becomes pyrexial.

ANTIEPILEPTIC DRUGS IN PREGNANCY

No antiepileptic drug has a proven safety record in pregnancy and the use of these drugs carries a risk of teratogenesis if the fetus is exposed in the first trimester (see Table 56.1). Fetal abnormalities are most frequent if more than one drug is used. Neural tube defects and other problems are particularly common with sodium valproate (malformations in about 10% of pregnancies) and to a lesser extent with carbamazepine and oxcarbazepine (2–4%). Developmental abnormalities also occur with phenobarbital, phenytoin, lamotrigine and topiramate, but there is too little information for many of the other drugs. There is also increasing evidence of neurodevelopmental effects leading to linguistic and cognitive deficits in children born to mothers who are taking antiepileptic drugs.

Women of childbearing age who are taking antiepileptic drugs should be given contraceptive advice. If they wish to become pregnant, they should be counselled about the risk and treatment should be slowly withdrawn if the seizure type or severity does not pose a serious threat. It is important to advise a potential mother with epilepsy that the risks of uncontrolled seizures during pregnancy, to both her and the fetus, may be greater than the risks associated with drug therapy. High-dose folic acid supplements may reduce the risk of neural tube defects and should be recommended before and during pregnancy.

The plasma concentration of antiepileptic drugs can change during pregnancy. The dose of carbamazepine, lamotrigine and phenytoin can be adjusted on the basis of plasma drug concentration monitoring.

When the mother is taking carbamazepine, phenobarbital or phenytoin, there is an increased risk of neonatal bleeding. Prophylactic vitamin K_1 should be given to the mother from 36 weeks of pregnancy and to the newborn immediately after birth.

SELF-ASSESSMENT

True/false questions

1. Generalised seizures include tonic-clonic and absence seizures.
2. Absence seizures occur mainly in adults.
3. Partial seizures cause motor, sensory or psychic symptoms without loss of consciousness.
4. Generalised muscle contractions do not occur in partial seizures.
5. The excitatory neurotransmitter glutamate is increased in some seizures.
6. There are currently no antiepileptic drugs that act by reducing excessive glutamatergic activity.
7. Antiepileptic drugs that stimulate GABA receptors or enhance GABA stability act by inhibiting Na^+ influx in neurons.
8. A major mechanism of antiepileptic drug action is the inhibition of Na^+ channels.
9. The metabolism of carbamazepine diminishes with regular use.
10. Activation of K^+ channels by retigabine hyperpolarises neurons.
11. Ethosuximide blocks neuronal Ca^{2+} channels.
12. The plasma concentrations of phenytoin increase in a linear manner with increasing dosage of the drug.
13. Vigabatrin is a first-line drug for the treatment of all types of epilepsy.
14. Tiagabine enhances GABA levels in synapses by reducing its reuptake.
15. The abrupt withdrawal of antiepileptics should be avoided.
16. The antiepileptic drug gabapentin is also used for neuropathic pain.

One-best-answer (OBA) question

Identify the *most accurate* statement about antiepileptic drugs.
A. Phenytoin causes hair loss.
B. The use of diazepam in epilepsy is confined to long-term prophylaxis in tonic-clonic seizures.
C. Valproate induces drug-metabolising enzymes in the liver.
D. The effectiveness of phenobarbital diminishes with time.
E. The risk of teratogenicity can be reduced in pregnancy by combining antiepileptic drugs.

Case-based questions

Case 1

A 7-year-old boy was described as "dreamy" by his mother. He was making slow progress at school and his mother and teachers commented that he could not concentrate and had frequent episodes of staring vacantly for a few seconds, then carrying on as normal. Following an electroencephalogram (EEG), a synchronised electrical discharge characteristic of an absence form of epilepsy was demonstrated.

1. Which of the following would be suitable as a drug of first choice: phenytoin, phenobarbital, sodium valproate or ethosuximide?
2. What are the major unwanted effects of the drug have chosen?
3. If control of absence seizures is inadequate with your chosen treatment, can combination therapy be given?

Case 2

A 19-year-old woman had a long-term history of epilepsy of the complex partial seizure type, which often gravitated to generalised seizures. For several years her epilepsy had been well controlled with a stable drug regimen. She now sought advice on contraception.

1. What antiepileptic drugs might be effective in the type of epilepsy this woman has?
2. What suitable options are available for contraception in this case?
3. What potential problems can arise if the woman takes the combined oral hormonal contraceptive?
4. Would an injected progestogen contraceptive be worth considering?
5. If the combined oral hormonal contraceptive were the chosen method, what strategies should be adopted to ensure its efficacy?
6. Would the oral progestogen-only contraceptive be a suitable method of contraception?

ANSWERS

True/false answers

1. **True.** Tonic-clonic seizures (formerly termed *grand mal*) and absence seizures (formerly *petit mal*) are two types of generalised seizure affecting the whole brain.
2. **False.** Absences, manifested by transient unawareness of surroundings and generally without motor disturbance, occur in children.
3. **False.** Simple partial (or focal) seizures do not cause loss of consciousness, but consciousness can be impaired in complex partial seizures and in secondary generalised seizures that arise from partial seizures.
4. **False.** In "Jacksonian" epilepsy an epileptic focus in the primary motor cortex causes jerking localised to a specific group of muscles; this gradually spreads to involve many other muscle groups.
5. **True.** Glutamatergic overactivity is implicated in some types of epilepsy and may cause neuronal excitotoxicity.
6. **False.** Reducing glutamatergic activity may account in part or in whole for the action of antiepileptic drugs such as perampanel and topiramate, which can block AMPA glutamate receptors, and others such as lamotrigine,

levetiracetam and retigabine, which decrease glutamate release.

7. **False**. GABA hyperpolarises neurons by increasing the influx of Cl^- ions via $GABA_A$ receptors.
8. **True**. Na^+ channel blockade that holds the channel in an inactivated state reduces repetitive neuronal firing; this is a major mechanism of action of many antiepileptic drugs.
9. **False**. The Na^+ channel blocker carbamazepine induces its own metabolism (autoinduction), so its elimination is accelerated with regular use.
10. **True**. The K^+ channel activator retigabine hyperpolarises neurons and modulates GABA and glutamate release.
11. **True**. The action of ethosuximide in absence seizures rests on its blockade of T-type Ca^{2+} channels in thalamocortical relay neurons.
12. **False**. Phenytoin exhibits first-order kinetics at low doses, but at higher doses it has zero-order kinetics because the liver's drug-metabolising enzymes become saturated; there is also substantial interindividual variability in phenytoin metabolism.
13. **False**. Vigabatrin inhibits the breakdown of GABA by GABA-T and is effective in all types of epilepsy; but because of the risk of irreversible narrowing of the visual field, it is reserved for specialist use for epilepsy that is resistant to other drugs.
14. **True**. Tiagabine reduces GABA reuptake by glial cells and presynaptic neurons by inhibiting the GABA transporter GAT-1.
15. **True**. Withdrawal of an antiepileptic drug should be gradual over 2–3 months to prevent rebound seizures.
16. **True**. Gabapentin is now thought to act by blocking the $\alpha 2\delta$ subunit of P/Q-type voltage-gated Ca^{2+} channels; it is used for epilepsy, neuropathic pain and (unlicensed use) migraine.

One-best-answer (OBA) answers

Answer D is correct.
A. Incorrect. Phenytoin causes hair growth (hirsutism); other unwanted effects include gingival hyperplasia, acne and facial coarsening.
B. Incorrect. Diazepam is used intravenously or rectally for status epilepticus, febrile convulsions and convulsions due to poisoning.
C. Incorrect. Valproate *inhibits* drug-metabolising enzymes in the liver, thus increasing plasma concentrations of many other drugs.
D. **Correct**. Tolerance to the therapeutic and unwanted effects of phenobarbital develops with time.

E. Incorrect. The risk of teratogenesis is increased if more than one drug is given.

Case-based answers

Case 1
1. The absence seizures experienced by this boy should respond well to sodium valproate or ethosuximide; phenytoin and phenobarbital are ineffective in absence seizures.
2. Sodium valproate causes nausea, reversible hair loss and weight gain. Uncommonly, liver damage can occur. Ethosuximide causes nausea, anorexia and headache.
3. Adherence with ethosuximide or sodium valproate monotherapy should be checked before combining drugs. Clonazepam and lamotrigine are suitable alternatives.

Case 2
1. A variety of antiepileptic drugs could be used by this woman with complex partial seizures. First-line drugs usually include carbamazepine, oxcarbazepine, lamotrigine or sodium valproate.
2. Nonhormonal contraceptives such as barrier methods or intrauterine devices are effective and do not carry the risk of drug interactions. However, many women will want to use a hormonal method.
3. Carbamazepine, phenytoin, phenobarbital and topiramate all induce liver enzymes that increase the metabolism of sex steroids and reduce the efficacy of oral contraceptives.
4. The metabolism of injected medroxyprogesterone acetate (MPA) is affected less than that of sex steroids taken orally. The interval between MPA injections should nevertheless be reduced to 10 weeks. MPA may also reduce the incidence of seizures.
5. Because oestrogen metabolism is enhanced by several antiepileptic drugs, it is recommended that if one of these drugs needs to be prescribed, formulations containing a high concentration of oestrogen (at least 50 µg) should be used. Sometimes more than 100 µg oestrogen daily in split doses may be required to prevent breakthrough bleeding. The pill-free period can also be reduced. If any change in medication for the woman's epilepsy is made, additional barrier methods of contraception should be used until the medication is stabilised.
6. The progestogen-only oral contraceptive would be unsafe as its metabolism is increased.

FURTHER READING

Betjeman, J.P., Lowenstein, D.H., 2015. Status epilepticus in adults. Lancet Neurol. 14, 615–624.

Brodie, M.J., Kwan, P., 2012. Newer drugs for epilepsy in adults. Br. Med. J. 344, e345.

Guerrini, R., 2006. Epilepsy in children. Lancet 367, 499–524.

Kinney, M.O., Morow, J., 2016. Epilepsy in pregnancy. Br. Med. J. 353, i2880.

Moshé, S.L., Perrucca, E., Ryvlin, P., et al., 2015. Epilepsy: new advances. Lancet 385, 884–898.

Rugg-Gunn, F.J., Sander, J.W., 2012. Management of chronic epilepsy. Br. Med. J. 345, e4576.

Schmidt, D., Schachter, S.C., 2014. Drug treatment of epilepsy in adults. Br. Med. J. 348, g2546.

Viale, L., Allotey, J., Chong-See, F., et al., 2015. Epilepsy in pregnancy and reproductive outcomes: a review and meta-analysis. Lancet 386, 1845–1852.

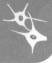

Compendium: drugs used to treat epilepsy and status epilepticus

Drug	Characteristics
Drugs used for the control of epilepsy	
Drugs given orally unless otherwise stated.	
Acetazolamide	Carbonic anhydrase inhibitor. Low efficacy but has a specific role in epilepsy associated with menstruation; also used as adjunctive drug for partial and tonic-clonic seizures. Half-life 6–15 h
Carbamazepine	Sodium channel blocker. Drug of choice for simple and complex partial (focal) seizures and as adjunctive drug when monotherapy is ineffective; also a first-line drug for generalised tonic-clonic seizures. Not recommended in tonic, atonic, absence or myoclonic seizures owing to the risk of seizure exacerbation. Also used to control neuropathic pain (see Chapter 19) and for bipolar disorder unresponsive to lithium (see Chapter 21). Given orally or rectally. Half-life 12–17 h
Clobazam	Benzodiazepine; GABA$_A$ receptor agonist. Used as adjunctive therapy in generalised tonic-clonic and refractory partial seizures; also specialist use for refractory absence and myoclonic seizures. Also used short term for anxiety. Half-life 10–50 h
Clonazepam	Benzodiazepine; GABA$_A$ receptor agonist. Specialist use for refractory absence and myoclonic seizures. Half-life 18–45 h
Eslicarbazepine acetate	Sodium channel blocker; deacetylated derivative is active metabolite of oxcarbazepine. Used for adjunctive treatment in adults with partial seizures with or without secondary generalisation. Half-life 20–24 h
Ethosuximide	Blocks neuronal T-type Ca^{2+} channels. First-line monotherapy and also used as adjunctive treatment for absence seizures. Also licensed for myoclonic seizures. Half-life 40–60 h (adults), 30 h (children)
Gabapentin	Inhibits the α2δ subunit of P/Q-type voltage-gated Ca^{2+} channels in neocortex and hippocampus. Used as monotherapy and as an adjunct for partial seizures with or without secondary generalisation; not recommended if tonic, atonic, absence or myoclonic seizures are present. Also used for peripheral neuropathic pain (see Chapter 19) and for migraine prophylaxis (unlicensed) (see Chapter 26). Half-life 5–7 h
Lacosamide	Mechanism unclear, but slowly inactivates voltage-gated Na$^+$ channels in vitro. Used as adjunctive treatment of partial seizures with or without secondary generalisation. Given orally or intravenously. Half-life 13 h
Lamotrigine	Sodium channel blocker. First-line drug for partial seizures and primary and secondary generalised tonic-clonic seizures; also used for typical absence seizures in children; has unlicensed uses as adjunctive treatment in adults if first-line treatments have failed. May exacerbate myoclonic seizures; can cause severe skin reactions. Also used in bipolar disorder (see Chapter 21). Half-life 15–60 h
Levetiracetam	Mechanism unclear but may reduce neurotransmitter release by binding to synaptic vesicle protein 2A, a transmembrane transporter on presynaptic cells. Used for partial seizures with or without secondary generalisation and as an adjunct for myoclonic seizures in patients with juvenile myoclonic epilepsy and primary generalised tonic-clonic seizures. Unlicensed use alone or in combination for myoclonic seizures and absence seizures. Given orally or by intravenous infusion. Half-life 6–8 h
Oxcarbazepine	Sodium channel blocker; analogue of carbamazepine, converted (half-life 2 h) to active S-licarbazepine. Used as monotherapy or adjunctive therapy for partial seizures with or without secondary generalised tonic-clonic seizures. Unlicensed use for primary generalised tonic-clonic seizures; not recommended in tonic, atonic, absence or myoclonic seizures owing to the risk of seizure exacerbation
Perampanel	Noncompetitive antagonist of postsynaptic AMPA glutamate receptors. Used as adjunctive treatment for partial seizures with or without secondary generalised seizures. Half-life 105 h (shortens to 25 h in combination with strong CYP3A inducers)
Phenobarbital	Barbiturate; GABA$_A$ receptor agonist. Effective for all forms of epilepsy except typical absence seizures; also for status epilepticus. No longer a front-line drug owing to sedation in adults, behavioural disturbances in children and drug interactions (potent CYP450 inducer). Half-life 50–150 h
Phenytoin	Sodium channel blockade and other antiepileptic actions. Effective for all forms of epilepsy except absence seizures but now little used. Potent inducer of CYP450 isoenzymes. Elimination is variable, saturable and dose-dependent; half-life 7–60 h

Compendium: drugs used to treat epilepsy and status epilepticus (cont'd)

Drug	Characteristics
Pregabalin	Structural analogue of gabapentin. Used for partial seizures with or without secondary generalisation; not recommended if tonic, atonic, absence or myoclonic seizures are present. Also used for neuropathic pain (see Chapter 19) and generalised anxiety disorder (see Chapter 20). Half-life 6 h
Primidone	Prodrug of phenobarbital. Used for all forms of epilepsy except absence seizures. Also used for essential tremor. Potent inducer of CYP450 isoenzymes. Half-life 4–22 h
Retigabine	Activator of neuronal K^+ channels KCNQ 2 and 3. Used for adjunctive treatment of drug-resistant partial seizures with or without secondary generalisation. Half-life 6–10 h
Rufinamide	Sodium channel blocker. Used as adjunctive drug in Lennox-Gastaut epilepsy syndrome in children and adults. Also specialist use in refractory tonic or atonic seizures (unlicensed). Half-life 6–10 h
Tiagabine	Inhibits GABA reuptake transporter GAT-1 in neurons and glial cells. Used as adjunctive treatment for partial seizures with or without secondary generalisation not satisfactorily controlled by other antiepileptics. May exacerbate absence, myoclonic, tonic and atonic seizures. Half-life 7–9 h
Topiramate	Mechanism unclear but blocks neuronal Na^+ channels and activates a subset of $GABA_A$ receptors; may also block glutamate kainate/AMPA receptors and inhibit carbonic anhydrase. Used alone or as adjunct in generalised tonic-clonic seizures or partial seizures with or without secondary generalisation; also used as adjunctive treatment for Lennox-Gastaut syndrome and specialist use for absence, myoclonic, tonic and atonic seizures (unlicensed). Also used in migraine. Half-life 21 h
Valproate sodium	Mechanism unclear, but blocks neuronal Na^+ channels, enhances GABA synthesis by GAD, reduces GABA breakdown by GABA-T, and inhibits HDAC. Drug of choice in primary generalised tonic-clonic seizures, partial seizures, generalised absences, and myoclonic seizures; also used in atypical absence seizures and as a first-line option in atonic and tonic seizures. Given orally or intravenously (see Chapter 26). Half-life 9–21 h
Vigabatrin	Reduces GABA breakdown by irreversibly inhibiting GABA-T. Specialist use as adjunctive treatment in refractory partial epilepsy with or without secondary generalised tonic-clonic seizures. Given orally or rectally (unlicensed route). Half-life 5–8 h
Zonisamide	Sodium channel and T-type Ca^{2+} channel blocker. Used as an adjunct for refractory partial seizures. Half-life 60 h

Drugs used primarily for status epilepticus

These drugs may also be used for other forms of epilepsy.

Clonazepam	Benzodiazepine; $GABA_A$ receptor agonist. Given by intravenous injection or infusion; see earlier for other information
Diazepam	Benzodiazepine; $GABA_A$ receptor agonist. Given intravenously or rectally for status epilepticus, febrile convulsions and convulsions due to poisoning; see Chapter 20 for other details
Fosphenytoin sodium	Ester prodrug of phenytoin. Given intravenously or by intramuscular injection. Half-life 0.2 h
Lorazepam	Benzodiazepine $GABA_A$ receptor agonist. Drug of choice for seizures lasting more than 5 minutes. Given by intravenous injection; see Chapter 20
Midazolam	Benzodiazepine; $GABA_A$ receptor agonist. Given by buccal administration; see Chapter 20
Paraldehyde	Trimer of acetaldehyde; sedative but with little respiratory depression. Given rectally; oxidises in air and reacts with plastic and rubber. Half-life 4–10 h
Phenobarbital sodium	Barbiturate. Given by intravenous injection; see earlier
Phenytoin sodium	Sodium channel blocker. Given by intravenous injection or infusion; see earlier

GABA-T, GABA transaminase; *GAD*, glutamic acid decarboxylase; *HDAC*, histone deacetylase.

24 Extrapyramidal movement disorders and spasticity

THE BASAL GANGLIA AND CONTROL OF MOTOR FUNCTION

The area of the brain known as the basal ganglia (Fig. 24.1) is part of an integrative motor circuit, the cortico-basal ganglia-thalamo-cortical loop. This neuronal loop is intimately involved in the coordination of motor function. Nuclei in the basal ganglia feed neuronal output to the cortex and receive input from the cortex.

The basal ganglia system includes several nuclei, such as the substantia nigra, the striatum, the globus pallidus and the subthalamic nucleus (see Fig. 24.1). Between these nuclei there are many complex internal neuronal loop circuits that use glutamate, dopamine, acetylcholine or γ-aminobutyric acid (GABA) as neurotransmitters. In addition, there are external neuronal loop circuits that integrate neurons outside of the basal ganglia with the internal circuits of the basal ganglia. The details of the complex interplay between the neuronal circuits are beyond the scope of this book, and only general principles are given.

Degeneration of vital neurons in the basal ganglia produces disordered regulation of neuronal activity and dysfunctional motor activity. Treatment for these disorders is directed at restoring the balance among the neurotransmitters in the basal ganglia.

PARKINSON'S DISEASE AND RELATED SYNDROMES

Parkinson's disease arises from dysfunction in the basal ganglia. It is characterised by a symptom triad of:

- resting tremor,
- skeletal muscle rigidity,
- bradykinesia (poverty of movement).

There are three clinical subtypes of Parkinson's disease: the akinetic-rigid subtype, the tremor-dominant subtype and the mixed subtype. However, it is now recognised that a variety of nonmotor symptoms of Parkinson's disease may precede the motor symptoms by several years. These include bowel dysfunction, mood disorders, sleep disorders and reduced sense of smell. A classification based on the presence of nonmotor symptoms has been proposed as this may predict progression and guide treatment.

The trigger for Parkinson's disease is unknown, but environmental toxins and specific gene mutations may be responsible in a small proportion of cases. The underlying pathology of Parkinson's disease involves loss of dopaminergic neurons in the substantia nigra pars compacta that projects to the striatum. This results from deposition of intraneuronal Lewy bodies and intraneuritic Lewy neurites, which are deposits of misfolded protein fibrillary aggregates mainly comprising α-synuclein. The aggregates in conjunction with neuroinflammation, possibly involving impaired handling of free radicals generated during dopamine metabolism, produce functional changes in dopaminergic neurons of the nigrostriatal pathway. This ultimately leads to progressive neuronal death and degeneration of the nigrostriatal pathway (see Fig. 24.1). More than 50% of substantia nigra pars compacta neurons must be lost before symptoms are apparent. Degeneration of the nigrostriatal dopaminergic pathways destabilises the motor control networks. α-Synuclein aggregates in nondopaminergic neurons in the brainstem,

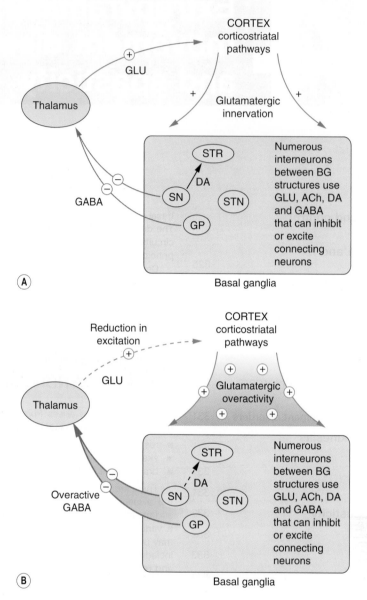

Fig. 24.1 **The cortico-basal ganglia-thalamo-cortical loop.** (A) Main pathways connecting the basal ganglia, the thalamus and the cortex involved in movement; (B) indicates how they are disordered in Parkinson's disease relative to (A). In Parkinson's disease the pathological changes in the basal ganglia, principally the loss of dopaminergic activity required to initiate movement, result in increased inhibitory γ-aminobutyric acid (GABA) transmission in pathways from the substantia nigra and the globus pallidus to the thalamus. Consequently there is excessive inhibition of thalamic-cortical brainstem motor networks. Hyperactivity in the glutamatergic cortico-basal ganglia pathways and also in cholinergic pathways within the basal ganglia exacerbates the predominant inhibitory influence of the basal ganglia on movement. *ACh*, acetylcholine; *BG*, basal ganglia; *DA*, dopamine; *GLU*, glutamate; *GP*, globus pallidus; *SN*, substantia nigra; *STN*, subthalamic nucleus; *STR*, striatum; –, inhibition; +, stimulation; dashed line, reduced activity compared to normal function in control (A).

olfactory-limbic region or neocortex are responsible for the nonmotor manifestations of Parkinson's disease.

The basal ganglia normally provide a persistent inhibitory influence on the initiation of movement through GABAergic inhibition of the thalamus. When movement is initiated, activity increases in the nigrostriatal dopaminergic pathways. Acting through D$_1$ and D$_2$ receptors in the striatum, dopamine releases

inhibition of glutamatergic neurotransmission in thalamic and cortical motor systems. In Parkinson's disease, denervation of the substantia nigra results in reduced stimulation of the striatum and failure to remove the GABAergic inhibition of the thalamus. Fig. 24.1B shows functional changes in Parkinson's disease relative to normal function in Fig. 24.1A. At the same time, hyperactivity in the glutamatergic pathways projecting from the cortex to the basal ganglia reinforces the inhibitory influence of the basal ganglia on movement. Cholinergic transmission in the basal ganglia is also enhanced in Parkinson's disease, contributing particularly to tremor.

There are several parkinsonian disorders that have clinical similarities to Parkinson's disease but have different underlying pathology. Examples are the Steele–Richardson–Olszewski (progressive supranuclear palsy) and Shy–Drager syndromes, in which the GABA neurons also degenerate. This explains the poor response of these conditions to treatment with dopamine-replacement therapy. Drugs that block striatal dopamine receptors, such as antipsychotic drugs (see Chapter 21), can produce a parkinsonian syndrome which also responds poorly to dopamine-replacement therapy.

DRUGS FOR PARKINSON'S DISEASE

The main target for drug therapy in Parkinson's disease is to enhance nigrostriatal dopaminergic activity, with a lesser role for inhibition of cholinergic activity. Glutamatergic dysregulation has not yet provided suitable targets for drug therapy.

DOPAMINERGIC DRUGS

Levodopa

Mechanism of action

Dopamine cannot be used to replace the underlying neurotransmitter deficiency in the basal ganglia because it does not cross the blood–brain barrier. Levodopa (L-3,4-dihydroxyphenylalanine [L-DOPA]) is the immediate precursor of dopamine in its synthetic pathway and is carried by the large neutral amino acid transporter into the brain. It is taken up into dopaminergic neurons and converted to dopamine by L-aromatic amino acid decarboxylase, also known as DOPA decarboxylase. This provides additional dopamine for release by the surviving nigrostriatal neurons.

Pharmacokinetics

Levodopa is absorbed from the small intestine by the active transport mechanism for large neutral amino acids. A similar transport system transfers levodopa across the blood–brain barrier. Levodopa is extensively decarboxylated to dopamine in peripheral tissues such as the gut wall, liver and kidney. This reduces the amount of levodopa that reaches the brain to about 1% of an oral dose, while the peripheral dopamine that is generated produces unwanted effects. To minimise peripheral metabolism, levodopa is given in combination with a DOPA decarboxylase inhibitor that does not cross the blood–brain barrier. The two available inhibitors are carbidopa (combined with levodopa as co-careldopa) and benserazide (combined with levodopa as co-beneldopa). Inhibition of the peripheral metabolism of levodopa increases the amount that crosses the blood–brain barrier to 5–10% of the oral dose. Since the DOPA decarboxylase inhibitor does not cross the blood–brain barrier, it has no effect on the required conversion of levodopa to dopamine by DOPA decarboxylase within the central nervous system (CNS).

The half-life of levodopa is short (about 1 hour). In the early stages of Parkinson's disease, synthesis and storage of dopamine in striatal neurons are sufficient to ensure a stable response despite infrequent doses of levodopa. This becomes less reliable as the disease progresses and more neurons are lost. Modified-release formulations of levodopa are then used to provide a more continuous supply of drug to the neurons. Transition from an immediate-release levodopa formulation to a modified-release formulation is not straightforward, because the latter has a lower bioavailability, which makes it difficult to estimate the equivalent dose.

Unwanted effects

- Peripheral formation of dopamine produces nausea and vomiting due to stimulation of the chemoreceptor trigger zone (CTZ) of the medullary vomiting centre, which lies outside the blood–brain barrier. Nausea and vomiting are rarely dose-limiting but can be reduced by domperidone, a peripheral dopamine antagonist (see Chapter 32). Peripheral dopamine generation can cause arrhythmias and also vasodilation, which may cause postural hypotension and flushing.
- Excessive dopamine generation within the CNS produces dyskinetic involuntary movements, especially of the face and neck, or akathisia (restlessness). Psychological disturbance can also occur, including hallucinations, anxiety, abnormal dreams, confusion, impulse control disorders (such as pathological gambling and hypersexuality) and psychosis.
- Sedation, sudden onset of sleep, dizziness.

Dopamine receptor agonists

apomorphine, pramipexole, ropinirole, rotigotine

Mechanism of action

In contrast to levodopa, these drugs are direct agonists at central dopaminergic receptors (see Chapter 4). They have a longer duration of action than levodopa. Dopamine agonists have different patterns of selectivity at dopamine receptor subtypes, but activity at receptors of the D_2-like family is thought to underlie their therapeutic effect in Parkinson's disease (Fig. 24.2). Bromocriptine and pergolide are dopamine agonists that are structurally related to ergot alkaloids (see Chapter 26) and have been associated with fibrotic reactions (discussed later). These drugs are now rarely used. The nonergot drugs ropinirole, pramipexole and rotigotine are also used to treat restless legs syndrome. Dopamine receptor agonists are also used for treatment of hyperprolactinaemia and acromegaly (see Chapter 42).

Pharmacokinetics

Pramipexole is eliminated by hepatic metabolism and has a half-life of 8–12 hours. Ropinirole is eliminated by the kidneys, with a half-life of 6 hours. Rotigotine is only formulated for delivery via a transdermal patch to provide a more continuous

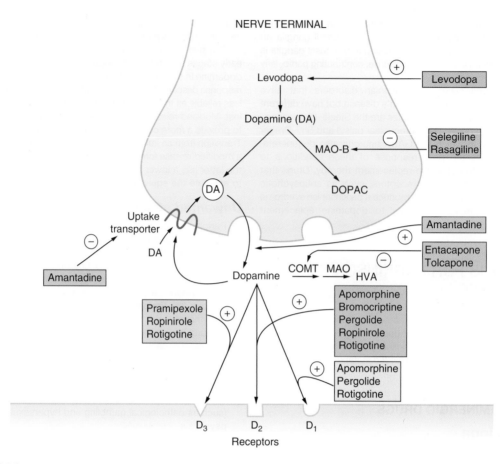

Fig. 24.2 **The major effects of drugs on the dopaminergic nerve terminal in the central nervous system.** Drugs act at a number of different sites to amplify dopaminergic signalling. *COMT,* catechol-O-methyltransferase; *DA,* dopamine; *DOPAC,* 3,4-dihydroxyphenylacetic acid; *HVA,* homovanillic acid; *MAO-B,* monoamine oxidase B; +, stimulation; −, inhibition.

supply of the drug. Its duration of action is determined by the rate of absorption of the patch rather than the intrinsic half-life of the drug.

Apomorphine is given parenterally by subcutaneous injection or continuous infusion, giving a very rapid onset of action. It has a short duration of action because of rapid hepatic metabolism with a half-life of 30 minutes.

Unwanted effects

Gradual dosage titration may limit unwanted effects.

- Nausea, vomiting, decreased appetite, abdominal pain, constipation;
- Dyskinesias, dizziness, nervousness, fatigue, sedation, sudden onset of sleep;
- Hallucinations and confusion, which are more frequent than with levodopa;
- Skin reactions (with rotigotine transdermal patches);
- Postural hypotension, peripheral oedema;
- Ergot-derived drugs such as bromocriptine and pergolide (now rarely used) may cause peripheral vasospasm (especially in people with Raynaud's phenomenon), pulmonary, pericardial and retroperitoneal fibrosis, and fibrotic cardiac valve lesions (leading to valve regurgitation).

Amantadine

Mechanism of action and uses

Amantadine is believed to act in Parkinson's disease as a weak glutamate *N*-methyl-D-aspartate (NMDA) receptor antagonist, reducing glutamatergic overactivity (see Fig. 24.1). It also stimulates release of dopamine stored in nerve terminals, reduces reuptake of released dopamine by the presynaptic neuron (see Fig. 24.2) and blocks muscarinic receptors. Its effectiveness is low and often short-lived because of the development of tolerance. Amantadine is also used as an antiviral drug (see Chapter 51).

Pharmacokinetics

Amantadine is excreted unchanged by the kidneys. It has a long half-life (10–15 hours).

Unwanted effects

Most are mild and dose-related.

- Anorexia, nausea, dry mouth;
- Peripheral oedema, postural hypotension;
- Headache, mood changes, hallucinations, slurred speech;
- Livedo reticularis.

Selective monoamine oxidase type B inhibitors

Examples

rasagiline, selegiline

Mechanism of action and effects

These drugs are irreversible inhibitors of the enzyme monoamine oxidase (MAO), which is responsible for the intraneuronal degradation of monoamine neurotransmitters (see Chapter 4 and Fig. 22.3). At low doses, they are relatively selective for the isoenzyme (MAO-B) found in the striatum. This isoenzyme is distinct from MAO-A, which is also present in the gut wall and other peripheral tissues. Interactions with drugs and foods containing tyramine, which is a problem with conventional nonselective MAO inhibitor (MAOI) antidepressants but do not occur with these MAO-B-selective drugs (see Chapter 22 for explanation). Selective MAO-B inhibitors prolong the duration of action of dopamine and reduce levodopa dosage requirement by about one-third, but only produce modest clinical benefit when used alone.

Pharmacokinetics

Selegiline and rasagiline have short half-lives (1–3 hours) due to rapid hepatic metabolism, but their duration of action is longer due to irreversible inhibition of their enzyme target. Selegiline undergoes metabolism in part to the L-isomers of amphetamine and metamphetamine, which have long half-lives and may contribute to unwanted neuropsychiatric effects.

Unwanted effects

- Nausea, dry mouth, dyspepsia, constipation, diarrhoea.
- Insomnia, agitation, confusion, hallucinations, headache, dizziness, vertigo.
- Arthralgia, myalgia.

Catechol-O-methyltransferase inhibitors

Examples

entacapone, tolcapone

Mechanism of action and effects

Catechol-O-methyltransferase (COMT) is normally responsible for metabolism of 10–30% of levodopa, both peripherally and in the CNS, converting it to the inactive compound 3-O-methyldopa (see Chapter 4). In the presence of a peripheral DOPA decarboxylase inhibitor, COMT is responsible for most of the peripheral metabolism of levodopa. Inhibition of COMT produces a 50% increase in the motor response to levodopa combined with a peripheral decarboxylase inhibitor. The dose of levodopa may therefore need to be reduced when a COMT inhibitor is started.

Pharmacokinetics

Entacapone and tolcapone are rapidly but variably absorbed from the gut. They are metabolised in the liver and have short half-lives of 2–3 hours. Entacapone does not cross the blood–brain barrier, and therefore only inhibits peripheral COMT. Tolcapone crosses the blood–brain barrier and has greater efficacy but causes more unwanted effects.

Unwanted effects

- Dry mouth, nausea, abdominal pain, diarrhoea, constipation.
- Dyskinesias, dystonias, hallucinations, confusion, insomnia.
- Reddish-brown discoloration of urine.
- Sweating.
- Risk of hepatotoxicity limits tolcapone to specialist use.

ANTIMUSCARINIC DRUGS

Examples

orphenadrine, procyclidine, trihexyphenidyl hydrochloride

Mechanism of action and effects

Drugs that block central muscarinic receptors (see Chapter 4) help restore the balance between CNS cholinergic and dopaminergic activity. They have little effect on bradykinesia, and are less effective than levodopa for treating tremor and rigidity.

Pharmacokinetics

Antimuscarinic drugs used for parkinsonian symptoms undergo hepatic metabolism and have half-lives in the range of 3–16 hours.

Unwanted effects

Tolerability of the antimuscarinic drugs varies, and changing to an alternative may be helpful if there are unwanted effects.

- Blockade of peripheral muscarinic receptors (see Chapter 4) causes constipation, dry mouth, urinary retention and blurred vision. Reduced saliva production can be helpful in some people with Parkinson's disease, in whom sialorrhoea is a problem.
- Blockade of CNS muscarinic receptors can produce confusion, memory impairment and restlessness in the elderly.

MANAGEMENT OF PARKINSON'S DISEASE AND RELATED SYNDROMES

Treatment is usually delayed in Parkinson's disease until symptoms affect quality of life. Levodopa (with a peripheral decarboxylase inhibitor) is still widely used for the initial treatment, and about 70% of people will have a useful

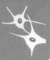

clinical response. Levodopa is particularly effective for reducing bradykinesia. Poor responses to individual doses of levodopa may be due to interference with its absorption by a high-protein meal or by delayed gastric emptying, and the response can be improved by taking the drug before meals. There is increasing reluctance to use levodopa in the early stages of Parkinson's disease, since it is possible that pulsatile dopaminergic stimulation produced by oral doses of levodopa may increase the risk of dyskinesias and response fluctuations developing later in treatment. Various strategies to reduce this problem are under investigation.

A dopamine receptor agonist such as pramipexole is an alternative option for initial treatment of Parkinson's disease. There is significantly less risk of response fluctuation or dyskinesias when the disease becomes advanced, and a dopamine receptor agonist is often preferred for treatment of younger people. Levodopa is still preferred to a dopamine receptor agonist for older people (over 65 years) or those with cognitive impairment, because of its lower propensity to cause confusion.

Fluctuating motor responses with prolonged use of levodopa are due to a change from a long-duration response to a short-duration response to each dose as the population of dopaminergic neurons reduces and their dopamine storage capacity is limited. There are several patterns of motor complication:

- the duration of symptomatic benefit after each dose may be reduced ('wearing off'),
- the dose may take longer to work ('delayed on'),
- the dose may sometimes fail to produce any improvement ('no on'),
- rapid swings between severe bradykinesia and toxic dyskinesias ('on–off').

Variations in motor performance should be treated by a reduction in total levodopa dosage and adding another drug, with the aim of maintaining more stable delivery of levodopa to the neurons. Successful combinations include:

- levodopa and a peripheral decarboxylase inhibitor with either an MAO-B inhibitor such as selegiline or a COMT inhibitor such as entacapone.
- adding a dopaminergic receptor agonist.
- subcutaneous apomorphine, which can be invaluable to abort the 'off' state in advanced disease. Apomorphine is highly emetogenic and may need to be given with domperidone, an antiemetic dopamine receptor blocker that does not cross the blood–brain barrier (see Chapter 32). Domperidone should be taken 30 minutes before apomorphine, but it is often necessary to 'load' with domperidone for 24 hours before starting apomorphine.
- infusion of levodopa gel into the jejunum via a gastrostomy tube can improve motor function in late-stage disease.
- addition of amantadine may reduce levodopa-associated dyskinesias.

For people who respond to levodopa but continue to have marked motor complications despite optimising therapy, high-frequency bilateral electrical stimulation of the subthalamic nuclei via implanted electrodes can be used to switch off their activity. It is preferred to surgical ablation of the nuclei since it allows the clinician to vary the site and area of the stimulation with time. Depression may be a problem with this treatment. Surgical treatment is sometimes advocated in advanced Parkinson's disease. Severe tremor

may respond to stereotactic thalamotomy or pallidotomy. Pallidotomy can also be helpful for severe dyskinesias.

Antimuscarinic agents are rarely used for idiopathic Parkinson's disease, but may be given for tremor that responds inadequately to levodopa. They can also be helpful in reducing excessive salivation.

Symptomatic treatment for a variety of associated symptoms may be necessary in Parkinson's disease. These include treatment of autonomic symptoms such as postural hypotension, vomiting, constipation, urinary frequency and impotence. Parkinsonian psychosis affects 70% of those who have had the disorder for 10 years. It should be treated with an atypical antipsychotic drug, such as quetiapine (see Chapter 21).

Drugs improve symptoms and quality of life in idiopathic Parkinson's disease, but there is little evidence that they alter the underlying rate of neuronal degeneration. Levodopa therapy increases life expectancy, probably by reducing complications such as aspiration pneumonia. Several studies are underway to look at a potential neuroprotective effect of dopamine receptor agonists. However, neuroprotective strategies have so far proved disappointing.

Drug-induced parkinsonism (e.g. with antipsychotics; see Chapter 21) responds poorly to levodopa because the causative drug occupies the D_2 receptors. Parkinsonism resulting from antipsychotic drug therapy responds best to withdrawal of the drug. If this is not possible, then an atypical antipsychotic drug should be used and an antimuscarinic drug used to treat residual symptoms.

OTHER INVOLUNTARY MOVEMENT DISORDERS (DYSKINESIAS)

Dyskinesias are abnormal involuntary movement disorders that can present in several ways.

- **Tremor** is a rhythmic sinusoidal movement caused by repetitive muscle contractions. Tremors are classified by the frequency of oscillations and by the context in which they occur – for example, a rest tremor (usually parkinsonian) or a postural tremor which may be worse on movement (kinetic tremor).
- **Akathisia** is a compulsive need to move, often in stereotyped patterns.
- **Chorea** is irregular, unpredictable, jerky and nonstereotyped movement that involves several different parts of the body.
- **Myoclonus** is rapid shock-like movements that are often repetitive.
- **Tics** are rapid repetitive movements that can sometimes be controlled voluntarily, but with difficulty, for short periods.
- **Dystonias** are sustained spasms of muscle contraction that distort a part of the body into a dystonic posture. Dystonias are often exaggerated by voluntary movement. Examples include spasmodic torticollis (twisted neck) and oculogyric crisis.

Involuntary movement disorders have numerous causes, and can be precipitated by drug therapy. For example, a tremor can be caused by lithium, sodium valproate, tricyclic antidepressants and sympathomimetics. Antipsychotic drugs (see Chapter 21) are associated with a wide variety of movement disorders, ranging from acute dystonia to akathisia, and tardive dyskinesias (involving choreodystonic movements often of the face and mouth). The dopamine receptor antagonist metoclopramide (see Chapter 32) can produce acute dystonias, especially in children and young adults, and occasionally tardive dyskinesias.

Some movement disorders have a genetic origin. An example is Huntington's disease, an autosomal dominant hereditary condition, which presents in adult life with progressive impairment of motor coordination, bizarre limb movements and dementia. The pathology is a loss of GABA inhibitory neurons projecting from the neostriatum to the substantia nigra. This reduces inhibitory activity on dopaminergic cells in the substantia nigra and the globus pallidus. These cells generate uncoordinated discharges that produce bursts of excess motor activity.

MONOAMINE DEPLETOR FOR MOVEMENT DISORDERS

Tetrabenazine

Mechanism of action

Tetrabenazine inhibits the vesicular monoamine transporter 2 protein (VMAT2) in CNS neurons that transport newly synthesised monoamines from the cytosol into synaptic vesicles for storage and later release. The cytosolic monoamines, including dopamine, are degraded prematurely by MAO. Tetrabenazine is mainly used for Huntington's disease, hemiballismus, senile chorea and related disorders.

Pharmacokinetics

Tetrabenazine is extensively metabolised by first-pass metabolism in the liver to an active derivative. The half-lives of parent drug and metabolite are 7 and 12 hours, respectively.

Unwanted effects

- Vomiting, dysphagia, constipation, diarrhoea.
- Postural hypotension.
- Anxiety, depression, drowsiness, insomnia, parkinsonism.

MANAGEMENT OF DYSKINESIAS AND DYSTONIAS

Treatment options depend on the cause. Drug-induced tremor will usually resolve rapidly on discontinuation of the medication. Some common strategies for other conditions are listed here.

- **Tardive dyskinesias** associated with antipsychotic treatment (see Chapter 21) may become worse on drug withdrawal, but then slowly improve over many months. There is no effective treatment.
- **Enhanced physiological tremor** (e.g. anxiety tremor or tremor of thyrotoxicosis) is a postural tremor that may respond to a nonselective β-adrenoceptor antagonist such as propranolol (see Chapter 5).
- **Essential tremor** is a postural tremor that usually presents later in life and can also affect the head and jaw. It can be suppressed by a β-adrenoceptor antagonist

or by primidone (see Chapter 23). Gabapentin or topiramate are alternative second-line treatments (see Chapter 23).

- **Dystonic tremor** is a jerky tremor that affects dystonic body parts or is task-specific (such as writing or playing a musical instrument). It can respond to drugs that are effective for essential tremor.
- **Choreiform movements** sometimes respond to tetrabenazine or an atypical antipsychotic drug (see Chapter 21). Carbamazepine or valproate (see Chapter 23) are also used but are generally less effective.
- **Tics** that do not respond to psychological therapy can be treated clonidine (see Chapter 6) or tetrabenazine. An atypical antipsychotic drug such as risperidone (see Chapter 21) may be effective. Injection of botulinum toxin can be helpful, or deep brain stimulation for severe disabling tics.
- **Myoclonus** has multiple causes which may need specific treatment. If a drug is required to suppress myoclonus, the first choices are clonazepam or sodium valproate (see Chapter 23). Alternatives are levetiracetam, phenytoin and primidone.
- **Acute dystonias** often respond to an antimuscarinic drug such as trihexyphenidyl given orally, or procyclidine given by intramuscular or intravenous injection for more severe symptoms.
- **Persistent dystonias** may respond to an antimuscarinic drug or to enhanced inhibitory GABA neurotransmitter activity with baclofen (discussed later), sodium valproate or clonazepam (see Chapter 23). A small number of early-onset dystonias will respond to levodopa. Focal dystonias can be treated by botulinum toxin (see Chapter 27) injected into the dystonic muscles to provide temporary relief by blocking transmission at the neuromuscular junction. Spread of the paralytic effect to adjacent muscles can cause problems; for example, dysphagia after injection of neck muscles for torticollis. Deep brain stimulation is considered for refractory disabling dystonia.

SPASTICITY

Spasticity is a state of sustained skeletal muscle tone or tension which is often associated with an increase in stretch reflexes. The increase in muscle tone arises from continued spinal reflex activity in the absence of inhibitory input from the motor cortex, such as resulting from a stroke, spinal cord injury or multiple sclerosis. Spasticity is often associated with partial or complete loss of voluntary movement and can produce painful and deforming shortening of the muscle (contractures).

DRUGS FOR SPASTICITY

Diazepam

Diazepam and other benzodiazepines enhance spinal inhibitory pathways by facilitating GABA-mediated inhibitory neurotransmission (see Chapter 20). The main disadvantages are sedation, a result of inhibitory activity in higher centres at the doses necessary for a spasmolytic action, and dependence.

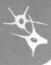

Baclofen

Mechanism of action

Baclofen is an analogue of GABA that inhibits reflex excitatory activity in the spinal cord. It is an agonist at GABA$_B$ receptors and hyperpolarises excitatory glutamatergic neurons by increasing K$^+$ conductance, which inhibits neurotransmitter release. Baclofen also has an analgesic effect, probably by inhibition of the release of substance P in pain pathways (see Chapter 19).

Pharmacokinetics

Baclofen is eliminated by the kidneys and has a short half-life (3–4 hours). It can be given by intrathecal infusion using an implantable pump for severe spasticity that is resistant to oral therapy.

Unwanted effects

- Sedation, drowsiness, confusion, depression, dizziness, ataxia, seizure, headache.
- Nausea, gastrointestinal disturbances.
- Urinary disturbances.
- Sudden withdrawal can precipitate hyperactivity, autonomic dysfunction and seizures.

Tizanidine

Mechanisms of action

Tizanidine is an α_2-adrenoceptor and imidazoline receptor agonist that decreases activity in excitatory descending pathways in the spinal cord. This inhibits reflex activity in motor neurons.

Pharmacokinetics

Tizanidine is well absorbed from the gut but undergoes extensive first-pass metabolism in the liver. Its elimination half-life is 2–4 hours.

Unwanted effects

These are mainly dose-related, and can be minimised by slow dose titration. They include:

- Drowsiness, fatigue, dizziness.
- Dry mouth, nausea, gastrointestinal disturbances.
- Hypotension. Tizanidine has only 10% of the antihypertensive activity of the α_2-adrenoceptor agonist clonidine (see Chapter 6).

Dantrolene

Mechanism of action and uses

Dantrolene is an antagonist at the ryanodine receptor (RyR1) that inhibits the release of Ca^{2+} from the sarcoplasmic reticulum of skeletal muscles (see Chapter 5) and uncouples muscle excitation from activation of the contractile apparatus.

Dantrolene is also used for the treatment of malignant hyperthermia (see Chapter 17) and as an adjunctive treatment in neuroleptic malignant syndrome (see Chapter 21).

Pharmacokinetics

Dantrolene is metabolised in the liver. It has a variable and unpredictable half-life (2–24 hours).

Unwanted effects

- Drowsiness, dizziness, weakness, malaise.
- Anorexia, nausea, diarrhoea, abdominal pain.
- Headache, drowsiness, dizziness, seizures.
- Pericarditis, pleural effusion.
- Rash.
- Dose-related risk of hepatitis.

MANAGEMENT OF SPASTICITY

Mild spasticity can be useful in a weak limb since the increased tone can provide postural stability or aid function. In this situation drug therapy can be detrimental by producing muscle hypotonia. Contractions from excessive spasticity following a stroke or in multiple sclerosis are most effectively prevented by physiotherapy, and can be helped with orthoses that support the limb and correct deformities.

Drugs are most useful for deforming or painful spasticity, particularly if the person is not ambulant. Baclofen is usually the drug of first choice, and is most often required for spasticity associated with multiple sclerosis or spinal cord injury. Tizanidine or dantrolene are alternative options. Cannabis extract (see Chapter 54) has modest benefit for spasticity in multiple sclerosis that does not respond to standard treatments. Intramuscular injection of botulinum toxin (discussed previously, and in Chapter 27) produces 'chemodenervation' and is used for severe focal spasticity. It produces an effect after 24–72 hours, which is maximal after 2 weeks and lasts for 2–3 months. Severe spasticity that fails to respond to standard treatments can be treated with intrathecal baclofen infusion.

SELF-ASSESSMENT

True/false questions

1. In Parkinson's disease, there is abnormally low dopaminergic activity and increased GABAergic, glutamatergic and cholinergic activity.
2. Symptoms of Parkinson's disease become apparent when approximately 25% of striatal dopaminergic neurons have been lost.
3. Glutamate receptor antagonists are being investigated for use in Parkinson's disease.
4. Levodopa has a half-life of over 24 hours.
5. Treatment with levodopa may lead to dyskinesias and on–off fluctuations.
6. In early Parkinson's disease, the dopamine receptor agonist ropinirole is as effective as levodopa.
7. Antimuscarinic drugs such as trihexyphenidyl have a low incidence of unwanted effects.
8. Pramipexole is a potent agonist at dopamine D$_3$ receptors.
9. Some of the movement disorder in Parkinson's disease arises from abnormalities in nondopaminergic innervated areas of the brain.
10. The chemoreceptor trigger zone (CTZ) is stimulated by peripheral dopamine generated from levodopa.

11. Selegiline inhibits monoamine oxidase and causes the 'cheese' reaction with ingestion of tyramine-containing foods.
12. Entacapone is a direct dopamine receptor agonist.
13. Tetrabenazine may cause depression.
14. Dantrolene is useful in spasticity, as it reduces the Ca^{2+} release that contributes to contraction of skeletal muscle.
15. Baclofen enhances muscle tone.
16. Botulinum toxin has a duration of action of up to 3 months.

One-best-answer (OBA) questions

1. Which is the *most accurate* statement about drugs used for Parkinson's disease?
   A. Levodopa slows the progress of Parkinson's disease.
   B. Bromocriptine can cause fibrosis.
   C. More than 50% of oral levodopa enters the brain unaltered.
   D. Currently used drugs for Parkinson's disease selectively stimulate D_1-type dopamine receptors.
   E. Carbidopa inhibits DOPA decarboxylase in the CNS.
2. Which adjunctive therapy *will not* increase dopamine levels in the brain when given together with levodopa?
   A. Entacapone
   B. Benserazide
   C. Carbidopa
   D. Procyclidine
   E. Rasagiline
3. Which unwanted effect is *least likely* to occur following levodopa administration?
   A. Nausea and vomiting
   B. Arrhythmias
   C. Orthostatic hypotension in the elderly
   D. Slowing of heart rate
   E. Dyskinesia

Case-based questions

Case 1: A 75-year-old woman has been suffering from progressive symptoms of Parkinson's disease for 5 years. From the outset she has been treated continuously with levodopa, but problems have developed in controlling the symptoms with this drug.
1. What is the cause of Parkinson's disease?
2. What symptoms is this woman likely to have?
3. Levodopa was given as co-beneldopa; what are the benefits of this formulation compared with levodopa alone?
4. What difficulties can arise in controlling symptoms with co-beneldopa in the later stages of treatment?
5. What changes in therapy could then be considered?

Case 2: A married man aged 40 years is newly diagnosed as suffering from Parkinson's disease. His symptoms are tremor, bradykinesia, hypokinesia and rigidity, which are sufficiently mild so that he is still able to carry out his work and pursue his hobbies. He was a security guard and had previously fought as a relatively unsuccessful professional boxer for 10 years, before retiring from the ring at the age of 35.
1. What are the optimal treatment regimens for this man?

ANSWERS

True/false answers

1. **True.** Loss of dopaminergic neurons in the nigrostriatal pathway creates abnormal activity within GABAergic, glutamatergic and cholinergic pathways.
2. **False.** Symptoms usually develop when more than 50% of neurons have been lost.
3. **True.** There is overactivity of some glutamatergic neurons in parkinsonism; weak antagonism of glutamate NMDA receptors may contribute to the action of amantadine.
4. **False.** The short half-life of levodopa (1–2 hours) may contribute to end-of-dose deterioration; modified-release formulations provide a more continuous supply of the drug.
5. **True.** About 50% of people will experience these complications after 5 years of treatment with levodopa.
6. **True.** In very early Parkinson's disease clinical trials, up to 6 months' duration indicate ropinirole is as effective as levodopa.
7. **False.** Trihexyphenidyl can cause minor unwanted effects but also severe confusion, particularly in the elderly.
8. **True.** Pramipexole is a high-affinity D_3 agonist, but also an agonist at other members of the D_2-like receptor subfamily.
9. **True.** Tremor and rigidity in particular may occur because of transmitters other than dopamine.
10. **True.** The CTZ in the area postrema of the medulla is outside the blood–brain barrier and can be activated by dopamine synthesised peripherally from levodopa.
11. **False.** Selegiline (and rasagiline) selectively inhibit MAO-B, leaving MAO-A active to metabolise tyramine in cheese and other foods (see Figure 22.3).
12. **False.** Entacapone is a peripheral inhibitor of catechol-O-methyltransferase (COMT), so it preserves levodopa for access to the brain and subsequent conversion to dopamine; tolcapone crosses the blood–brain barrier and also blocks COMT in the CNS.
13. **True.** The risk of depression with tetrabenazene is consistent with its depletion of CNS monoamines (see Chapter 22).
14. **True.** Dantrolene is a ryanodine receptor (RyR1) antagonist that blocks Ca^{2+} release from sarcoplasmic reticulum; it therefore reduces excitation–contraction coupling in skeletal muscle.
15. **False.** Baclofen improves spasticity by inhibiting excitatory synapses, probably acting at $GABA_B$ receptors.
16. **True.** Botulinum toxin is used in spasticity by intramuscular injection and inhibits local acetylcholine release for up to 3 months.

One-best-answer (OBA) answers

1. **Answer B is correct.**
   A. Incorrect. Use of levodopa in the early stages of Parkinson's disease may increase the risk of dyskinesias and response fluctuations in the later stages.
   B. **Correct.** Bromocriptine and the other ergot-derived dopamine receptor agonists can cause pulmonary, retroperitoneal and pericardial fibrosis.

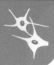

C. Incorrect. Only 1–2% of an oral dose of levodopa enters the brain in the absence of a peripheral decarboxylase inhibitor.

D. Incorrect. Drugs for Parkinson's disease are thought to act mainly by agonist activity at the D_2-like receptor family (D_2, D_3, D_4).

E. Incorrect. Carbidopa is a peripheral DOPA decarboxylase inhibitor; it does not cross the blood–brain barrier.

2. **Answer D is correct.**

A. Incorrect. Entacapone inhibits peripheral catechol-O-methyltransferase (COMT), increasing the amount of levodopa crossing into the brain and its subsequent conversion to dopamine.

B. Incorrect. Benserazide is a peripheral decarboxylase inhibitor that increases the amount of levodopa crossing into the brain and its subsequent conversion to dopamine.

C. Incorrect. Carbidopa is a peripheral decarboxylase inhibitor that increases the amount of levodopa crossing into the brain and its subsequent conversion to dopamine.

D. **Correct.** Procyclidine is a muscarinic receptor antagonist and will not affect dopamine levels.

E. Incorrect. Rasagiline is an irreversible selective MAO-B inhibitor that will reduce the breakdown of dopamine within the brain.

3. **Answer D is correct.**

A. Incorrect. Dopamine is a neurotransmitter in the chemoreceptor trigger zone and stimulates nausea and vomiting.

B. Incorrect. Dopamine can stimulate β-adrenoceptors in the heart, increasing the likelihood of arrhythmias.

C. Incorrect. Orthostatic hypotension is common, particularly in the elderly.

D. **Correct.** Dopamine may increase myocardial contractility, but without affecting the heart rate.

E. Incorrect. Excessive CNS dopamine concentrations are associated with involuntary movements.

Case-based answers

Case 1:

1. Parkinson's disease results from degeneration of more than 50% of dopaminergic neurons in the substantia nigra. The cause of this degeneration is unknown, but hypotheses include the actions of reactive oxygen species, neurotoxins, immune disturbances and specific gene mutations. The consequent neurochemical disturbances include overactivity of cholinergic, GABAergic and glutamatergic pathways. Current therapies aim to supplement dopaminergic activity or decrease cholinergic activity.

2. People with Parkinson's disease have akinesia, rigidity and tremor, possibly from inhibition of the motor cortical system, whereas the descending inhibition of the brainstem locomotor areas may contribute to abnormalities of gait and posture.

3. Levodopa is the immediate precursor of dopamine and is transported into the CNS by the large neutral amino acid transporter and converted into dopamine, while dopamine itself cannot cross the blood–brain barrier.

Levodopa causes nausea and vomiting because it also metabolises to dopamine in the periphery, which activates the chemoreceptor trigger zone (CTZ). Co-beneldopa is a combination of levodopa with benserazide, a peripheral decarboxylase inhibitor, which prevents the breakdown of levodopa to dopamine in the periphery. The peripheral dopamine receptor antagonist domperidone can also be used to protect against nausea and vomiting.

4. Levodopa remains the most effective treatment for Parkinson's disease, but there is considerable debate about when to start levodopa therapy. There is no convincing evidence that levodopa accelerates neurodegeneration, and survival is reduced if treatment is delayed until greater disability is present. In time, and despite long-term treatment with levodopa, there is an increasing incidence of dyskinesias and on–off fluctuations of effect, although most people continue to derive benefit throughout the duration of their illness. At the end of 5 years of treatment, approximately 50% of those treated will experience reduced effectiveness with levodopa. These motor fluctuations can be a result of unpredictable pharmacokinetic changes, such as unpredictable absorption across the blood–brain barrier or delayed gastric emptying, or because further loss of dopaminergic neurons during disease progression further reduces neuronal storage capacity for dopamine.

5. Resolving these problems is highly individual, but dyskinesia and on–off effects may be helped by dosage adjustment (up or down), by shortening the dose interval or by using modified-release formulations. An antimuscarinic drug can be given with levodopa and may be useful in the treatment of tremor, but could cause confusion and hallucinations, particularly in this elderly person. Other drugs which inhibit dopamine metabolism can also be introduced. The selective MAO-B inhibitors selegiline or rasagiline are far more effective as adjuncts to levodopa than as monotherapy. The COMT inhibitor entacapone reduces the peripheral breakdown of levodopa and dopamine and prolongs the benefits of levodopa therapy. A direct dopamine receptor agonist could also be added to levodopa treatment for this woman; nonergot derivatives including ropinirole, rotigotine (as a transdermal patch) or pramipexole are preferred. Apomorphine, a D_1/D_2 receptor agonist, given subcutaneously, can also be used to counteract the 'off' periods in advanced disease, with domperidone given to reduce its emetic effects.

Case 2:

1. There is considerable debate about when to commence levodopa therapy in early-onset Parkinson's disease. The goal should be to improve quality of life and limit long-term unwanted effects. If the degree of disability is not severe, there may be no immediate need for therapy, but this is controversial because survival is reduced if treatment with levodopa is delayed until disability develops. If treatment is required in this patient, dopamine receptor agonists could be started. These are less likely to produce dyskinesias and could delay the need for levodopa until progressive disabilities start to occur. The possibility of brain damage caused by boxing injury should also be considered; this responds poorly to standard treatments for Parkinson's disease.

FURTHER READING

Parkinson's disease

Connolly, B.S., Lang, A.E., 2014. Pharmacological treatment of Parkinson's disease: a review. J. Am. Med. Assoc. 311, 1670–1683.

Goetz, C.G., Pal, G., 2014. Initial management of Parkinson's disease. Br. Med. J. 349, 6258.

Guridi, J., Gonzalez-Redondo, R., Obeso, J.A., 2012. Clinical features, pathophysiology and treatment of levodopa-induced dyskinesias in Parkinson's disease. Parkinsons Dis. 943159. doi:10.1155/2012/943159.

Kalia, L.V., Lang, A.E., 2015. Parkinson's disease. Lancet 386, 896–912.

Other movement disorders and spasticity

Marcerollo, A., Martino, D., 2016. What is new in tics, dystonia and chorea? Clin. Med. 16, 383–389.

Mink, J.W., Zinner, S.H., 2010. Movement disorders I: tics and stereotypies. Paediatr. Rev. 31, 223–233.

Mink, J.W., Zinner, S.H., 2010. Movement disorders II: chorea, dystonia, myoclonus and tremor. Paediatr. Rev. 31, 287–295.

Nair, K.P.S., Marsden, J., 2014. The management of spasticity in adults. Br. Med. J. 349, g4737.

Waln, O., Jankovic, J., 2013. An update on tardive dyskinesia: from phenomenology to treatment. Tremor Other Hyperkinet. Mov. (N. Y.) 3, tre-03-161-4138-1. doi: 10.7916/D88P5Z71.

Waln, O., Jankovic, J., 2015. Paroxysmal movement disorders. Neurol. Clin. 33, 137–152.

Compendium: drugs used to treat extrapyramidal movement disorders

Drug	Characteristics
Drugs used for Parkinson's disease	
Given orally unless otherwise stated.	
Dopamine receptor agonists	
Apomorphine	D_2 and D_1 receptor agonist; opioid derivative. Given by subcutaneous injection; not effective orally. Half-life: 0.5–1 h
Bromocriptine	D_2 receptor agonist. Ergot derivative; risk of fibrotic reaction. Half-life: 3 h
Cabergoline	D_2 receptor agonist. Ergot derivative; risk of fibrotic reactions. Used as an adjunct to levodopa. Half-life: 60–90 h
Levodopa (L-DOPA)	Metabolised by DOPA decarboxylase to dopamine. Normally given with carbidopa or benserazide (see peripheral decarboxylase inhibitors, listed later) to reduce peripheral metabolism. Half-life: 1.3 h
Pergolide	D_2 and D_1 receptor agonist. Ergot derivative; risk of fibrotic reactions. Half-life: 27 h
Pramipexole	Selective D_3 receptor agonist, some activity at D_2 receptors. Half-life: 8–12 h
Ropinirole	D_3 and D_2 receptor agonist. Half-life: 6 h
Rotigotine	D_3, D_2 and D_1 receptor agonist. Administered via a transdermal patch. Half-life: 5–7 h
Peripheral decarboxylase inhibitors (used in combination with oral levodopa therapy)	
Benserazide	Combination of benserazide with levodopa (in ratio 1 : 4) is co-beneldopa
Carbidopa	Combination of carbidopa with levodopa (in ratio of 1 : 4 or 1 : 10) is co-careldopa
Monoamine oxidase (MAO) type B inhibitors	
Rasagiline	Irreversible MAO-B inhibitor. Used alone or in combination with levodopa. Half-life: 3 h
Selegiline	Irreversible MAO-B inhibitor. Used alone or in combination with levodopa. Amphetamine metabolites may contribute to unwanted neuropsychiatric effects. Oral and buccal formulations. Half-life: 1–2 h
Catechol-O-methyltransferase (COMT) inhibitors	
Entacapone	Does not cross blood–brain barrier. Used as adjunct to levodopa for end-of-dose deterioration. Half-life: 2–3 h
Tolcapone	Crosses blood–brain barrier. Specialist use as adjunct to levodopa for end-of-dose deterioration. Risk of hepatotoxicity. Half-life: 2–3 h
Other dopaminergic drugs	
Amantadine	Enhances dopamine release, blocks dopamine reuptake; weak dopamine receptor agonist and glutamate NMDA receptor antagonist. Also used as antiviral agent. Half-life: 10–15 h

Compendium: drugs used to treat extrapyramidal movement disorders (cont'd)

Drug	Characteristics
Antimuscarinic drugs	
Efficacy of the antimuscarinic drugs used in Parkinson's disease is similar; little effect on bradykinesia.	
Orphenadrine	Half-life: 14–16 h
Procyclidine	Given orally or by intramuscular or intravenous injection. Half-life: 3 h
Trihexyphenidyl hydrochloride	Also known as benzhexol. Half-life: 3–7 h
Drugs used for essential tremor, chorea, tics and related neurological disorders	
Given orally.	
Chlorpromazine	Antipsychotic; see Chapter 21
Clonidine	α_2-Adrenoceptor agonist; see Chapter 6
Haloperidol	Antipsychotic; see Chapter 21
Pimozide	Antipsychotic; see Chapter 21
Piracetam	Mechanism uncertain; used as adjunctive treatment for cortical myoclonus. Half-life: 4 h
Primidone	Barbiturate; see Chapter 23
Propranolol	β-Adrenoceptor antagonist; see Chapter 8
Sulpiride	Antipsychotic; see Chapter 21
Tafamidis meglumine	Inhibits amyloid formation. Specialists use for treatment of transthyretin familial amyloid polyneuropathy (TTR-FAP) to delay peripheral neurological impairment. Half-life: 59 h
Tetrabenazine	Vesicular monoamine transporter (VMAT2) inhibitor; depletes monoamines from central nervous system neurons. Half-life: 7 h
Trihexyphenidyl	Antimuscarinic; discussed previously
Drugs used to treat spasticity	
Given orally.	
Baclofen	GABA$_B$ receptor agonist; suppresses spinal reflexes. Given orally or by intrathecal injection. Half-life: 3–4 h
Dantrolene	Ryanodine receptor antagonist; blocks excitation/contraction coupling in skeletal muscle. Also used for malignant hyperthermia and neuroleptic malignant syndrome. Half-life: 4–24 h
Diazepam	Benzodiazepine; see Chapter 20
Tizanidine	α_2-Adrenoceptor agonist; inhibits polysynaptic motor neuron transmission. Half-life: 2–4 h
Other drugs affecting movement	
Botulinum toxins A and B	Block acetylcholine release. Specialist use for torsional dystonias and other involuntary movements. Given by local intramuscular injection
Methocarbamol	Carbamate; centrally acting muscle relaxant. Given orally for short-term symptomatic relief of muscle spasm. Half-life: 1 h
Quinine	Given orally for nocturnal leg cramps. Half-life: 8–21 h

25 Other neurological disorders: multiple sclerosis, motor neuron disease and Guillain–Barré syndrome

MULTIPLE SCLEROSIS

Multiple sclerosis is a chronic autoimmune, inflammatory neurological disease of the central nervous system (CNS). It is characterised by an immunologically mediated demyelination of the myelin sheath of neurons in the CNS. The cause is unknown, but it may be initiated by exposure of genetically susceptible individuals to an infective agent with an antigenic structure similar to myelin basic protein (molecular mimicry). The trigger initiates a peripheral immune response, and the blood–brain barrier is then breached by primed T- and B-lymphocytes and macrophages. The inflammation in the brain has the characteristics of a Th1-cell autoimmune response (see Chapter 38), with the T-cells secreting inflammatory cytokines such as interferon-γ, interleukin (IL)-17 and lymphotoxin (or tumour necrosis factor β, TNF β).

The destruction of myelin is probably initiated by B-cell-derived autoantibodies. The T-cell cytokines activate macrophages that phagocytose myelin coated with antimyelin antibody, and destroy the myelin sheath around nerves, particularly in white matter. The immunological damage also affects oligodendrocytes, the cells that produce the myelin. The result of these processes is the generation of demyelinated plaques that disturb normal conduction of electrical impulses in the CNS. However, the long-term disability in multiple sclerosis is mainly due to secondary axonal damage, which occurs most extensively in the acute stages of the disease.

Multiple sclerosis usually begins in the second or third decades of life and in 85% of cases presents with relapsing and remitting symptoms, along with signs of multifocal CNS dysfunction. In this form of the condition, the usual clinical course is initially one of stepwise deterioration, but eventually there is progressive deterioration (secondary progressive multiple sclerosis). In 10% of cases the course is slowly progressive from the outset (primary progressive multiple sclerosis). The remaining 5% have progressive-relapsing disease, with steady progression interrupted by intermittent flares. To secure the diagnosis, episodes of neurological dysfunction must be separated in both time and place (more than one episode in more than one area of the brain). A single clinical episode of demyelination with several areas of demyelination on magnetic resonance scanning of the brain that have not caused symptoms is known as clinically isolated syndrome. The areas of the CNS most often involved in multiple sclerosis are the optic nerves, spinal cord, brainstem and cerebellum. Common clinical presentations are optic neuritis, weakness with spasticity, ataxia and bladder and bowel dysfunction.

DISEASE-MODIFYING THERAPIES

There is no cure for multiple sclerosis, but in relapsing–remitting disease there is increasing evidence that modulating the immune response as early as possible in the disease process can reduce disability. By contrast, most treatments are ineffective in primary or secondary progressive multiple sclerosis.

- Corticosteroids (see Chapter 44) are often used to treat an acute relapse (e.g. intravenous methylprednisolone for 3 days or oral prednisolone for 3 weeks). They probably shorten the duration of a relapse, but have no effect on long-term outcome.
- Interferon beta-1a or -1b are naturally occurring cytokines that can reduce relapses by about one-third; they do not prevent ultimate disability. After translocation to cell nuclei they act as transcription factors by binding to enhancer elements, where they stimulate gene expression. Possible mechanisms for the clinical effect in multiple sclerosis include reduced disruption of the blood–brain barrier and modulation of T- and B-cell and cytokine function. After a single episode of demyelination, about 50% of people will subsequently develop the clinical syndrome of multiple sclerosis. The use of interferon beta at the time of this clinically isolated syndrome significantly reduces the risk

of developing multiple sclerosis 2 years after treatment. Otherwise, the use of interferon beta is reserved for ambulant individuals who have had at least two attacks of relapsing and remitting disease over the previous 2 or 3 years. Interferon beta is given by intramuscular or subcutaneous injection. The most frequent unwanted effects are influenza-like symptoms, which may persist for several months, and pain or ulceration at the injection site. About 25% of those who start treatment discontinue within 1–2 years. Neutralising antibodies are produced during repeated administration in 5% of people, which leads to treatment failure within 2 years of starting treatment.

■ Glatiramer acetate is a synthetic tetrapeptide immu-nomodulator that has some structural similarities to myelin basic protein. It may produce immunological tolerance by stimulating regulatory T-cells. It reduces the frequency of relapses, but like interferon beta, it does not influence long-term disability. Glatiramer acetate is mainly used when antibodies reduce the effectiveness of interferon beta. It is given by subcutaneous injection. Unwanted effects include flushing, chest pain, palpitation and dyspnoea immediately after injection, and reactions at the injection site.

■ Natalizumab is a humanised monoclonal antibody that selectively inhibits the α_4-integrin adhesion molecule on the surface of T-cells. This prevents T-cells from interacting with receptors on the vascular endothelium and crossing the blood–brain barrier. Natalizumab reduces the relapse rate in relapsing–remitting multiple sclerosis. It increases the risk of infection, and there is a small risk of developing the brain disease progressive multifocal leukoencephalopathy (PML), particularly if there has been previous use of immunosup-pressant drugs or if natalizumab is used for longer than 2 years. PML is caused by the John Cunningham virus, which is found dormant in up to 60% of the population. Serological testing for the virus should be carried out before and regularly during use of the drug.

■ Fingolimod is an oral prodrug that undergoes reversible phosphorylation to create an agonist of sphingosine 1-phosphate receptors on lymphocytes, causing receptor internalisation. The receptors are essential for lymphocytes to leave lymph nodes, and therefore fingolimod traps the cells and reduces their migration to demyelinating lesions in the CNS. It is more effective than interferon beta, reducing relapses by about 50%. Fingolimod can produce bradycardia and heart block after a single dose and should not be used in people at high risk of heart block. It can also cause cough, dyspnoea and macular oedema and increases the risk of viral infections.

■ Dimethyl fumarate is fully discussed under fumaric acid esters in Chapter 49. Its efficacy in multiple sclerosis is similar to glatiramer acetate.

■ Teriflunamide is the active metabolite of leflunomide, and full details are found in Chapter 30. Its efficacy in multiple sclerosis is similar to interferon beta.

■ Alemtuzumab is a humanised monoclonal antibody against the cell surface marker CD52 on the surface of monocytes and lymphocytes. Full details are found in Chapter 52. A single dose depletes B-cells for 5–6 months and T-cells for up to a year. It carries an increased risk of autoimmune thyroid disease and idiopathic thrombocytopenic purpura. There is also an increased risk of viral infections, especially with the herpes virus. Alemtuzumab may be particularly useful for breakthrough disease during treatment with other disease-modifying drugs or for induction in aggressive disease.

Management of multiple sclerosis

There are two principal aims of treatment. The first is to reduce the frequency of relapses in the relapsing–remitting form of the disease. There are no disease-modifying drugs that are effective for the progressive forms of the condition. The second aim is to treat residual disability.

The first-choice disease-modifying drug is either interferon beta or glatiramer acetate. The others are used if the first choice drugs are contraindicated, poorly tolerated or ineffective.

Relapses are new signs and symptoms caused by a new focal demyelinating lesion in the CNS. Infection should also be considered if new symptoms develop. Once infection is excluded or treated, significant relapse can be managed with a high-dose corticosteroid, such as methylprednisolone, given for 3–5 days. This shortens the duration of a relapse but does not affect the long-term outcome. Most recovery from a relapse occurs in the first 2–3 months, but with residual disability in up to 50% of cases.

Fampridine is a voltage-gated potassium channel blocker that targets exposed K^+ channels in demyelinated axons and inhibits repolarisation of the neuron. This prolongs the nerve action potential and may improve walking speed and mobility. However, fewer than 50% of people with multiple sclerosis will respond, and it should be discontinued if there is no improvement in 2 weeks.

Symptomatic treatment of spasticity may be necessary, for example with baclofen (see Chapter 24) or gabapentin (see Chapter 23), and physiotherapy has an important role. A multidisciplinary team approach is essential for the management of the numerous disabling symptoms that may occur in multiple sclerosis.

MOTOR NEURON DISEASE

Motor neuron disease is an uncommon, rapidly progres-sive disorder of motor neurons that occurs most often in middle-aged males. The pathophysiology involves neuronal loss among the anterior horn cells of the spinal cord, motor cortex and hypoglossal nucleus in the lower medulla. The cause is unknown, but recent evidence suggests that there is underlying dysfunction in a nuclear RNA splicing factor known as transactive response DNA-binding protein (TAR)-43, leading to aberrant mRNA splicing. There is evidence of excessive activation of excitatory glutamate receptors in the CNS, which may lead to neuronal Ca^{2+} overload and cell death (excitotoxicity). Mutations of genes coding for the free radical-scavenging enzyme, superoxide dismutase, may also lead to excessive free radical activity.

The most common form of motor neuron disease, amyotrophic lateral sclerosis, produces both upper motor neuron signs and symptoms (hypertonia, impaired fine movement and hyperreflexia) and lower motor neuron signs and symptoms (fasciculations, muscle cramps, weakness and muscle atrophy). Other forms affect either upper or lower motor neurons. Up to half of affected people develop cognitive impairment. Death from respiratory failure usually occurs 2–5 years from the onset of symptoms.

DRUG TREATMENT

Riluzole is the only available agent that alters the course of motor neuron disease. It crosses the blood–brain barrier and inhibits the release of glutamate, as well as acting as an antagonist at glutamate *N*-methyl-D-aspartate (NMDA) receptors on damaged neurons. These actions may inhibit glutamate-induced excitotoxicity. Treatment with riluzole does not arrest the disease, but may slow its progression to a modest extent, improving survival by an average of 3 months after 18 months of treatment. Unwanted effects of riluzole include nausea, vomiting, diarrhoea, lethargy and dizziness.

Physiotherapists can help with advice on posture and exercise early in the disease, and later with passive movement to reduce musculoskeletal pain. Symptomatic treatment is often necessary for complications, particularly spasticity and associated pain. Bulbar involvement often causes dysphagia that requires enteral feeding. Late in the progression of the condition, chest wall weakness leads to type II respiratory failure that may require artificial ventilation.

GUILLAIN–BARRÉ SYNDROME

Guillain–Barré syndrome is an autoimmune acute inflammatory demyelinating polyradiculopathy that only affects the peripheral nervous system. It is triggered in about 40% of cases by infection, of which *Campylobacter jejuni* infection followed by cytomegalovirus are the most frequent. The most typical presentation is rapid symmetrical onset of lower limb weakness, with loss of tendon reflexes and autonomic dysfunction, accompanied by variable sensory signs. The weakness then rapidly progresses upward over hours or days. Bulbar weakness and respiratory difficulties are common with respiratory failure in 20–30% of cases. Symptoms usually progress for up to 2 weeks, plateau for 2–4 weeks, and then improve. About 5% of affected people die in the acute-illness phase, and up to 10% have incomplete recovery and are left with severe long-term disability.

The immunological response is probably due to shared antigens on the infecting organism and the peripheral nerve tissue. In most cases, the target of immune attack is gangliosides, found in large quantities in peripheral nerves. The autoantibodies fix complement, and attract lymphocytes and then macrophages, which invade the myelin sheaths (acute inflammatory demyelinating polyneuropathy). In about 5% of cases the problem arises from primary autoimmune injury to axons, known as acute motor (or motor and sensory) axonal neuropathy. Axonal degeneration frequently results in greater long-term disability.

EARLY MANAGEMENT

There are several aspects to the early management of Guillain–Barré syndrome:

- Supportive treatment may be life-saving and is the cornerstone of management. For example, ventilatory support is necessary for respiratory muscle weakness or paralysis in 30% of cases. Haemodynamic disturbance, including significant tachycardia or bradycardia and asystole, can result from autonomic involvement and may require cardiovascular support. Prophylaxis for deep venous thrombosis with subcutaneous heparin (see Chapter 11) should be given. Neuropathic pain may require analgesia, or the use of tricyclic antidepressants, gabapentin or carbamazepine (see Chapters 22 and 23), and can be reduced by passive limb movement.
- High-dose intravenous immunoglobulin (IgG) given within the first 2 weeks is usually the preferred treatment. It may work by neutralising the pathological antibodies and interfering with the function of both T- and B-cells. Unwanted effects include malaise, chills and fever. IgG reduces the need for supported ventilation, and the time taken to recover walking.
- Plasma exchange is an alternative to intravenous IgG. When used within 4 weeks of the onset of symptoms, it improves the long-term outcome. The benefit is probably due to removal of autoantibodies.
- Corticosteroids are of no benefit, either alone or in combination with IgG.

Physiotherapy and other supportive management become increasingly important to aid long-term recovery. Overall mortality is about 5%, and about 20% of people cannot walk unaided 6 months after onset. Most people are left with persistent pain and fatigue.

SELF-ASSESSMENT

True/false questions

1. Treatment with interferon beta is of benefit in reducing relapses in multiple sclerosis.
2. Multiple sclerosis is characterised in the early years by a steady progressive worsening of symptoms in the majority of people.
3. Glutamate can cause neuronal damage.
4. Riluzole is of benefit in motor neuron disease by blocking the release of γ-aminobutyric acid (GABA).
5. Natalizumab is used in multiple sclerosis, as it enhances the action of adhesion molecules, increasing the passage of lymphocytes into the CNS.
6. Fingolimod is a produg activated by phosphorylation.

One-best-answer (OBA) question

1. Which is the *most accurate* statement about the treatment of multiple sclerosis?
   A. Interferon beta causes influenza-like symptoms in 1% of those who receive it.
   B. Expert opinion does not support the use of glatiramer acetate as a first-line drug for use in multiple sclerosis.
   C. Glatiramer acetate causes few unwanted effects following injection.
   D. Corticosteroid treatment is of benefit in reducing the progression of multiple sclerosis.
   E. Neuronal conduction is unimpaired in multiple sclerosis.

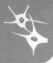

ANSWERS

True/false answers

1. **False.** Interferon beta is used in multiple sclerosis and may diminish the production of inflammatory interferon-γ.
2. **False.** Multiple sclerosis is usually characterised by relapses and remissions over a number of years, although after about 10 years a steady decline sets in.
3. **True.** Glutamate is an excitatory amino acid neurotransmitter but can cause cell damage and death (excitotoxicity) by a number of mechanisms, including an uncontrolled increase in intracellular Ca^{2+}.
4. **False.** Riluzole is the only drug that will alter the course of motor neuron disease; it inhibits glutamate release and action, thereby reducing its toxicity.
5. **False.** Natalizumab is an inhibitor of the α_4-integrin adhesion molecule and reduces the migration of lymphocytes into the CNS.
6. **True.** Fingolimod is rapidly phosphorylated by sphingosine kinases.

One-best-answer (OBA) answer

1. **Answer B** is correct.
   A. Incorrect. Influenza-like symptoms can occur in about 50% of people.
   B. **Correct**. The use of glatiramer acetate is usually restricted to people who cannot tolerate interferon beta, or who have developed antibodies to interferon beta.
   C. Incorrect. Glatiramer acetate can cause flushing, chest tightness, palpitations, anxiety and breathlessness.
   D. Incorrect. Corticosteroids may shorten the duration of acute attacks but have no effect on progression or eventual disability in multiple sclerosis.
   E. Incorrect. Long-term disability is due to demyelination of nerves and consequent further axonal damage. Demyelination of nerves results in disordered neuronal conduction.

FURTHER READING

El-Said, A.M., 2014. Emergent management of Guillain–Barré syndrome. Ain-Shams J. Anesthesiol. 7, 88–95.

Galea, I., Ward-Abel, N., Heesen, C., 2015. Relapse in multiple sclerosis. Br. Med. J. 350, h1765.

Kiernan, M.C., Vucic, S., Cheah, B., et al., 2011. Amyotrophic lateral sclerosis. Lancet 377, 942–955.

Nageshwaran, S., Davies, L.M., Rafi, I., et al., 2014. Motor neurone disease. Br. Med. J. 349, g4052.

Willison, H.J., Jacobs, B.C., van Doorn, P.A., 2016. Guillain–Barré syndrome. Lancet 388, 717–727.

Wingerchuk, D.M., Weinshenker, B.G., 2016. Disease-modifying therapies for relapsing multiple sclerosis. Br. Med. J. 354, i3518.

Yuki, N., Hartung, H.-P., 2014. Guillain–Barré syndrome. N. Engl. J. Med. 366, 2294–2304.

Compendium: drugs used to treat multiple sclerosis, motor neuron disease and Guillain–Barré syndrome

Drug	Characteristics
Corticosteroids	Corticosteroids such as methylprednisolone or prednisolone may be of benefit for acute relapse in people with multiple sclerosis (see Chapter 44)
Fampridine	Potassium channel blocker that prolongs action potentials. Given orally to adults with multiple sclerosis with walking disability. Half-life: 6 h
Glatiramer acetate	Hydrolysed rapidly to a tetrapeptide that may act as an immunological decoy for myelin basic protein. Given by subcutaneous injection to treat multiple sclerosis. Half-life of the tetrapeptide is not known.
Fingolimod	Prodrug of a sphingosine analogue; phosphorylated form prevents lymphocyte egress from lymph nodes; given orally for multiple sclerosis. Half-life: 4–9 days
Interferon beta	Antiinflammatory cytokine. Given by subcutaneous or intramuscular injection for relapsing–remitting multiple sclerosis. Half-life: 2–4 h
Natalizumab	A monoclonal antibody that blocks lymphocyte adhesion. Given as an intravenous infusion for relapsing–remitting multiple sclerosis. Half-life: 11 days
Riluzole	Glutamate receptor antagonist. Given orally for motor neuron disease. Half-life: 12 h

26 Migraine and other headaches

Headaches have many causes; most headaches have no underlying structural abnormality or metabolic disturbance and are known as primary headaches (Box 26.1). Tension headache is by far the most common primary headache, accounting for about two-thirds of cases, while migraine is the second most frequent cause. When headache is present for a prolonged time, or is recurrent, secondary causes may need to be excluded by a full history and examination to elicit any associated neurological symptoms and signs.

MIGRAINE

Migraine is an episodic headache, typically lasting 4–72 hours. The diagnostic features of migraine are listed in Box 26.2. These are the only symptoms in the majority of migraineurs. However, in about 15% of cases, the headache is preceded or accompanied by focal neurological symptoms (migraine with aura), usually visual disturbances (such as flashing or jagged lights), but occasionally sensory disturbance or more severe focal neurological episodes such as hemiparesis.

PATHOGENESIS OF MIGRAINE

The pathogenesis of migraine is incompletely understood, but it is now believed that the primary driver is neuronal dysfunction in the trigeminovascular system (Fig. 26.1). Vascular changes (vasoconstriction and vasodilation) are probably secondary to the neuronal trigger. Genetic predisposition is a factor in migraine, and abnormal function of voltage-dependent ion channels in cortical and brainstem structures may provide the basis for increased glutamatergic neurotransmission and hyperexcitability in the neuronal circuits that are responsible for the headache.

A migraine aura is probably caused by a slowly propagated wave of cortical depolarisation that transiently depresses spontaneous and evoked neuronal activity (cortical spreading depression). The depressant wave is associated with intracranial vasoconstriction, which can produce focal neurological symptoms and signs. The majority of migraineurs who do not experience an aura appear to have 'silent' cortical spreading depression, and this suppression of electrical activity may therefore be the trigger for the migraine headache. The trigger for cortical spreading depression is unknown.

Cortical spreading depression activates meningeal nociceptors in the trigeminovascular pathway, which carries nociceptive information from the meninges to the brain. The pathway is coordinated by the trigeminal ganglion, which has peripheral neuronal projections to the pia, dura and large cerebral arteries, and central projections to the trigeminal nucleus in the brainstem. The trigeminal nucleus also receives nociceptive afferents from various intracranial structures, periorbital skin and pericranial muscles. Activation of the trigeminovascular pathway may be through release of vasoactive peptides such as calcitonin gene-related peptide (CGRP) from the perivascular axons in the dura mater. CGRP promotes vasodilation and release of proinflammatory molecules such as serotonin, histamine, bradykinin and prostaglandin E_2. The result is neurogenic inflammation of the dural blood vessels with plasma protein extravasation, platelet aggregation and mast cell degranulation.

Headache in patients with migraine is associated with sensitisation of the pain pathways (decreased response threshold and increased magnitude of response) produced by the inflammation. Sensitisation occurs in the meninges (peripheral sensitisation) and also in the processing of sensory stimuli in the spinal cord and brain (central sensitisation). Sensitisation makes the pathways increasingly responsive

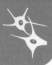

Primary headache
Tension-type headache
Migraine
Idiopathic stabbing headache
Exertional headache
Cluster headache

Secondary headache
Systemic infection
Head injury
Drug-induced headache
Vascular disorders
Brain tumour

Box 26.2 | **Diagnostic features of migraine**

Two or more of the following features:
- unilateral pain,
- throbbing,
- aggravation on movement,
- pain of moderate or severe intensity.
Also, one of the following:
- nausea or vomiting,
- light or noise sensitivity (photophobia or phonophobia).

to nociceptive stimuli but also non-nociceptive stimuli such as light, noise and smell. Nociceptive impulses are relayed through the trigeminovascular pathway to the thalamus and brainstem, leading to pain, nausea and vomiting. The trigeminovascular pathway is rich in serotonin 5-HT$_{1B}$ receptors on vascular smooth muscle and 5-HT$_{1D}$ receptors on the perivascular nerve terminals and in the dorsal horn. Stimulation of these receptors blocks the release of vasoactive peptides and inhibits neurotransmitter release.

DRUGS FOR MIGRAINE

SPECIFIC DRUGS FOR THE ACUTE MIGRAINE ATTACK

Triptans

frovatriptan, sumatriptan, zolmitriptan

Mechanisms of action and effects

The triptans are serotonin 5-HT$_{1B/1D}$ receptor agonists, which may alter the pathophysiology of migraine (Fig. 26.2) by:
- intracranial vasoconstriction (5-HT$_{1B}$),
- inhibition of neurotransmission in the trigeminovascular pathway and inhibition of release of proinflammatory and vasoactive mediators from perivascular trigeminal neurons (5-HT$_{1B/1D}$).

Sumatriptan does not easily cross the blood–brain barrier since it is water-soluble, but this barrier appears to be impaired during a migraine attack. Zolmitriptan and frovatriptan penetrate the blood–brain barrier more readily. Triptans relieve both the pain and nausea associated with migraine.

Pharmacokinetics

Absorption of sumatriptan from the gut is rapid but erratic, whereas other triptans have better absorption. Effective plasma concentrations of all triptans are usually reached in 30–60 minutes after oral administration, although the onset of action of frovatriptan may be longer. Sumatriptan can also be delivered by subcutaneous injection or intranasal spray, and zolmitriptan by nasal spray or an orally disintegrating tablet. These routes relieve symptoms within 15 minutes and can also be more effective if headache is accompanied by nausea, when gastric stasis delays oral drug absorption. Elimination of most triptans is partially by hepatic metabolism and partially by renal excretion. Most triptans have short half-lives of between 2 and 6 hours, but the half-life of frovatriptan is longer, at 26 hours.

Unwanted effects

The frequency and intensity of unwanted effects are highest after subcutaneous use of sumatriptan.

- Tingling, pressure, tightness, heaviness or sensation of warmth in the head, neck, chest and limbs.
- Flushing;
- Dizziness or vertigo;
- Drowsiness;
- Nausea or vomiting;
- Angina caused by coronary artery vasoconstriction (via 5-HT$_{1B}$ receptor stimulation);
- Pain or irritation at the injection site, or in the nose after local use.

Ergotamine

Mechanism of action

Ergotamine probably has an antimigraine action similar to the triptans by stimulating 5-HT$_1$ receptors. Unwanted effects arise from agonist activity at several other receptors, including α_1-adrenoceptors and dopamine D$_2$ receptors.

Pharmacokinetics

Oral administration is often accompanied by nausea, and absorption is poor, erratic and delayed. Ergotamine undergoes extensive metabolism in the liver and has a short half-life (2 hours). However, tight receptor binding produces a longer duration of action.

Unwanted effects

- Nausea and vomiting are caused by dopamine receptor stimulation at the chemoreceptor trigger zone (see Chapter 32).
- Abdominal cramps.
- Dizziness.
- Severe vasoconstriction as a result of α_1-adrenoceptor stimulation can lead to peripheral gangrene (acute ergotism). Ergotamine should be avoided in people with

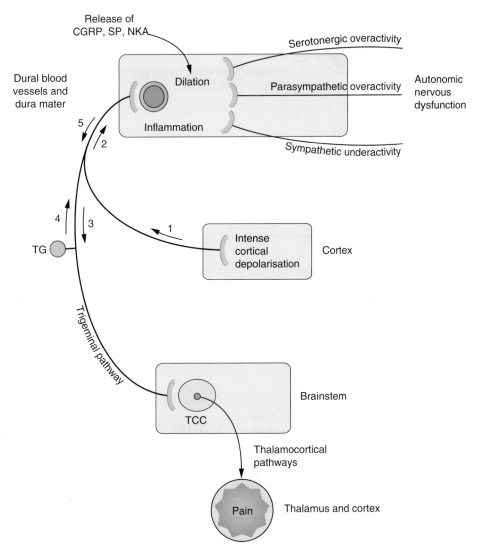

Fig. 26.1 Proposed mechanisms associated with the processes of migraine. The sequence and nature of neurogenic and vascular involvement in migraine are vigorously debated and may vary in different kinds of migraine-type headache. One scenario is that the trigger is a wave of cortical depression *(1)* which sensitises and stimulates the trigeminal pathway in either direction *(2, 3)*. This results in stimulation of the trigeminocervical complex (TCC) *(3)* in the brainstem, and onward stimulation of the thalamus and other areas can cause pain and nausea. Other reflex pathways from the brainstem via the superior salivatory nucleus to the dural blood vessels, which result in vasodilation, can also be activated at this stage. The stimulation of trigeminal nerves innervating the dural blood vessels *(2, 4)* results in the release of mediators such as calcitonin gene-related peptide (CGRP), substance P (SP) and neurokinin A (NKA), which cause vasodilation and contribute to inflammation. CGRP and possibly other mediators are able to stimulate nociceptors in the trigeminal nerve endings, resulting in further activation of the pathways to the TCC and thalamus *(5)* and consequently further pain. The control of vascular tone in the dural blood vessels is complex, with sympathetic, parasympathetic and serotonergic systems contributing to the migraine process. Vasoconstrictor innervation of these vessels is by sympathetic nerves, and vasodilation occurs by parasympathetic innervation. Serotonergic pathways produce vasoconstriction by stimulation of 5-HT$_{1B}$ receptors and vasodilation via 5-HT$_2$ receptors. *TG*, Trigeminal ganglion.

known atheromatous vascular disease (including ischaemic heart disease).

■ Chronic intoxication with dependence can occur after prolonged use. Withdrawal then produces nausea and headache similar to an acute migraine attack. For this reason, treatment with ergotamine should not be repeated at intervals of less than 4 days.

PROPHYLACTIC DRUGS

Beta-adrenoceptor antagonists

Several β-adrenoceptor antagonists, such as propranolol, timolol and metoprolol, are effective for prophylaxis of migraine. Drugs with partial agonist activity that cause

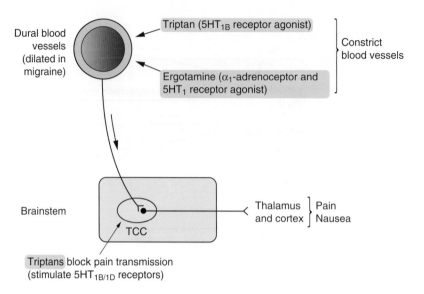

Fig. 26.2 Possible mechanisms of action of 5-HT receptor agonists in migraine. The trigeminocervical complex (TCC) is rich in 5-HT$_{1B/1D}$ receptors, and stimulation of these receptors by so-called second-generation triptans inhibits neurotransmission to the thalamus and cortex. Triptans also cause vasoconstriction, acting at 5-HT$_{1B}$ receptors on blood vessels.

vasodilation (e.g. pindolol) are ineffective. Effects on central nervous system functions include reduced neuronal firing in noradrenergic neurons in the locus coeruleus and inhibition of cortical potentials evoked by auditory and visual stimuli, suggesting a modulation of neuronal excitability. Full details of β-adrenoceptor antagonists can be found in Chapter 5.

Antiepileptic drugs

Sodium valproate, gabapentin and topiramate are effective in the prophylaxis of migraine and almost certainly work by multiple mechanisms, including γ-aminobutyric acid (GABA)-mediated suppression of neurotransmission through the trigeminovascular pathway, and modulation of neuronal excitability through effects on voltage-gated Na$^+$ channels. Blockade of P/Q-type Ca^{2+} channels may also contribute by reducing glutamate release. Antiepileptic drugs with a predominant single mechanism of action are ineffective in treatment of migraine. Full details of antiepileptic drugs can be found in Chapter 23.

Amitriptyline

The mechanism of action of amitryptyline in migraine is unknown but probably relates to multiple neurotransmitter–receptor interactions that modulate the processing of nociceptive impulses. Prophylactic doses of amitriptyline for migraine and tension headache are similar to those used for neuropathic pain and are lower than those used to treat depression. Other antidepressants are ineffective. Full details of amitriptyline can be found in Chapter 22.

MANAGEMENT OF MIGRAINE AND OTHER HEADACHES

THE ACUTE MIGRAINE ATTACK

Withdrawal of possible triggers such as cheese, chocolate, citrus fruits or alcoholic drinks may reduce the frequency of migraine attacks by up to 50%. The combined oral hormonal contraceptive is a potential exacerbating factor, although it can be helpful for prevention of menstrual-related migraine.

Simple analgesia with a nonsteroidal antiinflammatory drug (NSAID) such as ibuprofen (see Chapter 29) may be sufficient for the relief of a mild acute attack of migraine. Nausea frequently accompanies a migraine attack and delays gastric emptying. If this occurs, absorption of the analgesic will be more rapid if an antiemetic such as metoclopramide or domperidone (see Chapter 32) is given concurrently. If the person is vomiting, rectal or intramuscular analgesia, for example with an NSAID such as diclofenac or naproxen, can be used together with rectal domperidone. Analgesics are usually more effective when given early after the onset of pain. Opioid analgesics are not recommended for treatment of migraine, as they are short-acting, produce dependence and frequent use can promote medication-overuse headache (discussed later).

If migraine attacks are poorly controlled by simple analgesics or are moderate to severe in intensity, a triptan is usually highly effective. Triptans can relieve pain, even if taken more than 4 hours after the onset of an attack, but are less effective in those migraineurs who have developed cutaneous allodynia (a form of neuropathic pain; see Chapter 19) in the trigeminal nerve distribution in association with the headache. Subcutaneous sumatriptan, intranasal sumatriptan or zolmitriptan, or an orally disintegrating tablet of zolmitriptan are useful if a rapid response is required or if nausea precludes oral therapy. The response of individuals varies to the different triptans, and it is worth changing to an alternative after two unsuccessful attempts at treatment with one drug. Headache recurs in about 40% of those who initially gain relief from a triptan, although the risk of recurrence may be less with frovatriptan, which has a long duration of action. A second dose of a triptan can be used for recurrent headache if there was a good response to the first dose. If migraine headaches are prolonged or recur frequently despite treatment with a triptan, then the combination of a triptan with an NSAID can be tried.

Ergotamine has been used to treat acute attacks, but the risk of vasospasm and habituation means that ergotamine should be avoided in older people (who may have cardiovascular disease) and in those with frequent attacks. Ergotamine is now infrequently used and should not be used concurrently with a triptan.

PROPHYLAXIS OF MIGRAINE

Prophylaxis is usually recommended for people experiencing at least two migraine attacks each month that significantly interfere with their daily routine. β-Adrenoceptor antagonists are widely held to be the best choice, providing there are no contraindications. The antiepileptic drugs sodium valproate and topiramate are effective second-line alternatives. There is less consistent evidence for the use of gabapentin, which is used as a third-line option. The major disadvantage of antiepileptic drugs is the risk of teratogenicity in women of childbearing age. Amitriptyline can be particularly effective when tension headache coexists with migraine. Pizotifen (see the compendium at the end of this chapter) is infrequently used.

Botulinum toxin type A (see Chapter 24) given by injection into sites such as the forehead, temporalis, cervical and trapezius muscles may reduce migraine attacks for up to 3 months. The mechanism is unclear, but inhibition of peripheral sensory neurons may reduce central neuronal sensitisation. Some evidence suggests that people who describe their migraine headache as 'being crushed from the outside' or who have 'eye-popping' headaches (imploding or ocular headaches) respond better than those who describe a build-up of pressure inside the head (exploding headache). Botulinum toxin may therefore work best if there is an extracranial trigger for the pain.

The efficacy of all current prophylactic treatments is limited. Although the response to an individual drug is unpredictable, only about half of all migraineurs can expect to have a 50% reduction in the frequency of attacks.

MEDICATION-OVERUSE HEADACHE

Regular use of opioids or compound analgesic drugs, especially those containing caffeine, to treat any type of headache or regular use of triptans to treat migraine can lead to a chronic daily headache known as medication-overuse headache. It is the third most common cause of headache.

The mechanisms underlying medication-overuse headache are not well understood, but probably involve downregulation of receptor or enzyme targets of the drugs, with consequent sensitisation of the pain pathways. Medication-overuse headache is most common in women aged between 30 and 60 years, and is diagnosed when headache is present for at least 15 days each month over a period of at least 3 months in someone who is taking regular medication to treat headache. The person experiencing the headache is often reluctant to consider that the drugs are the cause, but abrupt withdrawal of the causative treatment is advised to achieve resolution. NSAIDs can be used for withdrawal headaches, along with prophylactic treatment for the underlying tension or migrainous headache given prior to withdrawal.

MANAGEMENT OF OTHER HEADACHES

Most other primary headaches are managed just as any other form of acute pain, usually using medications at step 1 of the World Health Organization (WHO) analgesic ladder (see Chapter 19). Care must be taken to avoid medication-overuse headache.

Tension-type headache is usually bilateral and not disabling. Frequent tension headaches may respond to prophylactic treatment with amitriptyline at low dosage.

Cluster headache is characterised by severe attacks of unilateral pain in the distribution of the trigeminal nerve that are associated with autonomic features on the side of the headache (such as ptosis, miosis, conjunctival injection, lacrimation, and rhinorrhoea). Cluster headache usually responds to a triptan, but if prophylaxis is needed for recurrent episodes, then the calcium channel blocker verapamil (see Chapter 5) is the drug of choice.

Suspected secondary headache requires treatment of the precipitating cause. Red flag features include thunderclap headache with peak severity achieved in seconds or minutes (usually primary headache, but consider subarachnoid haemorrhage), focal neurological signs or new cognitive disturbance (possible intracranial pathology), and headache that worsens on standing (possible low-pressure headache due to cerebrospinal fluid leak). Other features suggesting raised intracranial pressure are headache that wakes the person from sleep or worsening of headache with coughing, laughing or straining. Headache due to an intracerebral tumour that is causing raised intracranial pressure is often alleviated by dexamethasone (see Chapter 44), which reduces cerebral oedema around the tumour.

SELF-ASSESSMENT

True/false questions

1. Diet plays little part in the precipitation of migraine attacks.
2. Serotonin is released in a migraine attack.
3. Agonists at 5-HT$_{1B/1D}$ receptors are used for the treatment of migraine.
4. Ergotamine is used prophylactically for migraine.
5. Sumatriptan is not useful for acute migraine attacks, as it is slow-acting.

6. Sumatriptan causes chest discomfort in 40% of people as a result of coronary vasoconstriction.
7. Regular use of triptans can cause rebound headache.
8. Pizotifen is used prophylactically and blocks 5-HT$_2$ receptors.
9. Ergotamine is safe to use in ischaemic heart disease.
10. Tricyclic antidepressants and β-adrenoceptor antagonists may be useful in prophylaxis of migraine.
11. Where migraine is associated with vomiting, metoclopramide and paracetamol given together is a useful combination.
12. Pindolol is effective in prophylaxis of migraine.
13. The combined oral hormonal contraceptive reduces the frequency of migraine attacks in women.
14. Prophylactic treatment for migraine is highly effective.
15. Injections of botulinum toxin may reduce migraine symptoms.

ANSWERS

True/false answers

1. **False.** In some people, stress and dietary items like chocolate, cheese and alcohol may provoke migraine attacks.
2. **True.** Serotonin, histamine, nitric oxide and other vasoactive mediators contribute to neurogenic inflammation in migraine.
3. **True.** The triptans are 5-HT$_{1B/1D}$ agonists used in acute migraine. Stimulation of 5-HT$_{1B/1D}$ receptors inhibits neurotransmission in the trigeminovascular pathway and inhibits release of vasoactive and proinflammatory mediators, while 5-HT$_{1B}$ stimulation produces intracranial vasoconstriction.
4. **False.** Because of unwanted effects, ergotamine should not be used prophylactically, or more than twice a month for acute attacks.
5. **False.** Oral sumatriptan acts within 30 minutes, and more quickly when given by subcutaneous or nasal routes of administration.
6. **False.** Although sumatriptan causes chest discomfort and is contraindicated in people with ischaemic heart disease, chest discomfort in people without ischaemic heart disease is probably caused by oesophageal spasm, not myocardial ischaemia.
7. **True.** Medication-overuse headache may occur with triptans, opioids and compound analgesics when used regularly for headache.
8. **True.** Pizotifen is not commonly used but reduces perivascular inflammation, vasodilation and pain by antagonist activity at 5-HT$_2$ receptors.
9. **False.** Ergotamine causes vasoconstriction and should be avoided in people with vascular diseases.
10. **True.** β-Adrenoceptor antagonists like propranolol are first-line drugs for migraine prophylaxis, with antiepileptic drugs such as sodium valproate, topiramate and gabapentin also commonly used. The tricyclic antidepressant amitryptiline is useful when tension headache co-exists with migraine.
11. **True.** Metoclopramide is an antiemetic and increases gastric emptying, thus improving the rate of absorption of paracetamol.
12. **False.** β-Adrenoceptor antagonists with partial agonist activity like pindolol are not effective, as they may exacerbate vasodilation.
13. **False.** The combined oral hormonal contraceptive may exacerbate migraine, although it can be helpful in women with menstrual-related migraine.
14. **False.** The prophylaxis of migraine is effective in only about half of those who are treated.
15. **True.** Pericranial injections of botulinum toxin type A can reduce the frequency of migraine attacks.

FURTHER READING

Burstein, R., Noseda, R., Borsook, D., 2015. Migraine: multiple processes, complex pathophysiology. J. Neurosci. 35, 6619–6629.

Drug and Therapeutics Bulletin, 2010. Management of medication overuse headache. Br. Med. J. 340, 968–972.

Fenstermacher, N., Levin, M., Ward, T., 2011. Pharmacological prevention of migraine. Br. Med. J. 342, 540–543.

Nesbitt, A.D., Goadsby, P.J., 2012. Cluster headache. Br. Med. J. 344, e2407.

Pringsheim, T., Becker, W.J., 2014. Triptans for symptomatic treatment of migraine headache. Br. Med. J. 348, g2285.

Compendium: drugs used to treat migraine

Drug	Characteristics
Analgesics	
Most migraine headaches respond to nonsteroidal antiinflammatory drugs, but reduced gastric emptying may slow the rate of oral absorption; tolfenamic acid is licensed specifically for oral treatment of acute attacks; diclofenac potassium, flurbiprofen and ibuprofen are also licensed for migraine; see Chapter 29.	
Antiemetics	
Antiemetics (see Chapter 32) such as metoclopramide or domperidone are often given to relieve the nausea associated with migraine attacks.	
5-HT$_1$ receptor agonists (triptans)	
Act on 5-HT$_{1B}$ and 5-HT$_{1D}$ receptors. May be used during the acute headache phase; preferred treatment for those who fail to respond to analgesics.	
Almotriptan	Given orally. Half-life: 3–4 h
Eletriptan	Given orally. Half-life: 4–5 h
Frovatriptan	Given orally; long-acting. Half-life: 26 h
Naratriptan	Given orally; long-acting. Half-life: 6 h
Rizatriptan	Given orally. Half-life: 2–3 h
Sumatriptan	First-generation triptan. Given orally, intranasally or by subcutaneous injection; also used for cluster headaches. Half-life: 2 h
Zolmitriptan	Given orally or intranasally; also used intranasally for cluster headaches. Half-life: 3 h
Ergot alkaloids and related compounds	
Ergotamine	5-HT$_1$ and α_1-adrenoceptor agonist. Given orally or as suppositories. Half-life: 2 h
Other drugs for migraine	
Amitriptyline	Tricyclic antidepressant used for migraine prophylaxis; see Chapter 22
Antiepileptic drugs	Some antiepileptic drugs such as sodium valproate, topiramate and gabapentin are used for migraine prophylaxis; see Chapter 23
β-Adrenoceptor antagonists	Some β-adrenoceptor antagonists such as propranolol are used for migraine prophylaxis; see Chapter 8
Clonidine	Used orally for prophylaxis but not recommended; see Chapter 6
Isometheptene	Indirectly-acting sympathomimetic that constricts dilated cranial and cerebral arterioles. Used orally for acute attacks in combination with paracetamol, but other drugs usually preferred. Half-life: not known
Pizotifen	5-HT$_2$ antagonist and antihistamine; given orally for prophylaxis, but rarely used. Half-life: 26 h

6

The musculoskeletal system

27

The neuromuscular junction and neuromuscular blockade

NEUROMUSCULAR TRANSMISSION

The neuromuscular junction is a specialised synapse of a somatic neuron with skeletal muscle, termed the motor endplate (Fig. 27.1A). Depolarisation of the postsynaptic membrane at the motor endplate causes contraction of the muscle fibre in an all-or-nothing response.

The neurotransmitter at the neuromuscular junction is acetylcholine (ACh), acting at postsynaptic N_2 (or 'muscle-type') nicotinic receptors. The processes of synthesis and release of ACh are described in Chapter 4 in relation to the general properties of neurotransmitters in the nervous system. The presynaptic nerve terminal at the neuromuscular junction contains 300,000 or more vesicles. In response to an action potential, about 60 vesicles discharge their contents (up to 10,000 molecules of ACh each) into the synapse over 0.5 ms; this is 10 times the amount of Ach required to depolarise the motor endplate. Nicotinic acetylcholine receptors are also present on the pre-synaptic neuronal membrane (mobilisation receptors), which modulate the synthesis, storage and release

of ACh and augment ACh release in response to an action potential in the neuron.

Each N_2 receptor has two binding sites for ACh, and the Na^+ channel in the centre of the receptor opens when both sites are occupied (see Fig. 1.1). This triggers an influx of Na^+ into the muscle cell and depolarisation of the motor endplate, generating a local current, the endplate potential. When the endplate potential reaches a threshold, then voltage-gated Na^+ channels open, leading to full depolarisation of the muscle cell. This generates an action potential which is propagated along the postsynaptic membrane (sarcolemma) to the T tubules, where Ca^{2+} is released from the sarcoplasmic reticulum. The increased availability of intracellular Ca^{2+} brings about the processes that result in muscle contraction (see Fig. 27.1B). The voltage-gated Na^+ channels close and become inactive after depolarisation, requiring the membrane potential to be reset before they can be reactivated.

The action of ACh on N_2 receptors is very short-lived (about 0.6 ms) because the synaptic cleft contains large amounts of the enzyme acetylcholinesterase (AChE), which rapidly degrades ACh (see Chapter 4). Butyrylcholinesterase in plasma (also called pseudocholinesterase or plasma cholinesterase) hydrolyses any ACh that escapes from the synaptic cleft. Butyrylcholinesterase is important pharmacologically because of its ability to metabolise several drugs with ester bonds. Tissue esterases that break down ACh are also present in many cells, notably in the liver.

Although ACh is the neurotransmitter responsible for contraction of both skeletal muscle and most smooth muscles, the basic organisation and functioning of these neuroeffector systems are very different, as shown in Table 27.1.

DRUGS ACTING AT THE NEUROMUSCULAR JUNCTION

ACETYLCHOLINESTERASE INHIBITORS (ANTICHOLINESTERASES)

AChE inhibitors (such as pyridostigmine and neostigmine) block the breakdown of ACh following its release in neuronal synapses and at neuroeffector junctions. The mechanisms of action of different types of AChE inhibitor are described in Chapter 4; they are nonselective and prolong the availability and actions of ACh at all its receptors (nicotinic N_1 and N_2 and muscarinic). Their main use is in the treatment of myasthenia gravis (see Chapter 28).

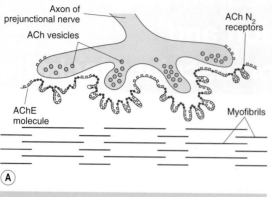

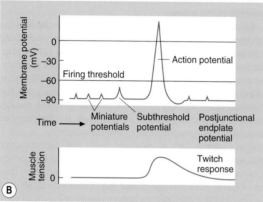

Fig. 27.1 Acetylcholine (ACh) at the neuromuscular junction. (A) The released ACh acts upon postsynaptic nicotinic N_2 receptors on the motor endplate, opening cation channels; an influx of Na^+ then occurs, resulting in depolarisation. (B) At rest, insignificant amounts of ACh are released and the miniature endplate potentials generated are insufficient to reach the threshold potential to cause a propagated action potential. If sufficient ACh is released, an action potential is propagated, causing muscle contraction. Nondepolarising muscle relaxants prevent the generation of the action potential by blocking N_2 receptors. *AChE*, Acetylcholinesterase.

INHIBITORS OF ACETYLCHOLINE RELEASE

Botulinum toxin from the anaerobic bacillus *Clostridium botulinum* decreases the release of ACh from neuronal vesicles. It binds selectively to a receptor on the presynaptic membrane of cholinergic nerve terminals and is endocytosed inside synaptic vesicles responsible for re-uptake of neurotransmitter. Inside the cell, botulinum toxin is released into the cytosol, where it cleaves cytoplasmic synaptosomal-associated protein 25 (SNAP-25) on the cell membrane, a protein that is essential for docking and fusion of vesicles with the neuronal membrane. Therefore botulinum toxin inhibits neurotransmitter release. This chemical denervation stimulates the growth of collateral axons which eventually results in the formation of a new neuromuscular junction. Botulinum toxin is extremely dangerous, as evidenced by the consequences of botulinum poisoning, but it also has clinical roles when injected locally. Two toxin serotypes, A and B, are used in clinical practice as botulinum toxin–haemagglutinin complex. They are therapeutically equivalent but the doses are not interchangeable. Injection into skeletal muscles produces local muscle paralysis for 3–4 months until new nerve terminals develop. Botulinum toxin is used to treat involuntary movements such as blepharospasm (spasm of the eyelids), hemifacial spasm or spasmodic torticollis (wry-neck), strabismus (misalignment of the eyes that prevents binocular vision) and to relieve focal spasticity (see Chapter 24). It is also used by local injection to reduce excessive axillary sweating (hyperhidrosis), because it inhibits ACh release at sweat glands and can be injected into facial muscles for the prophylaxis of migraine (see Chapter 26). Intravesical injection of botulinum toxin is sometimes used to treat severe overactive bladder syndrome. Botulinum toxin is frequently used by local injection for cosmetic reasons to temporarily remove frown lines and wrinkles.

NEUROMUSCULAR JUNCTION BLOCKERS

Skeletal muscle relaxation is achieved by drugs that reversibly block the actions of ACh on nicotinic N_2 receptors at the neuromuscular junction. Drugs that block the neuromuscular

Table 27.1 Comparison of skeletal and smooth muscle innervation

Property	Skeletal muscle fibre	Smooth muscle fibre
Nerves supplying fibre	Single	Multiple
Junction	Highly organised motor endplate	Simple
Neurotransmitter	Acetylcholine	Acetylcholine
Receptor subtype	Nicotinic N_2 (muscle-type)	Muscarinic (mainly M_3)
Receptor distribution	Only at motor endplate; only one motor endplate per muscle fibre	Widely on the muscle surface
Effects of stimulation	Single nerve contracts the whole muscle fibre (all-or-none response)	Each nerve contracts part of muscle fibre (graded response)
Effect of overdose with acetylcholinesterase inhibitor	Flaccid paralysis	Spasticity

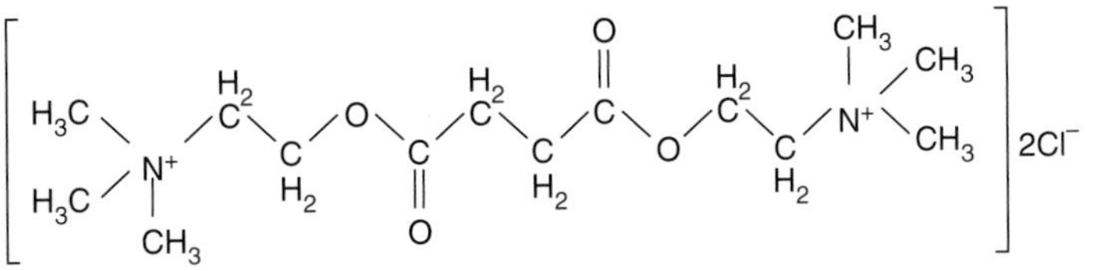

Fig. 27.2 Structures of pancuronium, a nondepolarising blocking drug, and suxamethonium (succinylcholine), a depolarising blocker. Suxamethonium resembles two molecules of acetylcholine, each with a quaternary ammonium (N^+) group, linked back to back. Pancuronium was designed to have a similar spatial arrangement of quaternary nitrogens but held rigidly in place by a steroid bridge that is resistant to butyrylcholinesterase.

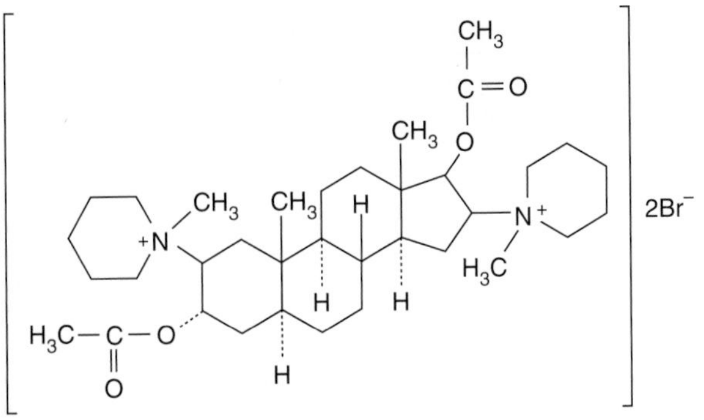

junction almost all resemble ACh in that they have a quaternary ammonium (N^+) group that binds strongly to the anionic site of the nicotinic N_2 receptor (Fig. 27.2).

A neuromuscular blocker must occupy 70–80% of postsynaptic N_2 receptors before it can start to produce neuromuscular blockade and must occupy at least 92% of receptors to produce complete blockade. The potency of a neuromuscular blocker is measured by the ED_{95}, which is the dose required to produce 95% depression of the height of muscular twitch. About twice this dose is required for muscle relaxation adequate to permit tracheal intubation. The laryngeal muscles are more rapidly paralysed than other skeletal muscle groups, but the effect is often of shorter duration. This may reflect either the higher blood flow to laryngeal muscles or their greater density of N_2 receptors. Recovery of muscle action depends on the rate of clearance of the drug from the synapse.

Competitive N_2 receptor antagonists (nondepolarising blockers)

Examples

atracurium, cisatracurium, mivacurium, pancuronium, rocuronium, vecuronium

Mechanism of action and effects

Competitive N_2 receptor antagonists bind to the nicotinic N_2 receptor at the neuromuscular junction without causing depolarisation of the postsynaptic membrane. This blocks the depolarising effect of ACh and leads to muscle relaxation. These drugs also hold the receptors in their inactive state (desensitisation block). Presynaptic receptor block further

contributes to their action by reducing the synthesis and mobilisation of ACh. Whereas it takes two ACh molecules to activate the N_2 receptor, only one molecule of a nondepolarising neuromuscular blocker at each receptor will prevent neurotransmission. Inhibition of ACh hydrolysis by an AChE inhibitor (such as neostigmine; see Chapter 28) will prolong the action of ACh and rapidly reverse competitive neuromuscular junction blockade. This principle is used at the end of an operation to aid recovery of the neuromuscular block.

Pharmacokinetics

Nondepolarising neuromuscular blockers are highly polar molecules and are given by intravenous injection. They have a low apparent volume of distribution and do not cross the blood–brain barrier. Vecuronium, pancuronium and rocuronium are aminosteroids that depend, at least in part, on metabolism for their elimination. Vecuronium is partially metabolised in the liver but largely excreted unchanged in the bile. Pancuronium and rocuronium are eliminated by a combination of metabolism and renal excretion of unchanged drug.

Atracurium, cisatracurium and mivacurium are benzylisoquinolinium compounds that are degraded in plasma. Atracurium (a racemic mixture of 10 isomers) and cisatracurium (a single isomer of atracurium) undergo nonenzymatic spontaneous degradation as well as hydrolysis by nonspecific esterases in the plasma, which is an advantage in hepatic or renal impairment. Mivacurium, like the depolarising blocker suxamethonium (see below), is metabolised by butyrylcholinesterase.

The speed of onset and duration of action and unwanted effects of competitive blockers differ (Table 27.2). A fast onset of action can be useful during rapid sequence intubation (see below). After a bolus injection of an aminosteroid

Table 27.2 Properties of some neuromuscular junction-blocking drugs

Muscle relaxant	ED$_{95}$ (mg/kg)[a]	Time to maximum block (min)[b]	Duration (min)[c]	Unwanted effects
Pancuronium	0.06	4–5	90	Tachycardia, hypertension due to sympathetic stimulation; increase in cardiac output
Vecuronium	0.05	3–4	45	Allergy
Atracurium	0.25	3–4	40	Histamine release; increase in heart rate and decrease in systemic vascular resistance, tachycardia, bronchospasm
Cisatracurium	0.05	4.5–5.5	30–40	Low incidence of unwanted effects
Rocuronium	0.4	2–3	30	Increase in heart rate; allergy
Mivacurium	0.08	2–3	15–20	Histamine release; increase in heart rate and decrease in systemic vascular resistance, tachycardia, bronchospasm; prolonged block in people lacking butyrylcholinesterase
Suxamethonium (succinylcholine)		Fast	3–12	Muscle fasciculation; postoperative muscle pain; bradycardia, hyperkalaemia, malignant hyperthermia; prolonged block in people lacking butyrylcholinesterase

[a]ED$_{95}$ is the effective dose required to suppress muscle twitch by 95%.
[b]Time to maximum block following administration of the dose used for intubation (double the ED$_{95}$).
[c]Time taken to recover to 25% of the original twitch height after an intubation dose.

neuromuscular blocker, the action is terminated largely as a result of redistribution to tissues rather than metabolism. Redistribution lowers the plasma concentration and consequently the concentration at the motor endplate. The clinically effective duration of neuromuscular blockade will be more prolonged after repeated boluses or infusions because when equilibrium between plasma and tissue concentrations has been reached, the duration of effect becomes mainly dependent on metabolism.

Unwanted effects

See Table 27.2.

Depolarising neuromuscular-blocking drugs

suxamethonium (succinylcholine)

Mechanism of action and effects

Suxamethonium is the only agent of this class in clinical use, but it is now largely replaced by rapid-acting nondepolarising blockers. Suxamethonium is succinic acid with a choline molecule attached at each carboxylic acid group; it therefore resembles two ACh molecules joined back to back (see Fig. 27.2). When two molecules of suxamethonium bind to the nicotinic N$_2$ receptor it acts as an agonist and depolarises the motor endplate. However, suxamethonium is not hydrolysed by AChE and therefore produces more prolonged depolarisation than ACh. The voltage-gated Na$^+$ channels are kept in their inactive state, producing depolarising (Phase 1) block and muscle flaccidity. Prolonged exposure to suxamethonium promotes the transition of voltage-gated Na$^+$ channels to a desensitised state, in which they are insensitive to ACh – a state called desensitisation block. Although the muscle can respond to direct electrical stimulation, it can no longer be stimulated via the neuronal release of ACh. After repeated boluses or continuous infusion, suxamethonium also produces a nondepolarising competitive type of blockade (Phase 2 block). Phase 2 block can be partially reversed by an AChE inhibitor, although this is unreliable.

Pharmacokinetics

Suxamethonium is a highly polar molecule, which is given intravenously. It has a low volume of distribution and does not cross the blood–brain barrier. Suxamethonium has an onset of action within 1 minute but is rapidly hydrolysed by butyrylcholinesterase, which results in a very short duration of action (about 3–12 minutes). An infusion is therefore necessary to produce a prolonged effect. A very prolonged paralysis occurs in the approximately 1 in 3000–5000 individuals who have a genetically determined deficiency of butyrylcholinesterase. In this population, the action of suxamethonium is terminated after some 2–3 hours by nonspecific tissue esterases.

Unwanted effects

- There is an initial depolarisation of the motor endplates prior to blockade, which results in muscle fasciculation. This may in part be due to the pre-synaptic receptor action of suxamethonium, which stimulates ACh release.
- Postoperative muscle pain is common, especially on the day after surgery, possibly as a consequence of muscle fasciculation. It usually affects the diaphragm, intercostal muscles and interscapular muscles.

- Prolonged neuromuscular blockade and apnoea occur if there is a low circulating concentration of butyrylcholinesterase through either a genetic deficiency or a decreased synthesis of the enzyme in severe liver disease.
- The use of suxamethonium during anaesthesia is a trigger for the development of a rare but potentially fatal disorder of muscles known as malignant hyperthermia, with a rapid rise in temperature, muscle rigidity, tachycardia and acidosis. The predisposition to this condition has an autosomal dominant inheritance and is associated with mutations in the ryanodine receptor (RyR1). Treatment is with intravenous dantrolene (see Chapter 24).
- Stimulation of nicotinic N_1 receptors at autonomic ganglia and muscarinic receptors produces bradycardia, especially with repeated doses.
- Hyperkalaemia, probably due to persistent activation of N_2 receptors, results in the escape of intracellular K^+ ions from skeletal muscle fibres. This is especially marked in the presence of prolonged immobilisation, major tissue trauma and severe burns.
- Anaphylaxis with repeated use due to type 1 hypersensitivity.

INDICATIONS FOR NEUROMUSCULAR-BLOCKING DRUGS

The neuromuscular-blocking drugs are used in both surgical procedures and intensive care. Their administration forms part of the achievement of balanced anaesthesia described in Chapter 17.

ENDOTRACHEAL INTUBATION

Relaxation of the vocal cords by a neuromuscular blocker allows easy passage of an endotracheal tube. In emergency surgery, when the stomach may contain food, a rapid onset of action is essential to minimise the risk of aspiration of gastric contents (rapid sequence intubation). Pre-oxygenation is followed by a rapidly acting neuromuscular blocker and then intubation before any artificial ventilation. This minimises insufflation of air into the stomach and regurgitation of gastric contents. Rapid sequence intubation is the only current use for suxamethonium. However, because of frequent unwanted effects, suxamethonium is largely superseded by rapidly acting nondepolarising blockers such as rocuronium or vecuronium.

DURING SURGICAL PROCEDURES

Neuromuscular blockade produces muscle relaxation for procedures such as abdominal incisions. Selective skeletal muscle relaxation reduces the amount of general anaesthetic needed for deep anaesthesia. It can be achieved by a single injection of a neuromuscular blocker for short procedures or either repeated bolus injections or intravenous infusion for more prolonged surgery. At the end of the operation the effect of a nondepolarising blocker can be reversed within 1 minute by the intravenous injection of neostigmine. A muscarinic

receptor blocker such as glycopyrrolate or atropine (see Chapter 4) is given before neostigmine to prevent bradycardia or the excessive salivation produced by the stimulation of muscarinic receptors.

The response to a neuromuscular blocker can be assessed by peripheral nerve stimulation, often the ulnar nerve. This may be necessary when complete paralysis is essential, such as for ophthalmic surgery or neurosurgery. It is also used when the pharmacokinetic profile of the drug or the pharmacodynamic response to the drug may be abnormal.

IN INTENSIVE CARE

Neuromuscular blockade is used in addition to analgesia and sedation during mechanical ventilation, particularly if respiratory drive is inadequate to maintain oxygenation (e.g. in adult respiratory distress syndrome or status asthmaticus), for status epilepticus or tetanus and for people with raised intracranial pressure.

ANTAGONISING NEUROMUSCULAR BLOCK

The term *postoperative residual curarisation* describes residual paralysis from neuromuscular blockade after anaesthesia. It is more common with continuous infusion of a neuromuscular blocker than with repeated boluses and with longer-acting drugs. It is detected by perioperative neuromuscular monitoring with acceleromyography.

The action of competitive neuromuscular-blocking agents can be terminated by intravenous injection of the anticholinesterase neostigmine, given with an antimuscarinic agent (usually glycopyrronium, which has a similar time course of action) to prevent bradycardia. Anticholinesterases only reverse residual neuromuscular block once recovery has started.

Sugammadex is a cyclodextrin with a hydrophilic outer surface and a lipophilic core. It is a specific antagonist for the aminosteroids rocuronium and vecuronium (but not pancuronium) by chelating them in the core and reducing their plasma concentration. The complex is then eliminated by the kidneys.

SELF-ASSESSMENT

For a case-based question on the use of neuromuscular junction-blocking drugs in surgery, see the case-based self-assessment section of Chapter 17.

True/false questions

1. A skeletal muscle fibre is innervated by a single motor endplate.
2. The nicotinic receptors at skeletal muscle and autonomic ganglia are identical.
3. Suxamethonium is a competitive antagonist of nicotinic N_2 receptors.
4. Vecuronium has no haemodynamic effects.

5. Malignant hyperthermia is a rare, genetically determined reaction to suxamethonium.
6. The duration of action of all nondepolarising neuromuscular junction-blocking drugs is limited by redistribution.
7. Suxamethonium is the only muscle relaxant used for tracheal intubation.
8. All nondepolarising neuromuscular junction (NMJ) blockers can be used for long-term muscle relaxation in intensive care.
9. Botulinum toxin acts post-synaptically to block the neuromuscular junction.
10. Botulinum toxin can be used to treat excessive sweating.

One-best-answer (OBA) question

Which statement about neuromuscular junction-blocking drugs is the *most accurate*?
A. Rocuronium crosses the blood–brain barrier and has direct effects on the central nervous system.
B. Pancuronium is the neuromuscular-blocking drug of choice for a surgical procedure that will take less than 30 minutes.
C. Suxamethonium is the only muscle relaxant that can be used for electroconvulsive therapy.
D. About 50% of nicotinic N_2 receptors must be occupied by a nondepolarising neuromuscular-blocking drug to produce complete block of an evoked twitch.
E. Atracurium causes the release of histamine.

ANSWERS

True/false answers

1. **True.** Contraction of a skeletal muscle fibre is an all-or-none response to nerve stimulation at the motor endplate.
2. **False.** The nicotinic N_2 receptor at skeletal muscle is selectively blocked by nondepolarising and depolarising muscle relaxants, while the N_1 receptor at autonomic ganglia is selectively blocked by ganglion-blocking drugs (which now have little clinical application).

3. **False.** Suxamethonium is a nicotinic N_2 receptor *agonist* that causes persistent depolarisation and then desensitisation of the receptor.
4. **True.** Unlike atracurium and mivacurium, vecuronium does not cause histamine release, so it does not have significant haemodynamic effects.
5. **True.** Malignant hyperthermia in response to suxamethonium, halothane and some other drugs is associated with mutations in the ryanodine receptor (RyR1) and is treated with dantrolene, a RyR1 antagonist.
6. **False.** Atracurium and cisatracurium undergo spontaneous hydrolysis, and mivacurium is hydrolysed by pseudocholinesterase.
7. **False.** Short-acting nondepolarising neuromuscular blockers such as rocuronium can also be used for intubation. The use of suxamethonium is declining because of the occurrence of malignant hyperthermia.
8. **False.** Some nondepolarising blockers (e.g. mivacurium) are too short-acting for this purpose.
9. **False.** Botulinum toxin acts pre-synaptically to cause long-lasting blockade of ACh release.
10. **True.** Local injections of botulinum toxin can reduce the activity of sweat glands, which are innervated by postsynaptic cholinergic fibres of the *sympathetic* nervous system.

One-best-answer (OBA) answer

Answer E is correct.
A. Incorrect. All nondepolarising neuromuscular-blocking drugs have a quaternary ammonium in their structure and will not cross the blood–brain barrier.
B. Incorrect. Pancuronium is a long-acting blocking drug and is used for procedures taking longer than 90 minutes.
C. Incorrect. Short-acting nondepolarising blocking drugs such as rocuronium or mivacurium are viable alternatives.
D. Incorrect. More than 92% of receptors must be occupied to produce a complete block of skeletal muscle contractility.
E. **Correct.** Atracurium is one of the most potent neuromuscular-blocking drugs, causing the release of histamine.

FURTHER READING

Appiah-Ankram, J., Hunter, J.M., 2004. Pharmacology of neuromuscular blocking drugs. Contin. Educ. Anaesth. Crit. Care Pain 4, 1–27.

Jankovic, J., 2004. Botulinum toxin in clinical practice. J. Neurol. Neurosurg. Psychiatry 75, 951–957.

Khirwadkar, R., Hunter, J.M., 2012. Neuromuscular physiology and pharmacology: an update. Contin. Educ. Anaesth. Crit. Care Pain 12, 237–244.

McGrath, C.D., Hunter, J.M., 2006. Monitoring of neuromuscular block. Contin. Educ. Anaesth. Crit. Care Pain 6, 7–12.

Nair, V.P., Hunter, J.M., 2004. Anticholinesterases and anticholinergic drugs. Contin. Educ. Anaesth. Crit. Care Pain 4, 164–168.

Rosenberg, H., Pollock, N., Schiemann, A., et al., 2015. Malignant hyperthermia: a review. Orphanet J. Rare Dis. 10, 93. doi:10.1186/s13023-015-0310-1.

Compendium: drugs acting at the neuromuscular junction

Drug	Characteristics[a]
Drugs for reversal of neuromuscular blockade	
Acetylcholinesterase inhibitors	
Edrophonium	Very short-acting. Used in myasthenia gravis (see Chapter 28)
Neostigmine	Given intravenously to reverse the effects of a nondepolarising blocker (with an antimuscarinic to minimise parasympathetic effects of enhanced acetylcholine); also used in myasthenia gravis (see Chapter 28)
Pyridostigmine	Slower onset and longer duration of action than neostigmine. Given orally in myasthenia gravis (Chapter 28)
Other drugs for reversal of neuromuscular blockade	
Sugammadex	A modified gamma cyclodextrin used intravenously for rapid reversal of neuromuscular blockade induced by rocuronium or vecuronium, usually in an emergency. Half-life: 2 h
Neuromuscular junction-blocking drugs	
Nondepolarising (competitive) blockers	
All are used for muscle relaxation for surgery, given by intravenous injection or infusion.	
Atracurium	A complex mixture of 10 isomers. Short to intermediate duration, used for muscle relaxation during surgery and in intensive care. Breaks down by spontaneous hydrolysis within blood (0.3 h)
Cisatracurium	A single isomer of atracurium. Intermediate duration, used for surgery and in intensive care. Spontaneous degradation (0.5 h)
Mivacurium	Two active isomers; used for surgery. Short duration because hydrolysed by butyrylcholinesterase (half-life: 2–60 min), but prolonged effect in rare individuals with genetic deficiency of this enzyme
Pancuronium	Long duration; used during surgery and for long-term muscle relaxation during mechanical ventilation in intensive care. Half-life: 0.5–2.0 h
Rocuronium	Intermediate duration, used for surgery and in intensive care; most rapid onset of action of drugs in this class (<2 min). Half-life: 1.2 h
Vecuronium	Intermediate duration, used for surgery. Half-life: 1 h
Depolarising blocker	
Suxamethonium (succinylcholine)	Given intravenously for NMJ blockade of rapid onset and short duration of action (e.g. intubation); paralysis preceded by painful fasciculations. Hydrolysed by butyrylcholinesterase (half-life: 1–2 min); prolonged effect in rare individuals with genetic deficiency of this enzyme

[a]See also Table 27.2 for additional drug properties of key NMJ blockers.

28 Myasthenia gravis

Myasthenia gravis is a comparatively rare autoimmune disease; in the majority of cases there is an autoantibody to the nicotinic N_2 acetylcholine receptor (AChR) system at the neuromuscular junction on skeletal muscle (see Chapter 27). Fewer functional receptors are available, so acetylcholine (ACh) is less likely to depolarise the muscle cell sufficiently to reach its threshold firing potential. In healthy skeletal muscle, a larger number of receptors are depolarised than the threshold required for generation of an endplate potential. Repetitive nerve stimulation leads to a rapid reduction in the numbers of sensitive receptors, but there are sufficient remaining receptors to ensure that there is no reduction in muscle activity. However, in myasthenia gravis, with repetitive stimulation, the reduction of an already small receptor pool reduces receptor availability to a level at which increasing numbers of muscle fibres fail to fire. Consequently there is characteristic rapid muscle fatigue on exertion. If the number of available receptors falls further, there is skeletal muscle weakness at rest. About 15% of people with myasthenia gravis do not have detectable antibodies to AChRs. Many of these individuals have antibodies to other postsynaptic proteins, such as MuSK or LRP4. The clinical presentation is often atypical compared with classic myasthenia gravis.

The thymus gland plays a part in the genesis of the immune response in myasthenia gravis, although its precise role remains uncertain. About 80% of people with myasthenia gravis have an abnormality in the thymus, which is usually lymphoreticular hyperplasia (especially in females and when the condition has its onset before 50 years of age) or a thymoma.

The earliest symptom of myasthenia gravis is often diplopia, which arises from weakness of the extraocular muscles, or ptosis. In 85% of cases the symptoms progress to involve many other muscle groups, particularly producing bulbar, facial and proximal limb weakness. Atypical presentations of myasthenia gravis involve the eyes less often.

Symptomatic treatment of the weakness in myasthenia gravis is achieved by prolongation of the action of ACh through the inhibition of acetylcholinesterase (AChE), the enzyme responsible for its hydrolysis. However, immunosuppression is also important for disease control.

ACETYLCHOLINESTERASE INHIBITORS

Examples

edrophonium, neostigmine, pyridostigmine

MECHANISM OF ACTION AND EFFECTS

AChE inhibitors block the breakdown of ACh released from presynaptic neurons. Details of their mechanisms of action are found in Chapter 4. Their therapeutic actions in myasthenia gravis are achieved by increasing the duration of action of ACh at nicotinic N_2 (muscle-type) receptors. However, they enhance the effect of ACh at all synaptic connections at which ACh is the neurotransmitter. Unwanted effects arise from the excessive actions of ACh at nicotinic N_1 receptors in autonomic ganglia and at muscarinic receptors in postganglionic nerve endings in the parasympathetic nervous system and in sweat glands in the sympathetic nervous system.

PHARMACOKINETICS AND CLINICAL USES

Neostigmine and pyridostigmine are quaternary amines that are incompletely absorbed from the gut. As a result, oral doses must be approximately 10 times greater than parenteral doses to be effective. They have short elimination half-lives (1–2 hours) and do not readily cross the blood–brain barrier (see Chapter 9 for AChE inhibitors that cross the blood–brain barrier and are used in Alzheimer's disease). Pyridostigmine is preferred for the treatment of myasthenia gravis because it has a longer duration of action and is less likely to cause unwanted effects.

Neostigmine is given by intravenous injection to reverse the effect of competitive neuromuscular blockers (see Chapter 27).

Edrophonium has a very short duration of action (2–5 minutes) owing largely to rapid tissue distribution. It is given as an intravenous bolus to test the therapeutic response to AChE inhibitors in myasthenia gravis (see below) but is of no value in treatment.

UNWANTED EFFECTS

Unwanted effects are experienced by up to one-third of people. Peripheral muscarinic effects, which can be blocked by co-administration of a muscarinic receptor antagonist such as propantheline, include

- nausea, diarrhoea, abdominal cramps, excessive salivation;
- bradycardia, hypotension (uncommon);
- miosis and lacrimation;
- bronchoconstriction.

Excessive dosage of AChE inhibitors will lead to a depolarising neuromuscular blockade by ACh. Initially there may be muscle twitching and cramps, followed by weakness through the buildup of excess ACh (see below).

MANAGEMENT OF MYASTHENIA GRAVIS

DIAGNOSIS

When the diagnosis of myasthenia gravis is suspected, useful diagnostic information can be obtained rapidly by pharmacological testing. In untreated people with myasthenia, an intravenous injection of the short-acting AChE inhibitor edrophonium will produce clinical improvement within 1 minute, lasting for about 5 minutes. Pre-treatment with atropine will prevent profound bradycardia. Detection of circulating N_2 receptor antibodies and single-fibre electromyography are used to confirm the diagnosis.

TREATMENT

Symptomatic treatment of myasthenia gravis is with an AChE inhibitor, usually pyridostigmine, which inhibits the normal rapid breakdown of ACh and thereby enhances the activity of ACh released by nerve stimulation. The onset of action of pyridostigmine is delayed for about 15–30 minutes after oral dosing, with a duration of action of 3–6 hours. An antimuscarinic agent (such as propantheline) may be necessary to block any parasympathomimetic actions of pyridostigmine, especially if large doses are given. Some individuals do not respond well to AChE inhibitors, while unwanted effects may preclude the use of adequate doses in others. In addition, muscle groups do not all respond equally well to AChE inhibitors; ptosis and diplopia are the most resistant to treatment.

Excessive dosage of an AChE inhibitor can lead to prolonged stimulation of the N_2 receptors by ACh, resulting in a depolarising blockade of the neuromuscular junction similar to that produced by suxamethonium (see Chapter 27). Therefore muscle weakness in myasthenia gravis can be the result of either inadequate dosage ('myasthenic crisis') or excessive dosage ('cholinergic crisis') with an AChE inhibitor. The safest way to distinguish these problems is to use assisted ventilation and temporarily withdraw the AChE inhibitor.

Generalised myasthenia is usually treated by immunosuppression with a corticosteroid, such as prednisolone (see Chapter 44). Corticosteroids are also used for patients who are severely ill. They probably act by suppressing T-cell proliferation and reducing antibody synthesis. Initial high-dose corticosteroid therapy can make the weakness worse, particularly in the first 7–10 days, possibly owing to a direct effect on neuromuscular transmission. A clinical response is usually apparent after 1 month, but maximum benefit is delayed for up to 9 months. Azathioprine (see Chapter 38) is added if there is a poor response to a corticosteroid alone. Methotrexate, mycophenolate mofetil or tacrolimus (see Chapter 38) are alternatives to azathioprine. Cyclophosphamide or rituximab has been used successfully for resistant disease. Long-term immunosuppression is usually necessary since relapse frequently occurs on withdrawal of therapy.

Plasma exchange to remove circulating ACh receptor antibodies can produce a short-term response in severe disease. With repeated plasma exchanges, improvement is seen after 1 day, with a maximum response after 1–2 weeks that is sustained for 2–8 weeks. An alternative is the use of intravenous immunoglobulin, of which IgG is the active component. It produces improvement after about 4 days and an optimal response after 1–2 weeks that is sustained for 6–15 weeks. Immunoglobulin treatment is usually better tolerated than plasma exchange.

Thymectomy can induce remission in myasthenia gravis, although this can be delayed for up to 5 years. Thymectomy is most effective early in the disease in those with lymphoreticular hyperplasia and positive AChR antibodies, when it produces complete remission within 5 years in about 40% and significant improvement in a further 35%. Thymomas should be surgically removed because of the potential for malignant change, although the clinical benefit for myasthenia gravis is less clear-cut.

Some drugs can interfere with neuromuscular transmission and exacerbate the symptoms of myasthenia gravis. Those most often implicated include aminoglycoside antibiotics (see Chapter 51), β-adrenoceptor antagonists (see Chapter 5), phenytoin (see Chapter 23) and chloroquine and penicillamine (see Chapter 30). There is also altered sensitivity to neuromuscular junction blockers, with increased response to competitive (nondepolarising) neuromuscular junction blockers but resistance to depolarising neuromuscular junction blockers (see Chapter 27).

LAMBERT–EATON MYASTHENIC SYNDROME

Lambert–Eaton myasthenic syndrome (LEMS) is a clinical syndrome resembling myasthenia gravis. It is often a paraneoplastic syndrome, with about 60% of cases associated with malignancy (often small-cell lung cancer). LEMS is caused by antibodies to P/Q-type voltage-gated Ca^{2+} channels on the presynaptic membrane of motor nerves at the neuromuscular junction. These channels are responsible for Ca^{2+} influx into the neuron that initiates ACh release. LEMS presents with leg and arm weakness and autonomic disturbance such as postural hypotension. While it can involve bulbar muscles, eye muscles are less often affected.

When LEMS is related to cancer, treatment of the malignancy leads to resolution. The potassium channel blocker amifampridine is the first-choice drug for symptom relief. It delays repolarisation of the nerve terminal after an action potential, giving more time for Ca^{2+} to accumulate in the neuron. The prolonged depolarisation allows greater ACh release. Pyridostigmine can help the symptoms by prolonging the action of released ACh at the motor endplate. Immunosuppression is relatively ineffective in the treatment of LEMS.

SELF-ASSESSMENT

True/false questions

1. In myasthenia gravis, autoantibodies develop to nicotinic N_1 receptors.
2. AChE inhibitors may cause bronchoconstriction.
3. Pyridostigmine produces fewer muscarinic effects than neostigmine.
4. In myasthenia gravis, there is increased sensitivity to suxamethonium.
5. A cholinergic crisis should be confirmed by giving pyridostigmine.

One-best-answer (OBA) question

1. Which statement about myasthenia gravis is the *most accurate*?
   A. People diagnosed with myasthenia gravis invariably have a thymoma.
   B. AChE inhibitors used to treat myasthenia gravis increase activity in the motor cortex of the brain.
   C. Glucocorticoids can be of benefit in myasthenia gravis because of their antiinflammatory actions.
   D. The unwanted effects of acetylcholinesterase (AChE) inhibitors include diarrhoea, urination, miosis, bradycardia, nausea, lacrimation and salivation.
   E. Plasmapheresis reduces plasma levels of butyrylcholinesterase, thereby reducing breakdown of acetylcholine.

Case-based questions

A 35-year-old woman with no previous illness noticed that she had ptosis and occasional diplopia. Over time she became aware that she suffered from leg weakness on exertion, although her coordination was normal. Following a sustained upward gaze for 1 minute, ptosis and diplopia could be elicited. Myasthenia gravis was suspected.
1. What tests could be performed to verify the diagnosis?
2. What is the pathogenesis of myasthenia gravis?
3. Why is edrophonium injection used as a test for myasthenia gravis?
4. If myasthenia gravis is confirmed, what principles should treatment follow?

ANSWERS

True/false answers

1. **False.** Skeletal muscle weakness in myasthenia gravis is due to autoimmunity to nicotinic N_2 receptors in the neuromuscular junction.
2. **True.** Increased ACh at muscarinic receptors in the parasympathetic nervous system can cause bronchoconstriction; such effects can be blocked with antimuscarinic drugs such as propantheline.
3. **True.** Neostigmine has greater potency and a shorter duration of action than pyridostigmine, so is more likely to cause muscarinic effects; pyridostigmine is therefore preferred in the treatment of myasthenia gravis.
4. **False.** Owing to the loss of nicotinic N_2 receptor function, people with myasthenia gravis are less sensitive to the depolarising neuromuscular junction blocker suxamethonium but more sensitive to competitive blockers such as vecuronium.
5. **False.** The cholinergic crisis results from the excessive effects of an AChE inhibitor and would be exacerbated by pyridostigmine, which is long-acting; assisted ventilation and withdrawal of the treatment should be performed.

One-best-answer (OBA) answer

1. **Answer D** is the most accurate.
   A. Incorrect. About 15% have a thymoma and 60–80% have hyperplasia of the thymus.
   B. Incorrect. The main anticholinesterases used in treating myasthenia gravis are quaternary amines and do not cross the blood–brain barrier; they act at the neuromuscular junction.
   C. Incorrect. Glucocorticoids work by suppressing the production of autoantibodies to nicotinic N_2 receptors.
   D. **Correct.** These parasympathomimetic effects are caused by excess ACh activity at muscarinic receptors.
   E. Incorrect. Plasmapheresis reduces the levels of circulating autoantibodies to nicotinic N_2 receptors.

Case-based answers

1. Tests include electromyography (Jolly test), single-muscle-fibre electromyography (SFEMG), anti-AChR antibody titres and injection of a short-acting inhibitor of AChE (the Tensilon test, named after the proprietary name of edrophonium).
2. Autoantibody blocks nicotinic N_2 receptors; receptors are destroyed by complement activation and receptors are cross-linked, which causes them to be destroyed more rapidly. The decrease in functional receptors impairs motor endplate potentials and reduces the likelihood of the muscle contracting.

3. Edrophonium is used because it is rapid in onset and short-acting, producing an improvement in muscle strength within 30–60 seconds that subsides in 4–5 minutes.

4. An AChE inhibitor, most commonly pyridostigmine, is used for symptomatic treatment; an antimuscarinic drug may be needed to reduce unwanted parasympathetic effects. Immunosuppression may be required with a corticosteroid or with immunosuppressants such as ciclosporin or azathioprine. Plasmapheresis, intravenous immunoglobulins or thymectomy may also be considered.

FURTHER READING

Sathasivam, S., 2014. Diagnosis and management of myasthenia gravis. Prog. Neurol. Psych. 18, 6–14.

Trouth, A.J., Dabi, A., Solieman, N., et al., 2012. Myasthenia gravis: a review. Autoimmune. Dis. 2012, 874680. doi:10.1155/2012/874680.

Compendium: drugs used in myasthenia gravis and Lambert–Easton myasthenic syndrome

Drug	Characteristics
AChE inhibitors used in myasthenia gravis	
Edrophonium	Very short duration of action (<5 min), so mainly used for diagnosis. Given intravenously over 30 s. Half-life: 1.8 h
Neostigmine	Short-acting with pronounced unwanted muscarinic effects; often given simultaneously with an antimuscarinic (atropine or glycopyrronium). Given orally or by subcutaneous or intravenous injection for myasthenia gravis; also used for reversal of neuromuscular block (see Chapter 27). Half-life: 0.4–1.7 h
Pyridostigmine	Preferable to neostigmine in myasthenia gravis owing to a smoother onset and longer duration of action. Given orally. Half-life: 0.4–1.9 h
Drug used for LEMS	
Amifampridine	Acetylcholine release-enhancer. Specialist use for symptomatic LEMS. Given orally. Half-life: 6 h

AChE, Acetylcholinesterase; LEMS, Lambert–Easton myasthenic syndrome.

29 Nonsteroidal antiinflammatory drugs

THE ROLE OF CYCLO-OXYGENASE ENZYMES IN THE ACTIONS OF NONSTEROIDAL ANTIINFLAMMATORY DRUGS

The major therapeutic and unwanted actions of nonsteroidal antiinflammatory drugs (NSAIDs) result from inhibition of cyclo-oxygenase (COX) enzymes. COX enzymes are essential in the production of the prostanoids (prostaglandins, prostacyclin and thromboxanes), the most active of which are generated from the 20-carbon, polyunsaturated (ω-6) fatty acid arachidonic acid (Fig. 29.1). Arachidonic acid can also be converted via arachidonate 5-lipoxygenase to leukotrienes, some of the actions of which are blocked by leukotriene receptor antagonists (see Chapter 12) and via arachidonate 15-lipoxygenase to the related eoxins. Together these form the classical eicosanoid families (oxygenated derivatives of arachidonate). They are local mediators that are generally synthesised and catabolised close to their site of action, and have numerous physiological actions. Arachidonic acid and related fatty acids (such as dihomo-γ-linoleic acid) are also the precursors of several other families of lipid mediators such as lipoxins, resolvins, hepoxilins and endocannabinoids.

Arachidonic acid is mostly derived from dietary linoleic acid, which is found in vegetable oils such as sunflower oil. Linoleic acid is converted in the liver to arachidonic acid in several steps; the arachidonic acid is then incorporated into phospholipids in cell membranes, and consequently released from membrane phospholipids by the action of phospholipase A_2.

The action of COX on arachidonic acid generates unstable cyclic endoperoxide intermediates which are converted by cell-specific synthases and isomerases to various receptor-active prostanoids (see Fig. 29.1). The products of the COX pathway differ among various tissues, depending upon the enzymes present. This ensures that prostanoids are formed with actions tailored to the individual requirements of each cell type. Most cells can form different prostanoids simultaneously and vary the amount of each that they produce, with the pattern of production modulated by regulatory influences on the cell.

There are two COX isoenzymes, COX-1 and COX-2. They have long been considered to have distinct roles:

- COX-1 is constitutively expressed in the endoplasmic reticulum of most tissues, mainly in blood vessels, smooth muscle cells and mesothelial cells. It is the only isoform expressed in platelets. Prostanoids generated via COX-1 are produced in small amounts by these cells in the resting state and contribute to the regulation of several homeostatic processes such as renal and gastric blood flow, gastric cytoprotection and platelet aggregation (Table 29.1). However, there is evidence for induction of COX-1 during the lipopolysaccharide-mediated inflammatory response.
- COX-2 is present in greater concentrations in the nuclear envelope than in the endoplasmic reticulum and is found principally in parenchymal cells. COX-2 shows constitutive expression in the brain, kidney and female reproductive tract, but is a highly inducible enzyme in response to cytokines and other inflammatory stimuli, so that COX-2-derived prostanoids are formed in large amounts in response to inflammation, pain and fever.

The original concept that there is only a pathological role for inducible COX-2-derived prostanoids and a 'housekeeping' physiological role for the constitutive COX-1 enzyme is too simplistic. It is now clear that either isoform may be

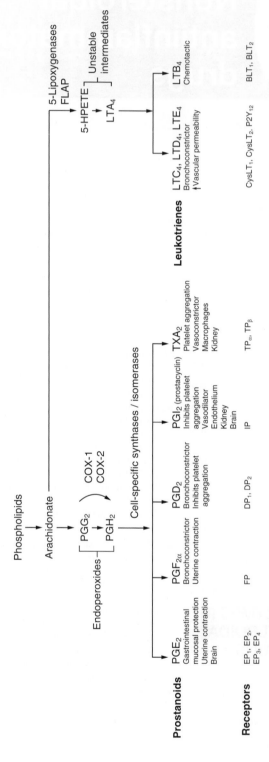

Fig. 29.1 The arachidonic acid cascade of eicosanoid synthesis. Arachidonic acid liberated from membrane phospholipids can be utilised by cyclo-oxygenases (COX-1, COX-2) to form prostanoids (prostaglandins, prostacyclin and thromboxane) or by the 5-lipoxygenase pathway to form leukotrienes. The types and amounts of these eicosanoid products that are generated depend on the relative expression of the COX isoenzymes, 5-lipoxygenase and their respective downstream synthases in different cell types. After release from the cell, the eicosanoids have a multitude of actions via their selective G-protein-coupled receptors on the surface of target cells, such as bronchial, uterine and vascular smooth muscle cells, endothelial cells, platelets and leucocytes (see Table 29.2). FLAP, Five-lipoxygenase activating protein; 5-HPETE, 5-hydroperoxyeicosatetraenoic acid; LT, leukotriene; PG, prostaglandin; TX, thromboxane.

Table 29.1 Some biological roles of cyclo-oxygenase 1 and 2

COX-1 homeostatic roles	COX-2 homeostatic roles
Gastrointestinal protection	Renal function
Platelet aggregation	CNS function
Blood flow regulation	Tissue repair and healing (including gastrointestinal)
CNS function	Reproduction
	Uterine contraction
	Blood vessel dilation
	Pancreas
	Inhibition of platelet aggregation
	Airways
COX-1 pathological roles	**COX-2 pathological roles**
Chronic inflammation	Chronic inflammation
Chronic pain	Chronic pain
Raised blood pressure	Fever
	Blood vessel permeability
	Reproduction
	Alzheimer's disease
	Angiogenesis, inhibition of apoptosis
	Tumour cell growth

COX, cyclo-oxygenase; CNS, central nervous system.

involved in the production of 'physiological' or 'pathological' prostanoids, and that the role of each enzyme subtype may vary among different tissues (see Table 29.1). Nevertheless, there is considerable evidence that the two enzyme subtypes are not functionally interchangeable within individual cells.

The actions of prostaglandins and thromboxanes depend upon the circumstances and site of their formation, and whether they are formed in physiological or excessive amounts. This is often more important than the COX isoform responsible for their production. For example, prostaglandin E_2 (PGE$_2$) is generated in low physiological amounts in gastric mucosa, where it is important for maintaining mucosal integrity by a variety of mechanisms (see Chapter 33). However, damage to many tissues leads to increased PGE$_2$ synthesis, which contributes to inflammation by vasodilation and increased vascular permeability. PGE$_2$ also sensitises Aδ and C pain fibre nerve endings in peripheral tissues to the nociceptive action of bradykinin, serotonin and substance P (see Chapter 19). By contrast, following tissue damage enhanced prostanoid generation may contribute to the processes of wound healing.

Prostanoids act via five main classes of G-protein-coupled receptors on cell surfaces (see Fig. 29.1). Some of the actions of prostaglandins are shown in Table 29.2.

NONSTEROIDAL ANTIINFLAMMATORY DRUGS

NSAIDs have three major therapeutic actions: antiinflammatory, analgesic and antipyretic.

MECHANISMS OF ACTION

Most NSAIDs reversibly bind to the site in the COX enzymes that accepts arachidonic acid. Aspirin (acetylsalicylic acid) produces irreversible inactivation of COX by acetylation of a serine residue in the enzyme. This irreversible mechanism of action is important in the use of aspirin as an antiplatelet drug (discussed later and in Chapter 11).

NSAIDs are differentiated by their specificity for inhibition of the two COX isoenzymes. The degree of COX selectivity of each NSAID will also depend on the dosage used, with less selectivity at higher doses. Highly selective inhibitors of COX-2 (coxibs) were developed with the aim of reducing the unwanted effects associated with inhibition of COX-1, but with limited success (discussed later).

Neither the nonselective NSAIDs nor the selective COX-2 inhibitors directly affect the production of leukotrienes by 5-lipoxygenase. However, PGE$_2$ normally inhibits leukotriene synthesis and reduced PGE$_2$ generation as a consequence of NSAID use may increase leukotriene synthesis (for leukotriene receptor antagonists, see Chapter 12).

NSAIDs have additional actions that appear to be independent of prostaglandin inhibition. These include altered expression of cell cycle regulators and induction of cell cycle arrest, as well as reduced production of reactive oxygen species. It is unclear whether these actions contribute to the antiinflammatory actions of these drugs or to their ability to reduce the risk of developing some cancers.

CLASSIFICATION OF NONSTEROIDAL ANTIINFLAMMATORY DRUGS

Table 29.3 shows the principal chemical types of NSAIDs, with an indication of their selectivity in inhibiting COX-1 or COX-2. Many nonselective NSAIDs produce greater inhibition of COX-1 than of COX-2, although at usual doses this selectivity may not be apparent and both isoenzymes will be effectively inhibited. The coxibs are highly selective inhibitors of COX-2 at clinically relevant doses.

ACTIONS AND EFFECTS OF NONSELECTIVE NONSTEROIDAL ANTIINFLAMMATORY DRUGS

Some of the properties and actions of a selection of commonly used analgesic drugs are compared in Table 29.4.

Analgesic effect

The analgesic action of NSAIDs is in part a peripheral action at the site of pain and is most effective when the pain has an inflammatory origin (see Chapter 19). It is achieved predominantly through inhibition of PGE$_2$ in inflamed or injured tissues, which reduces stimulation of pain fibre nerve endings.

Table 29.2 Main biological actions of the eicosanoids

Tissue	Effect	Eicosanoid
Platelets	Increased aggregation	TXA_2
	Decreased aggregation	PGI_2, PGD_2
Vascular smooth muscle	Vasodilation	PGI_2, PGE_2, PGD_2
	Vasoconstriction	TXA_2, LTC_4, LTD_4
Other smooth muscle	Bronchodilation	PGE_2
	Bronchoconstriction	LTC_4, LTD_4, LTE_4, PGD_2, PGF_2, TXA_2
	Gastrointestinal tract (contraction/relaxation, depends on muscle type)	PGF_2, PGE_2, PGI_2, PGD_2
	Uterine contraction	PGE_2, $PGF_{2\alpha}$
Vascular endothelium	Increased permeability	LTC_4, LTD_4, LTB_4
	Potentiates histamine/bradykinin	PGE_2, PGI_2
Leucocytes	Chemotaxis of neutrophils, monocytes, lymphocytes	LTB_4
	Chemotaxis of eosinophils, basophils	LTE_4, PGD_2
Gastrointestinal mucosa	Reduced acid secretion	PGE_2, PGI_2
	Increased mucus secretion	PGE_2
	Increased blood flow	PGE_2, PGI_2
Nervous system	Inhibition of noradrenaline release	PGD_2, PGE_2, PGI_2
	Endogenous pyrogen in hypothalamus	PGE_2
	Sedation, sleep	PGD_2
Endocrine/metabolic	Secretion of ACTH, GH, prolactin, gonadotrophins	PGE_2
	Inhibition of lipolysis	PGE_2
Kidney	Increased renal blood flow	PGE_2, PGI_2
	Antagonism of ADH	PGE_2
	Renin release	PGI_2, PGE_2, PGD_2
Pain	Potentiates pain through bradykinin, serotonin	PGE_2, PGD_2

Only the main eicosanoids are shown. Inhibition of COX isoenzymes by NSAIDs reduces the synthesis only of prostanoids. Synthesis of leukotrienes is reduced by 5-lipoxygenase inhibitors (zileuton, not available in the UK). Antagonists of the cysteinyl-leukotriene (LTC_4, LTD_4, LTE_4) receptor 1 are used in asthma prophylaxis (see Chapter 12). *ACTH*, Adrenocorticotrophic hormone (corticotropin); *ADH*, antidiuretic hormone (vasopressin); *GH*, growth hormone; *LT*, leukotriene; *PG*, prostaglandin; *TX*, thromboxane.

There is also a central nervous system (CNS) component to the analgesic action of NSAIDs, which is due to reduction of PGE_2 synthesis in the dorsal horn of the spinal cord. This inhibits neurotransmitter release and reduces the excitability of neurons in the pain relay pathway. The analgesic action of NSAIDs is apparent after the first dose, but does not reach its maximal effect until about 1 week with repeated dosing.

Antiinflammatory effect

Inhibition of vasodilation and vasogenic oedema is related to a reduction in peripheral prostaglandin synthesis and possibly effects on other inflammatory processes. The antiinflammatory effects of NSAIDs increase gradually over about 3 weeks.

Antipyretic effect

Fever is reduced through inhibition of hypothalamic COX-2. Circulating pyrogens such as interleukin-1 enhance PGE_2 production in the hypothalamus, which depresses the response of temperature-sensitive neurons. NSAIDs do not affect normal body temperature.

Reduction of platelet aggregation

This action is mediated by inhibition of the synthesis of the potent platelet-aggregating agent thromboxane A_2 (TXA_2) by platelet COX-1 (see Chapter 11). Aspirin is the most effective antiplatelet NSAID because it has an irreversible action on COX-1, and since platelets do not have nuclei,

Table 29.3 Selectivity of some nonsteroidal antiinflammatory drugs for inhibition of cyclo-oxygenase-1 compared with cyclo-oxygenase-2

Drug	Class
Flurbiprofen	Propionic acid
Ketoprofen	Propionic acid
Ketorolac	Heterocyclic acetic acid
Aspirin	Salicylate
Indometacin	Indole
Ibuprofen	Propionic acid
Naproxen	Propionic acid
Fenoprofen	Propionic acid
Salicylate	Salicylate
Meloxicam	Enolic acid
Proxicam	Enolic acid
Sulindac	Indole
Diclofenac	Phenyl acetic acid
Celecoxib	Sulphonamide (coxib)
Etoricoxib	Bipyridine (coxib)

Increasing selectivity for inhibition of COX-1 compared with COX-2

Approximately equal inhibition of COX-1 and COX-2

Increasing selectivity for inhibition of COX-2 compared with COX-1

Table 29.4 Properties of some commonly used analgesic drugs

	Aspirin (moderate doses)	Paracetamol	Indometacin	Ibuprofen	Celecoxib
Analgesic	++	++	++	+	+
Antiinflammatory	+	−	+++	+	+
Antipyretic	+	+	+	+	+
Gastrointestinal bleeding	+	−	+	Low	Low

they are unable to synthesise more enzymes during their life span. Selective COX-2 inhibitors do not inhibit platelet aggregation (see Table 29.3).

PHARMACOKINETICS

Most NSAIDs are weak acids that undergo some absorption from the stomach due to pH partitioning (see Chapter 2). This explains the relatively high drug concentration in cells of the gastric mucosa. However, the majority of the drug is absorbed via the larger surface area of the small bowel.

Absorption of NSAIDs from the gut is usually fairly rapid from conventional formulations. Some NSAIDs with short half-lives, such as diclofenac, are available as modified-release formulations to prolong their duration of action. Certain NSAIDs can be given by intramuscular or intravenous injection for rapid onset of analgesia (such as ketorolac), or rectally to achieve a prolonged action (such as diclofenac and ketoprofen). Transcutaneous delivery of several NSAIDs, usually as a gel formulation, was introduced with the intention of providing high local drug concentrations while attempting to minimise systemic unwanted effects. Systemic toxicity will depend on the amount absorbed from the site of application.

Most NSAIDs undergo hepatic metabolism to inactive compounds. NSAIDs differ widely in their elimination half-lives, and short-acting drugs require frequent dosing to maintain continuous therapeutic effects, although synovial fluid concentrations in joint disease fluctuate less than plasma concentrations. Piroxicam undergoes enterohepatic cycling, which contributes to its long half-life.

Aspirin (acetylsalicylic acid) is initially converted to an active metabolite, salicylic acid, and finally inactivated by conjugation with glycine and, to some extent, glucuronic acid.

Conjugation with glycine is saturable at higher doses, and the metabolism of salicylate then changes from first-order to zero-order elimination kinetics (see Chapter 2). This has important implications for aspirin overdose (see Chapter 53).

UNWANTED EFFECTS

Most unwanted effects arise in part from the inhibition of prostaglandin synthesis throughout the body. They are usually dose-related.

Gastrointestinal effects

- Nausea, dyspepsia, gastric irritation, peptic ulceration and bleeding and perforation are the most frequent unwanted effects of NSAIDs. Dyspepsia does not predict the risk of more serious upper gastrointestinal complications. The more serious gastric effects occur principally as a result of inhibition of mucosal production PGE_2 and PGI_2. PGE_2 has several actions that confer cytoprotection in the stomach (see Chapter 33). It is likely that inhibition of both COX-1 and COX-2 is necessary for the development of much of the gastric toxicity. There are many mechanisms by which NSAIDs cause gastric irritation.
  - Mucus secretion and bicarbonate secretion are reduced, and acid secretion is increased due to inhibition of prostaglandin production.
  - Reduced mucosal blood flow due to inhibition of prostaglandin production, which probably enhances cytotoxicity by producing tissue hypoxia and enhanced local generation of free radicals.
  - The mucus gel layer is rendered less hydrophobic due to the acidic nature of NSAIDs and their local concentration in gastric mucosal cells; this reduces the barrier effect of the surface layer.
  - Uncoupling of cellular oxidative phosphorylation by NSAIDs increases mucosal cell permeability, with consequent back-diffusion of H^+ ions, which are trapped in the mucosal epithelium and lead to cytotoxicity.
  - NSAIDs accumulate within gastric mucosal cells by direct absorption of the drug from the gastric lumen and also by systemic delivery of the drug to the mucosa. Therefore rectal or transdermal administration or the use of a prodrug may reduce but will not eliminate the risk of gastric damage. Occult blood loss from the bowel is increased during regular treatment with NSAIDs, and the risk of overt gastrointestinal bleeding is greater. The highest risk of gastrointestinal bleeding is with piroxicam and ketoprofen, while indometacin, diclofenac and naproxen carry an intermediate risk. Ibuprofen has the lowest risk. Prevention and management of NSAID-induced gastric damage is considered in Chapter 33.
- Exacerbation of inflammatory bowel disease.
- Lower gastrointestinal bleeding or perforation.
- Local irritation and bleeding from rectal administration.

Renal effects

- NSAIDs can produce a reversible decline in glomerular filtration rate, with a rise in serum creatinine. Inhibition of prostaglandins (PGE_2, PGI_2) reduces renal medullary blood flow (see Chapter 14). NSAIDs are more likely to impair renal function if there is underlying chronic kidney disease (as is often the case in the elderly) or acute kidney injury. There is also an increased risk in the presence of heart failure or cirrhosis, conditions that are associated with reduced effective circulating blood volume, when prostaglandins play a greater role in the maintenance of renal blood flow. NSAIDs are the second most common cause of drug-induced acute kidney injury after aminoglycoside antimicrobials, and this most often occurs during the first few weeks of treatment.
- NSAIDs can produce renal salt and water retention, even when renal function is normal. Reduced prostaglandin synthesis in the ascending limb of the loop of Henle increases expression of the $Na^+/K^+/2Cl^-$ co-transporter complex, and prostaglandins antagonise the action of vasopressin (antidiuretic hormone, ADH; see Chapter 14). Salt and water retention produced by NSAIDs can exacerbate heart failure and raises blood pressure by an average of 3–5 mm Hg. In addition, the efficacy of drug treatments for heart failure and hypertension (e.g. diuretics, angiotensin-converting enzyme inhibitors, β-adrenoceptor antagonists) is blunted by NSAIDs.
- Suppression of prostaglandin-mediated renin secretion by NSAIDs can lead to hypoaldosteronism and hyperkalaemia.
- Acute interstitial nephritis is a less common cause of renal impairment and can occur with any NSAID. It often becomes apparent after several months of NSAID use.

Hypersensitivity

Hypersensitivity reactions occasionally produce asthma, urticaria, angioedema and rhinitis. People with nasal polyps and known allergic disorders appear to be most susceptible. NSAIDs can also precipitate a 'pseudo-allergic' asthmatic attack in a subgroup of people with asthma, through inhibition of PGE_2 production in the lung. PGE_2 has an inhibitory effect on leukotriene synthesis and mast cell degranulation. A reduction in PGE_2 leads to an increased synthesis of bronchoconstrictor cysteinyl-leukotrienes (LTC_4, LTD_4, LTE_4; see Chapter 12). As many as one in seven people with asthma may be sensitive to NSAIDs.

Other unwanted effects

Other unwanted effects are unrelated to prostaglandin inhibition and are sometimes specific for individual compounds.

- CNS unwanted effects such as headache, dizziness, drowsiness, insomnia and confusion, particularly in the elderly.
- Rashes.
- Aspirin can cause Reye's syndrome in children, a rare condition producing acute encephalopathy and fatty degeneration of the liver. Aspirin should be avoided in children under the age of 12 years.
- The risk of myocardial infarction is increased by most NSAIDs (and particularly diclofenac). A similar proportional increase in risk is found in people with no risk factors for coronary artery disease and those with known ischaemic heart disease. It may be related to reduced production of PGI_2 in coronary arteries. Low-dose naproxen may be

associated with a lower risk than other NSAIDs. There is no definite increased risk of stroke with NSAIDs.

- NSAIDs taken in pregnancy can delay labour, increase blood loss at delivery and cause premature closure of the ductus arteriosus in the fetus.

CYCLO-OXYGENASE-2-SELECTIVE INHIBITORS

celecoxib, etoricoxib, parecoxib

Mechanism of action

Selective COX-2 inhibitors have less inhibitory action on COX-1, but the degree of selectivity for COX-2 varies among the drugs in this class. Selective COX-2 inhibitors have antiinflammatory actions similar to conventional nonselective NSAIDs, but there is some evidence that they may be less effective analgesics. Selective COX-2 inhibitors do not affect platelet TXA$_2$ production and therefore do not directly impair platelet aggregation. However, they suppress the production of the antiaggregatory and vasodilator PGI$_2$ by blood vessels, which may allow TXA$_2$ to exert unopposed aggregatory effects on platelets. Selective COX-2 inhibitors may also have antiinflammatory actions unrelated to reduced prostaglandin production.

Pharmacokinetics

Celecoxib and etoricoxib are well absorbed from the gut. They are eliminated by hepatic metabolism. The half-life of celecoxib is 11 hours, while that of etoricoxib is longer (25 hours). Parecoxib can be given by intramuscular or intravenous injection for control of postoperative pain and has a half-life of 5–9 hours.

Unwanted effects

- COX-2-selective inhibitors produce fewer upper gastrointestinal unwanted effects and celecoxib, but not etoricoxib, reduces the risk of gastric ulcers and ulcer complications by up to 50%, compared with conventional NSAIDs. However, if low-dose aspirin is taken concurrently, this negates any benefits of coxibs on the gastric mucosa.
- Exacerbation of inflammatory bowel disease.
- Stomatitis or mouth ulcers.
- Fatigue, influenza-like symptoms.
- Palpitation.
- Selective COX-2 inhibitors rarely induce asthma attacks in NSAID-sensitive individuals.
- Selective COX-2 inhibitors increase the risk of myocardial infarction. The risk is similar to most nonselective NSAIDs.
- Renal effects, including salt and water retention and acute kidney injury, are similar for selective COX-2 inhibitors and nonselective NSAIDs.

PARACETAMOL
Mechanism of action

Paracetamol (acetaminophen in the United States) is an analgesic and antipyretic without antiinflammatory activity. Its mechanisms of action remain incompletely understood, but it has a highly selective inhibitory effect on COX-2 in the spinal cord by reducing the availability of an essential co-substrate for the enzymatic action of COX-2. This inhibits the transmission of pain impulses to higher centres. In peripheral tissues, peroxides present in inflammatory lesions usually impair the action of paracetamol on COX-2, which may explain the lack of antiinflammatory activity.

Metabolites of paracetamol may have additional analgesic actions. One metabolite of paracetamol, AM404, inhibits neuronal reuptake of the endogenous cannabinoid, anandamide. Anandamide is an agonist at cannabinoid CB$_1$ receptors and transient receptor potential vanilloid 1 (TRPV$_1$) receptors that are involved in the transmission and modulation of pain. A second active metabolite of paracetamol (*N*-acetyl-*p*-benzoquinone imine [NAPQI]) stimulates transient receptor potential ankyrin 1 (TRPA$_1$) receptors in the spinal cord to suppress pain signal transmission. NAPQI may also inhibit cysteine proteases involved in the generation of inflammatory interleukins IL-1β and IL-6.

Pharmacokinetics

Paracetamol is rapidly absorbed from the gut. It is metabolised mainly by conjugation, but the minor metabolite NAPQI is produced by cytochrome P450 in the liver and kidneys. NAPQI is detoxified by the limited supply of glutathione in these organs.

Unwanted effects

- Paracetamol is usually well tolerated, and because it does not inhibit peripheral prostaglandin synthesis, it does not cause problems with homeostatic functions of prostanoids (e.g. gastrointestinal disturbances).
- Hepatic damage and renal failure in overdose due to failure to conjugate NAPQI (see Chapter 53).

INDICATIONS FOR USING NONSTEROIDAL ANTIINFLAMMATORY DRUGS

NSAIDs are useful for pain relief, particularly for:

- Inflammatory conditions affecting joints, soft tissues, etc. Their use for inflammatory arthritis is discussed in Chapter 30 and for gout in Chapter 31; for osteoarthritis, paracetamol or topical NSAIDs (alone or in combination) should be tried before considering oral NSAIDs (see Chapter 30).
- Postoperative pain, intravenously or orally.
- Renal colic.
- Headache.
- Primary dysmenorrhoea; stimulation of the uterus by prostaglandins can be responsible for the pain in this condition.
- Topical use on the cornea of the eye after cataract or corneal surgery.

About 60% of people will achieve adequate pain relief with any one NSAID, but those who fail to respond to one may derive benefit from another. Adequate time must be allowed for the full analgesic or antiinflammatory effect to develop (as noted previously). The initial choice of NSAID is mainly determined by unwanted effects, particularly on the stomach and the cardiovascular system. For these reasons, low-dose ibuprofen is often the oral NSAID of first choice. Selective COX-2 inhibitors should be used in preference to standard NSAIDs only in people who are at high risk of developing serious gastrointestinal adverse effects, and when an NSAID is clearly indicated as part of the management. In older people or those at high risk of gastrointestinal complications, a proton pump inhibitor should be taken with an NSAID or a selective COX-2 inhibitor (see Chapter 33).

NSAIDs are also used for other conditions not associated with pain:

- As an antipyretic in febrile conditions.
- To achieve closure of a patent ductus arteriosus in a neonate where patency may be inappropriately maintained by prostaglandin production. NSAIDs should not be given to a pregnant mother in the third trimester, to avoid premature closure of the ductus.
- For modest reduction of menstrual blood loss in menorrhagia (excessive blood loss at menstruation).
- Low-dose aspirin for prevention of vascular occlusion by inhibition of platelet aggregation in atherosclerotic arterial disease (see Chapter 11).
- Aspirin and other NSAIDs reduce the risk of developing colorectal cancer, oesophageal and gastric cancer, breast cancer, bladder cancer and adenocarcinoma of the lung by about 30%. Aspirin also reduces the risk of metastasis from adenocarcinoma by about 50%. The effect of NSAIDs may result from inhibition of COX isoenzymes or actions on other nuclear transcription and cell signalling pathways that result in reduced cellular proliferation, migration and angiogenesis, and enhanced apoptosis.

SELF-ASSESSMENT

True/false questions

1. Two COX isoenzymes can synthesise prostanoids.
2. Gastrointestinal complications are the most common unwanted effects of NSAIDs.
3. COX-2 is not expressed constitutively in cells.
4. PGE_2 does not cause pain directly.
5. NSAIDs inhibit COX-1 and COX-2 isoenzymes with equal potency.
6. Paracetamol is a potent analgesic and antiinflammatory drug.
7. Aspirin is a suitable analgesic for infants.
8. NSAIDs reduce gastric blood flow.
9. Celecoxib causes a greater incidence of gastrointestinal symptoms than naproxen.
10. Antiplatelet doses of aspirin (75 mg per day) can compromise renal function.
11. The elderly have a greater risk of gastrointestinal adverse events when given NSAIDs.
12. Ibuprofen is an effective first-choice NSAID in severe rheumatoid arthritis.
13. Celecoxib is an antipyretic.
14. NSAIDs increase the risk of colorectal cancer.

Extended-matching-item questions

Choose the *most appropriate* NSAID from options A–E to be given initially in the case scenarios (1–3) provided.
A. Aspirin
B. Celecoxib
C. Diclofenac plus a proton pump inhibitor
D. Paracetamol
E. Indometacin

Case 1. An elderly man with a long history of hypertension, congestive heart failure with oedema and chronic gastritis has chronic mild knee pain due to osteoarthritic changes. The pain is interrupting his sleep.

Case 2. A 38-year-old woman with poorly controlled asthma and a history of nasal polyposis and recurrent dyspepsia has rheumatoid arthritis and no history of heart disease.

Case 3. A 45-year-old man who recently had a myocardial infarction is taking an angiotensin-converting enzyme (ACE) inhibitor and simvastatin.

ANSWERS

True/false answers

1. **True.** The two isoenzymes are COX-1 and COX-2.
2. **True.** Gastric irritation, ulceration and bleeding caused by inhibition of gastroprotective prostanoid synthesis are common unwanted effects of NSAID use.
3. **False.** COX-2 is present constitutively in some tissues such as renal arterioles, but can be markedly induced in many cell types by cytokines and inflammatory stimuli.
4. **True.** PGE_2 does not directly stimulate nociceptors, but sensitises them to bradykinin and other stimuli.
5. **False.** There is a wide range in the selectivity of NSAIDs for inhibition of COX-1 and COX-2. Their anti-inflammatory potency relates broadly to their potency in inhibiting COX-2, and their unwanted gastrointestinal effects to their potency in inhibiting COX-1.
6. **False.** Paracetamol is analgesic and antipyretic but has only a weak antiinflammatory effect. The reasons for this are imperfectly understood, but it may act on pain pathways within the CNS.
7. **False.** Aspirin can precipitate Reye's syndrome and should not be used in children under 12 years old. Other NSAIDs are also preferred to aspirin for analgesia and antiinflammatory effects in older children and adults, such as for rheumatoid disease.
8. **True.** Reduced blood flow contributes to the gastric damage caused by NSAIDs; they also inhibit bicarbonate and mucus secretion.
9. **False.** The COX-2-selective inhibitor celecoxib is associated with fewer gastrointestinal unwanted effects than the nonselective NSAID naproxen, although this difference declines with continued use.
10. **False.** Low doses of aspirin are safe, but long-term use of high doses can result in renal ischaemia, sodium and water retention, papillary necrosis and chronic renal failure.

11. **True.** Gastrointestinal unwanted effects are particularly common in those older than 75 years of age and in those with a history of peptic ulcer.

12. **False.** Ibuprofen is effective in mild-to-moderate arthritis, but other NSAIDs such as indometacin or diclofenac have greater antiinflammatory potential, albeit a greater propensity to cause unwanted side effects.

13. **True.** Pyrexia is caused by elevation of PGE_2 levels synthesised in the CNS by COX-2.

14. **False.** Increasing evidence suggests that NSAIDs reduce the risk of many cancers, most probably by inhibiting PGE_2 synthesis by COX-2, or by COX-independent pathways.

Extended-matching-item answers

Case 1: **Answer D** is correct. Paracetamol is a good choice for this man's mild osteoarthritic pain. His hypertension and heart failure mean that he should not be given an NSAID that may result in salt and water retention. Both the COX-2-selective and nonselective NSAIDs contribute to salt and water retention.

Case 2: **Answer B** is correct. The selective COX-2 inhibitor celecoxib could be prescribed, as these are less likely than nonselective NSAIDs such as aspirin or diclofenac to precipitate a hypersensitive asthmatic attack. Paracetamol would not be useful, as it has little antiinflammatory action.

Case 3: **Answer A** is correct. This man should be given low-dose aspirin (75 mg daily), as it prevents platelet aggregation by inhibiting TXA_2 synthesis while having a minimal effect on the production of the vasodilator and antiaggregatory PGI_2 (prostacyclin). This low dose has been shown to reduce the risk of another infarction.

FURTHER READING

Burian, M., Geisslinger, G., 2005. COX-dependent mechanisms involved in the antinociceptive action of NSAIDs at central and peripheral sites. Pharmacol. Ther. 107, 139–154.

Day, R.O., Graham, G.G., 2013. Nonsteroidal anti-inflammatory drugs (NSAIDs). Br. Med. J. 346, f3195.

Farooque, S.P., Lee, T.H., 2009. Aspirin-sensitive respiratory disease. Annu. Rev. Physiol. 71, 465–487.

Trelle, S., Reichenbach, S., Wandel, S., et al., 2011. Cardiovascular safety of nonsteroidal anti-inflammatory drugs: network meta-analysis. Br. Med. J. 342, c7086.

Compendium: nonsteroidal antiinflammatory drugs and related drugs

Drug	Characteristics
NSAIDs (including selective COX-2 inhibitors)	
Aceclofenac	Analogue of diclofenac. Given orally for pain and inflammation in rheumatoid arthritis, osteoarthritis and ankylosing spondylitis. Half-life: 4 h
Acemetacin	Prodrug of indometacin. Given orally for pain and inflammation in rheumatic disease and other musculoskeletal disorders, and for postoperative analgesia. Half-life: 1 h
Aspirin	Not suitable for children younger than 12 years due to the risk of Reye's syndrome. Aspirin is now generally restricted to antiplatelet use (see Chapter 11). Hydrolysed rapidly to active salicylic acid, which has a half-life of 3–20 h
Celecoxib	Selective COX-2 inhibitor. Given orally for pain and inflammation in rheumatoid arthritis, osteoarthritis and ankylosing spondylitis. Half-life: 11 h
Dexibuprofen	Active enantiomer of ibuprofen. Given orally for mild to moderate pain and inflammation, and for osteoarthritis and other musculoskeletal disorders. Half-life: 2–4 h
Dexketoprofen	Isomer of ketoprofen. Given orally for short-term treatment of mild to moderate pain. Half-life: 1–3 h
Diclofenac	Similar in efficacy to naproxen. Given orally, rectally, by deep intramuscular injection or intravenous infusion, transdermally, or topically. Used for pain and inflammation in rheumatic disease and other musculoskeletal disorders, acute gout, postoperative pain, migraine, fever in ear, nose or throat infection in children; available in combined formulation with misoprostol for gastric protection (see Chapter 33). Diclofenac potassium is more quickly absorbed than diclofenac sodium. Half-life: 1–2 h
Etodolac	Similar efficacy to naproxen. Given orally for pain and inflammation in osteoarthritis and rheumatoid arthritis. Half-life: 6–7 h
Etoricoxib	Selective COX-2 inhibitor. Given orally for pain and inflammation in osteoarthritis, rheumatoid arthritis and acute gout; not approved for use in the United States. Half-life: 25 h
Felbinac	Given topically for musculoskeletal pain and inflammation. Half-life: 10–17 h
Fenoprofen	Efficacy similar to naproxen, but higher risk of gastrointestinal side effects; given orally for pain and inflammation in osteoarthritis and rheumatoid arthritis. Half-life: 2–3 h

Compendium: nonsteroidal anti-inflammatory drugs and related drugs (cont'd)

Drug	Characteristics
Flurbiprofen	May be slightly more effective than naproxen, but there is a slightly higher risk of gastrointestinal side effects. Used for pain and inflammation in rheumatic disease and other musculoskeletal disorders, mild to moderate pain including dysmenorrhea, migraine, postoperative analgesia, sore throat. Given orally, rectally, as lozenge for sore throat, or topically to the eye. Half-life: 3–9 h
Ibuprofen	Relatively weak antiinflammatory action, but low risk of adverse effects. Used for pain and inflammation in rheumatic disease and other musculoskeletal disorders; mild to moderate pain including dysmenorrhea, postoperative analgesia, migraine, dental pain, fever with discomfort and pain in children, and postimmunisation pyrexia. Given orally or transdermally. Half-life: 2–4 h
Indometacin	Used for pain and moderate to severe inflammation in rheumatic disease and other acute musculoskeletal disorders, acute gout, dysmenorrhea, and in premature labour (see Chapter 45). Given orally or rectally. Half-life: 3–5 h
Ketoprofen	Used for pain and mild inflammation in rheumatic disease and other musculoskeletal disorders, after orthopaedic surgery, in acute gout and for dysmenorrhea. Given orally, rectally, by deep intramuscular injection or transdermally; also available in oral formulation with omeprazole. Half-life: 1–3 h
Ketorolac	Used in short-term management of moderate to severe acute postoperative pain. Given orally, or by intramuscular or slow intravenous injection. Half-life: 3–9 h
Mefenamic acid	Weak antiinflammatory action. Used for pain and inflammation in rheumatoid arthritis and osteoarthritis, postoperative pain, mild to moderate pain, dysmenorrhoea and menorrhagia. Half-life: 3–4 h
Meloxicam	Given orally for pain and inflammation in rheumatoid arthritis, osteoarthritis (short-term) and in ankylosing spondylitis. Half-life: 12–20 h
Nabumetone	Similar efficacy to naproxen. Given orally for pain and inflammation in osteoarthritis and rheumatoid arthritis. Half-life: 24 h
Naproxen	Good efficacy with low incidence of adverse effects. Used for pain and inflammation in rheumatic disease (including juvenile idiopathic arthritis) and other musculoskeletal disorders, dysmenorrhea and acute gout. Given orally or rectally; also available in combined formulation with misoprostol or esomeprazole (see Chapter 33). Half-life: 12–15 h
Parecoxib	Selective COX-2 inhibitor. Licensed for short-term management of postoperative pain. Given by deep intramuscular or intravenous injection. Half-life: 5–9 h
Piroxicam	Similar efficacy to naproxen, but long duration of action allows once daily dosage. Restricted use because of gastrointestinal unwanted effects and serious skin reactions. Given orally, rectally or by deep intramuscular injection for rheumatoid arthritis, osteoarthritis and ankylosing spondylitis; also unrestricted transdermal use. Half-life: 30–60 h
Sulindac	Prodrug with active metabolite. Similar profile to naproxen; given orally for pain and inflammation in rheumatic disease and other musculoskeletal disorders, and acute gout. Half-life: 7–8 h
Tenoxicam	Similar profile to naproxen. Given orally (once daily) or by intramuscular or intravenous injection for pain and inflammation in rheumatic disease and other musculoskeletal disorders. Half-life: 44–100 h
Tiaprofenic acid	Similar profile to naproxen. Given orally for pain and inflammation in rheumatic disease and other musculoskeletal disorders. Not suitable for people with urinary tract disorders due to risk of cystitis. Half-life: 2–4 h
Tolfenamic acid	Licensed for the treatment of acute migraine (see Chapter 26). Given orally. Half-life: 2 h
Related drug	
Paracetamol (acetaminophen)	The most widely used nonopioid analgesic. Given orally, rectally or intravenously. Also available in compound formulations with codeine or dihydrocodeine (see Chapter 19). Hepatotoxicity in overdose due to NAPQI metabolite (see Chapter 53). Half-life: 3–4 h

30 Rheumatoid arthritis, other inflammatory arthritides and osteoarthritis

RHEUMATOID ARTHRITIS

Rheumatoid arthritis is a chronic systemic inflammatory condition with an underlying genetic predisposition to immune dysregulation. Autoimmune processes contribute to the maintenance of rheumatoid arthritis, but it is uncertain how these are initiated. Two autoantibodies, rheumatoid factor (immunoglobulin M [IgM] autoantibodies reactive with IgG) and anticyclic citrullinated peptide (CCP) antibodies, are often detected in plasma before symptoms arise. The initiating antigen is believed to bind to Toll-like receptors (TLRs) – pattern-recognition molecules that bind to both foreign and self-structures – on dendritic cells and macrophages (antigen-presenting cells), which then activate naïve T-cells (see Chapter 38). Antigen-presenting cells express CD80 and CD86 co-stimulatory molecules which provide further signals for the activation of T-cells (Fig. 30.1).

The primary response to T-cell activation is lymphoid cell infiltration of the synovium around joints, formation of new blood vessels and a proliferation of mesenchymal cells in the synovial membrane. The synovium becomes locally invasive at the junction of the joint cartilage and bone (pannus), and osteoclasts then destroy both joint cartilage and bone. Apart from psoriatic arthritis, other forms of inflammatory arthritis do not produce erosive changes in periarticular bone or joint destruction to the same degree.

The chronic inflammatory process in joints is initiated by T-helper 1 (Th1) lymphocytes that migrate into the joint. Failure of suppression of Th1 cells by regulatory T-cells may be important in the pathogenesis of rheumatoid arthritis. Activated T-cells produce proinflammatory cytokines such as interferon-γ. These cytokines stimulate B-lymphocytes, macrophages, fibroblasts, chondrocytes and osteoclasts (see Fig. 30.1). Macrophages and fibroblasts in the inflammatory tissue produce tumour necrosis factor α (TNFα), interleukin-1 (IL-1), IL-6 and granulocyte macrophage colony stimulating factor (GM-CSF), as well as numerous chemokines that attract other inflammatory cells. B-cells play an important role in the pathology of rheumatoid arthritis. They act as antigen-presenting cells that co-stimulate T-cells, generate inflammatory cytokines such as TNFα and produce rheumatoid factor antibody and anti-CCP. The pattern of inflammation in rheumatoid arthritis differs from that in most other immune-mediated diseases.

TNFα has a prominent role in the recruitment of immune and inflammatory cells into the joint by increasing the expression of adhesion molecules (integrins) on vascular endothelial cells. It also orchestrates the production of other inflammatory mediators. Activated synovial fibroblasts, osteoclasts and chondrocytes release tissue-destroying matrix metalloproteinases (MMPs). Activated macrophages, lymphocytes and fibroblasts stimulate angiogenesis in the synovium. Activated osteoclasts increase bone resorption. Rheumatoid factor forms complexes with collagen in damaged cartilage, causing activation of the complement pathway. The relevance of this to joint damage is unknown. The plethora of cells that enter the

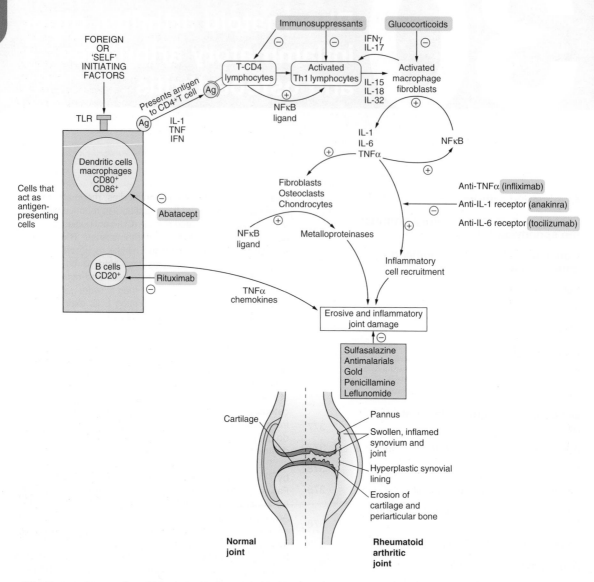

Fig. 30.1 **The biology of rheumatoid arthritis and sites of drug action.** The affected synovial joint is characterised by inflamed and swollen synovium, with angiogenesis and increased presence of fibroblasts, osteoclasts, plasma cells, mast cells and B-lymphocytes. The synovial fluid contains increased numbers of neutrophil leucocytes, and there is erosion of cartilage and adjacent bone. The cascade of self-perpetuating inflammatory events involves many factors, including upregulation of the ubiquitous nuclear transcription factor NF-κB and generation of cytokines including IL-1, IL-6 and TNFα. Some of the drugs shown act at multiple sites. *APCs*, Antigen presenting cells; *IFN*, interferon; *IL*, interleukin; *NF-κB*, nuclear factor κB; *TLR*, toll-like receptor; *TNFα*, tumour necrosis factor α.

synovium and the array of cytokines that are involved provide a large number of potential targets for disease-modifying antirheumatic drugs (DMARDs; see Fig. 30.1).

Rheumatoid arthritis usually presents as a symmetrical polyarthritis, with a peak incidence age of 60–70 years. Symptoms usually appear gradually and most often involve the proximal interphalangeal joints of the fingers, metacarpophalangeal joints and wrists. Inflammation of other joints such as the ankles and hips may be the presenting complaint, or they may become involved later. The affected joints are warm, swollen and painful. Stiffness is troublesome, particularly for longer than 30 minutes in the morning, as a result of an increase in extracellular fluid in and around the joint. Systemic disturbance is common, including general fatigue, malaise and weight loss, while extra-articular manifestations such as vasculitis and neuropathy can occur.

OTHER TYPES OF INFLAMMATORY ARTHRITIS: THE SPONDYLOARTHRITIDES

There are many types of inflammatory arthritis with a pattern of joint involvement different from that of rheumatoid arthritis. They involve the sacroiliac joints (sacroiliitis) and can affect small or large joints peripherally. They are characterised by co-occurrence with acute anterior uveitis, inflammatory bowel disease and psoriasis. Collectively they are called the spondyloarthritides, and include ankylosing spondylitis, psoriatic arthritis, arthritis associated with inflammatory bowel disease, reactive arthritis and some juvenile idiopathic arthritis.

There is a genetic predisposition to spondyloarthritides, notably possession of the human leukocyte antigen (HLA)-B27 gene in axial spondyloarthritides (that affect the spine), with additional polygenic influences in the other disorders. It is possible that spondylitis is initiated by binding of an antigenic peptide to HLA-B27 on antigen-presenting cells.

Spondyloarthritides are considered to be autoinflammatory syndromes and probably arise from activation of innate immune processes in response to as yet unknown triggers. However, the adaptive immune system is also involved in the genesis of psoriatic arthropathy. A variety of cytokines appear to be involved in the inflammatory response, including those derived from macrophages (TNFα, and various interleukins such as IL-1, IL-6, IL-8, IL-18), Th1-cells (IL-2, interferon α [IFNα]), antigen-presenting cells (IL-23) and Th17 cells (IL-17). The inflammation is characteristically associated with enthesopathy (inflammation at the bone insertion of tendons and ligaments) and formation of new endochondral bone.

The presence of different pathophysiological mechanisms in rheumatoid arthritis and the spondyloarthritides probably explains their different responses to treatments designed to modify disease progression.

CONVENTIONAL DISEASE-MODIFYING ANTIRHEUMATIC DRUGS

Nonsteroidal antiinflammatory drugs (NSAIDs; see Chapter 29) provide symptomatic relief in inflammatory arthritis but do not alter the long-term progression of joint destruction in rheumatoid arthritis. A diverse group of compounds can reduce the rate of progression of joint erosion and destruction, leading to improvement both in symptoms and in the clinical and serological markers of rheumatoid arthritis activity. These drugs produce long-term depression of the inflammatory response, even though they have little direct antiinflammatory effect. They all have a slow onset of action, with many producing little improvement until about 3 months after starting treatment. Such drugs are grouped together and known as DMARDs.

SULFASALAZINE

The action of sulfasalazine in arthritis is poorly understood. It is cleaved in the colon by bacterial enzymes to 5-aminosalicylic acid and sulfapyridine. Sulfapyridine in the colon may reduce the absorption of antigens that promote joint inflammation. However, both sulfasalazine and sulfapyridine are absorbed from the gut and are found at similar concentrations in synovial fluid. Sulfasalazine inhibits an enzyme involved in the biosynthesis of purines, 5-aminoimidazole-4-carboxamide ribonucleotide (AICAR) transformylase, in a similar manner to methotrexate (see Chapter 38) and may have an antiinflammatory effect by increasing the extracellular concentration of adenosine.

High doses of sulfasalazine are required for the treatment of rheumatoid arthritis, and these often produce gastrointestinal upset. This can be minimised by increasing the dose slowly and by using an enteric-coated formulation. Other problems include reversible oligospermia (and therefore sulfasalazine should be avoided in males who wish to have a family) and blood dyscrasias. Sulfasalazine is discussed more fully in Chapter 34.

ANTIMALARIALS

Hydroxychloroquine

Mechanism of action

Hydroxychloroquine is weakly basic, which permits its uptake and concentration in a nonionised form within cells. Having entered the lysosomes inside the cell, the acidic environment traps and concentrates the drug in its ionised state. Macrophages depend on acid proteases in their lysosomes for digestion of phagocytosed protein. Hydroxychloroquine slightly increases the pH inside the macrophage lysosomes, which alters the processing of peptide antigens and reduces their subsequent presentation on the cell surface. Thus the interaction between T-helper cells and antigen-presenting macrophages responsible for joint inflammation is reduced, with a reduction in the inflammatory response. Hydroxychloroquine also reduces the activation of antigen-presenting dendritic cells by blocking TLRs on their cell membrane. Antioxidant activity has also been demonstrated, but the relevance of this to rheumatoid disease is unknown.

Monitoring and prevention of unwanted effects

Retinal toxicity is a potential problem, due to selective binding to melanin in photoreceptor cells in the macula and subsequent disruption of lysosomal function. It is rare with recommended doses of hydroxychloroquine, but specialist assessment of the eyes is recommended before treatment and again during treatment if there is a change in visual acuity or blurring of vision or if treatment continues for more than 5 years.

The other unwanted effects and pharmacokinetics of hydroxychloroquine can be found in Chapter 51.

LEFLUNOMIDE

Mechanism of action

Leflunomide is an isoxazole derivative prodrug that is converted to an active derivative, teriflunomide. Teriflunomide inhibits dihydro-orotate dehydrogenase, a key mitochondrial enzyme in the de novo synthesis of the pyrimidine ribonucleotide uridine monophosphate (rUMP). Activated lymphocytes require at least an eightfold increase in their pyrimidine pool to proliferate. Inadequate provision of rUMP increases the expression of the tumour-suppressor molecule p53 which translocates to the cell nucleus and arrests the cell cycle in the G_1 phase. This cytostatic action reduces the population of Th1-cells in rheumatoid arthritis and shifts the balance in favour of Th2-cells. Dividing cells other than lymphocytes can obtain pyrimidines from a separate salvage pathway that reuses existing ribonucleotides, so these cells are not affected by leflunomide. Leflunomide also reduces T-cell-mediated B-cell activation by inhibition of tyrosine kinases, thereby suppressing immunoglobulin production.

Pharmacokinetics

Leflunomide is a prodrug that is well absorbed from the gut and is converted nonenzymatically, mainly in the intestinal mucosa and plasma, to its active metabolite teriflunomide. The metabolite is excreted via the bile, and enterohepatic circulation contributes to its very long plasma half-life (15 days).

Unwanted effects

- Anorexia, abdominal pain, nausea, diarrhoea.
- Increased blood pressure.
- Headache, dizziness, lethargy.
- Leucopenia, or less frequently anaemia or thrombocytopenia.
- Rash, dry skin and pruritus.
- Alopecia.
- Hepatotoxicity, which is potentially life-threatening, especially in the first 6 months of use.
- Teratogenicity: It is advised that conception should be avoided for 2 years after stopping treatment in women and for 3 months in men.

Monitoring and prevention of unwanted effects

Monitoring of full blood count and liver function should be carried out regularly during treatment with leflunomide. If serious unwanted effects occur, elimination of the drug can be increased by the use of colestyramine (see Chapter 48) or activated charcoal to bind the active metabolite present in the gut after biliary excretion, thereby interrupting its enterohepatic circulation.

IMMUNOSUPPRESSANT DRUGS

Several drugs with immunosuppressant actions have been shown to be effective in rheumatoid arthritis. These include:

- antimetabolites: methotrexate, azathioprine (see Chapter 38),
- calcineurin inhibitor: ciclosporin (see Chapter 38).

Methotrexate is one of the most effective antirheumatic drugs. Although methotrexate is a folate antagonist, co-administration of folic acid supplements does not reduce its immunomodulatory effect, but it does prevent much of the mucosal and gastrointestinal toxicity of the drug. A more important mechanism of action of methotrexate in arthritis is inhibition of the deamination of adenosine, causing its extracellular accumulation (see Chapter 38). Methotrexate is usually given orally once a week for the treatment of inflammatory arthritis. It can be given intramuscularly if oral use produces intractable gastrointestinal symptoms or if absorption by the oral route is inadequate.

GOLD

sodium aurothiomalate

Mechanism of action

The precise mechanism by which gold compounds act is unknown. A popular concept is that the compound is taken up by mononuclear cells and inhibits their phagocytic function. This will reduce the release of inflammatory mediators and inhibit inflammatory cell proliferation. It has also been suggested that the thiol group in sodium aurothiomalate sequesters reactive aldehydes produced by inflammatory cells that contribute to destruction of cartilage.

The advent of more effective and less toxic drugs has reduced the use of gold salts in current clinical practice.

Pharmacokinetics

Sodium aurothiomalate is given by deep intramuscular injection. An initial test dose is given to screen for acute toxicity (discussed later), followed by injections at weekly intervals to gradually achieve a therapeutic concentration in the tissues. Subsequently, a smaller dose is used to maintain remission. Sodium aurothiomalate dissociates in plasma to gold and free thiomalate. The gold binds readily to albumin and several tissue proteins, and accumulates in many tissues such as the liver, kidney, bone marrow, lymph nodes and spleen. Elimination is largely renal. Gold has a half-life of several weeks, probably as a result of its extensive tissue binding.

Unwanted effects

The unwanted effects can be serious, and all but the most minor effects should lead to immediate cessation of treatment:

- Oral ulceration.
- Proteinuria from membranous glomerulonephritis. This can develop after several weeks of treatment, sometimes progressing to nephrotic syndrome; recovery can take up to 2 years following drug withdrawal.
- Blood disorders, especially thrombocytopenia but also agranulocytosis and aplastic anaemia.
- Rashes.
- Pulmonary fibrosis.

Monitoring and prevention of unwanted effects

Urine should be checked for protein and a full blood count obtained before each injection of gold, and regularly during oral therapy. Major complications may require treatment with dimercaprol or penicillamine to chelate the gold (see Chapter 53) and increase its elimination. Corticosteroids can be helpful to treat blood dyscrasias. Gold should not be used if there is a history of renal or hepatic disease, blood dyscrasias or severe rashes. Gold should be stopped if stomatitis, a pruritic rash, neutropenia, thrombocytopenia or significant proteinuria (>1 g in 24 hours) develops.

PENICILLAMINE

Mechanism of action and uses

The mechanisms of action of penicillamine are uncertain, but modulation of the immune system is believed to be important. The thiol group may also have a similar function to sodium aurothiomalate (described previously). Penicillamine does not slow the progression of joint erosions and is now rarely used for rheumatoid arthritis.

The thiol moiety in penicillamine can chelate many metals, which has given the drug a role in the management of poisoning (see Chapter 53) and in Wilson's disease, a genetically determined illness that is associated with copper overload.

Pharmacokinetics

Penicillamine is well absorbed from the gut, although oral iron supplements substantially reduce its absorption. It is excreted by the kidneys and has a very long half-life of 4 days due to tissue binding.

Unwanted effects

Unwanted effects occur frequently and are responsible for about 30% of people stopping treatment. They can be reduced by slow increases in dose. Many unwanted effects resemble those of gold.

- Nausea, vomiting, abdominal discomfort and rashes (often with fever), especially early in treatment.
- Loss of taste is common, but may resolve despite continued treatment.
- Oral ulceration.
- Proteinuria, which is caused by immune-complex glomerulonephritis and is dose-related. Nephrotic syndrome can also occur.
- Blood disorders, especially thrombocytopenia, but also neutropenia and, rarely, aplastic anaemia.

Monitoring and prevention of unwanted effects

Regular monitoring of urine, protein and blood counts should be carried out during treatment.

BIOLOGICAL DRUGS FOR INFLAMMATORY ARTHRITIS

ANTIBODIES AGAINST TUMOUR NECROSIS FACTOR α

 Examples

adalimumab, certolizumab, etanercept, golimumab, infliximab

Mechanism of action

TNFα stimulates several inflammatory processes (see previous discussion and Fig. 30.1). It acts by binding to one of two cell surface receptors, type 1 (TNFR1; widely expressed in many tissues) and type 2 (TNFR2; found only on cells of the immune system). There are several antibody derivatives available that block the action of TNFα.

- Adalimumab and golimumab are fully humanised monoclonal antibodies specific for TNFα.
- Certolizumab pegol is a pegylated Fab fragment of a humanised monoclonal antibody specific for TNFα.
- Etanercept is a fusion protein consisting of two recombinant soluble extracellular portions of the human TNFR2, fused to the constant (Fc) domain of human immunoglobulin (IgG₁). It binds to TNFα and also to the cytokine lymphotoxin α (also known as TNFβ).
- Infliximab is a chimaeric monoclonal antibody comprising the variable region of a murine antibody, which neutralises TNFα, spliced to the constant region of a human antibody.

Pharmacokinetics

Adalimumab, certolizumab pegol, etanercept and golimumab are given by subcutaneous injection, and infliximab is given by intravenous infusion. The mechanism of elimination of these recombinant compounds is poorly defined but likely to be via the endosomal degradation pathway. Degradation is reduced by the presence of a human immunoglobulin Fc domain and can be further reduced by pegylation of the molecule. All antibodies to TNFα have very long half-lives between 5 and 20 days, enabling dosing at frequencies ranging from twice weekly to monthly.

Unwanted effects

- All biological drugs can produce gastrointestinal upset, hypertension, hypersensitivity reactions, injection-site reactions, fever, headache and depression. Blood disorders, including anaemia, leucopenia and thrombocytopenia, also occur.
- Worsening heart failure.
- Increased risk of pulmonary tuberculosis: Screening for evidence of tuberculosis is recommended before initiation of therapy. Septicaemia and reactivation of hepatitis B virus occur more frequently.

INTERLEUKIN-1 RECEPTOR ANTAGONIST

Anakinra

Mechanism of action

Anakinra is a recombinant human IL-1 receptor antagonist (see Fig. 30.1). IL-1 is actually a family of cytokines, including two IL-1 receptor agonists (IL-1α and IL-1β) and a natural IL-1 receptor antagonist (IL-Ra). The theoretical basis for the use of anakinra is that joint destruction arises from an imbalance between the agonists and the antagonist. IL-1 agonists are proinflammatory cytokines released by macrophages and fibroblasts in inflamed synovium, and by neutrophils in synovial fluid. The IL-1 peptides compete for occupancy of the IL-1 receptor on the membrane of synovial cells, and as little as 2–3% occupancy by the agonists produces maximal proinflammatory cell activation. Anakinra blocks the IL-1 receptor and suppresses the inflammatory response.

Pharmacokinetics

Anakinra is given by daily subcutaneous injection. Elimination is via the kidneys, and it has a short half-life (4–6 hours).

Unwanted effects

- Injection-site reactions.
- Increased risk of serious infections, particularly in people with asthma.
- Neutropenia.

INTERLEUKIN-6 RECEPTOR ANTAGONIST

tocilizumab

Mechanism of action

Tocilizumab is a recombinant humanised monoclonal antibody that acts as a competitive antagonist at the IL-6 receptor. IL-6 is a proinflammatory cytokine produced by a variety of cell types, including T- and B-lymphocytes, monocytes and fibroblasts. It is also produced by synovial and endothelial cells in joints affected by inflammatory processes such as rheumatoid arthritis. IL-6 is involved in T-cell activation, immunoglobulin secretion, and stimulation of hematopoietic precursor cell proliferation and differentiation.

Pharmacokinetics

Tocilizumab is given by intravenous infusion every 4 weeks. It has a long half-life of 6 days, and is probably cleared by proteolysis.

Unwanted effects

- Abdominal pain, mouth ulceration, dyspepsia, raised liver enzymes.
- Increased risk of infections, particularly upper respiratory tract infections.
- Oedema, hypertension.
- Dizziness, headache.
- Leucopenia.

INTERLEUKIN-12 AND INTERLEUKIN-23 RECEPTOR ANTAGONIST

ustekinumab

Mechanism of action and uses

Ustekinumab is a human monoclonal antibody that binds to a subunit present on both IL-12 and IL-23. These interleukins are involved in natural killer cell activation and Th-cell differentiation and activation. It is used for treatment of psoriasis and psoriatic arthritis.

Pharmacokinetics

Ustekinumab is given by subcutaneous injection, initially every 4 weeks then every 12 weeks. It has a long half-life of 15–45 days, and is probably cleared by proteolysis.

Unwanted effects

- Oropharyngeal pain, nausea, diarrhoea.
- Increased risk of infections.
- Injection site reactions.
- Dizziness, headache.
- Arthralgia, myalgia.
- Malaise, pruritis.

T-CELL CO-STIMULATION MODULATOR

abatacept

Mechanism of action and uses

T-lymphocyte activation requires recognition of a specific antigen carried by an antigen-presenting cell, and a second co-stimulatory signal. A major co-stimulatory signal involves binding of CD80 and CD86 molecules on the surface of antigen-presenting cells to the CD28 receptor on T-cells. Abatacept is a monoclonal antibody that selectively binds to CD80 and CD86 and blocks the co-stimulatory signal. Abatacept therefore reduces the subsequent production of inflammatory mediators and proinflammatory cytokines.

A related co-stimulation inhibitor, belatacept, is used as an immunosuppressant in renal transplantation (see Chapter 38).

Pharmacokinetics

Abatacept is given by intravenous infusion. Its metabolism is unknown, and it has a very long half-life of about 14 days.

Unwanted effects

- Headache, dizziness, fatigue, paraesthesia.
- Nausea, stomatitis, abdominal pain, diarrhoea.
- Conjunctivitis.
- Leucopenia.
- Upper respiratory tract infection and, less commonly, other infections.

ANTI-CD20 B-CELL DEPLETER

rituximab

Mechanism of action and uses

Rituximab specifically depletes CD20+ B-cells by binding to the CD20 antigen expressed on the cell surface (see Fig. 30.1). The depletion of mature and differentiating B-cells will reduce antigen presentation, stimulation of T-cells, cytokine production and production of autoantibodies. Responses in rheumatoid arthritis usually last for up to 6 months, and relapse corresponds with B-cell repopulation.

Pharmacokinetics

Rituximab is given by intravenous infusion. Its metabolism is unknown, and it has a very long half-life of about 3–8 days.

Unwanted effects

- Cytokine release syndrome with fever, chills, nausea, vomiting and allergic reactions occurs in about one-third of people with the first infusion. Premedication with an antihistamine and sometimes a corticosteroid will reduce these reactions.
- Abdominal pain, dyspepsia.
- Severe rashes.
- Headache, depression.
- Pancytopenia.
- Exacerbation of angina, arrhythmia or heart failure can occur in people with cardiovascular disease.
- Reactivation of hepatitis B infection.

MANAGEMENT OF RHEUMATOID ARTHRITIS

Progressive joint damage is common in rheumatoid arthritis, and much of this damage occurs early in the disease. There is now a substantial body of evidence that early use of DMARDs (within 3 months of the onset of symptoms) leads to a better long-term outcome. DMARDs do not have significant antiinflammatory action and require 2–3 months before an effect is established. Therefore they are almost always used initially in combination with a corticosteroid or an NSAID.

Methotrexate, given with folic acid supplementation separated by 2–3 days, is the most commonly used DMARD. It is usually taken orally once a week, but subcutaneous use can be considered if gastrointestinal tolerability is a problem. A combination of two DMARDs is now recommended as standard first-line therapy and is more effective than a single drug. Sulfasalazine, leflunomide or hydroxychloroquine are the drugs most frequently used in combination with methotrexate. In early rheumatoid disease, a low dose of corticosteroid, given for up to 6 months in combination with DMARDs, provides early symptomatic relief. It also retards bone destruction and slows disease progression. Because of unwanted effects, corticosteroids should be withdrawn as soon as disease control is achieved. Intramuscular methylprednisone is often used and is preferred over oral prednisolone, which can be difficult to withdraw (see Chapter 44). Pulsed intramuscular corticosteroid therapy can also be given for disease flares. Intra-articular injections of corticosteroid are used for individual inflamed joints (especially the knee and shoulder). If disease activity cannot be suppressed by two DMARDs, then a combination of three DMARDs (such as methotrexate, sulfasalazine and hydroxychloroquine) can be tried. Relapse is common if DMARD therapy is stopped, and restarting treatment may not produce remission. Therefore it is often recommended that treatment is continued long term with the lowest DMARD dose that maintains clinical remission.

Biologic therapies are usually given when disease fails to respond to conventional DMARDs. TNFα inhibitors such as etanercept, abatacept or toculizumab are often used. They are typically used in combination with methotrexate, or with leflunomide if methotrexate is not tolerated, which produces a better response than the biological agent given alone. The combination produces remission and halts disease progression in up to 70% of people who are treated. If one anti-TNFα drug is ineffective or poorly tolerated, then a different drug from the same class should be tried. Rituximab is used for those who fail to respond to, or who cannot tolerate, a first-line biologic therapy. Anakinra is less effective than anti-TNFα drugs and is currently not recommended in the United Kingdom.

Immunosuppressant drugs such as ciclosporin or azathioprine are generally reserved as third-line agents. Gold and penicillamine are less widely used due to toxicity and, in the case of penicillamine, limited efficacy. Cyclophosphamide is useful for the management of extra-articular manifestations of rheumatoid disease, such as vasculitis, pericarditis or pleurisy.

NSAIDs (see Chapter 29) are useful for symptomatic treatment of all types of inflammatory arthritis, since they reduce both pain and stiffness. However, they do not affect the long-term course of the disease, and DMARDs have superseded them as the mainstay of treatment of rheumatoid arthritis. NSAIDs should usually be stopped as soon as DMARDs are effective. There is considerable variation in responses to different NSAIDs, and there is no way of predicting effectiveness in an individual. Propionic acid derivatives, such as ibuprofen, are often used first. They have weaker antiinflammatory activity than other classes of NSAID, but generally have fewer unwanted effects. More powerful drugs such as naproxen can be used when ibuprofen fails to control symptoms, although the increased risk of gastrointestinal irritation and cardiovascular events limit their use, especially in the elderly. Morning stiffness is often disabling in inflammatory arthritis. This is helped by giving a late-evening dose of an NSAID with a long half-life, a modified-release formulation of a compound with a short half-life or an NSAID suppository. Topical NSAIDs applied over the affected joint(s) are not usually recommended. Selective cyclo-oxygenase (COX)-2 inhibitors are usually reserved for people who are intolerant of nonselective NSAIDs, or who have a higher risk of serious gastrointestinal complications with an NSAID (see Chapter 29).

Physical aids such as splinting and bed rest can help acute flares of joint inflammation. There is an increased risk of cardiovascular disease in people with rheumatoid arthritis, and attention to the conventional risk factors for prevention of atherosclerosis is important (see Chapter 5).

MANAGEMENT OF SPONDYLOARTHRITIDES

NSAIDs are the first-line treatment for spondyloarthritides, and will relieve pain and improve function. They should be avoided in enteropathic arthritis, as they can exacerbate bowel disease. NSAIDs should be combined with a tailored exercise regimen. Although most evidence for the use of DMARDs has been obtained in the treatment of rheumatoid arthritis, there is limited evidence for their efficacy in the seronegative spondyloarthritides. Sulfasalazine, methotrexate and leflunomide give some benefit for peripheral joint disease in these forms of inflammatory arthritis, but do not improve axial joint inflammation or enthesitis. The place of apremilast in therapy of psoriatic arthritis is not well established.

Anti-TNFα agents can produce remission of disease in ankylosing spondylitis, enteropathic arthritis and psoriatic arthritis in about one-third of those treated, with considerable symptomatic benefit in others. Ustekinumab is an option in psoriatic arthritis when an anti-TNFα agent is ineffective or poorly tolerated, and will also improve the skin lesions. Biologic therapies were thought to have little effect on new bone formation in spondyloarthritides, but recent evidence suggests that this may be improved if treatment is started early. If treatment with an anti-TNFα agent is stopped after remission is achieved, then relapse usually occurs within 6–12 months.

OSTEOARTHRITIS

Osteoarthritis is the clinical manifestation of joint degeneration that results from loss of articular cartilage and becomes more common with increasing age. Osteoarthritis is either age-related (when it can be localised or generalised) or premature due to a single strong risk factor such as joint injury or chondrocalcinosis. The cardinal symptom of osteoarthritis is pain in the affected joint during physical activity, which is relieved by rest. Pain also occurs at rest with advanced

disease. Stiffness may be troublesome for a few minutes after rest, but is not prolonged, as in inflammatory arthritis. Various small joints can be involved, particularly the distal interphalangeal joints of the fingers and the carpometacarpal joint of the thumb. Large joints such as the knee, hip, elbow and shoulder are often asymmetrically affected.

The integrity of articular cartilage depends on the balance of synthetic and catabolic activity of the chondrocytes embedded in the cartilage matrix. Mechanical stress is the single most important factor in the development of osteoarthritis, and this can be an abnormal load on a normal joint or a normal load on a joint that has impaired protection against mechanical stress. There is a strong polygenic predisposition to osteoarthritis, which accounts for up to 60% of risk. Compression of cartilage produces many physical and biochemical stimuli that influence chondrocyte metabolism and promote matrix destruction and apoptotic chondrocyte death. Osteoarthritis is caused by an imbalance of cartilage degradation compared with synthesis of cartilage, with loss of the normal cartilage matrix. This is more common with increasing age because ageing cartilage has less synthesis of new matrix, activated degradative pathways and impaired removal of damaged cells. Obesity increases mechanical load on joints but is also associated with release from adipocytes of inflammatory cytokines that degrade the matrix. Synovial inflammation results from release of cartilage debris into the joint, accompanied by catabolic mediators, which results in joint swelling.

Cartilage is an avascular tissue, and chondrocytes rely on a hypoxic environment for optimal function. Chondrocytes do not proliferate in adult cartilage but promote synthesis of cartilage matrix by the expression of growth factors, particularly insulin-like growth factor 1 and transforming growth factor β (TGFβ). Chondrocytes normally maintain cartilage homeostasis by autophagy, a housekeeping process that removes damaged cells and eliminates inflammatory cells. Autophagy is impaired with ageing and under mechanical or inflammatory stress. This allows mechanical stress and increased reactive oxygen species to combine with chronic low-grade inflammation to disrupt the pericellular cartilage matrix. Degradation of cartilage matrix proteins is carried out initially by aggrecanases which degrade the proteoglycan aggrecan and expose collagen to breakdown by MMPs. Aggrecanases and MMPs are synthesised by chondrocytes in response to stimulation by the proinflammatory cytokines IL-1β and TNFα released by inflammatory cells. Loss of collagen matrix leads to swelling and fissuring of the surface of the cartilage and loss of surface lubrication.

Subchondral bone develops microcracks in response to mechanical stress and becomes increasingly vascular with new bone being laid down. It is uncertain whether the initiating factors for osteoarthritis originate in the articular cartilage or subchondral bone. However, recent evidence suggests that stiffening of subchondral bone, with less effective shock absorption, may be the trigger for cartilage loss.

MANAGEMENT OF OSTEOARTHRITIS

Treatment of osteoarthritis currently remains symptomatic. Despite the role of inflammatory mediators in initiating damage to collagen, modulation of the effect of these mediators or inhibition of the enzymes involved in cartilage degradation have not shown any ability to modify the progression of the osteoarthritis. Nonpharmacological therapies such as weight loss, exercise and orthotics are the mainstay of initial treatment.

Glucosamine sulphate or chondroitin sulphate supplements (over-the-counter preparations in the United Kingdom) are often used by people with osteoarthritis to limit progression, but there is conflicting evidence of benefit. If pain is troublesome, simple analgesics such as paracetamol should usually be considered as first-line treatment. NSAIDs may be helpful for inflammatory episodes or if paracetamol is ineffective. In vitro studies suggest that some NSAIDs may accelerate the loss of articular cartilage in osteoarthritis. Clinical studies are inconclusive, but avoidance of powerful NSAIDs is probably desirable. The risks of gastrointestinal and cardiac toxicity may limit the use of NSAIDs.

Intra-articular or periarticular injection of a corticosteroid (see Chapter 44) can provide short-term symptomatic relief in osteoarthritis, even if there is little clinical evidence of joint inflammation. Corticosteroids inhibit proinflammatory mediators in synovial tissue, such as IL-1 and TNFα. Joint injection with hyaluronic acid remains a controversial treatment, with conflicting evidence of efficacy from clinical trials. Long-term management of osteoarthritis may eventually require surgical joint resurfacing or replacement.

SELF-ASSESSMENT

True/false questions

1. The action of most DMARDs is slow in onset.
2. NSAIDs reduce the symptoms of rheumatoid disease and retard its progress.
3. If penicillamine does not lead to clinical benefit within 6 months, it should be stopped.
4. Intramuscular gold can cause proteinuria.
5. Methotrexate has a relatively rapid onset of action compared with other DMARDS.
6. During methotrexate therapy, folic acid is contraindicated.
7. Methotrexate has relatively few unwanted effects compared with other DMARDs.
8. The active component of sulfasalazine in rheumatoid disease is 5-aminosalicylic acid.
9. Combination therapy with DMARDs should not be used in rheumatoid arthritis.
10. Leflunomide selectively inhibits pyrimidine synthesis in lymphocytes.
11. Intra-articular injections of corticosteroids slow the progression of erosions.
12. Prolonged treatment with high doses of corticosteroids can cause adrenal atrophy.
13. The antimalarial hydroxychloroquine is of little benefit in rheumatoid arthritis.
14. Rituximab depletes B-lymphocytes.
15. Adalimumab and golimumab are fully humanised anti-TNFα monoclonal antibodies.
16. Abatacept blocks antigen presentation to T-lymphocytes
17. Anakinra and tocilizumab activate cytokine receptors.
18. DMARDs are effective treatments for ankylosing spondylitis.

Case-based questions

1. A 30-year-old woman had developed painful wrists gradually over 4 weeks; she had not experienced similar episodes of pain before. On examination, both wrists and the metacarpophalangeal joints of both hands were tender but not deformed. What course of treatment would you suggest?
2. There was some initial symptomatic improvement, but subsequently the pain, stiffness and swelling of the hands persisted, and 8 weeks later both knees became similarly affected. She saw a rheumatologist, who confirmed that she was suffering from rheumatoid arthritis and altered her treatment. What treatment option would now be appropriate?
3. She commenced treatment that required folic acid supplements to counteract folate depletion. What drug treatment had been started?

ANSWERS

True/false answers

1. **True.** Most DMARDs take several weeks to show a clinical improvement.
2. **False.** NSAIDs do not slow disease progression; indeed, some evidence suggests they may hasten progress of the disease.
3. **True.** The second-line drugs take a long time to act (4–6 months), but they should be discontinued if there is no sign of improvement by that time.
4. **True.** Proteinuria occurs associated with immune-complex nephritis. Only 15% of people continue with gold treatment after 5–6 years because of unwanted effects.
5. **True.** Methotrexate is an immunosuppressant often chosen as initial disease-modifying therapy for rheumatoid arthritis because of its relatively rapid onset of action (4–6 weeks).
6. **False.** The mode of action of methotrexate in arthritis is inhibition of the deamination of adenosine, but it also inhibits reduction of folic acid to dihydrofolate and tetrahydrofolate, which are essential for nucleotide synthesis. Folic acid can be given daily to prevent the resulting gastrointestinal and haematological complications.
7. **True.** More than 50% of people who take methotrexate for rheumatoid arthritis continue taking the drug for 5 years or more, but a similar proportion have to cease treatment with most other DMARDs within 2 years.
8. **True.** Sulfasalazine is converted in the colon to 5-aminosalicylic acid, which is the active moiety in the treatment of inflammatory bowel disease, and to sulfapyridine, which is probably the main active moiety in rheumatoid arthritis.
9. **False.** The combination of methotrexate with ciclosporin, sulfasalazine or hydroxychloroquine has shown significant benefit in people with severe rheumatoid disease.
10. **True.** The active metabolite of leflunomide inhibits synthesis of uridine monophosphate, and this slows the proliferation of T- and B-lymphocytes.

11. **False.** Corticosteroids can give dramatic relief of symptoms in rheumatoid arthritis, but there is no evidence they slow progression of the disease.

12. **True.** Adrenal atrophy caused by negative feedback on the hypothalamo–pituitary–adrenal axis can last for many months following prolonged treatment.

13. **False.** Hydroxychloroquine can cause remission of rheumatoid arthritis but does not slow the progression of joint damage.

14. **True.** Rituximab depletes B-lymphocytes by binding to their CD20 surface antigen.

15. **True.** Adalimumab, golimumab and other TNFα inhibitors are the most commonly used biological agents for moderate–severe rheumatoid arthritis, usually in combination with methotrexate or other DMARDs.

16. **True.** Abatacept blocks the CD80 and CD86 co-stimulatory molecules on antigen-presenting cells, preventing their interaction with CD28 on T-lymphocytes.

17. **False.** They are cytokine receptor antagonists; anakinra is an IL-1 receptor antagonist, and tocilizumab blocks IL-6 receptors.

18. **False.** There is limited evidence proving the efficacy of DMARDs in the spondyloarthritides; TNFα inhibitors may be effective in inducing remission.

Case-based answers

1. The brief duration of the symptoms and their mild nature warrant the initial administration of an NSAID, such as ibuprofen, and follow-up.

2. The persistence of the symptoms and their spread to the knees suggest that a DMARD should be started. Guidelines now advise that DMARDs should be considered for persistent inflammatory joint disease of more than 8 weeks' duration.

3. Methotrexate is a DMARD that requires folate supplements (see the answer to the OBA question 6, given previously). Methotrexate takes 4–6 weeks for its onset of action. Methotrexate and an NSAID (or a corticosteroid) should be given together to cover this interim period.

FURTHER READING

Rheumatoid arthritis and other inflammatory arthritides

Donahue, K.E., Gartlehner, G., Jonas, D.E., et al., 2008. Systematic review: comparative effectiveness and harms of disease-modifying medications for rheumatoid arthritis. Ann. Intern. Med. 148, 162–163.

Dougados, M., Baeten, D., 2011. Spondyloarthritis. Lancet 377, 2127–2137.

Goldblatt, F., O'Neill, S.G., 2013. Clinical aspects of autoimmune rheumatic disease. Lancet 382, 797–808.

Klarenbeek, N.B., Kerstens, P.J., Huizinga, T.W., et al., 2010. Recent advances in the management of rheumatoid arthritis. BMJ 341, c6942.

Murphy, G., Lisnevskaia, L., Isenberg, D., 2013. Systemic lupus erythematosus and other autoimmune rheumatic diseases: challenges to treatment. Lancet 382, 809–831.

Palazzi, C., D'Angelo, S., Gilio, M., et al., 2015. Pharmacological therapy of spondyloarthritis. Expert Opin. Pharmacother. 16, 1495–1504.

Smolen, J.S., Aletaha, D., McInnes, I.B., 2016. Rheumatoid arthritis. Lancet 388, 2023–2038.

Osteoarthritis

Gallagher, B., Tjoumakaris, F.P., Harwood, M.I., et al., 2015. Chondroprotection and the prevention of osteoarthritis progression of the knee: a systematic review of treatment agents. Am. J. Sports Med. 43, 734–744.

Glyn-Jones, S., Palmer, A.J.R., Agricola, R., et al., 2015. Osteoarthritis. Lancet 386, 376–387.

Hunter, D.J., Felson, D.T., 2006. Osteoarthritis. BMJ 332, 639–642.

Compendium: disease-modifying antirheumatic drugs

Drug	Characteristics
For NSAIDs see Chapter 29, and for corticosteroids see Chapter 44.	
Aurothiomalate (sodium salt)	Gold compound. Given by deep intramuscular injection for active progressive rheumatoid arthritis and juvenile arthritis. Half-life: 250 days
Chloroquine	Antimalarial drug (see Chapter 51). Given orally for moderate active rheumatoid arthritis and juvenile arthritis. Half-life: 1–3 weeks
Hydroxychloroquine	Antimalarial drug (see Chapter 51). Given orally for moderate active rheumatoid arthritis and juvenile arthritis. Half-life: 18 days
Penicillamine	Given orally for active progressive rheumatoid arthritis. Half-life: 1–6 h
Sulfasalazine	Antiinflammatory drug. Given orally for active rheumatoid arthritis; also used for ulcerative colitis (see Chapter 34). Converted in the gut to 5-aminosalicylate (half-life: 4–10 h) and sulfapyridine (half-life: 6–17 h)

Compendium: disease-modifying antirheumatic drugs (cont'd)

Drug	Characteristics
Drugs suppressing the immune response	
Azathioprine	Immunosuppressant. Given orally for moderate to severe rheumatoid arthritis in people who have not responded to other DMARDs; more toxic than methotrexate and used for those who have not responded to methotrexate. See Chapter 38 for more details
Ciclosporin	Calcineurin inhibitor. Given orally or intravenously for severe active rheumatoid arthritis when conventional second-line therapy is inappropriate or ineffective. See Chapter 38 for more details
Cyclophosphamide	Given orally for rheumatoid arthritis with severe systemic manifestations when response to other DMARDs has been inadequate; also used in cancer treatment (see Chapter 52)
Leflunomide	Given orally for moderate to severe rheumatoid arthritis; more toxic than methotrexate and used for people who have not responded to methotrexate. Prodrug converted to active metabolite, which has a half-life of 2 weeks
Methotrexate	Front-line DMARD for moderate to severe rheumatoid arthritis; given orally, subcutaneously or intramuscularly; also used in cancer (see Chapter 52)
Cytokine modulators and other immunobiological drugs	
Recombinant human proteins; should be used under specialised supervision.	
Abatacept	Monoclonal antibody against CD80/CD86 co-stimulatory molecules. Given by intravenous infusion in severe rheumatoid arthritis in those uncontrolled by other DMARDs, including a TNFα inhibitor and rituximab. Half-life: 14 days
Adalimumab	Fully humanised monoclonal antibody against TNFα; used in combination with methotrexate for moderate to severe active rheumatoid arthritis when response to other DMARDs has been inadequate. Given by subcutaneous injection. Half-life: 12 days
Anakinra	IL-1 receptor antagonist. Licensed for rheumatoid arthritis, but not recommended for routine use in United Kingdom. Given by daily subcutaneous injection. Half-life: 4–6 h
Apremilast	Phosphodiesterase type-4 inhibitor with antiinflammatory activity. Given orally as monotherapy or in combination with DMARDs in psoriatic arthritis. Half-life: 9 h
Belimumab	Inhibitor of BLyS. Licensed as adjunctive therapy for arthritis in active, severe, poorly controlled systemic lupus erythematosus. Given by monthly intravenous infusion. Half-life: 19 days
Certolizumab pegol	Pegylated Fab fragment of monoclonal antibody against TNFα; used in combination with methotrexate for moderate to severe active rheumatoid arthritis when response to other DMARDs has been inadequate. Given by subcutaneous injection every 2 or 4 weeks. Half-life: 14 days
Etanercept	Fusion protein of TNFα receptor components with IgG. Used for severe, active and progressive rheumatoid arthritis which has failed to respond to at least two standard DMARDs. Given by subcutaneous injection weekly or twice weekly. Half-life: 5 days
Golimumab	Fully humanised monoclonal antibody against TNFα; used with methotrexate for moderate to severe active rheumatoid arthritis when response to other DMARDs has been inadequate. Given by monthly subcutaneous injection. Half-life: 7–20 days
Infliximab	Monoclonal antibody against TNFα; used for severe, active and progressive rheumatoid arthritis which has failed to respond to at least two standard DMARDs. Given by intravenous infusion every 8 weeks. Half-life: 8–10 days
Rituximab	Monoclonal antibody against CD20 that depletes B-lymphocyte precursors and mature B-cells; used in people with moderate–severe active rheumatoid arthritis who have an inadequate response to DMARDs and a TNFα inhibitor. Given by intravenous infusion at a 2-week interval. Half-life: 3–8 days
Tocilizumab	Monoclonal antibody against IL-6 receptors; used in people with moderate–severe rheumatoid arthritis when response to at least one DMARD or TNFα inhibitor has been inadequate. Given by monthly intravenous infusion. Half-life: 6 days

BLyS, B-lymphocyte stimulator; *DMARDs*, disease-modifying antirheumatic drugs; *IFNα*, interferon α; *IgG*, immunoglobulin G; *IL*, interleukin; *NSAIDs*, nonsteroidal antiinflammatory drugs; *TNFα*, tumour necrosis factor α.

31

Hyperuricaemia and gout

THE PATHOPHYSIOLOGY OF GOUT

Gout is the most common inflammatory arthritis which arises when monosodium urate crystals are deposited in cartilage, bone and periarticular tissues and subsequently shed into the joint space. Gout is associated with a persistently raised plasma uric acid (urate) concentration (although the concentration may be normal during an acute attack). The major source of plasma uric acid is catabolism of the nucleic acid purine bases guanine and adenine (Fig. 31.1), with about 30% derived from dietary purines. Uric acid is relatively insoluble in water. Its immediate metabolic precursors are xanthine and hypoxanthine, which are more water-soluble. Most uric acid is normally eliminated by the kidney, with about 30% lost through the gut. Uric acid is filtered at the glomerulus, but more than 90% is reabsorbed in the early proximal tubule. An amount equivalent to 6–10% of the filtered load is secreted into tubular fluid by an active organic acid transporter in the second part of the proximal tubule.

Hyperuricaemia has many causes:

- Overproduction of uric acid due to:
  - excessive cell destruction (e.g. treatment of lymphoproliferative or myeloproliferative disorders);
  - inherited defects that increase purine synthesis;
  - high purine intake (such as red meat, fish, beer and spirits);
  - metabolic syndrome (obesity, insulin resistance, hypertension and hyperlipidaemia).
- Reduced renal excretion of uric acid accounts for at least 80% of cases of gout and may be caused by:
  - reduced tubular uric acid secretion, which may have a genetic component;
  - renal failure;
  - drugs that compete for the tubular transporter for uric acid (e.g. loop and thiazide-type diuretics, ciclosporin). Low-dose aspirin also reduces uric acid excretion, but the effect is probably clinically insignificant.

A high plasma concentration of uric acid is often an incidental finding and does not always lead to symptoms; only 10% of people with hyperuricaemia will develop gout. Monosodium urate crystal deposition in tissues begins when the plasma uric acid concentration exceeds about 0.42 mmol/L. However, gout only develops when the crystals are shed into the joint space, where they are phagocytosed by neutrophils, macrophages, mast cells and dendritic cells within the synovium, which release inflammatory cytokines such as interleukin-1β. These mediators activate mast cells and endothelial cells, which express adhesion molecules and release inflammatory chemokines. Uric acid crystals also provide a surface on which complement C5 is cleaved, with formation of complement membrane attack complex. Activated endothelial cells and complement membrane attack complex attract neutrophil leucocytes, which release proteolytic and lysosomal enzymes that enhance tissue inflammation, destroy cartilage and damage the joint. Most attacks of gout are self-limiting, probably in part due to coating of the uric acid crystals with protein, which reduces their irritant properties.

Gout is more common with increasing age. In younger people, it usually affects a single joint (often initially the first metatarsalphalangeal joint), with repeated acute attacks of arthritis affecting other joints if the underlying cause is not treated. Acute gout usually presents with rapid onset of severe joint pain that reaches maximum intensity within 24 hours. In the elderly, a chronic arthritis affecting multiple joints (midfoot, ankle, knee, finger joints, wrist and elbow) with progressive joint damage can occur. A definitive diagnosis of gout requires the demonstration of monosodium urate crystals in the affected joint, but a clinical diagnosis is usually adequate if symptoms are classical.

With persistent hyperuricaemia, impacted uric acid crystal deposits (tophi) are sometimes found in tendon sheaths and

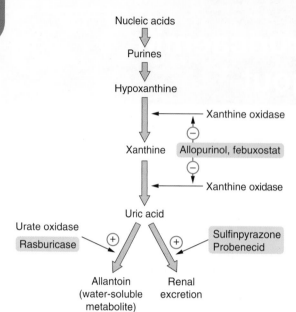

Nucleic acids

↓

Purines

↓

Hypoxanthine

← Xanthine oxidase

⊖

Xanthine   Allopurinol, febuxostat

⊖

← Xanthine oxidase

Uric acid

Urate oxidase

Rasburicase → ⊕   ⊕ ← Sulfinpyrazone
                                    Probenecid

Allantoin   Renal
(water-soluble   excretion
metabolite)

Fig. 31.1 The pathway for production of uric acid from purines and the sites of action of some of the drugs used in gout and hyperuricaemia.

soft tissues. Excess uric acid can also be deposited in the interstitium of the kidney or can form stones in the renal calyces, both of which can produce progressive renal damage.

Pseudogout, due to deposition of calcium pyrophosphate crystals in the joint space, has a similar clinical presentation to acute gout.

There are two components of drug treatment for gout:

- treatment of an acute attack of gout;
- reduction of plasma uric acid concentration for prophylaxis against recurrent attacks of gout or to prevent kidney damage.

DRUGS FOR THE TREATMENT OF GOUT AND PREVENTION OF HYPERURICAEMIA

COLCHICINE

Mechanism of action and uses

Colchicine interferes with recruitment and function of neutrophil leucocytes in the gouty joint. It disrupts the assembly of microtubules in neutrophil leucocytes by forming a complex with tubulin in the cell. Microtubules have many functions in the cell, and the action of colchicine impairs the adhesion of neutrophils to endothelial cells, which reduces their recruitment into the inflamed joint, and also impairs phagocytosis of crystals if the neutrophil does enter the joint. In addition, if crystals are phagocytosed into the neutrophil, then the effect

of colchicine inhibits the subsequent release of enzymes and free radicals that damage the joint. Colchicine has other actions that probably contribute to its effects in gout, such as increased production of antiinflammatory molecules and increased activity of the antioxidant redox system.

All of these actions give colchicine a specific antiinflammatory effect in the gouty joint. Colchicine is also effective in pseudogout, which has a mechanism of inflammation similar to gout, but it is ineffective in other forms of inflammatory arthritis. Other uses of colchicine include the management of recurrent pericarditis and familial Mediterranean fever.

Pharmacokinetics

Colchicine is well absorbed from the gut. It is usually given every 6–12 hours until symptomatic relief is achieved or unwanted effects occur. Pain relief usually begins after about 18 hours and is maximal by 48 hours.

Unwanted effects

Colchicine has a low therapeutic index, so unwanted effects are common and often dose-limiting. These include:

- Gut toxicity caused by inhibition of mucosal cell division, which produces abdominal pain, nausea, vomiting and diarrhoea.
- Rash.

XANTHINE OXIDASE INHIBITORS

allopurinol, febuxostat

Mechanism of action

Allopurinol is an analogue of hypoxanthine, which is an intermediate in the pathway that generates uric acid. Both allopurinol and its major metabolite (oxipurinol) competitively inhibit the enzyme xanthine oxidase for which hypoxanthine is the natural substrate, thereby reducing uric acid formation (see Fig. 31.1). Febuxostat is a nonpurine, selective xanthine oxidase inhibitor. Although plasma xanthine and hypoxanthine concentrations increase when these drugs are given, they do not crystallise. Because of their greater water solubility, their concentrations remain well below saturation levels, even with maximal xanthine oxidase inhibition. Xanthine and hypoxanthine are reincorporated into the purine synthetic cycle, which decreases the need for de novo purine formation.

Pharmacokinetics

Allopurinol is well absorbed from the gut and converted in the liver to an active metabolite with a long half-life, oxipurinol (alloxanthine). Both allopurinol and its metabolite undergo renal excretion. Febuxostat is well absorbed from the gut and eliminated by both metabolism and renal excretion with a variable half-life (1–15 hours).

Unwanted effects

- Gastrointestinal upset.
- An increased risk of acute gout during the first few weeks of treatment; this may be caused by fluctuations in plasma uric acid, possibly through uric acid release from tissue deposits.
- Hypersensitivity reactions with allopurinol, especially in people with renal impairment. These reactions include serious rashes such as Stevens–Johnson syndrome or toxic epidermal necrolysis.
- Drug interactions: Allopurinol and febuxostat inhibit the metabolism of the cytotoxic drugs mercaptopurine and azathioprine (see Chapter 52) because these are also metabolised by xanthine oxidase.

RASBURICASE

Mechanism of action

Rasburicase is a recombinant version of the enzyme urate oxidase, which catalyses the oxidation of uric acid to a soluble metabolite, allantoin. This enzyme is present in mammals other than humans; the recombinant version is produced by a genetically modified strain of the fungus *Aspergillus flavus*. Rasburicase is used for prophylaxis of hyperuricaemia during treatment of malignancies with chemotherapy.

Pharmacokinetics

Rasburicase is given intravenously and is metabolised by peptide hydrolysis in plasma.

Unwanted effects

- Fever.
- Nausea, vomiting, diarrhoea.
- Hypersensitivity reactions: Rasburicase induces antibody responses in about 10% of those treated, although allergic reactions such as rash, bronchospasm and anaphylaxis are rare.
- Haemolysis from the production of hydrogen peroxide as a by-product of the formation of allantoin.

URICOSURIC AGENTS

 Examples

lesinurad, sulfinpyrazone

Mechanism of action

Sulfinpyrazone and lesinurad competitively inhibit the urate anion transporter (URAT1) responsible for reabsorption of uric acid in the proximal tubule. They increase urate excretion in urine and reduce the concentration in plasma. There is a risk of precipitation of uric acid crystals in the kidney, particularly during the early stages of treatment, which can be prevented by maintaining a high fluid intake and alkaline urine (using potassium citrate or sodium bicarbonate) and by slowly titrating the dose. Aspirin and other salicylates should not be given with uricosuric drugs, because low doses of salicylates inhibit tubular uric acid secretion.

Pharmacokinetics

Sulfinpyrazone and lesinurad are eliminated by hepatic metabolism and have half-lives of 4–5 hours.

Unwanted effects

- Gastrointestinal upset.
- Renal uric acid deposition; deterioration of renal function can occur, especially if there is preexisting renal impairment.
- Allergic rashes.
- Headache with lesinurad.

TREATMENT OF GOUT

ACUTE GOUT

For acute attacks of gout, nonsteroidal antiinflammatory drugs (NSAIDs; see Chapter 29) are the treatment of choice. Cyclo-oxygenase 2 (COX-2)-selective antiinflammatory drugs are as effective as nonselective NSAIDs (see Chapter 29). Colchicine is usually reserved for people who are intolerant of NSAIDs, or who have a contraindication to their use. Colchicine was once used in high doses, which often produce vomiting or diarrhoea, but smaller doses are better tolerated and equally effective.

Intra-articular injection of a corticosteroid can be very effective if a single joint is involved, especially if other treatments are contraindicated. Oral corticosteroids (e.g. prednisolone; see Chapter 44) are reserved for resistant episodes of gout. A 5-day high-dose regimen can be used, or alternatively 2 days of a high dose followed by a gradual reduction over 8–12 days to minimise the risk of a rebound flare of symptoms.

Rest and joint cooling with ice can provide benefits in addition to drug therapy.

PREVENTION OF GOUT ATTACKS

The long-term aim of the treatment of gout is to prevent uric acid crystal formation and dissolve existing crystals by lowering the serum uric acid concentration. Efforts should always be made to identify and remove precipitating causes, particularly enquiring about diet and alcohol intake and reviewing concurrent drug therapy.

Allopurinol is the first-line drug for prophylaxis against recurrent attacks of acute gout, for chronic tophus formation in the tissues, or for the prevention of uric acid-induced renal damage. It is also given prophylactically before cytotoxic chemotherapy, when tissue breakdown releases purines which generate large amounts of uric acid. To prevent gout, the serum uric acid concentration should be reduced to less than 0.36 mmol/L, although it may be necessary to go below 0.30 mmol/L to reabsorb gouty tophi.

Allopurinol is often started 2–4 weeks after an acute attack of gout to reduce the risk of exacerbating the attack, but delaying treatment is probably not necessary. There are two strategies that will reduce the risk of provoking an attack when allopurinol is started in someone with hyperuricaemia. First, a low dosage of allopurinol can be given initially with slow dose titration until the target plasma uric acid concentration is achieved. Secondly, low dosage of an NSAID or colchicine can be given during the first 3–6 months of treatment. Febuxostat and sulfinpyrazone are reserved for people who do not tolerate allopurinol. Sulfinpyrazone is also used in combination with allopurinol for resistant hyperuricaemia. The latest option for management of resistant hyperuricaemia is the renal urate transport inhibitor lesinurad, used together with allopurinol. Low-dose NSAIDs or colchicine are sometimes used long-term to prevent gout, although good data on their efficacy are lacking. Rasburicase is used when intravenous prophylaxis against gout is required during cancer chemotherapy.

Prophylactic treatment should usually be lifelong, since recurrence of gout or tophi frequently occurs if treatment is stopped. However, during cytotoxic chemotherapy, only short-term prophylaxis is needed to prevent gout.

SELF-ASSESSMENT

One-best-answer (OBA) question

Choose the *most appropriate* statement concerning drugs used in the treatment of gout.
A. Sodium urate is more water-soluble than its precursor, hypoxanthine.
B. Febuxostat is a purine analogue.
C. Allopurinol enhances the renal secretion of uric acid.
D. Colchicine inhibits the release of neutrophil proteases that cause joint damage.
E. Celecoxib is more effective in reducing pain and inflammation in acute attacks of gout than naproxen.

Case-based questions

A 56-year-old man awoke in the night with sudden severe pain in his first metatarsophalangeal joint, which lasted for 1 week. Over the next few months, he had similar acute episodes of pain in his ankles and knees, as well as his big toe. He had hypertension but no other vascular disease. The general practitioner (GP) suspected gout and referred him to a specialist.
1. What treatment should the GP institute for the acute attacks, prior to the specialist diagnosis?
2. What test could the rheumatologist do to confirm the suspected diagnosis?
3. The diagnosis of gout was confirmed. What is the cause of gout?
4. What would you prescribe for prophylaxis to reduce recurrent attacks, and how does this agent act?

5. The chosen treatment was only partially effective; what additional treatment could you prescribe?
6. What might be the consequences of inadequate treatment of this man?

ANSWERS

One-best-answer (OBA) answer

Answer D is correct.
A. Incorrect. Hypoxanthine is more water-soluble than urate; this is the rationale for the use of allopurinol, which inhibits conversion of hypoxanthine to urate by inhibiting xanthine oxidase.
B. Incorrect. Febuxostat is a nonpurine inhibitor of xanthine oxidase.
C. Incorrect. Allopurinol prevents uric acid formation; the renal secretion of urate is enhanced by sulfinpyrazone and lesinurad, which inhibit the URAT1 transporter responsible for its renal reabsorption.
D. **Correct.** Reducing neutrophil leucocyte activity is one of the antiinflammatory mechanisms of colchicine in gout.
E. Incorrect. The COX-2 selective inhibitor celecoxib is no more effective than NSAIDs such as naproxen in acute gout.

Case-based answers

1. The treatment of choice for an acute attack is an NSAID to reduce pain and inflammation. Indometacin is often used and is effective within 2 days. Colchicine or corticosteroids can be used in people intolerant to NSAIDs, but both have significant unwanted effects.
2. Plasma uric acid will be raised. An arthrocentesis sample will show sodium urate crystals. Infection should be excluded in an acutely inflamed joint.
3. Gout is caused by relatively insoluble sodium urate, a product of purine metabolism, crystallising in the joint space. People who develop gout have had hyperuricaemia for years. Overproduction of uric acid due to dietary purines (e.g. in meat and fish) or excessive alcohol consumption can contribute to gout, but in most people hyperuricaemia is caused by impaired renal clearance of uric acid.
4. Hyperuricaemia is treated after resolution of the acute attack. People who overproduce uric acid are best treated with allopurinol, which reduces plasma uric acid by inhibiting xanthine oxidase. This increases concentrations of hypoxanthine and xanthine, which are more water-soluble than urate.
5. A low renal excretion of uric acid may be treated with a uricosuric drug (sulfinpyrazone); this inhibits the reabsorption of uric acid in the proximal convoluted tubule.
6. Untreated gout can lead to chronic joint damage and the formation of kidney stones. A significant number of people with gout will have hypertension and increased risk of cardiovascular and renal disease.

FURTHER READING

Dalbeth, N., Merriman, T.R., Stamp, L.K., 2016. Gout. Lancet 388, 2039–2052.

Rees, F., Hui, M., Doherty, M., 2014. Optimizing current treatment of gout. Nat. Rev. Rheumatol. 10, 271–283.

Roddy, E., Mallen, C.D., Doherty, M., 2013. Gout. Br. Med. J. 347, f5648.

Compendium: drugs used for gout and hyperuricaemia

Drug	Characteristics
For nonsteroidal antiinflammatory drugs used in gout, see Chapter 29.	
Allopurinol	Xanthine oxidase inhibitor. Given orally for prophylaxis of gout and of hyperuricaemia associated with cancer chemotherapy. Rapidly converted to active metabolite (oxipurinol) which has a long half-life (10–40 h)
Colchicine	Anti-inflammatory drug. Given orally for acute gout and short-term prophylaxis during initial therapy with other drugs. Half-life: <1 h
Febuxostat	Nonpurine xanthine oxidase inhibitor. Given as oral prophylaxis in people who are intolerant to allopurinol or when allupurinol is contraindicated. Half-life: 1–15 h
Lesinurad	New uricosuric drug (URAT1 inhibitor). Given orally (with allopurinol) for resistant hyperuricaemia. Half-life: 5 h
Probenecid	Uricosuric drug. Given orally to prevent nephrotoxicity associated with use of the antiretroviral drug cidofovir; only available on special order in the United Kingdom. Half-life: 4–17 h
Rasburicase	Recombinant form of fungal urate oxidase which converts urate to soluble allantoin. Given intravenously for hyperuricaemia during initial chemotherapy of haematological malignancy. Half-life: 18–22 h
Sulfinpyrazone	Uricosuric drug (URAT1 inhibitor). Given orally for gout prophylaxis and hyperuricaemia. Half-life: 4–5 h

7

The gastrointestinal system

32

Nausea and vomiting

NAUSEA AND VOMITING

Nausea, retching and vomiting (emesis) are part of the body's defence against ingested toxins. Vomiting is a protective reflex that removes toxic agents from the gut before absorption. The reflex is integrated by a loose neuronal network known as the *vomiting centre* (VC) in the medulla oblongata of the brain stem. Afferent input to the VC comes from several sources (Fig. 32.1):

- Pro-emetic abdominal and cardiac vagal afferents, which are activated by mechano- or chemosensory receptors. Chemosensory receptors respond to several agonists released from enterochromaffin cells or mast cells in response to emetogenic stimuli. These include acetylcholine, dopamine, serotonin, prostaglandins, histamine and various neurokinins.
- The chemoreceptor trigger zone (CTZ), which is located in the area postrema in the floor of the fourth ventricle. It lies outside the blood–brain barrier and responds to stimuli from both the cerebrospinal fluid and the systemic circulation including drugs (Box 32.1), metabolic products and bacterial toxins. The CTZ has receptors for neurotransmitters such as dopamine (D_2), serotonin ($5HT_3$) and substance P (NK_1); it has numerous afferent and efferent connections with the underlying nucleus tractus solitarius.
- The vestibular nuclei, which are involved in the emetic response to motion (muscarinic and histamine H_1 receptors).
- Other brainstem structures, such as the amygdala.

- Higher centres of the cortex and intracranial pressure receptors.

Vomiting can result from the summation of several subemetic stimuli – for example, in the genesis of postoperative nausea and vomiting. Several neurotransmitter receptors are found in the VC, including those for dopamine (D_2), serotonin ($5HT_2$), acetylcholine (muscarinic) and histamine (H_1) (see Fig. 32.1). The roles of these multiple receptors in the triggering of nausea and vomiting are complex.

Efferent connections from the VC include the vagus and phrenic nerves. When stimulated, these nerves relax the fundus and body of the stomach and the lower oesophageal sphincter; then retrograde giant contractions occur in the small intestine. Contractions of the diaphragmatic and abdominal muscle compress the stomach, and together these factors produce vomiting.

ANTI-EMETIC AGENTS

The efficacy of anti-emetic agents varies according to the trigger for vomiting. All anti-emetic drugs are relatively ineffective for treating nausea and retching.

Antihistamines

Examples

cyclizine, promethazine

Mechanism of action and clinical use

Antihistamines prevent and treat vomiting by their antagonist action at histamine H_1 receptors (see Chapter 39), and many also have antimuscarinic effects. Promethazine also blocks some 5-HT receptor subtypes. Antihistamines are effective against most causes of vomiting but, apart from the use of cyclizine for drug-induced vomiting, they are rarely treatments of choice. Promethazine is used to treat vomiting in pregnancy, since it appears to be free from teratogenic effects.

Pharmacokinetics

These drugs are well absorbed orally; both promethazine and cyclizine can also be given by intramuscular or intravenous injection. After oral dosing, promethazine undergoes extensive first-pass metabolism. The half-life of promethazine is 7–14 hours and that of cyclizine 20 hours.

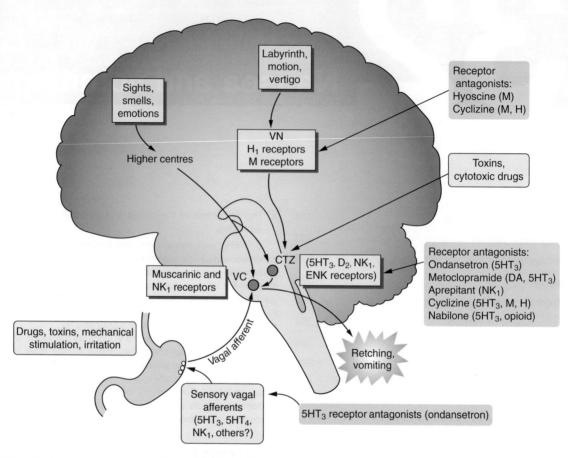

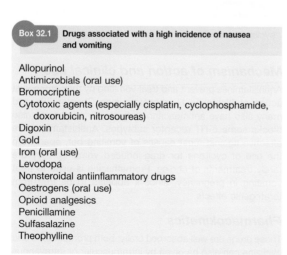

Fig. 32.1 **Neuronal pathways and receptors involved in the control of nausea and vomiting.** The pathways and neurotransmitter receptors involved in nausea and vomiting are complex; only those underpinning the mechanisms of action of the anti-emetic drugs are shown. The chemoreceptor trigger zone (CTZ) has neuronal connections to the vomiting centre (VC), which is a collection of nuclei including the dorsal motor nucleus of the vagus and the nucleus tractus solitarius. *5HT₃,* 5-Hydroxytryptamine type 3 receptor; *DA,* dopamine receptor; *ENK,* enkephalin (opioid) receptor; *H₁,* histamine type 1 receptor; *M,* muscarinic receptor (possibly M₂); *NK₁,* neurokinin 1 receptor; *VN,* vestibular nuclei. Other mediators such as glutamate may also be involved.

Box 32.1	Drugs associated with a high incidence of nausea and vomiting

Allopurinol
Antimicrobials (oral use)
Bromocriptine
Cytotoxic agents (especially cisplatin, cyclophosphamide, doxorubicin, nitrosoureas)
Digoxin
Gold
Iron (oral use)
Levodopa
Nonsteroidal antiinflammatory drugs
Oestrogens (oral use)
Opioid analgesics
Penicillamine
Sulfasalazine
Theophylline

Unwanted effects

- Sedation (particularly with promethazine) and headache.
- Antimuscarinic effects (see Chapter 4), especially dry mouth, urinary retention and blurred vision.

Antimuscarinic agent

Example

hyoscine

Mechanism of action and clinical use

Muscarinic receptors are involved in the visceral afferent input from the gut to the VC and in the eighth cranial nerve connection from the labyrinth to the CTZ via the vestibular nucleus. Hyoscine (scopolamine in the United States) is used for the treatment of motion sickness and postoperative vomiting. Some antihistamines such as promethazine and cyclizine (see earlier) and dopamine receptor antagonists such as prochlorperazine (see below) also have antimuscarinic activity.

Pharmacokinetics

Hyoscine is available for oral, parenteral or transdermal use. Oral absorption is good and the half-life is 8 hours. The adhesive patch for transdermal delivery is usually placed behind the ear and delivers a therapeutic dose for 72 hours.

Unwanted effects

- Typical antimuscarinic actions such as dry mouth, urinary retention and blurred vision (see Chapter 4).
- Sedation.

Dopamine receptor antagonists

 Examples

domperidone, levomepromazine, metoclopramide, prochlorperazine

Mechanism of action and clinical use

Domperidone, metoclopramide and the antipsychotic drugs are antagonists at dopamine D_2 receptors and inhibit dopaminergic stimulation of the CTZ (see Fig. 32.1). Anti-emetic doses of antipsychotic drugs are generally less than one third of those used to treat psychoses. The pharmacology of the antipsychotic drugs is discussed in Chapter 21.

Domperidone acts solely by dopamine receptor blockade and does not readily cross the blood–brain barrier. Metoclopramide is a dopamine receptor antagonist at usual oral doses but also acts as a 5-HT_3 receptor antagonist at higher doses. Metoclopramide also has prokinetic actions on the gut due to agonist activity at the 5-HT_4 receptor subtype in the enteric nervous system. It increases tone in the gastro-oesophageal sphincter and enhances both gastric emptying and small intestinal motility.

Dopamine receptor antagonists are mainly used to reduce vomiting induced by radiotherapy, drugs and surgery. The dual-receptor action of metoclopramide gives enhanced efficacy; it is used at high doses intravenously to treat delayed vomiting induced by emetogenic cytotoxic agents such as cisplatin. Levomepromazine is used to relieve vomiting in palliative care. Domperidone and metoclopramide are ineffective for vomiting arising from stimulation of the vestibular system. Antipsychotic drugs such as prochlorperazine are effective for vestibular disorders and motion sickness owing to their antimuscarinic activity.

Pharmacokinetics

Metoclopramide and domperidone are well absorbed orally and undergo extensive first-pass metabolism in the liver. Metoclopramide is also available for intravenous or intramuscular use, while domperidone can be given rectally by suppository. Metoclopramide has a shorter half-life (3–5 hours) than domperidone (12–16 hours).

Unwanted effects

Unwanted effects on the central nervous system (CNS) are produced by metoclopramide and the antipsychotics and to a lesser extent by domperidone as a result of its lower CNS penetration.

- Acute and chronic extrapyramidal effects from dopamine receptor blockade in the basal ganglia can lead to acute dystonias (especially in girls, young women and the very elderly), akathisia and a parkinsonian-like syndrome. Tardive dyskinesias can develop with prolonged use (see also Chapter 24). Because of the risk of neurological adverse effects, metoclopramide should not be taken for more than 5 days.
- Galactorrhoea, gynaecomastia and amenorrhoea caused by hyperprolactinaemia from pituitary dopamine receptor blockade.
- Dry mouth (with domperidone), diarrhoea.
- Domperidone can cause serious ventricular arrhythmias due to QT prolongation on the electrocardiogram (ECG). Its use should be limited to no more than 7 days.

5-HT₃ receptor antagonists

 Examples

granisetron, ondansetron, palonosetron

Mechanism of action and clinical use

The 5-HT_3 receptor antagonists act at receptors in the CTZ and the gut (see Fig. 32.1). They are particularly effective against the acute vomiting induced by highly emetogenic chemotherapeutic agents used for treating cancer (e.g. cisplatin; see Chapter 52) and for postoperative vomiting. They are also used for prophylaxis before surgery when the consequences of retching and vomiting could be particularly deleterious, as after eye surgery.

Pharmacokinetics

Oral absorption of ondansetron is rapid; it has a short half-life of 3 hours. It can also be given by intravenous or intramuscular injection or by rectal suppository. Granisetron has a similar profile and is available for oral, intravenous or transdermal use. Palonosetron has a long half-life of 40 hours and is given orally or intravenously.

Unwanted effects

- Headache, insomnia dizziness, drowsiness.
- Constipation, probably caused by 5-HT_3 receptor blockade in the gut.
- Flushing.
- Prolongation of the Q–T interval on the ECG at high doses, which predisposes to arrhythmias.

Neurokinin 1 receptor antagonists

 Examples

aprepitant, fosaprepitant

Mechanism of action

Aprepitant and its prodrug fosaprepitant are antagonists at NK_1 receptors in the CNS, inhibiting the action of substance P. They augment the effects of 5-HT_3 receptor antagonists and corticosteroids in preventing the acute and delayed emetic response to the cancer chemotherapeutic agent cisplatin.

Pharmacokinetics

Aprepitant is well absorbed from the gut and has a long half-life of 9–13 hours. Fosaprepitant is rapidly converted to aprepitant in the liver and several other tissues. It is given by intravenous infusion.

Unwanted effects

- Fatigue, dizziness, headache, hiccups.
- Anorexia, dyspepsia, constipation, diarrhoea.

Cannabinoids

nabilone

Mechanism of action and clinical use

Nabilone, a synthetic derivative of tetrahydrocannabinol (a psychoactive substance in cannabis; see Chapter 54), is effective in combating vomiting induced by cytotoxic drugs provided that it is given before chemotherapy is started. The mechanism is uncertain but may involve inhibition of cortical activity and anxiolysis. Cannabinoid CB_1 receptors are found in several areas of the CNS and the action of nabilone at these receptors may inhibit neuronal serotonin release in the dorsal vagal nucleus.

Pharmacokinetics

Nabilone is well absorbed from the gut. It is metabolised extensively in the liver and has a short half-life, but some of its metabolites have long half-lives and may contribute to the activity.

Unwanted effects

- Sedation, dizziness, ataxia, sleep disturbance.
- Dry mouth.
- Dysphoric reactions with hallucinations and disorientation are most disturbing to older people. These may be reduced by the concurrent use of prochlorperazine (see dopamine receptor antagonists, discussed previously).

Corticosteroids

Dexamethasone and methylprednisolone are weak anti-emetics. However, they produce additive effects when given with other anti-emetic drugs. High doses of dexamethasone can be given intravenously before cancer chemotherapy, with subsequent oral doses to prevent delayed emesis. The mechanism of action is unknown but may involve the reduction of prostaglandin synthesis or release of endorphins. The pharmacology of corticosteroids is discussed in Chapter 44.

Table 32.1 Common indications for various anti-emetic agents

Cause of vomiting	Treatment
Motion sickness	Hyoscine, cyclizine, promethazine
Postoperative vomiting	Hyoscine, metoclopramide, domperidone, prochlorperazine, ondansetron (reserved for resistant vomiting)
Drug-induced vomiting	Prochlorperazine, metoclopramide, cyclizine (particularly for opioid-induced vomiting)
Cytotoxic drug-induced vomiting	Prochlorperazine, metoclopramide, nabilone, ondansetron, aprepitant Adjunctive treatment (e.g. dexamethasone, benzodiazepines)
Pregnancy-induced vomiting	Promethazine, metoclopramide, pyridoxine

Benzodiazepines

Benzodiazepines, such as lorazepam, have no intrinsic anti-emetic activity. They are given orally or intravenously before cancer chemotherapy to produce sedation and amnesia. They are especially useful if there has previously been vomiting with a cytotoxic treatment, since anticipatory nausea and vomiting are then common with subsequent courses. Benzodiazepines are discussed in Chapter 20.

MANAGEMENT OF NAUSEA AND VOMITING

Anti-emetics are used in a number of situations where nausea and vomiting can be troublesome. Some specific clinical uses are considered in more detail in Table 32.1.

Drug-induced vomiting

It is sometimes necessary to use drugs that carry a high risk of inducing nausea and vomiting (see Box 32.1). Cyclizine, prochlorperazine and metoclopramide are often effective for prevention of opioid-induced vomiting.

More problematic are the highly emetogenic agents used for cancer treatment. Consideration must be given to the risk associated with the agent and risk factors in the person receiving treatment. Factors increasing the probability of experiencing chemotherapy-induced nausea and vomiting include young age, female gender, history of low alcohol intake, motion sickness, emesis during pregnancy, impaired quality of life and previous chemotherapy. For treatments or associated factors that predict a low risk of vomiting, routine prophylaxis is not needed. For moderately emetogenic treatments, a 5-HT_3 receptor antagonist such as ondansetron, possibly combined with a corticosteroid (such as dexamethasone), is usually recommended. For highly emetogenic chemotherapy or when standard treatments are ineffective, a 5-HT_3 receptor antagonist combined with dexamethasone and aprepitant can achieve control in up to 80% of cases. Prochlorperazine, domperidone or nabilone can be used when there is intolerance of 5-HT$_3$ receptor antagonists or corticosteroids.

Delayed emesis, occurring at least 16 hours after chemotherapy, may be mediated by CNS 5-HT$_3$ and NK$_1$ receptors. Dexamethasone combined with aprepitant is recommended for control of delayed emesis, with a 5-HT$_3$ receptor antagonist being an alternative to aprepitant.

Anticipatory vomiting prior to cycles of chemotherapy usually occurs if previous cycles have been accompanied by nausea and vomiting. It is most effectively prevented by including a benzodiazepine such as lorazepam with the chemotherapy regimen from the start of treatment in order to produce amnesia.

Postoperative vomiting

Postoperative nausea and vomiting frequently occur in the first 24 hours after anaesthesia and surgery. They are more common in women, in nonsmokers and when there has been a previous episode of postoperative nausea and vomiting. They are provoked by inhalational rather than intravenous anaesthesia; more often by abdominal, ophthalmic or ear-nose-throat procedures; by the concurrent use of opioid analgesics, and by postoperative pain, hypotension and gastric stasis.

Dexamethasone, prochlorperazine, hyoscine (using a transdermal patch), cyclizine and 5-HT$_3$ receptor antagonists are all effective for preventing postoperative vomiting. Combination of drugs from more than one class is often effective when a single drug has failed or as prophylaxis when the consequences of vomiting are dangerous (such as after eye surgery).

Motion sickness

Motion sickness arises from a mismatch between sensory inputs from the visual and vestibular systems. Behavioural treatments such as habituation or coping strategies involving distraction can be effective. If a drug is needed an antimuscarinic such as hyoscine or an antihistamine such as cyclizine are effective, with promethazine as an alternative if more sedation is desirable. Antimuscarinic unwanted effects may be troublesome with each of these agents.

Vomiting in pregnancy

Nausea is common in pregnancy. High doses of pyridoxine (vitamin B$_6$) or ground ginger may be effective; counselling or hypnotism can also be tried.

Hyperemesis gravidarum, severe morning sickness which begins in the first trimester, can lead to marked maternal weight loss, dehydration, electrolyte disturbances and vitamin deficiencies. There is a natural desire to avoid drugs whenever possible if vomiting arises in pregnancy. Promethazine, prochlorperazine or metoclopramide are used for short-term treatment. All these drugs appear to be safe in early pregnancy. For more severe vomiting, intravenous rehydration and nutritional supplementation (particularly thiamine in hyperemesis gravidarum) will be necessary.

Box 32.2	Causes of vertigo

Ménière's disease
Benign positional vertigo
Migraine
Vestibular neuronitis
Multiple sclerosis
Brainstem ischaemia
Temporal lobe epilepsy
Cerebellopontine angle tumours

VERTIGO

Vertigo is a hallucination of motion, usually perceived as spinning, which is generated in the vestibular system of the inner ear. It is frequently accompanied by nausea and vomiting. There are several causes of vertigo (Box 32.2), but the mechanisms of vertigo are poorly understood. Treatment is empirical and involves modulation of neurotransmitters and receptors involved in the vestibular sensory pathway to the oculomotor nucleus. The neurochemistry of vertigo therefore overlaps with that of vomiting.

Ménière's disease is one of the causes of vertigo for which the pathogenesis is better understood. It usually presents with episodic vertigo and associated signs of vagal overactivity such as pallor, sweating, nausea and vomiting. Tinnitus and eventually sensorineural deafness are common. The underlying problem is excess endolymph in the membranous labyrinth of the middle ear. The condition may have a genetic predisposition, while anatomical abnormalities in the middle ear and various immunological, vascular or viral precipitating insults can be involved.

DRUGS FOR TREATMENT OF VERTIGO

- Antihistamines (histamine H$_1$ receptor antagonists; e.g. cyclizine, promethazine). These are the most widely used drugs for vertigo.
- Antimuscarinic agents. Vestibular suppression can be achieved with hyoscine; the mechanism of action may be similar to that involved in the treatment of motion sickness.
- Benzodiazepines. The use of these agents for short periods may help in severe attacks of vertigo.
- Cimetidine. This drug probably produces symptom relief by histamine H$_2$ receptor antagonism in the CNS (see Chapter 33).
- Histamine receptor agonists. The use of betahistine to treat Ménière's disease illustrates the paradox that both histaminergic and antihistaminic drugs have been advocated for treatment of this condition. Betahistine is an analogue of L-histidine, the metabolic precursor of histamine. It is a partial agonist at postsynaptic histamine H$_1$ receptors and an antagonist at presynaptic H$_3$ receptors, an action that facilitates central histaminergic neurotransmission. Betahistine also increases blood flow to the inner ear. It is metabolised to an active derivative in the liver. The main unwanted effects are headache and nausea.

- Dopamine receptor antagonists. Several antipsychotic drugs such as prochlorperazine are used in vertigo, mainly to treat the associated nausea.

MANAGEMENT OF VERTIGO

Many causes of vertigo are brief and self-limiting. Acute vertigo, such as that caused by vestibular neuronitis, is often treated with anti-emetic agents until vestibular compensation occurs, which is usually encouraged by maintaining activity. The anti-emetic drug should usually be withdrawn as soon as the acute symptoms subside.

Benign paroxysmal positional vertigo responds poorly to drugs and is most effectively treated by vestibular exercises. Drug therapy should be avoided if possible, since it can blunt the effectiveness of the exercises by inhibiting vestibular compensation.

Ménière's disease is often treated initially with lifestyle changes, such as avoidance of excess caffeine, chocolate, alcohol and salt. Modification of the endolymph production in the inner ear with diuretics such as bendroflumethiazide (see Chapter 14) is advocated for persistent symptoms, although clear evidence of efficacy is lacking. Betahistine is often co-prescribed with a diuretic, again with little evidence of benefit. Oral or intratympanic injection of corticosteroid is an alternative to a diuretic. Sedative anti-emetic drugs such as promethazine or prochlorperazine should only be used for very short periods since they impair vestibular rehabilitation and have potentially serious neurological unwanted effects. For refractory symptoms, the vestibular apparatus can be ablated – for example, by using local delivery of gentamicin (see Chapter 51), which is toxic to the inner ear. Surgical treatment is also used for refractory disease.

Several drugs can cause dizziness or a sensation similar to vertigo; recent changes in drug therapy should be considered when a person presents with a new onset of dizziness. Examples of drugs that commonly cause dizziness are antihypertensive agents, vasodilators and antiparkinsonian agents. A more serious degree of vestibular toxicity can be produced by aminoglycoside antimicrobials (see Chapter 51) and high doses of loop diuretics such as furosemide (see Chapter 14). This type of vestibular toxicity can be permanent.

SELF-ASSESSMENT

True/false questions

1. Emetogenic toxins cross the blood–brain barrier to stimulate the CTZ.
2. Some antihistamines are useful for motion sickness.
3. Dopamine antagonists such as metoclopramide can cause movement abnormalities.
4. Metoclopramide decreases intestinal motility.
5. Aminoglycoside antibiotics may cause vertigo.

One-best-answer (OBA) question

1. Which statement concerning nausea and vomiting is the *most accurate*?
   A. Afferents from the stomach to the VC inhibit vomiting when stimulated.
   B. Selective 5-HT$_3$ receptor antagonists are effective against motion sickness.
   C. Nabilone is derived from a psychoactive component of cannabis.
   D. Stimulation of neurokinin 1 (NK$_1$) receptors in the CTZ inhibits nausea.
   E. Digoxin inhibits nausea.

Case-based questions

A 35-year-old man was diagnosed with non-Hodgkin's lymphoma requiring many sessions of treatment with combined cytotoxic therapy, including cyclophosphamide and vincristine.
1. Why was this man likely to experience nausea and vomiting?
2. Nausea and vomiting started several hours after each course of treatment and continued for 4–5 days. What planned anti-emetic treatments prior to the first course of chemotherapy could be beneficial, and how do they work?
3. This man became very distressed by the severity of the nausea and vomiting and developed intense nausea and vomiting prior to the administration of the chemotherapeutic agents. What treatment could be given to reduce the anticipatory nausea and vomiting?

ANSWERS

True/false answers

1. **False.** Emetogenic toxins act on the CTZ (area postrema) outside the blood–brain barrier. Some toxins can also cause vomiting by stimulating vagal afferents in the stomach.
2. **True.** Common antihistamines like promethazine have antimuscarinic activity and inhibit activity in the VC and the vestibular nuclei. It is not certain whether the antihistamine activity plays a role.
3. **True.** Dopamine receptor antagonists used as anti-emetics are given at lower doses than in antipsychotic treatment, but they carry a risk of extrapyramidal movement disorders, particularly in the elderly.
4. **False.** Metoclopramide *increases* stomach and intestinal motility (prokinetic activity), which can add to its anti-emetic effects.
5. **True.** Aminoglycosides (such as gentamicin) and also loop diuretics (furosemide) may cause vestibular damage, leading to vertigo.

One-best-answer (OBA) answer

1. **Answer C** is correct.
   A. Incorrect. The vagal afferents from the stomach respond to toxins and are emetogenic.
   B. Incorrect. Selective 5-HT$_3$ receptor antagonists are not effective against motion sickness, for which a drug with antimuscarinic actions (e.g. hyoscine or promethazine) should be used.
   C. **Correct**. Nabilone is a derivative of tetrahydrocannabinol and an agonist at cannabinoid CB$_1$ receptors.

D. Incorrect. The effect of stimulating NK$_1$ receptors in the CTZ is to cause vomiting.

E. Incorrect. Digoxin may cause nausea and vomiting.

Case-based answers

1. Cyclophosphamide induces nausea and vomiting in almost all people, but vincristine is much less emetogenic. The vomiting arises from stimulation of the CTZ.

2. A selective 5-HT$_3$ receptor antagonist such as ondansetron, alone or together with a corticosteroid, would be beneficial.

Ondansetron inhibits 5-HT$_3$ receptors in the CTZ and also in the stomach. In the stomach, some cancer chemotherapeutic agents can cause damage and the release of serotonin, which stimulates vagal afferents to the VC. It is uncertain how corticosteroids work, but they have an anti-emetic effect that is additive with ondansetron.

3. Anticipatory nausea and vomiting is poorly treated with anti-emetic drugs. Treatment with benzodiazepine anxiolytic drugs prior to the course of chemotherapy can be helpful.

FURTHER READING

Collis, E., Mather, H., 2015. Nausea and vomiting in palliative care. Br. Med. J. 351, h6249.

Harcourt, J., Barraclough, K., Bronstein, A.M., 2014. Ménière's disease. Br. Med. J. 349, g6544.

Jordan, K., Jahn, F., Aapro, M., 2015. Recent developments in the prevention of chemotherapy-induced nausea and vomiting (CINV): a comprehensive review. Ann. Oncol. 26, 1081–1090. doi:10.1093/annonc/mdv138.

McParlin, C., O'Donnell, A., Robson, S.C., 2016. Treatments for hyperemesis gravidarum and nausea and vomiting in pregnancy: a systematic review. JAMA 316, 1392–1401.

Nurdin, L., Golding, J., Bronstein, A., 2011. Managing motion sickness. Br. Med. J. 343, d7430.

Sébastien, P., Whelan, R., 2012. Nausea and vomiting after surgery. Contin. Educ. Anaesth. Crit. Care. Pain. doi:10.1093/bjaceaccp/mks046.

Thompson, T.L., Amedee, R., 2009. Vertigo: a review of common peripheral and central disorders. Ochsner J. 9, 20–26.

Compendium: anti-emetic agents

Drug	Characteristics
Antihistamines	
These drugs have sedating properties.	
Cinnarizine	Used for vestibular disorders and motion sickness; also used for peripheral vascular disease. Given orally. Half-life: 3 h
Cyclizine	Used for a wide range of indications; given orally or by intramuscular or intravenous injection. Half-life: 20 h
Promethazine	Given orally, by deep intramuscular injection or by slow intravenous injection for a wide range of indications. Half-life: 7–14 h
Dopamine receptor antagonists	
Phenothiazine and related drugs (see also Chapter 21)	
Chlorpromazine	Used for nausea and vomiting associated with terminal illness. Given orally, rectally or by deep intramuscular injection. Half-life: 8–35 h
Droperidol	Used for postoperative nausea and vomiting; given by intravenous injection. Half-life: 2 h
Perphenazine	Given orally for severe nausea and vomiting. Half-life: 9 h
Prochlorperazine	Given orally or by deep intramuscular injection for severe nausea and vomiting. Half-life: 6–7 h
Trifluoperazine	Given orally for severe nausea and vomiting. Half-life: 7–18 h
Domperidone and metoclopramide	
Domperidone	Used for a wide range of indications. Treatment limited to 7 days because of risk of arrhythmias. Given orally or rectally. Half-life: 12–16 h
Metoclopramide	Used for a wide range of indications. Treatment limited to 5 days because of risk of extrapyramidal movement disorders. Given orally or by intramuscular injection or intravenous injection over 1–2 min. Half-life: 3–5 h

Compendium: anti-emetic agents (cont'd)

Drug	Characteristics
5-HT$_3$ receptor antagonists	
Granisetron	Used to prevent nausea and vomiting induced by cytotoxic chemotherapy or radiotherapy. Given orally or by intravenous injection or infusion. Half-life: 3–9 h
Ondansetron	Used to prevent nausea and vomiting induced by cytotoxic chemotherapy or radiotherapy. Given orally, rectally, by intramuscular injection or by slow intravenous infusion. Half-life: 3 h
Palonosetron	Given orally or by intravenous injection for nausea and vomiting associated with severely emetogenic chemotherapy. Half-life: 40 h
NK$_1$ receptor antagonists	
Aprepitant	Given orally as an adjunct for preventing nausea and vomiting associated with severely emetogenic chemotherapy. Half-life: 9–13 h
Fosaprepitant	Prodrug of aprepitant. Given by intravenous infusion as an adjunct for preventing nausea and vomiting associated with severely emetogenic chemotherapy
Cannabinoids	
Nabilone	Given orally to prevent nausea and vomiting induced by cytotoxic chemotherapy that is unresponsive to conventional anti-emetics. Half-life: 2 h
Antimuscarinics	
Hyoscine (scopolamine)	Given orally or as a transdermal patch for motion sickness and as premedication; also given by subcutaneous or intramuscular injection. Half-life: 8 h
Other drugs used for treatment and prevention of nausea and vomiting	
Benzodiazepines	See Chapter 20
Betahistine	Mixed actions at histamine receptors. Given orally for vertigo and tinnitus associated with Ménière's disease. Active product has a half-life of 5 h
Corticosteroids	See Chapter 44

NK$_1$, Neurokinin 1.

33

Dyspepsia and peptic ulcer disease

THE SPECTRUM OF DISEASE

Dyspepsia is the term used for a group of symptoms that arise from the upper gastrointestinal tract. They include heartburn, abdominal pain or discomfort, fullness, bloating, early satiety, belching and nausea. Dyspepsia can occur alone (nonulcer dyspepsia) or in association with various upper gastrointestinal disorders such as gastritis, peptic ulcer disease or gastro-oesophageal reflux disease (GORD).

NONULCER DYSPEPSIA

Nonulcer dyspepsia is probably caused by a combination of abnormalities in gastrointestinal motility, increased gastroduodenal sensitivity to mechanical distention and increased acid sensitivity in the duodenum.

PEPTIC ULCER DISEASE

Peptic ulceration describes both gastric and duodenal ulcers. The characteristic symptom of peptic ulceration is epigastric pain, but other dyspeptic symptoms also occur. Symptoms are not a reliable guide to the location of an ulcer. However, pain with duodenal ulceration is usually worse during fasting and at night and is relieved by antacids or by food. By contrast, pain with gastric ulcer may be made worse by food and gastric ulcer is more likely than duodenal ulcer to be associated with weight loss, anorexia and nausea. Chronic ulcers at either site can also be asymptomatic. Complications of peptic ulcers include bleeding, perforation and, if close to the pylorus, scarring with gastric outlet obstruction.

Mechanisms of protection of gastric and duodenal mucosa

The healthy gastric mucosa is able to resist acid digestion. There is an adherent layer of viscoelastic mucus that acts as a physical barrier to acid, and HCO_3^- is secreted into the mucus to neutralise acid locally. In addition, there is a high electrical resistance of, and tight junctions between, gastric mucosal cells, which make the mucosa relatively impermeable to luminal contents. Gastric mucosal blood flow provides an extra layer of defence, delivering HCO_3^- to buffer any H^+ ions that penetrate the mucosa and also regulating acid secretion. Many of these protective functions are dependent on synthesis of the prostaglandins PGE_2 and PGI_2 by gastric mucosal cells (see Chapter 29; Table 33.1).

The duodenal mucosa is protected by a layer of viscoelastic mucus, but the mucosal cells are highly permeable, permitting absorption of luminal nutrients. The mucosal cells secrete HCO_3^-, which accumulates in the mucus layer and buffers the pulses of gastric acid released from the stomach.

Aetiology of peptic ulceration

The aetiology of peptic ulceration is not fully understood, but many contributory factors have been identified. Gastric acid

Table 33.1 Factors associated with protection and damage of the intestinal mucosa

Factors associated with peptic ulcer disease	Factors associated with peptic ulcer protection and healing
Thin or breached mucus layer	Intact mucus layer
Helicobacter pylori and host immune response	Adequate blood flow
Reduced bicarbonate secretion	Bicarbonate in mucus layer
Reduced mucosal blood flow	Prostaglandins (generated by COX-1 and COX-2 isoenzymes)
Stress	Hydrophobicity of phospholipid layer of epithelial cells
Smoking	Regrowth of epithelial cell layer following damage (restitution)
Alcohol	Growth factors
Acid	Nitric oxide
Pepsin	
Iatrogenic (e.g. NSAIDs)	

NSAIDs, nonsteroidal antiinflammatory drugs.

is essential for ulceration to arise, and there is often failure of the normal luminal acid concentration to inhibit further gastric acid secretion. Pepsin secretion is also enhanced in people with peptic ulceration. Accelerated gastric emptying is a factor in promoting duodenal ulceration, with entry of gastric contents at a lower pH into the duodenum. Prostaglandins enhance mucosal protection against ulceration, and deficient production of prostaglandin E_1 is a factor in reducing resistance to mucosal erosion in both the stomach and duodenum.

Helicobacter pylori *and peptic ulceration*

A major risk factor associated with peptic ulceration is gastric and duodenal infection with the Gram-negative bacterium *Helicobacter pylori*. The incidence of *H. pylori* colonisation in the gastric mucosa varies widely in the adult population in different countries, being highest in those who have poorer living conditions. About 10–15% of the United Kingdom population is infected. Infection is usually acquired in childhood and persists unless it is treated. Infection with *H. pylori* is a risk factor for gastritis, peptic ulcer, gastric cancer and mucosa-associated lymphoid tissue (MALT) lymphoma. However, only a small percentage of those who carry the bacterium develop *H. pylori*-associated disease, perhaps reflecting different host responses to the infection and whether the infecting strain carries particular factors for high virulence. *H. pylori* penetrates the mucus lining of the stomach and attaches to epithelial cells. It secretes the enzyme urease, which contributes to its survival during exposure to gastric acid by producing ammonia from urea. Ammonia is toxic to mucosal cells, and an immune response

to the bacterial proteins also contributes to development of chronic inflammation.

Helicobacter pylori *and gastric ulceration*

Gastric ulceration is associated in about 70% of cases with *H. pylori* infection of the corpus of the stomach or both the corpus and antrum. In contrast to duodenal ulceration, there is no excess gastric acid secretion and often a reduction. *H. pylori* infection of the corpus is associated with the atrophy of acid-secreting cells and metaplasia of the gastric mucosa, which predisposes to gastric ulceration and gastric cancer.

Helicobacter pylori *and duodenal ulceration*

Infection with *H. pylori* is present in about 80% of people with duodenal ulcer, in whom it is predominantly found in the stomach but confined to the antral mucosa. The infection impairs secretion of somatostatin and therefore promotes secretion of gastrin from antral mucosal cells, which stimulates excess acid secretion from the body of the stomach. Exposure of duodenal cells to excess acid makes them more like gastric mucosal cells (gastric metaplasia) and allows duodenal colonisation by *H. pylori*.

Drugs and peptic ulceration

There is a higher incidence of peptic ulcer in people who use nonsteroidal antiinflammatory drugs (NSAIDs), including low-dose aspirin (see Chapter 29). NSAIDs are the most frequent cause of peptic ulceration in the absence of *H. pylori* infection. However, the prevalence of non-*H. pylori*, non-NSAID-associated gastric ulcers appears to be increasing in Western societies. Other drugs that are much less commonly associated with peptic ulcers include bisphosphonates, selective serotonin reuptake inhibitors (SSRIs) and spironolactone. Smoking and a high alcohol intake delay the healing of peptic ulcers, but there is less evidence that they are involved in the genesis of the ulcer.

GASTRO-OESOPHAGEAL REFLUX DISEASE

GORD can produce heartburn from regurgitation of gastric contents into the oesophagus (reflux), pain or difficulty in swallowing and even the regurgitation of gastric contents into the mouth. If reflux produces inflammation of the oesophageal mucosa (oesophagitis), there may be more prolonged chest pain and even chronic bleeding. Symptoms in GORD are usually chronic and relapsing, with at least two-thirds of those diagnosed still taking continuous or intermittent treatment after 10 years. GORD can precipitate asthma through the micro-aspiration of gastric contents into the lungs and triggering of vagal oesophago-bronchial reflexes. Micro-aspiration is also associated with chronic cough.

It is now believed that there are three distinct clinical groups of GORD rather than a steady progression of severity. These are possibly determined by genetic factors and the immunological response to reflux. The groups are

- Nonerosive reflux disease.
- Erosive oesophagitis, an acute inflammatory T-helper cell 1 (Th1) response (see Chapter 38).

■ Barrett's oesophagus (intestinal metaplasia of oesophageal mucosal cells) with increased risk of cancer; this is a Th2-type immunological response (see Chapter 38).

Gastro-oesophageal reflux is produced by the generation of transient lower oesophageal sphincter relaxations (TLOSRs) in the absence of swallowing. TLSORs arise from stimulation of gastric vagal mechanoreceptors and allow gastric acid, pepsin and bile to come into contact with the vulnerable epithelium of the oesophagus. Oesophageal hypomotility and abnormal patterns of oesophageal contractility often coexist with GORD, which reduces the clearance of refluxed material. The disturbance of motility may reflect a sensory abnormality in the oesophageal mucosa. There is little correlation between the extent of oesophagitis at endoscopy and the severity of symptoms. Up to 50% of people with symptoms of GORD have no apparent oesophagitis, whereas severe oesophagitis can be asymptomatic unless complications such as stricture or anaemia arise.

The relationship of *H. pylori* infection to GORD is not straightforward. Antral infection predisposes to GORD by promoting greater amounts of gastric acid secretion, while corporal gastritis is protective partly because the acid content of the stomach may be reduced.

OESOPHAGEAL SPASM

Oesophageal spasm is a distinct disorder in which oesophageal pain is often not accompanied by any change in luminal pH. However, acid can induce spasm in some people with symptoms of reflux. The pain frequently occurs without evidence of oesophageal dysmotility, when the symptoms arise from a combination of local mucosal sensory disturbances and psychological factors.

CONTROL OF GASTRIC ACID SECRETION

Acid secretion into the canaliculi of gastric parietal cells is initiated by the activity of a membrane-bound proton pump that exchanges H^+ and K^+ across the cell membrane (H^+/K^+-ATPase). Hydrogen ions are obtained from carbonic acid (H_2CO_3) by carbonic anhydrase, and HCO_3^- enters the plasma in exchange for Cl^- ions. Chloride ions are then secreted into the stomach lumen with H^+ via a symport carrier. The activity of the proton pump is enhanced by several mediators, including histamine, gastrin and acetylcholine (Fig. 33.1).

DRUGS FOR TREATING DYSPEPSIA, PEPTIC ULCER AND GASTRO-OESOPHAGEAL REFLUX DISEASE

ANTISECRETORY DRUGS

Antisecretory drugs reduce production of gastric acid. It is only necessary to raise intragastric pH above 3 for a few hours each day to promote healing of most peptic ulcers. However, rapid healing requires acid suppression for a minimum of 18–20 hours/day. The duration of acid suppression determines the rate of healing but not the eventual proportion of ulcers healed. Several classes of drug have antisecretory actions on the gastric mucosa.

Proton pump inhibitors

esomeprazole, lansoprazole, omeprazole, pantoprazole

Mechanism of action

The proton pump (H^+/K^+-ATPase) is the final common pathway for acid secretion in gastric parietal cells, and inhibition of the pump blocks acid secretion almost completely (see Fig. 33.1). Proton pump inhibitors are pro-drugs that are rapidly absorbed from the small intestine. As weak bases, they are selectively concentrated from the circulation into the acid environment of the secretory canaliculi of the gastric parietal cells. The drugs are then converted to active derivatives by protonation and covalently bind to and irreversibly inhibit the proton pump. The return of acid secretion is dependent on the synthesis of new proton pumps. Because protonation only takes place at acid pH, these drugs have a selective action on gastric parietal cells, and proton pumps elsewhere in the body are not inhibited. A single dose of a proton pump inhibitor inhibits acid production by up to 90% for approximately 24 hours.

Pharmacokinetics

Proton pump inhibitors are unstable in acid and are given orally as enteric-coated formulations. Esomeprazole, omeprazole and pantoprazole are also available as intravenous formulations. Elimination is by hepatic metabolism. They have short plasma half-lives, but because of the irreversible mechanism of action, these bear no relationship to the long duration of action.

Unwanted effects

■ Gastrointestinal upset, such as nausea, vomiting, abdominal pain, diarrhoea, constipation.
■ Headache.
■ All proton pump inhibitors inhibit CYP2C9 and CYP2C19 in the liver to varying extents. This can give rise to drug interactions with other substrates of these isoenzymes – for example, decreasing the metabolism and increasing the clinical effects of warfarin, clopidogrel, phenytoin and several antiviral drugs (see Table 2.7). Esomeprazole may be less likely to cause such interactions than other proton pump inhibitors.

Concerns that substantial reductions of gastric acid, and the associated rise in gastrin secretion, might increase the risk of gastric cancer (comparable to the increased risk in pernicious anaemia) are unfounded. Proton pump inhibitors do not completely abolish acid secretion, and intragastric pH can still fall below 4 during part of the day, the critical pH below which bacterial populations that predispose to cancer cannot become established. However, symptomatic improvement following treatment with a proton pump inhibitor can mask the symptoms of pre-existing gastric cancer.

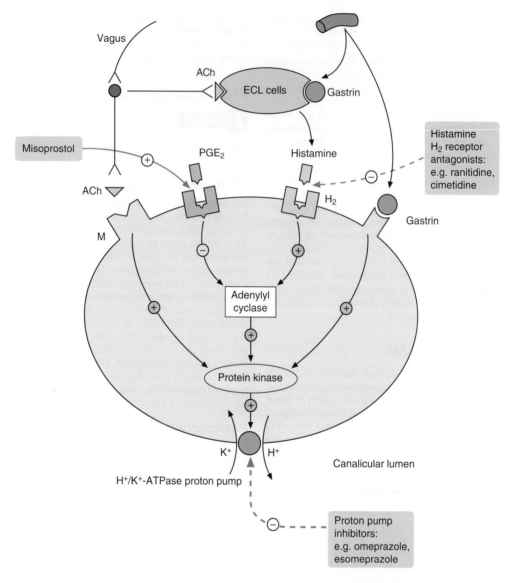

Fig. 33.1 Control of gastric acid secretion from the parietal cell. Acid secretion from the parietal cell is stimulated by acetylcholine (ACh), histamine and gastrin. Gastrin and ACh also reinforce acid secretion by causing the release of histamine from the enterochromaffin-like (ECL) cells, which lie close to the parietal cells in the gastric pits. Prostaglandin E_2 (PGE$_2$) reduces acid secretion. The sites of action of the main drugs used to inhibit acid secretion from the parietal cell are shown. There are no useful inhibitors of gastrin action, and the gastric-selective muscarinic receptor (M$_1$) antagonist pirenzepine is no longer available in the United Kingdom. H_2, Histamine type 2 receptor.

Histamine H$_2$ receptor antagonists

cimetidine, ranitidine

Mechanism of action

Histamine H$_2$ receptor antagonists act competitively with histamine at receptors on gastric parietal cells. They reduce basal acid secretion and pepsin production and prevent the increase in secretion that occurs in response to several secretory stimuli. Overall, acid secretion is reduced by about 60% (see Fig. 33.1).

Pharmacokinetics

Cimetidine and ranitidine are mainly eliminated unchanged by the kidney and have short half-lives between 1 and 4 hours.

Unwanted effects

- Diarrhoea and other gastrointestinal disturbances.
- Headache, dizziness, tiredness.

- Rash.
- Drug interactions: cimetidine is an inhibitor of hepatic P450 isoenzymes (see Table 2.7) and can increase the plasma concentrations and actions of drugs such as warfarin, phenytoin and theophylline. Other histamine H_2 receptor antagonists do not inhibit P450 isoenzymes.

ANTACIDS

aluminium hydroxide, magnesium trisilicate

Mechanism of action

Antacids neutralise gastric acid. They have a more prolonged effect if taken after food. If used without food, the effect lasts no more than an hour because of rapid gastric emptying. Antacids rapidly relieve symptoms in peptic ulcer disease, but large doses are required to heal ulcers. Liquid preparations work more rapidly, but tablets are more convenient to use. Most antacids are relatively poorly absorbed from the gut. Simeticone is sometimes added to an antacid as an antifoaming agent. The combination may reduce flatulence or relieve hiccups in palliative care.

Unwanted effects

- Constipation can occur with aluminium salts and diarrhoea with magnesium salts; mixtures of aluminium and magnesium salts may have less effect on stool consistency.
- Systemic alkalosis can occur with very large doses.
- In advanced renal failure, retention of absorbed aluminium may contribute to metabolic bone disease and encephalopathy. Magnesium salts can also cause hypermagnesia with weakness and confusion in renal failure.
- Drug interactions: aluminium salts can bind to NSAIDs and tetracyclines in the gut and reduce their absorption.

Antacids with alginic acid

Alginic acid is an inert substance. It is claimed that it forms a raft of high-pH foam that floats on the gastric contents and protects the oesophageal mucosa during reflux. All proprietary preparations combine alginic acid with an antacid, which is probably responsible for much of the clinical effect. Some formulations contain a high Na^+ concentration, which can be undesirable in people with fluid retention or hypertension.

CYTOPROTECTIVE DRUGS

Sucralfate

Mechanism of action

Sucralfate is a complex of aluminium hydroxide and sucrose octasulfate. It dissociates in the acid environment of the stomach to its anionic form, which binds to the ulcer base. This creates a protective barrier to pepsin and bile and inhibits the diffusion of gastric acid. Sucralfate also stimulates the gastric secretion of bicarbonate and prostaglandins.

Pharmacokinetics

Sucralfate is only slightly absorbed from the gut (<2%).

Unwanted effects

- Constipation.
- Bezoar formation (a mass trapped in the gut, usually the stomach), especially if gastric emptying is delayed.

Prostaglandin analogues

misoprostol

Mechanism of action

Misoprostol is an analogue of PGE_1 and has several actions that protect the gastric and duodenal mucosae. It is most widely used to prevent NSAID-associated ulcers and is available in combination products with diclofenac or naproxen (see Chapter 29).

Pharmacokinetics

Misoprostol undergoes first-pass metabolism to active misoprostolic acid. Elimination is mainly by hepatic metabolism and it has a very short half-life (<1 hour).

Unwanted effects

- Diarrhoea and abdominal cramps are common.
- Uterine contractions: therefore misprostol is to be avoided in pregnancy. It can, however, be used to induce labour (see Chapter 45).
- Menorrhagia and postmenopausal bleeding.

MANAGEMENT OF DYSPEPSIA, PEPTIC ULCER AND GASTRO-OESOPHAGEAL REFLUX DISEASE

NONULCER DYSPEPSIA

Most people with dyspepsia do not have significant underlying disease (i.e. they have nonulcer or functional dyspepsia). In all cases, efforts should be made to remove exacerbating agents, for example smoking, excess alcohol or NSAIDs. Upper gastrointestinal endoscopy may be indicated to assess the cause of symptoms. However, younger people (especially those under 55 years of age) who do not have ALARM symptoms (**a**naemia, **l**oss of weight, **a**norexia, **r**ecent onset of progressive symptoms, **m**elaena, haematemesis or dysphagia) are often treated initially without investigation.

A proton pump inhibitor is more effective than a histamine H_2 receptor antagonist for symptom relief in nonulcer dyspepsia. Treatment should be given for 4–6 weeks, followed by clinical review with the intention of reducing the dose of drug or moving to intermittent or on-demand therapy for symptom relief. Eradication of *H. pylori* does not usually reduce symptoms. On the occasions it is effective (about 15% of people with suspected nonulcer dyspepsia), symptoms are probably due to undiagnosed peptic ulceration. Recurrent symptoms may prompt further investigation to exclude peptic ulceration or GORD.

CONFIRMED PEPTIC ULCERATION

Proton pump inhibitors produce the fastest rate of ulcer healing (over 90% of ulcers heal within 4 weeks). Histamine H_2 receptor antagonists usually give symptomatic relief for both gastric and duodenal ulcers within a week, but healing of the ulcer is much slower, requiring up to 8 weeks for duodenal ulcer or 12 weeks for gastric ulcer. Other agents such as sucralfate will heal ulcers in a similar proportion of people but are used less often, since they do not improve symptoms as quickly.

Eradication of *H. pylori* infection enhances ulcer healing and reduces relapse, so that maintenance therapy with acid-suppressing drugs is often unnecessary for uncomplicated ulcers. If *H. pylori* is not eradicated, 80% of ulcers will reoccur within a year; following successful eradication, the recurrence is less than 20%.

ERADICATION OF *HELICOBACTER PYLORI* INFECTION

Several indications for *H. pylori* eradication have been proposed based on acid suppression and antibacterial treatment (Box 33.1). Many eradication regimens are available: the most widely used is a high dose of proton pump inhibitor combined with two antibacterials (to maximise efficacy and minimise resistance) given for 1 week. The first choice antibacterials are clarithromycin with either amoxicillin or metronidazole, but it is important to avoid an antibacterial that has been used recently for treatment of other infections. Treatment for 2 weeks has a higher eradication rate, but unwanted effects often reduce adherence to the regimen, which limits the success rate. The incidence of in vitro resistance of *H. pylori* to metronidazole and clarithromycin is increasing. If in vitro clarithromycin resistance is detected, it is always reflected in a reduced ability to eliminate the bacterium clinically. By contrast, eradication may be successful even when laboratory resistance to metronidazole is demonstrated.

Box 33.1   Indications for eradication of *Helicobacter pylori*

Eradication recommended
Proven peptic ulcer
Low-grade mucosa-associated lymphoid tissue gastric lymphoma
Severe gastritis
After resection of early gastric cancer

Eradication suggested (less certain indications)
Functional dyspepsia
Family history of gastric cancer
Nonsteroidal antiinflammatory drug therapy
Intended long-term proton pump inhibitor therapy

Resistance to amoxicillin is less common, and resistance to tinidazole is currently lower than to metronidazole. Concurrent use of probiotic yoghurts can improve both tolerability and the outcome of eradication therapy.

H. pylori eradication with a triple regimen is successful in about 85% of cases in the United Kingdom and reinfection is rare. Testing to confirm eradication is required only if the indication for treatment was MALT lymphoma or peptic ulcer disease. Failure of eradication usually reflects antibacterial resistance or poor adherence to treatment. However, resistance to standard triple therapy is more common in some parts of the world, with a failure to eradicate *H. pylori* in up to 20% of people adherent to treatment. Further treatment should then be guided by the results of microbiological sensitivity tests on biopsy specimens or a third antimicrobial drug may be considered as part of the regimen.

After *H. pylori* eradication, it is usually possible to stop acid-suppression treatment for peptic ulcers, although it is normally continued for up to 3 weeks if the ulcer is large, has bled or has perforated. Longer-term therapy with acid-suppressant treatment is required only if symptoms continue and after exclusion of more serious conditions.

BLEEDING FROM PEPTIC ULCERS

Active bleeding from a peptic ulcer is a medical emergency. Endoscopic treatment applied to a visible vessel in the ulcer base using diathermy, clipping, laser coagulation or injection with adrenaline may stop the bleeding. Even after achieving haemostasis, recurrent bleeding occurs in up to 20% of cases. Endoscopic treatment should be followed by intravenous infusion of a high dose of proton pump inhibitor for 72 hours before changing to oral therapy. This reduces the rebleeding rate and the need for surgery by 30–40%. Proton pump inhibitors reverse the deactivation of the coagulation system and platelet aggregation in the gut mucosa that occurs when the local pH falls below 4.

PEPTIC ULCERATION ASSOCIATED WITH NONSTEROIDAL ANTIINFLAMMATORY DRUGS

Ideally, the NSAID should be stopped. If continued treatment is essential, then NSAID-associated ulcers will usually heal if an ulcer-healing agent is co-prescribed. Continued use of NSAIDs can slow ulcer healing by histamine H_2 receptor antagonists but probably not by proton pump inhibitors. Eradication of *H. pylori* infection is recommended if an NSAID must be continued in someone who has had previous peptic ulceration, although this may prevent further ulcers only early in treatment with NSAIDs and is less effective during long-term use.

When an NSAID is first used, careful assessment is recommended to determine whether prophylaxis against ulceration should be given in the absence of upper gastrointestinal symptoms. Those at higher risk of NSAID-induced ulceration include people over 65 years of age, smokers, heavy alcohol users and those taking concomitant treatment with medicines that cause gastrointestinal irritation, such as corticosteroids. There is also an increased risk in people with a history of previous ulceration or those who have serious comorbidities, such as cardiovascular disease, diabetes mellitus or renal or hepatic impairment.

Misoprostol provides effective prophylaxis against NSAID-induced gastric or duodenal ulceration. However, a high dosage is necessary for prevention of ulcer recurrence, and this is often poorly tolerated because of colic or diarrhoea. Standard doses of a histamine H_2 receptor antagonist protect against NSAID-induced duodenal ulcers but not against gastric ulceration. Double the usual doses of a histamine H_2 receptor antagonist or standard doses of a proton pump inhibitor protects against both gastric and duodenal ulceration; these are better tolerated than misoprostol. There is limited evidence to support the use of a cyclo-oxygenase-2 (COX-2)-selective inhibitor with a proton pump inhibitor as a strategy to further reduce the risk of peptic ulceration in people at highest risk of ulceration. The combination of a COX-2-selective inhibitor with low-dose aspirin carries the same risk of ulceration as a conventional NSAID and should be avoided.

GASTRO-OESOPHAGEAL REFLUX DISEASE

Initial measures for GORD include avoidance of tight clothing around the waist, smoking, and the use of alcohol and caffeine and encouraging weight loss. Raising the head of the bed on wooden blocks by 15 cm can promote symptom relief and mucosal healing. For mild persistent symptoms, reduction of gastric acid with antacids, with or without the addition of an alginate to provide a mechanical barrier, is often helpful. Alginates should be taken after meals to reduce their clearance by rapid gastric emptying. Eradication of *H. pylori* in GORD has no effect on symptoms.

Proton pump inhibitors are the most effective treatment for severe resistant or relapsing GORD. They will rapidly ease symptoms and heal oesophagitis within 8 weeks in up to 85% of those treated. Acid secretion can break through at night during treatment with a proton pump inhibitor. This may be important in severe erosive oesophagitis or Barrett's oesophagus; in this situation esomeprazole may be more effective than other proton pump inhibitors. Failure to heal oesophagitis with a proton pump inhibitor often indicates bile reflux rather than acid reflux.

Histamine H_2 receptor antagonists usually relieve heartburn in up to 50% of people after 4 weeks of treatment. However, oesophagitis heals in only about 20% of cases. Better healing rates can be achieved by using double the standard dosages, with healing in 70–80% of cases by 8–12 weeks.

Intermittent therapy with healing agents or the use of an alginate after healing often controls recurrent symptoms. For severe or resistant reflux disease, long-term use of a proton pump inhibitor is the only effective drug treatment, although about 60% of people will need only a low maintenance dose after healing has occurred. Laparoscopic antireflux surgery is increasingly used for resistant GORD, particularly if there is high-volume reflux.

OESOPHAGEAL SPASM

The frequency of oesophageal spasm can be reduced by regular use of a proton pump inhibitor when it is induced by oesophageal reflux. Pain due to oesophageal spasm, with or without associated reflux, can respond to smooth muscle relaxants such as calcium channel blockers (see Chapter 5), nitrates (see Chapter 5) or sildenafil (see Chapter 16). Local injection of botulinum toxin (see Chapter 24) has also been successful in limited studies.

SELF-ASSESSMENT

True/false questions

1. Histamine acts on H_1 receptors on the parietal cell to stimulate acid secretion.
2. Vagal stimulation of the parietal cell increases acid secretion.
3. An unwanted effect of antacids containing magnesium salts is diarrhoea.
4. Antacids are not effective in healing peptic ulcers.
5. Cimetidine can potentiate the effects of other drugs by inhibiting cytochrome P450 enzymes.
6. Ranitidine is associated with a lower incidence of gynaecomastia than cimetidine.
7. Cimetidine reduces acid secretion by more than 90%.
8. Esomeprazole is a prodrug.
9. The active metabolite of lansoprazole is a reversible proton pump inhibitor.
10. Omeprazole inhibits the cytochrome P450 system in the liver.
11. Prostacyclin (prostaglandin I_2, PGI_2) reduces gastric mucosal blood flow.
12. Misoprostol causes constipation.
13. Histamine H_2 receptor antagonists and proton pump inhibitors are not useful for treatment of ulcers induced by NSAIDs.
14. Sucralfate binds to the ulcer base and promotes ulcer healing.

One-best-answer (OBA) question

1. Identify the least accurate statement about *H. pylori*.
   A. *H. pylori* infection in the gastric antrum reduces acid secretion.
   B. *H. pylori* infection can be found in the duodenum in people with duodenal ulcers.
   C. If *H. pylori* is not eliminated, a duodenal ulcer is likely to recur.
   D. *H. pylori* is a risk factor for the development of gastric cancer.
   E. *H. pylori* frequently develops resistance to antibacterial treatment.

Case-based questions

A 56-year-old man, Mr T.K., was newly appointed as headmaster of a large comprehensive school and was experiencing some difficulties with the increasing demands of the job. He increased his smoking from 5 to 20 cigarettes a day and drank 10 units of alcohol a week. He had a good, varied diet. He had suffered intermittently from dyspepsia for some years, taking proprietary antacids when required. His symptoms then increased and the pain caused him to waken most nights. He bought a supply of ranitidine from the local chemist without consultation with the pharmacist. Following 2 weeks of treatment, his symptoms were successfully relieved and he was symptom-free for 3 months. His symptoms then returned and he took further treatment with ranitidine for 2 weeks. He was symptom-free for a further month, but when symptoms returned again he consulted his general practitioner (GP).

1. Why did his symptoms return?
2. Would his symptoms have been less likely to return following a short course of a proton pump inhibitor?
3. What should be the GP's course of action?
   An endoscopic examination revealed a duodenal ulcer.
4. Why do some people infected with *H. pylori* develop gastric ulcers and some duodenal ulcers?
5. What eradication therapy for *H. pylori* should be given, and is a proton pump inhibitor beneficial when given with antibacterial therapy?
   The eradication therapy given was 7 days with omeprazole, amoxicillin and clarithromycin. Mr T.K. was symptom-free for 6 weeks but then his symptoms returned.
6. What were the possible reasons for the return of the symptoms?
7. What treatment could be given?

ANSWERS

True/false answers

1. **False.** The histamine receptors on parietal cells that stimulate acid secretion are H_2 receptors, which are selectively antagonised by ranitidine and cimetidine.
2. **True.** The vagal neurotransmitter acetylcholine stimulates muscarinic receptors, which increases acid secretion.
3. **True.** Magnesium salts may cause diarrhoea, and antacids containing aluminium salts may cause constipation.
4. **False.** Antacids can heal peptic ulcers, but their effects are slower than those of proton pump inhibitors or histamine H_2 receptor antagonists.
5. **True.** Cimetidine – but not famotidine, nizatidine or ranitidine – inhibits cytochrome P450 isozymes and should be avoided in people taking warfarin, phenytoin or theophylline.
6. **True.** Cimetidine is more likely than other histamine H_2 receptor antagonists to cause galactorrhoea in women or gynaecomastia in men by inhibiting oestrogen metabolism.
7. **False.** Histamine H_2 antagonists reduce acid secretion by only about 60% because these drugs do not block other stimuli for acid secretion, such as gastrin and acetylcholine.
8. **True.** Like other proton pump inhibitors, esomeprazole is converted to its active form by protonation in acid conditions. It is therefore selectively active on the proton pump in the gastric parietal cell but not on proton pumps in other tissues that operate at higher pH.
9. **False.** The active metabolites of proton pump inhibitor prodrugs are irreversible inhibitors and fresh protein must be synthesised to replace the inhibited proton pump.

10. **True.** Omeprazole can inhibit the metabolism of drugs such as warfarin or phenytoin by both CYP2C9 and CYP2C19. Proton pump inhibitors differ in their inhibitory activity on cytochrome P450 isozymes, with pantoprazole and rabeprazole thought to have the least effect.
11. **False.** Part of the gastroprotective action of PGI_2 and PGE_2 is by increasing gastric mucosal blood flow, removing back-secreted H^+ and providing HCO_3^- to buffer the H^+ ions. They also increase mucus secretion and decrease acid secretion.
12. **False.** Misoprostol is a prostaglandin analogue. Prostaglandins can increase gastrointestinal motility and secretions and cause diarrhoea.
13. **False.** Both histamine H_2 antagonists and proton pump inhibitors can cause healing of NSAID-induced ulcers. Proton pump inhibitors may produce more rapid healing as this is probably related to the degree of acid suppression.
14. **True.** The mucosal protectants sucralfate and bismuth salts have been largely superseded, although bismuth chelates (with low bismuth content) still have a place as quadruple therapy with PPIs and antibacterial drugs when triple therapy fails.

One-best-answer (OBA) answer

1. **Answer A** is the *least accurate* statement.
   A. **Incorrect.** Acid secretion is *enhanced* by *H. pylori* infection in the antrum, while infection in the corpus is associated with reduced or unchanged acid secretion.
   B. Correct. Increased acid secretion caused by antral infection produces changes in the duodenal mucosa that enable duodenal colonisation by *H. pylori*.
   C. Correct. Following healing with a proton pump inhibitor, approximately 80% of duodenal ulcers will recur within a year if *H. pylori* is not eradicated.
   D. Correct. *H. pylori* infection increases the risk of developing gastric adenocarcinoma by five- to sixfold.
   E. Correct. In some countries *H. pylori* resistance to metronidazole is as high as 90%.

Case-based answers

1. This man could have nonulcer dyspepsia or peptic ulceration. Ranitidine for only 2 weeks of treatment is available without prescription; if it had been continued, the symptoms would probably have been suppressed longer. If he is *H. pylori*-positive and has nonulcer dyspepsia, it is likely that he will develop peptic ulcer disease in the future. If he is *H. pylori*-positive and has peptic ulceration, failure to eradicate *H. pylori* is likely to result in a recurrence of peptic ulcer within a year.
2. If *H. pylori* is present, the symptoms will still recur in a high percentage of individuals.
3. It is recommended that any person over 55 years of age, such as Mr T.K., be referred for endoscopic examination. *H. pylori* infection can be detected noninvasively using a blood test (antibody to urease), a stool antigen test or a radiolabelled (^{13}C) urea breath test. In a gastric antral biopsy, it can be detected using bacterial culture, histopathology or a rapid urease (CLO) test. Use of

NSAIDs, tobacco and alcohol consumption should be assessed, as these are strongly contributory to ulcer disease and/or will prevent healing.

4. The reasons why some people develop gastric ulcers and others develop duodenal ulcers are imperfectly understood. If there is only antral inflammation and *H. pylori* is present, more gastrin and therefore excess acid is produced, resulting in duodenal ulcers. If a pangastritis exists, it is associated with corporal atrophy, lower levels of acid secretion and gastric ulcers.

5. Numerous treatment regimens have been evaluated. One week of therapy with a proton pump inhibitor (or ranitidine, if intolerant) plus two antimicrobials (clarithromycin and either metronidazole or amoxicillin, in a combination dictated by local sensitivities) results in a 70%–90% eradication rate.

6. It is possible that the strain of *H. pylori* was resistant to the antibiotics used. Tests should be carried out to see whether *H. pylori* is still present after treatment. If necessary, quadruple therapy or longer treatment periods should be used.

7. Culture sensitivities of the *H. pylori* in a biopsy specimen could be sought. Quadruple therapy, which has 93%–98% success, could be used; for example, a proton pump inhibitor (or histamine H$_2$ receptor antagonist) plus bismuth chelate plus metronidazole (or tinidazole) plus tetracycline (Fig. 33.2).

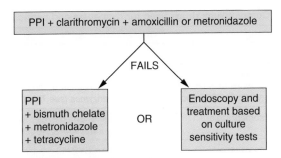

Fig. 33.2 **Recommended regimens for the eradication of** *H. pylori*. Many regimens exist, dictated by local patterns of sensitivity and resistance. Increasing resistance to metronidazole and clarithromycin is reducing the success rate of the triple regimen. If the proton pump inhibitor (PPI) is not tolerated, a histamine H$_2$ receptor antagonist can be substituted. If initial eradication fails, quadruple therapy with a PPI (or histamine H$_2$ antagonist), bismuth chelate (tripotassium dicitratobismuthate), metronidazole (or tinidazole) and tetracycline can be used, or the person can be referred for endoscopy and treatment based on the results of culture and sensitivity testing.

FURTHER READING

Bredenoord, A.J., Pandolfino, J.E., Smout, A.J.P.M., 2013. Gastro-esophageal reflux disease. Lancet 381, 1933–1942.

Ford, A.C., Moayyedi, P., 2013. Dyspepsia. Br. Med. J. 347, f5059.

Katz, P.O., Gerson, L.B., Vela, M.F., 2013. Diagnosis and management of gastroesophageal reflux disease. Am. J. Gastroenterol. 108, 308–328.

Lau, J.Y.W., Barkun, A., Fan, D.-M., et al., 2013. Challenges in the management of acute peptic ulcer bleeding. Lancet 381, 2033–2043.

Li, B.-Z., Threapleton, D.-E., Wang, J.-Y., et al., 2015. Comparative effectiveness and tolerance of treatments for *Helicobacter pylori*: systematic review and network analysis. Br. Med. J. 351, h4052.

Malfertheiner, P., Chan, F.K.L., McColl, K.E.L., 2009. Peptic ulcer disease. Lancet 374, 1449–1461.

McColl, K.E.L., 2010. *Helicobacter pylori* infection. N. Engl. J. Med. 362, 1597–1604.

Sinha, M., Gautam, L., Shukla, P.K., et al., 2013. Current perspectives in NSAID-induced gastropathy. Mediators Inflamm. 2013, 258209.

Talley, N.J., Ford, A.C., 2015. Functional dyspepsia. N. Engl. J. Med. 373, 1853–1863.

Tutuian, R., Castell, D.O., 2006. Oesophageal spasm—diagnosis and management. Aliment. Pharmacol. Ther. 23, 1393–1402.

Compendium: drugs used for dyspepsia and peptic ulcer disease

Drug	Characteristics
Antisecretory agents	
H$_2$ receptor antagonists	
Cimetidine	May cause drug interactions by inhibiting cytochrome P450 enzymes. Given orally. Half-life: 1–3 h
Famotidine	Does not affect cytochrome P450 enzymes. Given orally. Half-life: 3–4 h
Nizatidine	Does not affect cytochrome P450 enzymes. Given orally or by intravenous infusion. Half-life: 1–2 h
Ranitidine	No effect on cytochrome P450 enzymes. May be given orally, by intramuscular injection, or by slow intravenous injection or infusion. Half-life: 2–3 h

Compendium: drugs used for dyspepsia and peptic ulcer disease (cont'd)

Drug	Characteristics
Proton pump inhibitors	
Because of the irreversible mechanism of action of the active metabolites, the proton pump inhibitors have much longer durations of action than indicated by the half-life of the parent compound. All may cause drug interactions by inhibiting hepatic CYP2C9 and/or CYP2C19 isoenzymes (see Table 2.7).	
Esomeprazole	The S-isomer of omeprazole; may cause fewer CYP450 drug interactions than omeprazole. Given orally, or by intravenous injection or infusion. Half-life: 1–2 h
Lansoprazole	Possibly fewer CYP450 drug interactions than omeprazole. Given orally. Half-life: 1–2 h
Omeprazole	Potent inhibition of CYP450 isoenzymes may cause drug interactions. Given orally or by slow intravenous injection (over 5 min) or infusion. Half-life: 1 h
Pantoprazole	Possibly fewer CYP450 drug interactions than omeprazole. Given orally or by slow intravenous injection (over 2 min) or infusion. Half-life: 1 h
Rabeprazole	Fewer CYP450 drug interactions than omeprazole. Given orally. Half-life: 1–2 h
Cytoprotective agents	
Given orally	
Misoprostol	Prostaglandin E_1 analogue; pro-drug of misoprostolic acid. Used to prevent NSAID-associated ulcers in the frail or very elderly from whom NSAIDs cannot be withdrawn. Half-life: 0.3 h
Sucralfate	Mucosal protectant that forms ulcer-adherent complex. Minimal absorption (<2%)
Tripotassium dicitratobismuthate	A chelate of bismuth that acts as a mucosal protectant. Low bismuth content is not associated with encephalopathy seen with older, high-bismuth preparations (no longer recommended). Used in gastric and duodenal ulcers and in *Helicobacter pylori* eradication when initial treatment fails
Other drugs	
Alginic acid	Alginates form a viscous gel ('raft') that floats on the surface of the stomach contents, reducing acid reflux. Usually combined with antacids
Antacids	Antacids include aluminium hydroxide, sodium carbonate, and magnesium trisilicate, carbonate or hydroxide. Antacids neutralise acid within the stomach. May be combined with simeticone, an antifoaming agent
Antimicrobials	Used with a PPI to eradicate *H. pylori* infection. See Chapter 51

PPI, proton pump inhibitors.

34 Inflammatory bowel disease

● ●

Crohn's disease and *ulcerative colitis* are chronic inflammatory disorders of the gastrointestinal tract which together are termed 'inflammatory bowel disease' (IBD). However, there are many differences in predisposition and pathogenesis between the two conditions. It is also likely that within each category there are different phenotypes. There are other uncommon, atypical forms of inflammatory bowel disease, such as collagenous colitis and lymphocytic colitis, which will not be considered in this chapter.

Ulcerative colitis is a disorder with inflammation usually confined to the large bowel, although when the whole of the colon is involved, there can also be inflammation in the terminal ileum. The extent of colonic involvement varies, but the rectum is always involved and mucosal inflammation is continuous, not patchy. Inflammation is superficial and confined to the mucosa and submucosa. Symptoms include bloody diarrhoea, urgency, tenesmus and, if severe, fever and weight loss (Box 34.1). Ulcerative colitis can be associated with extracolonic manifestations such as primary sclerosing cholangitis, autoimmune liver disease, uveitis, seronegative spondyloarthritis and skin disorders.

Crohn's disease can involve any part of the gut. The bowel involvement is discontinuous and segmental, most frequently found in the terminal ileum and colon but often sparing the rectum. Fistula formation, small-bowel strictures and perianal disease such as abscesses and fissures are common. In the gut, inflammation is transmural with granuloma formation. Clinical features of colonic involvement include diarrhoea (with or without blood), abdominal pain and weight loss. Malaise, fever and anorexia are also common. Involvement of more proximal parts of the gut produces various symptoms, depending on the site of the disease, and diarrhoea need not be present (see Box 34.1). In the gut, inflammation is a transmural granulomatous condition. Extraintestinal manifestations include aphthous mouth ulcers, pyoderma gangrenosum, erythema nodosum and seronegative spondyloarthritis.

Exact diagnosis of the type of IBD may be difficult at presentation if the disease is confined to the colon, as the initial histological findings may not be typical of either ulcerative colitis or Crohn's disease (indeterminate colitis).

The aetiologies of IBD are unclear, although many susceptibility genes have been identified. Some of these may disrupt the colonic epithelial barrier and expose dendritic cells to commensal bacteria, while others alter several innate and adaptive immune responses to the bacteria (Fig. 34.1). Having breached the mucosa, colonic bacteria promote excessive activation of the host immune system. Cells involved in innate immunity contribute to the inflammation, including natural killer T-cells, neutrophil leucocytes, macrophages and dendritic cells. These secrete tumour necrosis factor α (TNFα) and a variety of proinflammatory interleukins and chemokines. The abnormal immune response also involves an excess number of adaptive immune cells. In Crohn's disease these are T-helper type 1 (Th1) lymphocytes, while in ulcerative colitis they are T-helper type 2 (Th2) lymphocytes, leading to different patterns of cytokine release (see Chapter 38). T-helper type 17 (Th17) lymphocytes are involved in the pathogenesis of both conditions. Regulatory T-cells are probably deficient in IBD.

There is a close interaction between the immune system and the enteric nervous system that contributes to motility disturbance in the bowel and pain. Cigarette smoking increases the risk of acquiring Crohn's disease and the frequency of exacerbations, but slightly decreases the risk of developing ulcerative colitis.

Inflammatory bowel disease can undergo periods of relapse and remission over many years. Treatment of both types of IBD is intended to induce and maintain remission but does not cure the condition.

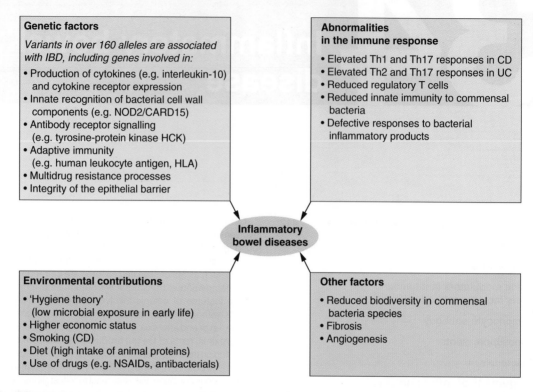

Genetic factors

Variants in over 160 alleles are associated with IBD, including genes involved in:
- Production of cytokines (e.g. interleukin-10) and cytokine receptor expression
- Innate recognition of bacterial cell wall components (e.g. NOD2/CARD15)
- Antibody receptor signalling (e.g. tyrosine-protein kinase HCK)
- Adaptive immunity (e.g. human leukocyte antigen, HLA)
- Multidrug resistance processes
- Integrity of the epithelial barrier

Abnormalities in the immune response
- Elevated Th1 and Th17 responses in CD
- Elevated Th2 and Th17 responses in UC
- Reduced regulatory T cells
- Reduced innate immunity to commensal bacteria
- Defective responses to bacterial inflammatory products

Inflammatory bowel diseases

Environmental contributions
- 'Hygiene theory' (low microbial exposure in early life)
- Higher economic status
- Smoking (CD)
- Diet (high intake of animal proteins)
- Use of drugs (e.g. NSAIDs, antibacterials)

Other factors
- Reduced biodiversity in commensal bacteria species
- Fibrosis
- Angiogenesis

Fig. 34.1 Factors associated with inflammatory bowel disease. Investigations into the aetiology of inflammatory bowel disease have confirmed the multiplicity of factors that might be involved. The association of some events is strong, while others are weak. Some changes may occur as a consequence of the disease rather than being involved in the cause. *CD*, Crohn's disease; *IBD*, inflammatory bowel disease; *IL*, interleukin; *Th*, T-helper; *TNFα*, tumour necrosis factor α; *UC*, ulcerative colitis.

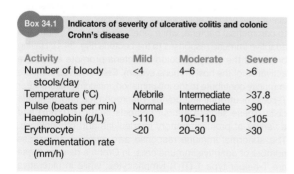

Box 34.1	Indicators of severity of ulcerative colitis and colonic Crohn's disease		
Activity	**Mild**	**Moderate**	**Severe**
Number of bloody stools/day	<4	4–6	>6
Temperature (°C)	Afebrile	Intermediate	>37.8
Pulse (beats per min)	Normal	Intermediate	>90
Haemoglobin (g/L)	>110	105–110	<105
Erythrocyte sedimentation rate (mm/h)	<20	20–30	>30

DRUGS FOR INFLAMMATORY BOWEL DISEASE

AMINOSALICYLATES

xamples

balsalazide, mesalazine, olsalazine, sulfasalazine

Mechanism of action and effects

The active antiinflammatory constituent of all the aminosalicylates is 5-aminosalicylic acid (5-ASA). All the different compounds are designed to deliver 5-ASA to the lumen of the colon (see the following section on pharmacokinetics). Sulfasalazine, a combination of 5-ASA and sulfapyridine, was the first aminosalicylate shown to be effective in treating IBD. Sulfapyridine is responsible for many of the unwanted effects of sulfasalazine, but in contrast to its role in inflammatory arthritis (see Chapter 30), sulfapyridine has no therapeutic value in IBD. The mechanisms of action of aminosalicylates are not clear, but they may involve inhibition of leucocyte chemotaxis by reducing cytokine formation, reduced free radical generation and inhibition of the production of lipid inflammatory mediators (such as prostanoids, leukotrienes and platelet-activating factor). Aminosalicylates are most effective for reducing relapse in ulcerative colitis. Their efficacy in Crohn's disease is less well established, particularly for noncolonic disease. They are less effective in treatment of acute exacerbations of IBD.

Pharmacokinetics

Sulfasalazine is partially absorbed from the gut intact, but most reaches the colon where it undergoes reduction by gut bacteria to sulfapyridine and 5-ASA. Sulfapyridine and about 20% of the 5-ASA are absorbed from the colon, and then metabolised in the liver. There are several formulations of 5-ASA that deliver the drug to the mucosa of the lower gut without requiring sulfapyridine. Mesalazine (the 5-ASA molecule itself) is given as an enteric-coated or modified-release formulation to limit absorption from the small bowel. Olsalazine is two 5-ASA molecules joined by an azo bond. It is not absorbed from the upper gut, and 5-ASA is released after lysis of the azo bond by colonic flora. Balsalazide is a prodrug in which 5-ASA is linked to a carrier molecule (4-amino-benzoyl-β-alanine) by an azo bond, which is cleaved by bacterial reduction in the large bowel.

Mesalazine and sulfasalazine can be given rectally (by suppository or enema) to treat distal disease in the colon.

Unwanted effects

These occur in up to 45% of people treated with sulfasalazine, but only 15% of those who take mesalazine.

- Nausea, vomiting, diarrhoea, abdominal pain.
- Headache.
- Rashes.
- Blood dyscrasias, especially agranulocytosis and thrombocytopenia.
- Cough, insomnia, fever and oligospermia with sulfasalazine.

CORTICOSTEROIDS

budesonide, hydrocortisone, prednisolone

Corticosteroids (see Chapter 44) are very effective for inducing remission in active IBD; however, there is little evidence that they prevent relapse when used at doses that do not produce significant unwanted effects. Budesonide used topically on the rectal mucosa is less well absorbed than prednisolone or hydrocortisone and has fewer systemic unwanted effects. Liquid or foam corticosteroid enemas or suppositories are useful for localised rectal disease, but oral or parenteral administration is needed for more severe or extensive disease.

CYTOKINE MODULATORS (ANTITUMOUR NECROSIS FACTOR α ANTIBODIES)

adalimumab, golimumab, infliximab

Mechanism of action and uses

These are monoclonal antibodies that inhibit the binding of TNFα to its receptors, which in turn reduces production of proinflammatory cytokines (e.g. IL-1 and IL-6), leucocyte migration and infiltration, and activation of neutrophils and eosinophils. Infliximab was the first monoclonal antibody to be approved for the treatment of Crohn's disease. Adalimumab is effective when infliximab is poorly tolerated, or for those

who have become refractory to treatment. Infliximab may also be useful for treatment of severe attacks of ulcerative colitis. Unwanted effects of anti-TNFα antibodies are discussed in Chapter 30.

ANTILYMPHOCYTE ANTIBODY

vedolizumab

Mechanism of action and uses

Vedolizumab is a monoclonal antibody to integrin α4β7, which is expressed on a subset of memory T-lymphocytes, and inhibits binding of these lymphocytes to mucosal addressin cell adhesion molecule 1 (MADCAM1), found on gut mucosal cells. Vedolizumab does not inhibit T-cell binding to vascular cell adhesion molecules and selectively reduces inflammation in the gut. It can be used to induce and maintain remission in ulcerative colitis or Crohn's disease that is refractory to conventional treatments and to anti-TNFα antibodies. Unwanted effects include infusion-related reactions, arthralgia, nausea, headache, cough, fatigue and upper respiratory tract infections.

IMMUNOSUPPRESSANTS

Azathioprine and, less often, mercaptopurine, have a 'corticosteroid-sparing' action in active IBD that may enable corticosteroid doses to be reduced. Maximal efficacy is not achieved for about 6–12 weeks. Nausea, vomiting, rashes and a hypersensitivity syndrome affect about 10% of people during the first 6 weeks of therapy. Pancreatitis and liver toxicity are rare but serious complications.

Methotrexate is useful in Crohn's disease. It is given subcutaneously or intramuscularly and is used when azathioprine has failed. Ciclosporin can induce remission in corticosteroid-resistant acute exacerbation of ulcerative colitis but has no long-term efficacy. More details of these drugs are found in Chapters 38 and 52.

ANTIBACTERIALS

Metronidazole (see Chapter 51) is moderately effective for treatment of some aspects of Crohn's disease, particularly perianal disease, although the mechanism of action is uncertain. Ciprofloxacin probably has similar efficacy.

MANAGEMENT OF INFLAMMATORY BOWEL DISEASE

ULCERATIVE COLITIS

Nonsteroidal antiinflammatory drugs (NSAIDs) and also selective cyclo-oxygenase 2 (COX-2) inhibitors (see Chapter

29) can exacerbate symptoms in severe colitis and should be avoided. Opioids (see Chapter 35) should not be used in the treatment of diarrhoea in extensive colitis, since they can precipitate the life-threatening complication of toxic megacolon. The goals of treatment are control of symptoms and endoscopic mucosal healing, since the latter reduces the risk of relapse or subsequent colectomy. The choice of treatment depends on the severity and extent of the colitis.

For mild symptoms, mesalazine is often the treatment of choice. Rectal delivery of mesalazine is usually successful if the disease is limited to the rectum or left side of the colon (distal colitis). Foam enemas or suppositories will treat inflammation up to 12–20 cm from the anus, while liquid enemas are effective up to 30–60 cm (i.e. to the splenic flexure). Oral aminosalicylate can be combined with rectal administration to improve efficacy, and oral treatment alone may be preferred by some people. More extensive colitis with mild to moderate symptoms is usually treated with an oral aminosalicylate. The disadvantage of aminosalicylates is that they may not produce a response for up to 4 weeks, so for more severe disease or when there is a lack of improvement after 2 weeks, an oral corticosteroid is used to induce remission. To minimise unwanted effects, the dose of corticosteroid should be quickly reduced once control is achieved and then stopped as soon as possible. If repeated courses of corticosteroid are needed, then azathioprine can be effective although it has a slow onset of action over 12–16 weeks.

Acute severe colitis requires intensive fluid and electrolyte replacement; anaemia should be corrected by transfusion, and large doses of parenteral corticosteroid should be given. Infliximab, adalimumab or cyclosporin induce remission in about 40% of cases of corticosteroid refractory disease. Golimumab or vedolizumab are alternative options if there is no response to, or poor tolerability of, the first-line agents. Colectomy is required in about 10% of people with ulcerative colitis that does not settle with conservative treatment.

Once remission is achieved, maintenance treatment with topical mesalazine or an oral aminosalicylate should be lifelong and reduces the relapse rate by two-thirds. It also reduces the risk of developing colorectal cancer, a complication of long-standing extensive colitis, by up to 75%. If disease flares occur despite the regular use of an aminosalicylate, then addition of an immunosuppressant drug such as azathioprine can be effective.

CROHN'S DISEASE

Corticosteroid therapy is the mainstay of medical treatment for active Crohn's disease, usually with oral prednisolone. Remission occurs in over 60% of those treated, but maintenance corticosteroid therapy does not reduce the risk of relapse. Every effort should be made to withdraw the drug once the disease activity has been controlled. Disease confined to the distal colon can respond to topical therapy with a corticosteroid, and an oral aminosalicylate such as mesalazine can also have a modest benefit in colonic Crohn's disease (see the previous section on the management of ulcerative colitis). For Crohn's disease outside the colon, aminosalicylates are ineffective. Infliximab or adalimumab are used to induce remission in Crohn's disease that is resistant to conventional therapy. A single infusion can induce remission for up to 3 months. Vedolizumab should be considered if there is no response to infliximab or adalimumab, or these drugs

are poorly tolerated. The antibacterial drugs ciprofloxacin and metronidazole are particularly useful for treating perianal fistulas, but rarely result in complete healing. Azathioprine or infliximab are usually required for fistulating disease.

Aminosalicylates are ineffective for maintaining remission in Crohn's disease. Azathioprine should be considered if control of Crohn's disease requires more than two 6-week courses of oral corticosteroid therapy per year, or if the disease relapses as the dose of corticosteroid is reduced. Infliximab or adalimumab can be used to maintain remission if they were used to induce remission. Methotrexate is effective for maintaining remission in Crohn's disease but is often poorly tolerated, so it is used when there is intolerance to azathioprine or anti-TNFα drugs. Smoking cessation reduces the risk of relapse in Crohn's disease by 65%, an effect comparable in size to that achieved with an immunosuppressant.

Surgery may be necessary for disease that is refractory to medical therapy – for example, bowel resection for intestinal obstruction from fibro-stenotic disease, drainage of perianal abscesses or control of penetrating disease with fistulas. A defunctioning ileostomy to 'rest' the bowel may allow active inflammation to settle with medical therapy in refractory disease, but colonic disease usually recurs after closure of the stoma. Surgery should always be an integral part of the management plan, and is required at some time in up to 80% of people with Crohn's disease.

SELF-ASSESSMENT

True/false questions

1. Crohn's disease lesions are transmural and confined to the small bowel.
2. Cigarette smoking increases the risk of Crohn's disease.
3. In IBD the main active constituent of sulfasalazine is sulfapyridine.
4. Mesalazine (5-ASA) can be given rectally.
5. Mesalazine is equally useful in the treatment of Crohn's disease involving the colon or the small bowel.
6. Corticosteroids are effective for maintaining remission in ulcerative colitis.
7. Immunosuppressants such as azathioprine are ineffective for the treatment of Crohn's disease.
8. Infliximab can induce remission even in refractory IBD.
9. NSAIDs should be avoided in IBD.
10. Diarrhoea in IBD can be treated with the opioid loperamide.

One-best-answer (OBA) question

Choose the *most accurate* statement concerning IBD drugs from A–E.
A. 5-Aminosalicylic acid given orally or rectally is well absorbed.
B. Balsalazide comprises two molecules of 5-ASA joined by an azo bond.
C. Azathioprine is the first-line drug of choice in treating mild Crohn's disease.
D. Adalimumab is an antibody directed against interleukin-6.
E. Vedolizumab selectively impairs lymphocyte activity in gut inflammation.

Case-based questions

A 35-year-old man presented with a 3-week period of frequent diarrhoea with mucus but no blood in the stool. Stool analysis for infective agents was negative. Sigmoidoscopy indicated gross thickening of the mucosa, with inflammation and linear ulcers. Changes were present in restricted areas (skip lesions), with intervening normal mucosa. Histology was diagnostic of Crohn's disease, and investigation suggested that the condition was confined to the sigmoid and part of the ascending colon.

1. What is the cause of Crohn's disease?
2. How should this man be treated initially?
3. How do corticosteroids act in Crohn's disease?
4. How should the corticosteroid be given, and why?
5. Why should the corticosteroid dosage be reduced slowly at the end of treatment?
6. How can remission be maintained in this man?
7. What alternative therapies can be given to try to reduce the risk of corticosteroid dependence?

ANSWERS

True/false answers

1. **False.** Crohn's disease is transmural but can affect any part of the gastrointestinal tract.
2. **True.** There is increased risk of Crohn's disease in smokers but a slightly decreased risk of ulcerative colitis.
3. **False.** Sulfasalazine is broken down in the colon to 5-ASA, which is responsible for the beneficial effects in IBD, and sulfapyridine, which is inactive in IBD but causes most of the unwanted effects.
4. **True.** Modified-release formulations of mesalazine are available for rectal administration to deliver the drug to the distal colonic mucosa.
5. **False.** Although mesalazine may be of some benefit in colonic Crohn's disease, it is not very effective for small-bowel Crohn's disease.
6. **False.** Although they are effective for inducing remission, there is little evidence that corticosteroids prevent relapse.
7. **False.** People with chronic Crohn's disease can become corticosteroid-dependent, and immunosuppressants such as azathioprine can be useful in reducing this dependence. Many months of treatment are required before they are fully effective.
8. **True.** A single infusion of infliximab can induce remission for up to 3 months; remission may be maintained by further infusions at twice-monthly intervals.
9. **True.** NSAIDs and selective COX-2 inhibitors (coxibs) can exacerbate symptoms in severe disease.
10. **False.** Opioids should be avoided, as they can precipitate toxic megacolon.

One-best-answer (OBA) answer

Answer E is the most accurate.
A. Incorrect. 5-ASA is poorly absorbed by either route and acts locally within the gut.
B. Incorrect. The 5-ASA dimer is olsalazine, while balsalazide is a molecule of 5-ASA linked to an inert carrier molecule; in both cases the active 5-ASA is released by colonic bacterial reduction.
C. Incorrect. Azathioprine is usually given in corticosteroid-refractory disease or when people are having frequent courses of corticosteroids for treatment (more than two 6-week courses per year).
D. Incorrect. Adalimumab is a fully humanised monoclonal antibody against TNFα and is given subcutaneously for the treatment of refractory disease; inhibition of IL-6 (and IL-1) is secondary to its action on TNFα.
E. **Correct.** Vedolizumab is an antibody to integrin α4β7 that blocks adhesion of memory T-lymphocytes to MADCAM1 found on gut mucosal cells.

Case-based answers

1. The cause of Crohn's disease is unknown, although there is a central role of Th1 lymphocytes while Th2 lymphocytes predominate in ulcerative colitis. Several hypotheses have implicated a number of risk factors, including infection, altered immune response to infection and environmental factors (see Fig. 34.1).
2. Initial treatment is with corticosteroids. Because Crohn's disease is confined to the distal colon, topical treatment with a corticosteroid such as budesonide could be used to limit systemic unwanted effects. If, however, there was involvement of the proximal large bowel or small bowel, it would be necessary to give an oral corticosteroid, such as prednisolone.
3. Corticosteroids have a variety of actions. They can alter the release of inflammatory mediators such as arachidonic acid metabolites, kinins and cytokines. They can alter cell-mediated cytotoxicity, antibody production, adhesion molecule expression, phagocytic function, leucocyte chemotaxis and leucocyte adherence.
4. Corticosteroids should be given until remission occurs. If possible, the corticosteroid should be administered locally to keep the plasma concentration low, but for individuals who experience systemic symptoms of IBD (such as fatigue, anorexia or weight loss), oral therapy is indicated.
5. Systemic corticosteroids suppress the hypothalamo–pituitary–adrenal axis and can reduce the circulating levels of endogenous adrenal glucocorticoids (see Chapter 44). Gradual reduction of the dose of therapeutic corticosteroid allows recovery of the production of endogenous glucocorticoids.
6. If the colitis is restricted to the distal colon, topical administration of mesalazine or an oral formulation that delivers 5-ASA to the colon could be used. 5-ASA is, however, less effective in Crohn's disease, particularly if it involves the small bowel.
7. Continuous corticosteroid therapy for periods of 6 months or longer is eventually required in 40–50% of people with Crohn's disease. If more than two 6-week courses of corticosteroid per year are required to maintain control of symptoms, immunosuppressive therapy should be considered. Immunosuppressive therapy is usually with azathioprine, or 6-mercaptopurine; prolonged treatment with these drugs is usually required (up to 6 months) before a clinical response occurs. Anti-TNFα antibody treatment is also of benefit in severe disease that is not responsive to other therapies.

FURTHER READING

Danese, S., Fiocchi, C., 2011. Ulcerative colitis. N. Engl. J. Med. 365, 1713–1725.

Ford, A.C., Moayyedi, P., Hanauer, S.B., 2013. Ulcerative colitis. Br. Med. J. 346, f432.

Kalla, R., Ventham, N.T., Arnott, I.D., 2014. Crohn's disease. Br. Med. J. 349, g6670.

Park, S.C., Jeen, Y.T., 2015. Current and emerging biologics for ulcerative colitis. Gut Liver 9, 18–27.

Compendium: drugs used in inflammatory bowel disease

Drug	Characteristics
Aminosalicylates	
Balsalazide	Prodrug cleaved by the colonic flora to 5-ASA and an inactive metabolite. Given orally for mild to moderate ulcerative colitis and maintenance of remission
5-ASA	Used for mild to moderate ulcerative colitis and maintenance of remission. Given orally, or rectally as a foam or retention enema or suppository. Absorbed in upper intestine; may be more effective than sulfasalazine in the presence of diarrhoea, because there is no requirement for reduction by the gut flora. Half-life: 0.5–1 h
Olsalazine	Dimer of 5-ASA; colonic flora generates free 5-ASA. Given orally for mild ulcerative colitis and maintenance of remission. Half-life: 1 h
Sulfasalazine	Converted by colonic flora to 5-ASA, which has local actions, and sulfapyridine, which has no therapeutic action but causes many of the unwanted effects. Used for mild to moderate and severe ulcerative colitis and for Crohn's disease. Given orally, or rectally as a suppository. 5-ASA half-life 4–10 h
Cytokine modulators	
Other than the drugs listed below, anti-TNFα antibodies used for rheumatoid arthritis (see Chapter 30) are not currently approved for IBD.	
Adalimumab	Monoclonal antibody against TNFα. Given by subcutaneous injection in severe Crohn's disease and ulcerative colitis unresponsive to other treatments. Half-life: 12 days
Golimumab	Monoclonal antibody against TNFα. Given by subcutaneous injection in severe ulcerative colitis unresponsive or intolerant to conventional therapy. Half-life: 12 days
Infliximab	Monoclonal antibody against TNFα. Given by intravenous infusion in severe Crohn's disease and ulcerative colitis unresponsive to other treatments. Half-life: 8–10 days
Antilymphocyte antibody	
Vedolizumab	Monoclonal antibody against the $\alpha_4\beta_7$ integrin preferentially expressed on gut-homing T helper lymphocytes. Given by intravenous infusion in moderate to severe Crohn's disease and ulcerative colitis unresponsive or intolerant to conventional medication or to a TNFα inhibitor. Half-life: 25 days
Immunosuppressants	
Azathioprine	Prodrug of 6-mercaptopurine. Given orally in resistant and frequently relapsing cases of ulcerative colitis or Crohn's disease. See Chapter 38
Ciclosporin	Given intravenously for short-term treatment of severe acute ulcerative colitis (an unlicensed indication in the United Kingdom). See Chapter 38
Corticosteroids	Beclometasone dipropionate, budesonide, hydrocortisone and prednisolone. Given orally by intravenous injection and locally by enema or suppository, as adjuncts to aminosalicylates in moderate or refractory Crohn's disease and ulcerative colitis. See Chapter 44
Mercaptopurine	A thiopurine antimetabolite; main use is as an anticancer drug (see Chapter 52). Given orally in resistant and frequently relapsing cases of ulcerative colitis or Crohn's disease. Half-life: 1–1.5 h
Methotrexate	Folate analogue. Given weekly by mouth or by intramuscular injection in unresponsive or chronically active Crohn's disease. See Chapter 52
Antibiotics	
Metronidazole	May be beneficial for the treatment of active Crohn's disease; used in people who fail to respond to sulfasalazine. See Chapter 51

5-ASA, Mesalazine or 5-aminosalicylic acid; *IBD,* inflammatory bowel disease; *TNFα,* tumour necrosis factor α.

35 Constipation, diarrhoea and irritable bowel syndrome

CONSTIPATION

The frequency of normal defaecation ranges from three times a day to once every 3 days, although for some it may be less often. Maintenance of 'regular' bowel habits is a preoccupation of Western societies and is best achieved by increasing dietary fibre. Nevertheless, laxative drugs are widely prescribed or taken without prescription.

Frequent constipation affects 10% of the population. It is defined as the passage of hard, small stools less frequently than the person's own normal function and is often associated with straining. Constipation has many causes (Box 35.1). Underlying organic disease should be excluded when there is persistent constipation or if there has been a recent change in bowel habit.

LAXATIVES

Laxatives are drugs that increase the frequency of defaecation or ease the passage of stool. The mechanisms of action of common laxatives are shown in Fig. 35.1. Some drugs have more than one mechanism; they are classified by their principal action.

Bulk-forming laxatives

Examples

bran, ispaghula husk, methylcellulose, sterculia

Bulking agents include various natural polysaccharides, usually of plant origin, such as unprocessed wheat bran, ispaghula husk, methylcellulose and sterculia, all of which are poorly broken down by digestive processes. They have several mechanisms of action:

- a hydrophilic action causing retention of water in the gut lumen, which expands and softens the faeces,
- proliferation of colonic bacteria, which further increases faecal bulk,
- stimulation of colonic mucosal receptors by the increased faecal bulk, promoting peristalsis,
- degradation of polysaccharides in sterculia to substances that have an osmotic laxative effect.

Bulking agents take at least 24 hours after ingestion to work. A liberal fluid intake is important to lubricate the colon and minimise the risk of obstruction. Bulking agents are useful for establishing a regular bowel habit in chronic constipation, diverticular disease and irritable bowel syndrome (IBS), but they should be avoided if the colon is atonic or there is faecal impaction.

Unwanted effects include a sensation of bloating, flatulence or griping abdominal pain.

Osmotic laxatives

Examples

lactulose, macrogols, magnesium salts, sodium acid phosphate

Osmotic laxatives draw water into stool, which becomes softer and easier to pass. Lactulose is a disaccharide of fructose and galactose. In the colon, bacterial action releases the fructose and galactose, which are fermented to lactic and acetic acids with release of gas. The fermentation products are osmotically active. They also lower intestinal pH, which favours overgrowth of some selected colonic flora but inhibits the proliferation of ammonia-producing bacteria. This is useful in the treatment of hepatic encephalopathy (see Chapter 36). Unwanted effects include flatulence and abdominal cramps. Lactulose can take more than 24 hours to act.

Diet low in fibre or fluid
Disease-induced – e.g. colonic cancer, myxoedema,
　　hypercalcaemia
Drug-induced – frequent causes include:
　　opioid analgesics (this chapter and Chapter 19)
　　antimuscarinic agents – e.g. oxybutynin (Chapter 15),
　　　orphenadrine (Chapter 24), cyclizine (Chapter 32)
　　antacids containing calcium or aluminium salts
　　　(Chapter 33)
　　calcium channel blockers (Chapter 5)
　　iron salts (Chapter 47)
　　tricyclic antidepressants (Chapter 22)
　　phenothiazines (Chapter 21)
Slow gut transit, especially in young women
Immobility
Hypotonic colon in the elderly

**Fig. 35.1 Sites of action of the major classes of
laxative drug.** Some laxative drugs have more than one
mechanism of action. For mechanisms of some other drugs
used in constipation, see the drug compendium. *CCK*,
Cholecystokinin.

Macrogol 3350 is a large, inert polymer of ethylene glycol
that is not absorbed from the gut and exerts an osmotic
effect in the colon. It is formulated in combination with sodium
and potassium salts. Macrogol 3350 is as effective as other
osmotic agents, but its Na^+ content may be hazardous for
people with impaired cardiac function.

Magnesium salts such as the sulfate (Epsom salts) and
the hydroxide are poorly absorbed from the gut and act as
osmotically active solutes that retain water in the colonic
lumen. They may also stimulate cholecystokinin release
from the small-intestinal mucosa, which increases intestinal
secretions and enhances colonic motility (see Fig. 35.1). These
actions result in more rapid transit of gut contents into the

large bowel, where distension promotes evacuation within
2–4 hours. About 20% of ingested magnesium is absorbed
and excreted by the kidneys. In renal failure, this can result in
hypermagnesaemia with muscle weakness, hypotension and
bradycardia. Magnesium hydroxide is a mild laxative, while the
action of magnesium sulfate can be quite fierce, associated
with considerable abdominal discomfort. Magnesium salts
are recommended only for occasional use.

Sodium acid phosphate is an osmotic preparation given
orally or as an enema, usually for bowel preparation before
local procedures or surgery.

Irritant and stimulant laxatives

Examples

bisacodyl, dantron, docusate sodium, senna, sodium
picosulphate

Irritant and stimulant laxatives include the anthraquinones
senna and dantron and the polyphenolic compounds
bisacodyl and sodium picosulphate. They act by a variety
of mechanisms, including stimulation of local reflexes through
myenteric nerve plexuses in the gut, which enhances gut
motility and increases water and electrolyte transfer into the
lower gut. Stimulant laxatives are useful for more severe
forms of constipation, but tolerance is common with regular
use and they can produce abdominal cramps. Given orally,
they stimulate defecation after about 6–12 hours.

- Senna has the most gentle purgative action of this group.
　Given orally, it is hydrolysed by colonic bacteria to release
　the irritant derivatives sennosides A and B.
- Bisacodyl can be given orally or as a rectal suppository
　for a more rapid action in 15–30 minutes.
- Dantron is available as co-danthramer, a combination
　with the surface wetting agent poloxamer 188, and as
　co-danthrusate, a combination with the faecal-softening
　agent docusate (see below). Dantron is carcinogenic at
　high doses in animals; it is recommended that its use
　be limited to the elderly or terminally ill.
- Sodium picosulphate is a powerful irritant and is given
　orally to prepare the bowel for surgery or colonoscopy.
　It usually acts in less than 6 hours.

The chronic use of stimulant laxatives has been suspected
to cause progressive deterioration of normal colonic function,
with eventual atony ('cathartic colon'). It is now recognised
that the condition probably arises from severe, refractory
constipation rather than from the treatment.

Faecal softeners

Example

arachis oil, co-danthrusate, docusate sodium

Arachis oil can be given rectally to soften impacted
faeces. Other drugs with faecal-softening actions include
bulk-forming laxatives and docusate sodium. Liquid paraffin
can be given orally but is not recommended, since it impairs

the absorption of fat-soluble vitamins, can cause anal seepage with anal pruritus and carries a risk of lipoid pneumonia after accidental inhalation.

Docusate sodium has mild stimulant activity as well as detergent properties that may soften stools by increasing fluid and fat penetration into hard stool. It is a relatively ineffective laxative that is given rectally by enema or orally. It is also used in combination with dantron as co-danthrusate (see above).

MANAGEMENT OF CONSTIPATION

For simple constipation, adopting a high-fibre diet is recommended. Exercise and an adequate fluid intake are also important. A stimulant laxative such as senna or bisacodyl can be taken orally at night to give a morning bowel action. Suppositories will give a more rapid effect. For longer-term therapy, regular macrogol 3350 is usually well tolerated and effective, or lactulose can be considered. Bulk laxatives are generally less effective.

Certain laxatives may be useful in specific situations:

- Senna, magnesium salts and docusate appear to be safe in pregnancy.
- Bisacodyl, co-danthramer and co-danthrusate are suitable for the elderly or for the terminally ill with opioid-induced constipation.
- For opioid-induced constipation when other laxatives are ineffective, the peripheral opioid receptor antagonist methylnaltrexone can be used (see Chapter 19).
- Lactulose is useful specifically to treat constipation associated with hepatic encephalopathy (see Chapter 36).
- For people in whom neurological disease affecting bowel motility is the cause of constipation, a faecal softener should be used, with regular enemas or rectal washouts.

Refractory idiopathic constipation is a condition almost exclusively found in women, starting at a young age. Long-term use of stimulant laxatives, often at high dosage, may be necessary. Bulk-forming laxatives are ineffective, and a high-fibre diet usually increases abdominal distension and discomfort. Biofeedback can help in up to 80% of people with the condition. Prucalopride, a 5-HT$_4$ receptor agonist, or lubiprostone, a chloride-channel activator, is used for refractory chronic idiopathic constipation when other measures have failed. Surgical intervention with colectomy may be the only option for the most severely affected people.

DIARRHOEA

Diarrhoea is frequent watery bowel movements, with or without cramping. Acute diarrhoea is usually caused by gastrointestinal infection, when it can be the consequence of both reduced absorption of fluid and an increase in intestinal secretions. Locally released bacterial enterotoxins have a variety of actions on gut mucosal cells, including stimulation of intracellular cyclic adenosine monophosphate synthesis, which causes excess Cl$^-$ secretion into the bowel. Enteropathic viruses, such as rotavirus and norovirus, damage enterocytes, resulting in proliferation of immature cells with greater secretory capacity. Viral gastroenteritis is much more common than bacterial causes of acute diarrhoea in children, but both viruses and bacteria are important in adults. Traveller's diarrhoea is a particularly common problem because the person is exposed to organisms

that have not been encountered before. Common causes include enterotoxin-producing *Escherichia coli*, *Clostridium jejuni* and *Salmonella* and *Shigella* species. Parasites such as *Giardia lamblia*, *Cryptosporidium* species and *Cyclospora cayetanensis* are less commonly involved.

Drugs that can produce diarrhoea include magnesium salts (see previous), cytotoxic agents (see Chapter 52), α- and β-adrenoceptor antagonists (see Chapters 5 and 6) and broad-spectrum antibacterial drugs, which alter colonic flora (see Chapter 51). Antibacterial treatment can also be associated with *Clostridium difficile* colitis.

Chronic diarrhoea requires full investigation for non-infectious causes such as carcinoma of the colon, inflammatory bowel disease and coeliac disease. Irritable bowel syndrome (IBS) is often accompanied by increased frequency of defaecation, loose stool and a sensation of incomplete evacuation (see below).

DRUGS FOR TREATING DIARRHOEA

Opioids

codeine phosphate, diphenoxylate, loperamide

The antimotility action of opioids is a result of binding to μ-opioid receptors on neurons in the submucosal neural plexus of the intestinal wall (see Chapter 19). They enhance segmental contractions in the colon, inhibit propulsive movements of the small intestine and colon and prolong the transit time of intestinal contents. Prolonged contact of intestinal contents with the gut mucosa provides the opportunity for enhanced absorption of fluid.

The opioids most often used to treat diarrhoea are codeine, loperamide and diphenoxylate (used in combination with atropine as co-phenotrope). Codeine and diphenoxylate have short half-lives (<5 hours). Loperamide has a more rapid onset of action and a longer half-life (11 hours), giving it a longer duration of action. It is relatively selective for the gut since efflux mediated by P-glycoprotein prevents loperamide crossing the blood-brain barrier. Therefore, in contrast to other opioids, dependence is not a problem. Loperamide has additional antimuscarinic activity that also inhibits peristalsis (also achieved by atropine in co-phenotrope) and increases anal tone. Morphine is licensed to treat diarrhoea in combination with kaolin (see below) but is not generally recommended. Unwanted effects of opioid drugs are discussed in Chapter 19.

Adsorbent and bulk-forming agents

Kaolin is an adsorbent that is relatively ineffective and is not recommended for the treatment of acute diarrhoea. Ispaghula, methylcellulose and sterculia are bulking agents that can help to control faecal consistency in diarrhoea-predominant IBS or for people with an ileostomy or colostomy. They are not recommended for treatment of acute diarrhoea.

MANAGEMENT OF DIARRHOEA

In developed countries, most people with acute infective diarrhoea who are otherwise fit generally require only high oral fluid and electrolyte intake. Fluid and electrolyte balance are particularly important in young children and the elderly, as they can dehydrate more quickly. Specially formulated powders containing electrolytes (particularly Na^+ and K^+) and glucose (to enhance electrolyte absorption) are available as oral rehydration therapy (ORT). When correctly reconstituted with clean water, they provide a balanced rehydration solution that should be given rapidly over 3–4 hours, after which the need for further treatment should be reassessed. Intravenous fluids may be required for severe dehydration.

If drug treatment is required, an opioid is useful for mild to moderate diarrhoea. Opioids should be avoided in dysentery, when prolonging contact of the organism with the gut mucosa can be detrimental. In young children, ileus with severe abdominal distension can occur with opioids; it is recommended that they should not be used in this age group.

Antibacterial prophylaxis can be used to prevent traveller's diarrhoea in people visiting high-risk areas. Ciprofloxacin or azithromycin are most often recommended (see Chapter 51), depending on the area to which the person is travelling. Alternatively, an antibacterial can be taken at the first sign of illness, when it will usually shorten the duration of the attack to less than 24 hours. Ciprofloxacin is often recommended for empirical treatment if there is fever or bloody diarrhoea, suggesting invasive disease (such as that produced by *Campylobacter* or *Shigella* species). If these are not present, rifaximin, a nonabsorbable antimicrobial, can be used.

Diarrhoea in inflammatory bowel disease should be treated by management of the underlying condition. Antidiarrhoeals should not be used in active inflammatory bowel disease because of the risk of precipitating toxic megacolon (see Chapter 34).

Clostridium difficile-associated diarrhoea

Antibacterial-induced diarrhoea usually resolves rapidly on stopping the provoking drug. However, overgrowth of *C. difficile* produces more prolonged and severe diarrhoea. Any broad-spectrum antibacterial can promote colonisation with *C. difficile* in the colon, but cephalosporins, penicillins and quinolones are the most frequent causes. Symptoms from *C. difficile* colonisation arise from production of toxin by the bacteria; the diagnosis is confirmed by detection of toxin in the stool. *C. difficile*-associated diarrhoea fails to settle with conservative treatment in 80% of cases and can produce fatal colitis. The organism can usually be eliminated with oral metronidazole or oral vancomycin (see Chapter 51).

IRRITABLE BOWEL SYNDROME

IBS is common, occurring in 15% of the population. It is characterised by abdominal pain or discomfort, bloating and change in bowel habit. There are two overlapping clinical presentations: constipation-predominant and diarrhoea-predominant. Abdominal discomfort may be relieved by defecation, but there is often a sensation of incomplete evacuation and mucus is often passed per rectum. The cause is unknown, but altered processing of visceral pain (gut hypersensitivity) is a factor. A strong psychological component, particularly stress, is also evident.

Confirming the diagnosis of IBS involves exclusion of more serious bowel pathology. Screening should include inflammatory markers, coeliac disease immunology, and the exclusion of anaemia, which may indicate alternative diagnoses. Faecal calprotectin (a marker of inflammatory bowel disease) may also be part of a screening workup.

DRUGS FOR TREATING IRRITABLE BOWEL SYNDROME

Antimuscarinic drugs

 Examples

dicycloverine, propantheline

Mechanism of action

Antimuscarinic drugs reduce colonic motility by inhibiting parasympathetic stimulation of the myenteric and submucosal neural plexuses. They also inhibit gastric emptying.

Pharmacokinetics

Oral absorption of dicycloverine is good, and it is metabolised in the liver with a half-life of 10 hours. Propantheline is a poorly absorbed quaternary amine and most is hydrolysed in the bowel.

Unwanted effects

- Constipation.
- Transient bradycardia followed by tachycardia.
- Urinary retention.
- Blurred vision.
- Dry mouth.

Other antispasmodic agents

 Examples

alverine citrate, mebeverine, peppermint oil

Mechanism of action

These antispasmodic agents have direct smooth muscle-relaxant properties (possibly by phosphodiesterase inhibition). They can relieve gut spasm and the associated pain.

Pharmacokinetics

Oral absorption of mebeverine is rapid and it undergoes extensive first-pass metabolism, so little reaches the circulation. Little is known about the pharmacokinetics of alverine citrate and peppermint oil.

Unwanted effects

Unwanted effects are rare.

- Nausea with alverine citrate,
- Heartburn and perianal irritation with peppermint oil,
- Headache,
- Allergic reactions.

MANAGEMENT OF IRRITABLE BOWEL SYNDROME

Drug therapy should form only part of the treatment of IBS, supplemented by cognitive behavioural therapy, relaxation and hypnotherapy where appropriate. Hypnotherapy is effective in up to 60% of people but should be given by a properly trained therapist. Reductions in tea and coffee consumption and smoking as well as modification of diet with exclusion of trigger foods may be helpful.

Constipation can be treated with bulking agents such as ispaghula husk or, if colonic transit time is very prolonged, an osmotic laxative may be effective. Lactulose is not recommended as it can promote bloating and stimulant laxatives can cause abdominal cramps. Prucalopride is a selective 5-HT$_4$ receptor antagonist that improves colonic motility in constipation-predominant IBS that has responded inadequately to standard treatments. Linaclotide is a guanylate cyclase 2C receptor agonist that activates the enzyme on the luminal surface of intestinal epithelial cells and increases anion and fluid secretion. It is used to treat constipation and reduce abdominal pain in refractory constipation-predominant IBS.

Loperamide is the first-choice drug for treatment of diarrhoea because it has a rapid onset of action and enables people to control their bowels, particularly when out of their normal environment or in other circumstances where diarrhoea would be socially disruptive. Care must be taken with other opioids because of the risks of dependency. Regular use of small doses of an antidiarrhoeal drug may be preferable to intermittent use. Colestyramine (see Chapter 48) may reduce diarrhoea when there is terminal ileal dysfunction by chelating bile salts. Bacterial overgrowth has been demonstrated in many people with IBS; 2 weeks' treatment with the non-absorbable antibacterial rifaximin can reduce bloating.

Treatments for diarrhoea in IBS do not usually reduce the abdominal pain. There may be benefit from antispasmodic agents or a low dose of a tricyclic antidepressant for analgesic effect (see Chapter 19). An antidepressant may also be useful for management of co-existing depression, which is frequently present. Selective serotonin reuptake inhibitors are recommended only if a tricyclic antidepressant is ineffective, as they have no analgesic action (see Chapter 22).

SELF-ASSESSMENT

True/false questions

1. Constipation is defined as defecation occurring less often than once daily.
2. Most cases of simple constipation can be treated by lifestyle changes.
3. Chronic intake of senna causes progressive hyperactivity of colonic motility.
4. Antacids containing aluminium salts cause constipation.
5. Laxatives invariably induce bowel movements within 6 hours.
6. Diarrhoea is largely of psychological origin in some people.
7. In infants (<2 years old) diarrhoea is mainly caused by bacterial infection.
8. Broad-spectrum antibacterial drugs may cause pseudomembranous colitis.
9. The use of antibacterial drugs to treat acute episodes of diarrhoea is rarely necessary.
10. Oral rehydration powders are reconstituted to give a hypertonic solution.

One-best-answer (OBA) questions

1. Choose the *correct* statement below concerning drugs used for constipation.
    A. Use of bulk laxatives should be accompanied by ample fluid intake.
    B. Prucalopride blocks serotonin 5-HT$_4$ receptors in the gut.
    C. Lactulose acts by stimulating the enteric nerves.
    D. Lubiprostone is an activator of guanylate cyclase 2C.
    E. Sterculia acts as a laxative within 12 hours.
2. Which statement about diarrhoea is the *least accurate*?
    A. Rotavirus is an uncommon cause of diarrhoea in adults.
    B. Kaolin is not recommended for acute diarrhoea.
    C. *Campylobacter jejuni* is a common cause of bacterial gastroenteritis in the United Kingdom.
    D. Loperamide decreases the gut residence time of the infective organism.
    E. Antibacterial drugs can be used prophylactically for traveller's diarrhoea.

ANSWERS

True/false answers

1. **False.** Normal bowel habit varies widely, with defecation between three times daily and once every 3 days (or longer) regarded as normal.
2. **True.** Increased fibre intake and exercise help most cases of 'simple' constipation.
3. **False.** Chronic use of senna has been associated with loss of colonic function and damage to the myenteric plexus ('cathartic colon'), although it is now thought to be due to the refractory constipation itself rather than to inappropriate use of stimulant laxatives.
4. **True.** Aluminium salts can cause constipation, as do other drugs including opioid analgesics, calcium channel blockers and some antidepressants.
5. **False.** Some laxatives (such as magnesium salts) can act within 6 hours, whereas others including lactulose and docusate take considerably longer to exert their activity.
6. **True.** There is a psychological component to diarrhoea and other symptoms in irritable bowel syndrome that may respond to counselling or hypnotherapy.
7. **False.** Viral gastroenteritis, especially rotavirus, is the major cause of infant diarrhoea.
8. **True.** Broad-spectrum antibacterials may cause colitis due to overgrowth of the anaerobe *C. difficile*; it is treated with metronidazole or vancomycin.
9. **True.** In developed countries antibacterial drugs are rarely necessary for acute diarrhoea in otherwise healthy individuals; fluid and electrolyte replacement are appropriate.
10. **False.** The osmotic action of a hypertonic solution would draw water into the bowel, exacerbating diarrhoea; oral rehydration solution should be isotonic or slightly hypotonic.

One-best-answer (OBA) answers

1. **Answer A** is correct.
   A. **Correct.** Adequate water intake is necessary to hydrate bulk-forming laxatives.
   B. Incorrect. Prucalopride promotes colonic motility by its highly selective *agonism* of serotonin 5-HT₄ receptors.
   C. Incorrect. Lactulose is an osmotic laxative.
   D. Incorrect. Lubiprostone increases intestinal secretions by activating **c**hloride (CLCN2) channels.
   E. Incorrect. The bulk-forming laxative sterculia takes more than 24 hours to act.
2. **Answer D** is the *least accurate*.
   A. Correct. Rotavirus causes diarrhoea in young children but very rarely in adults.
   B. Correct. Kaolin is an adsorbent with limited effectiveness.
   C. Correct. *C. jejuni* is one of the commonest causes of gastroenteritis in adults in developed countries.
   D. **Incorrect.** Loperamide inhibits gut contractility by its opioid and antimuscarinic actions, and this may *increase* the residence of invasive organisms.
   E. Correct. Ciprofloxacin or azathioprine can be used prophylactically in travellers to high-risk areas.

FURTHER READING

DuPont, H.L., 2009. Bacterial diarrhea. N. Engl. J. Med. 361, 1560–1569.

Ford, A.C., Talley, N.J., 2012. Laxatives for chronic constipation in adults. Br. Med. J. 345, e6168.

Halland, M., Saito, Y.A., 2015. Irritable bowel syndrome: new and emerging treatments. Br. Med. J. 350, h1622.

Kelly, C.P., LaMont, J.T., 2008. *Clostridium difficile*—more difficult than ever. N. Engl. J. Med. 359, 1932–1940.

Sayuk, G.S., Gyawali, C.P., 2015. Irritable bowel syndrome: modern concepts and management choices. Am. J. Med. 128, 817–827.

Thielman, N.M., 2004. Acute infectious diarrhea. N. Engl. J. Med. 350, 38–47.

Compendium: drugs used in constipation, diarrhoea and irritable bowel syndrome

Drug	Characteristics
Constipation	
Laxatives	
Bulk-forming laxatives	Wheat bran, ispaghula husk, methylcellulose (also a faecal softener), sterculia. Generally not absorbed, but may affect the absorption of nutrients and minerals
Osmotic laxatives	Lactulose, macrogols, magnesium salts. Generally not absorbed but may affect the absorption of nutrients and minerals. Also phosphates and sodium citrate (rectal), for specialist use
Irritant and stimulant laxatives	Bisacodyl (oral or rectal), dantron, docusate sodium (oral or rectal), glycerol (rectal), senna, sodium picosulphate
Faecal-softening agents	Arachis oil, used rectally. Glycerol (rectal), bulk-forming laxatives and docusate sodium (see earlier) also have faecal-softening properties. Oral liquid paraffin is not recommended
Other drugs used for constipation	
Linaclotide	Peptide agonist of guanylate cyclase 2C; increases intracellular cyclic guanosine monophosphate in intestinal epithelial cells and stimulates fluid secretion; also desensitises colonic sensory neurons. Used orally for constipation and associated pain in irritable bowel syndrome (IBS). Minimal absorption
Lubiprostone	Chloride-channel (CLCN2) activator; increases intestinal fluid secretion, which improves motility. Specialist use for chronic idiopathic constipation in adults unresponsive to lifestyle changes. Not significantly absorbed
Methylnaltrexone	Peripherally acting opioid receptor antagonist (see Chapter 19). Used for opioid-induced constipation in terminal care when other laxatives are ineffective
Prucalopride	Serotonin 5-HT₄ receptor agonist; enhances colonic motility. Specialist use for chronic constipation in women when other laxatives fail to provide an adequate response. Half-life: 24–30 h
Diarrhoea	
Antimotility drugs such as opioids can be used for treatment of acute uncomplicated diarrhoea in adults but not in young children.	
Codeine phosphate	Opioid (see Chapter 19)
Diphenoxylate	Opioid (see Chapter 19); given as co-formulation with atropine (co-phenotrope). Half-life: 2–3 h

Compendium: drugs used in constipation, diarrhoea and irritable bowel syndrome (cont'd)

Drug	Characteristics
Kaolin	Adsorbs fluid within gut; not absorbed systemically
Loperamide	Opioid (see Chapter 19), with some antimuscarinic activity. Acts within gut with little central nervous system activity. Half-life: 11 h
Morphine	Opioid (see Chapter 19); available in combination with kaolin for short-term treatment of diarrhoea. Half-life: 1–5 h

Antispasmodic and antimuscarinic drugs

Some drugs listed below are used for IBS.

Alverine citrate	Smooth muscle relaxant used for IBS and as an adjunct in disorders characterised by spasm, also for dysmenorrhea
Atropine	Antimuscarinic used in disorders characterised by gastrointestinal spasm; also used in the eye (see Chapter 50) and as a surgical premedication (see Chapter 17); unwanted effects limit use. Half-life: 12 h
Dicycloverine	Antimuscarinic used for disorders characterised by gastrointestinal spasm, including IBS; less severe unwanted effects than atropine. Half-life: 9–10 h
Hyoscine	Antimuscarinic used for disorders characterised by gastrointestinal spasm and for smooth muscle spasm in genitourinary disorders; also used as surgical premedication (see Chapter 50) and for motion sickness (see Chapter 32); unwanted effects limit use. Half-life: 8 h
Linaclotide	See drugs used for constipation above
Mebeverine	Smooth muscle relaxant used in disorders characterised by gastrointestinal spasm, including IBS. Minimal systemic absorption
Peppermint oil	Smooth muscle relaxant used for gastrointestinal spasm in IBS; local irritant if enteric-coated capsule not swallowed whole
Propantheline	Antimuscarinic used in disorders characterised by gastrointestinal spasm including IBS; also used in urinary incontinence (see Chapter 15). Half-life: 1.5–2 h

All drugs given orally unless otherwise indicated.

36 Liver disease

ACUTE LIVER FAILURE

Acute liver failure usually occurs in people who do not have preexisting liver disease. It can arise from a number of insults to liver cells, the most frequent being viral infections or the toxic effects of drugs and chemicals. In the United Kingdom, paracetamol poisoning (see Chapter 53) is the most common cause of acute liver failure.

Presenting symptoms of liver failure are often nonspecific, with malaise, nausea and abdominal pain. As the syndrome progresses, signs of impairment of brain function occur (hepatic encephalopathy), with initial confusion followed by drowsiness and coma. These clinical features reflect alterations in neurotransmitter synthesis and increased central nervous system neuroinhibition with astrocyte swelling. The major cause is failure of the liver to metabolise ammonia and glutamate generated by bacteria in the gut, which therefore reach the systemic circulation. Both ammonia and glutamate are neurotoxins that lead to cerebral oedema. Their effects are compounded when there is a systemic inflammatory response to infection.

The syndrome of acute liver failure is usually categorised by the speed of onset of encephalopathy after the onset of jaundice. One frequently used classification, the O'Grady system, recognises three subsets:

- Hyperacute liver failure: Onset within 7 days, most often due to paracetamol or hepatitis A or E virus infection.
- Acute liver failure: Onset between 7 and 28 days, typically due to hepatitis B virus (HBV) infection.
- Subacute liver failure: Onset between 29 days and 12 weeks; in this form, ascites and renal failure may also be prominent. It is typically due to nonparacetamol drug-induced injury.

MANAGEMENT OF ACUTE AND SUBACUTE LIVER FAILURE

- Acetylcysteine should be given if paracetamol was the precipitant (see Chapter 53). It has antioxidant and immunological actions that may also improve survival in acute liver failure from other causes if treatment is started early when there is only low-grade encephalopathy.
- Restoration of intravascular volume to maintain organ perfusion. Peripheral vasodilation with low blood pressure is common even in the absence of sepsis. Persistent hypotension can be treated with a vasoconstrictor such as terlipressin (discussed later).
- Broad-spectrum antibacterial agents are often used to prevent sepsis, since functional immunosuppression is common.
- Cerebral oedema is most marked if there is concurrent systemic infection. The risk of cerebral oedema can be reduced by avoiding hyponatraemia and the consequent plasma hypo-osmolality. When the risk of cerebral oedema is high, sedation and mechanical ventilation are used to maintain a low arterial carbon dioxide concentration, and intracranial pressure can be reduced by intravenous mannitol (see Chapter 14) or hypertonic saline.
- Intravenous glucose is used to correct hypoglycaemia.
- Bleeding is uncommon, since synthesis of both coagulant and anticoagulant factors is impaired. If bleeding is a problem, intravenous vitamin K (see Chapter 11), or fresh frozen plasma or cryoprecipitate may be necessary.
- Emergency liver transplantation may be considered for severe liver failure.

CHRONIC LIVER DISEASE AND LIVER CIRRHOSIS

There are many causes of chronic liver injury that produce necrosis with inflammation followed by fibrosis and nodular regeneration. These processes eventually alter the liver architecture and lead to distortion of the vasculature within the liver. This advanced structural change is called cirrhosis, and in developed countries is most often caused by alcohol, hepatitis C virus (HCV) or nonalcoholic fatty liver disease. By contrast, HBV is the most common cause in many developing countries. Other causes include autoimmune liver disease, haemochromatosis, Wilson's disease and α_1-antitrypsin deficiency. The diagnosis of liver cirrhosis is often made when complications arise (often referred to as decompensated cirrhosis), which include development of ascites, variceal haemorrhage, spontaneous bacterial peritonitis, hepatic encephalopathy and renal failure (discussed later).

AUTOIMMUNE HEPATITIS

The pathogenesis of autoimmune hepatitis (AIH) is poorly understood, but the occurrence of circulating autoantibodies (antinuclear antibodies and smooth muscle antibodies, antibodies to liver/kidney microsome type 1) and T-lymphocytes in the inflammatory infiltrate in the liver has encouraged the use of immunosuppressant treatments. Without immunosuppression, AIH usually progresses to cirrhosis.

MANAGEMENT OF AUTOIMMUNE HEPATITIS

- Corticosteroids, usually prednisolone (see Chapter 44), induce remission in 85% of people with AIH, but when used alone, up to 50% of those treated will still have developed cirrhosis after 10 years.
- Azathioprine (see Chapter 38) has a corticosteroid-sparing action in AIH and is widely used in combination with corticosteroids, both to induce remission and for maintenance therapy. Treatment is usually required for up to 2 years.
- Mycophenolate mofetil or ciclosporin (see Chapter 38) is used for the 10–15% of cases of AIH that do not respond to corticosteroids. Evidence for their effectiveness is limited.
- Liver transplantation is necessary for end-stage disease.

PRIMARY BILIARY CIRRHOSIS

Primary biliary cirrhosis (PBC) is characterised by interlobular bile duct destruction. Although antimitochondrial antibodies are present and an autoimmune origin seems likely, immunosuppression is ineffective. Common symptoms include fatigue, itching and in the later stages jaundice and portal hypertension.

MANAGEMENT OF PRIMARY BILIARY CIRRHOSIS

- Ursodeoxycholic acid is a bile acid that is produced by bacterial oxidation of chenodeoxycholic acid, and is the only effective treatment. It retards progression of the disease possibly by reducing apoptosis of hepatocytes and suppression of the cytotoxic effects of other bile acids. The main unwanted effect is diarrhoea. About one-third of people treated will have a response, with reduction in serum liver enzymes, and a reduced risk of either death or the need for liver transplantation.
- Supportive therapy is necessary to reduce the complications that can arise from malabsorption of fat-soluble vitamins. Vitamin D (see Chapter 42) and calcium supplements should be given to reduce the risk of osteomalacia and osteoporosis.
- Treatment of pruritis with colestyramine (see Chapter 48), which binds bile acids in the gut.
- Liver transplantation is offered for end-stage disease.

CHRONIC VIRAL HEPATITIS

There are two important hepatic viral infections that can cause chronic hepatitis: HBV (a DNA virus) and HCV (an RNA virus). The eventual consequence of the chronic inflammation produced by the host response to viruses is cirrhosis. Serological evidence of hepatitis B infection is found in 30% of the world's population.

DRUGS FOR TREATMENT OF CHRONIC VIRAL HEPATITIS

Interferon alpha

Mechanism of action and effects

Interferons are glycoprotein cytokines that are naturally produced by virus-infected cells and protect uninfected cells of the same type. When given therapeutically, interferon alpha binds to host cell surface receptors and stimulates production of enzymes that impair viral mRNA translation by host ribosomes. This inhibits viral replication and augments viral clearance from infected hepatocytes (see Chapter 51). There are two forms of interferon alpha, interferon alpha-2a and interferon alpha-2b, which differ in structure by a single amino acid. Interferons are obtained either by recombinant DNA technology or from virus-stimulated leucocytes.

Pharmacokinetics

Interferon alpha is given by subcutaneous injection three times a week for 4–6 months. It is metabolised in the kidney and has a short half-life (3–4 hours). The polyethylene glycol-conjugated (pegylated) form (peginterferon alpha) has more persistence levels in the blood and is given once weekly.

Unwanted effects

- Immediate effects are almost universal and include headache, myalgia, fever and rigors, usually occurring 4–6 hours after injection. Tolerance to these effects occurs with repeated use.

- Delayed effects include fatigue, anorexia, nausea and diarrhoea.
- Depression.
- Bone marrow suppression, especially affecting granulocytes.
- Unmasking or exacerbation of autoimmune conditions.

Nucleoside and nucleotide analogues

entecavir, lamivudine, ribavirin, tenofovir disoproxil

Mechanism of action and uses

These drugs are analogues of either nucleosides or nucleotides (phosphorylated nucleosides). Those that inhibit reverse transcriptase are effective against HBV; inhibitors of RNA synthesis or transcription are effective against HCV.

- Entecavir is a guanosine nucleoside analogue that inhibits the viral enzyme reverse transcriptase, reduces DNA copies of the viral RNA and suppress viral replication (see Chapter 51).
- Lamivudine is a cytidine nucleoside analogue that inhibits reverse transcriptase.
- Ribavirin is a guanosine nucleoside analogue that inhibits viral RNA synthesis by blocking incorporation of uridine and cytidine. It also increases the production of antiviral cytokines. Ribavirin has little effect on viral replication when used alone, but it enhances the efficacy of interferon alpha against HCV. Ribavirin is also used by inhalation to treat respiratory syncytial virus infection.
- Sofosbuvir is a uridine nucleotide analogue that inhibits RNA polymerase, reduces RNA transcription and viral replication.
- Tenofovir is an adenosine 5′-monophosphate nucleotide analogue that inhibits reverse transcriptase.

Resistance

Viral resistance is due to emergence of mutations that interfere with the binding of the analogue to the enzyme. Resistance to reverse transcriptase inhibitors can also arise through development of hydrolytic processes that remove the drug from the DNA chain.

Pharmacokinetics

Nucleos(t)ide analogues are inactive prodrugs that are phosphorylated intracellularly to the active nucleotide derivatives, and then eliminated by the kidney. See the drug compendium at the end of this chapter for further details.

Unwanted effects

- Anorexia, abdominal pain, nausea, vomiting, diarrhoea.
- Cough, dyspnoea.
- Headache, dizziness, insomnia, fatigue.
- Rashes.
- Lactic acidosis with hepatic steatosis.
- Accumulation of ribavirin in red cells produces haemolysis.
- Interstitial pneumonitis, palpitation, chest pain, syncope with ribavirin.

Protease inhibitors

boceprevir, simeprevir, telaprevir

Mechanism of action

HCV protease inhibitors are specific inhibitors of a serine protease (nonstructural protein NS3) responsible for the cleavage of viral polyprotein, which is an essential process in viral replication. The protease may also aid the virus in evading the normal inflammatory response of the host cell, so protease inhibitors may enhance the host response to infection.

Resistance

Viral resistance is due to emergence of mutations that interfere with the ligand-binding site on the protease.

Pharmacokinetics

Boceprevir and telaprevir are metabolised in the liver with half-lives of about 3 and 10 hours, respectively. Simeprevir has a longer half-life (41 hours) in people with HCV infection.

Unwanted effects

- Nausea, vomiting, anorectal discomfort, diarrhoea. Altered taste with boceprevir.
- Severe dermatitis with telaprevir.
- Anaemia.
- Paraesthesia, dizziness, headache, anxiety, depression, insomnia with boceprevir.
- Drug interactions: Inhibition of the P450 enzyme CYP3A4 and P-glycoprotein by these drugs can lead to several potential drug interactions. Drugs that inhibit the activity of CYP3A4 can enhance the unwanted effects of protease inhibitors, whereas the concurrent use of inducers of CYP3A4 can lower plasma concentrations of the protease inhibitor and encourage viral resistance.

Nonstructural protein NS5A inhibitors

daclatasvir

Mechanism of action

Nonstructural protein NS5A plays a key role in regulating HCV replication and assembly. Inhibition by daclatasvir rapidly prevents HCV replication.

Resistance

Viral resistance is due to emergence of mutations that interfere with the ligand-binding site on NS5A.

Pharmacokinetics

Daclatasvir is metabolised in the liver and has a half-life of about 12 hours.

Unwanted effects

- Nausea, vomiting, abdominal pain, diarrhoea.
- Alopecia, dry skin.
- Anaemia.
- Anxiety, headache, insomnia.

MANAGEMENT OF CHRONIC VIRAL HEPATITIS

Chronic hepatitis B infection

There is no role for drug treatment in acute hepatitis B infection, which usually resolves spontaneously. Chronic infection is characterised by persistence of hepatitis B surface antigen (HBsAg) and other immunological markers at least 6 months after the acute infection. Antiviral treatment should be used if there is evidence of active chronic infection with ongoing liver damage (persistently raised serum alanine aminotransferase) and high viral replication (high titre of HBV DNA). This is usually, but not always, associated with hepatitis B antigen (HBeAg) in plasma as a marker of active viral replication. The criteria for successful treatment are a matter of debate. Seroconversion to HBe antibody only occurs in a minority of those who are treated, and even fewer seroconvert to HBs antibody, which is the ideal outcome. Measurement of HBV DNA is a sensitive way to monitor treatment and detect drug resistance.

Pegylated interferon alpha-2a is recommended as first-line therapy for 48–52 weeks. It achieves seroconversion in about one-third of cases, with no difference between the pegylated and nonpegylated forms of the drug. About 30% of those who are HBeAg-positive will seroconvert, and a similar proportion of those who are HSeAg-negative have a sustained reduction in HBV DNA.

If the person has a suboptimal response to interferon, then second-line therapy is advocated. Tenofovir is the most common choice, with entecavir as an alternative if tenofovir is poorly tolerated. Hepatitis B is rarely resistant to either of these nucleos(t)ide analogues. Treatment with a nucleos(t)ide analogue is usually lifelong as relapse is high on cessation.

Lamivudine is used as prophylaxis against vertical transmission in HBsAg-positive mothers or in HBsAg- or HBcAg-positive people about to start immunosuppressant chemotherapy.

Chronic hepatitis C

The aim of treatment is eradication of the virus. If left untreated, about 85% of people who are infected develop chronic infection and of these up to 30% will develop cirrhosis. Treatment with pegylated interferon alpha and ribavirin is standard treatment if tolerated. Treatment duration and success depend on the viral strain, or genotype, of which there are six worldwide, with three found commonly in Europe. Interferon with ribavirin produces an overall response rate of 45% for genotype 1 and 80% for genotypes 2 or 3. For genotypes 2 or 3, treatment for 24 weeks is sufficient for a maximal response, while treatment for genotype 1 (the most common type in developed countries) should be continued for 48 weeks in those who have a response in the first 24 weeks. Pegylated interferon produces up to a 10% higher response rate than the conventional interferon.

The addition of viral protease inhibitors such as boceprevir or telaprevir to the combination of interferon alpha and ribavirin is more effective than dual therapy in genotype 1 infection and produces a rapid virological response in 50–60% of those treated. The triple therapy combination has a higher incidence of anaemia and other unwanted effects.

Most recently, several regimen options for oral treatment without interferon have been introduced. Choice is determined by the HCV genotype and the presence or absence of cirrhosis. Examples are sofosbuvir combined with daclatasvir or simeprevir.

COMPLICATIONS OF CIRRHOSIS

Decompensation of cirrhosis can present with encephalopathy, gastrointestinal bleeding or ascites.

CHRONIC HEPATIC ENCEPHALOPATHY

Liver cirrhosis predisposes to the neuropsychiatric disturbance known as chronic hepatic encephalopathy. Encephalopathy can also result from portal venous bypass with porto-systemic shunting (including iatrogenic transjugular intrahepatic portosystemic shunting [TIPS] procedures). Hepatic encephalopathy is the core feature of chronic liver failure and is associated with a 3-year survival of 23%. The clinical features of chronic hepatic encephalopathy are similar to those occurring in acute liver failure. Spontaneous bacterial peritonitis is a common cause of acute deterioration in previously compensated liver failure. In people with chronic encephalopathy, nutritional support may be necessary, and malabsorption of fat-soluble vitamins can be a particular problem if there is cholestasis. Osteoporosis can result, made worse by the use of corticosteroids.

Management of chronic hepatic encephalopathy

Chronic hepatic encephalopathy only requires treatment if it is adversely affecting quality of life. Treatment is generally directed at shortening episodes of acute encephalopathy and preventing further events.

- Prompt treatment of infections, constipation and it electrolyte disturbances (particularly hypokalaemia), and avoidance of sedative drugs will help prevent symptomatic encephalopathy. Sepsis, including spontaneous bacterial peritonitis, is often due to bowel flora and should be treated with intravenous broad-spectrum antibacterial drugs, such as cefuroxime with metronidazole (see Chapter 51)
- Lactulose (see Chapter 35) is given orally to reduce colonic production of neurotoxins (particularly ammonia) by shortening intestinal transit time and increasing nitrogen fixation by colonic bacteria. It may also reduce bacterial translocation from the colon and reduce the risk of spontaneous bacterial peritonitis. Lactulose is effective for both treatment and prevention of acute episodes of encephalopathy.
- Low-absorption oral antibacterials, such as rifaximin (see Chapter 51), reduce bacterial ammonia production in the colon. Rifaximin is used together with lactulose to

prevent episodes of acute encephalopathy. Neomycin is now less commonly used because of its potential to cause nephrotoxicity and ototoxicity, even though little is absorbed from the gut.

- Careful attention to nutrition is required, especially a balanced carbohydrate and protein intake. Branched-chain amino acids should be consumed in preference to aromatic amino acids.

- Fat malabsorption can be treated with medium-chain triglyceride supplements, and sufficient calorie intake should be ensured. Supplements of fat-soluble vitamins (A, D, E, K) may be needed. Metabolic bone disease may require treatment with bisphosphonates (see Chapter 42).

VARICEAL HAEMORRHAGE

Varices are large collateral venous communications that develop in portal hypertension, most frequently at the gastro-oesophageal junction but also at other places such as the rectum. Gastropathy (friable gastric mucosa with ectatic superficial blood vessels) is also commonly associated with raised portal pressure. Varices arise from a combination of increased splanchnic blood flow and increased resistance to portal blood flow within the liver. Varices are found in 70% of people with cirrhosis, and they carry a high risk of haemorrhage, from which mortality is 30–50%. The normal pressure gradient between the portal vein and the inferior vena cava is less than 5 mm Hg and varices form when the hepatic-venous pressure gradient rises above 10 mm Hg. The probability of rupture is increased when the pressure gradient reaches 12 mm Hg, and is greatly increased when above 20 mm Hg.

Management of bleeding gastro-oesophageal varices

- Repletion of blood volume can be carried out with colloid solution, or preferably with whole blood to maintain a haemoglobin concentration of 70–90 g/L. Impaired coagulation and thrombocytopenia are common findings in advanced liver disease, and transfusion of platelet concentrates and fresh frozen plasma may be necessary.

- The risk of bacterial infections is high in acute variceal bleeding, and short-term antibacterial prophylaxis with an agent such as ciprofloxacin or ceftriaxone (see Chapter 51) should be given.

- Endoscopic variceal band ligation or injection with a sclerosant successfully occludes varices in up to 95% of cases. The main complications are oesophageal ulceration, increased risk of infections and pleural effusions.

- Endoscopic variceal injection of a cyanoacrylate tissue adhesive is effective for bleeding gastric varices, and is successful in 80% of cases. It is also an option for oesophageal varices. These compounds are tissue glues that polymerise on contact with water or blood.

- Balloon tamponade to compress the bleeding point achieves control in 80–90% of bleeding varices. It can be used to treat rebleeding after endoscopic sclerosant therapy or as a holding measure, but is rarely used as a first-line treatment.

- A TIPS is used as rescue therapy in the 10–20% of cases when sclerosant therapy has failed.

- Terlipressin (N-triglycyl-8-lysine-vasopressin) is a splanchnic vasoconstrictor that reduces portal pressure and limits bleeding from varices. Terlipressin is a prodrug that is slowly converted to lysine-vasopressin, a synthetic vasopressin analogue (see Chapter 43). It is given intravenously by bolus injection for 2–5 days. Unwanted effects are uncommon. It is mainly used as an adjunct to endoscopic band ligation. Vasopressin is rarely used, as it has a shorter duration of action than terlipressin, must be given by intravenous infusion and systemic vasoconstriction causes ischaemic complications in up to 50% of those treated. Octreotide (see Chapter 43) and somatostatin (see Chapter 43) are splanchnic vasoconstrictors that are as effective as vasopressin for stopping haemorrhage, but there is less convincing evidence compared with terlipressin.

Prevention of variceal bleeding and rebleeding

- Splanchnic vasoconstrictors that lower portal blood flow and reduce the hepatic-venous portal pressure gradient by at least 20% will reduce the risk of bleeding. A nonselective β-adrenoceptor antagonist such as propranolol is often used. The β-adrenoceptor antagonist carvedilol has vasodilator activity by antagonism of α_1-adrenoceptors (see Chapter 5); it produces a greater reduction in the pressure gradient than propranolol and may be more effective for reducing bleeding.

- Endoscopic band ligation or sclerosant therapy of the varices will reduce the risk of rebleeding but does not reduce portal pressure, and bleeding can still occur from gastropathy. In about 50% of cases, the varices will recur within 2 years. Banding should therefore be followed by drug therapy to lower portal pressure.

- A TIPS procedure can be used when rebleeding occurs, despite endoscopic band ligation or sclerosant therapy together with drug therapy to lower portal pressure.

ASCITES IN CHRONIC LIVER DISEASE

Ascites in chronic liver disease arises largely as a result of splanchnic vasodilation from increased production of nitric oxide. Effective circulating blood volume is initially maintained by an increase in cardiac output, but eventually activation of the renin–angiotensin system promotes salt and water retention in the kidney. The increased portal pressure leads to transudation of fluid into the peritoneal cavity. Spontaneous bacterial peritonitis due to translocation of colonic bacteria can complicate ascites associated with liver disease and make the ascites resistant to treatment. Renal vasoconstriction in end-stage liver disease with ascites leads to hepatorenal syndrome and onset of renal impairment.

Management of ascites

The presence of ascites in chronic liver disease is associated with a poor prognosis, with a 5-year survival of 30–40%, unless liver transplantation is carried out. Management of ascites involves several options.

- Screening for and treating underlying infection.
- Reduction of salt intake to 80–120 mmol/day.
- Diuretic therapy, starting with the potassium-sparing diuretic spironolactone (see Chapter 14) alone or together

with a low dose of furosemide, with care taken to avoid hypovolaemia and consequent prerenal failure.

- Drainage by paracentesis is usually required in large-volume ascites in addition to diuretics as maintenance therapy; paracentesis should be accompanied by plasma expansion with intravenous albumin to maintain circulating blood volume when the volume drained exceeds 5 L.
- A TIPS procedure can be used to lower portal pressure for refractory ascites.
- Prophylaxis with norfloxacin (see Chapter 51) should be considered if there has been an episode of spontaneous bacterial peritonitis associated with ascites. Proton pump inhibitors should preferably be avoided, as they increase the risk of spontaneous bacterial peritonitis in people with ascites. By contrast, nonselective β-adrenoceptor antagonists reduce the risk.

SELF-ASSESSMENT

One-best-answer (OBA) questions

1. Which antiviral drug is a specific inhibitor of the HCV serine protease NS3?
   A. Adefovir
   B. Boceprevir
   C. Daclatasvir
   D. Entecavir
   E. Sofosbuvir
2. A 45-year-old woman was admitted to the emergency department with acute liver failure. Identify the *least* accurate statement concerning her condition.
   A. Paracetamol overdose should be excluded.
   B. Paracetamol-induced hepatocellular liver damage is not reversible.
   C. Mannitol could be used to reduce the cerebral oedema associated with acute liver failure.
   D. Warfarin could be used to manage coagulopathy.
   E. Terlipressin could be given as a vasoconstrictor to treat shock.

Case-based questions

Mr. S.A. was a 61-year-old publican who presented 'feeling as though I am 9 months pregnant'. His abdominal swelling was caused by ascites, which was drained. A liver biopsy was performed, which showed micronodular cirrhosis. He commenced treatment with oral spironolactone.

1. Was this a good choice of diuretic?

He remained well on this regimen for 5 years but continued to imbibe large quantities of alcohol. He re-presented as an emergency, having haematemesis and melaena. At the time he was slightly jaundiced and demonstrated signs of hepatic encephalopathy. In addition, there was gynaecomastia and testicular atrophy. The liver edge was palpable 8 cm below the right costal margin. Investigations showed a bilirubin level of 27 mmol/L (normal <17 mmol/L) and albumin of 30 g/L (normal 32–50 g/L). A gastroscopy was performed under sedation with intravenous diazepam and revealed oesophageal varices.

2. What evidence was there to indicate diminished hepatic reserve in this man?
3. Was diazepam a good choice during gastroscopy?
4. It has been shown that the incidence of rebleeding from oesophageal varices can be reduced by oral propranolol (by reducing portal venous pressure). What effect is this man's liver disease likely to have on the pharmacodynamics and pharmacokinetics of propranolol?
5. People with hepatic cirrhosis are often treated with colestyramine and/or lactulose. How do these drugs work, and what benefits are produced?
6. What would you use for pain relief in someone with established liver cirrhosis?

ANSWERS

One-best-answer (OBA) answers

1. **Answer B** is correct.
   A. False. Adefovir is a nucleotide analogue used in chronic hepatitis B viral infection.
   B. **True**. Boceprevir specifically inhibits HCV serine protease NS3.
   C. False. Daclatasvir inhibits the HCV nonstructural protein NS5A.
   D. False. Entecavir is a nucleoside analogue used in chronic hepatitis B viral infection.
   E. False. Sofosbuvir inhibits HCV RNA polymerase (NS5B).
2. **Answer D** is the least accurate statement.
   A. True. Paracetamol poisoning is the most common cause of acute liver failure in the UK.
   B. True. Liver damage induced by paracetamol is irreversible.
   C. True. Mannitol is an osmotic diuretic with relatively few uses, but is effective for the reduction of cerebral oedema (see Chapter 14).
   D. **False**. The coagulopathy is due to a reduction in vitamin K-dependent clotting factors. Warfarin, a vitamin K antagonist, would make the problem worse, and vitamin K should be given.
   E. True. Terlipressin, an analogue of vasopressin that causes vasoconstriction, can be given to treat shock.

Case-based answers

1. Mr. S.A. is at risk of encephalopathy/coma from electrolyte imbalances. Spironolactone, a potassium-sparing diuretic, would avoid changes in serum K^+ such as might be caused by loop diuretics; a loop diuretic could be given cautiously after a few days of treatment with spironolactone. There is an increase in circulating aldosterone probably contributing to fluid retention, so spironolactone is usually chosen.
2. Diminished hepatic reserve is indicated by (i) increased plasma bilirubin, which will be a combination of unconjugated bilirubin due to impaired glucuronidation, plus conjugated bilirubin due to impaired biliary excretion; (ii) decreased plasma albumin, caused by decreased synthesis, which will lower the osmotic pressure of blood and lead to oedema/ascites; (iii) decreased clotting factors, caused by decreased synthesis, which may contribute to oesophageal bleeding; (iv) increased

oestrogenic activity, as evidenced by gynaecomastia and testicular atrophy, possibly caused by decreased sex steroid inactivation in the liver.

3. Reduced hepatic cytochrome P450 metabolism might cause increased plasma levels of diazepam, a long-acting benzodiazepine. A shorter-acting benzodiazepine without active metabolites, such as midazolam, would be a better choice.

4. Reduced plasma protein concentration means that less propranolol is bound and the free drug is increased. This will result in an increased response. Reduced hepatic CYP450 activity will decrease first-pass metabolism of propranolol and increase its bioavailability, while reduced clearance will increase its elimination half-life.

5. In liver cirrhosis, decreased bile outflow leads to accumulation of bile salts in the blood and their deposition in the skin, which causes itching. Colestyramine, an anion-exchange resin, adsorbs bile salts within the gut and reduces their enterohepatic circulation. Lactulose is a laxative (see Chapter 35), and its fermentation products in the lower gastrointestinal tract reduce microbial formation of ammonia and tyramine, which may otherwise contribute to encephalopathy.

6. Analgesia in cirrhosis can be difficult. Opioids should usually be avoided because of the risk of encephalopathy, but low doses could be given. Nonsteroidal antiinflammatory drugs (NSAIDs) are best avoided to reduce the risk of haemorrhage from oesophageal varices. Paracetamol is potentially hepatotoxic, but it is well tolerated in cirrhosis, probably because decreased perfusion of hepatocytes and reduced activity of cytochrome P450 outweigh the impaired inactivation by conjugation.

FURTHER READING

Bernal, W., Jalan, R., Quaglia, A., et al., 2015. Acute-on-chronic liver failure. Lancet 386, 1567–1587.

Carey, E.J., Ali, A.H., Lindor, K.D., 2015. Primary biliary cirrhosis. Lancet 386, 1565–1575.

Ellul, M.A., Gholkar, S.A., Cross, T.J., 2015. Hepatic encephalopathy due to liver cirrhosis. Br. Med. J. 351, h4187.

Garcia-Tsao, G., Bosch, J., 2010. Management of varices and variceal hemorrhage in cirrhosis. N. Engl. J. Med. 362, 823–832.

Ge, P.S., Runyon, B.A., 2016. Treatment of patients with cirrhosis. N. Engl. J. Med. 375, 767–777.

Heneghan, M.A., Yeoman, A.D., Verma, S., et al., 2013. Autoimmune hepatitis. Lancet 382, 1433–1444.

Rosen, H.R., 2011. Chronic hepatitis C infection. N. Engl. J. Med. 364, 2429–2438.

Sundaram, V., Kowdley, K.V., 2015. Management of chronic hepatitis B infection. Br. Med. J. 351, h4263.

Trépa, C., Chan, H.L.Y., Lok, A., 2014. Hepatitis B virus infection. Lancet 384, 2053–2063.

Tsochatzis, E.A., Bosch, J., Burroughs, A.K., 2014. Liver cirrhosis. Lancet 383, 1749–1761.

Webster, D.P., Klenerman, P., Dusheiko, G.M., 2015. Hepatitis C. Lancet 385, 1124–1135.

Wijdicks, E.F.M., 2016. Hepatic encephalopathy. N. Engl. J. Med. 375, 1660–1670.

Compendium: drugs used in liver disease

Drug	Characteristics
Autoimmune liver disease	
Azathioprine	Prodrug of 6-mercaptopurine, a thiopurine immunosuppressant (see Chapter 38). Corticosteroid-sparing action. Given orally or intravenously in combination with corticosteroids. Half-life: (azathioprine) 3–5 h
Corticosteroids	Usually prednisolone is used. See Chapter 44
Ursodeoxycholic acid	Secondary bile acid. The only drug licensed for use in primary biliary cirrhosis. Given orally; undergoes enterohepatic circulation. Half-life: several days
Other drugs	Ciclosporin, tacrolimus or mycophenolate (see Chapter 38) are used for autoimmune hepatitis unresponsive to corticosteroids
Viral hepatitis	
Interferons	
Interferon alpha	Antiviral cytokine. Used in the treatment of chronic hepatitis B virus (HBV) infection. Given by subcutaneous, intramuscular or intravenous injection. Half-life: 3–4 h
Peginterferon alpha	Polyethylene glycol-conjugated form of interferon alpha; the pegylated form gives more prolonged duration of action. Used in combination with ribavirin for chronic hepatitis C virus (HCV) infection. Given by subcutaneous injection. Half-life: 80 h

Compendium: drugs used in liver disease (cont'd)

Drug	Characteristics
Nucleoside and nucleotide analogues	
Adefovir dipivoxil	Prodrug of adefovir, a nucleotide reverse transcriptase inhibitor. Used in chronic HBV infection with *either* compensated liver disease with evidence of viral replication and histologically documented active liver inflammation and fibrosis, *or* decompensated liver disease. Given orally. Half-life: 8 h
Entecavir	Guanosine nucleoside reverse transcriptase inhibitor. Used in chronic HBV infection with compensated liver disease, evidence of viral replication and histologically documented active liver inflammation or fibrosis. Given orally. Half-life: 130 h
Dasabuvir	Inhibitor of hepatitis C viral RNA polymerase (nonstructural protein 5B). Used in chronic HCV infection in combination with other antiviral drugs (ombitasvir with paritaprevir and ritonavir, with or without ribavirin). Given orally. Half-life: 6 h
Lamivudine	Cytosine nucleoside reverse transcriptase inhibitor. Used in the initial treatment of HBV infection, and for decompensated liver disease. Given orally. Half-life: 5–7 h
Ribavirin (tribavirin)	Nucleoside analogue. Used with pegylated interferon alpha for chronic HCV infection. Given orally. Half-life: 7–21 days
Sofosbuvir	Uridine analogue; specific inhibitor of hepatitis C viral RNA polymerase (nonstructural protein 5B). Used in combination with ribavirin with or without peginterferon alpha, or in combination with daclatasvir, for chronic HCV infection. Given orally. Half-life: 27 h
Tenofovir disoproxil	Prodrug; nucleotide reverse transcriptase inhibitor. Used for people requiring treatment for both HIV and chronic HCV infection. Given orally. Half-life: 17 h
HCV protease inhibitors	
Boceprevir	Specific inhibitor of hepatitis C viral protease (nonstructural protein NS3). Used with ribavirin and pegylated interferon alpha for HCV genotype 1. Given orally. Half-life: 3–4 h
Simeprevir	Specific inhibitor of HCV protease (nonstructural proteins NS3/4A). Used in combination with ribavirin and peginterferon alpha for chronic HCV infection of genotypes 1 or 4, and in combination with sofosbuvir (with or without ribavirin) for urgent treatment when intolerant to peginterferon alpha. Given orally. Half-life: 10–13 h in healthy subjects, but 41 h in HCV patients
Telaprevir	Specific inhibitor of HCV protease (nonstructural proteins NS3/4A). Used with ribavirin and pegylated interferon alpha for HCV genotype 1. Given orally. Half-life: 10 h
HCV nonstructural protein NS5A inhibitors	
Specific inhibitors of HCV nonstructural protein NS5A that regulates viral replication and assembly.	
Daclatasvir	Used in permutations with sofosbuvir, ribavirin, peginterferon alpha in chronic infection with specific HCV genotypes. Given orally. Half-life: 12 h
Ledipasvir	Used in combination with sofosbuvir, with or without ribavirin, for chronic infection with specific HCV genotypes. Given orally. Half-life: 47 h
Ombitasvir (with paritaprevir and ritonavir)	Used in combination with dasabuvir, with or without ribavirin, for chronic infection with specific HCV genotypes. Given orally. Half-life: 21–25 h
Drugs used for oesophageal varices	
Octreotide	Somatostatin analogue. Given by subcutaneous injection, or by intravenous injection if a more rapid response is required. Half-life: 1.7 h
Terlipressin	Prodrug hydrolysed to active lysine-vasopressin. Given by intravenous injection. Half-life: 0.5 h

HBV, Hepatitis B virus; *HCV*, Hepatitis C virus.

37

Obesity

• •

Obesity is defined as a body mass index (BMI) greater than 30 kg/m², compared with the ideal range of 18.5–24.9 kg/m². A BMI of 25–29.9 kg/m² is considered overweight. The prevalence of obesity is increasing in the Western world; it varies from less than 10% in the Netherlands to about 50% in some parts of eastern Europe. In the United Kingdom it is currently about 15%, but over half the British population is now overweight.

The health consequences of obesity are considerable (Box 37.1). Obesity decreases life expectancy by 7 years at the age of 40 years. Recent data suggest that waist circumference greater than 102 cm in males or 88 cm in females is more closely correlated than BMI with the cluster of atherogenic risk factors known as the metabolic syndrome. Metabolic syndrome is the presence of at least two of the following characteristic features in association with large waist circumference:

■ abnormally raised triglyceride,
■ decreased high-density lipoprotein (HDL) cholesterol,
■ raised fasting blood glucose (as a result of insulin resistance),
■ hypertension.

Excess dietary calories are stored as fat in adipose tissue. Intra-abdominal (visceral) fat is most closely associated with the metabolic and atherothrombotic consequences of obesity. Enlarged visceral adipocytes secrete numerous inflammatory, proatherogenic and procoagulant cytokines such as interleukin-6, tumour necrosis factor α and plasminogen activator inhibitor-1, but secrete reduced amounts of the antiinflammatory and antiatherogenic hormone adiponectin.

PATHOGENESIS OF OBESITY

Food intake is controlled by numerous hormonal, societal, genetic and psychological factors. Obesity usually develops gradually, and results when energy input exceeds output for a prolonged period. A small imbalance between energy intake and exercise or muscular work is all that is required for progressive weight gain. There are polygenic influences that determine who is more susceptible to weight gain. However, the recent epidemic of obesity in the Western world suggests that major environmental factors (reduced activity and dietary changes) are responsible, rather than biological causes.

For a few individuals, obesity arises from hormonal disturbances, or from neurological conditions that lead to behavioural change. Several drugs can produce weight gain, such as antipsychotics, tricyclic antidepressants, corticosteroids, antiepileptics, antihistamines and antidiabetic drugs.

There are two types of adipose tissue: brown adipose tissue is responsible for thermogenesis and white adipose tissue for energy storage. White adipose tissue is a target for insulin, and in obese people there is resistance to the action of insulin, leading to accumulation of intracellular fat.

Energy balance is regulated in the hypothalamus, which integrates neural, hormonal and circulating nutrient stimuli, and sends signals to higher centres to trigger feelings of satiety or hunger. The hypothalamus regulates sympathetic nervous system function, which controls lipolysis to release fatty acids as an energy source and also modulates thermogenesis. It also regulates pituitary hormones that help determine energy expenditure.

The biochemical factors that underlie the regulation of weight are complex (Fig. 37.1). Signals to the hypothalamus that reduce food intake (satiety signals) are provided by a number of hormones produced by endocrine cells of the gut, adipose tissue and pancreas. Leptin, which is released from adipocytes, and insulin both signal via specific hypothalamic receptors to indicate the degree of filling of adipocytes and induce the sensation of satiety. Several gut-derived peptides act as short-term appetite regulators. Ghrelin is released by the stomach preprandially and *stimulates* orexigenic (appetite-stimulating) peptide hormones in the hypothalamus. Oxyntomodulin, glucagon-like peptide-1 (GLP-1), cholecystokinin and peptide YY (PYY) are released from the small intestine and colon in response to the presence of carbohydrates and lipids, and *inhibit* release of orexigenic peptides in the hypothalamus.

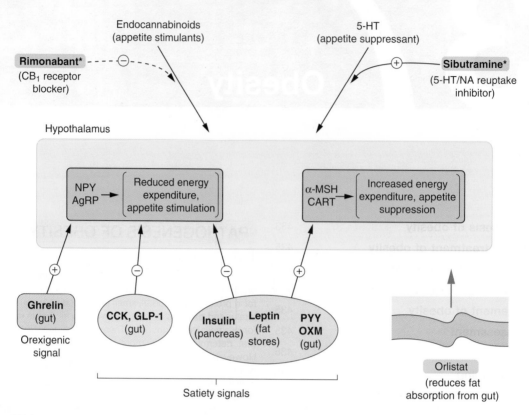

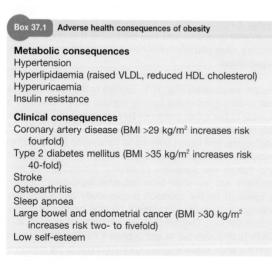

Fig. 37.1 Factors involved in the regulation of food intake. Feedback loops between the periphery and the brain control food intake. Peripheral signals stimulate or inhibit transmitters in the arcuate nucleus of the hypothalamus (shown in yellow) that control appetite and energy expenditure. The hypothalamus sends signals to higher centres, indicating satiety or hunger. The peripheral orexigenic (appetite-stimulating) signals include ghrelin, released preprandially from the gut, and satiety signals include insulin, leptin, peptide YY$_{3-36}$ (PYY) and oxyntomodulin (OXM). Other hypothalamic signalling mechanisms are described in the text. Endocannabinoid pathways are involved in stimulating appetite, and serotonin acts on the hypothalamus to suppress appetite. Note: Centrally acting appetite-suppressant drugs have been withdrawn in the United Kingdom due to unwanted effects, but rimonabant and sibutramine are shown to illustrate mechanisms. Orlistat reduces fat absorption from the gut by inhibiting pancreatic lipase. *AgRP*, Agouti-related protein; *CART*, cocaine- and amphetamine-regulated transcript; *CCK*, cholecystokinin; *GLP-1*, glucagon-like peptide-1; α-MSH, α melanocyte-stimulating hormone; *NA*, noradrenaline; *NPY*, neuropeptide Y.

Box 37.1 Adverse health consequences of obesity

Metabolic consequences
Hypertension
Hyperlipidaemia (raised VLDL, reduced HDL cholesterol)
Hyperuricaemia
Insulin resistance

Clinical consequences
Coronary artery disease (BMI >29 kg/m² increases risk
  fourfold)
Type 2 diabetes mellitus (BMI >35 kg/m² increases risk
  40-fold)
Stroke
Osteoarthritis
Sleep apnoea
Large bowel and endometrial cancer (BMI >30 kg/m²
  increases risk two- to fivefold)
Low self-esteem

BMI, Body mass index; *HDL*, high-density lipoprotein;
VLDL, very-low-density lipoprotein.

When energy levels are low, ghrelin release and suppression of leptin, insulin and other gut-derived peptides promote release of key hypothalamic neurotransmitters, including neuropeptide Y (NPY) and agouti-related protein (AgRP). NPY and AgRP decrease activity in the melanocortin system, which in turn permits signalling by the orexigenic hormones melanin-concentrating hormone (MCH) and orexin (ORX) to stimulate appetite.

Following a meal, high plasma concentrations of insulin, glucose, cholecystokinin and leptin stimulate the hypothalamic appetite-suppressing substances pro-opiomelanocortin (POMC) and cocaine- and amphetamine-regulated transcript (CART). These mediators increase α-melanocyte-stimulating hormone (α-MSH) release, which inhibits MCH/ORX activity and signal satiety.

Paradoxically, the circulating concentration of leptin is usually high in obesity. This probably reflects the combination of leptin release from excess fat deposits and hypothalamic resistance to satiety cues such as leptin. Other factors that influence appetite include the appetite inhibitors serotonin and dopamine, and the appetite stimulators cannabinoids, cortisol and growth hormone-releasing hormone.

Improved understanding of the biochemical signals that regulate appetite has led to a search for more effective appetite-suppressant drugs. So far there has been little translation of this research into clinical practice.

DRUGS FOR TREATMENT OF OBESITY

DRUGS ACTING ON THE GASTROINTESTINAL TRACT

Example

orlistat

Mechanism of action

Orlistat acts by binding to pancreatic lipase in the gut and inhibiting its action. It reduces triglyceride digestion and therefore energy intake from dietary fat. However, when used as an adjunct to dietary restriction (particularly a low-fat diet) and exercise, only about 20% of people will lose more than 5% of body weight. Continuous use of orlistat for more than 2 years is not recommended.

Pharmacokinetics

Orlistat undergoes minimal absorption after oral administration and is largely excreted unchanged in the faeces.

Unwanted effects

- Orlistat produces gastrointestinal upset, including flatulence, steatorrhoea, faecal urgency and faecal soiling. These symptoms are most common if there is poor adherence to a low-fat diet while taking the drug, and result in discontinuation of treatment by one-third of people. There is also impaired absorption of fat-soluble vitamins, especially vitamin D.

CENTRALLY ACTING APPETITE SUPPRESSANTS

The centrally acting appetite suppressants dexfenfluramine, fenfluramine and sibutramine were withdrawn because of the increased risks of valvular heart disease and pulmonary hypertension. The selective CB_1 receptor antagonist rimonabant that suppresses appetite by an effect on the hypothalamus was also withdrawn due to psychological disturbances.

There are two other drugs licensed in the United States but not in Europe for the management of obesity. Phentermine is an amphetamine analogue that increases hypothalamic noradrenaline concentration. It is formulated in combination with topiramate, which may reduce weight by suppressing appetite and decreasing lipogenesis. Lorcaserin is a selective $5HT_{2c}$ receptor agonist that stimulates production of α-melanocortin in the hypothalamus and suppresses appetite.

MANAGEMENT OF OBESITY

Weight loss reduces the morbidity associated with obesity, but it is not known whether it prolongs life. Obesity is not usually caused by psychological disturbances, but these commonly arise in obese people. The social prejudice against obesity, concern about body image, and the depression and irritability that arise from dieting are all contributory factors.

Weight loss can be difficult to achieve and to maintain. The management of obesity should be carried out by a multidisciplinary team who can advise on lifestyle and other treatment options. The cornerstone of management is to reduce energy intake to 500–600 kcal below daily requirements. Fat is 'energy dense' and should be particularly restricted. However, dietary restriction alone is usually inadequate to achieve weight loss, and increased exercise combined with diet is more effective than either alone. Exercise need not be vigorous, provided it is maintained long-term; walking or cycling is usually enough if performed daily. Behaviour modification is essential for long-term adherence to treatment and maintenance of weight loss.

Drug treatment should be restricted to individuals with a BMI of more than 30 kg/m^2, or a BMI of more than 28 kg/m^2 in the presence of diabetes, hypertension or hypercholesterolaemia. Currently orlistat is the only licensed available agent. A major disadvantage of its use is that weight gain often follows cessation of therapy. The use of levothyroxine to encourage weight loss by increasing metabolic rate is not recommended, due to long-term risks such as osteoporosis. Bulking agents such as methylcellulose are usually ineffective for reducing food intake. Specialist clinics may consider the use of metformin (see Chapter 40), selective serotonin reuptake inhibitors (see Chapter 22), synthetic incretin mimetics (GLP-1 agonists) such as liraglutide (see Chapter 40), or topiramate (see Chapter 23).

Bariatric surgery to restrict the size of the stomach (gastroplasty, gastric banding or vertical sleeve gastrectomy) or gastric bypass (such as Roux-en-Y) are used in the morbidly obese (BMI >40 kg/m^2), or those with a BMI greater than 35 kg/m^2 and an obesity-related medical condition.

Current drug and lifestyle treatments for obesity can be expected to produce weight loss of about 10–15%, which is often enough to ameliorate obesity-related metabolic disorders and their accompanying clinical manifestations. Bariatric surgery produces an average weight loss of 25–30%.

SELF-ASSESSMENT

True/false questions

1. The posterior pituitary is the main central nervous system site of appetite control.
2. Ghrelin is an orexigenic hormone.

3. Satiety signals include insulin and leptin.
4. Orlistat acts centrally to inhibit release of orexigenic neurotransmitters.
5. Vitamin D deficiency can occur with orlistat treatment.
6. Orlistat treatment for obesity should be restricted to individuals with a body mass index (BMI) of more than 30 kg/m^2.
7. Weight loss is usually sustained after 12 months of orlistat treatment.

ANSWERS

True/false answers

1. **False.** The hypothalamus and higher brain centres are most important in regulating food intake.
2. **True.** Ghrelin is produced by the gut preprandially and has an orexigenic (appetite-stimulating) action on the hypothalamus.
3. **True.** Satiety signals to the hypothalamus include insulin (from the pancreas), leptin (from fat stores) and gut peptides such as cholecystokinin, oxyntomodulin and peptide YY$_{3-36}$.
4. **False.** Orlistat reduces fat absorption in the gut by inhibiting pancreatic lipase.
5. **True.** People taking orlistat may unduly restrict their fat intake to avoid steatorrhoea, leading to reduced absorption of fat-soluble vitamin D.
6. **True.** Drug treatment should be restricted to obese people with BMI greater than 30 kg/m^2 (or >28 kg/m^2 in those with type 2 diabetes, hypertension or hypercholesterolaemia).
7. **False.** Weight loss with orlistat often reverses gradually after stopping the drug; lifestyle measures including diet and exercise are important in long-term weight control.

FURTHER READING

Bray, G.A., Frühbeck, G., Ryan, D.H., et al., 2016. Management of obesity. Lancet 387, 1947–1956.

McGavigan, A.K., Murphy, K.G., 2012. Gut hormones: the future of obesity treatment? Br. J. Clin. Pharmacol. 74, 911–919.

Rueda-Clausen, C.F., Padwal, R.S., 2014. Pharmacotherapy for weight loss. Br. Med. J. 348, g3526.

Compendium: drugs used in obesity

Drug	Characteristics
Orlistat	Pancreatic lipase inhibitor; acts within intestine to reduce fat absorption. Taken orally before, during or immediately after a meal. Minimal systemic absorption of drug

8

The immune system

38

The immune response and immunosuppressant drugs

BIOLOGICAL BASIS OF THE IMMUNE RESPONSE

Immunity is the balance between adequate defences to fight infection, disease and tumour cells and having sufficient tolerance to avoid inflammation, allergy and autoimmune disease. To achieve this, the immune system has the ability to distinguish between self and nonself proteins. The immune system is composed of innate (natural) and acquired (adaptive) components. Acquired immunity is further divided into humoral and cell-mediated immunity.

INNATE IMMUNITY

The term *innate immunity* is used because it is an inherited system. It comprises several generally *nonspecific* protective mechanisms, some of which do not involve the immune system. Innate immunity provides a rapid response to pathogens and is the first line of defence. It does not require previous exposure to a pathogen to mount a response. Pattern-recognition receptors on cells involved in the innate immune system recognise all pathogens approximately equally. They identify pathogenic 'groups' such as bacterial lipopolysaccharides and bacterial DNA, rather than responding to individual antigens. The innate immune system has an important role in processing pathogens and triggering the highly selective adaptive system, which is described later.

The innate immune system incorporates the following processes:

- Physicochemical barriers provide an initial external defence – for example, skin and mucous membranes, low stomach pH, antibacterial agents (lysozyme) in skin and tear secretions, cough, sneeze, vomiting, flushing of the urinary tract to prevent stasis.
- Macrophages and dendritic cells, particularly in lungs, liver, lymph nodes and spleen, phagocytose pathogenic material and degrade it to produce antigen fragments (short peptides of approximately 8–25 amino acids), which they then display on their surfaces within the cleft of major histocompatibility complex (MHC) class II molecules. The cells are then described as professional antigen-presenting cells (APCs). APCs are necessary for the presentation of the antigen to T-lymphocytes and the subsequent triggering of the adaptive immune system.
- Phagocytosis of bacteria and parasites by neutrophils, monocytes and macrophages.
- Actions of natural killer cells (large granular lymphocytes).
- Binding of antigens to IgE antibody on mast cells and basophils and the subsequent release of inflammatory mediators from the cell.
- Attraction of immune cells to sites of inflammation by autacoids, chemokines and cytokines released from cells involved in the innate immune response.
- Complement activation by the alternate pathway, initiated by microbial carbohydrate chains. Complement produces membrane attack complexes that lyse microorganisms.
- Acute-phase proteins and interferon. Interferon is a viral-related response that is released from virally infected cells and triggers neighbouring cells to produce antiviral enzymes.

The innate immune system may be an adequate defence to deal with many pathogens but, unlike adaptive immunity, long-term specific immune protection following initial exposure to a pathogen does not occur.

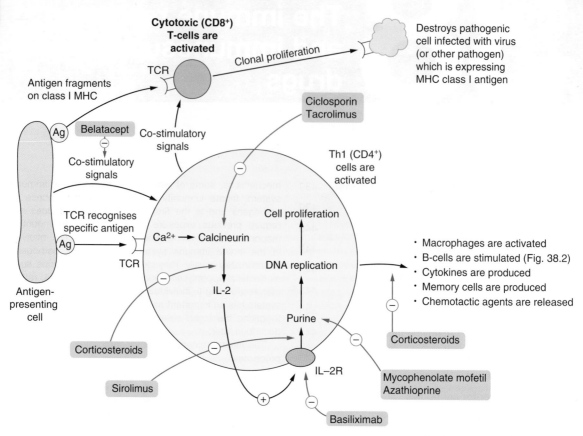

Fig. 38.1 **Aspects of cell-mediated immunity.** This shows in simplified form some steps in T-cell activation following antigen presentation to the T-cell receptor (TCR). Pathogenic antigens are presented by antigen-presenting cells (APCs) to the uncommitted CD4⁺ lymphocyte, which carries the specific receptor to the antigen, in association with major histocompatibility complex (MHC) class I and co-stimulatory molecules. Under the influence of interleukin-2 (IL-2), Th1 cells undergo clonal proliferation and play a variety of roles in cell-mediated immunity, including activation of macrophages and other cells. Antigens can also be presented to CD8⁺ lymphocytes, which mature into cytotoxic T-cells. Drugs used as immunosuppressants *(red arrows)* act at the sites shown. Corticosteroids act at many sites (see also Fig. 38.2 and Chapter 44). *Ag,* antigen; *IL-2R,* interleukin-2 receptor; *Th,* T-helper cell.

ADAPTIVE IMMUNITY

Adaptive immunity is superimposed upon the innate mechanisms. It differs from innate immunity in that it is slower to respond, offers long-term specific protection and has exquisite specificity in recognising individual nonself antigens. Adaptive immunity has two basic complementary and interacting mechanisms: *cell-mediated immunity* and *humoral immunity* (Figs 38.1 and 38.2).

Essential components of the adaptive system are the two populations of lymphocytes:

- *T-lymphocytes* (T-cells) are produced in the bone marrow and migrate to the thymus, where they mature, express receptors for antigens and interact with immunogenic self-peptides. T-cells are selected in the thymus for low or high avidity for self-peptides, and those showing high avidity are destroyed. The surviving T-cells retain the potential to recognise multiple foreign nonself-antigens but not self-antigens. The T-cells then leave the thymus and spread through the body including lymph nodes.

- *B-lymphocytes* (B-cells) make up about 10% of the lymphocyte population and mature in the bone marrow. Similar selection of B-cells occurs in the bone marrow, with elimination of those B-cells that bind self-antigens strongly. B-cells mature after migrating from the bone marrow to the spleen. After maturation, they either remain in the spleen or migrate through the blood to lymph nodes, where they encounter antigen delivered by circulating lymph.

T-cells and B-cells are coated with numerous proteins which act as receptors or as ligands for other receptors. These proteins are defined by antibody typing (immunophenotyping) and are given cluster of differentiation (CD) numbers such as CD4, CD8, and so on. When T-cells leave the thymus or B-cells mature in the spleen, they have not yet been exposed to nonself-antigens, and they are considered to be naïve or uncommitted.

Naïve T-cells comprise two major populations:

- T-helper (CD4⁺) (Th)-cells have surface receptors with a high affinity for class II MHC on professional APCs. Th-cells modulate responses of other immune cells

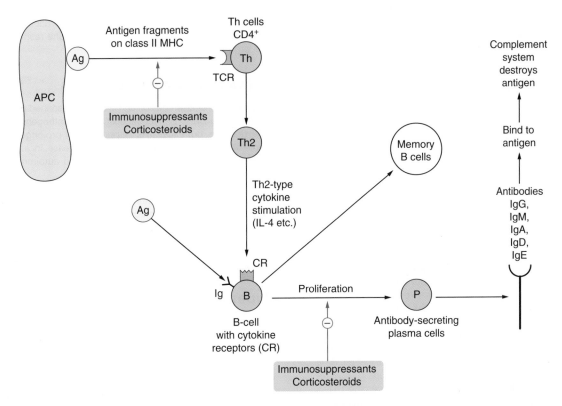

Fig. 38.2 Aspects of humoral immunity. Adaptive immunity can result in production of antibodies (humoral response) or a cell-mediated response (see Fig. 38.1). Antigens on bacteria or bacterial toxins bind to immunoglobulins on B-cells. Before proliferation and antibody production can occur, the B-cell also has to be stimulated by activated T-cell cytokine production, usually of the Th2 type. Antigen fragments can be presented with major histocompatibility complex (MHC) class II molecules to T-cells via a T-cell receptor (TCR) that recognises the antigen. T-cells undergo clonal proliferation and produce cytokines that stimulate B-cells to produce humoral antibodies (IgG, IgM, IgA, IgD and IgE). In atopic individuals, the T-cells are tipped toward the Th2 type and produce interleukins IL-4, IL-5, IL-10 and transforming growth factor β (TGFβ), which induce the B-cells to produce IgE. *Ag,* Antigen; *APC,* antigen-presenting cell; *CR,* cytokine receptor; *P,* plasma cell; *Th,* T-helper cell.

- T-cytotoxic or killer (CD8⁺) (Tc)-cells have an affinity for class I MHC, which displays specific antigens on the surface of infected host cells, tissue graft cells or tumour cells (see Fig. 38.1). Their action destroys cells harbouring the foreign antigen.

The Th-cell is activated when its receptors recognise and bind avidly to an antigen that has been processed and presented on an APC. This triggers a series of complex pathways which prepare the Th-cell for its immune role. Activated Th-cells secrete the T-cell growth factor interleukin-2 (IL-2), which acts in an autocrine fashion on the Th-cells and stimulates them to proliferate and mature into three cell types:

- effector Th-cells,
- memory Th-cells that retain the antigen affinity of the original cell,
- regulatory T-cells (T reg) that self-limit immune responses.

The effector Th-cells differentiate into two major subtypes: type 1 Th-cell (Th1) or a type 2 Th-cell (Th2), with smaller populations of other Th-cells such as Th17. The pattern of subtype differentiation may be determined by the type of antigen or possibly the concentration of antigen presented to the Th-cell. Differentiated Th-cells orchestrate the immune response by secretion of specific cytokines (see Figs 38.1 and 38.2).

- Th1-cell responses are triggered by IL-2, and the cells secrete interferon-γ (with other cytokines), which enhances the phagocytic activity of macrophages and stimulates the proliferation of cytotoxic Tc-cells. Th1-cells are the main host immunity effectors against intracellular bacteria and protozoa. Excessive Th1-cell activation against autoantigens produces type 4 delayed hypersensitivity (discussed later).
- Th2-cell responses are triggered by IL-4 and the cells secrete various interleukins. The main effector cells that respond to Th2-cell activation are eosinophils, basophils and mast cells, as well as B-cells, which initiate humoral immune responses. Th2-cells are the main host immunity effectors against extracellular parasites, such as helminths. Excessive Th2 activation produces type 1 IgE-mediated allergy (discussed later).

Co-stimulatory signals involving cell surface CD proteins are important processes in immune cell function. For example, the CD80 and CD86 proteins on professional APCs interact with CD28 proteins on Th- and Tc-cells to co-activate them together with Th-cell cytokines. CD28 activation confirms that the antigen is foreign and plays an important role in decreasing the risk of T-cell autoimmune responses. The expression of CD20 protein on B-cells enhances differentiation of B-cells into plasma cells and enables an optimum immune response against T-cell-independent antigens (antigens that elicit a full humoral immune response without participation of T-cell cytokines).

Immature B-cells can bind antigen with the cooperation of T-cells, but on subsequent exposure, antigen binds directly to specific immunoglobulins on the B-cell (see Fig. 38.2).

Cell-mediated immunity

Cell-mediated immunity is largely T-cell-driven, utilising Th1 (CD4⁺) and Tc-cell (CD8⁺) subtypes, and is involved in responses to viral infection, graft rejection, chronic inflammation and tumour immunity. Activated T-cells can take several days to initiate a cell-mediated attack after exposure to a novel antigen, but memory T-cells respond rapidly if primed by previous exposure. Fig. 38.1 shows schematically the basic processes occurring in cell-mediated immunity. T-cells that possess the receptor for the antigen of the invasive pathogen that is presented on professional APCs are stimulated to express IL-2 and the IL-2 receptor. For clarity, the many co-stimulatory processes that are described in this chapter are not shown in the figure.

Stimulation of the IL-2 receptor induces the Th1-cell to:

- attract macrophages and neutrophils to the site;
- activate macrophages that phagocytose the pathogen;
- stimulate Tc-cells to proliferate. Tc-cells recognise foreign antigen presented on nonprofessional APCs (all nucleated cells in the body) and attack pathogens expressing the antigen by releasing a variety of proteases or lysins to destroy the cell.

In addition, Th1-cells:

- stimulate IgG-producing B-cells to proliferate,
- prepare memory B-cells that respond rapidly to the pathogen on future exposure.

Humoral immunity

Fig. 38.2 illustrates the basic processes in humoral immunity. The foreign antigen is recognised by specific receptors to that antigen on the surface of a clone of B-cells and taken up into the cell by endocytosis. The presence of nearby Th2-cells that have been activated to secrete interleukins is required for initial antigen recognition by B-cells. Activated Th2-cells also express CD40L, a co-stimulatory factor for B-cell activation that binds to CD40 receptors on B-cells. Th2-cell interleukins also induce B-cell clonal proliferation, and convert B-cells into active plasma cells that can secrete antibodies which bind to and destroy pathogenic antigens.

B-cells can also be activated by foreign polysaccharides independently of Th2-cells. The response to these antigens is more rapid than to T-cell-dependent activation, but the antibodies have lower affinity for the antigens and are less functionally versatile.

On encountering an antigen, the primary immune response consists of IgM, replaced later by IgG. Some B-cells that are primed to produce specific antibodies survive as memory B-cells. On a further encounter with the antigen, reactivation of the memory B-cells produces a rapid immune response with large amounts of immunoglobulin.

UNWANTED IMMUNE REACTIONS

The processes of inflammation and immunity described previously are essential to protect the host against pathogens and other damage, but excessive, inappropriately prolonged or misdirected immune responses can cause disease, including hypersensitivity reactions, graft rejection and autoimmune diseases.

It is not always easy to decide whether predominantly Th1- or Th2-mediated immune responses are involved in a particular disease. Th1-mediated immune responses are prominent in rheumatoid arthritis and in the formation of atheroma. Th2-mediated responses are important in mild to moderate asthma but with increasing participation of Th1-mediated responses in severe asthma.

Hypersensitivity reactions

Hypersensitivity reactions were classified by Gell and Coombs in the late 1950s.

Type 1 (allergy, immediate)

In type 1 reactions, Th2-cells secrete interleukins, which promote eosinophilic inflammation and overproduction of IgE by B-cells. IgE molecules bind to high-affinity IgE receptors on the surface of mast cells and basophils, where they can be crosslinked by normally harmless antigens (such as pollens or house dust mites), leading to the synthesis and/or release of inflammatory mediators. These include cysteinyl-leukotrienes, prostaglandins, histamine, platelet-activating factor, proteases and cytokines. Examples of type 1 reactions include anaphylaxis, hay fever and acute asthma.

Type 2 (cytotoxic, antibody-dependent)

Cell surface antigens, including microbial proteins and drug molecules haptenised onto cell surfaces, are recognised and bound by IgG and IgM antibodies (opsonisation), leading to activation of complement (classic pathway) and cytolysis of the target cell by membrane attack complexes. Examples of type 2 reactions include destruction of red cells after incompatible blood transfusion. In some cases, the initiating antigen for the reaction is unknown, such as in autoimmune haemolytic anaemia, myasthenia gravis and Graves' disease.

Type 3 (immune complex disease)

Soluble antigens react with excess circulating antibodies to form complexes that precipitate in small blood vessels, causing a local inflammatory reaction with vasculitis and consequent organ damage. Serum sickness, systemic lupus erythematosus and the various forms of extrinsic allergic alveolitis, caused by exposure to animal or vegetable dusts, are systemic type 3 reactions, while the Arthus reaction is a local type 3 response to an injected antigen (e.g. nonhuman insulins).

Type 4 (cell-mediated, delayed-type hypersensitivity)

Inappropriate regulation of cell-mediated immunity may cause damaging chronic inflammation, leading to fibrosis and granuloma formation. Cell-mediated immunity misdirected against harmless foreign proteins (allergens) can lead to chronic allergic inflammation (such as occurs in eczema), or cause contact dermatitis in the skin in response to exposure to haptenising metals and chemicals.

Autoimmunity

Normally the immune system is tolerant of self-antigens. T-cells that express receptors with high avidity for self-peptides are normally destroyed before release from the thymus in a process known as negative selection (discussed previously). If this self-tolerance breaks down, autoimmune disorders result. Numerous mechanisms can trigger autoimmune diseases, including viral infection of host cells, binding of drug molecules to host cells (e.g. penicillin), sharing of antigens between host cells and microbes, and sequestration of antigens liberated by cell damage. Examples of autoimmune disease include autoimmune haemolytic anaemia, type 1 diabetes mellitus, Addison's disease, rheumatoid arthritis, myasthenia gravis, systemic lupus erythematosus and Graves' disease.

Blood transfusion and transplant rejection

Rejection of transfused blood usually occurs because non-self antigens on the transfused red blood cells (ABO system) trigger a type 2 hypersensitivity reaction in the recipient. By contrast, in people with immunodeficiency, transfused T-cells react against recipient antigens (graft-versus-host reactions).

Organ transplants always contain foreign antigens, and rejection will occur unless the immune response to these antigens is suppressed. The severity of the rejection reaction is dependent on how closely important antigens on the transplanted tissue match those of the recipient. Rejection can be immediate or hyperacute (minutes to hours), acute (days or weeks) or chronic (years).

- *Hyperacute rejection* is antibody-mediated, with preexisting antibodies leading to massive thrombosis in the graft. It can occur if, for example, there is ABO incompatibility.
- *Acute rejection* most commonly occurs in the first 6 months. If it occurs in the first week, it is usually antibody-mediated. Later rejection develops with formation of cellular immunity to foreign MHC molecules (human leucocyte antigens [HLA]). The latter can be reduced by HLA tissue typing to increase the chance of selecting a graft that is compatible with the host tissues.
- *Chronic rejection* can be antibody- or cell-mediated and appears as fibrosis or scarring in the graft. Frequently, it is not prevented by immunosuppressant drugs.

IMMUNOSUPPRESSANT DRUGS

The immune system presents a large number of potential molecular targets for therapeutic intervention to suppress the immune response. Most drugs currently used are nonspecific immunosuppressants with a range of unwanted effects. The following drugs are primarily used for their immunosuppressant action.

CORTICOSTEROIDS

Corticosteroids are the mainstay of many immunosuppressant regimens. They have direct lymphotoxic effects at high dosage, and at smaller doses they have a wide range of immunosuppressive and antiinflammatory actions. Examples of drugs that are widely used for immunosuppression are methylprednisolone and prednisolone. Corticosteroids are discussed in more detail in Chapter 44.

CALCINEURIN INHIBITORS

Examples

ciclosporin, tacrolimus

Ciclosporin

Mechanism of action

Ciclosporin is a fungal cyclic peptide which selectively inhibits T-cell division. It binds in the cell cytoplasm to the protein cyclophilin to form a complex that inhibits the action of calcineurin, a key component in T-cell activation (see Fig. 38.1). Calcineurin is a phosphatase produced in response to an antigenic signal at T-cell receptors (TCRs), and it dephosphorylates nuclear factor of activation in T-cells (NFAT). NFAT then enters the cell nucleus and binds to a promoter region of the IL-2 gene. Production of IL-2 stimulates T-cell division. By preventing dephosphorylation of NFAT, cyclosporin inhibits IL-2 production, and the T-cell division cycle is reversibly arrested between the G_0 and G_1 phases of the cell cycle.

Ciclosporin also inhibits the mitogen-activated protein kinase (MAPK) pathway, a part of the signaling cascade in T-cells connecting cell surface receptors to the cell nucleus. It is unclear how important this is in the action of the drug. An additional action of ciclosporin is increased production of transforming growth factor β (TGFβ), a fibrogenic cytokine which is probably responsible for some of the nephrotoxicity that occurs with the drug.

Pharmacokinetics

Oral absorption of ciclosporin is variable and incomplete, requiring initial dispersion by bile salts. To overcome this, a microemulsion formulation is used, which disperses when it comes into contact with water in the gut so that absorption is independent of bile production and more consistent. However, different microemulsion formulations do not have the same absorption characteristics, and switching formulations should be avoided. Ciclosporin can also be given by intravenous infusion. It is extensively metabolised in the liver by the CYP3A4 isoenzyme and has a half-life of about 8 hours. Monitoring of plasma drug concentration is essential to guide dosage for optimal effectiveness and to minimise toxicity. For most uses a trough (predose) concentration is measured. However, after renal transplantation, a blood concentration 2 hours postdose may be a better guide to graft survival and minimising toxicity.

Unwanted effects

- Nephrotoxicity almost always occurs, with a dose-dependent increase in serum creatinine in the first few weeks of use. The acute effect is due to intrarenal vasoconstriction that may persist and contribute to the less common long-term sequelae, which include interstitial fibrosis and tubular atrophy. The decline in glomerular filtration rate is usually reversible, but permanent renal impairment can result.

- Hypertension, often associated with fluid retention, occurs in up to 50% of people, and especially after heart transplantation. It usually responds to standard antihypertensive drug treatment.
- Hepatic dysfunction.
- Tremor, headache, paraesthesia, fatigue, myalgia.
- Hypertrichosis (excessive hair growth) and gingival hyperplasia.
- Gastrointestinal disturbances, including anorexia, nausea and vomiting, abdominal pain.
- Hyperlipidaemia, hyperuricaemia, hypomagnesaemia, hyperkalaemia.
- Drug interactions can be dangerous, especially drugs that inhibit or induce hepatic CYP3A4, which can affect the plasma concentrations of ciclosporin. Caution should also be taken when ciclosporin is used with other nephrotoxic drugs.

Tacrolimus

Mechanism of action and effects

Tacrolimus inhibits calcineurin, and therefore T-cell proliferation, by arresting the cell cycle between G_0 and G_1 in a similar manner to ciclosporin. After binding to a receptor protein called FK-binding protein-12, the complex binds to calcineurin and inhibits Ca^{2+}-dependent calcineurin activation. Tacrolimus also inhibits the MAPK pathway in a similar manner to ciclosporin. Unlike ciclosporin, tacrolimus does not stimulate production of TGFβ.

Pharmacokinetics

Tacrolimus is more water-soluble than ciclosporin and undergoes more predictable, though poor, absorption from the gut. It is metabolised by the liver and has a highly variable half-life (4–41 hours). Monitoring of the trough blood concentration of tacrolimus is essential for appropriate dose adjustment, especially early in treatment.

Unwanted effects

These are similar to those of ciclosporin, except that tacrolimus causes less hypertension, hirsutism and gingival hyperplasia. Effects that are more common with tacrolimus include:

- pleural and pericardial effusions;
- cardiomyopathy in children, who should be monitored by echocardiography.

MECHANISTIC TARGET OF RAPAMYCIN INHIBITORS

 xample

sirolimus

Mechanism of action and effects

Sirolimus is a natural fungal fermentation product that binds to intracellular FK-binding protein-12. The complex inhibits the action of the cytoplasmic kinase mechanistic target of rapamycin (mTOR), a key step in transducing signals from the cell surface IL-2 receptor and other cytokine receptors to cell-cycle regulators that promote DNA and protein synthesis and mitogenesis. The action of sirolimus therefore differs from that of tacrolimus, despite binding to the same intracellular receptor. Sirolimus inhibits T-cell proliferation by arresting the cell between the G_1 and S phases.

Pharmacokinetics

Sirolimus is rapidly absorbed from the gut and is a substrate for P-glycoprotein. It is metabolised by intestinal and hepatic CYP3A4 and has a very long half-life (60 hours).

Unwanted effects

- Oedema, ascites, pleural effusion, tachycardia, hypertension, venous thromboembolism.
- Abdominal pain, nausea, diarrhoea, stomatitis.
- Anaemia, thrombocytopenia, neutropenia.
- Hyperlipidaemia, hypokalaemia, hypophosphataemia, hyperglycaemia.
- Arthralgia, osteonecrosis.
- Lymphocele (a complication of renal transplantation that is more common if sirolimus is used; it can cause ureteric compression).
- Rash, acne.
- Drug interactions: Plasma sirolimus concentrations are affected by drugs that induce or inhibit CYP3A4 or P-glycoprotein.

ANTIPROLIFERATIVE AGENTS

 xamples

azathioprine, cyclophosphamide, mycophenolate mofetil

Azathioprine

Mechanism of action

Azathioprine is a prodrug that is converted by nonenzymatic degradation to 6-mercaptopurine in the erythrocytes and various tissues and then enzymatically to the active derivative 6-thioinosine monophosphate (TIMP), a purine analogue. TIMP is an unstable base that is incorporated into DNA and disrupts the function of endogenous purines. This particularly affects lymphocytes which depend on de novo purine synthesis and arrest division in the S-phase of the cell cycle (see Figs 52.1 and 52.2). Both cell- and antibody-mediated immune reactions are suppressed (see Figs 38.1 and 38.2).

Pharmacokinetics

Oral absorption is almost complete. The half-lives of azathioprine and its 6-mercaptopurine metabolite are short (3–5 hours). The enzyme that degrades the active metabolite, thiopurine methyltransferase (TPMT), is found mainly in haematopoietic cells. Deficiency of TPMT prolongs the duration of action and increases toxicity of azathioprine. It is often recommended that erythrocyte TPMT activity should be assessed before treatment is started and a lower dose of azathioprine used if activity is low or undetectable. Azathioprine can be given by intravenous injection, but the solution is alkaline and very irritant.

Unwanted effects

- Dose-dependent bone marrow suppression, especially leucopenia and thrombocytopenia. Regular monitoring of the full blood count (at least every 3 months) is essential.
- Hypersensitivity reactions, with malaise, dizziness, vomiting, diarrhoea, fever, myalgia, arthralgia, rash and hypotension. The drug should be stopped immediately if these arise.
- Increased susceptibility to infection, often with 'opportunistic' organisms (especially if used with a corticosteroid).
- Alopecia.
- Drug interactions: The most important interaction is with allopurinol. Allopurinol inhibits xanthine oxidase, which is involved in the catabolism of 6-mercaptopurine, and the dose of azathioprine should be reduced by 75% if the drugs are used together.

Cyclophosphamide

Cyclophosphamide is an alkylating drug that is less commonly used as an immunosuppressant. It has immunosuppressant actions at lower doses than those required to treat malignancy. Cyclophosphamide is discussed in detail in Chapter 52.

Mycophenolate mofetil and mycophenolic acid

Mechanism of action and effects

Mycophenolate mofetil is a prodrug of mycophenolic acid, which reduces purine synthesis by reversible noncompetitive inhibition of inosine monophosphate (IMP) dehydrogenase. This enzyme is involved in the conversion of IMP to guanosine triphosphate that is involved in RNA, DNA and protein synthesis. Inhibition of IMP dehydrogenase depletes the cell of guanine nucleotides, inhibits cellular DNA synthesis and therefore reduces cell proliferation. T- and B-cells rely on *de novo* purine nucleotide synthesis, unlike neutrophils and other cells, which can use preformed guanine released from the breakdown of preformed nucleic acids (the salvage pathway). Mycophenolate therefore is a selective inhibitor of lymphocyte proliferation and function.

Pharmacokinetics

Mycophenolate mofetil is a prodrug ester which is almost completely absorbed from the gut and hydrolysed rapidly to mycophenolic acid. Elimination of mycophenolic acid is via hepatic metabolism, and it has a long half-life (18 hours) due to enterohepatic circulation. Mycophenolate mofetil and mycophenolic acid can also be given by intravenous infusion.

Unwanted effects

- Gastrointestinal upset is very common, including nausea, vomiting, diarrhoea, abdominal cramps and, occasionally,

hepatitis or pancreatitis. Tolerance to the gastrointestinal symptoms often occurs.
- Hypertension, oedema, tachycardia, chest pain.
- Dyspnoea, cough.
- Dizziness, insomnia, headache, tremor, paraesthesia, seizures, confusion, depression, anxiety.
- Bone marrow suppression resulting in leucopenia, thrombocytopenia and anaemia.
- Opportunistic infections may be increased, especially with cytomegalovirus, herpes simplex, *Aspergillus* and *Candida*, as well as bacterial urinary tract infection and pneumonia.
- Increased risk of skin cancer.

FOLIC ACID ANTAGONIST

Example

methotrexate

Mechanism of action and uses

Methotrexate (as polyglutamate derivatives) inhibits dihydrofolate reductase and thymidylate synthase, competing with folate for the enzyme and reducing synthesis of tetrahydrofolate (THF). THF is essential for *de novo* purine and pyrimidine synthesis, so methotrexate inhibits the synthesis of DNA, RNA and ultimately protein. It is specific for the S-phase of cell division and slows G_1- to S-phase (see Chapter 52).

In inflammatory disease, low-dose methotrexate may have a different action by inhibiting 5-aminoimidazole-4-carboxamide ribonucleotide (AICAR) transformylase, which uses THF as a substrate and participates in purine synthesis. Inhibition of this enzyme leads to the release of adenosine from cells, which acts on specific cell surface receptors to suppress the expression of adhesion molecules on T-cells and neutrophils, thus inhibiting their proliferation. Adenosine also reduces phagocytosis by monocytes and cytokine release from a variety of inflammatory cells.

Pharmacokinetics

Methotrexate is well absorbed from the gut but can also be given intravenously, intramuscularly or subcutaneously. Excretion is via the kidney with a plasma half-life of about 10 hours, but it is converted to various polyglutamated forms that accumulate in cells over several weeks and are eliminated slowly over 1–4 weeks. Methotrexate is used by intermittent administration orally, subcutaneously or intramuscularly once a week in many conditions, such as inflammatory joint disease, Crohn's disease and psoriasis.

Unwanted effects

- Mucositis, nausea, abdominal discomfort, anorexia, diarrhoea.
- Rash, acne, alopecia.
- Drowsiness, dizziness, mood changes, headache.
- Pneumonitis, pulmonary fibrosis

- Myelosuppression.
- Hepatotoxicity during chronic therapy.

Toxicity is increased in the presence of reduced renal excretion and methotrexate should be avoided if there is significant renal impairment. Folic acid is frequently taken after methotrexate to reduce mucositis and myelosuppression. Nonsteroidal antiinflammatory drugs (NSAIDs) such as aspirin can reduce the renal excretion of methotrexate and increase its toxicity.

INTERLEUKIN-2 RECEPTOR ANTIBODIES

basiliximab

Mechanism of action and uses

Basiliximab is a chimaeric mouse-human monoclonal antibody that binds to the IL-2 receptor (IL-2R) on activated T-cells and prevents T-cell proliferation. It is used for initial induction therapy prior to transplantation, or for treatment of acute transplant rejection.

Pharmacokinetics

Basiliximab is given by intravenous infusion immediately before and again 4 days after surgery. It has a very long half-life of about 1 week.

Unwanted effects

- Arrhythmias.
- Hypersensitivity reactions.

SELECTIVE CO-STIMULATION BLOCKER

belatacept

Mechanism of action and uses

Belatacept is a fusion protein that binds to the CD80 and CD86 molecules on APCs and blocks their co-stimulatory action with CD28 on T-cell activation. It is used to prevent rejection in adults undergoing renal transplantation who are seropositive for the Epstein–Barr virus.

Pharmacokinetics

Belatacept is given by intravenous infusion and has a very long half-life (8–10 days).

Unwanted effects

- Anaemia, neutropenia, diarrhoea, constipation, oedema, cough, headache, pyrexia.

- Increased risk of skin cancer and progressive multifocal leucoencephalopathy.
- Lymphoproliferative disorder, especially in those with no prior exposure to Epstein–Barr virus.

IMMUNOSUPPRESSION IN INFLAMMATORY AND AUTOIMMUNE DISEASE

Immunosuppressant therapy is used for several diseases in which autoimmunity may contribute to the pathogenesis. Examples include connective tissue diseases such as vasculitis and systemic lupus erythematosus, inflammatory arthritis, polymyalgia rheumatica, glomerulonephritis, autoimmune hepatitis, psoriasis, inflammatory bowel disease and myasthenia gravis. Immunosuppressants are effective in these conditions through modulation of the immune system and, in some cases, through their antiinflammatory properties. Corticosteroids are highly effective antiinflammatory drugs that can be used systemically to suppress type 4 hypersensitivity reactions and autoimmune diseases. They are also used topically for inflammatory skin disease, inflammatory bowel disease and allergic rhinitis, and by inhalation for asthma (e.g. beclometasone, fluticasone; see Chapter 12). The main limiting factor is the unwanted effects with prolonged use. Some conditions, such as asthma, respond to short courses of prednisolone, which can be stopped abruptly, but many conditions will relapse unless the drug is slowly tapered. Sometimes prolonged use of low doses of prednisolone will be necessary to maintain control. Azathioprine, methotrexate and cyclophosphamide are second-line immunosuppressant drugs for many conditions. These drugs can be combined with a corticosteroid for their 'steroid-sparing' effect during maintenance treatment, which permits a lower dose of the corticosteroid to be used or the corticosteroid to be withdrawn.

Ciclosporin has been used in disorders such as nephritic syndrome, inflammatory bowel disease, atopic eczema and psoriasis, with some success. Mycophenolate mofetil is effective for some forms of vasculitis and for systemic lupus erythematosus.

Biological therapies, usually immunoglobulin derivatives directed against receptors on immunologically competent cells or against cytokines released from these cells, are increasingly used in inflammatory disorders, with evidence of immunological dysregulation. Many of these are discussed in the chapter on inflammatory arthritis (see Chapter 30), but they are also used for the treatment of inflammatory bowel disease and psoriasis.

In some conditions in which inflammation is triggered by an immune reaction but there is no autoimmune attack, inflammatory mediators released during the reaction can be blocked by antagonists at their receptors on target cells, or by inhibiting their synthesis. This is a useful strategy for management of allergic disorders and some inflammatory conditions. Antimediator drugs include histamine H1 receptor antagonists (antihistamines; see Chapter 39), cysteinyl-leukotriene receptor antagonists (LTRAs; see Chapter 12) and cyclo-oxygenase inhibitors (NSAIDs; see Chapter 29).

IMMUNOSUPPRESSION IN ORGAN TRANSPLANTATION

Immunosuppressant drugs block solid organ transplant rejection at the steps of T-cell activation, T-cell proliferation and cytokine production (see Figs 38.1 and 38.2). A major direction of current research is to find regimens that will induce immune tolerance and allow eventual withdrawal of immunosuppressant drugs.

Effective immunosuppression has improved the early survival of kidney, liver, pancreas, heart, heart–lung, intestinal and haematopoietic stem cell transplants. Suppression of acute rejection is more effective than prevention of chronic rejection, which usually responds poorly to immunosuppressant therapy. Regimens for immunosuppression vary among transplant units and according to the immunogenicity of the transplanted tissue. Combination therapy with a corticosteroid, calcineurin inhibitor and an antiproliferative agent is commonly used.

Kidney transplantation has some of the best outcomes, and is used here as an example of immunosuppressive regimens. Induction therapy is given at the time of transplantation to reduce initial acute rejection. Antithymocyte immunoglobulin, which inhibits T-cell activation in the thymus, is used for high immunological risk transplants. An IL-2R antibody such as basiliximab is given for low or moderate risk transplants or a corticosteroid for very low-risk transplants. Immunosuppression is then maintained with oral agents such as the corticosteroid prednisolone (see Chapter 44), together with a calcineurin inhibitor (tacrolimus is now preferred) and mycophenolate mofetil. An mTOR inhibitor (such as sirolimus) is used if calcineurin inhibitors are poorly tolerated, and azathioprine is used if there is intolerance to mycophenolate. In low-risk grafts, prednisolone is gradually withdrawn, and over the first year the doses of all immunosuppressant drugs are usually slowly reduced to maintenance regimens. There is some evidence that the use of belatacept in place of tacrolimus may confer fewer long-term complications. With such regimens, more than 90% of cadaveric kidney grafts will survive beyond 1 year. Only half of those that fail are lost due to rejection, and the rest from thrombosis of the graft blood supply. Progressive graft loss continues after the first year, with only 43% of grafts from deceased donors surviving at 10 years. Grafts from living donors have better survival rates of 96% at 1 year and 60% at 10 years. Most of the late graft losses are as a result of chronic vascular rejection, which can be confused with nephrotoxicity from long-term use of calcineurin inhibitors. Chronic rejection can also result from inadequate immunosuppression. If this occurs, increasing the dosages of the primary immunosuppressant drugs may help. Late acute rejection is a less common problem, which can be antibody- or cell-mediated. Regimens to treat acute rejection vary and include high-dose corticosteroid or polyclonal antilymphocytic globulin or monoclonal antilymphocytic globulin for cell-mediated rejection. Antibody-mediated rejection is treated with a variety of drugs that include combinations of corticosteroid, antithymocyte immunoglobulin, rituximab (see Chapter 30), bortezomib (see Chapter 52) and plasmapheresis.

Immunosuppressant therapy is essential for all solid organ transplants, such as heart (70% 5-year survival), heart–lung (40% 5-year survival), liver (70% 5-year survival), intestinal (80% 5-year survival) and pancreas (60% 5-year survival). After initial use of antilymphocytic globulin or an IL-2 receptor antibody (basiliximab), triple immunosuppressant regimens are widely used, but a corticosteroid is avoided in some centres unless there is acute rejection.

With haematopoietic stem cell transplantation, graft-versus-host disease (GVHD) is the major barrier. This usually begins at least 3 months after the transplant and has three phases. The first phase involves damage to intestinal mucosa and the liver, with activation of host cells and release of inflammatory cytokines. These cytokines upregulate MHC proteins on the host cells, which are then recognised by the donor T-cells. The second phase involves activation and proliferation of donor T-cells, and the third phase includes tissue destruction by monocytes primed by inflammatory cytokines and lipopolysaccharide from T-cells and damaged intestinal mucosa. Initial induction therapy before the transplant often uses cyclophosphamide and antithymocyte immunoglobulin. GVHD can then be prevented by inhibition of the first phase, with a calcineurin inhibitor such as ciclosporin or tacrolimus, or possibly mycophenolate mofetil with methotrexate. Acute GVHD can be treated by a corticosteroid with ciclosporin.

LONG-TERM EFFECTS OF IMMUNOSUPPRESSION

Immunosuppression increases the risk of infection. These are frequently bacterial in the first 1–2 months of treatment, most often affecting the lungs, renal tract or wounds. Later, opportunistic infections with viruses (particularly herpesviruses), *Pneumocystis jirovecii*, fungi and atypical mycobacteria become more common. Vaccination against influenza and pneumococcus are recommended with prolonged immunosuppression.

There is an increased risk of malignancy with prolonged immunosuppression. Early cancers are often viral-induced, especially lymphoproliferative disorders, cervical cancer and eventually skin cancer.

SELF-ASSESSMENT

True/false questions

1. Immunosuppression requires higher doses of methotrexate than used for cancer chemotherapy.
2. Ciclosporin and tacrolimus reduce IL-2 gene transcription in lymphocytes.
3. Ciclosporin causes bone marrow suppression.
4. Careful assessment of renal function is required with ciclosporin administration.
5. Azathioprine suppresses antibody-mediated immune responses.
6. Azathioprine interacts with allopurinol.
7. Sirolimus and tacrolimus share a common mechanism of action.
8. Corticosteroids have a narrow spectrum of immunosuppressant activity.
9. Mycophenolate is an alternative to azathioprine for preventing acute rejection.
10. Basiliximab is an antibody that blocks the IL-2 receptor.

Case-based questions

A 35-year-old woman was about to receive her second kidney transplant. The previous transplant had lasted 5 years, but despite immunosuppression with prednisolone and ciclosporin, it was eventually rejected.

1. How might the chances of acute rejection of the second transplant be reduced?
2. What could be the long-term risks of combination chemotherapy with corticosteroids, tacrolimus and azathioprine?

ANSWERS

True/false answers

1. **False.** Immunosuppressant doses of drugs such as methotrexate, cyclophosphamide and azathioprine are lower than those used for cancer chemotherapy.
2. **True.** These calcineurin inhibitors reduce the transcriptional effects of NFAT on IL-2; the loss of IL-2 suppresses T-cell maturation and proliferation.
3. **False.** The calcineurin inhibitors are selective suppressors of lymphocyte proliferation.
4. **True.** Ciclosporin is nephrotoxic and renal monitoring is necessary.
5. **True.** Azathioprine has a cytotoxic action by inhibiting purine metabolism, and the proliferation of lymphocytes and other immunocompetent cells is inhibited.
6. **True.** Allopurinol inhibits xanthine oxidase, which is involved in deactivating metabolites of azathioprine; doses of azathioprine should be reduced when given with allopurinol.
7. **False.** Sirolimus (rapamycin) binds to FK-binding protein-12, but the complex inhibits mTOR, a protein kinase involved in IL-2 signalling, unlike the calcineurin inhibitors that reduce IL-2 gene transcription.
8. **False.** Corticosteroids modulate the transcription of hundreds of immune and inflammatory genes encoding cytokines, mediators, adhesion molecules and apoptotic proteins.
9. **True.** Mycophenolate may have fewer toxic effects than azathioprine and is increasingly used in preventing acute rejection, but its place in preventing chronic rejection is less clear.
10. **True.** Basiliximab is a chimaeric monoclonal antibody that blocks the IL-2 receptor.

Case-based answers

1. Basiliximab given before and 4 days after renal transplant surgery reduces acute rejection by 35%. This is maintained typically by oral combination therapy of a corticosteroid (usually prednisolone) with a calcineurin inhibitor or mTOR inhibitor (such as ciclosporin, tacrolimus or sirolimus), and an antiproliferative immunosuppressant (such as azathioprine or mycophenolate). When used in combination, lower doses of the drugs can be administered than when giving the drugs alone. Intensive monitoring of liver and renal functions is important.
2. Oversuppression of the immune response brings problems of opportunistic infections. Additional 'steroid effects', as described for iatrogenic Cushing-like syndrome, may be also apparent (see Chapter 44).

FURTHER READING

Ferrara, J.L.M., Levine, J.E., Reddy, P., et al., 2009. Graft-versus-host disease. Lancet 373, 1550–1561.

Thiruchelvam, P.T.R., Willicombe, M., Hakim, N., et al., 2011. Renal transplantation. Br. Med. J. 343, d7300.

Zhang, R., 2013. Modern immunosuppressive therapy in kidney transplantation. Open J. Organ Transpl. Surg. 3, 22–31.

Zhang, R., 2014. Clinical management of kidney allograft dysfunction. Open J. Organ Transpl. Surg. 4, 7–14.

Compendium: immunosuppressant drugs

Drug	Characteristics
For the immunosuppressant activity of corticosteroids, see Chapter 44. See also the inflammatory arthritides (Chapter 30) and chemotherapy of malignancies (Chapter 52).	
Calcineurin inhibitors	
Ciclosporin	Lipid-soluble cyclic peptide. Used for prevention of graft rejection following bone marrow, kidney, liver, pancreas, heart, lung, and heart–lung transplantation, and for prophylaxis and treatment of GVHD. Given orally or intravenously. Half-life: 10–40 h
Tacrolimus	Similar to ciclosporin. Used to prevent kidney and liver transplant rejection. Given orally or intravenously. Half-life: 4–41 h
mTOR inhibitors	
Sirolimus	Potent noncalcineurin-inhibiting immunosuppressant. Used to prevent kidney transplant rejection. Given orally as an oil solution. Half-life: 60 h

Compendium: immunosuppressant drugs (cont'd)

Drug	Characteristics
Antiproliferative agents	
Azathioprine	Used for transplant recipients, for autoimmune conditions and for rheumatoid arthritis. Given orally or intravenously. Converted to active metabolite 6-mercaptopurine. Half-life: 3–5 h
Mycophenolate mofetil	Rapidly converted to active metabolite, mycophenolic acid. Used to prevent acute transplant rejection. Given orally or intravenously
Mycophenolic acid	Active metabolite of mycophenolate mofetil. Used to prevent acute transplant rejection. Given orally as enteric-coated formulation. Half-life: 12 h
IL-2 receptor antibodies	
Basiliximab	Monoclonal IL-2 receptor antibody that prevents T-lymphocyte proliferation. Given by intravenous infusion to prevent acute kidney transplant rejection. Half-life: 10 days
Co-stimulation blocker	
Belatacept	Fusion protein that blocks CD80/CD86 co-stimulatory molecules. Given by intravenous infusion to prevent renal transplant rejection in adults seropositive for Epstein–Barr virus. Half-life: 8–10 days

GVHD, Graft-versus-host disease; *IL-2*, interleukin-2; *mTOR*, mechanistic target of rapamycin.

39 Antihistamines and allergic disease

ATOPY, ALLERGIC DISORDERS AND ANAPHYLAXIS

Allergic responses occur in atopic individuals (people who are genetically predisposed to develop allergy), who produce antigen-specific immunoglobulin E (IgE) when exposed to common, normally harmless environmental allergens such as house dust mites, grass pollen or animal dander, usually in early life. Immunological memory takes about 7 days to develop, and subsequent re-exposure to the allergen triggers an allergic response, as explained below. Many atopic individuals have coexisting allergic diseases such as asthma, hay fever and eczema, although these are not invariably associated with atopy. Some allergies arise later in life, such as allergy to drugs.

The control of antibody production in the immune response is shown in Fig. 38.2. In people with allergies, initial challenge with allergens promotes an increase in the number of dendritic cells at the site of the challenge. In response to the presence of allergen and a co-stimulatory signal, such as viruses or compounds derived from viruses or bacteria, dendritic cells produce chemokines that enhance the T-helper type 2 (Th2) lymphocyte response rather than the usually dominant Th1-cell response (see Chapter 38). The release of the Th2 profile of interleukins, including IL-4, IL-5 and IL-13, stimulates B-lymphocytes to produce specific IgE rather than IgG, a phenomenon known as *class switching*. The IgE produced by these cells then binds to high-affinity IgE receptors on the surface of mast cells and basophils.

Most allergic reactions are of the type 1 (immediate) hypersensitivity category (see Chapter 38 for definitions). After the allergen cross-links allergen-specific IgE on mast cells and basophils, pre-formed and newly synthesised mediators of the allergic response are released. Histamine is the predominant pre-formed mediator. Newly synthesised mediators include platelet-activating factor, prostaglandin D_2 and the cysteinyl-leukotriene, LTC_4, which is converted to LTD_4 and LTE_4 extracellularly (see Chapter 29). All these mediators act at selective G protein-coupled receptors on smooth muscle cells, endothelial cells, epithelial cells, mucus glands and leucocytes in various tissues. Tryptase is also released from mast cells and stimulates protease-activated receptors (see Chapter 1).

Immediate hypersensitivity to an allergen in a person with atopy produces a wheal-and-flare reaction in the skin, sneezing and a runny nose or wheezing within minutes. A prolonged inflammatory reaction (delayed-type hypersensitivity) may follow the initial allergic response, reaching a peak 6–9 hours later. Depending on the site of the reaction, this produces an oedematous, red, indurated swelling in the skin (urticarial wheals), a sustained blockage in the nose or recurrent wheezing. This delayed reaction is associated with an initial accumulation of eosinophils and neutrophils in the affected tissues, followed by T cells and basophils.

At the most severe end of the spectrum of allergic response is anaphylaxis, a systemic allergic reaction that is life-threatening because of upper airway swelling and obstruction and/or hypotension. Severe anaphylactic reactions can occur within minutes of exposure to the allergen, or may be delayed by several hours after exposure. There are several causes of anaphylaxis (Box 39.1). About 80–90% of people experiencing anaphylaxis will have skin symptoms and signs, such as flushing, itching, urticaria, angioedema or morbiliform rash. If the allergen exposure is via systemic injection, hypotension and shock usually predominate. Foods are more likely to cause facial and laryngeal oedema with prominent respiratory problems. However, the constellation of symptoms and signs can vary between attacks in the same person.

Not all anaphylactic reactions are IgE-mediated; a few are IgG-mediated, such as anaphylaxis associated with infliximab.

Foods: especially peanuts, tree nuts, fish, shellfish, eggs, milk
Drugs: especially penicillin, intravenous anaesthetic agents, aspirin and other nonsteroidal anti-inflammatory drugs, intravenous contrast media, morphine
Bee and wasp stings
Latex rubber

Other similar reactions involve direct mast-cell and basophil activation, such as episodes triggered by exposure to cold or opioids. These nonimmunological reactions are often called anaphylactoid, but they present in the same way as true anaphylaxis.

Some allergic reactions, such as those that produce contact dermatitis, are driven by T cell-mediated inflammatory processes. These reactions can result from involvement of Th1 or Th2 cells or sometimes cytotoxic T cells. Delayed reactions can also arise without an immediate phase and may be triggered by primary activation of T cells rather than mast cells. Chronic allergic inflammation is maintained by continuing release of several Th2-type cytokines that promote the proliferation of mast cells and eosinophils, stimulate the expression of adhesion molecules and enhance the synthesis of IgE. Eosinophils release toxic basic proteins, cysteinyl-leukotrienes and platelet-activating factor. T cells, mast cells and eosinophils also produce neurotrophins that release neuropeptides such as substance P, calcitonin gene-related peptide and neurokinin A from sensory neurons. These various mediators contribute to the inflammatory response by producing vasodilation with increased vascular permeability; in the lung they promote smooth muscle contraction and mucus secretion.

HISTAMINE AS AN AUTACOID IN HOST DEFENCE

Histamine is a heterocyclic amine that is synthesised by decarboxylation of the dietary amino acid L-histidine in many different cells and functions as a local hormone (autacoid) and in the brain, where it acts as a neurotransmitter.

The autacoid function of histamine is important in host defence. Histamine is found in mast cells, which are prominent in tissues that come into contact with the outside world – for example, in the skin, lungs and gut they form part of the tissue defence mechanisms. Histamine is also present in circulating basophils, where it may also participate in tissue defence.

Histamine is released from mast cells and basophils by degranulation after activation of the cell either by a direct physical or chemical injury or by cross-linking of attached IgE molecules or complement proteins. After release from these cells, histamine is rapidly metabolised (see Chapter 4). The effects of histamine are mediated by four distinct types of G protein-coupled receptor known as H_1, H_2, H_3 and H_4 (see the table of receptors at the end of Chapter 1). In general, H_1 receptors are involved in the 'defensive'

actions of histamine and contribute to immune regulation and acute and chronic allergic inflammation.

Histamine H_1 receptors are normally in equilibrium between the active and inactive state. At rest, even in the absence of histamine, the H_1 receptor exerts a basal or constitutive level of activity. Histamine preferentially binds to the receptor in its active state and shifts the equilibrium further towards the active state. Histamine H_1 receptors act through intracellular Ca^{2+} as a second messenger and are coupled to inositol phospholipid intracellular signalling pathways. This activates the ubiquitous gene transcription factor nuclear factor κB (NF-κB; see Chapter 30), which stimulates production of pro-inflammatory cytokines (particularly tumour necrosis factor α and interleukins IL-6 and IL-8) and increases expression of epithelial and endothelial adhesion molecules. The following are the major consequences of H_1 receptor stimulation:

- Capillary and venous dilation, which can produce marked hypotension. In the skin, histamine contributes to the wheal-and-flare response; an axon reflex via H_1 receptors is responsible for the spread of vasodilation or flare from the oedematous wheal.
- Increased capillary permeability, which produces local oedema. This can lead to urticaria, angioedema and laryngeal oedema. The consequent loss of fluid from the circulating blood volume contributes to hypotension.
- Smooth muscle contraction, especially in bronchioles (producing bronchospasm) and the intestine (producing abdominal pain).
- Skin itching (produced by histamine in combination with kinins and prostaglandins).
- Pain due to stimulation of nociceptors (see Chapter 19).
- Increased antigen-presenting cell capacity, upregulation of Th1 cells and chemotaxis of eosinophils and neutrophils into affected tissues.

HISTAMINE H₁ RECEPTOR ANTAGONISTS (ANTIHISTAMINES)

Examples

first-generation (sedating) antihistamines: chlorphenamine, clemastine, promethazine
second-generation (nonsedating) antihistamines: cetirizine, desloratidine, fexofenadine, levocetirizine, loratadine, mizolastine

MECHANISMS OF ACTION AND EFFECTS

Antihistamines are competitive inverse agonists at the H_1 receptor (see Chapter 1) that have preferential affinity for the inactive state of the receptor and stabilise it in this conformation. Therefore, they are 'inverse agonists' that reduce the basal level of constitutive activity at histamine H_1 receptors as well as blocking the agonist effects of histamine. Antagonists at other histamine receptors are traditionally not called antihistamines. Useful clinical effects of antihistamines include:

- suppression of many of the vascular effects of histamine, with a reduction of vasodilation and oedema,

- inhibition of the accumulation of inflammatory cells in tissues,
- suppression of the immune response to antigens.

Antihistamines are functionally classified into two groups:

- First-generation antihistamines are lipophilic drugs that cross the blood–brain barrier, producing sedation by an action on central H_1 receptors. This action is employed therapeutically for relief of insomnia. They also have central antimuscarinic effects that are responsible for suppressing nausea in motion sickness (e.g. cyclizine, promethazine; see Chapter 32).
- Second-generation (nonsedating) antihistamines such as cetirizine, fexofenadine, loratadine and mizolastine are more hydrophilic. They do not cross the blood–brain barrier well and have little sedative effect. They also have little antimuscarinic action. The newest drugs in this group are active metabolites or optical isomers of second-generation drugs, such as desloratadine and levocetirizine.

PHARMACOKINETICS

Chlorphenamine is more slowly absorbed from the gut than promethazine; both undergo considerable first-pass hepatic metabolism to inactive compounds and have half-lives of 10–20 hours. Formulations of chlorphenamine and promethazine are available for administration by intravenous or intramuscular injection in medical emergencies.

Most second-generation antihistamines are rapidly absorbed from the gut and metabolised in the liver to active compounds with half-lives ranging from 2 to 20 hours. Cetirizine and fexofenadine undergo little metabolism and are mainly eliminated unchanged by the kidneys.

There are several topical formulations of antihistamines, including eye drops for allergic conjunctivitis and topical skin preparations for insect stings (although the latter are relatively ineffective).

UNWANTED EFFECTS

- Drowsiness or psychomotor impairment (CNS H_1 receptor actions), especially with first-generation compounds, although paradoxical stimulation can occur in children and the elderly.
- Headache.
- Dry mouth, blurred vision, urinary retention and gastro-intestinal upset (antimuscarinic effects) with first-generation compounds.
- Arrhythmias are a rare complication with some antihista-mines, when they arise from prolongation of the QT interval on the electrocardiogram (ECG).
- Topical antihistamines for use on the skin can cause hypersensitivity reactions.

MANAGEMENT OF ALLERGIC DISORDERS

ANAPHYLAXIS

Anaphylaxis is a serious allergic reaction that is rapid in onset and can cause death. It is a medical emergency and requires rapidly acting treatments. The person should be laid flat with the feet raised if there is hypotension and the airway should be secured. The trigger, such as an intravenously administered drug, should be removed immediately if possible. Adrenaline (epinephrine; see Chapter 4) should be given intramuscularly into the mid-outer thigh as soon as possible. Further doses can be given after 5–15-minute intervals if needed. Intravenous adrenaline should be given only if there is profound shock and then in a very dilute solution with close cardiac monitoring. Intravenous use carries a risk of arrhythmias and intense coronary artery vasoconstriction with ischaemic myocardial damage. Early use of adrenaline reduces the risk of biphasic or prolonged anaphylaxis and death. Adrenaline produces vasoconstriction by its action at α_1-adrenoceptors, reduces oedema and bronchodilates via β_2-adrenoceptors. It also attenuates further release of mediators from mast cells by binding to cell-surface β_2-adrenoceptors. People known to have allergies that cause anaphylaxis can carry a preloaded adrenaline syringe for emergencies, accompanied by detailed instructions on its appropriate use.

Once adrenaline has been given, intramuscular or slow intravenous injection of chlorphenamine can be given to relieve skin or nasal symptoms. Late relapse or prolonged symptoms can be prevented by intravenous hydrocortisone (see Chapter 44). Oxygen should be given in high concentration; if marked bronchospasm is unresponsive to adrenaline, it can be treated with an inhaled β_2-adrenoceptor agonist such as salbutamol (see Chapter 12). If there is persistent hypotension, a high volume of intravenous isotonic saline should be given rapidly.

It is important to observe someone who has had anaphylaxis for 4–6 hours, or 8–10 hours if there has been respiratory or circulatory compromise in case there is a late relapse. Recurrence of anaphylaxis triggered by venom from stinging insects can be avoided by immunotherapy to desensitise the person to the allergen.

SEASONAL AND PERENNIAL RHINITIS

Allergic inflammation of the lining of the nose produces symptoms of rhinitis including rhinorrhoea, nasal obstruction, sneezing and itching. These result from increased glandular secretions and afferent nerve stimulation. The allergic response makes individuals more susceptible to the nasal irritant effects of other, nonallergenic stimuli, such as tobacco smoke and changes in temperature. Allergic rhinitis is classified as

- intermittent rhinitis (symptoms for < 4 days a week or < 4 consecutive weeks) due to exposure to infrequently encountered allergens such as animal dander, pollens and moulds,
- persistent rhinitis (symptoms for > 4 days a week or > 4 consecutive weeks) due to exposure to commonly encountered allergens such as house dust mites.

For treatment of allergic rhinitis, oral nonsedating antihista-mines are useful for reducing itching, sneezing and rhinorrhoea but are less effective for nasal obstruction. They can also suppress associated allergic conjunctivitis. For more severe allergic rhinitis, a topical intranasal corticosteroid spray (see Chapter 44) is the treatment of choice, providing relief from most symptoms. Topical sodium cromoglicate or nedocromil (see Chapter 12) is less effective than antihistamines or topical corticosteroids; these are no longer preferred treatments. An oral leukotriene receptor antagonist (montelukast) may be beneficial in allergic rhinitis with concomitant asthma. Topical nasal decongestants have a short-term role in treatment. These contain α_1-adrenoceptor agonists such as ephedrine or xylometazoline and produce local vasoconstriction. Prolonged use should be avoided since it impairs ciliary activity in the nasal mucosa and can be associated with rebound nasal congestion. Oral corticosteroids are reserved for the most severe symptoms.

Rhinitis also has several nonallergic causes; these include acute and chronic sinus infection, for which antibacterial treatment is indicated. The antimuscarinic drug ipratropium bromide (see Chapter 12) can be used topically for relief of nonallergic rhinorrhoea. Chronic rhinosinusitis is a combination of inflammation and infection in the nasal passages and paranasal sinuses. It is distinguished from acute rhinosinusitis by symptoms that persist for at least 12 weeks. Symptoms include nasal blockage, congestion or discharge (anterior or posterior nasal drip), with either facial pain or pressure or a reduction or loss of smell for more than 12 weeks. The condition may be associated with nasal polyps that obstruct the airway. The cause of chronic rhinosinusitis is unknown; there is a link with the presence of atopy, but it is unclear whether allergy is the initial trigger. Initial treatment is with an intranasal corticosteroid, but a short course of oral corticosteroid can be used for severe disease in the presence of nasal polyps. If drugs fail, surgery for structural abnormalities such as nasal polyposis, hypertrophied inferior turbinates or a deviated nasal septum should be considered.

Aspirin and other nonsteroidal antiinflammatory drugs (NSAIDs) can produce rhinitis (as well as asthma, see Chapter 12) in sensitive individuals, probably by enhancing cysteinyl-leukotriene generation. Less frequent causes include β-adrenoceptor antagonists and angiotensin-converting enzyme (ACE) inhibitors.

URTICARIA AND ANGIOEDEMA

Urticaria is characterised by red, raised itchy lesions with a pale centre (wheal) caused by vasodilation, increased blood flow and increased vascular permeability. Mast-cell activation is prominent, with initial release of histamine, leukotrienes and prostaglandins, followed by delayed release of various other cytokines and chemokines such as TNFα, IL-4 and IL-5. Angioedema is tissue swelling of the face, oropharynx, genitalia or gut due to a local increase in vascular permeability. It is frequently painful rather than itchy. Wheals usually resolve within 48 hours but angioedema often persists for a few days. Urticaria occurs alone in about 50% of cases and in combination with angioedema in 40% of cases; angioedema alone comprises the other 10% of cases. Angioedema without wheals can occur in hereditary angioedema when it is due to excess production of bradykinin. ACE inhibitors can cause isolated angioedema, which can arise months or years after starting treatment and may also be due to excess bradykinin. ACE inhibitors should be avoided in people with a history of angioedema.

The most common causes of acute urticarial reactions are medications, foods, viral or parasitic infections, insect venom and contact allergens including latex. However, in up to half of cases of acute urticaria, no trigger is identified (idiopathic urticaria). Having identified a trigger, avoidance strategies are important in management. Second-generation antihistamines

are the treatment of choice, with an oral corticosteroid (see Chapter 44) for more severe episodes. Attacks of swelling in hereditary angioedema can be controlled with tranexamic acid (see Chapter 11) or the selective bradykinin antagonist icatibant.

Chronic urticaria (wheals that are present most days of the week for >6 weeks) is often nonallergic in origin. It can be provoked by physical factors such as cold, sun, scratching the skin or exercise, or it can be caused by urticarial vasculitis in association with connective tissue diseases such as systemic lupus erythematosus. In many cases the cause may be autoimmune, with IgG autoantibodies to the IgE receptors on mast cells and basophils documented. Second-generation antihistamines can be helpful to suppress the itch from chronic urticaria but often have little effect on the wheal. Leukotriene receptor antagonists such as montelukast (see Chapter 12) are effective when the trigger is aspirin, another NSAID or a delayed response to pressure. Corticosteroids (see Chapter 44) can be used in high dosage for severe symptoms, but long-term use should be avoided because of the unwanted effects. Immunosuppression with ciclosporin, tacrolimus or mycophenolate mofetil (see Chapter 38) has been used successfully for some severe autoimmune urticarias. Omalizumab, an antibody to IgE, has also been effective in both spontaneous and autoimmune chronic urticaria.

ALLERGIC CONJUNCTIVITIS

Oral or topical treatment with antihistamines, such as azelastine or antazoline, or with mast-cell stabilisers such as sodium cromoglicate or nedocromil, can relieve the itching, erythema, tearing and swelling in response to allergen exposure. Topical formulations are effective within 15 minutes of application (see Chapter 50).

SELF-ASSESSMENT

True/false questions

1. Antihistamines do not reduce acid secretion from the gastric parietal cells.
2. Histamine is synthesised de novo when mast cell IgE receptors are cross-linked by allergen.
3. Loratadine is a nonsedating antihistamine.
4. Fexofenadine is associated with ECG changes.
5. Fexofenadine reduces the release of histamine from mast cells.
6. Corticosteroids are effective for treating allergic rhinitis.
7. Histamine is the only mediator that causes symptoms in rhinitis.
8. Antihistamines have a well-defined place in the management of asthma.

One-best-answer (OBA) questions

1. What contributes to an allergic response in an atopic individual?
   A. Increased production of cytokines from Th1-cells
   B. Increased production of IgM

C. Stabilisation of mast cells

D. Histamine acting on H_1 receptors

E. Reduction in leukotriene production from mast cells

2. Choose the most accurate statement concerning antihistamines.

A. Second-generation antihistamines readily cross the blood–brain barrier.

B. Second-generation antihistamines have fewer antimuscarinic effects than first-generation antihistamines.

C. First-generation antihistamines are the preferred first-line treatment for vomiting induced by cytotoxic drugs.

D. Topical antihistamines are free from unwanted effects.

E. Antihistamines cause vasodilation.

Case-based questions

A 10-year-old boy visited his doctor with his mother in the spring. His current symptoms of rhinorrhoea, nasal congestion, sneezing and itching eyes were interfering with his schoolwork. He gave a history of repeated episodes of recurrent otitis media, rhinorrhoea, nasal congestion, sneezing and itching eyes occurring over a 3-year period but predominantly in the spring and autumn. He had had three episodes of otitis media over the previous 2 years, the last being 6 months before, which were treated with antibiotics because of prolonged residence of fluid in the middle ear. The boy had atopic dermatitis as an infant. He had no history of asthma; his mother had allergic rhinitis; they had two cats. Other than antibacterial drug treatment for his otitis media, he had taken no medication. Examination of the ears revealed healthy tympanic membranes with no current otitis media. He had no hearing loss and was otherwise fit.

1. What was the likely diagnosis?

2. Were the boy's symptoms related to the history of otitis media?

3. Allergen skin testing showed him to be responsive to cat dander and house dust mites. What treatment would you give?

ANSWERS

True/false answers

1. **True.** The term antihistamine is traditionally confined to H_1 receptor antagonists; these drugs do not block H_2 histamine receptors on the gastric parietal cells; selective histamine H_2 receptor antagonists include cimetidine and ranitidine.

2. **False.** Histamine is synthesised and stored in mast cell granules ready for release by IgE-dependent stimuli; in contrast, lipid mediators such as leukotrienes and prostaglandins are synthesised de novo after stimulation.

3. **True.** Loratadine is a second-generation antihistamine, lacking the sedative action of first-generation antihistamines.

4. **False.** The parent drug of fexofenadine, terfenadine, was associated with ventricular arrhythmias in high doses and has been withdrawn; fexofenadine retains the antihistamine activity without the unwanted effects on the heart.

5. **False.** Like other antihistamines, fexofenadine reduces histamine activity only by blocking H_1 receptors.

6. **True.** Nasal corticosteroids are very effective in allergic rhinitis.

7. **False.** Mast cells also synthesise prostaglandins and leukotrienes that contribute to nasal symptoms.

8. **False.** Antihistamines are not effective in asthma and have no place in asthma management guidelines.

One-best-answer (OBA) answers

1. **Answer D** is correct.

A. Incorrect. In atopy there is a predominance of a Th2 response profile which is partly genetically determined and partly related to early life environment.

B. Incorrect. The Th2 response leads to increased production of IgE.

C. Incorrect. Mast cells degranulate following allergen cross-linking of IgE.

D. **Correct.** The main effect of histamine in allergy is on H_1 receptor.

E. Incorrect. Increased leukotriene synthesis in mast cells contributes to allergic responses.

2. **Answer B** is correct.

A. Incorrect. Second-generation drugs are less able to cross the blood–brain barrier than first-generation drugs and cause less sedation.

B. **Correct**. Second-generation antihistamines have less antagonist activity at muscarinic receptors.

C. Incorrect. Antihistamines can be effective in motion sickness but not in vomiting caused by cancer chemotherapeutic agents.

D. Incorrect. Topical antihistamines may cause hypersensitivity reactions.

E. Incorrect. Antihistamines reduce vasodilation induced by the action of histamine at the H_1 receptor.

Case-based answers

1. The family history of atopy and the child's atopic dermatitis as an infant increase the likelihood that he would have had allergies. He is likely to have had seasonal allergic rhinitis but may also have had sensitisation to cat dander and/or dust mites or other perennial allergens. His fitness and lack of current drug intake suggest that it is not nonallergic rhinitis, which may arise because of infections, drugs, etc.

2. Yes. As many as 50% of children older than 3 years with recurrent otitis media have confirmed allergic rhinitis.

3. It is important to carry out sensitivity testing, and sensitivity to cat dander and house dust mites was identified in this boy. Avoidance of exposure to allergens is advisable and should be actively pursued in the home and school environment. If pharmacological treatment is required, a nonsedating oral antihistamine should reduce rhinorrhoea, sneezing and itching but will have little effect on nasal congestion. A short course of nasal inhaled corticosteroids can be effective in controlling symptoms of allergic rhinitis, including congestion. Nasal sodium cromoglicate may also offer symptom relief but is not the preferred treatment.

FURTHER READING

Ah-See, K.L., MacKenzie, J., Ah-See, K.W., 2012. Management of chronic rhinosinusitis. Br. Med. J. 345, e7054.

Ardern-Jones, M.R., Friedmann, P.S., 2010. Skin manifestations of drug allergy. Br. J. Clin. Pharmacol. 71, 672–683.

Barr, J.G., Al-Reefy, H., Fox, A.T., et al., 2014. Allergic rhinitis in children. Br. Med. J. 348, g4153.

BSACI guideline for the management of chronic urticaria and angioedema, 2015. Clin. Exp. Allergy 45, 547–565.

Greiner, A.N., Hellings, P.W., Rotiroti, G., et al., 2011. Allergic rhinitis. Lancet 378, 2112–2122.

Simons, F.E.R., Sheik, A., 2013. Anaphylaxis: the acute episode and beyond. Br. Med. J. 346, f602.

Wheatley, L.M., Togias, A., 2015. Allergic rhinitis. N. Engl. J. Med. 372, 456–463.

Compendium: antihistamines

Drug	Characteristics
Antihistamines are given orally or topically in the eye (see Chapter 50), in the nose or on the skin. Drugs with antihistamine actions that are not used to treat allergic conditions, such as cyclizine and meclozine, are used for the treatment of vestibular disorders and nausea and vomiting, especially motion sickness (see Chapter 32).	
Nonsedating antihistamines	
Acrivastine	Used for symptomatic relief of allergy such as hay fever and chronic idiopathic urticaria. Half-life: 2 h
Azelastine	Used topically as nasal spray for allergic rhinitis and as eye drops for allergic conjunctivitis (see Chapter 50); also available in combination with fluticasone. Half-life: 17 h
Bilastine	Used for symptomatic relief of allergic rhinoconjunctivitis and urticarial. Half-life: 14.5 h
Cetirizine	Used for symptomatic relief of allergy such as allergic rhinitis and chronic idiopathic urticaria. Half-life: 6–10 h
Desloratadine	The active metabolite of loratadine. Used for symptomatic relief of allergic rhinitis and urticaria. Half-life: 20–30 h
Fexofenadine	Used for symptomatic relief of seasonal allergic rhinitis and chronic idiopathic urticaria. Half-life: 14 h
Levocetirizine	An isomer of cetirizine. Used for symptomatic relief of allergic rhinitis and urticaria. Half-life: 8–9 h
Loratadine	Prodrug of desloratadine. Used for symptomatic relief of allergic rhinitis and chronic idiopathic urticaria. Half-life: 8 h
Mizolastine	Used for symptomatic relief of allergy such as allergic rhinitis and urticarial. Half-life: 15 h
Sedating antihistamines	
Alimemazine	Used for urticaria and pruritus and as a premedication before surgical anaesthesia. Half-life: 4–7 h
Chlorphenamine (chlorpheniramine in the United States)	Used for symptomatic relief of allergy such as hay fever, urticaria, food allergy, drug reactions, for relief of itch associated with chickenpox and for emergency treatment of anaphylactic reactions. Half-life: 22 h
Clemastine	Used for symptomatic relief of hay fever and urticaria. Half-life: 21 h
Cyproheptadine	Used for symptomatic relief of hay fever, urticaria and pruritus. Half-life: 1–4 h
Hydroxyzine	Used for pruritus. Half-life: 20 h
Ketotifen	Used for allergic rhinitis, and for allergic conjunctivitis (see Chapter 50). Half-life: 22 h
Promethazine	Used for symptomatic relief of hay fever, urticaria, pruritus and for emergency treatment of anaphylaxis and angioedema; also used for motion sickness and as a sedative premedication before general anaesthesia. Half-life: 10–14 h

9

The endocrine system and metabolism

40 Diabetes mellitus

CONTROL OF BLOOD GLUCOSE

Blood glucose concentration is normally maintained within a narrow range despite marked variations in the availability of glucose absorbed from the gut. Two hormones have a central role in the regulation of blood glucose concentration, insulin and glucagon.

Insulin is a protein secreted rapidly from the β-cells of the islets of Langerhans in the pancreas in response to a small rise in blood glucose; its secretion is inhibited by a fall in blood glucose (Table 40.1). Insulin consists of two peptide chains, A and B, connected by two disulphide bridges. In the β-cell, insulin aggregates into hexamers with zinc; after release from the cell, it dissociates initially into dimers and eventually into the active monomeric form.

The presence of glucose and fat in the small intestine stimulates the release of peptide hormones, called incretins, from enteroendocrine cells; the incretins promote insulin secretion. The principal incretins are glucose-dependent insulinotropic peptide (GIP), secreted by K cells in the proximal small intestine, and glucagon-like peptide-1 (GLP-1), which is released from L cells in the distal small intestine. Release of incretins is triggered by direct interaction of glucose with the secretory cells and by neural signals from the proximal gut. Incretins have several actions that maintain glucose homeostasis:

- enhanced glucose-dependent insulin secretion through specific GLP-1 and GIP receptors on pancreatic islet β-cells. Incretins are responsible for about 60% of the insulin secreted in response to a meal.
- inhibition of glucagon release.
- promotion of satiety by an action on the hypothalamus.

Incretins also increase lipogenesis in adipose tissue. The actions of GLP-1 and GIP are brief as they have very short plasma half-lives of 1–2 minutes owing to their rapid degradation by dipeptidyl peptidase-4 (DPP-4). Insulin secretion is increased to a lesser extent by regulators other than glucose and incretins (see Table 40.1).

Insulin is secreted into the blood even during fasting, with pulses released every 3–6 minutes, thus preventing downregulation of insulin receptors in target cells. In response to a rise in plasma glucose (both the extent and the rate of change in concentration), there is a superimposed biphasic pattern of insulin release.

- The *first phase* of release occurs within seconds, peaks at 3–5 minutes and lasts for about 10 minutes. This is

Table 40.1 Control of insulin release from pancreatic islets of Langerhans β-cells

Stimulants of insulin release	Inhibitors of insulin release
Parasympathetic stimulation (muscarinic receptors)	Sympathetic stimulation (α_2-adrenoceptors)
Increased glucose	Decreased glucose
Amino acids	Somatostatin
Fatty acids	Cortisol
Incretins (GLP-1, GIP)	
Glucagon	
Gastrin	
Cholecystokinin	
Secretin	

GIP, glucose-dependent insulinotropic peptide; *GLP-1*, glucagon-like peptide.

Table 40.2 Metabolic effects of insulin

Site	Effect
Liver	Increased glucose storage as glycogen
	Decreased gluconeogenesis
	Increased protein synthesis
	Decreased protein catabolism
Muscle	Increased glucose uptake
	Increased glycogen synthesis
	Increased amino acid uptake
	Increased protein synthesis
Adipose tissue	Increased glucose uptake
	Increased glycerol synthesis
	Increased triglyceride storage
	Decreased lipolysis

achieved by the release of a small pool of insulin in secretory vesicles.

■ The *second phase* of release is more gradual, rising to a lower peak than in phase 1, and is due to synthesis of new insulin.

Insulin secretion from pancreatic β-cells is modulated by K^+ channels in the cell membrane that are sensitive to ATP (K_{ATP} channels), which has subunits known as sulfonylurea receptors (SURs). First-phase insulin release is triggered when glucose enters the β-cell via the glucose transporter 2 (GLUT2) and undergoes glycolysis and then further metabolism in the tricarboxylic acid (TCA) cycle with generation of intracellular ATP. ATP, augmented by TCA intermediates, activates the SUR1 receptor isoform, which closes the K_{ATP} channel. This reduces membrane K^+ efflux and depolarises the β-cell, which opens voltage-gated L-type Ca^{2+} channels in the cell membrane. Influx of Ca^{2+} ions into the cell triggers second messengers, leading to exocytosis of insulin granules. (See Fig. 5.4 for a description of the K_{ATP} and Ca^{2+} channels in vascular smooth muscle.)

Peripheral tissues (especially skeletal and cardiac muscle and adipose tissue) express cell-surface insulin receptors that are linked to a tyrosine kinase known as insulin receptor kinase (see Chapter 1). When insulin stimulates these receptors, the GLUT4 glucose transporter is translocated to the cell surface, allowing glucose uptake into the tissue. Insulin also activates pathways involved in glycogen synthesis, glycolysis and fatty acid synthesis. Insulin has several metabolic effects.

■ Glucose metabolism: promotion of active transport of glucose into cells, particularly in skeletal muscle and adipose tissue, accompanied by K^+ ions. Insulin enhances storage of glucose as glycogen in liver and muscle and inhibits the breakdown of glycogen (glycogenolysis). Insulin also inhibits gluconeogenesis from amino acids in the liver. The overall effect is to increase glycogen stores.

■ Lipid metabolism: reduced plasma free fatty acids and increased adipocyte triglyceride storage. Insulin increases

hydrolysis of circulating triglycerides from lipoproteins by enhancing the activity of lipoprotein lipase and promotes fatty acid uptake by adipose cells. Glucose entry into adipocytes provides glycerol phosphate for esterification of fatty acids to triglycerides, and lipolysis is reduced by inhibition of lipases, preventing triglyceride breakdown.

■ Protein metabolism: inhibition of the catabolism of amino acids in the liver and increased amino acid transport into muscle, with enhanced protein synthesis.

The effects of insulin on different tissues are summarised in Table 40.2.

Glucagon is a peptide hormone released from α-cells in the pancreas when plasma glucose levels fall. Glucagon accelerates glycogenolysis and gluconeogenesis to raise the plasma glucose concentration. Several other hormones inhibit the anabolic actions of insulin, particularly on carbohydrate metabolism, although effects on protein metabolism vary. These include growth hormone (mediated by somatostatin), cortisol and catecholamines. Most of these hormones are released in stressful situations that require the breakdown of glycogen reserves to provide energy.

DIABETES MELLITUS

Failure to secrete sufficient insulin to maintain blood glucose within the normal concentration range results in diabetes mellitus. This condition is diagnosed when there are symptoms such as polyuria, polydipsia and unexplained weight loss together with either fasting plasma glucose concentration above 7.0 mmol/L or random plasma glucose above 11.1 mmol/L. In the absence of symptoms, a single raised plasma glucose is insufficient to confirm the diagnosis. The long-term consequences of diabetes mellitus include increased risk of the development of vascular and neuropathic disease (Table 40.3). Two patterns of diabetes mellitus are recognised: type 1 and type 2. There is still dispute over whether they represent distinct entities or different

Table 40.3 Complications of diabetes

Complication	Consequences
Microvascular	
Nephropathy	Microalbuminuria, macroalbuminuria, renal failure
Retinopathy	Background retinopathy, proliferative retinopathy leading to visual impairment
Peripheral neuropathy	Loss of peripheral sensation
	Pain, ulceration
Autonomic neuropathy	Impotence
	Gastrointestinal disturbance
	Orthostatic hypotension
Macrovascular	
Cardiovascular disease	Hypertension
	Ischaemic heart disease
Cerebrovascular disease	Stroke

Box 40.1 Factors responsible for the pathophysiological disturbances in type 2 diabetes (the 'ominous octet')

1. Decreased incretin effect
2. Decreased insulin secretion
3. Decreased glucose uptake by muscles
4. Neurotransmitter dysfunction
5. Increased glucagon secretion
6. Increased renal glucose absorption
7. Increased lipolysis
8. Increased hepatic glucose output

See also Fig. 40.1 for sites of drug action.

manifestations of the same disease process. There is a strong genetic predisposition for both conditions.

TYPE 1 DIABETES MELLITUS

Type 1 diabetes mellitus arises from severe deficiency of insulin production caused by autoimmune destruction of pancreatic β-cells; it usually presents in younger people. These individuals typically present with a short history of feeling tired and unwell, together with weight loss, polyuria and polydipsia. There is a high risk of ketoacidosis because of the breakdown of fatty acids and amino acids in the liver to provide an energy source to replace glucose, which generates ketone bodies.

TYPE 2 DIABETES MELLITUS

Type 2 diabetes mellitus is the consequence of a relative deficiency of insulin. It more commonly presents later in life than type 1 and accounts for 90% of cases of diabetes mellitus in the Western world. In established type 2 diabetes mellitus, the first phase of insulin secretion is absent or attenuated and the second phase is slowed. Symptoms in people with type 2 diabetes mellitus arise slowly. The condition is often present for many years before being recognised and may first present with complications or be identified only by screening.

People with type 2 diabetes mellitus are often overweight (the average body mass index at diagnosis is 30 kg/m²). This increases cellular resistance to insulin in the liver, muscles and adipose tissue, so that less glucose is transported into cells despite a normal or raised plasma insulin concentration. Target-cell insulin resistance characteristically precedes overt diabetes by 10–12 years, but increased insulin secretion by the pancreas is sufficient to overcome cellular resistance. However, the increase in basal insulin secretion probably

exacerbates insulin resistance by downregulating insulin receptors. In type 2 diabetes mellitus there is reduced or absent GLP-1 secretion in response to oral glucose and a reduced sensitivity to the peptide at pancreatic β-cells. Over time, high circulating free fatty acids and the production of reactive oxygen species in response to a sustained high plasma glucose concentration ('glucotoxicity') progressively reduces β-cell mass and therefore insulin secretion. This leads to a state of β-cell dysfunction with a reduction in the first-phase insulin response to a glucose load and loss of compensation for insulin resistance. In those people with type 2 diabetes mellitus who are not obese, the major defect is β-cell dysfunction. Overall, eight factors have been identified that are responsible for the pathophysiological disturbances in type 2 diabetes, often referred to as the 'ominous octet' (Box 40.1).

In type 2 diabetes mellitus, postprandial hyperglycaemia is the most prominent defect in blood glucose control, with excess glucose outside the cells rather than a shortage inside. The ideal approach to treatment would be an intervention that restores the early phase of insulin secretion in response to a glucose load. People with type 2 diabetes mellitus do not usually develop ketoacidosis because sufficient glucose enters cells to permit adequate energy production for most situations. However, ketosis-prone type 2 diabetes mellitus is now well recognised as a subset of the condition, particularly in people of Afro-Caribbean origin.

INSULIN AND INSULIN ANALOGUES FOR TREATMENT OF DIABETES MELLITUS

Insulin secreted from the pancreas is released into the portal circulation, and its release is strictly regulated to meet metabolic needs. Some 60% of the insulin released from the pancreas is extracted by the liver before it reaches the systemic circulation. In contrast, therapeutic delivery of insulin is to the systemic circulation, and the relationship to metabolic needs can only be approximated by the dosages used and their timing in relation to meals.

NATURAL INSULIN FORMULATIONS

Insulins for therapeutic use were originally extracted from either bovine or porcine pancreas. Bovine insulin differs chemically from human insulin in three amino acid residues and porcine insulin in one, but their actions are very similar to those of human insulin. These insulins have a higher immunogenicity than human insulin, and bovine insulin in particular is rarely used. Human-sequence insulin is produced either by enzymatic modification of porcine insulin or by recombinant DNA technology using bacteria or yeast. All current insulin preparations have a low impurity content and low immunogenic potential.

Insulins must be given parenterally because insulin is a protein and would be digested in the gut. Insulins (and insulin analogues) are usually formulated at a standard strength of 100 U/mL to reduce confusion over doses. However, the increasing use of very large doses in obese people with insulin resistance has led to the marketing of higher-strength formulations with 300 or 500 U/mL to reduce the volume of injection required. There are various injection devices, usually a form of prefilled syringe to facilitate accurate dosing and for ease of use.

Pharmacokinetics

Subcutaneous injection of insulin is used for routine treatment, with intravenous infusion for emergency situations. Recommended subcutaneous injection sites include the upper arms, thighs, buttocks and abdomen. Absorption is faster from the abdomen than from the limbs, although strenuous exercise can increase absorption from the limbs.

The half-life of insulin in plasma is very short (about 4–6 minutes) owing to uptake and degradation in the kidneys and liver. To avoid the need for very frequent injections during maintenance treatment, the absorption of insulin from injection sites must be prolonged. This is achieved by formulating insulin either as a soluble preparation (also called *neutral insulin*) or as a complex with protamine and/or zinc (Table 40.4).

Soluble insulins aggregate to form hexamers, which delays their absorption from the injection site. After subcutaneous injection, the maximum plasma concentration of insulin is achieved about 2 hours later. Therefore, to limit the increase in plasma glucose concentration generated by a meal, subcutaneous soluble insulin must be given 15–30 minutes before eating. Continued absorption from a subcutaneous injection site prolongs the duration of action to about 5 hours after injection. The action of intravenous soluble insulin lasts less than an hour.

To generate intermediate- or long-acting formulations, insulin is formulated as a complex with:

- protamine: to create an intermediate-acting complex isophane insulin. Isophane insulin is also available mixed with a solution of soluble insulin (biphasic isophane insulin) in various ratios, the most common being 30% soluble with 70% isophane, to avoid multiple injections.
- zinc: to create the intermediate-acting insulin zinc suspension. Insulin molecules form hexamers, which are stabilised by zinc; the size of these molecular aggregates determines the rate of diffusion from the site of injection. Insulin zinc suspension is available only as bovine insulin and is therefore rarely used (see Table 40.4).
- protamine and zinc: to create the long-acting protamine–zinc insulin. This is available only as bovine insulin and is now rarely used. It binds soluble insulin, which cannot be given in the same syringe.

Unwanted effects

All people with diabetes mellitus who take insulin should carry a card with details of their treatment ('insulin passport').

- The main problem with insulin is an excessive action producing hypoglycaemia; neuroglycopenia can cause confusion and coma. Although most people experience warning symptoms of hypoglycaemia, some do not and are prone to sudden hypoglycaemia with loss of consciousness. Frequent hypoglycaemic attacks can

Table 40.4 Characteristics of insulins following subcutaneous administration

Type	Onset of action	Peak activity	Duration	
Insulin formulations				
Insulin (neutral or soluble)	30–60 min	2–5 h	5–8 h	Short-acting
Isophane insulin[a]	1–2 h	4–12 h	18–24 h	Intermediate-acting
Insulin zinc suspension	2 h	6–14 h	22 h	Long-acting
Protamine–zinc insulin	4 h	12–24 h	30 h	Long-acting
Insulin analogues				
Insulin lispro	15–30 min	30–90 min	3–5 h	Rapid-acting
Insulin aspart	10–20 min	40–50 min	3–5 h	Rapid-acting
Insulin glulisine	20–30 min	30–90 min	1–2.5 h	Rapid-acting
Insulin glargine	1–1.5 h	Plateau 2–20 h	20–24 h	Long-acting
Insulin degludec	1 h	Plateau 1–40 h	>42 h	Ultra-long-acting
Insulin detemir	1– h	Plateau 6–8 h	Up to 24 h	Long-acting

[a]Sometimes called NPH (neutral protamine Hagedorn) insulin.

reduce awareness of the onset of future symptoms. If the person is conscious, hypoglycaemia is treated with sugary foods or drinks. If unconscious, oral glucose or glucose gel (10–20 g) or an intravenous injection of 20% glucose is used. Glucagon (see below) can be given intramuscularly if venous access is not available, followed by a sugary drink on waking.

■ Rebound hyperglycaemia can occur after an episode of hypoglycaemia, especially at night (Somogyi effect). This results from the compensatory release of hormones such as adrenaline. It can produce ketonuria, leading to a mistaken belief that too little insulin has been given.

■ All insulins (including human insulin) are immunogenic and can produce circulating antibodies, although this is less common with current, highly purified preparations. Immunological resistance to insulin is rare but can produce lipoatrophy at injection sites.

■ Insulins can cause local fat hypertrophy at the injection site, which can be minimised by rotating the site of injection.

INSULIN ANALOGUES

short-acting: insulin aspart, insulin glulisine, insulin lispro
long-acting: insulin detemir, insulin glargine, insulin
   degludec

Mechanism of action and effects

The insulin analogues are recombinant modifications of natural insulin with one or two amino acid changes. These changes have no effect on the binding of the molecule to cellular insulin receptors.

Rapid-acting insulin analogues

Because of the amino acid modifications in rapid-acting insulin analogues, they do not readily form dimers and hexamers. Therefore they are more rapidly absorbed from an injection site than soluble insulin, with a faster onset and a shorter duration of action.

Insulin aspart and lispro are available as ready-mixed biphasic preparations in which some of the analogue is in a complex with protamine (similar to isophane insulin) to give the mixture an intermediate duration of action.

Long-acting insulin analogues

■ Insulin detemir has an amino acid modification and a fatty acid chain added to enhance formation of hexamers and increase binding to albumin. It is slowly absorbed from the injection site and, once in the circulation, insulin detemir dissociates from albumin only slowly.

■ Insulin glargine has two amino acid changes that make the molecule more soluble at acid pH, and less soluble at physiological pH. It precipitates after subcutaneous injection, slowly redissolves and is then absorbed.

■ Insulin degludec has a single amino acid change and is conjugated to hexadecanedioic acid, which forms multi-hexamers in subcutaneous tissue and delays absorption.

Pharmacokinetics

Rapid-acting insulin analogues are absorbed faster after subcutaneous injection and have an earlier peak plasma concentration compared with soluble insulin (see Table 40.4). The duration of action is also shorter at almost 3 hours. These insulin analogues should be given just before a meal. Although they can be used immediately after eating, this increases the risk of postprandial hyperglycaemia and late hypoglycaemia. They can be mixed with long-acting insulins or used as premixed biphasic formulations. Insulin analogues can also be given by subcutaneous infusion or by intravenous injection or infusion.

Long-acting insulin analogues are slowly and uniformly absorbed after subcutaneous injection, which avoids plasma insulin peaks.

Unwanted effects

■ Unwanted effects are similar to those of other insulins. Despite the structural modifications, there is no reported excess of immunogenic reactions compared with standard insulin.

■ There is a slightly reduced frequency of hypoglycaemia with rapid-acting insulin analogues compared with soluble insulin because of the shorter duration of action.

THERAPEUTIC REGIMENS FOR INSULIN AND INSULIN ANALOGUES

The choice of regimen for insulin administration depends on the age, lifestyle, circumstances and preference of the individual. The general principle is to maintain a background (basal) level of insulin and then give insulin boluses prior to meals to deal with the glucose load (basal-bolus regimens). Options for regular insulin regimens include the following.

■ **Multiple-injection basal-bolus regimen** is preferred in younger, active people who require flexibility in their lifestyles. Insulin analogues are widely used as first-line treatment. The most common regimen is a long-acting insulin analogue (such as insulin detemir) at breakfast and at bedtime to ensure a 'background' or basal insulin concentration and then a rapid-acting insulin analogue before breakfast, at midday and at the evening meal. If twice-daily basal insulin injections are considered unacceptable, once-daily, long-acting insulin glargine can be used. The dose of both basal and rapid-acting insulin is determined by the fasting blood glucose concentration just before injection.

■ **Twice-daily injections before breakfast and the evening meal** is suitable only for people who have a reasonably stable pattern of activity and eating habits. Short- and intermediate-acting insulins or insulin analogues are given together from the same syringe, either in fixed-ratio biphasic preparations provided by the manufacturer or in varying ratios according to individual requirements.

■ **Single daily injections before breakfast or at bedtime** are used mainly for elderly people with type 2 diabetes mellitus who require insulin and in whom the long-term complications of diabetes are less relevant. An intermediate- or long-acting insulin is used, which can be combined with a short-acting insulin to improve control.

There are also situations in which a subcutaneous insulin regimen is not appropriate:

- **Continuous subcutaneous infusion** of soluble insulin or a rapid-acting insulin analogue via a portable syringe pump and catheter ('insulin-pump therapy') is used if there is a problem with recurrent hypoglycaemia, unpredictable daily lives or hyperglycaemia before breakfast despite optimisation of a multiple-injection insulin regimen. The rate of infusion can be programmed and boluses given before meals.

- **Intravenous infusion** is used for treatment of ketoacidotic crises, in labour, during and after surgery, or at other times when the person's usual routine cannot be adhered to. Soluble insulin or a rapid-acting insulin analogue is infused in 5% glucose solution with added potassium chloride (unless there is hyperkalaemia). A basal dose of subcutaneous long-acting insulin should usually be continued.

- **Intraperitoneal infusion** is used for people being treated for end-stage renal disease by continuous ambulatory peritoneal dialysis; they can add their insulin to the dialysis fluid. Some implantable insulin pumps also use this route. This is the only therapeutic regimen in which insulin has direct access to the portal circulation.

OTHER PARENTERAL GLUCOSE-LOWERING DRUGS

GLUCAGON-LIKE PEPTIDE-1 RECEPTOR AGONISTS

exenatide, liraglutide

Mechanism of action

Exenatide and liraglutide are peptides that share part of their amino acid sequences with the naturally occurring incretin GLP-1. They bind to and activate the GLP-1 receptor, leading to an increase in glucose-dependent synthesis of insulin and its secretion from β-cells (Fig. 40.1). They restore the first-phase insulin response to an oral glucose load and,

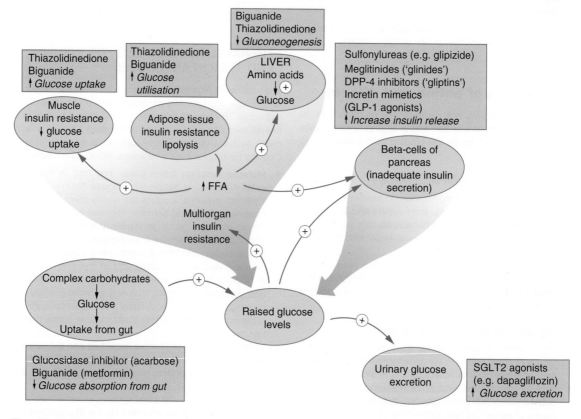

Fig. 40.1 Metabolic dysfunctions in type 2 diabetes and sites of drug action. The metabolic dysfunctions seen in type 2 diabetes result from inadequate insulin secretion from pancreatic β-cells and resistance of skeletal muscle and adipose tissue to the effects of insulin. The metabolic roles of free fatty acids (FFAs) are also indicated. Drugs that enhance insulin release include the sulfonylureas, meglitinides, dipeptidyl peptidase-4 (DPP-4) inhibitors (which inhibit breakdown of incretins) and synthetic incretin mimetics. The thiazolidinedione pioglitazone and the biguanide metformin act in tissues to enhance glucose uptake and utilisation and in the liver to reduce gluconeogenesis. Metformin also reduces glucose absorption from the gut, while inhibitors of sodium-glucose co-transporter 2 (SGLT-2) reduce renal glucose reabsorption and hence increase glucose excretion.

unlike insulin, promote weight loss. In contrast to GLP-1, they are resistant to the enzymatic action of DPP-4.

Pharmacokinetics

Exenatide and liraglutide are given by subcutaneous injection. Exenatide is eliminated by the kidney and has a short half-life of about 2 hours. It is also available as a modified-release formulation to prolong the duration of action. Liraglutide is eliminated by proteolysis and has a half-life of 11–15 hours. Liraglutide and modified-release exenatide are used once daily, within 1 hour of the first meal of the day or the evening meal. The standard formulation of exenatide is used twice daily.

Unwanted effects

- nausea, vomiting, diarrhoea, abdominal pain, decreased appetite with weight loss,
- dizziness, headache, fatigue, agitation,
- injection-site reactions.

ORAL GLUCOSE-LOWERING DRUGS

The main sites of action of oral glucose-lowering drugs are shown in Fig. 40.1.

SULFONYLUREAS

glibenclamide, gliclazide, glimepiride, glipizide, tolbutamide

Mechanism of action

Sulfonylureas act mainly by increasing the release of insulin from the pancreatic β-cells in response to stimulation by glucose (see Fig. 40.1). They bind to the sulfonylurea receptor SUR1, which closes the K_{ATP} channel in the β-cell membrane. The resultant membrane depolarisation opens voltage-gated Ca^{2+} channels and increases both first- and second-phase insulin secretion in response to a rise in plasma glucose. Compounds with a short duration of action are usually preferred to minimise the risk of hypoglycaemia, especially overnight. The long duration of action of glibenclamide carries a greater risk of hypoglycaemia, and it is not recommended for treatment of the elderly.

Pharmacokinetics

Sulfonylureas are structurally related to sulfonamide antimicrobials. They are absorbed rapidly (although the rate of absorption is reduced when taken with food), are highly protein-bound and are metabolised by the liver. Most sulfonylureas have half-lives of less than 10 hours and short durations of action. Glibenclamide has a longer duration of action because of slow dissociation from the SUR1 receptor.

Unwanted effects

- Gastrointestinal disturbance with nausea, vomiting, diarrhoea, constipation.
- Hypoglycaemia (particularly nocturnal) is most frequent with the longer-acting drugs or with excessive dosage, since the drugs continue to work at low plasma glucose concentrations.
- Weight gain is almost inevitable unless dietary restrictions are observed.
- Hypersensitivity reactions (usually in the first 6–8 weeks of therapy) include skin rashes and, rarely, blood disorders.
- Glipizide and glimepiride can increase renal sensitivity to antidiuretic hormone and produce water retention with dilutional hyponatraemia.
- Sulfonylureas (except glipizide) should be avoided in people with acute porphyria.
- Concerns have been raised that sulfonylureas might increase cardiovascular mortality in type 2 diabetes mellitus, possibly as a result of binding to SUR2 receptors in the heart, which could lead to arrhythmias in people who have ischaemic heart disease (see Chapter 5). However, recent clinical studies have failed to confirm the original concerns about cardiovascular mortality.
- There is some evidence that sulfonylureas may accelerate the rate of pancreatic β-cell loss.

MEGLITINIDES

nateglinide, repaglinide

Mechanism of action

Meglitinides (glinides) are based on the sulfonylurea moiety of glibenclamide (called meglitinide). They bind to the SUR1 receptor on the β-cell, although with lower affinity than sulfonylureas, and stimulate insulin release in the same way. Nateglinide, unlike repaglinide, has a greater effect on insulin secretion when plasma glucose levels are rising and therefore produces little stimulation of insulin secretion in the fasting state. These drugs have a rapid onset of action and a short duration of activity and are taken within 30 minutes of main meals.

Pharmacokinetics

Both nateglinide and repaglinide are metabolised in the liver and have short half-lives (1–2 h).

Unwanted effects

- Gastrointestinal upset, including nausea, vomiting, abdominal pain, diarrhoea or constipation with repaglinide.
- Hypoglycaemia is much less frequent than with sulfonylureas due to the short duration of action. This also reduces the desire to snack between meals, so weight gain is less common.
- Hypersensitivity reactions, urticaria.

BIGUANIDE

metformin

Mechanism of action and effects

Metformin does not affect insulin secretion. Its primary target is inhibition of mitochondrial respiratory chain complex 1, which reduces the cellular energy status. This activates the hepatic enzyme 5'-AMP-activated protein kinase (AMPK), a key regulator of the metabolism of fat and glucose, that protects cellular functions under conditions of energy restriction. Activated AMPK phosphorylates key synthetic enzymes and switches cells from an anabolic to a catabolic state by shutting down pathways that consume ATP.

The most important effect of metformin is decreased hepatic glucose production by inhibiting gluconeogenesis, an action that requires the presence of insulin. Since some gluconeogenic activity remains, the risk of hypoglycaemia is minimal. Metformin also increases fatty acid oxidation and reduces plasma triglycerides. A reduction in hepatic steatosis may be important in improving hepatic insulin sensitivity and the reduction in hepatic gluconeogenesis. Metformin has other actions that contribute to its ability to reduce plasma glucose. These include increased cell-surface expression and activity of the membrane insulin receptor and associated tyrosine kinase activity, which facilitates glucose uptake in skeletal muscle and adipocytes as well as increased synthesis of GLP-1.

Metformin can suppress appetite and causes less weight gain than the sulfonylureas, which is useful in overweight people with diabetes mellitus.

Pharmacokinetics

Metformin is excreted unchanged by the kidney and has a half-life of 2–4 hours. A modified-release formulation allows once-daily dosing.

Unwanted effects

- Gastrointestinal upset, including anorexia, nausea, taste disturbance, abdominal discomfort and diarrhoea. These can be minimised by initial use of low doses or a modified-release formulation.
- Decreased vitamin B_{12} absorption.
- Inhibition of pyruvate metabolism encourages lactate accumulation, especially in situations that lead to an increase in anaerobic metabolism, such as tissue hypoxaemia or renal impairment. Metformin should be avoided when the glomerular filtration rate is <30 mL/min per 1.73 m^2.

THIAZOLIDINEDIONE

pioglitazone

Mechanisms of action and effects

Pioglitazone has no effect on insulin secretion but is an insulin sensitiser. The effects are mediated through activation of peroxisome proliferator-activated receptor γ (PPAR-γ) on the cell nucleus. PPAR-γ is activated by specific natural ligands such as free fatty acids and eicosanoids and then associates as a heterodimer with the retinoid X receptor (RXR) in the cell nucleus. The heterodimer activates peroxisome proliferator response elements in the promoter domains of target genes. Pioglitazone replaces the natural ligands and transactivates genes that control adipocyte differentiation; it may increase the number of small adipocytes, which are more insulin-sensitive. It is also responsible for transrepression of several pro-inflammatory genes.

The actions of pioglitazone include:

- Enhanced insulin sensitivity and glucose utilisation in peripheral tissues, especially in adipocytes but also skeletal muscle and hepatocytes. Adipose tissue more readily takes up triglycerides from the blood, and the reduced availability of nonesterified fatty acids improves insulin sensitivity in muscle cells. Pioglitazone also reduces synthesis of pro-inflammatory cytokines that interfere with the insulin signalling cascade, such as interleukin-6, and increases secretion of the insulin-sensitising and antiinflammatory cytokine adiponectin from adipose tissue.
- The effect on plasma triglycerides improves diabetic dyslipidaemia. Plasma high-density lipoprotein (HDL) cholesterol concentration is increased due to increased lipolysis of triglycerides in very-low-density lipoprotein (VLDL).
- A small reduction in blood pressure, possibly by improving endothelial function and reducing sympathetic nervous system activity. Pioglitazone also reduces microalbuminuria associated with diabetic nephropathy.

Pharmacokinetics

Pioglitazone is metabolised in the liver. The half-life is not related to the action of the drug; since the mechanism of action involves gene transcription, the onset of the hypoglycaemic effect is gradual over 6–8 weeks.

Unwanted effects

- Gastrointestinal disturbances.
- Headache, dizziness, visual disturbances.
- Anaemia.
- Hypoglycaemia.
- Fluid retention leading to oedema. Pioglitazone should be avoided in people with heart failure.
- Weight gain because of fat-cell differentiation.
- Increased risk of fractures, especially in women.
- Increased risk of bladder cancer.
- Liver dysfunction has been reported rarely, and liver function tests should be monitored during treatment.

DIPEPTIDYL PEPTIDASE-4 INHIBITORS

linagliptin, sitagliptin, saxagliptin, vildagliptin

Mechanism of action

The 'gliptins' are competitive inhibitors of DPP-4 and reduce the ability of the enzyme to inactivate the incretin hormones GLP-1 and GIP. As a consequence, insulin synthesis and secretion are increased and glucagon secretion reduced.

Pharmacokinetics

Sitagliptin is excreted by the kidney and linagliptin is largely unchanged in faeces. Saxagliptin is cleared mainly by CYP450 metabolism in the liver, whereas vildagliptin undergoes CYP450-independent hydrolysis in the liver and kidney. The long duration of action of DPP-4 inhibitors is unrelated to the plasma half-life due to prolonged binding to the target enzyme.

Unwanted effects

- nausea, vomiting, dyspepsia,
- oedema,
- headache, dizziness, fatigue, nasopharyngitis.

GLUCOSIDASE INHIBITOR

 xample

acarbose

Mechanism of action and effects

Carbohydrate digestion in the intestine involves several enzymes that sequentially degrade complex polysaccharides, such as starch into monosaccharides like glucose. Initial digestion of carbohydrates in the gut lumen is carried out by amylases from the saliva and pancreas. The final digestion of oligosaccharides is carried out by β-galactosidases (including lactase) and various α-glucosidase enzymes (such as maltase, isomaltase, glucoamylase and sucrase, which hydrolyse oligosaccharides) in the small-intestinal brush border. Acarbose competes with dietary oligosaccharides for α-glucosidase enzymes and has a higher affinity for the enzymes. Binding to the enzymes is reversible, so that digestion and absorption of glucose after a meal is slower than usual but not prevented. As a result, the postprandial peak of blood glucose is reduced and blood glucose concentrations are more stable through the day. Acarbose has no effect on insulin secretion or its tissue action and is less effective for achieving glycaemic control than other oral hypoglycaemic agents.

Pharmacokinetics

Oral absorption of acarbose is very low, with only about 2% of the active parent drug reaching the circulation. Inactive metabolites are formed in the gut lumen by enzymic degradation.

Unwanted effects

Gastrointestinal effects include flatulence, abdominal distension and diarrhoea due to fermentation of unabsorbed carbohydrate in the bowel. These effects are dose-related and often transient.

SODIUM-GLUCOSE CO-TRANSPORTER 2 INHIBITORS

 xamples

canagliflozin, dapagliflozin

Mechanism of action

The dapagliflozin and canagliflozin are competitive reversible inhibitors of the sodium-glucose co-transporter type 2 (SGLT-2) in the proximal convoluted tubule of the kidney. Gliflozins reduce glucose absorption from the tubular filtrate and increase urinary glucose excretion. They do not block SGLT-1, so glucose absorption from the gut is not affected. Gliflozins produce modest weight loss and hypoglycaemia is unusual.

Pharmacokinetics

Dapagliflozin and canagliflozin are metabolised in the liver. They have half-lives of 13 hours.

Unwanted effects

- Constipation.
- Increased risk of urinary tract and genital infections.
- Thirst and polyuria with increased risk of hypovolaemia and electrolyte imbalance.
- Increased risk of diabetic ketoacidosis in type 2 diabetes mellitus.

DRUGS TO INCREASE PLASMA GLUCOSE LEVELS

GLUCAGON

Mechanism of action and use

Glucagon is a polypeptide synthesised by the α-cells of the pancreatic islets of Langerhans. It binds to specific hepatocyte receptors and activates membrane-bound adenylyl cyclase. The consequent increase in intracellular cyclic adenosine monophosphate (cAMP) leads to inhibition of glycogen synthase. This blocks the effect of insulin on hepatocytes and mobilises stored liver glycogen. Glucagon is used to raise blood glucose in severe insulin-induced hypoglycaemia.

Pharmacokinetics

Glucagon must be given by intramuscular, subcutaneous or intravenous injection and acts within 10–20 minutes. It is degraded rapidly by enzymes in the plasma, liver and kidney.

Unwanted effects

These are not usually troublesome with a single injection but include nausea, vomiting and diarrhoea.

MANAGEMENT OF TYPE 1 DIABETES MELLITUS

Insulin is essential for treatment of type 1 diabetes mellitus and the aim of treatment is to maintain a plasma glucose concentration as close to normal as possible. Hyperglycaemia leads to the glycosylation of proteins which inhibits their function and may promote vascular and neurological damage. In older people with type 1 diabetes, management of cardiovascular risk factors (see type 2 diabetes, below) becomes increasingly important. Advice should be given regarding an appropriate diet with a regulated carbohydrate intake distributed throughout the day ('carbohydrate counting'). Excess dietary saturated fat should be avoided.

The complications of type 1 diabetes mellitus can be reduced by close control of the blood glucose concentration ideally by giving insulin analogues (or insulin) in a basal-bolus regimen (see earlier). Regular measurement of the blood glucose concentration should be carried out on a finger-prick blood specimen using a blood glucose reagent strip. The insulin dose should be adjusted to maintain fasting plasma glucose between 5 and 7 mmol/L before breakfast, 4–7 mmol/L before meals at other times of the day and 5–9 mmol/L at least 90 minutes after eating. Long-term control of diabetes mellitus is usually assessed by the plasma concentration of glycosylated haemoglobin (HbA_{1c}). An HbA_{1c} concentration greater than 53 mmol/mol (the upper limit of normal is 42 mmol/mol) is associated with a higher risk of developing microvascular and neuropathic complications. The target should be 48 mmol/mol.

The most dramatic complication of untreated or poorly controlled type 1 diabetes mellitus is diabetic ketoacidosis (Fig. 40.2), which can lead to coma and death if it is severe. This may be the presenting problem with new-onset diabetes, while systemic infection, dietary indiscretion or inappropriate insulin dose reduction or omission can precipitate ketoacidosis in a person with treated type 1 diabetes mellitus. Apart from the treatment of any precipitating cause, the management of ketoacidosis includes:

- Restoration of extracellular volume: hyperglycaemia leads to an osmotic diuresis with excessive urinary salt and water loss. Replacement by isotonic (0.9%) saline is essential.
- Potassium replacement: the osmotic diuresis results in excessive urinary potassium loss. Potassium is also shifted from within cells into extracellular fluid in exchange for hydrogen ions in the ketoacidotic state. Correction of the extracellular acidosis reverses this shift and can produce profound hypokalaemia. Once a good urine flow has been established, intravenous potassium supplements are usually required.
- Intravenous insulin until the ketosis is abolished and the plasma glucose is below 15 mmol/L. An intermediate-acting insulin should be continued subcutaneously during the infusion to maintain a basal blood insulin concentration.
- The metabolic acidosis will usually correct with treatment of the hyperglycaemia and fluid replacement. Intravenous sodium bicarbonate is occasionally required if the arterial pH is less than 7.0, but it should be used with caution.

MANAGEMENT OF TYPE 1 DIABETES IN SPECIAL SITUATIONS

- Close attention to the control of diabetes mellitus is important before conception and during pregnancy because poor control will affect the fetus, leading to increased intra-uterine and perinatal mortality.
- At times of intercurrent illness, the dose of insulin will need to be increased, guided by blood glucose monitoring, to counteract the hyperglycaemic action of hormones released during stress reactions.

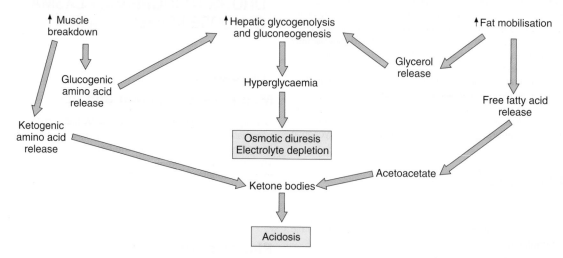

Fig. 40.2 **Pathophysiology of diabetic ketoacidosis.** Diabetic ketoacidosis is an emergency arising from the lack of insulin in type 1 diabetes mellitus. Breakdown of muscle proteins and accelerated fat metabolism produce hyperglycaemia, leading to osmotic diuresis and depletion of K^+ ions. Ketone bodies (acetoacetate and β-hydroxybutyric acid) generated from fatty acids and amino acids cause severe acidosis.

- During and immediately after surgery, soluble insulin should be given in 10% glucose solution by intravenous infusion, dosage being guided by the blood glucose concentrations. Subcutaneous insulin can be restarted as soon as the person is able to eat and drink.

MANAGEMENT OF TYPE 2 DIABETES MELLITUS

The mainstays of treatment are lifestyle and dietary modifications. As for type 1 diabetes mellitus, close control of the blood glucose concentration in type 2 diabetes mellitus reduces the risk of microvascular complications, although the effect on macrovascular complications such as myocardial infarction is less convincing. The target HbA_{1c} concentration is ≤48 mmol/mol, or ≤53 mmol/mol if more than one drug is prescribed to reduce the risk of hypoglycaemia.

More than 75% of people with newly diagnosed type 2 diabetes are obese. Weight reduction not only improves blood glucose levels but also reduces other cardiovascular disease risk factors. Dietary advice should include:

- Reducing energy intake if obese, with a target weight loss of 5–10% (an average weight loss of 18 kg is required to control blood glucose).
- Eating small, regular meals.
- Ensuring that more than half the total energy intake is from carbohydrates with controlled intake of saturated and trans fatty acids.
- Encouraging high-fibre, low-glycaemic-index sources of carbohydrate and also limiting sucrose and alcohol intake. Advice should also be given about regular exercise and stopping smoking to reduce vascular risk as appropriate.

If dietary management is insufficient, metformin is the treatment of choice, especially for overweight people, as it reduces appetite and can encourage weight loss. Metformin also reduces cardiovascular mortality, which has not been demonstrated for any other treatment in type 2 diabetes mellitus. If the target HbA_{1c} is not achieved after 3 months of treatment with metformin, a second drug should be added. The choice is guided by an assessment of the patient, disease and patient preference. Options include:

- metformin with pioglitazone (weight gain but low risk of hypoglycaemia),
- metformin with a DPP-4 inhibitor, such as sitagliptin (little effect on weight and low risk of hypoglycaemia),
- metformin with a sulfonylurea, such as glipizide (weight gain and moderate risk of hypoglycaemia).

Triple therapy may be necessary, with combinations of metformin and two additional drugs with a different mechanism of action. Recommended combinations include:

- metformin, DPP-4 inhibitor and a sulfonylurea,
- metformin, pioglitazone and a sulfonylurea.

If triple therapy with metformin and two other drugs is not effective, not tolerated or contraindicated, then metformin combined with a sulfonylurea and a GLP-1 receptor agonist should be considered. A GLP-1 receptor agonist should be continued only if there is a reduction in HbA1c of at least 11 mmol/mol and a loss of 3% of initial body weight after 6 months. Other drug combinations, such as those involving

SGLT-2 inhibitors, should usually be started only on the advice of a specialist. As an alternative to triple therapy, insulin can be considered either alone or in combination with an oral hypoglycaemic drug.

If standard-release metformin is poorly tolerated, then a modified-release formulation can be tried. As an alternative to metformin, obese people can be treated with pioglitazone or a DPP-4 inhibitor. People with type 2 diabetes mellitus who are not overweight often require early treatment with a sulfonylurea or repaglinide. Acarbose is of limited value when used alone or in combination with metformin. It may be most effective in early diabetes mellitus, when there is still sufficient insulin secretion for it to influence glycaemic control.

Within 3 years of diagnosis, 50% of people with type 2 diabetes mellitus will need combination therapy to achieve glycaemic control. Failure of oral treatment usually implies β-cell 'exhaustion', and up to 30% of those with type 2 diabetes mellitus require insulin. Insulin analogues are preferred to human insulin. A long-acting insulin analogue can be used as basal-only therapy with oral glucose-lowering drugs. Alternatively, a mixture of long-acting and rapid-acting insulin analogues given twice daily, possibly with additional rapid-acting insulin analogue before the midday meal, may be preferred, especially if the HbA1c is greater than 75 mmol/mol. There is some evidence that insulin therapy used early in type 2 diabetes mellitus may preserve β-cell function.

Intensive management of risk factors for cardiovascular disease is of crucial importance because the major complications of type 2 diabetes mellitus are vascular. In particular, control of raised blood pressure reduces both microvascular and macrovascular complications. The target blood pressure is less than 140/80 mm Hg or 130/80 mm Hg if there is kidney, eye or cerebrovascular damage. First-line therapy is with an angiotensin-converting enzyme (ACE) inhibitor or an angiotensin II receptor antagonist, which reduce the progression of diabetic nephropathy (see Chapter 6). In people of Afro-Caribbean origin, this should be combined with a diuretic or a calcium channel blocker. There is little to choose between other antihypertensive drugs for use in diabetes mellitus except that thiazides and β-adrenoceptor antagonists may cause hyperglycaemia and should probably be avoided in the few people who are managed with dietary control alone.

An atherogenic plasma lipid profile is common in type 2 diabetes mellitus, and statin therapy is recommended for people over the age of 40 years (see Chapter 48). Once a person with diabetes has developed coronary artery disease, management of all risk factors (see Chapter 48) will reduce the risk of subsequent myocardial infarction or death to the same extent as for someone without diabetes mellitus.

SELF-ASSESSMENT

True/false questions

1. Oral hypoglycaemic drugs are only used in type 2 diabetes mellitus.
2. Glipizide is the drug of choice when there is no residual insulin secretion.
3. Sulfonylureas should be administered in conjunction with a dietary regimen in obese people.

4. Glibenclamide can cause hypoglycaemia, particularly in the elderly.
5. Metformin and the sulfonylurea gliclazide cannot be taken together.
6. The meglitinides are structurally related to glibenclamide.
7. Oral hypoglycaemics given to a pregnant mother can cause hypoglycaemia in the fetus.
8. Sulfonylureas should not be given together with the antibacterial trimethoprim.
9. Insulin lispro has a longer duration of action than isophane insulin.
10. DPP-4 synthesises incretin hormones.
11. Synthetic incretin mimetics are given orally.
12. Acarbose is completely absorbed from the gut after oral administration.
13. Gliflozin drugs block absorption of glucose in the gut and in the renal tubule.
14. Glucagon mobilises glucose from glycogen in the liver.

One-best-answer (OBA) question

Ms. J.J. is a 55-year-old housewife with a body mass index (BMI) of 35 kg/m^2. She was diagnosed with type 2 diabetes mellitus. Choose the *correct* statement below.
A. The mainstay of treatment is diet and exercise.
B. Diabetes presenting in this way is a medical emergency.
C. A sulfonylurea would be the drug of first choice.
D. Pioglitazone would be the drug of first choice.
E. Treatment with metformin may increase her risk of heart disease.

Case-based questions

A 25-year-old teacher, Mr. J.A.H., was admitted to hospital as an emergency. He had developed a sore throat a week previously. His general practitioner (GP) prescribed penicillin, but the soreness persisted and Mr. J.A.H. noticed profuse white spots at the back of his throat. He drank fluids copiously and passed more urine than usual. Two days before admission, he began to vomit, and on the day before admission he became drowsy and confused. He had lost approximately 12 kg in weight despite eating more than usual. His great uncle had diabetes mellitus. Mr. J.A.H. was clinically dehydrated and ketones could be smelt on his breath. Results of blood tests indicated that he had diabetic ketoacidosis.
1. Which type of diabetes mellitus does Mr. J.A.H. have?
2. What was the significance of his sore throat?
3. Was it significant that his great uncle suffered from diabetes mellitus?
4. Explain his polyuria and polydipsia.
5. What treatments should have been instituted rapidly?
6. After he recovered from the acute illness, what general advice should he have been given about his diet?
7. Mr. J.A.H. was a 'three-meals-a-day' man whose only exercise was walking a mile to work and back each day. Although insulin regimens vary widely, suggest a possible regimen and the types of insulin that could be given.
8. How long before meals should subcutaneous injection of soluble insulin have been given?
9. In addition to blood glucose levels, what other indicator could have been measured to signify good control in diabetes mellitus?

Mr. J.A.H. became more active, joined a health club and met a partner who liked to party. His eating became more irregular, with hurried meals. His glycaemic control deteriorated.
10. What alterations to his insulin regimen could have been helpful?

ANSWERS

True/false answers

1. **True.** Oral hypoglycaemic drugs (sulfonylureas, biguanides, meglitinides, thiazolidinediones, dipeptidyl peptidase-4 inhibitors) are used only in type 2 diabetes mellitus and act by different mechanisms to control glucose levels.
2. **False.** Glipizide is a sulfonylureas that stimulates insulin secretion from the islet β-cells and would be ineffective in the absence of any insulin-secreting ability.
3. **True.** Sulfonylureas cause weight gain partly by stimulating appetite; metformin might be a better choice.
4. **True.** Glibenclamide has a long duration of action and active metabolites can accumulate when renal function declines; hypoglycaemia is a greater problem in the elderly.
5. **False.** These drugs act in part by different mechanisms and can be combined. Unlike the sulfonylureas, metformin has a neutral or suppressive effect on appetite.
6. **True.** Meglitinides (glinides) chemically resemble the sulfonylurea moiety of glibenclamide and act by a similar mechanism to enhance insulin release.
7. **True.** Neonates born to mothers with diabetes mellitus who are taking oral hypoglycaemics in pregnancy have problems with hypoglycaemia; insulin is normally substituted in pregnancy.
8. **True.** Sulphonylureas have some structural similarities to the sulfonamides, and trimethoprim and can produce severe hypoglycaemia when given together with sulfonylureas.
9. **False.** Isophane insulin is complexed with protamine and has a duration of action of 18 h, whereas synthetic insulin lispro is modified structurally and has a faster onset of action and shorter duration (2–5 hours).
10. **False.** DPP-4 breaks down the incretin GLP-1, so DPP-4 inhibitors such as sitagliptin enhance incretin activity on the pancreatic islet β-cells.
11. **False.** Incretin mimetics are peptides and can be administered only parenterally; the incretin mimetics are given subcutaneously with insulin or with oral hypoglycaemic drugs.
12. **True.** Acarbose is very poorly absorbed and acts within the gut to reduce the digestion of glucose by α-glucosidases.
13. **False.** Inhibitors of SGLT-2, such as canagliflozin and dapagliflozin, reduce the reabsorption of glucose in the proximal renal tubule and increase its excretion in urine but do not reduce glucose absorption in the gut, which is mediated by SGLT-1.
14. **True.** Glucagon reverses the effect of insulin on liver glycogen storage and is used to increase blood glucose in severe acute hypoglycaemia induced by insulin.

One-best-answer (OBA) answer

Answer A is correct.
A. **Correct.** Diet and exercise should be tried for 3 months before suggesting other treatments.
B. Incorrect. Treatment, support and advice should take place over many months.
C. Incorrect. Sulfonylureas can stimulate appetite by increasing insulin secretion and cause further weight gain.
D. Incorrect. The use of pioglitazone as second-line therapy added to either metformin or a sulfonylurea is not recommended except for people who are unable to tolerate metformin and sulfonylurea combination therapy or those in whom either drug is contraindicated; in such cases, the thiazolidinedione should replace the poorly tolerated or contraindicated drug.
E. Incorrect. Metformin has a cardioprotective effect which is not wholly explicable by its effects on glucose and may be due to improvements in the lipid profile.

Case-based answers

1. The ketoacidosis indicates that Mr. J.A.H. has type 1 diabetes mellitus.
2. An upper respiratory tract infection can be all that is necessary to precipitate ketoacidosis. Aggravating factors include the candidiasis in his throat and over-breathing, causing dryness.
3. There is a strong familial tendency, but neither type 1 nor type 2 diabetes mellitus is a single-gene disorder, so there is no classic pattern of inheritance.
4. Once the tubular transport maximum for glucose reabsorption in the kidneys is exceeded, the glucose in the distal tubules causes an osmotic diuresis, leading to polyuria and then to thirst.
5. Insulin, fluids and salts should be given to correct dehydration, glucose levels, ketoacidosis and electrolyte imbalances. Ketoacidosis can lead to coma.
6. A dietary regimen should be agreed to create a stable pattern of eating habits commensurate with his lifestyle. Diets low in animal fat and high in fibre are recommended, ideally with carbohydrate intake distributed throughout the day.
7. Initiate a stable pattern of eating habit and activity and twice-daily subcutaneous insulin injections before breakfast and the evening meal. The insulin regimen would contain a mixture of short- and long-acting insulins, the ratios of which vary depending upon Mr. J.A.H.'s glucose levels. Insulin analogues are frequently used.
8. The time to onset of activity of soluble insulin is 30 minutes, with peak activity at 1–3 hours.
9. The amount of glycosylated haemoglobin (HbA_{1c}) can be measured. High concentrations indicate an increased risk of microvascular and neuropathic complications.
10. Rapid-acting insulin analogues such as insulin lispro may be helpful. These have an onset of action of only 15 minutes and peak activity is reached at 0.5–1 hours, so they should be given immediately before a meal. Insulin lispro during the day with insulin isophane in the evening is a possible regimen, but education about eating and lifestyle would probably provide greater benefit than a change of insulin regimen.

FURTHER READING

Atkinson, M.A., Eisenbarth, G.S., Michels, A.W., 2014. Type 1 diabetes. Lancet 383, 69–82.

Bailey, C.J., 2011. The challenge of managing coexistent type 2 diabetes and obesity. Br. Med. J. 342, d1996.

Beigi, F.I., 2012. Glycemic management of type 2 diabetes mellitus. N. Engl. J. Med. 366, 1319–1327.

Chamberlain, J.J., Rhinehart, A.S., Shaefer, C.F., et al., 2016. Diagnosis and management of diabetes: synopsis of the 2016 American Diabetes Association standards of medical care in diabetes. Ann. Intern. Med. 164, 542–552.

Fu, Z., Gilbert, E.R., Lou, D., 2013. Regulation of insulin synthesis and secretion and pancreatic beta-cell dysfunction in diabetes. Curr. Diabetes Rev. 9, 25–53.

Gale, E.A.M., 2012. Newer insulins in type 2 diabetes. Br. Med. J. 345, e4611.

Holman, R.R., Sourij, H., Califf, R.M., 2014. Cardiovascular outcome trials of glucose-lowering drugs or strategies in type 2 diabetes. Lancet 383, 2008–2017.

Ley, S.H., Hamdy, O., Mohan, V., et al., 2014. Prevention and management of type 2 diabetes: dietary components and nutritional strategies. Lancet 383, 1999–2007.

Moghissi, E., King, A.B., 2014. Individualising insulin therapy in the management of type 2 diabetes. Am. J. Med. 127, S3–S10.

Pickup, J.C., 2012. Insulin-pump therapy for type 1 diabetes mellitus. N. Engl. J. Med. 366, 1616–1624.

Sorti, C., 2014. New developments in insulin therapy for type 2 diabetes. Am. J. Med. 127, S39–S48.

Compendium: drugs used in diabetes mellitus and in hypoglycaemia

Drug	Characteristics
Insulins	
Insulins are normally given subcutaneously, with the onset and duration of action depending on the formulation used (see Table 40.4). Many formulations are combinations containing bovine, porcine or human insulin. Short-acting insulins include soluble insulin and rapid-acting insulin analogues. Insulin complexes (such as isophane insulin) are intermediate-acting. Long-acting insulins include analogues formulated to be slowly absorbed from the subcutaneous injection site. Biphasic insulins combine short-acting and longer-acting insulins or insulin analogues to avoid multiple injections.	
Rapid- and short-acting insulins	
Insulin (neutral or soluble)	Short-acting bovine, porcine or human insulin; may also be given by intramuscular or intravenous injection or by intravenous infusion, depending on requirements

Compendium: drugs used in diabetes mellitus and in hypoglycaemia (cont'd)

Drug	Characteristics
Insulin aspart	Rapid-onset recombinant human insulin analogue; may also be given by intravenous injection or infusion, depending on requirements
Insulin glulisine	Rapid-onset recombinant human insulin analogue
Insulin lispro	Rapid-onset recombinant human insulin analogue; may also be given by intravenous injection or infusion, depending on requirements
Long-acting insulins	
Insulin detemir	Long-acting recombinant human insulin analogue
Insulin degludec	Ultra-long-acting (>40 h) human insulin analogue; less risk of nocturnal hypoglycaemia than with insulin glargine
Insulin glargine	Long-acting recombinant human insulin analogue
Insulin complexes	
Isophane insulin	Natural insulin complexed with protamine. Intermediate-acting
Insulin zinc suspension	Long-acting. Rarely used
Protamine-zinc insulin	Long-acting. Rarely used
Glucagon-like peptide-1 (GLP-1) agonists	
Synthetic peptide mimetics of the incretin GLP-1 that increase insulin release. Given by subcutaneous injection for type 2 diabetes.	
Albiglutide	Used either alone (if metformin is inappropriate) or in combination with other antidiabetic drugs if adequate glycaemic control has not been achieved with those drugs. Half-life: 5 days
Dulaglutide	Uses similar to albiglutide. Half-life: 4–5 days
Exenatide	Used with metformin, a sulfonylurea or both, or with pioglitazone, or with both metformin and pioglitazone. Half-life: 2.4 h
Liraglutide	Used with metformin or a sulfonylurea or both, or with pioglitazone, or with both metformin and pioglitazone. Half-life: 11–15 h
Lixisenatide	Used in combination with oral antidiabetic drugs (e.g. metformin, pioglitazone or a sulfonylurea) or basal insulin if adequate glycaemic control has not been achieved with those drugs. Half-life: 3 h
Sulfonylureas	
Sulfonylureas bind to the SUR1 receptor on pancreatic β-cells and increase insulin release. All are given orally for the treatment of type 2 diabetes.	
Glibenclamide (glyburide in the United States)	Long-acting sulfonylurea. Used for people who are not overweight or in whom metformin is contraindicated or not tolerated. Half-life: 10 h
Gliclazide	Used for people who are not overweight or in whom metformin is contraindicated or not tolerated. Half-life: 6–14 h
Glimepiride	Used for people who are not overweight or in whom metformin is contraindicated or not tolerated. Half-life: 5–9 h
Glipizide	Used for people who are not overweight or in whom metformin is contraindicated or not tolerated. Half-life: 2–4 h
Tolbutamide	Used for people who are not overweight or in whom metformin is contraindicated or not tolerated. Half-life: 4–6 h
Meglitinides ('glinides')	
Increase insulin release by similar mechanism to sulphonylureas. Given orally for the treatment of type 2 diabetes mellitus.	
Nateglinide	Used in combination with metformin when metformin alone is inadequate. Half-life: 1.5 h
Repaglinide	Used alone or in combination with metformin when metformin alone is inadequate. Half-life: 1 h

Compendium: drugs used in diabetes mellitus and in hypoglycaemia (cont'd)

Drug	Characteristics
Biguanide	
AMP kinase inhibitor; decreases hepatic glucose production, increases fatty acid oxidation and enhances glucose utilisation.	
Metformin	First-line treatment for type 2 diabetes mellitus; also available in combined formulations with pioglitazone, sitagliptin or vildagliptin. Given orally. Half-life: 2–4 h
Thiazolidinedione (glitazone)	
PPAR activator and insulin sensitiser.	
Pioglitazone	Used alone or in combination with metformin or a sulfonylurea or both for the treatment of type 2 diabetes mellitus. Given orally. Half-life 3–7 h
DPP-4 inhibitors (gliptins)	
Inhibitors of dipeptidyl peptidase-4 reduce breakdown of the incretins GLP-1 and GIP and enhance insulin release. Given orally in type 2 diabetes.	
Alogliptin	Used in combination with metformin, pioglitazone, a sulfonylurea or insulin or in combination with metformin and either pioglitazone or insulin. Half-life: 21 h
Linagliptin	Used if metformin is inappropriate or with metformin or with metformin and a sulfonylurea. Half-life: 12 h
Saxagliptin	Used with metformin or a sulfonylurea (if metformin inappropriate) or with pioglitazone. Half-life: 2.5–3 h
Sitagliptin	Used as monotherapy (if metformin inappropriate) or with metformin or a sulfonylurea or with metformin and pioglitazone. Half-life: 12 h
Vildagliptin	Uses similar to saxagliptin. Half-life: 3 h
Sodium-glucose co-transporter-2 (SGLT-2) inhibitors (gliflozins)	
SGLT-2 inhibitors increase glucose excretion by reducing its reabsorption in the renal proximal convoluted tubule. All are given orally in type 2 diabetes.	
Canagliflozin	Used alone or in combination with insulin or other antidiabetic drugs. Half-life: 10–13 h
Dapagliflozin	Used alone or in combination with insulin or other antidiabetic drugs. Not recommended in combination with pioglitazone. Half-life: 13 h
Empagliflozin	Used alone or in combination with insulin or other antidiabetic drugs. Half-life: 12 h
Glucosidase inhibitor	
Inhibition of α-glucosidase delays absorption of glucose from the gut.	
Acarbose	Given orally for diabetes mellitus inadequately controlled by diet with or without other hypoglycaemic drugs
Drug for treatment of hypoglycaemia	
Glucagon	Used for acute insulin-induced hypoglycaemia (*not* for chronic hypoglycaemia). Given by subcutaneous, intramuscular or intravenous injection. Half-life: 5–10 min

DPP-4, dipeptidyl peptidase-4; *GIP*, glucose-dependent insulinotropic peptide; *GLP-1*, glucagon-like peptide; *PPAR*, peroxisome proliferator-associated receptor; *SGLT-2*, sodium-glucose co-transporter 2.

41

The thyroid and control of metabolic rate

THYROID FUNCTION

The main functions of thyroid hormones are the control of metabolism, growth and development. The term 'basal metabolism' refers to the energy-utilising biochemical processes of the body at rest. Basal metabolic rate is controlled by thyroid hormones, acting together with other hormones such as insulin. Thyroid hormones have multiple actions:

- Stimulation of tissue oxygen consumption and regulation of energy and heat production, mainly through an increase in the metabolism of fats, carbohydrates and proteins.
- Thermogenic action on brown fat in infants, increasing synthesis of uncoupling proteins that divert the energy released during lipolysis into heat rather than high-energy phosphate synthesis.
- Promotion of gluconeogenesis, forming glucose from amino acids in tissues such as muscle and bone.
- Facilitating the development of the nervous system, somatic growth (synergistically with growth hormone) and puberty.
- Regulation of the synthesis of proteins involved in hepatic, cardiac, neurological and muscular functions.
- Enhancing tissue sensitivity to circulating catecholamines and sympathetic nervous system activation, in particular the effects of β-adrenoceptor stimulation.

THYROID HORMONES

There are two thyroid hormones, triiodothyronine (T_3) and thyroxine (T_4), both of which are synthesised in the thyroid gland (Fig. 41.1). T_3 is the main active hormone, while T_4 is considered to be a prohormone. Both hormones are partially composed of iodine. The thyroid gland actively traps inorganic iodide, which is then oxidised to iodine by thyroid peroxidase. Iodine is very reactive and attaches to tyrosyl residues of the glycoprotein thyroglobulin to form mono-iodotyrosine and di-iodotyrosine residues. When two adjacent di-iodinated tyrosine molecules are conjugated, this forms T_4, and one di-iodinated molecule with one mono-iodinated tyrosine molecule conjugate to form T_3 (see Fig. 41.1). Proteolytic enzymes from thyroid lysosomes then degrade thyroglobulin, and T_3 and T_4 are released into the circulation.

The synthesis and release of thyroid hormones are controlled by the anterior pituitary hormone thyrotropin (thyroid-stimulating hormone [TSH]). This in turn is controlled by the hypothalamus, which secretes thyrotropin-releasing hormone (TRH). Circulating T_3 and T_4 exert negative feedback on both TSH and TRH (Fig. 41.2).

The thyroid releases mainly T_4 and a small amount of T_3. Circulating thyroid hormones are highly protein-bound, mostly to thyroxine-binding globulin (TBG). Less than 0.03% of T_4 and less than 0.3% of T_3 circulate unbound and only this free fraction of hormone is available to enter cells and bind to specific intracellular receptors. Most T_3 is derived from peripheral deiodination of T_4 by tetraiodothyronine 5′ deiodinase, which is found in the liver, kidney, brain and brown adipose tissue. About 35% of T_4 is converted to T_3, while about 40% is converted to reverse T_3 (a metabolically inactive isomer of T_3). T_3 has a half-life in the circulation of about 1.5 days, compared with about 7 days for T_4. Elimination of T_3 and T_4 is by conjugation, mainly in the liver.

Thyroid hormones cross cell membranes via active transporters and bind to intracellular thyroid hormone receptors (TRs; see Chapter 1), which belong to the superfamily of nuclear receptors. Thyroid hormone receptors usually block gene transcription by forming a complex with corepressor molecules that binds to thyroid response elements close to genes. When thyroid hormone binds to the receptor it displaces the corepressor from the receptor/ DNA complex. The complex then recruits co-activators and activates gene transcription. Thyroid hormone receptors are expressed in most tissues, but there are three isoforms which differ in their tissue distribution and mediate different effects of thyroid hormones. T_3 also has nongenomic actions that

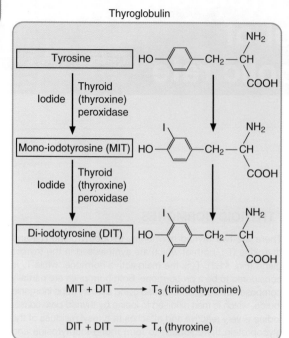

Thyroglobulin

MIT + DIT $\longrightarrow$ T$_3$ (triiodothyronine)

DIT + DIT $\longrightarrow$ T$_4$ (thyroxine)

Release of T$_4$ and T$_3$
from thyroglobulin by proteolysis

Fig. 41.1 The synthesis of thyroid hormones. Iodide is oxidised to iodine by thyroid peroxidase and incorporated into tyrosine residues of thyroglobulin, the colloidal substance that fills the lumen of the thyroid follicles. Conjugation of mono-iodotyrosine (MIT) and di-iodotyrosine (DIT) residues into T$_3$, or of two DIT residues to form T$_4$, is followed by the release of T$_3$ and T$_4$ when thyroglobulin is proteolysed.

include stimulation of cellular uptake of amino acids and glucose, and interactions with G-protein-coupled membrane receptors with activation of phosphatidylinositol 3-kinase and mitogen-activated protein kinase (MAPK) pathways.

HYPERTHYROIDISM

The commonest form of hyperthyroidism is Graves' disease, an autoimmune condition in which TSH receptor antibodies bind to thyroid cells and initiate signal transduction with increased production of thyroid hormone. This is often accompanied by an immunologically mediated inflammatory reaction in the extraocular muscles in the orbit, causing swelling and the characteristic exophthalmos. Toxic multinodular goitre, thyroid adenomas (toxic or 'hot' nodules) and various forms of thyroiditis are less common causes of hyperthyroidism. Rarely, hyperthyroidism arises from excess production of thyrotropin, or it can be induced by treatment with amiodarone (see Chapter 8).

The syndrome that arises from hyperthyroidism is called thyrotoxicosis. Symptoms include weight loss, palpitation, sweating, fatigue, nervousness, heat sensitivity and tremor. These are in part mediated by the action of excess thyroid hormone, and partly by excess sensitivity of tissues to β-adrenoceptor stimulation. Signs are often less marked in the elderly, who are more likely to present with atrial fibrillation that is resistant to treatment.

DRUGS FOR TREATMENT OF HYPERTHYROIDISM

Thionamides

Examples

carbimazole, propylthiouracil

Mechanism of action

Thionamides reduce the synthesis of thyroid hormone by inhibiting thyroid peroxidase (see Figs 41.1 and 41.2). The long half-life of T$_4$ means that changes in the rate of synthesis take 4–6 weeks to lower circulating T$_4$ and T$_3$ concentrations to within the normal range. Thionamides also reduce the levels of TSH receptor antibody in Graves' disease. Large doses of propylthiouracil inhibit tetraiodothyronine 5′ deiodinase and decrease peripheral conversion of T$_4$ to T$_3$.

Pharmacokinetics

Carbimazole is a prodrug that is converted to active methimazole (thiamazole). Propylthiouracil has about one-tenth of the activity of methimazole and a shorter half-life; it is usually reserved for individuals intolerant to carbimazole. Both drugs accumulate in the thyroid, which extends their duration of action beyond that expected from their short plasma half-lives.

Unwanted effects

- Gastrointestinal upset (especially nausea and epigastric discomfort), headache, arthralgia and pruritic rashes are common in the first 8 weeks of treatment.
- Allergic reactions, including vasculitis, a lupus-like syndrome, myopathy, cholestatic jaundice and nephritis. There is some cross-sensitivity between carbimazole and propylthiouracil.
- Bone marrow suppression, especially agranulocytosis, is an important unwanted effect and is more common with propylthiouracil than with carbimazole. A severe sore throat with fever is often the presenting complaint, and the occurrence of this, or any other infection, should

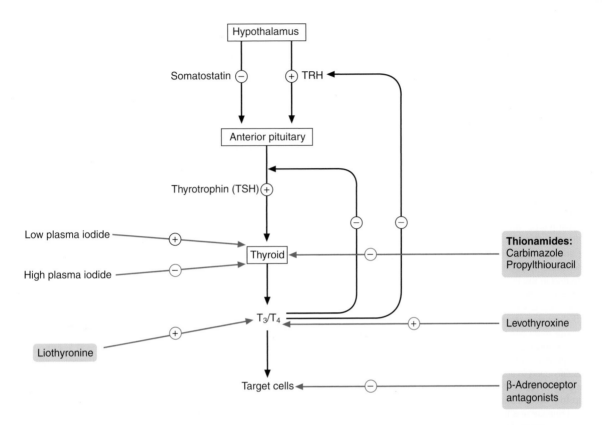

Fig. 41.2 Control of thyroid hormone synthesis and release. Thyrotropin (thyroid-stimulating hormone [TSH]) and thyrotropin-releasing hormone (TRH) are inhibited by circulating levels of T_3 and T_4. The sites of action of drugs acting on thyroid pathways are also shown.

be immediately reported to a doctor. The onset of agranulocytosis is sudden, and probably immunologically mediated, so that routine blood counts are unhelpful for monitoring. The blood count usually recovers about 3 weeks after drug withdrawal.

■ Carbimazole given to women who are pregnant has been associated with congenital defects, but not propylthiouracil. Carbimazole is secreted in breast milk but rarely produces hypothyroidism in the suckling infant.

MANAGEMENT OF HYPERTHYROIDISM

Graves' disease

Carbimazole is the drug of choice for Graves' hyperthyroidism, and will usually decrease the thyroid hormone concentration to normal levels over 4–8 weeks. Treatment is started with a high dose unless the thyrotoxicosis is mild, when smaller initial doses may control symptoms. Once the thyroid hormone concentration is normal, the dose is then gradually reduced every 4–6 weeks to reach the lowest possible dose that controls the serum free T_4. Treatment should be continued for 12–18 months. An alternative strategy is a 'block–replace' regimen, which involves giving a high dose of carbimazole and then adding levothyroxine replacement after 4 weeks. The dose of carbimazole is kept constant and the levothyroxine dose adjusted to maintain a normal serum free T_4 concentration.

The 'block–replace' regimen is given for 6 months and has a remission rate similar to the reducing regimen of carbimazole alone. Because of the risk of teratogenesis when carbimazole is used in pregnancy, propylthiouracil is preferred for treating thyrotoxicosis in the first trimester. Placental transfer of the active metabolite of carbimazole can produce neonatal hypothyroidism, but propylthiouracil does not transfer in large enough quantities to cause problems. However, in Graves' disease the thyroid-stimulating antibody crosses the placenta and causes fetal thyrotoxicosis; therefore carbimazole is the treatment of choice in the second and third trimester for maternal Graves' disease. Approximately 50% of people with Graves' disease have a single episode that is cured by drug treatment with a thionamide. This may be aided by suppression of TSH receptor antibody by the drug.

A β-adrenoceptor antagonist (especially propranolol because of its nonselective action; see Chapter 5) is particularly useful for symptomatic relief from tremor, anxiety or palpitation during the early period of treatment with carbimazole. It has immediate effects on symptoms but does not alter the rate of thyroid hormone synthesis or secretion. Exophthalmos associated with Graves' disease often responds poorly to treatment with antithyroid drugs. Severe thyroid eye disease can be helped by treatment with oral prednisolone if antithyroid treatment is not improving the condition. Decompressive surgery or radiotherapy may be needed for corneal exposure or visual impairment.

Radioiodine can be used as first-line treatment for Graves' disease, especially for people over 50 years of age, or for relapse after antithyroid drug treatment. Radioiodine can make thyroid ophthalmopathy worse, but this can be prevented by treatment with a corticosteroid such as prednisolone for 2–3 months. Before radioiodine treatment it is often recommended that the thyrotoxicosis should be stabilised with carbimazole. This reduces the risk of exacerbation of hyperthyroidism from radiation thyroiditis immediately after isotope treatment. However, carbimazole must be stopped for at least 2 days before radioactive iodine is given (2 weeks for propylthiouracil), or it will prevent uptake of the radioiodine by the thyroid cells. A β-adrenoceptor antagonist can be useful in this period to prevent symptomatic relapse. The antithyroid drug can be restarted 7 days after radioiodine, to cover the period of up to 8 weeks before radioiodine is fully effective. Between 10% and 20% of those treated will require a second dose of radioiodine to achieve euthyroid status. Permanent hypothyroidism occurs in at least 10% of those treated in the first year following radioiodine treatment, and thereafter the risk is 2–3% annually. There is no increase in risk of cancer or leukaemia following radioiodine treatment.

Surgery is recommended for Graves' disease if there is a poor response to antithyroid drugs, a very large goitre, for coexisting thyroid malignancy or if the person expresses a preference for this treatment. Before surgery, carbimazole is usually used to achieve a euthyroid state. If the thyrotoxicosis is drug-resistant, then oral potassium iodide can be given for up to 2 weeks before surgery to inhibit thyroxine synthesis and release and to reduce the vascularity of the hyperplastic thyroid gland. Hypothyroidism, often delayed by several months or years, occurs in up to 80% of people after surgery.

Toxic nodular goitre and toxic adenoma

Radioiodine is also used for toxic multinodular goitre and toxic adenoma. A solitary toxic thyroid nodule can be removed surgically, but radioactive iodine is extremely effective, because the isotope is taken up only by the abnormal nodule(s) (normal thyroid tissue is suppressed by the absence of thyrotropin in the circulation). Carbimazole is unsuitable as sole treatment for these conditions, since spontaneous remission does not occur. However, some elderly people may choose to continue treatment with a low dose of carbimazole for life.

Amiodarone-induced thyrotoxicosis

Amiodarone is an iodine-containing drug that interferes with deiodinase activity and reduces conversion of T_4 to T_3. Thyrotoxicosis results either from the excess iodide in the drug (type I thyrotoxicosis) or from destructive thyroiditis (type 2 thyrotoxicosis). Treatment of amiodarone-induced thyrotoxicosis (see Chapter 8) depends on the clinical subtype. Type 1 responds to antithyroid drug treatment. Type 2 responds well to treatment with a corticosteroid.

HYPOTHYROIDISM

Hypothyroidism is usually caused by primary thyroid failure, and the low circulating free T_4 concentration is accompanied by a raised serum thyrotropin (TSH) concentration. Autoimmune (Hashimoto's) thyroiditis is the most common cause, but hypothyroidism is occasionally congenital or due to iodine deficiency (the most common cause in mountainous regions of developing countries). Hypothyroidism can follow treatment for hyperthyroidism by surgery or radioiodine. Rarely, hypothyroidism can be secondary to pituitary or hypothalamic failure, when the circulating TSH concentration will be low. Drug therapy with lithium (see Chapter 22) or amiodarone (see Chapter 8) can produce hypothyroidism.

Typical symptoms of hypothyroidism in an adult are nonspecific and include lethargy, slowing of mental processes, cold intolerance, dry skin, hoarseness, weight gain, constipation and menorrhagia. Severe hypothyroidism (myxoedema) produces marked coarsening of the facial appearance and may ultimately lead to a hypothermic, comatose state. Maternal iodine deficiency in pregnancy can lead to permanent mental retardation in the infant, known as 'neurological' cretinism. In children, hypothyroidism stunts mental and physical development, resulting in 'myxoedematous' cretinism.

MANAGEMENT OF HYPOTHYROIDISM

Standard treatment is with oral levothyroxine (T_4). Although its absorption is incomplete and variable, sufficient T_3 will be formed by peripheral deiodination of T_4. The proportion of circulating T_3 is usually lower than normal, so the circulating concentration of T_4 will often need to be higher than those in healthy individuals in order to obtain a satisfactory response. In some people, particularly those with ischaemic heart disease, a rapid increase in metabolic activity with levothyroxine replacement can cause excessive cardiac stimulation, and therefore levothyroxine should be introduced gradually in those at risk of cardiac complications. In others, the anticipated weight-related maintenance dose can be given from the start. Because of its long half-life, a steady-state plasma concentration of levothyroxine will only be achieved with constant dosage after 4–5 weeks.

The adequacy of levothyroxine replacement therapy is best monitored by measurement of the serum TSH concentration 6–8 weeks after a change in levothyroxine dose. The TSH concentration should be in the lower third of the normal range, and then the plasma T_4 will usually be slightly high or in the upper part of the normal range. Once the dose of levothyroxine is correct, an annual check of serum TSH is sufficient, unless there are symptoms suggesting hypo- or hyperthyroidism.

When the hypothyroidism is caused by drug treatment, the precipitating drug can be continued while levothyroxine is given. Problems with levothyroxine replacement preparations are uncommon unless excessive doses are used, but allergic reactions have been reported, and transient scalp hair loss can occur in the first few weeks of treatment.

Some drugs interfere with the absorption of levothyroxine from the gut. These include iron, calcium carbonate, mineral supplements, colestyramine (see Chapter 48) and sucralfate (see Chapter 33). The metabolism of levothyroxine is accelerated by the concurrent use of the hepatic enzyme-inducing drugs phenobarbital, phenytoin, carbamazepine (see Chapter 23) and rifampicin (see Chapter 51). The therapeutic response to levothyroxine may be impaired in all of these situations.

Liothyronine (T_3) is usually reserved for intravenous use in severe hypothyroidism (myxoedema coma), when its potency, more rapid effect and shorter half-life allow more rapid attainment of a therapeutic blood concentration. However, even in this situation, a large dose of levothyroxine has been successfully used and may be associated with a lower mortality. An oral formulation of liothyronine is also available for rapid response in severe hypothyroid states.

SELF-ASSESSMENT

True/false questions

1. Secretion of T_3 and T_4 is controlled by anterior pituitary and hypothalamic hormones.
2. Circulating T_3 and T_4 are highly bound to plasma albumin.
3. T_4 has a long residence time in the body.
4. At target cells, T_3 binds to specific nuclear receptors.
5. Hyperthyroidism is made worse by iodine administration.
6. Severe hypothyroidism causes cretinism in children.
7. Therapy with ^{131}I can cause hypothyroidism.
8. Propylthiouracil is the drug of choice for Graves' disease.
9. Hypothyroidism is treated with levothyroxine.
10. Liothyronine is used in myxoedema coma.

One-best-answer (OBA) questions

1. Choose the *incorrect* statement about the treatment of thyrotoxicosis with carbimazole.
   A. Carbimazole takes several weeks to reduce circulating T_4 and T_3 to normal concentrations.
   B. Carbimazole is a prodrug.
   C. Carbimazole may cause bone marrow suppression.
   D. Carbimazole blocks thyrotropin (TSH) receptors on the thyroid.
   E. Carbimazole has a long duration of action.
2. Choose the *correct* statement about hypothyroidism and its treatment.
   A. Low circulating T_4 levels in hypothyroidism are accompanied by low levels of thyrotropin.
   B. Hepatic enzyme-inducing drugs reduce the response to levothyroxine.
   C. During regular dosing, steady-state plasma levels of levothyroxine are reached within 7 days.
   D. No precautions are required when prescribing levothyroxine in a person with hypothyroidism and ischaemic heart disease.
   E. Oxygen consumption in metabolically active tissues is unaffected by levothyroxine.

Case-based questions

A 45-year-old man suffered from weight loss, palpitations, tremor, anxiety and sweating, plus eyelid retraction and orbital and ocular inflammation. Blood tests showed increased levels of free and bound T_3 and T_4 and low levels of TSH. A diagnosis of Graves' thyrotoxicosis was made. An electrocardiogram showed atrial fibrillation.
1. What is Graves' disease, and why are T_3/T_4 levels high and TSH levels low?

2. What drug should be given to control the hyperthyroidism, and what other drugs might help control the symptoms in this man?
3. With treatment, he became euthyroid, but relapsed in the following year. A decision was made to treat him with ^{131}I. What treatment should be given before administering the ^{131}I, and what are the reasons for this?

ANSWERS

True/false answers

1. **True.** T_3 and T_4 synthesis and release are controlled by TRH from the hypothalamus, by thyrotropin TSH from the anterior pituitary, and by plasma iodide.
2. **False.** T_3 and T_4 in the plasma are largely bound to TBG, which should not be confused with thyroglobulin in the thyroid gland.
3. **True.** Thyroxine has a half-life of about 7 days.
4. **True.** The complex of T_3 and TR activates gene transcription and protein synthesis.
5. **False.** Iodine is converted to iodide and inhibits T_3 and T_4 release.
6. **True.** Severe hypothyroidism causes myxoedema in adults and cretinism in children.
7. **True.** Permanent hypothyroidism can occur after radioiodine treatment.
8. **False.** Propylthiouracil is usually reserved for people intolerant to carbimazole.
9. **True.** Oral levothyroxine is the standard treatment.
10. **True.** Liothyronine is more potent and has a more rapid effect than levothyroxine, so it is given intravenously in severe hypothyroidism (myxoedema coma).

One-best-answer (OBA) answers

1. **Answer D** is the incorrect statement.
   A. Correct. The long half-life of T_4 (about 7 days) means that carbimazole takes 5–6 weeks to reduce thyroid hormone levels to normal.
   B. Correct. Carbimazole is converted to methimazole, which is 10-fold more active.
   C. Correct. Bone marrow suppression is a serious unwanted effect of carbimazole; it can be indicated by infection, especially fever and a severe sore throat.
   D. **Incorrect**. Carbimazole does not block TSH receptors; it inhibits the oxidation of iodide by thyroid peroxidase and hence reduces incorporation of iodine into mono- and di-iodotyrosine.
   E. Correct. Carbimazole accumulates in the thyroid and is given only once daily.
2. **Answer B** is correct.
   A. Incorrect. If T_4 levels were low, then thyrotropin levels would be raised, as the negative-feedback effect of T_4 on thyrotropin release would be reduced.
   B. **Correct**. Hepatic metabolism of levothyroxine is accelerated by cytochrome P450 inducers such as phenobarbitone and phenytoin.
   C. Incorrect. The half-life of levothyroxine is 6–7 days; therefore the steady state would not be reached until about 5 weeks of administration.

D. Incorrect. Levothyroxine should be introduced gradually in ischaemic heart disease, as a rapid increase in metabolic activity can cause excessive heart stimulation.

E. Incorrect. Levothyroxine stimulates oxygen consumption in metabolically active tissues.

Case-based answers

1. Graves' disease is an autoimmune disease in which antibodies to TSH are generated which bind to and activate TSH receptors in the thyroid, promoting thyroid hormone (T_3/T_4) release. Thyrotropin (TSH) concentration is low due to the negative feedback effect of elevated T_3 and T_4.

2. Carbimazole is the drug of choice to control hyperthyroidism, given in a high dose, reducing over 4–6 weeks. Drugs for controlling symptoms include β-adrenoceptor antagonists (typically propranolol), although they do not improve fatigue and muscle weakness. Propranolol should also control a high ventricular rate due to the atrial fibrillation (see Chapter 8), and anticoagulation with warfarin should prevent thromboembolism, which has an increased incidence in people with both atrial fibrillation and thyrotoxicosis.

3. The clinical state should be stabilised with carbimazole and a β-adrenoceptor antagonist. Carbimazole is stopped at least 2 days before radioiodine is given, as it can prevent the uptake of iodine by thyroid cells. It can be restarted a week after radioiodine to cover the period of 8 weeks before radioiodine becomes effective.

FURTHER READING

De Leo, S., Braverman, L.E., 2016. Hyperthyroidism. Lancet 388, 906–918.

Smith, T.J., Hegedus, L., 2016. Graves' disease. N. Engl. J. Med. 375, 1552–1565.

Vaidya, B., Pearce, S.H.S., 2008. Management of hypothyroidism in adults. Br. Med. J. 337, a801.

Vaidya, B., Pearce, S.H.S., 2014. Diagnosis and management of thyrotoxicosis. Br. Med. J. 349, g5128.

Compendium: thyroid and antithyroid drugs

Drug	Characteristics
Thyroid hormones	
Levothyroxine/ thyroxine (T_4)	Deiodinated in peripheral tissues to T_3. Treatment of choice for maintenance therapy of hypothyroidism. Given orally. Half-life (T_3): 6–7 days
Liothyronine (L-triiodothyronine) (T_3)	Given orally or by slow intravenous injection for hypothyroid coma. More rapid onset of action than levothyroxine. Half-life: 1–2 days
Antithyroid drugs	
All antithyroid drugs are given orally once daily. Beta-adrenoceptor antagonists such as propranolol (see Chapter 5) can be used to treat the symptoms of thyrotoxicosis.	
Carbimazole	Thionamide inhibitor of thyroid peroxidase. Rapidly converted to more active derivative, methimazole (thiamazole). Treatment of choice for Graves' hyperthyroidism. Half-life: 5–6 h
Iodine and potassium iodide	Incorporated into thyroid hormones. Used as an adjunct to antithyroid drugs for 10–14 days before partial thyroidectomy, but should not be given for long-term treatment
Propylthiouracil	Thionamide inhibitor of thyroid peroxidase. Used in people intolerant to carbimazole. Half-life: 1–3 h

42

Calcium metabolism and metabolic bone disease

PHYSIOLOGY OF BONE TURNOVER

Bone is constantly undergoing remodelling (bone turnover), which involves resorption and replacement of small areas of bone. Up to 10% of bone undergoes remodelling every year, with trabecular bone (in the ends of long bones and in the vertebrae) undergoing greater turnover than cortical bone. Microdamage such as microcracks in bone allows the bone to dissipate energy during fatigue loading and avoids major fracture. Remodelling repairs microdamage and maintains bone strength. Osteocytes are the predominant cell in bone, and microdamage causes local osteocytes to undergo apoptosis, which signals osteoclasts to begin bone resorption. Resorption leaves trenches on the bone surface, and osteoclasts recruit osteoblasts to refill the trenches. The cycle of bone remodelling is essential for maintenance of Ca^{2+} homeostasis, replacement of apoptotic osteoclasts and repair of microfractures, and takes about 200 days.

There are many factors that regulate bone turnover, but the final pathway is the balance between receptor activator of nuclear factor-κB (RANK) expressed by osteoclasts and osteoprotegerin (OPG) secreted by osteoblasts. RANK is activated by RANK ligand (RANKL) secreted by stromal cells and osteoblasts. In the presence of macrophage colony stimulating factor (M-CSF), RANKL stimulates osteoclast activity and bone reabsorption and is the major paracrine factor activating bone remodelling. OPG secreted by osteoblasts acts as a soluble decoy receptor for binding RANKL and prevents osteoclast activation. The balance between osteoblast secretion of OPG and osteoclast expression of RANK is modulated by interactions among various hormones and cytokines, including sex steroids, interleukin-1 and prostaglandin E_2.

PLASMA CALCIUM HOMEOSTASIS

Calcium circulates in plasma partly bound to protein and the rest in the free ionised (and therefore 'active') form. The free Ca^{2+} concentration in plasma is maintained within narrow limits principally by the actions of parathyroid hormone (PTH) and 1,25-dihydroxyvitamin D_3 (calcitriol). Calcitonin secretion (discussed later) also responds to changing plasma Ca^{2+} concentrations, but it is less important in overall control of Ca^{2+} homeostasis. Calcium in plasma undergoes dynamic exchange with Ca^{2+} in the gut, renal tubules and bone. This is illustrated with the main controlling factors in Fig. 42.1.

PARATHYROID HORMONE AND CALCIUM HOMEOSTASIS

PTH is a polypeptide hormone which is the main physiological regulator of Ca^{2+} in blood. It is secreted from parathyroid chief cells in response to a reduction of ionised Ca^{2+} in plasma. PTH secretion is inhibited when the plasma Ca^{2+} concentration rises. The main actions of PTH relating to calcium homeostasis are:

- Stimulation of the synthesis of the biologically active form of vitamin D (calcitriol) in the kidney by upregulation of the enzyme responsible for 1α-hydroxylation.

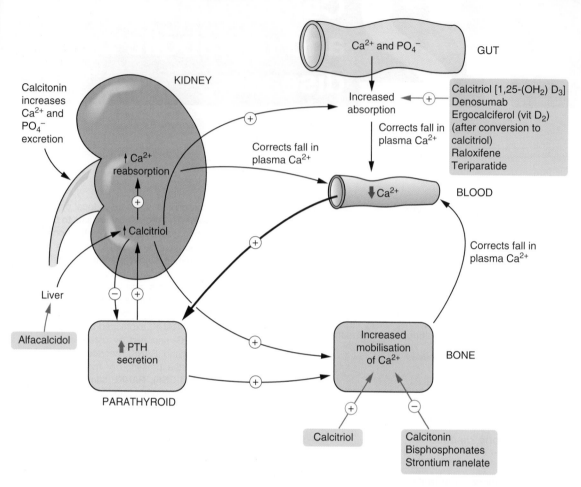

Fig. 42.1 **Regulation of calcium metabolism.** A fall in plasma Ca^{2+} leads to increased release of parathyroid hormone (PTH) from the parathyroid gland, which increases calcitriol [1,25-(OH_2)-D_3] formation in the kidney. This in turn increases gut absorption of Ca^{2+}. PTH further increases bone mobilisation of Ca^{2+} to return plasma Ca^{2+} to normal. An increase in plasma Ca^{2+}, conversely, decreases PTH secretion. Calcitonin, secreted by the thyroid, decreases Ca^{2+} reabsorption from the kidney and decreases bone turnover. Drugs used for hypercalcaemia are indicated by green arrows and drugs for hypocalcaemia by red arrows.

- Enhanced reabsorption of Ca^{2+} from the kidney distal tubules with increased urinary phosphate excretion. This increases the plasma Ca^{2+}/phosphate ratio and increases plasma free Ca^{2+}.
- Mobilisation of Ca^{2+} and phosphate from bone through stimulation of osteoclasts, which increases bone resorption. Osteoclasts do not have a receptor for PTH. PTH binds to osteoblasts and increases secretion of RANKL and decreases secretion of OPG which results in osteoclast activation.

The effect of PTH on the kidney occurs within minutes of PTH release, whereas that on bone begins after 1–2 hours.

VITAMIN D AND CALCIUM HOMEOSTASIS

Vitamin D (calciferol) is a group of compounds that have secosteroid nuclei (a steroid nucleus with one bond in the steroid ring broken). There are two precursors of active vitamin D: ergocalciferol and cholecalciferol. Ergocalciferol (vitamin D_2) is derived from food and absorbed from the gut. However, given adequate ultraviolet B sunlight, the major source of vitamin D is conversion of 7-dehydrocholesterol in the skin to cholecalciferol (vitamin D_3). Therefore vitamin D is really a skin-derived hormone rather than a vitamin, but this source was discovered after the dietary origins. Vitamins D_2 and D_3 are further metabolised in the liver to 25-hydroxyvitamin D_3 (calcidiol), and then in the kidney to 1,25-dihydroxyvitamin D_3 (calcitriol). 1α-Hydroxylation in the kidney is an essential step for activation of vitamin D. PTH stimulates 1α-hydroxylase activity in the kidney, increasing the formation of calcitriol. Calcitriol binds to specific vitamin D receptors, which belong to the nuclear receptor superfamily of steroid/thyroid hormone receptors, in the nuclei of target cells in most organs (see Chapter 1). The vitamin D–receptor complex acts as a transcription factor that activates various genes. Vitamin D increases the plasma concentration of Ca^{2+} by:

- facilitating absorption of Ca^{2+} from the small intestine;
- enhancing Ca^{2+} mobilisation from bone by increasing osteoclast numbers and activity.

In the kidney, vitamin D promotes phosphate retention, in contrast to the action of PTH. Overall, vitamin D maintains the plasma Ca^{2+} and phosphate concentrations to allow normal bone remodelling. Vitamin D has several other functions unrelated to plasma Ca^{2+} and phosphate homeostasis, such as immune cell proliferation and differentiation.

CALCITONIN AND CALCIUM HOMEOSTASIS

Calcitonin is a polypeptide hormone secreted by the parafollicular cells of the thyroid when its calcium-sensing receptors detect a rise in plasma Ca^{2+}. The calcitonin receptor is found on osteoclasts, in the kidney and the brain, and receptor activation stimulates adenylyl cyclase. Calcitonin inhibits osteoclasts and reduces bone turnover, inhibits Ca^{2+} absorption from the intestines, and also reduces Ca^{2+} and phosphate reabsorption by the kidney.

HYPERCALCAEMIA

The main causes of hypercalcaemia are:

- increased resorption of Ca^{2+} from bone (e.g. primary hyperparathyroidism, secretion of parathyroid-related hormone by cancer cells and osteolysis particularly in haematological malignancies);
- increased absorption of Ca^{2+} from the gut through excessive use of vitamin D or in sarcoidosis;
- reduced renal excretion of Ca^{2+}; for example, as caused by thiazide diuretics (see Chapter 14).

Hypercalcaemia occurs when the influx of Ca^{2+} into the extracellular space exceeds the capacity to remove it. Prolonged moderate hypercalcaemia leads to a progressive decline in renal function, formation of renal stones and ectopic calcification (e.g. cornea, blood vessels). Severe hypercalcaemia causes anorexia, nausea, vomiting, constipation, drowsiness and confusion, eventually leading to coma. Hypercalcaemia impairs the ability of the kidney to reabsorb salt and water which, in conjunction with vomiting, can lead to depletion of plasma volume and acute kidney injury from poor kidney perfusion. Urgent treatment is indicated when the plasma Ca^{2+} concentration rises above 3.5 mmol/L (normal <2.6 mmol/L), since sudden death from cardiac arrest can occur.

ANTIRESORPTIVE DRUGS FOR TREATING HYPERCALCAEMIA

Bisphosphonates

Examples

alendronic acid, sodium clodronate, pamidronate disodium, risedronate sodium, zoledronic acid

Bisphosphonates have a major role in the treatment of osteoporosis, Paget's disease of bone and pain from osteolytic bone metastases. Of the drugs considered here, sodium clodronate is only licensed in the UK for treatment of hypercalcaemia, and alendronic acid and risedronate sodium do not have a license for treatment of hypercalcaemia.

Mechanisms of action and effects

Bisphosphonates are pyrophosphate analogues that bind to hydroxyapatite crystals in the bone matrix. They are preferentially deposited under osteoclasts, and are taken up by these cells and inhibit their resorptive action on bone. There are two different cellular actions of the drugs on osteoclasts, depending on the structure of the bisphosphonate.

- Amino-bisphosphonates (nitrogen-containing drugs: alendronic acid, disodium pamidronate, risedronate sodium, zoledronic acid) act by inhibition of the ATP-dependent enzyme farnesyl diphosphate synthase in the 3-hydroxy-3-methyl-glutaryl-coenzyme A reductase (HMG-CoA) reductase synthetic pathway from mevalonic acid to cholesterol. This reduces the production of lipids that are essential for subcellular protein trafficking required for normal osteoclast function. As a result, differentiation of osteoclast precursors is impaired, and mature osteoclasts have a reduced ability to reabsorb bone. Eventually, osteoclast apoptosis is increased.
- Non-nitrogen-containing drugs (sodium clodronate) affect metabolism within the osteoclast by forming a nonfunctional analogue of ATP that induces apoptosis. Sodium clodronate has a relatively weak antiresorptive action.

Most bisphosphonates have a relatively short-lived action unless taken regularly, but zoledronic acid can suppress bone resorption for up to a year after a single dose.

Pharmacokinetics

Bisphosphonates are poorly absorbed from the gut, and oral formulations are best taken once weekly with the stomach empty to avoid binding by Ca^{2+} in food. Alendronic acid and risedronate sodium are only available in oral formulations, while pamidronate disodium and zoledronic acid are only formulated for intravenous use. Removal of most bisphosphonates from blood via the kidney is rapid, but their effect is prolonged since a fraction remains tightly bound to Ca^{2+} in bone for years.

Unwanted effects

- Gastrointestinal disturbance, particularly nausea, abdominal pain, diarrhoea or constipation with the oral treatments. Alendronic acid and risedronate sodium can cause severe oesophagitis and oesophageal strictures. Tablets should be swallowed intact with a full glass of water at least 30 minutes before food and followed by standing or sitting for at least 30 minutes. Once-weekly dosing reduces the risk of oesophageal damage.
- Headache, dizziness, vertigo, musculoskeletal pain.
- Transient pyrexia and influenza-like symptoms after intravenous infusion.
- Osteonecrosis of the jaw, especially after intravenous use in the treatment of cancer. Good oral hygiene will reduce the risk. Atypical femoral fractures and benign osteonecrosis of the external auditory canal are rare complications of prolonged treatment.

Calcitonin

Mechanism of action and effects

The actions of calcitonin on bone, gut and the kidneys to reduce plasma Ca^{2+} concentrations have been discussed previously. Calcitonin begins to act within a few hours of administration, with a maximum effect within 12–24 hours. However, the hypocalcaemic effect during repeated administrations only lasts between 2 and 3 days. The loss of clinical response results from downregulation of calcitonin receptors on osteoclasts, leading to a rebound increase in bone resorption.

Pharmacokinetics

Salmon calcitonin (salcatonin) is usually given by intramuscular or subcutaneous injection, although intravenous infusion can be used. The half-life is very short (about 20 minutes), as it is degraded to inactive fragments in the plasma and the kidney.

Unwanted effects

- Facial flushing occurs in most people.
- Headache, dizziness, fatigue.
- Nausea, vomiting, taste disturbance, abdominal pain, diarrhoea.

TREATMENT OF HYPERCALCAEMIA

When possible, the primary cause should be corrected, for example removal of a parathyroid adenoma or treatment of myeloma. Oral Ca^{2+} supplements, vitamin D and thiazide diuretics should be discontinued.

Mild hypercalcaemia (corrected serum Ca^{2+} <3.0 mmol/L) is usually caused by primary hyperparathyroidism. Immediate treatment to reduce the serum Ca^{2+} concentration is not required, but assessment of renal function and bone imaging for osteoporosis should be undertaken. Surgery to remove a parathyroid adenoma or hyperplastic parathyroid glands is indicated if the person is younger than 50 years old or there is renal involvement or osteoporosis. Cinacalcet is a calcimimetic agent that increases the sensitivity of Ca^{2+}-sensing receptors on chief cells of the parathyroid glands to extracellular Ca^{2+}, which reduces PTH secretion. Cinacalcet reduces the serum Ca^{2+} concentration in hyperparathyroidism but does not affect the bone or renal complications. Its main uses are in secondary hyperparathyroidism in end-stage renal failure treated by dialysis, or primary hyperparathyroidism when parathyroidectomy is not considered appropriate.

Oral bisphosphonate treatment may be sufficient for moderate hypercalcaemia (3.0–3.5 mmol/L). Corticosteroids such as prednisolone (see Chapter 44) are effective for lowering plasma Ca^{2+} when vitamin D excess is an important factor, for example in sarcoidosis and for acute treatment of vitamin D overdose, or for hypercalcaemia associated with haematological malignancy such as myeloma or lymphoma. Corticosteroids probably act by reducing the effect of vitamin D on intestinal Ca^{2+} transport, but can take several days to work.

Most people with severe hypercalcaemia (>3.5 mmol/L) are fluid-depleted at presentation. Rehydration with intravenous isotonic saline is essential; this also promotes a sodium-linked Ca^{2+} diuresis in the proximal and distal renal tubules. Loop diuretics such as furosemide (see Chapter 14) increase renal Ca^{2+} elimination, but there is only limited evidence to support their use, and they carry a risk of dehydration. Severe hypercalcaemia is usually due to increased bone resorption, and intravenous infusion of a bisphosphonate such as zoledronic acid or pamidronate disodium is the drug treatment of choice. Initial intravenous rehydration is essential to avoid precipitation of calcium bisphosphonate in the kidney. Following a single intravenous infusion of bisphosphonate, the plasma Ca^{2+} concentration falls gradually after 2–4 days, with a maximum effect after 4–7 days and a response that persists for 1–4 weeks after treatment. Because of the delay in onset of action of the bisphosphonates, calcitonin can be given concurrently for an early effect.

HYPOCALCAEMIA

There are two major underlying causes of hypocalcaemia:

- deficiency of PTH; for example, idiopathic hypoparathyroidism, after surgical parathyroid removal;
- deficiency of vitamin D (e.g. dietary deficiency, limited exposure to sunlight, renal failure [failure of 1α-hydroxylation]).

Hypocalcaemia produces neuromuscular irritability with paraesthesiae of the extremities or around the mouth, muscle cramps and tetany. When severe, it can produce seizures. Chronic hypocalcaemia, especially in congenital hypoparathyroidism, is associated with mental deficiency, seizures, intracranial calcification (e.g. choroid plexus) and ocular cataracts.

DRUGS FOR HYPOCALCAEMIA

Vitamin D compounds

alfacalcidol (1α-hydroxycholecalciferol),
calcitriol (1,25-dihydroxyvitamin D_3 or
1,25-dihydroxycholecalciferol), colecalciferol (vitamin D_3),
ergocalciferol (vitamin D_2), paricalcitol

Mechanism of action

The mechanism of action of vitamin D was discussed earlier. A dose-related increase in Ca^{2+} and phosphate absorption from the gut occurs at lower concentrations of vitamin D than those which stimulate bone resorption. Ergocalciferol is inactive and can only be used if 1α-hydroxylation by the kidney is intact. In chronic kidney disease, the hydroxylated active forms alfacalcidol or calcitriol should be used. Paricalcitol is a synthetic vitamin D analogue used in chronic kidney disease; it binds to the vitamin D receptor and inhibits PTH synthesis and secretion, but has less effect than natural vitamin D on the plasma Ca^{2+} concentration.

Pharmacokinetics

The fat-soluble D vitamins are well absorbed orally in the presence of bile. They can also be given intravenously. Alfacalcidol and calcitriol have short half-lives (about 3 hours) and are metabolised and excreted mainly in the bile. Paricalcitol requires intravenous injection.

Unwanted effects

- Excessive dosing will produce hypercalcaemia.
- Excretion of vitamin D supplements in breast milk can cause hypercalcaemia in a suckling infant.

TREATMENT OF HYPOCALCAEMIA

In addition to measures to correct hypocalcaemia, treatment should be directed to the underlying cause when possible. If there is concurrent hypomagnesaemia, it must be corrected; otherwise maintaining a normal serum Ca^{2+} will be difficult.

Acute severe hypocalcaemia (corrected serum Ca^{2+} <1.9 mmol/L) sometimes occurs after parathyroidectomy. It should initially be treated with intravenous Ca^{2+} gluconate, followed by oral Ca^{2+} supplements. If PTH is deficient, then vitamin D supplements are given.

Mild hypocalcaemia can be treated with oral Ca^{2+} supplements, taken between meals to avoid binding to dietary phosphate and oxalate, which forms salts that are poorly absorbed. In the absence of reversible pathology such as malabsorption due to coeliac disease, the mainstay of treatment for more severe hypocalcaemia is vitamin D supplements. Ergocalciferol or colecalciferol are given in large doses initially if there is vitamin D deficiency, and then at lower maintenance doses to maintain normocalcaemia. Oral Ca^{2+} supplements (as carbonate or citrate salts) are often used with vitamin D for the treatment of chronic hypocalcaemia.

For treatment of hypoparathyroidism, calcitriol or alfacalcidol is given, often with oral Ca^{2+} supplements during the early phase of treatment, because there is deficient renal hydroxylation of vitamin D in hypoparathyroidism. PTH is not licensed for replacement therapy, although injectable PTH and a synthetic PTH fragment, teriparatide, are now licensed for treatment of osteoporosis (discussed later). A thiazide diuretic is sometimes used to reduce urinary Ca^{2+} excretion during vitamin D therapy.

METABOLIC BONE DISEASE

OSTEOMALACIA

Osteomalacia is the bone disease resulting from failure of adequate bone mineralisation due to prolonged lack of vitamin D. Bone pain and tenderness is prominent, and low plasma concentrations of Ca^{2+} and phosphate produce proximal muscle weakness. In developing children whose growth plates have not fused, defective bone growth and shaping result in the bones becoming distorted (rickets). Treatment is with vitamin D (ergocalciferol or colecalciferol) supplements, but it will take at least a year to achieve a normal bone structure.

VITAMIN D DEFICIENCY AND REPLACEMENT THERAPY

Vitamin D deficiency is most common in people with pigmented skin. In adults there is an additional risk in the elderly who have less exposure to sunlight, obese people, those with malabsorption or renal disease, vegans or those who take certain anticonvulsants, rifampicin or antiretroviral drugs. Up to 50% of people in the United Kingdom are vitamin D deficient in the spring, but most are asymptomatic.

The rising incidence of vitamin D deficiency in infants has led to a recommendation that vitamin D supplements should be routinely given to children under 5 years old. For adults, vitamin D replacement is usually reserved for those with symptoms potentially due to deficiency and when vitamin D deficiency might interfere with treatment of osteoporosis. Initially, loading doses of ergocalciferol or colecalciferol can be used, but lower doses are usually adequate for initiation of treatment.

RENAL BONE DISEASE

Chronic renal disease (especially with an estimated glomerular filtration rate [GFR] <30 mL/minute per 1.73 m^2) is associated with deficient renal activation of vitamin D and hypocalcaemia. At the same time, reduced renal phosphate excretion leads to hyperphosphataemia. The low serum Ca^{2+} stimulates PTH secretion (secondary hyperparathyroidism) in an attempt to maintain the plasma Ca^{2+} concentration. The result is demineralisation of bone (renal bone disease) and soft tissue calcification from the increased plasma calcium–phosphate product. Vascular calcification is associated with increased cardiovascular disease and mortality.

Treatment of renal bone disease requires a 1α-hydroxylated vitamin D derivative (such as alfacalcidol or calcitriol). This will increase plasma Ca^{2+} but does not affect the plasma phosphate, and an oral phosphate binder such as aluminium hydroxide is necessary to reduce the plasma phosphate concentration if this is raised to avoid tissue calcification. People who are undergoing haemodialysis or ambulatory peritoneal dialysis cannot readily excrete absorbed aluminium, and an alternative phosphate binder such as sevelamer or lanthanum is used.

OSTEOPOROSIS

Osteoporosis is the loss of bone mass due to reduced organic bone matrix and, consequently, mineral content, which decreases the mechanical strength of bone. It results from an imbalance between bone resorption and formation, and affects trabecular bone more than cortical bone due to its higher natural remodelling. Osteoporosis is an inevitable part of the ageing process, beginning from age 30–35 years, with a marked acceleration in bone loss in females after the menopause. Predisposing factors to earlier osteoporosis include smoking, heavy alcohol intake, malnutrition, malabsorption and lack of exercise. Osteoporosis in younger people is associated with trabecular bone loss and predisposes to spontaneous vertebral fractures. In older people, cortical bone is also lost, increasing the risk of low-impact traumatic fracture, particularly of the forearm (Colles' fracture) and neck of the femur. Sometimes osteoporosis is secondary to other conditions such as myeloma or thyrotoxicosis, or occurs as a result of prolonged corticosteroid therapy (see Chapter 44).

The diagnosis of osteoporosis is usually made by estimating bone mineral density from dual-energy X-ray absorptiometry (DEXA) scanning. Bone mineral density is then compared with mean bone density in a young adult reference population, and a T-score calculated (standard deviations of bone mineral density from the mean of the reference population):

- T-score of −1.0 or above is normal.
- T-score between −1.0 and −2.5 is called osteopenia (reduced bone mass).
- T-score of −2.5 or below indicates osteoporosis.

Once established, osteoporosis is difficult to reverse, and emphasis should be placed on prevention where possible.

Prevention of osteoporosis

Preventive strategies are important in those identified as being at high risk of osteoporosis. Use of a prediction tool for calculating the risk of future fractures can help to target treatment. Early use of preventive treatments is important if prolonged corticosteroid treatment is planned (see Chapter 44).

- Oral calcium supplements increase bone mineral density in the spine in postmenopausal women, but with an uncertain effect on the risk of vertebral fractures. The addition of vitamin D (ergocalciferol) confers greater benefit, with a reduction in the risk of nonvertebral fractures. Recently, concern has been raised that high-dose Ca^{2+} supplements may increase the risk of myocardial infarction, but any increase in risk is modest.
- Oral bisphosphonates (discussed previously) are the treatment of choice for prevention of postmenopausal osteoporosis and corticosteroid-induced osteoporosis.
- Hormone-replacement therapy (HRT) with oestrogen (see Chapter 45) in peri- and postmenopausal women was once the mainstay of preventative treatment for osteoporosis. However, 5–10 years of oestrogen therapy may be required, and long-term use of HRT increases the risk of breast cancer and thromboembolic events. As a consequence, the use of HRT for this indication has declined.

Drugs for established osteoporosis

These fall into three categories. Antiresorptive therapies (bisphosphonates, raloxifene, oestrogen, denosumab) decrease markers of bone formation and bone resorption. Anabolic therapies (calcitonin, teriparatide) lay down new bone and produce an increase in markers of bone formation and bone resorption. Strontium ranelate does not conform to either of these patterns of effect on bone metabolism.

- Oral bisphosphonates (discussed previously) increase bone density, with the best evidence in postmenopausal women. Alendronic acid and risedronate sodium reduce hip, vertebral and wrist fractures. Intravenous bisphosphonates such as zoledronic acid once a year or ibandronic acid every 3 months are used when oral treatment is poorly tolerated.
- Raloxifene is a selective oestrogen receptor (ER) modulator (see Chapter 45). It is a partial agonist of ERα (which acts as a gene activator), but also an antagonist of ERβ by recruiting co-repressor molecules (which suppresses gene transcription). The distribution of the two receptors may explain the tissue specificity of raloxifene, which has ER agonist effects on bone and lipids (reducing low-density lipoprotein cholesterol) but acts as an anti-oestrogen on the breast and endometrium. Raloxifene reduces the risk of vertebral fractures by 40%, but has no effect on nonvertebral fractures, which may reflect the tissue distribution of ER subtypes. Raloxifene also reduces the risk of ER-positive breast cancer in postmenopausal women by 75%, but its effects on preexisting breast cancer are unknown. It does not affect menopausal vasomotor symptoms. Unwanted effects include hot flushes and leg cramps. In addition, raloxifene doubles the risk of venous thromboembolism, particularly during the first 4 months of treatment.
- Teriparatide is a synthetic recombinant fraction of PTH (amino acids 1–34) that is used mainly for the treatment of postmenopausal osteoporosis. It is given daily by subcutaneous injection. The most common unwanted effects are nausea, oesophageal reflux, postural hypotension, dyspnoea, depression and dizziness. Human recombinant PTH is an alternative option, also be given by subcutaneous injection.
- Strontium ranelate is preferentially taken up by trabecular bone and incorporated into bone in the same way as Ca^{2+}. It stimulates osteoblast activity and inhibits osteoclast differentiation and resorptive activity. Strontium ranelate reduces the risk of both hip and vertebral fractures. The pattern of bone remodelling, with increases in markers of bone formation and a decrease in bone resorption, differs from that seen with both antiresorptive and anabolic therapies. Minor unwanted effects include nausea, diarrhoea, headache and rashes. Severe allergic reactions with strontium ranelate include drug rash with eosinophilia and systemic symptoms (DRESS), such as fever, and lymphadenopathy. The most serious concern with the drug is an increased risk of myocardial infarction and strontium ranelate should not be given to people with a history of atherosclerotic arterial disease or who are at high risk of ischaemic heart disease. It also increases the risk of venous thromboembolic disease.
- Denosumab is a human monoclonal antibody which binds specifically to RANKL and prevents activation of the RANK receptor on osteoclasts. Maturation of osteoclasts is reduced, their function is inhibited and their survival reduced. Resorption of both cortical and trabecular bone is decreased, and denosumab reduces both vertebral and nonvertebral fractures. Denosumab has a very long half-life of about 26 days and is given subcutaneously twice a year. Unwanted effects include diarrhoea, constipation, dyspnoea, increased frequency of urinary tract and upper respiratory tract infections, limb pains, sciatica, hypocalcaemia, hypophosphataemia, rash, sweating and cataracts. Like bisphosphonates, denosumab can cause osteonecrosis of the jaw, particularly when used to treat bony metastases.
- Calcitriol is used when bisphosphonates are unsuitable, and is given for postmenopausal and corticosteroid-induced osteoporosis.
- Testosterone (see Chapter 46) is sometimes used for prophylaxis and treatment of corticosteroid-induced osteoporosis in men.

Management of osteoporosis

Management of osteoporosis includes nonpharmacological approaches, such as removing lifestyle and drug factors that increase the risk of demineralisation. Pain relief is important if there are fractures, and salmon calcitonin given subcutaneously can aid pain relief when used for up to 3 months after a vertebral fracture.

Drug treatment to prevent further bone loss can reduce the risk of further fractures by up to 50%. The choice of drug treatment depends on the clinical circumstances. Calcium and vitamin D supplements reduce hip fractures in house-bound elderly people and are often used together with other drug therapy. Bisphosphonates are the first-line treatment for prevention and treatment of established osteoporosis in men and women. They are also first choice for the prevention and management of corticosteroid-induced osteoporosis. If there has been a good response in bone mineral density after 5 years (3 years for zoledronic acid), then treatment is usually stopped for 3–5 years while monitoring markers of bone turnover. This strategy does not increase the risk of subsequent fractures.

For postmenopausal women who cannot tolerate a bisphosphonate, denosumab, teriparatide or strontium ranelate are options. Strontium ranelate should be avoided in those at high risk of myocardial infarction or venous thromboembolism. There is a rebound increase in bone turnover when denosumab is stopped, so another drug should be started if denosumab is withdrawn. Raloxifene is recommended for women who have had a vertebral fragility fracture and cannot take a bisphosphonate, or who have a fragility fracture after at least 1 year of treatment with a bisphosphonate. Hormone replacement therapy is not usually indicated as a treatment for preventing osteoporosis, but can be used if other treatments are not tolerated. It is most effective if started soon after the onset of the menopause.

Denosumab is effective for treatment of osteoporosis in men, including those undergoing androgen-depletion therapy for prostate cancer. Teriparatide or strontium ranelate can also be used for osteoporosis treatment in men and corticosteroid-induced osteoporosis. Testosterone is only used when there is evidence of hypogonadism.

PAGET'S DISEASE OF BONE

Paget's disease of bone is a disturbance of bone remodelling that is characterised by both excessive bone reabsorption by osteoclasts and an increase in formation of poor-quality bone that has a mosaic appearance on microscopy. The new bone matrix is nonlamellar woven bone (haphazard organisation of the collagen matrix due to rapid bone formation), with areas of osteosclerosis, leaving bone that is structurally weakened. Paget's disease mainly affects the skull and long bones. The aetiology is unknown, but there is a genetic predisposition and a viral infection may initiate the disease.

About a third of pagetic bone lesions are asymptomatic, but the remainder can produce bone pain and deformity, nerve entrapment and pathological fractures. Active treatment should be given if symptoms are present or a risk of complications is identified. Apart from symptomatic measures such as analgesics, bisphosphonates are used to inhibit bone resorption. Pamidronate disodium and risedronate sodium are the first-choice drugs, but zoledronic acid may be more effective for more severe disease. Bisphosphonates can relieve pain to a greater extent than analgesics but may not reduce bone deformity or decrease the risk of fractures. The indications for treatment are not agreed, but may include involvement of the skull (to reduce the risk of deafness), disease of the long bones (to reduce deformity) or disease of the spine (to reduce risk of spinal cord compression).

SELF-ASSESSMENT

True/false questions

1. Hypocalcaemia develops when there is a deficiency in PTH or vitamin D activity.
2. Vitamin D deficiency can lead to hypoparathyroidism.
3. Calcitonin decreases Ca^{2+} resorption in the kidney.
4. Bisphosphonates rapidly lower blood Ca^{2+} levels.
5. Oestrogens maintain bone density by directly enhancing Ca^{2+} absorption from the intestine.
6. Raloxifene stimulates ERs on bone, breast and uterine tissue.
7. Denosumab binds to RANKL and reduces osteoclast activity.
8. Teriparatide is used in the treatment of postmenopausal osteoporosis.

One-best-answer (OBA) questions

1. Identify the *accurate* statement below concerning drugs and osteoporosis.
   A. Oral prednisolone reduces the risk of osteoporosis.
   B. Strontium ranelate can cause fatal allergic reactions.
   C. Bisphosphonates enhance Ca^{2+} mobilisation in bone.
   D. Raloxifene reduces the risk of thromboembolism.
   E. Bisphosphonates have few adverse effects.
2. Identify the *inaccurate* statement below concerning osteomalacia and rickets.
   A. Lack of sunlight can contribute to osteomalacia.
   B. Renal failure reduces the effectiveness of ergocalciferol treatment in osteomalacia.
   C. Intestinal absorption of Ca^{2+} is decreased in osteomalacia.
   D. Vitamin D promotes bone mineralisation.
   E. Osteomalacia results in low circulating PTH.

ANSWERS

True/false answers

1. **True.** Deficiencies in the production of PTH or vitamin D, or in the responsiveness of their target tissues, cause hypocalcaemia.
2. **False.** Vitamin D deficiency leads to hyperparathyroidism, which may assist in reducing the worst effects of vitamin D deficiency. PTH increases calcitriol formation, and calcitriol has a negative feedback effect on PTH.
3. **True.** Calcitonin reduces Ca^{2+} resorption and inhibits bone turnover.
4. **False.** Bisphosphonates inhibit bone dissolution and their effects occur slowly; plasma Ca^{2+} concentrations fall slowly, with a maximum effect after about a week.
5. **False.** Oestrogens inhibit the cytokines that recruit the bone-resorbing osteoclasts. Oestrogens also inhibit the actions of PTH.

6. **False.** Raloxifene has been licensed to increase bone density in postmenopausal women. It is a selective oestrogen receptor modulator (SERM) active on ERs in bone but without stimulant effect on ERs in the breasts and uterus.

7. **True.** Denosumab prevents activation of RANK receptors on osteoclasts by RANKL, and reduces osteoclast proliferation, function and survival.

8. **True.** Teriparatide is a recombinant version of amino acids 1–34 of PTH and is given daily by subcutaneous injection for postmenopausal osteoporosis.

One-best-answer (OBA) answers

1. **Answer B** is the accurate statement.
   A. Incorrect. Long-term use of high doses of systemic corticosteroids can reduce the number of osteoclasts/osteoblasts, decrease Ca^{2+} absorption, increase renal Ca^{2+} excretion and increase bone resorption, enhancing osteoporosis risk.
   B. **Correct**. Strontium ranelate can cause DRESS, which may be fatal.
   C. Incorrect. Bisphosphonates reduce bone Ca^{2+} mobilisation and are particularly useful in corticosteroid-induced osteoporosis.

   D. Incorrect. Raloxifene is a partial agonist at oestrogen ERα receptors and an antagonist at ERβ receptors; it can result in hot flushes, leg cramps and thromboembolism in some women.
   E. Incorrect. Oral bisphosphonates can cause gastrointestinal disturbance and oesophageal damage; intravenous bisphosphonates cause transient pyrexia, and long-term use may lead to osteonecrosis of the jaw and atypical femoral fractures.

2. **Answer E** is the inaccurate statement.
   A. Correct. Sunlight is involved in the formation of cholecalciferol in the skin, which is then converted to active vitamin D compounds in the liver and kidneys.
   B. Correct. Ergocalciferol is 1α-hydroxylated in the kidney to calcitriol before it can exert its biological activity. In renal failure, if 1α-hydroxylase activity is defective, alfacalcidol or calcitriol may have to be substituted.
   C. Correct. Because of the lack of active vitamin D formed in the kidney, less Ca^{2+} and phosphate will be absorbed from the gut.
   D. Correct. Vitamin D promotes bone mineralisation by enhancing the laying down of hydroxyapatite on the collagen organic matrix.
   E. **Incorrect**. Vitamin D deficiency reduces plasma Ca^{2+} and results in higher levels of PTH (secondary hyperparathyroidism).

FURTHER READING

Ahmad, S., Kuraganti, G., Steenkamp, D., 2015. Hypercalcaemic crisis: a clinical review. Am. J. Med. 128, 239–245.

Black, D.M., Rosen, C.J., 2016. Postmenopausal osteoporosis. N. Engl. J. Med. 374, 254–262.

Cooper, M.S., Gittoes, N.J.L., 2008. Diagnosis and management of hypocalcaemia. B.M.J. 336, 1298–1302.

Elder, C.J., Bishop, N.J., 2014. Rickets. Lancet 383, 1665–1676.

Maraka, S., Kennel, K.A., 2015. Bisphosphonates for the prevention and treatment of osteoporosis. Br. Med. J. 351, h3783.

Marcocci, C., Cetani, F., 2011. Primary hyperparathyroidism. N. Engl. J. Med. 365, 2389–2397.

Mazziotti, G., Canalis, E., Giustina, A., 2010. Drug-induced osteoporosis: mechanisms and clinical implications. Am. J. Med. 123, 877–884.

Minisola, S., Pepe, J., Piemonte, S., et al., 2015. The diagnosis and management of hypercalcaemia. Br. Med. J. 350, h2723.

Pallan, S., Omair Rahman, M., Khan, A.A., 2012. Diagnosis and management of primary hyperparathyroidism. Br. Med. J. 344, e1013.

Pearce, S.H.S., Cheetham, T.D., 2010. Diagnosis and management of vitamin D deficiency. Br. Med. J. 340, b5664.

Rachner, T.D., Khosla, S., Hofbauer, L.C., 2011. Osteoporosis: now and the future. Lancet 377, 1276–1287.

Ralston, S.H., 2013. Paget's disease of bone. N. Engl. J. Med. 368, 644–650.

Rosen, C.J., 2011. Vitamin D insufficiency. N. Engl. J. Med. 364, 248–254.

Compendium: drugs used to regulate calcium metabolism and in metabolic bone disease

Drug	Characteristics
Calcitonin and parathyroid hormone	
Calcitonin (salmon)/salcatonin	Involved with parathyroid hormone in regulation of bone turnover. Used to lower plasma Ca^{2+} in hypercalcaemia and for treatment of Paget's disease. Given intranasally, by subcutaneous or intramuscular injection or by slow intravenous infusion. Half-life: 12–21 min
Parathyroid hormone	Human recombinant parathyroid hormone. Given by subcutaneous injection for the treatment of postmenopausal osteoporosis. Half-life: 1.5 h
Teriparatide	A recombinant fragment (amino acids 1–34) of parathyroid hormone. Given by subcutaneous injection for postmenopausal and corticosteroid-induced osteoporosis. Half-life: 1 h

Compendium: drugs used to regulate calcium metabolism and in metabolic bone disease (cont'd)

Drug	Characteristics
Bisphosphonates	
Bisphosphonates are tightly adsorbed onto hydroxyapatite crystals in bone and reduce bone turnover; the adsorbed fraction is eliminated very slowly (years).	
Alendronic acid (alendronate)	First-line option for the prevention and treatment of osteoporosis. Given orally
Clodronate (sodium)	Used for hypercalcaemia of malignancy. Given orally or by slow intravenous infusion
Ibandronic acid	Potent bisphosphonate. Used for osteoporosis, hypercalcaemia of malignancy, and for bone metastases in breast cancer. Given orally or intravenously
Pamidronate (disodium)	Used for hypercalcaemia of malignancy, Paget's disease and bone metastases of breast cancer or multiple myeloma. Given by slow intravenous infusion
Risedronate sodium	Potent bisphosphonate. Given orally for the prevention and treatment of osteoporosis and Paget's disease
Zoledronic acid	Used for prevention and treatment of osteoporosis, Paget's disease, hypercalcaemia of malignancy, and reduction of bone damage in advanced malignancies. Given by intravenous infusion (annually for osteoporosis)
Vitamin D	
Because vitamin D requires metabolic activation in the kidneys, alfacalcidol or calcitriol should be used in cases of severe renal impairment.	
Alfacalcidol	1α-Hydroxycholecalciferol; oxidised by a 25-hydroxylase to active calcitriol. Given orally or by intravenous injection Half-life: 3 h
Calcitriol	$1\alpha,25$-Dihydroxycholecalciferol. Given orally or by intravenous injection. Half-life: 3–6 h
Colecalciferol (vitamin D_3)	Oxidised to 25-hydroxycholecalciferol (calcidiol), then to active 1,25-dihydroxyvitamin D_3 (calcitriol) in the kidney. Given orally or by intravenous injection
Dihydrotachysterol	Synthetic analogue of vitamin D_2. Given orally
Ergocalciferol (calciferol; vitamin D_2)	Metabolised to cholecalciferol, then to active 1,25-dihydroxyvitamin D_3 (calcitriol) in liver and kidney. Given orally or by intravenous injection. Half-life: 19–24 h
Paricalcitol	Synthetic vitamin D analogue (19-nor-1α-25-dihydroxyvitamin D_2); binds to vitamin D receptor and inhibits parathyroid hormone synthesis. Used for secondary hyperparathyroidism in chronic renal failure. Given by slow intravenous injection. Half-life: 4–6 h
Other drugs affecting bone metabolism	
Denosumab	Human monoclonal antibody that blocks interaction of RANK and RANK ligand. Used for treatment of osteoporosis. Given subcutaneously twice yearly. Half-life: 26 days
Raloxifene	SERM. Used for the treatment and prevention of postmenopausal osteoporosis; does not affect menopausal vasomotor symptoms. Given orally. Half-life: 28 h
Strontium ranelate	Used for postmenopausal osteoporosis in women over 75 years if bisphosphonates are poorly tolerated. Given orally. Half-life: 60 h

RANK, Receptor activator of nuclear factor-κB; *SERM*, selective oestrogen receptor modulator.

43 Pituitary and hypothalamic hormones

ANTERIOR PITUITARY AND RELATED HYPOTHALAMIC HORMONES

The hypothalamus produces several hormones that control the release of hormones from the pituitary. Most are covered in this chapter, except thyrotropin and thyrotropin-releasing hormone, which are considered in Chapter 41.

GROWTH HORMONE

Growth hormone (GH), or somatotropin, is a peptide that is synthesised in specific somatotropic cells in the anterior pituitary. Its secretion is controlled by the hypothalamus by a balance between growth hormone-releasing hormone (GHRH) and somatostatin (SST), which is also called growth hormone release-inhibiting hormone (GHRIH; Fig. 43.1). The balance of GHRH and somatostatin is maintained by the stimulant effects of nutrition, sleep and exercise, with the inhibitory effects of free fatty acids, glucose and glucocorticoids.

GH is released in pulses repeatedly throughout the day and night. Like other peptide hormones, GH binds to cell surface receptors and activates several intracellular pathways, including production of insulin-like growth factor 1 (IGF-1, a somatomedin) in the liver. IGF-1 mediates many, but not all, of the effects of GH.

GH stimulates cell growth and division and has anabolic actions on protein metabolism that promote growth in most tissues, increasing skeletal muscle mass and stimulating epiphyseal cartilage growth (see Box 43.1). IGF-1 also binds to the insulin receptor and promotes hepatic gluconeogenesis. These actions have encouraged some athletes to misuse GH to increase muscle mass.

GH is also a stress hormone that mobilises glucose by reducing liver uptake and promotes lipolysis that increases circulating free fatty acids.

Growth hormone for therapeutic use

Example

somatropin (recombinant human GH)

Somatropin has several therapeutic uses in children with growth failure or short stature. These include:

- to improve linear growth in children with proven GH deficiency, which is usually due to lack of GHRH (pituitary dwarfism);
- chronic renal insufficiency before puberty;
- Turner syndrome and Prader–Willi syndrome.

To be effective, the hormone must be given before the closure of the epiphyses in long bones. Treatment should be stopped if growth velocity does not increase by at least 50% from baseline.

Adult GH deficiency may warrant treatment with somatropin if all the following criteria are fulfilled:

- severe GH deficiency;
- impaired quality of life;
- already receiving treatment for another pituitary hormone deficiency.

A recombinant form of IGF-1 (mecasermin) is now available for primary IGF-1 deficiency in children or for children with GH gene deletion who have developed neutralising antibodies to GH.

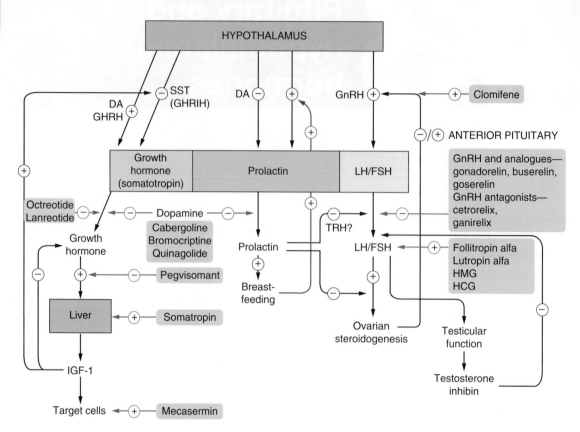

Fig. 43.1 Control mechanisms for the release of growth hormone, gonadotropins and prolactin from the anterior pituitary. For control of other hormones, see Chapter 41 (thyroid) and Chapter 44 (adrenocorticotropic hormones). Oestrogen effects on gonadotropin-releasing hormone (GnRH) are shown as both positive and negative, because oestrogen suppresses luteinizing hormone (LH) secretion in the early follicular phase but enhances secretion around ovulation (see Chapter 45). The actions of drugs are shown by red arrows. Gonadorelin is a synthetic GnRH, and buserelin and goserelin are GnRH analogues. Pulsatile administration of GnRH or its analogues enhances LH/follicle-stimulating hormone (FSH). On continuous administration, they downregulate the GnRH receptors, inhibiting LH/FSH release, an effect produced more rapidly by GnRH antagonists (cetrorelix, ganirelix). Somatropin is a synthetic growth hormone (GH), and mecasermin is a recombinant version of human insulin-like growth factor 1 (IGF-1), the somatomedin that mediates most of the somatotropic effects of GH. Octreotide and lanreotide are analogues of somatostatin (SST; also called GHRIH, growth hormone release-inhibiting hormone) that suppress GH release, and pegvisomant is a GH receptor antagonist. For details of dopamine (DA) agonists such as cabergoline, see Chapter 24. Dopamine stimulates GH release in healthy individuals, but paradoxically in acromegaly it inhibits release. *GHRH,* Growth hormone-releasing hormone; *HMG,* human menopausal gonadotropins (menotrophin); *HCG,* human chorionic gonadotropin.

> **Box 43.1 Effects of growth hormone**
>
> Anabolic effects on protein synthesis in muscle
> Increases bone growth and mineralisation
> Increases lipolysis
> Stimulates growth of most internal organs
> Reduces liver uptake of glucose and promotes gluconeogenesis
> Stimulates the immune system

Pharmacokinetics

Somatropin is given by subcutaneous injection. Intravenous somatropin has a short half-life (0.4 hours), but when given subcutaneously, its half-life is 2–3 hours due to slow absorption from the injection site.

Unwanted effects

- Headache, occasionally associated with visual problems, nausea and vomiting, and papilloedema from benign intracranial hypertension.
- Fluid retention with peripheral oedema.
- Arthralgia, myalgia, carpal tunnel syndrome.
- A transient insulin-like action occasionally produces hypoglycaemia.
- Pain at the injection site.

Acromegaly

Acromegaly results from excessive production of GH, almost always by an adenoma in the anterior pituitary, which also secretes prolactin in one-third of cases (see Fig. 43.1). The most common clinical features arise from excessive growth of bone and soft tissue. Metabolic consequences include insulin resistance with diabetes mellitus and hypertension.

If left untreated, people with acromegaly have a life expectancy approximately half that of the general population, due to an excess incidence of cardiovascular and respiratory disease and of carcinoma of the colon. Acromegaly is therefore usually treated actively.

Drugs for acromegaly

Somatostatin analogues

lanreotide, octreotide

Mechanisms of action and uses

The synthetic derivatives of SST are both more potent and longer-acting inhibitors of GH secretion than the native compound. Like SST, they also inhibit the release of gastrointestinal peptide hormones, such as insulin, enteroglucagon, cholecystokinin, gastrin, secretin, gastric inhibitory polypeptide (GIP) and vasoactive intestinal peptide (VIP). These actions make SST analogues useful for the treatment of a variety of conditions associated with excess secretion of gut hormones.

Uses of SST analogues include:

- Management of acromegaly.
- Management of other endocrine tumours – for example, carcinoid tumours (to reduce flushing and diarrhoea), VIPoma (to reduce diarrhoea) and glucagonoma (to improve the characteristic necrolytic rash).
- Management of medullary thyroid tumours (lanreotide) and prevention of complications following pancreatic surgery (octreotide).
- Octreotide is sometimes used to stop bleeding from oesophageal varices (see Chapter 36).

Pharmacokinetics

Octreotide is given by subcutaneous injection. It has a short half-life (1–2 hours) but suppresses GH secretion for up to 8 hours so it is used three times daily. An intramuscular depot preparation is available, which has a duration of action of about 4 weeks. Lanreotide also has a short half-life (1–2 hours) and is formulated as a sustained-release preparation given by subcutaneous or intramuscular injection every 1–4 weeks, depending on the indication.

Unwanted effects

- Gastrointestinal upset is common, especially anorexia, nausea, vomiting, abdominal pain, bloating and diarrhoea. These usually resolve with continued treatment.
- Impaired glucose tolerance.
- Gallstones, due to suppression of cholecystokinin secretion with decreased gallbladder motility. In addition, an increase in bowel transit time alters colonic flora and makes bile salts more lithogenic.
- Pain at the injection site.

Growth hormone receptor antagonist

pegvisomant

Mechanism of action

Pegvisomant is a pegylated synthetic analogue of GH that acts as a highly selective GH receptor antagonist.

Pharmacokinetics

Pegvisomant is given by subcutaneous injection. The addition of polyethylene glycol polymers slows clearance from the blood, and it has a very long half-life of 6 days.

Unwanted effects

- Nausea, vomiting, dyspepsia, abdominal distension, diarrhoea, constipation.
- Hypertension.
- Headache, dizziness, fatigue, drowsiness, tremor, sleep disturbance.
- Influenza-like symptoms, arthralgia, myalgia.
- Weight gain, hypo- or hyperglycaemia.
- Injection site reactions.

Dopamine receptor agonists

In healthy people, dopaminergic receptor stimulation increases the secretion of GH, but in acromegaly there is a paradoxical decrease. Bromocriptine was originally used to treat acromegaly, but the clinical response was unpredictable, and control of plasma IGF-1 was achieved in only about 20% of cases. It has been superseded by better-tolerated and more effective drugs such as cabergoline. Further details of these drugs can be found in Chapter 24.

Treatment of acromegaly

Surgery by the trans-sphenoidal route is the usual treatment of choice, sometimes followed by external radiotherapy if the tumour is large.

Three groups may be suitable for drug treatment:

- those in whom an excess of GH persists despite surgery and radiotherapy. After radiotherapy, the plasma GH concentration can take 1–2 years to fall.
- those with mild acromegaly.
- the elderly.

SST analogues are the first-line treatment, with pegvisomant used when there is intolerance or failure to respond. Cabergoline is sometimes used together with an SST analogue when there is resistance to other treatments. The effectiveness of treatment is monitored by the plasma concentration of IGF-1.

ADRENOCORTICOTROPIC HORMONE

Adrenocorticotropic hormone (ACTH; corticotropin) is a single-chain polypeptide with 39 amino acids, of which the 24 that form the N-terminal region are essential for full biological activity. It acts via cell surface receptors to promote steroidogenesis in adrenocortical cells. Release of ACTH occurs in response to the hypothalamic peptide corticotropin-releasing hormone (CRH). CRH secretion is pulsatile and has a diurnal rhythm, with maximal release in the morning around the time of waking (see further details in Chapter 44). The release of CRH is affected by other factors, including chemical (e.g. antidiuretic hormone, opioid peptides), physical (e.g. heat, cold, injury) and psychological influences. The main inhibitory influence on ACTH release is negative feedback control by circulating glucocorticoids. This occurs at both hypothalamic and pituitary levels. Adrenal androgens, although stimulated by ACTH, play no part in feedback control.

Adrenocorticotropic hormone for therapeutic use

tetracosactide

Tetracosactide is a synthetic peptide analogue which consists of the active N-terminal amino acids 1–24 of the ACTH molecule.

Pharmacokinetics

There are two formulations of tetracosactide: a rapid-acting formulation that can be given by intravenous or intramuscular injection, and a depot formulation given by intramuscular injection. Tetracosactide is metabolised rapidly with a very short half-life of about 10 minutes.

Unwanted effects

Prolonged use will produce all the features of corticosteroid excess (see Chapter 44).

Uses of tetracosactide

- The rapid-acting form increases steroidogenesis for about an hour and is suitable for tests of adrenocortical function. In adrenal insufficiency there is a subnormal or no rise of plasma cortisol 30 minutes after intramuscular or intravenous injection of tetracosactide.
- The depot formulation is absorbed slowly into the circulation over several hours and can be used as an alternative to exogenous corticosteroid therapy. However, the unpredictable corticosteroid response means that the therapeutic value is limited.

PROLACTIN

Prolactin is a glycoprotein similar in structure to GH but secreted by distinct lactotroph cells in the anterior pituitary (see Fig. 43.1). Release of prolactin is stimulated by eating, sexual intercourse, ovulation and nursing. Dopamine released by the hypothalamus inhibits prolactin secretion via D_2 receptors on lactotrophs. Thyrotropin-releasing hormone (TRH) and oestrogen increase prolactin secretion.

The main target tissue for prolactin is the breast, which secretes milk in response to prolactin if the mammary glands have been primed by ovarian and other hormones. At delivery,

maternal plasma prolactin concentration is high. Prolactin continues to be released as long as suckling continues. A high plasma concentration of prolactin suppresses follicle-stimulating hormone (FSH) release from the pituitary and leads to a failure of ovarian follicle growth. This may explain the relative subfertility of women who are breastfeeding.

Prolactin has several other functions, including sexual gratification after intercourse, contributing to production of surfactant in the fetal lung and proliferation of oligodendrocytes that form the neural myelin sheath in the central nervous system.

Hyperprolactinaemia

Persistent hyperprolactinaemia is usually caused by a microadenoma of the anterior pituitary or by the action of dopamine receptor antagonist drugs such as phenothiazines (see Chapter 21). In younger women, hyperprolactinaemia can produce amenorrhoea, infertility and signs and symptoms of oestrogen deficiency (e.g. vaginal dryness and dyspareunia, galactorrhoea and osteoporosis). In men it may cause hypogonadism.

Management should, when relevant, involve withdrawal of a provoking drug. For a microadenoma, a dopamine D_2 receptor agonist such as cabergoline (see Chapter 24) can be used to suppress prolactin secretion and shrink the adenoma. Normal plasma prolactin concentration is achieved in up to 90% of cases using cabergoline or quinagolide. Pituitary surgery may be considered for treatment failure, or when there is a large adenoma that is producing pressure effects.

GONADOTROPIN-RELEASING HORMONE

Gonadotropin-releasing hormone (GnRH) is a decapeptide that is synthesised in the hypothalamus. GnRH is released in pulses into the hypophysial portal circulation and reaches the anterior pituitary, where it stimulates the synthesis and release of both lutenising hormone (LH) and FSH (see Fig. 43.1). In males, pulse frequency remains constant, whereas in females it varies through the menstrual cycle with a surge just before ovulation (see Chapter 45). There are cell surface receptors for GnRH in many organs outside the pituitary, but their role is poorly understood.

Receptors on gonadotrophic cells are upregulated by repeated stimulation with GnRH, but pulsatile exposure is essential to maintain responsiveness. Low-frequency pulses stimulate FSH release, and high-frequency pulses stimulate LH release. There is rapid tolerance to constant-rate infusions of GnRH because of downregulation of cell surface receptors. Therapeutic administration of GnRH can be used to mimic pulsatile stimulation or produce receptor downregulation, and these regimens have different clinical uses, as described later. There is negative feedback control of GnRH release via neural pathways and sex steroids (see Fig. 43.1).

GnRH-related products for therapeutic use

Synthetic GnRH (gonadorelin)

Synthetic GnRH is available for assessing hypothalamic–pituitary function and is given as a subcutaneous or intravenous injection. Unwanted effects are unusual, but include nausea, headaches and abdominal pain.

Gonadorelin analogues

buserelin, goserelin, leuprorelin

Mechanism of action

Structurally similar to the natural hormone, gonadorelin analogues (see Chapter 52) initially stimulate GnRH receptors, but with regular use rapidly promote receptor downregulation, which inhibits further gonadotropin production. The result is reduced production of oestrogen or androgen. This latter action underlies their clinical uses.

Clinical uses of gonadorelin analogues

- The main use is to reduce testosterone secretion to castration levels in men with prostatic cancer. An initial rise in testosterone from receptor stimulation can produce tumour 'flare' in the first 1–2 weeks of treatment (see Chapter 52). An antiandrogen such as cyproterone acetate (see Chapter 46) is usually given to counteract this effect.
- Treatment of endometriosis by reducing oestrogen secretion (for up to 6 months only).
- Treatment of advanced breast cancer in women, by reducing oestrogen secretion.
- To reduce endometrial thickness for 3–4 months prior to intrauterine surgery.
- Preparation of women for assisted conception by methods such as in vitro fertilisation (IVF) (discussed later).
- Suppression of precocious puberty.
- 'Hormonal castration' of males with severe sexual deviation.

Pharmacokinetics

Buserelin can be given by either subcutaneous injection or intranasal spray and has a short half-life (1–1.5 hours). Goserelin also has a short half-life and must be given by subcutaneous injection. It is available as an oily depot preparation, which inhibits gonadotropin production for up to 4 weeks after a single injection. Leuprorelin is given as a depot preparation by subcutaneous or intramuscular injection and acts for 1–3 months, depending on the formulation.

Unwanted effects

- Menopause-like symptoms in women, with hot flushes, sweating, vaginal dryness and loss of libido.
- Orchidectomy-like effects in men, with loss of libido, gynaecomastia and vasomotor instability.
- Headache.
- Hypersensitivity reactions, including skin rashes, asthma and anaphylaxis.
- Osteoporosis with prolonged use.
- Local reactions at injection sites, or intranasally with spray.

GnRH receptor antagonists

cetrorelix, ganirelix

Mechanism of action and uses

These drugs are competitive GnRH receptor antagonists that produce immediate, reversible suppression of gonadotropin secretion. They are used for assisted reproduction in the management of female infertility (IVF; discussed later). They have advantages compared with gonadorelin analogues in this role, since there is no initial surge of LH release (which can lead to cancellation of the IVF in about 20% of cycles).

Pharmacokinetics

Both cetrorelix and ganirelix are given by subcutaneous injection and have long half-lives of greater than 12 hours.

Unwanted effects

- Nausea.
- Headache.
- Injection-site reactions.

GONADOTROPINS

LH and FSH are glycoproteins synthesised in the anterior pituitary. Release is stimulated by pulsatile exposure to GnRH. Negative feedback by inhibin, a hormone produced by the gonads, selectively inhibits FSH secretion. In addition, both gonadotropins are subject to negative feedback from gonadal steroids, including progesterone (see Chapter 45).

In males, LH acts on specific receptors on the surface of the Leydig cells in the testes, leading to the production of testosterone. FSH acts in a similar way on the Sertoli cells of the seminiferous tubules, stimulating the formation of a specific androgen-binding protein.

In females, receptors for FSH and LH are found in granulosa cells of ovarian follicles, and activation triggers production of oestrogen. FSH is responsible for development of the ovarian follicle. The control of ovulation by LH and FSH is discussed in Chapter 45. Both FSH and LH, like human chorionic gonadotropin (HCG), are also produced in large quantities by the placenta during pregnancy.

Prior to puberty, the hypothalamus and pituitary are very sensitive to negative feedback from sex hormones. This sensitivity decreases during puberty to adult levels, which allows increased production of oestrogen or testosterone.

Gonadotropins for therapeutic use

- Human menopausal gonadotropins (HMGs, or menotrophin) are a combination of FSH and LH in a 1:1 ratio that is extracted from urine obtained from postmenopausal women.
- HCG contains large quantities of LH with little FSH. It is secreted by the placenta and extracted from the urine of pregnant women. An alternative preparation is human choriogonadotropin alpha (recombinant human chorionic gonadotropin).
- Follitropin alpha and beta (recombinant human FSH; see Fig. 43.1) and corifollitropin alpha (modified recombinant FSH).
- Lutropin alpha (recombinant human LH; see Fig. 43.1).
- Gonadotropins are given by intramuscular or subcutaneous injection.

Unwanted effects

- Nausea and vomiting.
- Breast, abdominal and pelvic pain.
- Headache.
- In women the most serious problem during assisted conception is ovarian hyperstimulation syndrome, in which the ovaries can become grossly enlarged as a result of multiple follicle stimulation, leading to considerable abdominal pain, ascites and even pleural effusions.
- In men the most common problem is gynaecomastia or oedema with prolonged use.

Clinical uses of gonadotropins

- Treatment of infertility in women with hypopituitarism.
- Treatment of infertility in women after failure of clomifene treatment (discussed later).
- To create superovulation prior to assisted conception (such as *in vitro* fertilisation).
- In men with hypogonadotropic hypogonadism and oligospermia. This requires long courses of gonadotropin injections, initially to achieve external sexual maturation and then to maintain satisfactory sperm production. Spermatozoa take 70–80 days to mature, and a year or more of treatment may be needed to achieve optimal response. A combination of HMG and HCG is usually given.

INFERTILITY

Infertility is said to be present after 1 year of unprotected intercourse without conception. It has several causes, which requires full evaluation of both partners before treatment is given or assisted conception is considered.

Clomifene

Mechanism of action and use

Clomifene is a selective oestrogen receptor modulator that has both oestrogenic and antioestrogenic properties. It is an antagonist at hypothalamic oestrogen receptors and inhibits the negative feedback of oestrogen on gonadotropin release. It is used to stimulate ovulation in anovulatory infertility.

Pharmacokinetics

Clomifene is given orally and it has a very long half-life of 5 days.

Unwanted effects

- Reversible ovarian enlargement and cyst formation.
- Hot flushes.
- Abdominal or pelvic pain.
- Nausea, vomiting.
- Breast tenderness, weight gain.

Drug treatment of female infertility

When infertility is due to hyperprolactinaemia, then a dopamine agonist such as cabergoline should suppress prolactin levels and permit ovulation in 70–80% of women. The management of polycystic ovary syndrome is considered later.

When deficiency of gonadal stimulation by gonadotropin is the limiting factor, FSH (follitropin) can be given with LH (HMG), or in combination as HCG to encourage the development of a single mature ovarian follicle (see Chapter 45). Ovarian hyperstimulation can be a problem with this treatment.

If the hypothalamic–pituitary axis is functioning normally, clomifene is given from day 3 to day 5 of the menstrual cycle to decrease the negative feedback on FSH secretion (see Fig. 43.1). Increased FSH will stimulate ovarian follicle growth and oestrogen production. Since clomifene inhibits the negative feedback of oestrogen on the hypothalamus, more pulsatile GnRH secretion is promoted, with a relative increase in FSH which causes growth of the ovarian follicle. Ovulation usually occurs 6–7 days after the course of clomifene. There is a small risk of ovarian hyperstimulation, or multiple ovulation resulting in twins or triplets in about 10% of those who become pregnant.

Preparation for assisted conception (*in vitro* fertilisation)

When standard treatments for infertility are ineffective or not possible, then assisted conception with *in vitro* fertilisation of the ovum followed by embryo transfer into the uterus can be considered. There are many techniques to prepare the woman for IVF. Ovulation is usually targeted on a particular date, and a gonadorelin analogue or a GnRH antagonist is given to 'switch off' natural cyclical menstrual activity. Ovarian stimulation treatment is then begun to achieve maturation of oocytes at the time chosen for egg recovery prior to IVF. This involves giving HCG to stimulate the maturation of several follicles (superovulation treatment). These ova are then 'harvested' by transvaginal aspiration of the follicles.

Polycystic ovary syndrome

Polycystic ovary syndrome is a common cause of infertility, affecting 5–10% of women of reproductive age. It is characterised by abnormal ovarian function with hyperandrogenism. Menstrual disturbance, infertility, hirsutism, alopecia and acne are common. Polycystic ovary syndrome is often associated with obesity and insulin resistance in adipose and muscle tissue, conferring an increased risk of diabetes mellitus, hyperlipidaemia and cardiovascular disease in later life. Increased insulin secretion is also a factor in stimulating ovarian androgen production.

Management of polycystic ovary syndrome

Assessment and treatment of cardiovascular risk is an important component of management. If infertility is the main concern, weight loss (especially if the body mass index is > 29 kg/m^2) may restore ovulatory cycles. Metformin (see Chapter 40) can be used to improve fertility if weight loss is ineffective, as the resulting improvement in insulin sensitivity reduces the circulating androgen concentration. Metformin also encourages weight loss. Clomifene can be used to encourage ovulation if fertility is not restored.

Androgen-related symptoms are usually treated with a combined oral hormonal contraceptive if the woman does not wish to become pregnant, which can improve hirsutism and acne. Hormonal contraception will also improve menstrual irregularity. If androgen-related symptoms persist, antiandrogen therapy with cyproterone acetate (see Chapter 46) in combination with an oestrogen can be used. The aldosterone antagonist spironolactone (see Chapter 14) also has antiandrogenic activity and can be effective. Eflornithine cream (an ornithine decarboxylase inhibitor) can slow facial hair growth by inhibiting cell division in hair follicles. Topical minoxidil (see Chapter 6) may be helpful to reverse male-pattern hair loss on the scalp.

POSTERIOR PITUITARY HORMONES

VASOPRESSIN (ANTIDIURETIC HORMONE)

Vasopressin is a nonapeptide, sometimes referred to as arginine-vasopressin (AVP) because human vasopressin has an arginine residue in position 8. It is also known as the antidiuretic hormone (ADH). Vasopressin is produced in neurosecretory cells of the hypothalamus and transported down the axons of the nerve cells to the posterior pituitary. It is stored in the nerve endings in the posterior pituitary. Vasopressin is released in response to stimulation of the hypothalamus via osmoreceptors and baroreceptors in response to reduced plasma volume or increased plasma osmolality. Vasopressin has two main target tissues:

- Stimulation of V1 receptors in vascular smooth muscle leads to Ca^{2+} influx and vasoconstriction. Vasoconstriction sufficient to raise blood pressure only occurs at high plasma vasopressin concentrations and becomes important in hypovolaemic shock.
- Stimulation of V2 receptors in the distal convoluted tubule and collecting ducts of the kidney nephron leads to expression of aquaporin-2 channels that allow water reabsorption down an osmotic gradient to produce more concentrated urine. Enhanced expression of urea transporters in the connecting tubule and collecting duct increases urea reabsorption from the renal filtrate.

Vasopressin has a very short half-life of about 10 minutes. It is given therapeutically by subcutaneous or intramuscular injection or by intravenous infusion.

Vasopressin analogues

desmopressin, terlipressin

Desmopressin, des-amino-D-arginine-vasopressin (DDAVP), has a much longer duration of action, increased antidiuretic potency and reduced pressor activity, compared with vasopressin. An additional action of desmopressin is to increase clotting factor VIII concentration in blood (see Chapter 11).

Terlipressin is a vasopressin analogue with potent vasoconstrictor activity.

Pharmacokinetics

Desmopressin is administered via a nasal spray, orally or sublingually. It can also be given by subcutaneous, intramuscular or intravenous injection. Desmopressin has a longer half-life (0.5–2 hours) than vasopressin. Terlipressin is given intravenously. It is a prodrug that is hydrolysed to active lysine-vasopressin, which has a half-life of 0.5 hours.

Unwanted effects

- Excessive water retention, producing dilutional hyponatraemia.
- Headache.
- Nausea, vomiting and abdominal pain.

Clinical uses of vasopressin and its analogues

- Vasopressin can be given acutely for treatment of cranial diabetes insipidus (discussed later), using the longer-acting desmopressin orally, sublingually or intranasally for maintenance treatment.
- Desmopressin can be given orally or sublingually for primary nocturnal enuresis.
- Desmopressin given intranasally or by intravenous infusion is used to boost factor VIII concentration and reduce bleeding in mild to moderate haemophilia.
- Desmopressin is used by intramuscular or subcutaneous injection to treat lumbar puncture-associated headache.
- Desmopressin can be given to test for urine-concentrating ability in suspected diabetes insipidus (discussed later).
- Terlipressin given intravenously can control bleeding from oesophageal varices in portal hypertension (see Chapter 36). Vasopressin is sometimes used for this indication.
- Vasopressin is given for its pressor activity in the treatment of shock, when it also increases vascular sensitivity to noradrenaline.

Diabetes insipidus

Diabetes insipidus is usually caused by a failure of secretion of vasopressin in the hypothalamus ('cranial' diabetes insipidus). Tumours, inflammatory conditions, granulomatous conditions such as sarcoidosis, and trauma to the hypothalamus are the main causes. A distinct condition known as nephrogenic diabetes insipidus occurs when the kidney is less responsive or unresponsive to vasopressin. It can result from a hereditary deficiency of renal vasopressin receptors, or from drug therapy, particularly with lithium (see Chapter 22) or the tetracycline demeclocycline. Diabetes insipidus presents clinically with thirst, polyuria and a tendency to high plasma osmolality, together with an inappropriately low urine osmolality.

Management of diabetes insipidus

Vasopressin produces concentrated urine in people with cranial diabetes insipidus, but desmopressin is used for long-term treatment because of its longer duration of action. Treatment of nephrogenic diabetes insipidus is more difficult, because the kidney does not respond to vasopressin. If possible, a precipitating drug should be withdrawn. Paradoxically, thiazide diuretics (see Chapter 14) can reduce the polyuria. This may be due to initial contraction in extracellular volume, with subsequent increase in proximal tubular salt and water retention. Carbamazepine (see Chapter 23) is also effective, by sensitising the renal tubule to the effect of vasopressin.

Syndrome of inappropriate antidiuresis

This is a condition caused by inappropriately high secretion of vasopressin, resulting in excess water retention and a dilutional hyponatraemia. There are many causes, including malignant tumours that secrete vasopressin, pulmonary disorders (including infection) and various disorders of the central nervous system. Drugs such as antidepressants (see Chapter 22), carbamazepine (see Chapter 23) and various cytotoxic agents can also produce the syndrome.

Vasopressin V2 receptor antagonist

tolvaptan

Mechanism of action and uses

Tolvaptan is a competitive antagonist at vasopressin V2 receptors. Its major action is in the renal collecting ducts to reduce water reabsorption and produce aquaresis without sodium loss, thus increasing free water clearance and correcting dilutional hyponatraemia. Tolvaptan is effective for the treatment of hyponatraemia, secondary to inappropriate ADH secretion and also for correction of diuretic-induced hyponatraemia in cirrhosis and in heart failure.

Pharmacokinetics

Tolvaptan is given orally and has a half-life of about 8 hours.

Unwanted effects

- Thirst, dry mouth, polyuria.
- Hypotension.
- Hypernatraemia.
- Hypoglycaemia.

Treatment of syndrome of inappropriate antidiuresis

Severe hyponatraemia can cause confusion, seizures and coma, especially if it has an acute onset. In this situation, water moves into cells down the osmotic gradient, leading to cerebral oedema. If the hyponatraemia has been present for less than 48 hours, there will not have been time for neuronal adaptation, and rapid correction of the serum sodium, usually with intravenous saline 0.9%, is possible without causing harm. Less severe hyponatraemia may respond to fluid restriction.

Neuronal adaptation to hyponatraemia occurs over 48 hours, with loss of solutes from the neurons to prevent intracellular accumulation of water. Slow correction of the serum Na^+ concentration is then important, unless the hyponatraemia is producing severe symptoms, when more rapid initial correction may be required. With hyponatraemia that has been present for more than 48 hours, if the serum sodium is then raised to the point where extracellular fluid is more concentrated than the intracellular fluid before equilibration can occur across the cell membrane, the osmotic gradient draws water out of brain cells. The resulting cell shrinkage can produce a condition called central pontine myelinolysis, leading to dysarthria, spastic quadriparesis and pseudobulbar palsy. These symptoms can appear several days after the serum sodium is corrected and may be irreversible. Limiting any rise in serum Na^+ to 8–10 mmol/L in the first 24 hours will minimise the risk of osmotic demyelination.

In some situations, enhanced renal tubular water loss can be achieved by antagonising the effect of vasopressin on the kidney. Demeclocycline, a tetracycline antimicrobial agent, reduces the sensitivity of the collecting ducts to vasopressin and can be used to correct moderate hyponatraemia in addition to fluid restriction. The vasopressin V2 receptor antagonist tolvaptan is not suitable for urgent treatment of severe hyponatraemia, when there is a risk of significant neurological complications. When initiating treatment, it is important to monitor the rise in serum sodium to avoid rapid correction and precipitation of osmotic demyelination syndrome.

OXYTOCIN

Oxytocin is discussed in Chapter 45.

HYPOPITUITARISM

Pituitary insufficiency can arise from traumatic brain injury and subarachnoid haemorrhage, when a single hormonal axis is often affected. Pituitary irradiation or surgery, by contrast, often affects multiple hormones. Less common causes include both pituitary and nonpituitary intracranial tumours, and ischaemic damage.

Replacement of a deficiency of glucocorticoid (see Chapter 44) and thyroid (see Chapter 41) hormonal function is essential and urgent. Female sex hormone (see Chapter 45) or testosterone (see Chapter 46) replacement can be important at a later stage to restore libido and bone mass. In some individuals, deficiency of GH or vasopressin may also require replacement.

SELF-ASSESSMENT

True/false questions

1. The release of growth hormone (GH, somatotropin) is reduced by somatostatin.
2. Somatostatin is only produced by the hypothalamus.
3. Octreotide is a useful drug for the treatment of acromegaly.
4. Pegvisomant is a pegylated GH analogue that stimulates GH receptors.
5. Prolactin suppresses ovarian steroidogenesis.
6. Cabergoline reduces prolactin secretion.
7. Continuous administration of gonadorelin analogues stimulates synthesis of sex steroids.
8. The gonadorelin analogue buserelin stimulates gonadotropin-releasing hormone (GnRH) receptors

and is used for the treatment of endometriosis, but has no clinical use in males.

9. Cetrorelix and ganirelix are GnRH receptor antagonists used in female infertility.

10. Follitropin alpha is a recombinant follicle-stimulating hormone (FSH) analogue used in preparation for in vitro fertilisation.

11. The production of vasopressin is impaired in nephrogenic diabetes insipidus.

12. Vasopressin increases expression of aquaporin channels.

13. Desmopressin is administered by intranasal spray in cranial diabetes insipidus.

14. Tolvaptan is used in the urgent treatment of severe hyponatraemia.

15. In nephrogenic diabetes insipidus, thiazide diuretics increase the polyuria.

One-best-answer (OBA) question

Identify the *inaccurate* statement below about GH.
A. The release of GH is constant over a 24-hour period.
B. GH acts mainly by stimulating release of insulin-like growth factor 1 (IGF-1).
C. In acromegaly, cabergoline reduces GH levels.
D. IGF-1 has a negative feedback effect on GH release.
E. Somatropin is used for GH deficiency in children.

Case-based questions

An assessment of a 10-year-old girl with short stature shows that she has abnormally low levels of growth hormone-releasing hormone (GHRH) and GH.
1. Is this girl too old to benefit from treatment?
2. What treatment should be recommended and how should it be administered?
3. What unwanted effects might occur?

ANSWERS

True/false answers

1. **True.** Somatostatin is also known as growth hormone release-inhibiting hormone (GHRIH).

2. **False.** Somatostatin is also produced from intestinal and pancreatic cells.

3. **True.** Octreotide is a long-acting analogue of somatostatin and therefore inhibits GH release.

4. **False.** Pegvisomant is a pegylated analogue of GH, but it selectively blocks GH receptors; it is used when somatostatin analogues such as octreotide are poorly tolerated or ineffective.

5. **True.** Prolactin inhibits FSH release and suppresses ovarian follicle growth and steroidogenesis.

6. **True.** Cabergoline is a dopamine receptor agonist and inhibits prolactin release from the anterior pituitary; it can be used to improve fertility in women with hyperprolactinaemia.

7. **False.** Although brief administration of gonadorelin analogues stimulates sex steroid synthesis, on continued administration, gonadotropin receptors are rapidly downregulated and sex steroid synthesis declines.

8. **False.** Gonadorelin analogues downregulate GnRH receptors and are used to inhibit testosterone synthesis in prostate cancer, as well as reducing synthesis of ovarian hormones in endometriosis.

9. **True.** GnRH receptor antagonists produce immediate suppression of gonadotropin secretion without the initial surge in LH caused by gonadorelin analogues.

10. **True.** Follitropin alpha is a synthetic FSH analogue and promotes follicle development.

11. **False.** In nephrogenic diabetes insipidus, the kidney is unresponsive to vasopressin; the production of vasopressin is impaired in cranial diabetes insipidus.

12. **True.** Vasopressin (antidiuretic hormone) acting at V2 receptors enhances water reabsorption by increasing aquaporin-2 channels in the renal collecting duct.

13. **True.** Desmopressin is a modified vasopressin with a longer duration of action and selectivity for V2 receptors in the kidney.

14. **False.** The vasopressin V2 antagonist tolvaptan is licensed for maintenance treatment of hyponatraemia caused by excessive ADH secretion, but if used for acute treatment of severe hyponatraemia, it can cause neurological complications.

15. **False.** Paradoxically, in diabetes insipidus, the response to thiazide diuretics is a beneficial reduction in polyuria.

One-best-answer (OBA) answer

Answer A is the inaccurate statement.
A. **Incorrect.** GH is released in a pulsatile manner and its production is greater during deep sleep, particularly in children.
B. Correct. GH stimulates release of IGF-1 from the liver, which then acts as a somatomedin on receptors in many tissues and in concert with other hormones.
C. Correct. In normal individuals, dopamine receptor agonists such as cabergoline stimulate GH release, but in acromegaly they paradoxically inhibit GH release.
D. Correct. IGF-1 inhibits GH release and also stimulates somatostatin (GHRIH) release from the hypothalamus, which further inhibits GH release.
E. Correct. Somatropin is a recombinant GH used in growth failure. Growth failure due to primary deficiency of IGF-1 can be treated with mecasermin (rhIGF-1).

Case-based answers

1. Epiphyseal closure occurs much later than 10 years of age, so treatment of this patient with short stature can increase her growth.
2. Low levels of GHRH and GH suggest pituitary dwarfism, and therefore synthetic GH (somatropin) would be appropriate. Although somatropin has a half-life of only 25 minutes, it generates IGF-1, which is highly protein-bound, so three subcutaneous injections of somatropin a week are sufficient to maintain IGF-1 levels.
3. Transient insulin-like effects of somatropin can produce hypoglycaemia, and there may be pain at the site of injection. Headache and oedema can also occur.

FURTHER READING

Balen, A.H., Rutherford, A.J., 2007. Management of infertility. Br. Med. J. 335, 608–611.

Di Iorgi, N., Napoli, F., Allegri, A.E., et al., 2012. Diabetes insipidus—diagnosis and management. Horm. Res. Paediatr. 77, 69–84.

Giustina, A., Chanson, P., Kleinberg, D., et al., 2014. Expert consensus document: a consensus on the medical treatment of acromegaly. Nat. Rev. Endocrinol. 10, 243–248.

Gross, P., 2012. Clinical management of SIADH. Ther. Adv. Endocrinol. Metab. 3, 61–73.

Higham, C.E., Johannsson, G., Shalet, S.M., 2016. Hypopituitarism. Lancet 388, 2403–2415.

Hillier, S.G., 2013. IVF endocrinology: the Edwards era. Mol. Hum. Reprod. 19, 799–808.

Rogers, A., Karavitaki, N., Wass, J.A.H., 2014. Diagnosis and management of prolactinomas and non-functioning pituitary adenomas. Br. Med. J. 349, g5390.

Setji, T.L., Brown, A.J., 2014. Polycystic ovary syndrome: update on diagnosis and treatment. Am. J. Med. 127, 912–919.

Compendium: pituitary and hypothalamic hormones

Drug	Characteristics
Hypothalamic hormones and antagonists	
Gonadotropin-releasing hormone (GnRH)	
Gonadorelin	Synthetic preparation identical to GnRH. Used for endometriosis (see Chapter 45) and breast and prostate cancer (see Chapter 52). Given by subcutaneous or intravenous injection. Half-life: 4 min
Gonadorelin analogues	
Buserelin	Used for prostate cancer (see Chapter 52)
Goserelin	Used for prostate cancer (see Chapter 52)
Leuprorelin acetate	Used for prostate cancer (see Chapter 52)
Nafarelin	Used for endometriosis (see Chapter 45)
Triptorelin	Used for prostate cancer (see Chapter 52)
Gonadotropin-releasing hormone (GnRH) antagonists	
Inhibit the release of gonadotropins (LH and FSH); used to inhibit premature LH surges in the treatment of female infertility (under specialist supervision).	
Cetrorelix	Synthetic decapeptide. Given by subcutaneous injection. Half-life: 20–60 h
Ganirelix	Synthetic decapeptide. Given by subcutaneous injection. Half-life: 16 h
Drugs that interfere with gonadotropin release (antioestrogens)	
Antioestrogens used in the treatment of female infertility due to oligomenorrhoea or secondary amenorrhoea; they reduce negative feedback and induce gonadotropin release.	
Clomifene	Given orally. Half-life: 5 days
Tamoxifen	Main use is in breast cancer (see Chapter 52)
Somatostatin (growth hormone release-inhibiting hormone, GHRIH) analogues	
Lanreotide	Used for acromegaly and for neuroendocrine and thyroid tumours. Given by intramuscular or deep subcutaneous injection. Half-life: 1.3 h
Octreotide	Used for acromegaly and neuroendocrine tumours, and for reducing vomiting in palliative care and stopping oesophageal variceal bleeds. Given by subcutaneous injection or by intravenous injection. Half-life: 1.7 h
Pasireotide	Used for the treatment of Cushing's disease, when surgery has failed or is inappropriate. Given by subcutaneous injection. Half-life: 12 h
Anterior pituitary hormones and antagonists	
Corticotrophins	
Tetracosactide	Adrenocorticotropic hormone (ACTH) analogue. Used largely as a test of adrenocortical function. Given by intramuscular or intravenous injection. Half-life: 8 min

Compendium: pituitary and hypothalamic hormones (cont'd)

Drug	Characteristics
Gonadotropins (FSH, LH and HCG) and analogues	
Mainly used in the treatment of infertility in women with proven hypopituitarism or who have not responded to clomifene, or in superovulation treatment for assisted conception.	
Follitropin alpha and beta (FSH)	Recombinant human follicle-stimulating hormone (FSH). Given by subcutaneous or intramuscular injection. Half-life: 24–40 h
Lutropin alpha (LH)	Recombinant human luteinising hormone (LH). Given by subcutaneous injection. Half-life: 14 h
Human menopausal gonadotropins (menotrophin)	Contains a 1:1 mixture of FSH and LH. Given by deep intramuscular or subcutaneous injection. Half-life: 7–10 h (FSH) and 3 h (LH)
Human chorionic gonadotropin (HCG)	Mainly LH activity; extracted from urine of pregnant women. Given by subcutaneous or intramuscular injection. Half-life: 30–35 h
Choriogonadotropin alpha	Recombinant HCG. Given by subcutaneous injection. Half-life: 29 h
Corifollitropin alpha	Synthetic FSH (modified). Given by subcutaneous injection. Half-life: 59–79 h
Growth hormone and somatomedins	
Somatropin	Synthetic form of growth hormone (GH, somatotropin). Used to treat GH deficiency in children and in adults; also used in children for Prader-Willi syndrome, Turner syndrome, chronic renal insufficiency, short children considered small for gestational age at birth, and short stature homeobox-containing gene (SHOX) deficiency. Given by subcutaneous or intramuscular injection. Half-life: 2–3 h
Mecasermin	Recombinant version of human insulin-like growth factor 1 (IGF-1), the principal somatomedin mediating the somatotropic effects of human GH. Used to treat growth failure in children and adolescents with severe primary IGF-1 deficiency. Given by subcutaneous injection. Half-life: 6 h
Growth hormone receptor antagonists	
Pegvisomant	Pegylated synthetic antagonist of growth hormone receptors. Used for acromegaly in patients with inadequate response to surgery and/or radiation, and for treatment with GHRIH (somatostatin) analogues. Given by subcutaneous injection. Half-life: 6 days
Prolactin antagonists	
Used to suppress lactation. The ergot-derived drugs are associated with pulmonary, retroperitoneal and pericardial fibrosis.	
Bromocriptine	Ergot-derived D_2 receptor agonist. Given orally. See Chapter 24
Cabergoline	Ergot-derived D_2 receptor agonist. Given orally. See Chapter 24
Quinagolide	Nonergot D_2 receptor agonist. Given orally. Half-life: 17 h
Thyroid-stimulating hormone (TSH)	
Thyrotropin alpha	Recombinant TSH. Used to detect thyroid remnants post-thyroidectomy. Given by intramuscular injection. Half-life: 22 h
Posterior pituitary hormones and antagonists	
Demeclocycline	Tetracycline antibiotic with anti-ADH action in renal tubule. Used for treatment of hyponatraemia resulting from inappropriate secretion of ADH. Given orally. Half-life: 10–15 h
Desmopressin	Vasopressin analogue. Used for treatment of cranial diabetes insipidus. Given orally, intranasally, or by subcutaneous, intramuscular or intravenous injection. Half-life: 0.5–2 h
Terlipressin	Prodrug hydrolysed to active lysine-vasopressin. Used for treatment of oesophageal varices. Given by intravenous injection. Half-life: 0.5 h
Tolvaptan	Antagonist of vasopressin V2 receptors in renal collecting ducts. Used for treating hyponatraemia resulting from inappropriate secretion of ADH. Given orally. Half-life: 8 h
Vasopressin (ADH)	Used for treatment of cranial diabetes insipidus and bleeding oesophageal varices. Given by subcutaneous or intramuscular injection or by intravenous infusion. Half-life: 5–15 min

ACTH, Adrenocorticotropic hormone; *ADH*, antidiuretic hormone; *FSH*, follicle-stimulating hormone; *GHRIH*, growth hormone-release inhibiting hormone (somatostatin); *GnRH*, gonadotropin-releasing hormone; *HCG*, human chorionic gonadotropin; *IGF-1*, insulin-like growth factor 1; *LH*, luteinizing hormone.

44
Corticosteroids (glucocorticoids and mineralocorticoids)

- mineralocorticoid activity, which affects water and electrolyte balance.

The natural glucocorticoid is cortisol (also known as hydrocortisone), which has a hydroxyl grouping at position 17 and approximately equal affinity in vitro for glucocorticoid and mineralocorticoid receptors (but see further discussion later in this chapter). The natural mineralocorticoid is aldosterone, which has an aldehyde grouping at position 18 and has little glucocorticoid activity. Synthetic corticosteroids that have been modified structurally to enhance either the glucocorticoid or mineralocorticoid activity are widely used therapeutically.

Although hydrocortisone and various synthetic derivatives are used therapeutically for their glucocorticoid activity, they are frequently referred to as 'corticosteroids' or much less accurately as 'steroids'. In this chapter, the distinction between glucocorticoid and mineralocorticoid actions is emphasised. In the rest of the book, drugs with mainly glucocorticoid activity are usually referred to as corticosteroids.

CONTROL OF CORTICOSTEROID HORMONES

Cortisol (hydrocortisone) is released from the zona fasciculata of the adrenal cortex, and its secretion is controlled by the hypothalamo–pituitary–adrenal (HPA) axis (Fig. 44.3). Plasma glucocorticoid feeds back negatively to the hypothalamus and pituitary to reduce the release of corticotropin-releasing hormone (CRH) and adrenocorticotropic hormone (ACTH; corticotropin).

Aldosterone is secreted from the zona glomerulosa of the adrenal cortex. Aldosterone secretion is regulated by several factors, of which angiotensin II, low plasma Na^+ and high plasma K^+ are the most important. Angiotensin II acts via specific AT_1 receptors (see Chapter 6) to induce aldosterone release. ACTH has a modest stimulatory effect on aldosterone secretion.

MODE OF ACTION OF CORTICOSTEROID HORMONES

All steroid hormones have similar intracellular receptor mechanisms, but there are distinct receptors for the different structural variants (see Chapter 1). The distribution of the various receptors among tissues gives tissue specificity to each type of steroid hormone and defines its activity. Steroids are highly lipophilic and cross cell membranes by diffusion and bind to a specific cytoplasmic receptor. In the absence of a steroid molecule, the receptor is retained in the cytoplasm

CORTICOSTEROID HORMONES

Steroid hormones comprise several compounds that are synthesised mainly in the adrenal cortex and the gonads. They are derived from cholesterol and share a distinctive core structure of four conjoined rings (Fig. 44.1). The pathways of steroid hormone synthesis are shown in Fig. 44.2. The steroid hormones responsible for phenotypic gender differences are known as the sex hormones; these compounds are considered in Chapters 45 and 46.

This chapter considers steroid hormones derived predominantly from the adrenal cortex that are known as adrenal corticosteroids. They have two distinct classes of action (discussed later; see also Table 44.1):

- glucocorticoid activity, which affects carbohydrate and protein metabolism;

associated with a heat-shock protein (HSP), which prevents it from migrating to the cell nucleus. When the steroid binds to the receptor, the complex dissociates from the HSP, and the steroid–receptor complex then enters the nucleus and binds to a steroid-response element (SRE) in the promoter region of the target genes (see Fig. 1.8). SRE binding usually involves the presence of other proteins, called chaperone proteins, and can lead to either increased or decreased transcription of proteins, depending on the target cell. Some genes are activated by simple interaction of the steroid receptor with the SRE, but the rate of gene transcription is modulated by recruitment of various intranuclear co-regulator proteins and complexes. The corticosteroid receptor only interacts with the SRE for a matter of seconds before dissociating, and appears to have a 'hit-and-run' effect on gene transcription.

When corticosteroids are given for a therapeutic effect, the response is delayed by many hours, due to the time taken for modulation of protein synthesis. However, some actions of glucocorticoids are relatively rapid in onset and do not require gene transcription (nongenomic signalling pathways). Glucocorticoids may directly activate various kinases in the cell cytoplasm through a ligand-activated glucocorticoid receptor or through G-protein-coupled receptors, leading to effects such as vasodilation and regulation of cell growth.

Glucocorticoid receptors are found in most tissues, giving cortisol a wide range of actions. Mineralocorticoid receptors are found in several tissues, including the kidney, colon and heart. Important target cells are in the distal renal tubule and cortical collecting duct. Target cells for aldosterone,

Fig. 44.1 **The core structure of steroid hormones is derived from the cholesterol molecule shown.** The four rings are identified by a letter A–D, and each carbon atom by a number.

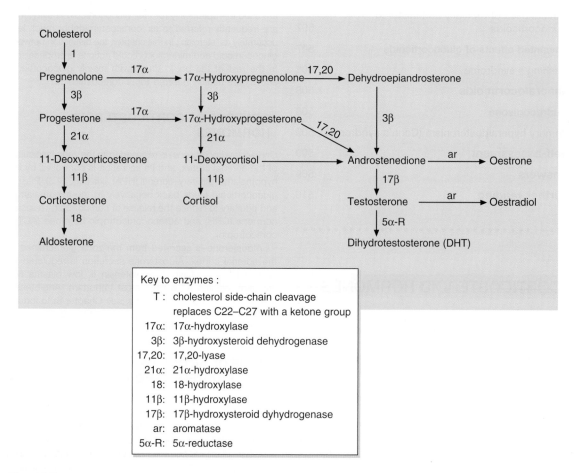

Fig. 44.2 Pathways of biosynthesis of steroid hormones, including progestogens, oestrogens, androgens, mineralocorticoids and glucocorticoids.

Table 44.1 Relative glucocorticoid and mineralocorticoid activities of some natural and synthetic corticosteroid hormones

	Glucocorticoid activity	Mineralocorticoid activity
Cortisol (hydrocortisone)	1	1
Prednisolone	4	0.8
Dexamethasone	30	Negligible
Betamethasone	30	Negligible
Aldosterone	0	80
Fludrocortisone	10	125

All potencies are relative to the glucocorticoid and mineralocorticoid activities of cortisol, each assigned an arbitrary value of 1. Due to intracellular metabolism by 11β-hydroxysteroid dehydrogenase in aldosterone-sensitive cells, cortisol has about one-thousandth of the mineralocorticoid activity of aldosterone in vivo.

especially in the renal tubule, contain 11β-hydroxysteroid dehydrogenase, which metabolises cortisol to cortisone. Cortisone has very low affinity for the mineralocorticoid receptor, and this ensures that most aldosterone-responsive tissues are not stimulated by endogenous glucocorticoid.

GLUCOCORTICOIDS

 Examples

betamethasone, dexamethasone, hydrocortisone, prednisolone

ACTIONS OF GLUCOCORTICOIDS

Immunosuppressant and antiinflammatory actions

Glucocorticoids have important immunomodulatory actions that underpin many of their therapeutic uses.

A major action of glucocorticoids is to silence proinflammatory genes (gene transrepression). Proinflammatory genes are activated by transcription factors such as nuclear factor κB (NF-κB) and activator protein 1 (AP-1), which are produced in response to inflammatory cytokines. NF-κB and AP-1 attach to the promoter region of the genes and recruit co-activator molecules such as cAMP response element-binding protein (CBP). CBP has histone acetyltransferase activity and acetylates core histones at the transcription complex. Acetylated core histones activate proinflammatory gene transcription, leading to the synthesis of inflammatory cytokines, chemokines, adhesion molecules, enzymes and receptors for inflammatory mediators. When glucocorticoid receptors enter the nucleus, they bind to CBP at the glucocorticoid response element of inflammatory genes and inhibit histone acetyltransferase activity by recruiting co-repressor

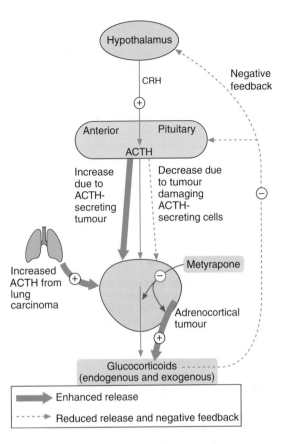

Fig. 44.3 Control of secretion of glucocorticoids. Corticotropin-releasing hormone (CRH) from the hypothalamus stimulates adrenocorticotropic hormone (ACTH; corticotropin) from the anterior pituitary, which increases the release of glucocorticoids from the adrenal cortex. The level of glucocorticoids in the blood feeds back negatively to control the release of CRH and ACTH. Synthetic glucocorticoids have the same suppressive action on the hypothalamo–pituitary–adrenal (HPA) axis. In conditions in which excess glucocorticoids are released (e.g. in ACTH-secreting tumours or adrenocortical tumours), glucocorticoid synthesis and release can be reduced by metyrapone *(red arrows)*. In people with tumours that result in hormone-induced reduction in glucocorticoids, synthetic glucocorticoids can be administered.

molecules. The glucocorticoid receptors also recruit histone deacetylase to suppress the proinflammatory genes.

Glucocorticoids also activate antiinflammatory genes (gene transactivation) by stimulation of core histone acetylation at their promoter regions.

Antiinflammatory effects

As a result of the above actions, glucocorticoids:

■ reduce T-lymphocyte proliferation and increase T-cell apoptosis, which impairs cell-mediated immunity (see Chapter 38). They also inhibit humoral immunity by reducing T-cell activation, B-lymphocyte proliferation and immunoglobulin production, particularly IgG (see Chapter 38).

- inhibit mononuclear cell and neutrophil leucocyte migration and their adhesion to inflamed capillary endothelium. The ability of these inflammatory cells to phagocytose and destroy micro-organisms and to release oxygen free radicals is also reduced through downregulation of their surface receptors (see Chapter 38).
- reduce the synthesis of inflammatory prostaglandins by inhibition of phospholipase A_2 activity and by suppression of cyclo-oxygenase expression (see Chapter 29).
- suppress fibroblast activity with reduced collagen synthesis and inhibition of matrix metalloproteinases, which impairs wound repair.
- decrease capillary permeability, which has a protective effect on blood volume and raises blood pressure. They also enhance the sensitivity of vascular walls to the vasoconstrictor actions of catecholamines and angiotensin II.

Metabolic effects

- Gluconeogenesis is increased, particularly in the liver, using amino acids and glycerol from triglycerides. Storage of glycogen in the liver and, to a lesser extent, in muscle is increased, and uptake and utilisation of glucose in muscle and adipose tissue are impaired. These actions promote hyperglycaemia.
- Protein is degraded, particularly in muscle, to release amino acids for synthesis of glucose while protein synthesis is inhibited. As a result, there is an overall negative nitrogen balance.
- Fat is redistributed from the glucocorticoid-sensitive fat stores in the limbs to the glucocorticoid-resistant stores in the face, neck and trunk. This action results from enhanced lipolytic response to catecholamines, and releases glycerol for glucose synthesis.

Effects on bone metabolism

- Osteoblast formation is decreased, and apoptosis of mature osteoblasts is increased. The function of mature osteoblasts is inhibited by reduced production of osteocalcin, a key extracellular matrix protein in bone that promotes bone mineralisation. Osteocyte apoptosis is increased, which stimulates osteoclast activity. By contrast, survival of osteoclasts is prolonged. These actions result in bone resorption and demineralisation.
- Inhibition of the proliferation and differentiation of chondrocytes at the epiphyseal end of the growth plate of long bones reduces bone growth in children.

Central nervous system effects

Plasma cortisol concentrations rise to a peak at the time of awakening and are lowest during sleep. In general, high circulating concentrations of cortisol are associated with alertness, but severe disturbances of mood may occur with abnormally high levels of glucocorticoid. Low concentrations produce a feeling of lethargy.

Mineralocorticoid effects

Mineralocorticoids act on cells in the distal renal tubule and cortical collecting duct, where they increase the permeability of the luminal tubular membrane to Na^+ by increasing the number of epithelial Na^+ channels (ENaC). They also stimulate the Na^+/K^+-ATPase pump in the basolateral membrane, which leads to active Na^+ reabsorption and loss of K^+ into tubular urine (see Chapter 14). Water is passively reabsorbed with Na^+, so that extracellular fluid volume and blood pressure are both increased. Natural glucocorticoids have some mineralocorticoid activity, although this has minimal impact at physiological doses (discussed previously). Synthetic glucocorticoid compounds are altered structurally to minimise the amount of mineralocorticoid activity (see Table 44.1).

PHARMACOKINETICS OF GLUCOCORTICOIDS

Both hydrocortisone and synthetic glucocorticoids are used in clinical practice. They are readily absorbed from the gut. Hydrocortisone binds to corticosteroid-binding globulin (transcortin) and to albumin in the blood, and is extensively metabolised in the gut wall and liver. Synthetic glucocorticoids bind to albumin but not to transcortin and are more slowly metabolised in the liver, giving them a longer duration of action. Of the many synthetic glucocorticoids, dexamethasone is the most potent and has the least mineralocorticoid activity.

Most glucocorticoids are available in formulations for parenteral use. This does not appreciably shorten the time to onset of action, since most effects are delayed by up to 8 hours while intracellular protein synthesis is modulated. Some glucocorticoids are available in formulations for topical use (e.g. beclometasone, budesonide and fluticasone by inhaler for asthma). Local delivery to the primary site of action reduces their systemic actions, although systemic unwanted effects can still occur, particularly with high doses.

The plasma half-lives of glucocorticoids vary, but because their mechanism of action depends on gene transcription and changes in protein synthesis, their biological (effective) half-lives are long (varying from 8 hours for hydrocortisone to 2 days for dexamethasone).

Physiological replacement therapy for corticosteroid deficiency

Addison's disease or pituitary insufficiency limits the ability of the adrenal glands to synthesise cortisol. Other conditions can give rise to glucocorticoid deficiency (Box 44.1). Acute adrenal insufficiency is life-threatening and requires immediate treatment with high-dose intravenous hydrocortisone. Replacement of deficient cortisol is usually with oral hydrocortisone, or an equivalent synthetic glucocorticoid is given orally twice or three times daily in doses as close as possible to the amount normally secreted by the adrenal cortex. The dose must be doubled or tripled in stressful situations – for example, intercurrent infection. If the cause of the corticosteroid deficiency is adrenal disease, replacement of deficient aldosterone production with fludrocortisone (discussed later) may also be necessary.

CLINICAL USES OF SYSTEMICALLY ADMINISTERED GLUCOCORTICOIDS

The antiinflammatory and immunosuppressant effects of glucocorticoids are used for control of various inflammatory

Box 44.1   Causes of glucocorticoid excess (Cushing's syndrome) and corticosteroid deficiency

Causes of Cushing's syndrome
- Excessive secretion of ACTH by the anterior pituitary (pituitary adenoma; Cushing's disease)
- Excessive secretion of ACTH from an ectopic source (most commonly carcinoma of the bronchus)
- A tumour of the adrenal cortex secreting predominantly cortisol
- Iatrogenic: administration of glucocorticoid or ACTH in pharmacological doses

Causes of corticosteroid deficiency
- Primary adrenal insufficiency (Addison's disease):
  - Autoimmune adrenalitis
  - Infections (e.g. tuberculosis, various fungi, opportunistic infections in AIDS)
  - Metastatic carcinoma
- Secondary adrenocortical failure (deficient ACTH from the anterior pituitary):
  - Pituitary tumour
  - Sarcoidosis
  - Suppression of the HPA axis by prolonged glucocorticoid treatment at pharmacological doses
  - Various enzyme defects in cortisol synthesis (congenital adrenal hyperplasia)

ACTH, Adrenocorticotropic hormone; *HPA,* hypothalamo–pituitary–adrenal.

Box 44.2   Examples of diseases for which systemic glucocorticoid therapy is useful

Replacement therapy in corticosteroid deficiency
Acute inflammatory disease:
 Bronchial asthma
 Anaphylaxis and angioedema
 Acute fibrosing alveolitis
Chronic inflammatory disease:
 Connective tissue disorders (e.g. systemic lupus erythematosus, polymyositis, vasculitis)
 Renal disorders (e.g. glomerulonephritis)
 Hepatic disorders (e.g. chronic active hepatitis)
 Bowel disorders (e.g. inflammatory bowel disease)
 Eye disorders (e.g. posterior uveitis)
Neoplastic disease:
 Myeloma
 Lymphomas
 Lymphocytic leukaemias
Miscellaneous disorders:
 Bell's palsy
 Sarcoidosis
 Organ transplantation
 Antiemetic therapy (for cytotoxic chemotherapy)

diseases (especially those which are immunologically mediated) and treatment of neoplastic conditions, particularly when they involve lymphoid tissue (Box 44.2). Powerful glucocorticoids with little mineralocorticoid activity, such as prednisolone, are usually chosen. Dexamethasone is used to reduce oedema around malignant tumours in the brain or compressing the spinal cord. It is also used in some antiemetic regimens during cancer chemotherapy (see Chapter 32).

Table 44.2 Examples of topical corticosteroid administration

Disease	Mode of administration	Chapter in this book
Asthma	Aerosol	12
Vasomotor rhinitis	Aerosol	39
Eczema	Ointment or cream	49
Superficial ocular inflammation	Aqueous solution	50
Ulcerative colitis	Aqueous solution or foam enema	34
Proctitis	Suppository	34
Arthritis	Aqueous solution by intra-articular injection	30

Resistance to the antiinflammatory and immunosuppressant effects of glucocorticoids occurs in some individuals. The mechanisms are complex, and arise from a variety of excessively activated intracellular inflammatory pathways. There are no reliable strategies to overcome glucocorticoid resistance, and alternative immunosuppressant drugs may need to be used (see Chapter 38).

For uses of ACTH and its analogues, see Chapter 43.

CLINICAL USES OF TOPICALLY ADMINISTERED GLUCOCORTICOIDS

Topical use of glucocorticoids can deliver high concentrations to a target site and reduce systemic unwanted effects. However, significant absorption into the blood occurs at higher doses. Examples of the clinical uses of topical glucocorticoids are given in Table 44.2.

UNWANTED EFFECTS OF GLUCOCORTICOIDS

Pharmacological doses of systemic glucocorticoids given over long periods will produce the typical features of adrenocortical overactivity (Cushing's syndrome). Unwanted glucocorticoid actions are shown in Box 44.3. These effects do not occur when physiological replacement doses of a glucocorticoid are used.

Cessation of glucocorticoid therapy

When a systemic pharmacological dose of glucocorticoid is used for a long period, it suppresses pituitary ACTH production and eventually causes adrenal atrophy. Sudden withdrawal can then lead to acute adrenal insufficiency, with hypotension and death. Less severe withdrawal symptoms include fever, myalgia, arthralgia, rhinitis, conjunctivitis and weight loss.

To avoid the consequences of sudden withdrawal, gradual reduction in dose is recommended, particularly if high doses have been used for more than 1 week or a lower therapeutic

---

Box 44.3 **Unwanted effects of glucocorticoids**

- Central obesity with 'buffalo hump', moon face and abdominal striae
- Loss of supporting tissue in skin with skin atrophy, bruising and poor wound healing; local atrophy can be marked at the site of topical corticosteroid application
- Osteoporosis due to catabolism of protein matrix in the bone and defective mineralisation
- Proximal (i.e. shoulder and hip girdle) muscle wasting and weakness
- Hyperglycaemia, which may lead to overt diabetes mellitus (see Chapter 40)
- Peptic ulceration due to inhibition of gastrointestinal prostaglandin (see Chapter 33)
- Mood changes, including euphoria and occasionally psychosis
- Posterior capsular cataracts in the eye, and exacerbation of glaucoma
- Increased susceptibility to infection with bacteria, viruses or fungi; activation of latent infections such as tuberculosis can also occur
- Growth retardation in children, with reduced linear bone growth and premature epiphyseal closure
- After long-term treatment, sudden withdrawal can produce an acute adrenal crisis due to suppression of the hypothalamic–pituitary–adrenal (HPA) axis and adrenal atrophy. Recovery of adrenal responsiveness can take several months. Basal cortisol secretion is restored before maximal responses, leaving patients at risk during stress and intercurrent infection
- Mineralocorticoid effects (which vary between the different drugs)

---

dose has been given for more than 3 weeks. The dose should be reduced quickly to physiological doses (equivalent to 7.5 mg of prednisolone) and then reduced more slowly until the drug is withdrawn.

CUSHING'S SYNDROME

Cushing's syndrome is characterised by excessive glucocorticoid effects (see Box 44.3). There are four possible causes (see Box 44.1), with 80% of cases being pituitary tumours.

Surgery is the definitive treatment for excessive pituitary secretion of ACTH (usually from an adenoma) and for unilateral adrenal tumours, with subsequent radiotherapy for some pituitary tumours.

Drug treatment to reduce glucocorticoid secretion is desirable for several weeks before surgery, in order to reverse the excessive tissue catabolism and correct the metabolic disturbances. This is usually achieved with metyrapone, which reduces glucocorticoid biosynthesis by competitive inhibition of 11β-hydroxylase (see Fig. 44.2). Metyrapone also inhibits cytochrome P450 in the liver, which can produce important drug interactions. Gastrointestinal upset is the main unwanted effect. The antifungal agent ketoconazole (see Chapter 51) also reduces cortisol synthesis by inhibition of 11β-hydroxylase, but its onset of action is slower than that of metyrapone. In addition, it inhibits sex steroid production

and therefore often causes gynaecomastia and decreased libido in males and hirsutism in females. Ketoconazole can be used alone or in combination with metyrapone prior to surgery. Both metyrapone and ketoconazole have relatively short-lived benefit, with rapid loss of control (escape) when increased ACTH secretion is the cause of the syndrome. Pasireotide is a multireceptor somatostatin analogue that reduces ACTH secretion and is effective in about 25% of cases unsuitable for surgery. Mifepristone has glucocorticoid receptor antagonist activity (see Chapter 45), and can also be considered.

Mitotane is a chemotherapeutic drug (see Chapter 52) that produces more profound suppression of glucocorticoid synthesis with no escape. It can be used for long-term control of symptoms for people with adrenal carcinoma. Glucocorticoid replacement therapy is usually necessary during treatment with mitotane.

Ectopic ACTH secretion is not usually amenable to surgical cure, but palliative drug treatment can be helpful (see Fig. 44.3).

MINERALOCORTICOIDS

Example

fludrocortisone

FLUDROCORTISONE

Pharmacokinetics

Aldosterone is almost completely inactivated on its first passage through the liver and is therefore unsuitable for oral use. Fludrocortisone (9α-fluorohydrocortisone) is a synthetic alternative, but only about 10% escapes first-pass metabolism. Its half-life is short (0.5 hours) due to rapid hepatic metabolism.

Unwanted effects

Excessive Na^+ retention and K^+ loss can occur with pharmacological doses of fludrocortisone. Hypertension can result, but the expansion of blood volume stimulates cardiac stretch receptors, leading to secretion of natriuretic peptides. This results in an 'escape' natriuresis, which establishes a new equilibrium between Na^+ intake and excretion at a higher blood volume. Consequently, oedema does not usually occur.

Clinical uses of fludrocortisone

- Fludrocortisone is given as replacement therapy for defective aldosterone production. This is usually the result of primary adrenal pathology with destruction of all three zones of the adrenal cortex (Addison's disease).
- Expansion of blood volume by fludrocortisone can be used to raise blood pressure in postural hypotension resulting from autonomic neuropathy. However, it often produces supine hypertension without fully eliminating the postural fall in blood pressure.

PRIMARY HYPERALDOSTERONISM (CONN'S SYNDROME)

Autonomous oversecretion of aldosterone causes hypertension and a hypokalaemic alkalosis. Some cases are caused by an adenoma in the zona glomerulosa of the adrenal cortex and are treated surgically. The majority are caused by hyperplasia of both zonae glomerulosae, which usually causes less marked metabolic disturbance. An aldosterone antagonist such as spironolactone is the treatment of choice to preserve the plasma K+ concentration and reduce blood pressure (see Chapter 14).

SELF-ASSESSMENT

True/false questions

1. Glucocorticoids take many hours to produce their clinical effects.
2. Inhaled glucocorticoids do not cause systemic unwanted effects.
3. Oral fludrocortisone is a useful antiinflammatory corticosteroid in severe asthma.
4. Fluticasone is not used orally.
5. Metyrapone inhibits glucocorticoid synthesis.
6. Hypoglycaemia is common during glucocorticoid administration.
7. If prolonged administration of prednisolone results in unwanted effects, it should be withdrawn immediately.
8. Mineralocorticoid secretion is decreased in Addison's disease.
9. Aldosterone secretion is inhibited by angiotensin II.
10. Glucocorticoids do not affect inflammatory responses provoked by infection.
11. Dexamethasone causes vomiting.
12. Glucocorticoids delay wound healing.

Case-based questions

Case 1

A 35-year-old woman showed signs of cortisol excess, including centripetal obesity, muscle weakness, easy bruising and amenorrhoea.

1. What are the possible causes?
2. She is not taking corticosteroids, eliminating an iatrogenic cause. The cortisol level in a 24-hour urine sample was elevated, and the plasma ACTH level was also high. What do these results indicate?
3. A single high dose of dexamethasone was administered and resulted in only marginal suppression of plasma cortisol. What does this result indicate?
4. A computed tomography scan and other tests showed an inoperable carcinoma of the bronchus.
   What treatment could be given?

Case 2

Mr B.F.G., a 69-year-old man, had late-onset asthma, which was poorly controlled by an inhaled β₂-adrenoceptor agonist.

His GP prescribed a low-dose inhaled corticosteroid that helped him initially.

1. Which glucocorticoids could have been given by aerosol inhaler?
2. What are the possible unwanted effects of the low-dose inhaled glucocorticoid?
3. Mr B.F.G. then had a particularly severe asthma episode, which led to his admission to hospital as an emergency. Among the drugs he was given was an intravenous corticosteroid. Which drug was likely to have been given, and what was the objective of its use?
4. Mr B.F.G.'s acute exacerbation resolved, and he was then prescribed a course of oral corticosteroid while in the hospital and subsequently sent home with high-dose inhaled corticosteroid. Which corticosteroid could have been used for oral therapy?
5. Mr B.F.G.'s asthma was poorly controlled by a higher dose of inhaled corticosteroid, and it was decided to recommence oral therapy. Why might oral therapy be more effective in controlling chronic severe asthma than inhaled therapy?
6. How would you have determined the dose to be used and monitored its appropriateness?
7. After many months of this therapy, Mr B.F.G. started to complain of apparently unrelated problems, including recurrent minor infections; minor epigastric discomfort, especially on an empty stomach; weight gain and increased appetite; a tendency to bruise easily and severe back pain after a minor fall. Examination revealed a cushingoid appearance, and investigation showed a raised plasma glucose level and a decreased plasma level of cortisol and ACTH. Discuss the reasons for Mr B.F.G.'s symptoms.

ANSWERS

True/false answers

1. **True.** Glucocorticoids act principally by modulating gene transcription so most of their clinical effects are not seen for several hours.
2. **False.** In maximum recommended doses, inhaled glucocorticoids can cause systemic effects.
3. **False.** Fludrocortisone is a synthetic mineralocorticoid with weak antiinflammatory effects; glucocorticoids such as prednisolone are used orally in severe asthma.
4. **True.** Inhaled fluticasone is used for topical effects on the airways in the treatment of asthma.
5. **True.** Metyrapone inhibits synthesis of cortisol, and to a lesser extent that of aldosterone, by inhibiting steroid 11β-hydroxylase.
6. **False.** Corticosteroids cause *hyper*glycaemia by reducing tissue uptake of glucose and increased gluconeogenesis.
7. **False.** Prolonged administration of a systemic glucocorticoid may suppress the HPA axis. The drug should be withdrawn slowly to allow the adrenals to recover their normal cortisol secretion and avoid corticosteroid deficiency.

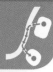

8. **True.** Addison's disease can be caused by autoimmune disease or drugs such as ketoconazole.
9. **False.** Angiotensin II is produced by the action of renin, which is secreted when plasma sodium concentrations are low; angiotensin II then stimulates aldosterone release from the adrenal cortex, and this increases Na^+ reabsorption in the renal tubule.
10. **False.** Glucocorticoids suppress all inflammatory responses, including those produced by infection.
11. **False.** Dexamethasone can inhibit vomiting and will add to the antiemetic actions of agents such as ondansetron, used in cancer chemotherapy.
12. **True.** Glucocorticoids delay wound healing because of their catabolic effect on protein synthesis.

Case-based answers

Case 1

1. Possible causes include a tumour of the adrenal cortex secreting cortisol; excess secretion of ACTH by a pituitary tumour, or by a nonpituitary tumour (commonly small-cell carcinoma of the lung, medullary or thyroid carcinoma); or therapeutic administration of glucocorticoids or ACTH (iatrogenic).
2. The cause could not be a primary cortisol-secreting adrenocortical tumour or glucocorticoid administration, as the plasma ACTH level would then be low due to negative feedback of glucocorticoid on the anterior pituitary and hypothalamus. The possibilities are an ACTH-secreting pituitary or nonpituitary tumour.
3. Dexamethasone suppresses ACTH of pituitary origin but not from ectopic ACTH-producing tumours or adrenocortical tumours. The result might therefore exclude a tumour of pituitary origin.

4. Metyrapone, an inhibitor of adrenal corticosteroid synthesis, could be given. She would probably also show signs of excess mineralocorticoid activity, which should be treated concomitantly with spironolactone.

Case 2

1. Inhaled glucocorticoids include beclometasone, budesonide and fluticasone.
2. Systemic unwanted effects are unlikely at low doses of inhaled glucocorticoids. Local problems such as oral candidiasis could be managed with a spacer device and good oral hygiene.
3. Intravenous hydrocortisone is likely to have been used to reduce airway inflammation in this acute exacerbation of asthma, although its onset of action would be delayed by several hours.
4. A short course (5 days) of oral prednisolone could have been used.
5. A high concentration of glucocorticoid is needed at inflammatory cells in the airways, and poor inhaler technique or airway obstruction by inflammation and mucus might prevent inhaled drugs from reaching their target. Systemic prednisolone reaches airway inflammatory leucocytes more effectively than after inhalation in these circumstances, and may also reduce bone marrow proliferation and airway recruitment of eosinophils.
6. The lowest possible doses of glucocorticoid should be used in chronic asthma management, using peak expiratory flow measurements and a symptom diary at home to monitor asthma control and to step the dosages up or down as appropriate.
7. Glucocorticoids have a wide range of metabolic effects in addition to their antiinflammatory and immunomodulatory actions. The cushingoid symptoms and signs described can all be attributed to actions on carbohydrate, protein and lipid metabolism, and suppression of the HPA axis.

FURTHER READING

Barnes, P.J., Adcock, I.M., 2009. Glucocorticoid resistance in inflammatory disease. Lancet 373, 1905–1917.

Charmandari, E., Nicolaides, N.C., Chrousos, G.P., 2014. Adrenal insufficiency. Lancet 383, 2152–2167.

Lacroix, A., Feelders, R.A., Stratakis, C.A., et al., 2015. Cushing's syndrome. Lancet 386, 913–927.

Weinstein, R.S., 2011. Glucocorticoid-induced bone disease. N. Engl. J. Med. 365, 62–70.

Wu, V.C., Chao, C.T., Kuo, C.C., et al., 2012. Diagnosis and management of primary aldosteronism. Acta Nephrol. 26, 111–120.

Compendium: corticosteroids

Drug	Characteristics
Glucocorticoids	
The durations of action of glucocorticoids greatly exceed their elimination half-lives because of their mechanism of action.	
Betamethasone	Used for suppression of inflammatory and allergic disorders, congenital adrenal hyperplasia and cerebral oedema. Given orally, topically, by intramuscular or slow intravenous injection, or by intravenous infusion; phosphate ester prodrug used for injections. Half-life: 35–55 h
Deflazacort	Rapidly hydrolysed to active 21-desacetyl metabolite. Used for suppression of inflammatory and allergic disorders. Given orally
Dexamethasone	Potent glucocorticoid with minimal mineralocorticoid activity. Used for suppression of inflammatory and allergic disorders, congenital adrenal hyperplasia and cerebral oedema, and diagnosis of Cushing's disease. Given orally, by intramuscular or slow intravenous injection, or by intravenous infusion; antiemetic; phosphate ester prodrug is used for injections. Half-life: 2–4 h
Hydrocortisone (cortisol)	Numerous antiinflammatory and antiallergic uses. Given orally, by intramuscular or slow intravenous injection, or by intravenous infusion; phosphate ester prodrug is used for injections. Half-life: 1–2 h
Methylprednisolone	Used for suppression of inflammatory and allergic disorders, cerebral oedema and connective tissue disease; given orally, by intramuscular or slow intravenous injection, or by intravenous infusion; injectable forms are lipid-soluble esters in solvents. Half-life: 1–3 h
Prednisolone	Used for suppression of numerous inflammatory and allergic disorders; given orally, topically and by intramuscular injection; injectable form is the acetate ester as an aqueous suspension. Half-life: 2–4 h
Prednisone	Mostly converted rapidly to prednisolone. Given orally for moderate to severe rheumatoid arthritis
Triamcinolone	Used for suppression of inflammatory and allergic disorders. Given by deep intramuscular injection as an aqueous suspension. Half-life: 2–5 h
Mineralocorticoids	
The durations of action of mineralocorticosteroids greatly exceed their chemical half-lives because of their mechanism of action.	
Fludrocortisone acetate	Mineralocorticoid used in combination with hydrocortisone for adrenocortical insufficiency. Given orally. Half-life: 0.5 h
Inhibitor of steroid metabolism	
Metyrapone	Inhibits synthesis of cortisol by 11β-hydroxylation in the adrenal cortex. Used to control the symptoms of Cushing's syndrome, especially prior to surgery. Given orally. Half-life: 2 h
Somatostatin analogue	
Pasireotide	Peptide analogue of somatostatin analogue (see Chapter 43); inhibits pituitary ACTH synthesis. Given subcutaneously for Cushing's syndrome when surgery has failed or is inappropriate

Additional corticosteroids used for specific purposes are covered in other chapters (see Table 44.2).

ACTH, Adrenocorticotropic hormone.

45

Female reproduction

PHYSIOLOGY OF THE MENSTRUAL CYCLE

The menstrual cycle prepares the female reproductive system for pregnancy. It is controlled by hormonal changes, driven by the endocrine function of the hypothalamo–pituitary–ovarian axis through a series of feedback loops (Fig. 45.1). Each cycle has three phases, according to events in the ovary and the uterus. The three phases of the ovarian cycle are the follicular phase, ovulation and the luteal phase. The uterine cycle consists of the menstruation, the proliferative phase and the secretory phase.

The menstrual cycle begins with *menstruation* (usually days 1 to 3–5 of the menstrual cycle), when the uterus sheds its lining. Following the shedding of the endometrium, a group of five to seven follicles in the ovary that have been growing for up to a year start to mature. This is the *follicular phase* of the *ovarian cycle* (approximately days 5–13 of the menstrual cycle) and is under the influence of follicle-stimulating hormone (FSH) secreted from the anterior pituitary. The secretion of FSH starts during menstruation and continues during the early follicular phase, controlled by pulsatile secretion of gonadotropin-releasing hormone (GnRH) from the hypothalamus (see also Chapter 43). GnRH increases because the low circulating concentration of oestrogen removes inhibitory feedback. FSH permits the growth of the small follicles and drives them to convert androgens produced by their thecal cells into oestradiol (see Fig. 44.2) within the granulosa cells. The follicles also produce inhibin, which increases sufficiently by about day 3 of menstruation to start to reduce FSH release. A single dominant ovarian follicle (or occasionally two) is selected and matures in preparation for ovulation at the expense of the remaining follicles which undergo atresia.

The small ovarian follicles produce a gonadotropin surge-attenuating factor (GnSAF) that, together with oestradiol, acts on the hypothalamus and pituitary to dampen surges in luteinising hormone (LH) release and provide the right environment for follicle growth. Oestradiol secretion from the follicle slowly rises as the follicle grows and matures. Eventually the plasma oestradiol reaches a critical concentration that, possibly with a decrease in GnSAF, triggers a switch from negative feedback to positive feedback of oestradiol on the pituitary and hypothalamus. This stimulates pulsatile release of GnRH, which combines with direct stimulation of the pituitary to produce a mid-cycle surge of LH for about 48 h, which is essential for ovulation. LH matures the egg and weakens the wall of the ovarian follicle. It also stimulates the granulosa cells in the follicle to secrete progesterone. Granulosa cells are destined to become the corpus luteum after ovulation.

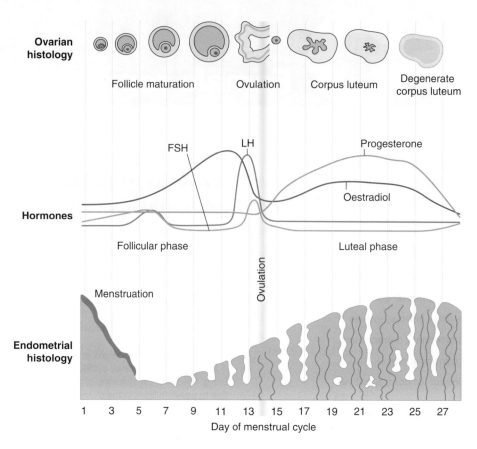

Fig. 45.1 Endocrine control of the menstrual cycle. *FSH*, Follicle-stimulating hormone; *LH*, luteinising hormone.

From day 5 to late in the menstrual cycle, the gradually increasing plasma concentrations of oestradiol cause the lining of the uterus to grow. This is the *proliferative phase* of the *uterine* cycle, during which there is proliferation and vascularisation of endometrial cells.

Ovulation is the second phase of the *ovarian* cycle (about day 14 of the menstrual cycle) and involves release of the secondary oocyte from the follicle, which rapidly matures into an ovum. Following ovulation, the residual follicle transforms into the corpus luteum under the influence of FSH and LH. The *luteal phase* of the *ovarian* cycle (days 15–26 of the menstrual cycle) results from proliferation of granulosa cells, expressing LH receptors in the corpus luteum, which produce increasing amounts of progesterone and well as some oestrogen. The increase in plasma progesterone stimulates the adrenals to produce oestrogen, but also suppresses LH and FSH production by negative feedback on the hypothalamus and pituitary. Progesterone causes the endometrial lining to enter the *secretory phase* of the *uterine* cycle (which therefore corresponds to the luteal phase of the ovarian cycle). The endometrial cells secrete a variety of fluids and nutrients that make the endometrium receptive for implantation. The temporal precision of the change in receptivity is critical if successful implantation of a fertilised oocyte is to occur.

If implantation of a fertilised ovum does not occur, the corpus luteum regresses after about 10 days, since it requires gonadotropins to maintain itself. Therefore the circulating

concentrations of progesterone and oestrogen eventually fall to levels that no longer support the endometrium. Deprived of hormonal support, the endometrial spiral arteries constrict and the endometrial cells become ischaemic and die, producing digestive enzymes (days 27–28 of the menstrual cycle). As a consequence of this and other changes, the endometrium is shed during menstruation.

The cervical mucus is influenced by oestrogen and progesterone concentrations. Under the dominant influence of progesterone, cervical mucus is viscid and acts as a barrier to penetration by sperm. At ovulation, the high plasma oestradiol concentration results in thinner and more serous and elastic mucus that is readily penetrable by sperm. Progesterone also inhibits the motility of the Fallopian tube and contractility of the uterine smooth muscle. Oestrogen has the opposite effect. At ovulation, oestradiol increases contraction of the Fallopian tubes, which brings the fimbria of the tubes closer to the ovaries. When progesterone levels rise 4–6 days after ovulation, the reduction in tubal motility allows passage of the ovum to the uterus by action of tubal cilia.

PHYSIOLOGY OF PREGNANCY

Pregnancy is accompanied by considerable hormonal changes. When a fertilised ovum implants in the uterine lining, the corpus luteum maintains the pregnancy during the first 6–8 weeks by the production of progesterone. After this, placental production of hormones takes over and the combined feto-placental unit produces progressively greater quantities of oestrogen and progesterone, which reach the maternal circulation. The dividing cells of the implanted ovum start to secrete human chorionic gonadotropin (HCG) from about 9 days after fertilisation. HCG prevents atrophy of the corpus luteum and stimulates it to continue to secrete progesterone and oestrogen. Eventually, the placenta takes over the production of HCG, progesterone and oestrogen. The placenta also produces human placental lactogen as pregnancy advances, which has metabolic actions that help to support fetal nutrition. The precise balance of sex steroids also contributes to quiescence of the uterus during pregnancy and the onset of labour at term.

CELLULAR ACTION OF OESTROGENS AND PROGESTOGENS

In common with other steroid hormones, both oestrogens and progestogens act by influencing gene transcription (see Chapter 44 for a detailed description of steroid receptor function). They passively diffuse into the cell and bind to specific receptors in the cytoplasm. When the hormone binds to the receptor, it displaces chaperone proteins, and the steroid–receptor complex is translocated by active transport to the cell nucleus. The steroid–receptor complex associates with hormone-response elements of numerous oestrogen- or progesterone-responsive genes. This leads to recruitment of co-activator molecules to the complex, and produces gene transcription (co-activation). There are two specific cytoplasmic receptors for oestrogen (ERα and ERβ), which have different tissue distributions. Progesterone also has two specific receptors (PR-A and PR-B) that regulate progesterone-responsive genes.

STEROIDAL CONTRACEPTIVES

Oral hormonal contraceptives ('the pill') are the most widely used form of contraception and contain either a combination of a synthetic oestrogen with a synthetic progestogen (a C19 synthetic progesterone derivative) or a progestogen alone.

MECHANISMS OF HORMONAL CONTRACEPTION

Persistently elevated circulating concentrations of synthetic oestrogen and progestogen prevent the precise cyclic pattern of hormone-related events seen in the normal menstrual cycle (Fig. 45.2), and can be used for contraception.

- The combination of oestrogen and progestogen exerts its contraceptive effect mainly through suppression of FSH release, which prevents development of the follicles in the ovary. The lack of a dominant follicle means that production of oestradiol is impaired. The failure of plasma oestradiol to rise, combined with negative feedback from the progestogen, prevents the midcycle LH surge that is essential for ovulation to occur.
- Progestogen produces asynchronous development of the endometrium with stromal thinning, which makes it less receptive to implantation of the fertilised ovum.

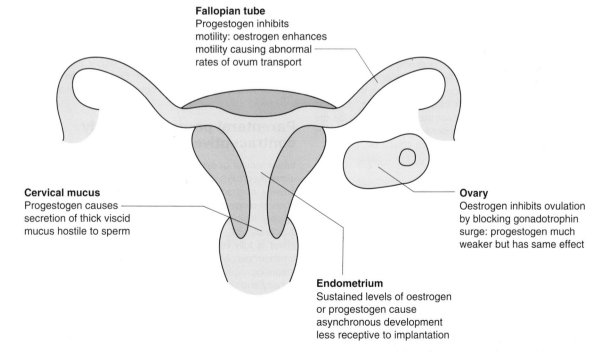

Fallopian tube
Progestogen inhibits motility: oestrogen enhances motility causing abnormal rates of ovum transport

Cervical mucus
Progestogen causes secretion of thick viscid mucus hostile to sperm

Ovary
Oestrogen inhibits ovulation by blocking gonadotrophin surge: progestogen much weaker but has same effect

Endometrium
Sustained levels of oestrogen or progestogen cause asynchronous development less receptive to implantation

Fig. 45.2 The main contraceptive actions of the synthetic oestrogens and progestogens in the combined oral hormonal contraceptive.

- Oestrogens increase Fallopian tube motility, while progestogens decrease motility; this may affect fertility by altering the rate of transport of the ovum.
- Progestogen reduces the amount of cervical mucus and makes it thicker, which impedes sperm penetration.

Progestogens can be used alone for contraception, when the mechanism depends on the dose of progestogen. Low-dose progestogen without oestrogen inhibits ovulation in only about 50% of cycles, and contraception relies upon the other actions of the hormone. With higher doses, inhibition of follicular development and ovulation becomes more important.

THE COMBINED HORMONAL CONTRACEPTIVE

Combined hormonal contraceptives contain both a synthetic oestrogen and a progestogen. The oestrogen component is most often ethinylestradiol (an oestrogen that is alkylated at C17 to slow its metabolism). In other combinations it is mestranol, which is metabolised to ethinylestradiol, or oestradiol (as oestradiol valerate or hemihydrate).

The progestogen component of many combined oral hormonal contraceptives is either levonorgestrel (the active isomer of norgestrel) or norethisterone; these compounds are testosterone analogues that also possess residual androgenic activity. Newer oral combined hormonal contraceptives contain modified progestogens that have less androgenic activity (desogestrel, gestodene, norgestimate, nomegestrel, which are all derivatives of norgestrel) or antiandrogenic activity (dienogest or drospirenone, a derivative of the aldosterone antagonist spironolactone with some antimineralocorticoid activity). Modified progestogens are used if there are unacceptable unwanted effects with levonorgestrel or norethisterone.

Monophasic preparations

Monophasic preparations contain fixed amounts of oestrogen and progestogen. Active tablets containing the hormones are taken daily, typically for the first 21 days of the menstrual cycle, followed by 7 hormone-free days when the woman takes tablets containing an inactive substance, such as lactose. The oestrogen concentration used should be the lowest that maintains good cycle control and produces minimal unwanted effects. There is a choice of:

- low-strength preparations that contain 20 µg ethinylestradiol;
- standard-strength preparations that contain 30 or 35 µg ethinylestradiol, or 50 µg mestranol, or 1.5 mg of oestradiol hemihydrate.

Monophasic oral combined hormonal contraceptives contain one of several progestogens. In some women it may be necessary to change the preparation to one containing a different progestogen to reduce unwanted effects, such as acne, headache, depression, breakthrough bleeding or breast symptoms during the menstrual cycle. The degree of androgenic activity possessed by different progestogens (see the previous section on combined hormonal contraceptives) may influence the suitability of an individual preparation for a particular woman.

A transdermal patch formulation of low-strength ethinylestradiol with the progestogen norelgestromin is also available; this is applied weekly for 3 weeks, followed by a 7-day patch-free interval. There is also a vaginal contraceptive ring that contains ethinylestradiol with the progestogen etonogestrel, which should remain in place for 3 weeks in each cycle.

Biphasic and triphasic preparations

Biphasic and triphasic preparations are designed to mimic more closely the changes in sex hormone concentrations that occur during the natural menstrual cycle. The total sex hormone intake through the cycle is no less than with monophasic preparations. Several preparations are available, which contain ethinylestradiol in combination with levonorgestrel, norethisterone or gestodene, or oestradiol valerate combined with dienogest. The dose of oestrogen is either kept constant throughout, as in the monophasic pills, or increased during days 7–12. Progestogen doses are increased once (biphasic) or twice (triphasic) as the menstrual cycle proceeds.

PROGESTOGEN-ONLY CONTRACEPTIVES

Oral progestogen-only contraceptives

The oral progestogen-only contraceptive (or 'progestogen-only pill'; POP) is particularly useful for women for whom the use of oestrogen is considered to be undesirable – for example, if there is a history of thromboembolic disorders or hypertension (discussed later). Progestogens used for oral preparations include desogestrel, levonorgestrel or norethisterone. The progestogen-only contraceptive must be taken daily, without a break, and within 3 hours of the usual time every day (see the discussion of efficacy later in the chapter). Because the dose of progestogen is low, bleeding does occur at monthly intervals but may be irregular. Breakthrough bleeding occurs in up to 40% of women; this is much higher than with the combined hormonal contraceptive. Some women become amenorrhoeic while using oral progestogen-only contraception.

Parenteral progestogen-only contraceptives

Intramuscular or subcutaneous injection of a progestogen, either medroxyprogesterone acetate or norethisterone, can provide contraception for up to 8–13 weeks. The higher dose of progestogen compared with the oral preparations reliably inhibits ovulation, and therefore there is a low incidence of ectopic pregnancy. The contraceptive effect is fully reversible, but there is a high incidence of amenorrhoea when its effect wears off. Prolonged use of medroxyprogesterone acetate can reduce bone mineral density and cause osteoporosis. The loss of bone mineral density occurs over the first 2–3 years of use and then stabilises. Prolonged use of medroxyprogesterone acetate beyond 2 years, or its use in adolescents or people with other risk factors for osteoporosis, is discouraged.

A subdermal implant of etonogestrel provides contraception for up to 3 years, after which time it should be replaced. The progestogen is released from a flexible rod inserted on the lower surface of the upper arm. Local irritation is experienced by some women. The implants are radio-opaque, so they can be easily located by radiography.

Intrauterine progestogen-only device

A plastic intrauterine contraceptive system (IUS) with a levonorgestrel-releasing system from a silicone reservoir provides effective contraception, with reduced menstrual blood loss compared with copper intrauterine contraceptive devices (IUCDs) that do not contain progestogen. It also carries less risk of pelvic inflammatory disease. The progestogen is released from the device for a period of 3–5 years, depending on the device chosen. The IUS is also used to control menstrual bleeding in women with primary menorrhagia by preventing endometrial proliferation.

EFFICACY OF HORMONAL CONTRACEPTION

When taken according to the recommended schedule, the failure rate for hormonal contraceptive (including the intrauterine progestogen-only device) is 0.2–0.3%. With the combined oral hormonal contraceptive, protection is reduced if there is a delay of more than 24 hours in taking the daily dose. In such circumstances the missed dose should be taken as soon as possible. If two doses are missed, then additional contraceptive measures should be used for 7 days.

With the oral progestogen-only contraceptive, if there is a delay of 3 hours or more after the normal time of taking the daily dose of oral progestogen-only contraceptive, other contraceptive precautions should be taken for 2 days.

EMERGENCY CONTRACEPTION

There are three methods of emergency contraception for use after unprotected sexual intercourse:

- oral levonorgestrel;
- oral ulipristal acetate;
- copper-containing IUCD.

A single large dose of levonorgestrel taken within 72 hours after unprotected intercourse, preferably within 12 hours, prevents pregnancy in up to 99% of cases. Levonorgestrel inhibits ovulation, but only if it is taken before the LH surge. Efficacy is greatly reduced if used between 72 and 120 hours after unprotected intercourse. Nausea is a frequent unwanted effect, occurring in up to 22% of women, and an antiemetic (e.g. domperidone; see Chapter 32) may be needed. Absorption takes 2 hours, and vomiting after this time will not affect the efficacy of treatment. A larger dose may be required if drugs that induce drug-metabolising enzymes in the liver are being taken. In the United Kingdom, levonorgestrel can be purchased without prescription by women over the age of 16 years.

Ulipristal acetate is a progesterone receptor modulator that suppresses the mature follicle up to and including the time of the LH surge, so it can be effective when taken up to 120 hours after unprotected intercourse.

Insertion of a copper IUCD up to 5 days after unprotected sexual intercourse is more effective as emergency

contraception than levonorgestrel, but it is not known whether it is more effective than ulipristal acetate.

PHARMACOKINETICS OF CONTRACEPTIVE SEX STEROIDS

The synthetic oestrogens, like the naturally occurring oestradiol-17β (oestradiol), and progestogens are highly lipid-soluble molecules. The synthetic sex steroids are metabolised more slowly than the natural hormones, with less first-pass metabolism and a longer half-life. For example, oestradiol has a half-life of 1–2 hours, while that of ethinylestradiol is 8–24 hours. Oestrogens and progestogens are eliminated by hepatic metabolism, often involving CYP3A4-mediated oxidation and/or conjugation with glucuronic acid or sulphate. Enterohepatic cycling of ethinylestradiol conjugates is responsible for maintaining effective plasma concentrations with low-dose oestrogen formulations.

Drug interactions

The pharmacokinetics of oestrogens and progestogens can be affected by the administration of other drugs. Contraceptive failure may occur if there is concomitant treatment with drugs that induce liver cytochrome P450 enzymes (see Table 2.7), such as anticonvulsants (e.g. barbiturates, carbamazepine or phenytoin), antiretroviral drugs (e.g. nelfinavir, nevirapine or ritonavir) or certain antibacterials (e.g. rifampicin and rifabutin; see Chapter 51). A higher dose of ethinylestradiol should be used during administration of these drugs and for 4 weeks after stopping. Alternatively, a form of contraception unaffected by enzyme-inducing drugs should be used (such as an IUS or parenteral progestogen).

UNWANTED EFFECTS OF CONTRACEPTIVE SEX STEROIDS

Both oestrogens and progestogens have a number of minor unwanted effects, but the incidence of the major unwanted effects, although important, is relatively low.

- Venous thromboembolism: The incidence of venous thromboembolic disease is increased in women taking the combined hormonal contraceptive, especially in the first year. The mechanisms are complex but include procoagulant activity from increased production of clotting factors X and II and decreased production of antithrombin. Fibrinolysis is impaired, while reduced prostacyclin generation enhances platelet aggregation (see Chapter 11). The baseline risk of venous thromboembolism in women of reproductive age not taking the combined oral hormonal contraceptive is about 2 per 10,000 per year. The risk in women taking combined oral hormonal contraceptives is related to oestrogen dose and also to the progestogen component, ranging from 5 to 7 per 10,000 per year with levonorgestrel and 9 to 12 per 10,000 per year with gestodene. It is important that these risks are put into context; for example, the risk of venous thromboembolism is 6 per 10,000 pregnancies. The risk of thromboembolism in all women increases with age, and is greater in women who smoke (because smoking increases the risk of thrombogenesis) or who are obese, and in those with a prothrombotic coagulation disorder, such as deficiency of protein C or protein S or the presence of factor V Leiden. Risk assessment and counselling about the use of a combined oral hormonal contraceptive should consider these additional factors. There is no increase in venous thromboembolism risk with progestogen-only contraception.

- Ischaemic heart disease and ischaemic stroke: There is an increased risk of myocardial infarction and stroke in women taking the combined hormonal contraceptive who smoke, are hypertensive, have diabetes mellitus or are obese, and those over the age of 35 years. The additional risk in those over 40 years is 20 per 100,000 for smokers and 29 per 100,000 for women with hypertension. Enhanced thrombogenesis rather than premature atherogenesis is probably responsible for the excess cardiovascular risk with the combined hormonal contraceptive. The lowest possible dose of oestrogen should be given to older women who use the combined hormonal contraceptive. There is no increase in risk of stroke or myocardial infarction with progestogen-only contraception.

- Increase in blood pressure: A small increase in blood pressure, typically 5/3 mm Hg, is common during use of the combined hormonal contraceptive, but not with progestogen-only contraceptives. A significant rise can occur in about 5% of women with previously normal blood pressure and in up to 15% of women with preexisting hypertension. The mechanism is probably an increase in plasma renin substrate (see Chapter 6) produced by oestrogen. Blood pressure may remain elevated for some months after the combined hormonal contraceptive has been stopped. Regular monitoring of blood pressure is advisable during use of the combined hormonal contraceptive, and it should be stopped if the blood pressure rises above 160 mm Hg systolic or 95 mm Hg diastolic.

- Breast and cervical cancer: It is uncertain whether the increase in risk of breast cancer during use of the combined hormonal contraceptive relates to earlier diagnosis. However, the rate of diagnosis remains higher for 10 years after the combined hormonal contraceptive is stopped. The incidence of cervical cancer is slightly increased by combined hormonal contraceptives after 5 years of use. By contrast, the combined oral contraceptive reduces the risk of ovarian cancer by 40% and endometrial cancer by 50% after 5 years of use, which persists for up to 15 years after stopping. Progestogen-only contraception has no effect on the risk of cancer.

- Nausea, mastalgia, depression, headache, weight gain and provocation of migraine. These effects may be reduced by prescribing preparations with low oestrogen content, or by replacing levonorgestrel and norethisterone with desogestrel, drospirenone or gestodene. The combined hormonal contraceptive should be avoided in women who have migraine with aura, because of an increased risk of stroke.

- Breakthrough intermenstrual bleeding occurs frequently in some women, whereas in others, withdrawal bleeding fails to occur at the end of a cycle. Gestodene-containing pills or triphasic preparations probably give the best cycle control. Amenorrhoea after stopping the combined hormonal contraceptive can last beyond a few months in

about 5% of women, and a small number can experience amenorrhoea for more than a year. A history of irregular periods before taking the combined hormonal contraceptive increases the chance of prolonged amenorrhoea.

- Metabolic effects: Oestrogens increase arterial prostacyclin and nitric oxide synthesis, inhibit platelet adhesion and suppress smooth muscle cell proliferation. Some progestogens such as norethisterone and medroxyprogesterone acetate may oppose the beneficial effects of oestrogens on the arterial wall. When oestrogen is used in combination with levonorgestrel or norethisterone, high density lipoprotein (HDL) cholesterol is reduced. By contrast, combined hormonal contraceptives containing gestodene and desogestrel increase plasma triglycerides but increase HDL cholesterol. The clinical relevance of these small changes is uncertain.

- Increased skin pigmentation can occur in some women who take oestrogens. The androgenic progestogens can sometimes cause or aggravate hirsutism and acne or induce weight gain. For women with hyperandrogenaemia (such as occurs with polycystic ovary syndrome), gestodene or desogestrel, which have little androgenic activity, are preferred.

- Cholestatic jaundice can be produced by progestogens, and oestrogens increase the risk of gallstones.

NONCONTRACEPTIVE USES OF STEROIDAL CONTRACEPTIVES

Combined hormonal contraceptives can be used:

- to reduce excessive blood loss from menorrhagia;
- to reduce the pain of dysmenorrhoea;
- to treat premenstrual tension;
- to treat endometriosis;
- to treat acne in women (see Chapter 49).

Menorrhagia

Excessive menstrual blood loss is a common gynaecological problem. Menstrual loss can be reduced to a variable extent by nonsteroidal antiinflammatory drugs (NSAIDs; see Chapter 29), taken only during the time of menstruation. Combined hormonal contraceptives and progestogen-only contraceptives can also reduce excessive menstrual loss. Progestogen-only contraceptives must be taken for 3 weeks in each cycle at a fairly high dose. A more effective way of giving the progestogen is from an intrauterine progestogen system (IUS), which reduces blood loss by up to 90%.

The antifibrinolytic agent tranexamic acid (see Chapter 11) can also reduce menstrual blood loss by up to 50%. Its effect is rapid, and therapy is only required during the time of menstruation.

Primary dysmenorrhoea

The cause of primary dysmenorrhoea (pain associated with menstruation) is unknown. Many explanations have been proposed, including uterine hyperactivity, excessive prostaglandin or leukotriene generation and excessive production of vasopressin. NSAIDs (see Chapter 29) relieve the pain of dysmenorrhoea in approximately 70% of women. There are differences in efficacy among the NSAIDs that do not seem to be simply related to their analgesic or antiinflammatory activity. NSAIDs with a license for this indication in the United Kingdom include ibuprofen, mefenamic acid and naproxen. If there is no response to NSAIDs after three menstrual cycles, a combined hormonal contraceptive or the progestogen-only contraceptive can be considered.

If symptoms do not respond to standard treatments, then laparoscopy to look for endometriosis, the most common cause of secondary dysmenorrhoea, should be undertaken.

Premenstrual syndrome

Many women experience a variety of symptoms precipitated by ovulation that may continue up to the end of menstruation. The term *premenstrual syndrome* is used to describe the symptom complex if a woman has at least 1 week free of symptoms every cycle. Physical symptoms include joint and muscle pains, breast tenderness, abdominal bloating, headaches, weight gain and oedema of the hands or feet. These are often accompanied by increased appetite, fatigue, mood swings, irritability and sleep disturbance. Combined hormonal contraceptives containing levonorgestrel or norethisterone can produce symptoms similar to premenstrual syndrome.

Treatment includes cognitive behavioural therapy, aerobic exercise and vitamin B6 for emotional symptoms. The diuretic spironolactone (see Chapter 14) taken in the luteal phase (days 15–28 of the menstrual cycle) can reduce abdominal bloating, breast discomfort and mood disturbance. Selective serotonin reuptake inhibitors, such as citalopram (see Chapter 22), can treat both physical symptoms and mood disturbance when used either continuously or in the luteal phase. They are often effective at lower doses than those required to treat depression. A combined hormonal contraceptive containing drospirenone is helpful if fertility is not an issue. For severe symptoms, ovulation can be suppressed with a GnRH analogue such as goserelin (see Chapter 43), but add-in hormone replacement therapy (HRT) will be required to prevent osteoporosis if treatment is continued for more than 6 months.

Endometriosis

Endometriosis is the presence and proliferation of endometrial tissue outside the uterine cavity. It may arise from retrograde menstrual flow through the fallopian tubes. The main consequences are pelvic pain, dysmenorrhoea, dyspareunia and infertility. Treatment is either medical or surgical. Medical treatment to relieve symptoms can be given to suppress ovarian activity and create a hypo-oestrogenic anovulatory state. This is not recommended for women who wish to conceive, as it delays fertility.

Symptoms often improve in pregnancy, and the combined hormonal contraceptive or a progestogen-only contraceptive are often effective treatments. An alternative strategy is induction of a pseudopostmenopausal state with the use of a GnRH analogue (see Chapter 43). Treatment is usually necessary for at least 6 months, but up to 50% of women have recurrence of painful symptoms in the 5 years after it is stopped.

If fertility is the major problem, then laparoscopic surgical excision or ablation of deposits can be considered, and in vitro fertilisation may be required (see Chapter 43).

HORMONE-REPLACEMENT THERAPY

The menopausal transition from regular periods to amenorrhoea begins at a median age of 51 years and takes place over about 4 years. It arises because there is a natural depletion of ovarian follicles, and as a result the plasma oestrogen concentration falls, with a consequent rise in plasma FSH. After menopause, the ovaries do not produce oestrogen or progesterone, but continue to produce testosterone. Some oestrogen is still produced by conversion of adrenal corticosteroids to oestradiol in peripheral adipose tissue. The consequences of hormonal changes during and after menopause include:

- Vasomotor instability (hot flushes and night sweats) that results from resetting of the hypothalamic temperature set-point so that it perceives that the body is warmer than it is. Vasodilation and sweating represent an attempt to disperse heat. The mechanism of hypothalamic disturbance may be either reduced oestrogen or increased FSH, leading to a reduction in noradrenergic or serotonergic neurotransmission.
- Altered sexual and urinary function. Loss of connective tissue in the vagina and trigone of the bladder, and a less acidic vaginal pH produce vaginal dryness, discomfort and itching, dyspareunia, and urinary urgency, frequency and incontinence. Breast atrophy and thinning of the skin also occur.
- Irritability and depression, which are less clearly related to oestrogen deficiency.
- Bone loss leading to osteoporosis (see Chapter 42) and an increased susceptibility to fragility fracture occur after menopause. Oestrogen deficiency increases bone turnover, with bone resorption increasing more than formation.
- Cardiovascular disease and cerebrovascular disease are increased. The cause is uncertain. Unfavourable changes in lipids may be part of the explanation, due to a reduced HDL_2 cholesterol subfraction and increased low density lipoprotein (LDL) cholesterol (see Chapter 48). However, loss of the action of oestrogen in reducing plasma fibrinogen (a factor in thrombogenesis) may be more important. Stimulation of oestrogen receptors on cells of the arterial wall decreases arterial resistance and increases vessel compliance, and loss of these effects may also be relevant.

Treatment with oestrogen replacement therapy during the peri- and postmenopausal period has the potential to reverse the effects of oestrogen deficiency.

HORMONE-REPLACEMENT THERAPY AND RELATED DRUGS

Oral oestrogens and progestogens

For HRT, oestrogens are given at much lower doses than are used for contraception. However, if oestrogen is given alone for more than a few weeks to a woman who has a uterus, then cystic hyperplasia of the endometrium can occur. Progestogen is given concurrently to avoid this, and is used for 12 days each calendar month or continuously if withdrawal bleeding is to be avoided. Oestrogen can be used alone if the woman has had a hysterectomy.

The majority of oral HRT preparations contain natural oestradiol as the oestrogen, although preparations with conjugated equine oestrogens are also available. Synthetic progestogens are used: dydrogesterone, medroxyprogesterone, norethisterone, levonorgestrel or drospirenone.

Oral oestrogen replacement will reduce the symptoms of postmenopausal oestrogen deficiency, although relief may take up to 3 months. Treatment for symptom relief probably should be given for at least 6 months to perimenopausal women, after which withdrawal can be attempted to see whether symptoms have resolved spontaneously.

Subcutaneous oestrogen implants

Oestradiol can be implanted surgically as pellets that release drug for up to 6 months. The major use for this option is when tolerance of oral oestrogen is poor, perhaps because of nausea. Oral progestogen must also be taken for 10–12 days each month if the woman has a uterus, and continued for up to 2 years after stopping oestrogen, to prevent vaginal bleeding from persistently high oestrogen levels.

Transdermal oestrogen and oestrogen with progestogen

A variety of transdermal patches that deliver sex steroids are available. In some preparations, oestrogen alone is delivered by patches applied twice weekly for 2 weeks, followed by patches delivering oestrogen plus progestogen for 2 weeks. In other regimens, progestogen is taken orally for at least 12 days of the cycle, while continuing with the patch-delivered oestrogen. Patches delivering continuous oestrogen plus progestogen (levonorgestrel or norethisterone) are also available. An alternative approach is oestradiol gel applied twice daily, which also requires co-administration of oral progestogen for 12 days per month in women with a uterus. It is recommended that oestrogen is applied below the waistline, and not close to the breasts, to avoid breast tenderness.

Vaginal oestrogen

Oestrogen cream (usually oestradiol) or pessaries can be used to treat vaginal atrophy and dyspareunia, and can relieve perimenopausal urinary symptoms such as frequency and dysuria. Considerable systemic absorption occurs with some formulations, and an oral progestogen may be needed to prevent endometrial hyperplasia. Creams or pessaries are used daily for 2–3 weeks initially and then applied twice weekly for as long as required.

Tibolone

Tibolone is a synthetic compound which is metabolised to compounds with either oestrogenic or progestogenic activity. Its effects are complex and tissue-specific:

- Oestrogenic metabolites have effects on bone that reduce postmenopausal bone loss.
- Oestrogenic effects on the brain and blood vessels.
- In breast tissue, tibolone inhibits one enzyme and activates another that prevents conversion to oestrogenic metabolites, giving a low incidence of breast tenderness.
- In the endometrium, an effect on the same enzymes prevents formation of the oestrogenic metabolite and leaves a progestogenic metabolite, which prevents stimulation of the endometrium.

Tibolone reduces postmenopausal symptoms and prevents postmenopausal bone loss. Vaginal bleeding can occur in women who still produce some endogenous oestrogen, and therefore tibolone is not usually given to women who are within 12 months of their last period.

Pharmacokinetics

Tibolone is a prodrug that is metabolised in the liver to active metabolites with half-lives of about 8 hours.

Unwanted effects

- Hot flushes.
- Leg cramps.
- Increased risk of stroke.
- Increased risk of breast cancer and endometrial cancer, but to a lesser extent than combined hormonal HRT.

Raloxifene

Raloxifene is a selective oestrogen receptor modulator with oestrogenic effects on bone but oestrogen antagonistic actions on breast and uterine receptors. This may be due to the way it binds to oestrogen receptors, with a side chain that prevents recruitment of activation factors in breast and uterine cells. Bone and other nonreproductive tissues contain 'raloxifene responding elements' in the nucleus that are stimulated by recruitment of helping proteins that differ from the activating factors in reproductive tissue. Raloxifene increases bone mineral density in postmenopausal osteoporosis, but does not treat menopausal symptoms. More details on raloxifene and osteoporosis are given in Chapter 42.

> ### UNWANTED EFFECTS OF HORMONE-REPLACEMENT THERAPY
>
> - Breakthrough bleeding can be troublesome, and regular withdrawal bleeds during the cycle are common unless continuous progestogen is used. These may be preceded by symptoms of premenstrual tension.
> - Headache, breast tenderness, bloating and muscle cramps are common but usually resolve over the first 3 months.
> - Nausea and vomiting.
> - Depression, irritability, loss of energy and poor concentration due to progestogen.
> - Transdermal delivery can cause contact sensitisation.
> - Increased risk of venous thromboembolism, especially in the first year and in those with other risk factors (obesity, smoking, immobility, previous thromboembolic disease). The risk after 5 years of use is increased by about 40% for combined HRT. This equates to an excess risk of 7 cases per 1000 for combined HRT, if aged 50–59 years, compared with a background incidence of 5 cases per 1000; the excess risk is more than doubled between

60 and 69 years. Transdermal oestrogen replacement is associated with a lower risk of venous thromboembolism.

- Increased risk of stroke (excess risk is 1 case per 1000 over 5 years if aged 50–59 years).
- HRT does not prevent coronary heart disease, and may increase the risk in the first year of treatment.
- Increased risk of dementia in women aged over 65 years.
- Increased risk of breast cancer within 1–2 years of starting use, increasing further with duration of use. The excess risk is lost 5 years after stopping HRT. Taking combined HRT for 10 years leads to a 40% increase in the risk of developing breast cancer in women aged 50–64 years (excess risk is 6 cases per 1000). Oestrogen-only HRT carries about one-quarter of this excess risk.
- The risk of endometrial cancer is increased by oestrogen-only HRT, which should always be combined with progestogen in women who have a uterus.
- The risk of cholecystitis is increased by oral but not transdermal oestrogen.

TREATMENTS FOR MENOPAUSAL SYMPTOMS

Oestrogen (used alone in women without a uterus or together with a progestogen) is by far the most effective treatment for menopausal symptoms, improving vasomotor symptoms and low mood. An initial low oral dose of oestrogen or transdermal delivery will minimise the risk of venous thromboembolism. It is important to emphasise that HRT does not provide contraceptive protection and to discuss the increased risk of breast cancer. HRT reduces the risk of vertebral and hip osteoporotic fractures. However, because of the potential risks of treatment, HRT is not considered to be first-line treatment to treat or prevent osteoporosis.

The benefits and risks of oestrogen-based HRT are highly individual for the patient. Unwanted effects are most likely to be troublesome in women who have been oestrogen deficient for some time, and usually resolve with continued use. There is a choice of continuous combined oestrogen and progestogen or sequential (cyclical) combined HRT with continuous oestrogen and added progestogen for 12–14 days a month. Continuous combined HRT is not suitable for women who are within 12 months of their last period, but will provide period-free HRT for older women. HRT should be reviewed annually, and women older than 50 years should be encouraged to use it for at least 3 years. If HRT is continued beyond 5 years or beyond age 54 years, then continuous combined HRT is desirable to avoid endometrial cystic hyperplasia. When a decision to stop is made, HRT should be withdrawn gradually. Women with premature natural or surgical menopause (before the age of 45 years) are recommended to continue treatment, at least until the average age of menopause at 51.4 years.

Tibolone is an option for women who have had amenorrhoea for at least 12 months. Atrophic vaginitis may respond to vaginal oestrogen, which is usually necessary long-term. There is limited evidence for the use of antidepressants that modulate monoaminergic neurotransmission, such as selective serotonin reuptake inhibitors (SSRIs) and serotonin and noradrenaline reuptake inhibitors (SNRIs; see Chapter 22) to treat perimenopausal symptoms. Clonidine (see Chapter 6) or the anticonvulsant gabapentin (see Chapter 23) can be used to treat hot flushes.

PREGNANCY AND LABOUR

THE ONSET AND INDUCTION OF LABOUR

Labour is the physiological process by which the fetus is expelled from the uterus (Fig. 45.3). The onset of labour is preceded by connective tissue changes in the cervix that allow it to dilate when uterine contractions start. The uterine muscle, the myometrium, must also be converted from a quiescent structure with dyssynchronous contractions to an active coordinated contractile unit, a process called activation. These events lead to spontaneous rupture of the fetal membranes.

The timing of the onset of labour is controlled by fetal–placental–maternal interactions. Activation of the uterine muscle is an inflammatory process mediated by several chemokines produced by the myometrium. These lead to gene expression for receptors for the myometrial contraction inducers (uterotonins) oxytocin and prostaglandin (PG)$F_{2\alpha}$.

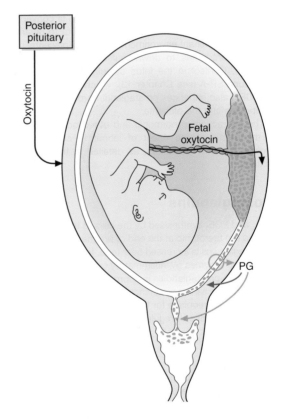

Fig. 45.3 **Induction of labour.** The mechanisms involved in the onset of labour in humans are uncertain but likely to be multifactorial. Prostaglandins (PG) are synthesised by the amnion and decidua and they stimulate the uterus and soften the cervix. Fetal and maternal oxytocin and prostaglandins may be involved in the processes of labour; their role in the initiation of labour is uncertain.

Contraction-associated proteins are also produced, which enhance the sensitivity of the uterus to uterotonins, and gap junctions between myometrial prostaglandin (PG)$F_{2\alpha}$ cells are increased. Together, these changes permit forceful and coordinated uterine contractions. The contractility of the uterus during labour commences at the uterotubular junction and progresses through the body of the uterus to the cervix, thus promoting efficient labour.

Pregnancy is maintained by the antiinflammatory effects of progesterone, and functional withdrawal of the effect of progesterone acts together with inflammatory signalling to induce labour. The inflammatory signal from the fetus that initiates labour includes production of surfactant protein-A (SP-A) and the inflammatory amniotic phospholipid platelet-activating factor (PAF).

Activation of the fetal hypothalamo–pituitary–adrenal (HPA) axis is the final common pathway toward labour. Placental expression of the gene for corticotropin-releasing hormone (CRH) is a crucial component of the biochemical signalling that precedes the inflammatory response. Placental CRH production is initially suppressed by progesterone, but increases exponentially at the end of pregnancy in response to maternal cortisol production. Activation of the fetal HPA axis by CRH leads to adrenocorticotropic hormone (ACTH) production and release of dehydroepiandrostenedione sulphate (DHEAS) and cortisol from the fetal adrenal glands. DHEAS is converted sequentially by the fetal liver and the placenta to oestriol. The cortisol-dominant environment of the feto-placental unit probably contributes to downregulation of progesterone receptors. Cortisol in the fetus stimulates the fetal lung to produce SP-A (see Chapter 13), which enters amniotic fluid. CRH also enhances prostaglandin production in fetal membranes and the placenta.

The interaction of hormonal and other local influences on the uterus at the onset of labour is complex and involves a variety of factors, as detailed in the following sections.

Prostaglandins

$PGF_{2\alpha}$ and PGE_2 synthesised by the cells of the amnion and decidua are uterotonic at the end of pregnancy. Production of prostaglandins is increased near term, following induction of synthetic enzymes by inflammatory cytokines. Myometrial sensitivity to prostaglandins is approximately 10-fold higher at term than in earlier pregnancy. PGE_2 softens the cervix, an essential prerequisite for the smooth passage of labour. Prostaglandins also upregulate oxytocin receptors.

Oxytocin

Oxytocin is a uterotonic peptide produced by the posterior pituitary (see Chapter 43). There is a marked increase in the expression of uterine oxytocin receptors from about 35 weeks of pregnancy onward. Oxytocin has a marked uterotonic action at term but is much less effective earlier in pregnancy. Oxytocin releases prostaglandins from fetal membranes and acts synergistically with prostaglandins to release Ca^{2+} from intracellular stores in the myometrial cells and promote muscle contraction. The oxytocin concentration in the maternal circulation does not increase until the second stage of labour when the cervix is fully dilated.

Oestradiol/oestriol

Oestrogen production increases in the last 4–6 weeks of pregnancy. Oestrogens increase the synthesis of prostaglandins and upregulate receptors for prostaglandins and oxytocin, which increases the sensitivity of the uterus to their effects. They increase myometrial gap junctions and promote fundal dominance of uterine contractility by an effect on the functional pacemaker at the uterotubular junction.

Progesterone

Progesterone is a major factor in uterine quiescence and maintaining cervical integrity. Progesterone decreases myometrial gap junctions, which reduces intrinsic contractility, diminishes uterine pacemaker activity and decreases the sensitivity of the uterus to oxytocin and prostaglandins. It also suppresses prostaglandin production. At the onset of labour there is reduced responsiveness of progesterone receptors, which blocks the cellular action of the hormone. This may be due to increased cortisol, which also antagonises the effects of progesterone on the feto-placental unit.

MYOMETRIAL RELAXANTS (TOCOLYTICS) AND PRETERM LABOUR

Preterm birth is a delivery that occurs before 37 weeks of gestation, and affects 7–10% of pregnancies. The causes include intrauterine growth restriction, preeclampsia, placenta previa, premature rupture of the membranes, intrauterine infection and uterine stretching from multiple birth pregnancy. Preterm birth may also be spontaneous.

Prematurity is the largest cause of neonatal morbidity and mortality, but relatively poor pharmacological tools are available currently to prevent it. This reflects our incomplete understanding of the underlying pathophysiology. Therapeutic strategies have concentrated on inhibition of myometrial contractions (tocolysis) when labour begins between 24 and 33 weeks gestation.

Atosiban

Mechanism of action

Atosiban is a peptide analogue of oxytocin that is an antagonist at oxytocin receptors in the decidua and myometrium, reducing the release of intracellular Ca^{2+}.

Pharmacokinetics

Atosiban is given initially by intravenous bolus injection followed by an infusion; it has a short half-life (0.2–1.7 h).

Unwanted effects

- Nausea, vomiting.
- Headache, dizziness.
- Tachycardia, hypotension, hot flushes.
- Hyperglycaemia.

Beta$_2$-adrenoceptor agonists

β_2-Adrenoceptor agonists inhibit uterine contractility by increasing the intracellular concentration of cyclic adenosine monophosphate. Salbutamol is given intravenously or orally for up to 48 hours following the start of preterm labour, after which the risks to the mother increase with no benefit to the fetus. Unwanted effects include nausea, vomiting, flushing, and maternal and fetal tachycardia with hypotension (see also Chapter 12).

Calcium channel blockers

Nifedipine (see Chapter 5) is used orally and is as effective as other tocolytics, with fewer unwanted effects than β_2-adrenoceptor agonists.

Nonsteroidal antiinflammatory drugs

NSAIDs (see Chapter 29) can delay delivery, but there are concerns about transient neonatal renal impairment and premature closure of the ductus arteriosus. They are not widely used.

Management of preterm labour

Tocolytics prolong pregnancy for up to 7 days, but do not improve fetal morbidity or mortality. However, they provide a limited time for treatment with a corticosteroid to enhance lung maturation (see Chapter 13), or for transfer of the mother to a specialist unit. When a tocolytic drug is indicated, then nifedipine or atosiban are preferred, since they have fewer unwanted effects on the mother than a β_2-adrenoceptor agonist. Nifedipine has the advantage of oral administration.

Intravenous magnesium sulphate is recommended for all women in preterm labour to reduce the risk of cerebral palsy, although it does not prolong pregnancy.

INDUCING AND AUGMENTING LABOUR

Induction of labour may be necessary if a woman has not entered spontaneous labour by 42 weeks gestation or if there has been spontaneous rupture of membranes after 34 weeks. Inadequate uterine contractions in the first stage of labour may respond to pharmacological augmentation.

Dinoprostone

Dinoprostone (the name for exogenous PGE_2) produces contractions in both the nonpregnant and the pregnant uterus. The sensitivity of the uterus to prostaglandins is higher than to oxytocin prior to term. Dinoprostone can produce contractions that are indistinguishable from spontaneous labour and have the added advantage of softening ('ripening') the cervix, so it can be used for induction of labour before term. Dinoprostone is given as vaginal tablets, pessaries or gels.

Unwanted effects

- Gastrointestinal disturbances, particularly nausea, vomiting and diarrhoea.
- Uterine hypertonus, amniotic fluid embolism, placental abruption.
- Maternal hypertension.
- Bronchospasm.

Oxytocin

Oxytocin is given by slow intravenous infusion to augment contractions in inadequate labour. The concentration given depends upon the response, and the aim is to produce regular coordinated contractions with complete relaxation between contractions. Oxytocin is an effective uterine stimulant in women at term, and labour will usually proceed well if the cervix is partially dilated and softened prior to its use. Oxytocin, unlike prostaglandins, does not soften the cervix.

Inappropriately high concentrations of oxytocin can cause uterine hypertonus, when the uterus does not relax between contractions, and fetal distress can occur. As labour progresses and the woman's 'endogenous' induction mechanisms come into play, the concentration of oxytocin may need to be reduced. Following delivery, oxytocin can also be useful to reduce postpartum haemorrhage (discussed later). Oxytocin in high doses has a weak antidiuretic activity, as it is related to vasopressin, and large doses can cause fluid retention (see Chapter 43).

Pharmacological induction and augmentation of labour

A membrane sweep is the initial approach to initiate labour if the membranes have not ruptured. Vaginal dinoprostone is used after premature rupture of membranes without spontaneous onset of labour, but only if the pregnancy has advanced beyond 34 weeks or there is infection or fetal compromise. Vaginal dinoprostone is also the preferred method for induction in prolonged gestation. Induced labour is often more painful than natural labour, and regional analgesia is more likely to be needed.

If there is delay in the first stage of labour (after the onset of regular painful contractions and progressive cervical dilation), then intravenous infusion of oxytocin can be considered to progress the delivery. Gradual incremental increase in the rate of infusion may be necessary, with the goal being to achieve 4–5 contractions in 10 minutes and to avoid uterine hyperstimulation.

MEDICAL ABORTION

Mifepristone

Mechanism of action and uses

Mifepristone is a potent progesterone receptor antagonist. It is given orally to soften the cervix and induce decidual necrosis, which encourages placental detachment. Mifepristone also sensitises the uterus to prostaglandin-induced contractions.

Mifepristone can be given alone to soften the cervix 36 hours before surgical termination of early pregnancy.

Pharmacokinetics

Mifepristone is metabolised in the liver and has a half-life of 18 hours.

Unwanted effects

- Abdominal cramps.
- Vaginal bleeding.
- Uterine pain, which can be severe.

Prostaglandin derivatives

Prostaglandins soften the cervix and produce prolonged uterine contraction. Misoprostol can be given orally or vaginally, and gemeprost (a PGE$_1$ analogue) is given as an intravaginal pessary.

Gemeprost is also given as a pessary to ripen and soften the cervix prior to early surgical abortion.

Induction of medical abortion

For medical termination of pregnancy up to 24 weeks' gestation or following spontaneous fetal death, mifepristone is given as a single oral dose followed 6–48 hours later by a prostaglandin. This can be either vaginal gemeprost, or misoprostol (see Chapter 33), which can be given orally but is more effective given vaginally. Early administration of the prostaglandin after mifepristone is only used for gestations up to 9 weeks. The abortion may be complete 4–5 hours after the prostaglandin, but can take up to a few days. Antibiotics, such as metronidazole with azithromycin, are given to reduce the risk of infection and NSAIDs for pain relief.

PAIN RELIEF IN LABOUR

Pain in labour can be alleviated by breathing and relaxation techniques, massage and undergoing labour in water. Inhalation of a 50:50 mixture of oxygen and nitrous oxide (see Chapter 17) is often helpful, but may cause nausea and lightheadedness. Opioids are sometimes used, but may cause drowsiness, nausea and vomiting for the mother, and respiratory depression and drowsiness in the baby.

Regional analgesia is increasingly used with either low-dose epidural analgesia or combined spinal-epidural analgesia. A combination of bupivacaine and fentanyl is often used (see Chapter 18).

POSTPARTUM HAEMORRHAGE

Excessive bleeding from the uterus can arise after incomplete abortion or after a normal delivery. It is more common in women who are morbidly obese, with multiple pregnancies, aged over 35 years, or who have had pregnancy induced or required the use of oxytocin to speed up labour.

Ergometrine maleate

Ergometrine causes hypertonic contractions of the uterus and is therefore not used for induction of labour, as it would result in fetal distress and poor progress in labour. It also causes vasoconstriction by α-adrenoceptor stimulation (see ergotamine, Chapter 26), which further limits haemorrhage.

Pharmacokinetics

Ergometrine is given intramuscularly and works within 2–7 minutes.

Unwanted effects

- Nausea, vomiting, abdominal pain.
- Headache, dizziness, tinnitus.
- Chest pain, peripheral vasoconstriction, hypertension, dyspnoea.

Prevention and management of postpartum haemorrhage

To minimise bleeding after delivery, a single intramuscular dose of oxytocin should be given to the mother on delivery of the anterior shoulder, unless the mother has requested a physiological birth. After placental separation, uterine hypertonus produced by oxytocin squeezes the uterine blood vessels and reduces blood loss. Use of oxytocin reduces the risk of significant postpartum haemorrhage by 55%.

Initial management of significant haemorrhage involves uterine massage, intravenous fluids and controlled cord traction if the placenta has not been delivered. First-line drug treatment is a bolus dose of either intravenous oxytocin, intramuscular ergometrine or combined intramuscular oxytocin and ergometrine. There are several options if bleeding continues, including a repeat bolus of the first-line treatment, one of the prostaglandin analogues (misoprostol vaginally or carboprost by intramuscular injection), or oxytocin infusion. Intravenous tranexamic acid (see Chapter 11) can be given as an adjuvant option.

SELF-ASSESSMENT

True/false questions

1. Oestrogen has a negative feedback effect on luteinising hormone (LH) and follicle-stimulating hormone (FSH) secretion from the anterior pituitary throughout the follicular phase of the menstrual cycle.
2. In the luteal phase, the elevated level of progesterone is controlled by gonadotropins.
3. Progesterone causes cervical mucus to be viscous and hostile to the passage of sperm.
4. The oral progestogen-only contraceptive reliably inhibits ovulation.
5. Both oestrogen and progesterone inhibit the motility of the Fallopian tube.
6. The functioning corpus luteum maintains pregnancy for the first 6–8 weeks after implantation.
7. Progestogens used in combined hormonal contraceptives do not differ in their androgenic activity.
8. Biphasic and triphasic formulations of combined oral hormonal contraceptives result in lower overall dosages of oestrogen and progestogen than monophasic formulations.
9. Effective protection is lost if there is a delay of more than 3 hours in taking the daily oral dose of a combined hormonal contraceptive.
10. Emergency contraception with ulipristal acetate is effective when taken up to 120 hours after unprotected intercourse.
11. An etonogestrel implant beneath the skin of the upper arm provides effective contraception for 5 years.
12. Antiepileptic drugs such as carbamazepine can reduce the plasma concentrations of oestrogens and progestogens.
13. Mortality from venous thromboembolism is increased in women using the oral combined hormonal contraceptive who smoke.

14. The combined hormonal contraceptive significantly increases blood pressure in most women.
15. Oestrogen used on its own as hormone-replacement therapy (HRT) may cause endometrial hyperplasia.
16. Postmenopausal women taking continuous HRT with both oestrogen and progestogens do not experience breakthrough bleeding.
17. Oestrogens and progestogens can be given transdermally.
18. Raloxifene blocks oestrogen receptors in bone.
19. Tibolone reduces bone loss in postmenopausal women.
20. Oxytocin is preferred to prostaglandins for the induction of labour at 34 weeks of gestation.
21. Progesterone increases the number of gap junctions in the uterus.
22. Ergometrine can be used for the induction of labour.
23. Atosiban is a tocolytic drug that acts by blocking oxytocin receptors.
24. Nonsteroidal antiinflammatory drugs (NSAIDs) are used in treating dysmenorrhoea.

One-best-answer (OBA) questions

1. Identify the *most accurate* statement below concerning the contraceptive options for a 35-year-old woman who smokes 40 cigarettes a day, but who, despite treatment, has not been able to stop smoking.
   A. The oral combined hormonal contraceptive would be suitable for her contraception.
   B. The oral combined hormonal contraceptive would increase her risk of endometrial cancer.
   C. The oral combined hormonal contraceptive would have a lower failure rate than an intrauterine contraceptive device (IUD).
   D. The oral progestogen-only contraceptive would provide adequate contraception without increasing the risk of venous thromboembolism.
   E. An intramuscular injection of medroxyprogesterone acetate would give contraceptive protection for at least 6 months.
2. Identify the *incorrect* statement concerning drugs used during labour and abortion.
   A. Mifepristone is a progesterone receptor antagonist used to induce abortion.
   B. Prostaglandin E_2 is preferred to oxytocin for induction of labour at 35 weeks of gestation.
   C. Oxytocin is less likely than prostaglandins to cause uterine hypertonus.
   D. β_2-Adrenoceptor agonists to prolong pregnancy do not reduce mortality in babies born preterm.
   E. Ergometrine reduces postpartum haemorrhage by constricting uterine blood vessels.

ANSWERS

True/false answers

1. **False.** The negative feedback in the early part of the follicular phase switches to positive feedback at an oestradiol level of approximately 200 pg/mL, resulting in the midcycle surge in LH and FSH.

2. **True.** The LH levels fall precipitously after the midcycle surge, but they are high enough to support the secretion of progesterone in the luteal phase.
3. **True.** The effect on cervical mucus is an important action of the oral progestogen-only contraceptive.
4. **False.** Ovulation occurs in up to 50% of women with the oral progestogen-only contraceptive, as other effects are responsible for its contraceptive action. Ovulation is reliably inhibited in women using parenteral progestogens.
5. **False.** Progesterone inhibits fallopian tube motility, and oestrogens enhance it. An imbalance may alter oocyte transport and the probability of fertilisation and implantation.
6. **True.** After 6–8 weeks of pregnancy maintained by the corpus luteum, the placenta takes over production of sex steroids under the influence of human chorionic gonadotropin (HCG).
7. **False.** Progestogens in second-generation combined hormonal contraceptives (such as levonorgestrel and norethisterone) have variable androgenic activity, but gestodene and desogestrel used in third-generation combined hormonal contraceptives have little or no androgenic activity.
8. **False.** Biphasic and triphasic formulations mimic more closely the steroidal changes in the menstrual cycle, but they do not reduce the overall administered dose of each component.
9. **False.** Protection is reduced if there is a delay of more than 12 hours in taking a daily dose of the combined oral hormonal contraceptive, but this can occur with a delay of only 3 hours in taking oral progesterone-only contraceptives.
10. **True.** The progesterone receptor modulator ulipristal acetate suppresses the follicle until the time of the LH surge and is effective for up to 120 hours after unprotected intercourse.
11. **False.** Etonogestrel implants must be replaced every 3 years.
12. **True.** By inducing liver microsomal enzymes, carbamazepine, phenytoin, rifampicin and other drugs lower the effective concentrations of oestrogens and progestogens as their metabolism is enhanced.
13. **True.** The excess risk of thromboembolic disease in women taking the combined hormonal contraceptive is significantly greater in smokers; other risk factors include age over 35 years, family history, obesity and long-term immobilisation.
14. **False.** A small increase in blood pressure is commonly seen with the combined contraceptive, but a significant rise occurs in only 5% of previously normotensive women.
15. **True.** The risk of endometrial hyperplasia with oestrogen is reduced by giving progestogens concurrently; oestrogens can be used alone in women who have had a hysterectomy.
16. **False.** Breakthrough bleeding frequently occurs, particularly in the first 6 months of treatment.
17. **True.** Both oestrogens and progestogens undergo extensive first-pass hepatic metabolism, and this can be avoided by transdermal absorption from patches.
18. **False.** Raloxifene is a selective oestrogen receptor modulator; it stimulates oestrogen receptors in bone but not in breast or uterine tissue.

19. **True.** Tibolone has weak oestrogenic and progestogenic activity and reduces bone loss.
20. **False.** Oxytocin is less effective in earlier pregnancy compared with full term. An intravaginal pessary of prostaglandin would increase uterine contractility and also soften the cervix.
21. **False.** Oestrogens increase uterine gap junctions in the uterus, facilitating uterine contractility, while progesterone opposes this action of oestrogens.
22. **False.** Ergometrine is given alone or together with oxytocin at the time of delivery to reduce postpartum haemorrhage; it should not be given for labour induction, as hypertonic uterine activity would delay labour and cause fetal distress.
23. **True.** Atosiban is a partial agonist of oxytocin receptors that acts as an antagonist in the presence of oxytocin, and reduces uterine contractility in preterm labour; other tocolytic drugs include β_2-adrenoceptor agonists and calcium channel blockers.
24. **True.** NSAIDs relieve dysmenorrhoea in approximately 70% of women; the combined and progestogen-only hormonal contraceptives may also be effective.

One-best-answer (OBA) answers

1. **Answer D** is the most accurate statement.
   A. Incorrect. In a 35-year-old woman who smokes, the oral combined hormonal contraceptive is not a good choice due to an increased risk of cardiovascular complications.
   B. Incorrect. The oral combined hormonal contraceptive reduces the risk of endometrial cancer.
   C. Incorrect. The IUD is as effective as the combined hormonal contraceptive.
   D. **Correct.** The risk of thromboembolic complications of the combined oral hormonal contraceptive is related to the oestrogen content; progestogen-only contraception does not increase thromboembolism risk.
   E. Incorrect. Intramuscular medroxyprogesterone acetate is effective for 8–12 weeks.
2. **Answer C** is the incorrect statement.
   A. Correct. Blockade of the actions of progesterone by mifepristone results in abortion, although the precise mechanisms are uncertain.
   B. Correct. Women should be given prostaglandins to soften the cervix prior to rupture of the membranes, and then intravenous oxytocin if required.
   C. **Incorrect.** Both oxytocin and prostaglandins can cause uterine hypertonus and fetal distress if given in inappropriate amounts.
   D. Correct. β_2-Adrenoceptor agonists may delay labour for up to 48 hours, but they have not been shown to decrease morbidity or mortality in the preterm newborn child.
   E. Correct. Ergometrine constricts uterine blood vessels via α_1-adrenoceptors, and uterine hypertonus further compresses blood vessels, reducing postpartum blood loss.

FURTHER READING

Bakour, S.H., Williamson, J., 2015. Latest evidence on using hormone replacement therapy in the menopause. Obstet. Gynaecol. 17, 20–28.

Haas, D.M., Caldwell, D.M., Kirkpatrick, P., et al., 2012. Tocolytic therapy for preterm delivery: systematic review and network meta-analysis. Br. Med. J. 345, e6226.

Harel, Z., 2012. Dysmenorrhea in adolescents and young adults: an update on pharmacological treatments and management strategies. Expert Opin. Pharmacother. 13, 2157–2170.

Hickey, M., Elliott, J., Davison, S.L., 2012. Hormone replacement therapy. Br. Med. J. 344, e763.

Hickey, M., Ballard, K., Farquhar, C., 2014. Endometriosis. Br. Med. J. 348, g1752.

Kaunitz, A.M., 2008. Hormonal contraception in women of older reproductive age. N. Engl. J. Med. 358, 1262–1270.

O'Brien, S., Rapkin, A., Dennerstein, L., et al., 2011. Diagnosis and management of premenstrual disorders. Br. Med. J. 342, d2994.

Prabakar, I., Webb, A., 2012. Emergency contraception. Br. Med. J. 344, e1492.

Ryu, A., Kim, T.-H., 2015. Premenstrual syndrome: a mini review. Maturitas 82, 436–440.

Compendium: drugs acting on the female reproductive system

Drug	Characteristics
Oestrogens	
Used as components of combined oral hormonal contraceptives and also for hormone-replacement therapy (HRT) for menopausal symptoms and osteoporosis prophylaxis; other uses are specified. Some oestrogens, progestogens and oestrogen receptor antagonists are used for the treatment of malignant disease (see Chapter 52).	
Conjugated oestrogen (equine)	Given as sulphate conjugates of >10 equine oestrogens. Used as a component of HRT
Oestradiol	Converted to oestrone and oestriol. Given alone as HRT, and also (as oestradiol hemihydrate) in combined oral hormonal contraceptive (with nomegestrol). Half-life: 1–2 h
Oestradiol valerate	Prodrug of oestradiol. Component of combined oral hormonal contraceptive (with dienogest). Half-life: 24 h

Compendium: drugs acting on the female reproductive system (cont'd)

Drug	Characteristics
Ethinylestradiol	Component of combined oral hormonal contraceptive (with desogestrel, drospirenone, gestodene, levonorgestrel, norethisterone or norgestimate); also used (with norelgestromin) in once-weekly transdermal patch, and (with etonogestrel) in vaginal ring. Also used in hereditary haemorrhagic telangiectasia. Half-life: 8–24 h
Mestranol	Mostly converted to ethinylestradiol. Component of oral combined hormonal contraceptive (with norethisterone). Half-life: 8–24 h

Progestogens

Used as components of oral, parenteral and intrauterine contraceptives and for HRT; other uses are specified.

Desogestrel	Third-generation progestogen, derived from norgestrel; converted to etonogestrel. Component of combined oral hormonal contraceptives and also as progestin-only oral contraceptive. Half-life: 30 h
Dienogest	Third-generation progestogen. Used (with oestradiol valerate) in combined oral hormonal contraceptive. Half-life: 11 h
Drospirenone	Third-generation progestogen with antimineralocorticoid and antiandrogen activity. Component of combined oral hormonal contraceptives (with ethinylestradiol) and as HRT (with oestrogens). Half-life: 36–42 h
Dydrogesterone	Progesterone analogue used in endometriosis, infertility, recurrent miscarriage, premenstrual syndrome, amenorrhoea and dysmenorrhea, and as HRT (with oestrogens). Half-life: 5–7 h
Etonogestrel	Third-generation progestogen. Slow-release etonogestrel implant inserted subdermally to give prolonged contraception; also used (with ethinylestradiol) in vaginal ring. Half-life: 29 h
Gestodene	Third-generation progestogen, derived from norgestrel. Component of oral hormonal contraceptives (with ethinylestradiol). Half-life: 18 h
Levonorgestrel	Second-generation progestogen; isomer of norgestrel. Used as component of oral combined hormonal contraceptive (with ethinylestradiol), and as progestin-only oral contraceptive; also used (with oestrogens) as HRT. Effective emergency contraception up to 72 h after unprotected sexual intercourse. Also used in an intrauterine device for contraception and primary menorrhagia. Half-life: 8–30 h
Medroxyprogesterone acetate	Long-acting progestogen. Given as deep intramuscular injection or subcutaneous injection for contraception; also used (with oestrogens) as HRT. Half-life: 30 days
Nomegestrol	Third-generation progestogen. Used (with oestradiol hemihydrate) in combined oral hormonal contraceptive. Half-life: 46 h
Norelgestromin	Third-generation progestogen. Used as a once-weekly transdermal patch (with ethinylestradiol); applied for 3 weeks in every four. Half-life: 28 h
Norethisterone	Testosterone-derived, first-generation progestogen. Used as component of oral hormonal contraceptives (with ethinylestradiol or mestranol) and as progestogen-only oral contraceptive, and (with oestrogens) as HRT. Also used for endometriosis, premenstrual syndrome, dysmenorrhoea and postponement of menstruation. Half-life: 5–12 h
Norethisterone acetate	Converted to norethisterone. Component of oral hormonal contraceptives and also used as HRT
Norethisterone enantate	Hydrolysed to norethisterone. Long-acting progestogen. Given as an oily solution by deep intramuscular injection
Norgestimate	Third-generation progestogen; derivative of norgestrel. Prodrug converted to active metabolites including norelgestromin and levonorgestrel (half-lives 8–30 h). Component of oral hormonal contraceptives (with ethinylestradiol)
Norgestrel	Second-generation progestogen. Used (with oestrogens) as HRT. Half-life: 20 h
Progesterone	Converted to pregnanediol. Given as rectal or vaginal pessaries for infertility, premenstrual syndrome and postnatal depression, or by injection for dysmenorrhea. Half-life: 5–20 min
Ulipristal acetete	Progesterone receptor modulator. Effective emergency contraception up to 120 h after unprotected sexual intercourse. Given orally. Half-life: 32 h

Compendium: drugs acting on the female reproductive system (cont'd)

Drug	Characteristics
Drugs used primarily for endometriosis	
Other uses are specified.	
Danazol	Antigonadotrophic drug with androgenic, antioestrogenic and antiprogestogenic effects. Also used for severe pain in benign fibrocystic breast disease and hereditary angioedema. Given orally. Half-life: 4–5 h
Gonadorelin	Gonadotropin-releasing hormone. Given by intravenous injection for assessment of pituitary function. See Chapter 43
Gonadorelin analogues	
Downregulate gonadotropin-releasing hormone (GnRH) receptors and thereby reduce the release of gonadotropins. Used for endometriosis and infertility, and before intrauterine surgery; other uses are specified.	
Buserelin	Used for prostate cancer (see Chapter 52). Given intranasally for endometriosis and by subcutaneous injection. Half-life: 1–1.5 h
Goserelin	Used for prostate cancer and early and advanced breast cancer (see Chapter 52). Given by subcutaneous implant. Half-life: 4 h
Leuprorelin acetate	Used for prostate cancer (see Chapter 52). Given by subcutaneous or intramuscular injection. Half-life: 3 h
Nafarelin	Used for endometriosis. Given intranasally. Half-life: 3–4 h
Triptorelin	Used for prostate cancer (see Chapter 52). Given by intramuscular injection. Half-life: 3 h
Drugs used for menopausal symptoms and/or osteoporosis	
Raloxifene	Selective oestrogen receptor modulator. Used in treatment of postmenopausal osteoporosis (Chapter 42). Given orally. Half-life: 28 h
Tibolone	Oestrogenic, progestogenic and weak androgenic activities. Used for the short-term treatment and prevention of menopausal vasomotor symptoms and postmenopausal osteoporosis. Given orally. Active metabolite half-lives: 4–14 h
Anti-oestrogens	
Induce gonadotropin release by suppressing negative feedback by oestrogen.	
Clomifene	Used for female infertility associated with oligomenorrhoea or secondary amenorrhoea. Given orally. See Chapter 43
Tamoxifen	Main use is in breast cancer. See Chapter 52
Drugs used to treat mastalgia	
Bromocriptine	See Chapters 24 and 43
Danazol	See drugs for endometriosis listed previously
Tamoxifen	See Chapter 52
Prostaglandins, oxytocics and drugs used to reduce postpartum haemorrhage	
Carbetocin	Oxytocin receptor agonist. Used for uterine atony and postpartum haemorrhage after caesarean section. Given by intravenous injection. Half-life: 40 min
Carboprost	15-Methyl derivative of $PGF_{2\alpha}$. Used for severe postpartum haemorrhage due to uterine atony. Given by deep intramuscular injection. Half-life: 8 min
Dinoprostone (PGE_2)	Used for induction of labour. Given intravaginally (or rarely by intravenous injection). Half-life: 30 s
Ergometrine (ergonovine)	Used to prevent and treat postpartum haemorrhage. Given by intramuscular injection. Half-life: 2 h
Gemeprost	Prostaglandin E_1 analogue. Used to soften the cervix in labour induction and to induce abortion. Given intravaginally. Hydrolysed locally in minutes
Oxytocin	Used for induction of labour. Given by slow intravenous injection or infusion. Half-life: 2–10 min

Compendium: drugs acting on the female reproductive system (cont'd)

Drug	Characteristics
Drugs used for effects on ductus arteriosus	
Alprostadil (PGE$_1$)	Used to maintain patency of the ductus arteriosus in neonates with congenital heart defects. Given by intravenous infusion. Half-life: 30 s
Indometacin	NSAID. Used to close the ductus arteriosus in premature babies. Given by intravenous injection. See Chapter 29
Drugs used primarily for therapeutic abortions	
Gemeprost	Prostaglandin E$_1$ analogue (noted previously). Used for the medical induction of late therapeutic abortion. Given as an intravaginal pessary
Mifepristone	Acts as a progesterone receptor antagonist. Given orally or vaginally prior to therapeutic abortion to sensitise uterus to actions of prostaglandins. Half-life: 18 h
Misoprostol	Prostaglandin E$_1$ analogue. Used for the induction of second trimester abortion. Given orally or vaginally. Half-life: 20–40 min
Myometrial relaxant drugs	
Atosiban	Peptide antagonist of oxytocin receptors. Used for inhibition of uncomplicated premature labour at 24–33 weeks of gestation. Given by intravenous injection or infusion. Half-life: 0.2–1.7 h
Nifedipine	Calcium channel blocker (Chapter 5). Given orally
Salbutamol	β_2-Adrenoceptor agonist (see Chapter 12); used for inhibition of uncomplicated premature labour at 24–33 weeks of gestation. Given by intravenous infusion and then orally
Terbutaline	β_2-Adrenoceptor agonist (see Chapter 12); used for inhibition of uncomplicated premature labour at 24–33 weeks of gestation. Given orally, subcutaneously or by intravenous infusion

HRT, hormone-replacement therapy; *NSAID*, nonsteroidal antiinflammatory drug; *PG*, prostaglandin.

46

Androgens, antiandrogens and anabolic steroids

ANDROGENS AND ANABOLIC STEROIDS

Naturally occurring androgens are 19-carbon steroid hormones (Fig. 44.1) that are synthesised in the adrenal cortex and gonads from cholesterol (Fig. 44.2). They have characteristic actions on the reproductive tract and other tissues, as well as an anabolic effect on metabolism, including inhibition of fat deposition and enlargement of skeletal muscles. A number of synthetic androgenic steroids have been developed. The term *anabolic steroid* is used when the predominant action of the compound is anabolic rather than reproductive. There are a few medical uses for anabolic steroids, but they have achieved notoriety because of their abuse by athletes to enhance muscle development.

Testosterone is secreted by the Leydig cells of the testis, and its synthesis and release are stimulated by the gonadotropin luteinising hormone (LH). In many tissues testosterone is aromatised to form oestradiol, which accelerates closure of bony epiphyses and contributes to brain development. It is oestradiol rather than testosterone that inhibits the release of gonadotropin-releasing hormone (GnRH) from the hypothalamus and LH via a negative-feedback loop (see Chapter 43). Two further androgens, dehydroepiandrosterone and androstenedione, are released from the adrenal cortex in response to stimulation by adrenocorticotropic hormone (ACTH; corticotropin; Fig. 44.2). Men produce large amounts of androgens and small amounts of oestrogens, while the reverse is the case in women.

The effects of testosterone are in part due to its metabolite dihydrotestosterone (DHT). This is produced from testosterone in the prostate, skin and reproductive tissues by the enzymatic action of 5α-reductase (Fig. 44.2). DHT has a higher affinity than testosterone for the androgen receptor, and is five times more potent as an androgen. DHT is mainly responsible for the development of secondary sexual characteristics in men.

The cellular mechanism of action of steroid hormones is discussed in Chapter 1. Androgens act mainly through genomic effects on protein synthesis. They form a complex with the cytoplasmic androgen receptor (AR), which then translocates to the cell nucleus. The androgen receptor also produces rapid-onset, nongenomic actions in the cytoplasm by affecting signal transduction and ion transport. This is responsible for effects such as vasodilation (see also Chapter 44).

Circulating androgens are bound largely to a specific transport protein, sex hormone-binding globulin (SHBG), which has a greater affinity for androgens than for oestrogen.

MALE SEX HORMONES

Examples

mesterolone (methyltestosterone), testosterone

Actions of testosterone

Actions of androgens include the following:

- sexual differentiation in the fetus.
- sexual development of the male testis, penis, epididymis, seminal vesicles and prostate at puberty, and maintenance of these tissues in adults.
- spermatogenesis in adults.
- stimulation and maintenance of sexual function and behaviour.
- metabolic actions. Testosterone is a powerful anabolic agent, producing a positive nitrogen balance with an increase in the bulk of tissues such as muscle and bone. In the skin, sebum production is increased, which can provoke acne. Growth of axillary, pubic, facial and chest

hair is stimulated. In the liver, testosterone increases the synthesis of several proteins, including clotting factors, but decreases high-density lipoprotein (HDL) synthesis (see Chapter 48). Testosterone also induces several liver enzymes, including steroid hydroxylases.

■ haematological actions. Testosterone stimulates the production of erythropoietin by the kidneys, leading to higher haemoglobin concentrations in men than in women.

Pharmacokinetics

■ Oral preparations. After oral administration, testosterone is almost completely degraded by first-pass metabolism in the gut wall and liver. Oral absorption can be enhanced by esterification of testosterone to create hydrophobic compounds, such as testosterone undecanoate, which are absorbed via lacteals into the lymphatic system, thus avoiding hepatic metabolism. Mesterolone is a synthetic testosterone derivative that has a greater oral bioavailability than testosterone, but less androgenic activity.

■ Depot injection. The most widely used therapy for hypogonadism in men is an intramuscular injection of a testosterone ester, usually in oily solution, given at intervals from 2–3 weeks up to 10–14 weeks, depending on the formulation. Testosterone is absorbed gradually after ester hydrolysis at the site of injection. Examples are testosterone enantate, propionate and undecanoate.

■ Transdermal delivery using testosterone gel.

Testosterone is metabolised in the liver to androstenedione, and then to inactive compounds. Some testosterone undergoes conversion in specific organs to dihydrotestosterone, and a small amount undergoes aromatisation to oestradiol (discussed previously). Mesterolone is not metabolised to oestrogenic compounds.

Unwanted effects

■ Prostate cancer.

■ In hypogonadal adolescents, initial nitrogen retention and a spurt in linear growth is followed by premature epiphyseal closure and short stature. A short course of testosterone can be used for the treatment of delayed puberty without inducing epiphyseal closure.

■ Headache.

■ Anxiety, depression.

■ Nausea, vomiting, gastrointestinal bleeding.

■ Sodium retention with oedema and hypertension.

■ Hirsutism, male-pattern baldness, acne.

■ Conversion to oestrogens by aromatase can produce gynaecomastia (see Fig. 44.2). This is less likely to occur with mesterolone.

■ Suppression of gonadotropin release with diminished testicular size and reduced spermatogenesis. Hypogonadal men will not regain fertility while taking androgens.

■ Cholestatic jaundice.

■ Local irritation from topical formulations.

Clinical uses of testosterone

■ The main clinical use is as hormone-replacement therapy for primary hypogonadism in adult males. Late-onset hypogonadism may present with erectile dysfunction, fatigue, depression, hot flushes, muscle weakness and reduced body hair. Testosterone replacement can improve quality of life in this situation.

■ It can be used briefly in constitutionally delayed puberty, even in the absence of hypogonadism.

■ Androgens are occasionally beneficial for promoting erythropoiesis in some forms of aplastic anaemia.

DANAZOL

Mechanism of action

Danazol is an androgen derivative described as an 'impeded' androgen, which is weakly androgenic on peripheral tissues. It has no oestrogenic activity as, unlike testosterone, it is not converted into an oestrogen by aromatases. Its main action is feedback inhibition of gonadotropin and GnRH secretion. It therefore has antioestrogenic and antiprogestogenic actions.

Pharmacokinetics

Danazol is metabolised in the liver and has a short half-life of 3 hours.

Unwanted effects

■ Nausea, epigastric pain.

■ Acne, hirsutism, oedema, hair loss or deepening of voice, due to androgenic effects.

■ Depression, anxiety.

■ Dizziness, headache.

■ In women, vaginal dryness, reduction in breast size, changes in libido, amenorrhoea, hot flushes.

Clinical uses of danazol

■ Treatment of endometriosis (see Chapter 45).

■ Treatment of menorrhagia (see Chapter 45).

■ Management of gynaecomastia (see Chapter 45).

■ Long-term management of hereditary angioedema.

ANABOLIC STEROIDS

Examples

nandrolone, oxymetholone

Anabolic steroids are most frequently encountered as drugs of abuse to improve athletic performance (doping). In medical practice there are few indications for these compounds, and there is little evidence for efficacy in many conditions where their use has been advocated.

PHARMACOKINETICS

Nandrolone is given as a decanoate ester depot formulation by intramuscular injection every 3 weeks. Oxymetholone is available as an oral formulation from specialist suppliers.

UNWANTED EFFECTS

Androgenic effects may be troublesome in women.

CLINICAL USES

- Oxymetholone is used to promote erythropoiesis in aplastic anaemias.
- Itching associated with chronic biliary obstruction in palliative care.

ABUSE OF ANABOLIC STEROIDS

The ability of androgens to promote an increase in muscle mass has led to their abuse to improve physical performance by athletes, weightlifters and bodybuilders. Often, several different androgens are used for prolonged periods, perhaps with a brief 'drug-free' period. Abused compounds include testosterone, nandrolone and oxymetholone, and many others that are licensed only for veterinary use. The consequences of abuse include:

- weight gain from muscle hypertrophy and fluid retention;
- acne in adolescent and young men;
- decreased testicular size and reduced sperm count;
- hepatotoxicity with cholestasis, hepatitis, or occasionally, hepatocellular tumours;
- atherogenic changes in the plasma lipids with a rise in plasma low density lipoprotein (LDL) cholesterol and a fall in high density lipoprotein (HDL) cholesterol (see Chapter 48), which may predispose to premature vascular disease;
- psychological disturbance, including changes in libido, increased aggression and psychotic symptoms.

ANTIANDROGENS

BICALUTAMIDE AND FLUTAMIDE

Mechanism of action

Bicalutamide and flutamide are nonsteroidal, relatively pure antiandrogens. They bind competitively to androgen receptors in the cell cytoplasm, producing distortion of the co-activator binding site, so that the receptor cannot initiate gene transcription.

Pharmacokinetics

Bicalutamide is metabolised in the liver and has a very long half-life of 7–10 days. Flutamide undergoes extensive first-pass metabolism and has a half-life of 8 h.

Unwanted effects

- Antiandrogenic effects (e.g. gynaecomastia, hot flushes, impotence, decreased libido and inhibition of spermatogenesis).
- Nausea, vomiting, diarrhoea, weight gain.
- Rash, pruritis, dry skin
- Cholestatic jaundice.

CYPROTERONE ACETATE

Mechanism of action

Cyproterone acetate, a 21-carbon steroid, is a progestogen and a weak glucocorticoid (see Chapter 44). Its progestational activity produces feedback inhibition of gonadotrophin (LH) secretion (see Chapter 45). At high doses cyproterone inhibits androgen binding to its receptors.

Pharmacokinetics

Cyproterone acetate is metabolised in the liver, and has a very long half-life of 2 days.

Unwanted effects

- Antiandrogenic effects (e.g. gynaecomastia, hot flushes, impotence, decreased libido and inhibition of spermatogenesis).
- Fatigue.
- Hepatotoxicity with long-term use, causing hepatitis and, occasionally, hepatic failure.

CLINICAL USES OF ANTIANDROGENS

- The main use of antiandrogens is in the treatment of carcinoma of the prostate (see Chapter 52), usually in conjunction with a gonadorelin analogue (see Chapter 43).
- Cyproterone acetate is used in male sexual offenders as 'chemical castration'.
- Cyproterone acetate can be given for manifestations of hyperandrogenisation in females, such as acne and hirsutism, in conjunction with ethinylestradiol in combined oral hormonal contraceptive (see Chapter 45).

5α-REDUCTASE INHIBITORS

dutasteride, finasteride

Mechanism of action and effects

Dutasteride and finasteride reduce the formation of dihydrotestosterone by inhibiting 5α-reductase. In men finasteride and dutasteride can reduce the size of the prostate in benign prostatic hypertrophy and improve the lower urinary tract symptoms. More details are found in Chapter 15.

SELF-ASSESSMENT

True/false questions

1. Androgen deficiency in adult men may cause decreased libido.
2. Testosterone cannot be given orally.

3. Testosterone alone is used to stimulate spermatogenesis.
4. Nandrolone causes less virilisation in women than testosterone.
5. Cyproterone acetate is used as an adjunct to the treatment of prostate cancer.
6. Antiandrogens can cause gynaecomastia.

One-best-answer (OBA) question

1. Choose the *most accurate* statement concerning drugs that affect androgenic and anabolic activities.
   A. 5α-Reductase inactivates dihydrotestosterone.
   B. Cyproterone acetate promotes spermatogenesis.
   C. Nandrolone reduces muscle mass.
   D. Danazol is used in the treatment of endometriosis.
   E. Dihydrotestosterone has marked antianabolic activity.

ANSWERS

True/false answers

1. **True.** Androgen deficiency may also cause impotence, reduced muscle mass, loss of body hair and other effects.
2. **True.** Testosterone is ineffective when given orally, as it undergoes very extensive first-pass metabolism; it is given as implants or transdermal patches, or as testosterone ester formulations by mouth or intramuscular depot injection.
3. **False.** Other treatments are required, including human chorionic gonadotropin (HCG) and other gonadotropins.
4. **True.** Nandrolone has fewer androgenic effects than testosterone, but has many other unwanted effects.
5. **True.** Cyproterone acetate is an antiandrogen used with a gonadorelin analogue in prostate cancer.
6. **True.** Antiandrogens can cause gynaecomastia, inhibition of spermatogenesis and other unwanted effects.

One-best-answer (OBA) answer

1. **Answer D** is correct.
   A. Incorrect. 5α-Reductase converts testosterone to active dihydrotestosterone.
   B. Incorrect. Cyproterone is an antiandrogen; it inhibits spermatogenesis.
   C. Incorrect. Nandrolone is an androgen and causes an increase in muscle mass.
   D. **Correct.** Danazol has antiandrogen, antioestrogen and antiprogesterone activity and is used in the treatment of endometriosis.
   E. Incorrect. Dihydrotestosterone is anabolic, increasing turnover and growth in many tissues and cells.

FURTHER READING

Di Luigi, L., Romanelli, F., Lenzi, A., 2005. Androgenic-anabolic steroid abuse in males. J. Endocrinol. Invest. 28 (Suppl. 3), 81–84.

Traish, A.M., Miner, M.M., Morgentaler, A., et al., 2011. Testosterone deficiency. Am. J. Med. 124, 578–587.

Compendium: drugs acting on the male reproductive system and anabolic agents

Drug	Characteristics
Androgens	
Danazol	Feedback inhibitor of pituitary gonadotropin release. Used for endometriosis (see Chapter 45)
Mesterolone (methyltestosterone)	Given orally for androgen deficiency and male infertility associated with hypogonadism. Half-life: 12–13 h
Testosterone and testosterone esters	Used for androgen deficiency, and for breast cancer in women. Testosterone undergoes extensive first-pass metabolism; it is also cleared rapidly from blood (half-life: 2–4 h). Testosterone esters, depot formulations, implants and patches improve bioavailability. Given orally (as undecanoate), by intramuscular injection (as enantate or propionate), or as an implant or transdermal patch (as testosterone). *Sustanon* is a mixture of testosterone esters, with a longer duration of action, given by intramuscular injection
Anabolic steroids	
Nandrolone decanoate	Used for aplastic anaemia; not used for effects on male reproductive system. Given as deep intramuscular injection. Half-life: 5–17 h
Oxymetholone	Given orally for 3–6 months for aplastic anaemia (see Chapter 47). Half-life: 9 h
Gonadorelin analogues	
Given for advanced prostate cancer (see Chapter 52) and for actions on the female reproductive system (see Chapter 45)	
Buserelin	Given by subcutaneous injection followed by intranasal dosage. See Chapter 45
Goserelin	Given by subcutaneous implant. See Chapter 45

Compendium: drugs acting on the male reproductive system and anabolic agents (cont'd)

Drug	Characteristics
Leuprorelin acetate	Given by subcutaneous or intramuscular injection. See Chapter 45
Triptorelin	Given by subcutaneous or intramuscular injection. See Chapter 45

Antiandrogens

Drug	Characteristics
Abiraterone acetate	Prodrug of abiraterone, a 17α-hydroxylase inhibitor that reduces androgen synthesis. Given orally for metastatic castration-resistant prostate cancer. Half-life: 12 h
Bicalutamide	Androgen receptor antagonist. Given orally for advanced prostate cancer. Half-life: 7–10 days
Cyproterone acetate	Steroidal antiandrogen, progestogen and antigonadotropin. Used as an adjunct for prostate cancer, for hirsutism and acne in women, and for severe hypersexuality and sexual deviation in men. Given orally. Half-life: 2 days
Flutamide	Rapidly hydroxylated to active derivative, which inhibits androgen receptors. Given orally for advanced prostate cancer. Half-life: 8 h
Enzalutamide	Potent inhibitor of androgen receptor binding and translocation. Given orally; used in metastatic castration-resistant prostate cancer resistant to docetaxel-containing chemotherapy

5α-Reductase inhibitors

Reduce conversion of testosterone to 5α-dihydrotestosterone (DHT), the primary androgen that stimulates prostate development, by inhibiting 5α-reductase.

Drug	Characteristics
Dutasteride	Inhibitor of type I and type II 5α-reductase. Given orally for benign prostatic hyperplasia. Half-life: 5 weeks
Finasteride	Selective inhibitor of type II 5α-reductase. Given orally for benign prostatic hyperplasia and male-pattern baldness. Half-life: 5–6 h

47 Anaemia and haematopoietic colony-stimulating factors

ANAEMIA

The definition of anaemia is rather arbitrary, and the absolute normal ranges for haemoglobin concentration in blood vary among laboratories. In adults, anaemia equates to a blood concentration of haemoglobin in males below about 130 g/L (normal is about 130–170 g/L) or in nonpregnant females below about 120 g/L (normal is about 120–150 g/L). Many individuals, however, have concentrations below these ranges without apparent detriment. Lower concentrations can be normal in children and during pregnancy. Anaemia can cause many symptoms, including shortness of breath, fatigue and worsening of angina or intermittent claudication. There are many causes of anaemia (Box 47.1), the forms of which are classified by red cell size and haemoglobin content (Box 47.2).

There are three key dietary factors that are required for normal red cell synthesis, referred to as haematinics:

- iron;
- folic acid;
- vitamin B$_{12}$.

IRON

Iron is important for cell respiration, energy production, DNA synthesis and cell proliferation. Dietary iron is absorbed from the duodenum and upper jejunum. In an omnivorous diet most iron is absorbed from meat, in which it is present as haem. Haem is the ferrous form of iron (Fe^{2+}), complexed with a porphyrin ring, and is readily absorbed from the gut. Nonhaem iron in a vegetarian diet, which is mainly in the ferric state (Fe^{3+}), is inefficiently absorbed. Absorption of ferric iron occurs mainly in the duodenum and is facilitated by several factors:

- gastric acid, which increases its solubility;
- conversion to ferrous iron by ferric reductase on the brush border of enterocytes, which is enhanced by dietary reducing agents such as ascorbic acid, fructose and some amino acids;
- expression of the divalent metal transporter 1 (DMT-1), mainly present in the duodenal enterocytes, which is increased in iron deficiency and in hereditary haemochromatosis.

After uptake into enterocytes, iron is oxidised to the ferric state and transported to the circulation by the protein ferroportin. Iron transport from enterocytes is regulated by the peptide hormone hepcidin, which is an acute-phase reactant synthesised in the liver. When circulating and tissue iron levels are high, or in the presence of systemic inflammation or infection, hepcidin is increased and binds to ferroportin, promoting its degradation. Conversely iron deficiency, increased erythropoiesis, and tissue hypoxia suppress hepcidin production and promote iron absorption.

In blood, ferric ions are bound to the globulin apotransferrin and transported to the bone marrow and iron stores as transferrin where cellular iron uptake occurs via transferrin receptors. In most cells, iron is complexed with the protein apoferritin and stored as ferritin. In some tissues iron is also found as relatively insoluble aggregates of degraded forms of ferritin, known as haemosiderin. Two-thirds of the iron in the body is present in circulating red cells, and about half of the remainder is found in macrophages, reticuloendothelial cells and hepatocytes. The rest is present in myoglobin in muscle cells or associated with various intracellular enzymes.

When ageing red cells are broken down by the reticuloendothelial system, most of the released iron is recycled via macrophages for further erythropoiesis. Iron loss from the body is normally low, and occurs through shedding of mucosal cells containing ferritin.

Iron deficiency

The main cause of iron deficiency in the United Kingdom is abnormal loss of blood, particularly from the gut or from exaggerated menstrual loss. Iron malabsorption can result

> **Box 47.1** **Causes of anaemia**
>
> Reduced red cell production:
> - Defective precursor proliferation (e.g. iron deficiency, anaemia of chronic disorder, marrow aplasia or infiltration)
> - Defective precursor maturation (e.g. vitamin B_{12} or folate deficiency, myelodysplastic syndrome, toxins)
>
> Increased rate of red cell destruction:
> - Haemolysis
>
> Loss of circulating red cells:
> - Bleeding

> **Box 47.2** **Classification of anaemias by red cell characteristics**
>
> Hypochromic, microcytic (small-size cells):
> - Genetic (e.g. thalassaemia, sideroblastic anaemia)
> - Acquired (e.g. iron deficiency, sideroblastic anaemia)
>
> Normochromic, macrocytic (large-size cells):
> - With megaloblastic marrow: Vitamin B_{12} or folate deficiency
> - With normoblastic marrow: Alcohol, myelodysplasia
>
> Polychromatophilic, macrocytic:
> - Haemolysis
>
> Normochromic, normocytic (normal-size cells):
> - Chronic disorders (e.g. infection, malignancy, autoimmune disease)
> - Renal failure
> - Bone marrow failure

from disease of the upper small intestine (e.g. coeliac disease), or following partial gastrectomy. Dietary deficiency is rarely a major cause in Western societies, although worldwide a vegetarian diet low in absorbable forms of iron is the commonest contributory cause to iron deficiency.

Therapeutic iron preparations

Oral iron

Oral iron supplements are preferred and are given as ferrous salts (e.g. ferrous sulphate, fumarate or gluconate). Tablets are normally used, but some people find that syrup is more palatable. In the presence of iron deficiency, a daily oral dose equivalent to 100–200 mg of elemental iron (of which about one-third will be absorbed) produces the maximum rate of rise of haemoglobin (200 mg ferrous sulfate contains 65 mg iron). Addition of ascorbic acid (vitamin C) to oral iron preparations has a minimal effect on absorption.

Unwanted effects

- Gastrointestinal intolerance is common, especially nausea and dyspepsia. The prevalence of these effects depends on the dose of elemental iron and psychological factors, rather than the iron salt used. Intolerance can be minimised by taking iron supplements with food (although this reduces absorption) or by reducing the dose. Modified-release iron formulations have been developed to improve tolerability, but much of the iron is released beyond the duodenum,

the site where it is best absorbed. These formulations should only be used when other methods for improving iron tolerance are ineffective. Diarrhoea or constipation also occur, but are not dose-related.
- Oral iron turns stools black.

Parenteral iron

Iron can be given by slow intravenous injection or infusion, or less commonly by deep intramuscular injection. Formulations involve complexing a ferric salt to a carrier to form:

- iron dextran (by intravenous infusion in one or two doses; can be used by deep intramuscular injection);
- iron sucrose (by intravenous infusion twice weekly for 2–10 doses);
- ferric carboxymaltose (by two short intravenous infusions);
- iron isomaltoside 1000 (by one or two short intravenous infusions).

The iron in these formulations is not bound to transferrin in plasma but accumulates in reticuloendothelial cells. When calculating the amount of iron to give, the approximate total body iron deficit (haemoglobin and body stores) is estimated from the person's size and haemoglobin concentration. Oral iron should not be given until at least 5 days after parenteral iron.

Unwanted effects

- Nausea, vomiting, diarrhoea, abdominal pain.
- Flushing, fever.
- Rash.
- Increased risk of infection since parenteral iron promotes bacterial growth.
- Anaphylactoid/anaphylactic reactions, including cardiovascular collapse, particularly with iron dextran; facilities for resuscitation should always be available.

Therapeutic use of iron

The cause of iron deficiency should always be sought when starting symptomatic treatment with iron. If this is not done, then serious disorders such as gastrointestinal malignancy can be overlooked. Oral iron supplements are adequate for most mild or moderate iron-deficiency anaemias. After an initial delay of a few days while new red cells are formed, oral iron supplements should raise the blood haemoglobin concentration by about 20 g/L over the first 3–4 weeks, and about 10 g/L per week thereafter. Oral iron supplements should be continued for 3 months after the haemoglobin concentration has been restored, in order to replenish tissue iron stores.

Failure to respond to oral iron can be caused by several factors:

- incorrect diagnosis (e.g. anaemia of chronic disease, as the hepcidin blocks its absorption, or thalassaemia);
- poor adherence to oral iron therapy;
- inadequate iron dosage (e.g. in some modified-release formulations);
- continuing excessive blood loss;
- malabsorption;
- concurrent deficiency of other substances necessary for haemoglobin synthesis.

Parenteral iron preparations are used if there are intractable unwanted effects from oral preparations, if there is severe uncorrectable malabsorption, continuing heavy blood loss, during renal haemodialysis when epoetin is given and when adherence to oral treatment is poor. Parenteral iron can raise the haemoglobin concentration faster than oral iron, especially in renal impairment.

Oral iron supplements are occasionally given for prophylaxis against iron deficiency at times of high demand for iron – for example, pregnancy (given together with folic acid), menorrhagia or if there is a poor dietary intake. The reduced iron absorption after subtotal or total gastrectomy can also be overcome by long-term iron supplements.

FOLIC ACID

Folate is essential for cell growth and development, including maintenance of normal erythropoeisis, through its involvement in multiple biochemical processes. Folic acid (pteroylglutamic acid) is ingested as conjugated folate polyglutamates, found mainly in fresh leaf vegetables (in which it is heat-labile) and in liver (where it is more heat-stable). Before absorption, the polyglutamates are deconjugated to the monoglutamate. Folate monoglutamate is absorbed principally in the duodenum and jejunum, and the majority is then methylated. Dihydrofolate reductase then generates 5-methyltetrahydrofolate during absorption. 5-Methyltetrahydrofolate enters cells by receptor-mediated endocytosis, where it is demethylated. Tetrahydrofolate is a coenzyme in the synthesis of nonessential amino acids and purine and thymidylate nucleic acids, and therefore of DNA and RNA (see also Chapter 52).

Folate deficiency

The most obvious consequence of folate deficiency is a macrocytic anaemia with the presence of megaloblasts in the marrow, a feature it shares with vitamin B_{12} deficiency. Folate deficiency can arise for a number of reasons (Box 47.3). Unlike iron, folate cannot be recycled from old red cells that are removed from the circulation.

Therapeutic use of folic acid

Folate deficiency almost always responds to oral folic acid supplements. Folic acid is a poor substrate for dihydrofolate

reductase, and is largely absorbed unchanged and then converted to tetrahydrofolic acid in plasma and the liver. Most causes of folate deficiency are self-limiting, and folic acid treatment is usually given for 4 months to correct the anaemia and replace folate stores.

Folic acid is given prophylactically in pregnancy. It is given in higher doses if there is an increased risk of conceiving a child with a neural tube defect. Those at higher risk include a partner with a neural tube defect, history of neural tube defect in a previous pregnancy, or if the woman has coeliac disease, diabetes mellitus, sickle-cell anaemia or is taking antiepileptic drugs (see Chapter 23). Folic acid is also given prophylactically to premature infants, during renal dialysis, and for chronic haemolytic anaemia.

Treatment of deficiency of both vitamin B_{12} and folate using only folic acid may correct anaemia but precipitate neurological damage (discussed later). Therefore vitamin B_{12} deficiency must be excluded before folic acid is used, or both vitamin B_{12} followed by folic acid should be given if there is a possibility of vitamin B_{12} deficiency.

For folate deficiency produced by drugs that inhibit dihydrofolate reductase (e.g. methotrexate; see Chapter 52 and Fig. 51.4), it is necessary to 'bypass' this enzyme blockade by giving the synthetic tetrahydrofolic acid, folinic acid (5-formyl tetrahydrofolic acid). This is the basis of 'folinic acid rescue' to reduce the toxic effects on healthy tissues of high-dose methotrexate used for treatment of malignancy (see Chapter 52). Folinic acid is formulated as a salt and given orally, usually as calcium folinate. When low-dose methotrexate is used in a once-a-week regimen for immunosuppression, folic acid can be given on a separate day to reduce toxicity.

VITAMIN B_{12}

Vitamin B_{12} is essential as a coenzyme in nucleic acid synthesis, and in other metabolic pathways such as fatty acid synthesis in conjunction with folate. Many functions of vitamin B_{12} can be performed by folate, but there are two enzyme families that only vitamin B_{12} can facilitate. These are responsible for homeostasis of methylmalonic acid and homocysteine.

The term *vitamin B_{12}* refers to a group of cobalt-containing compounds, also known as cobalamins. Bacteria are the only organisms that can synthesise cobalamins de novo. Humans obtain vitamin B_{12} from meat (particularly liver), fish and shellfish, or from animal products (milk, cheese, eggs, etc.) or vegetables contaminated by bacteria. Absorption is by an unusual mechanism. Dietary vitamin B_{12} is released by proteases from food and binds to haptocorrin, produced in salivary glands, which protects the vitamin from degradation by gastric acid. In the duodenum, haptocorrin is digested and the vitamin B_{12} then binds to a glycoprotein in the stomach called *intrinsic factor* that is produced by gastric parietal cells. The vitamin B_{12}-intrinsic factor is absorbed principally from the terminal ileum, where it undergoes receptor-mediated endocytosis and then binds to transcobalamin II in the enterocytes. Most vitamin B_{12} in plasma is bound to the glycoproteins haptocorrin and transcobalamin II. Transcobalamin II is responsible for delivery of vitamin B_{12} to tissues where it undergoes receptor-mediated endocytosis. The liver stores about 50% of the body content of vitamin B_{12}.

Box 47.3   Causes of folate deficiency

■ Poor diet: Folate stores are adequate for a few weeks only. Lack of folate is uncommon in Western diets, but may be more common in the diet of elderly people or in alcoholism.
■ Increased requirements (e.g. pregnancy, malignancies, haemolytic anaemias, exfoliative dermatitis).
■ Malabsorption (e.g. coeliac disease, tropical sprue).
■ Drugs that interfere with folate metabolism: Anticonvulsants (especially phenytoin; see Chapter 23), methotrexate (see Chapter 52), pyrimethamine (see Chapter 51).

Vitamin B₁₂ deficiency

Impairment of vitamin B_{12}-dependent enzyme reactions affects DNA synthesis. The major organs affected by vitamin B_{12} deficiency are those with a rapid cell turnover, particularly the bone marrow and the gastrointestinal tract.

Vitamin B_{12} deficiency presents with a macrocytic anaemia and a megaloblastic bone marrow, neutropenia and thrombocytopenia. The tongue becomes smooth and painful. With severe deficiency, demyelination of the posterior and lateral neuronal tracts in the spinal cord can also occur, leading to a condition known as subacute combined degeneration of the cord. Symptoms of the latter include motor and sensory disturbances and abnormal balance. Cognitive impairment occurs from cerebral damage. The neurological damage may not be fully reversible after correction of vitamin B_{12} deficiency, due to axonal loss.

Causes of vitamin B_{12} deficiency include:

- diet: Strict vegetarians (vegans) only;
- intestinal malabsorption due to damage to the terminal ileum – for example, Crohn's disease, lymphoma;
- deficiency of intrinsic factor: Pernicious anaemia (destruction of gastric parietal cells with achlorhydria and failure of intrinsic factor production), total and subtotal gastrectomy.

Therapeutic use of vitamin B₁₂

Most people with vitamin B_{12} deficiency have problems absorbing it from the gut, and treatment is usually by intramuscular injection of vitamin B_{12} in aqueous solution. Hydroxocobalamin, the form of vitamin B_{12} produced by bacteria, is used for treatment of deficiency. Following initial injections on alternate days for 2 weeks to replenish stores, maintenance injections every 3 months for life are adequate. In the rare dietary causes of vitamin B_{12} deficiency, oral cyanocobalamin supplements can be given, but otherwise oral treatment is never indicated.

If there is concurrent folate deficiency, hydroxocobalamin replacement should always be started first (as noted previously).

ERYTHROPOIETIN

darbepoetin, epoetin

Erythropoietin is a glycosylated protein hormone produced mainly by the kidney. It regulates red cell production by reducing apoptosis and stimulating differentiation and proliferation of erythroid progenitor cells. Erythropoietin binds to its receptor which is found in high concentration on erythroid precursors, and enables the receptor to activate several intracellular signalling pathways. Deficiency of erythropoietin in end-stage renal disease contributes to the anaemia that characterises this disorder. Interestingly, the hormone has also been found to have a protective effect on ischaemic neurons in the brain. Human erythropoietin for therapeutic use has been synthesised using recombinant DNA technology (epoetin); it is produced in three forms – alpha, beta and zeta – which have similar clinical effects. Erythropoietin is also available as two longer-acting derivatives: a hyperglycosylated derivative, darbepoetin alpha, and methoxy polyethylene glycol-epoetin beta.

Pharmacokinetics

Epoetin can be given intravenously or, more conveniently, subcutaneously, when a 25–50% lower dose can be used. The red cell response is more rapid after intravenous use, but ultimately greater after subcutaneous injection. Epoetin has a half-life of about 4–6 hours, and is normally given two or three times a week. Darbepoetin has a longer half-life and is given once a week, and methoxy polyethylene glycol-epoetin beta is given every 2–4 weeks. The route of elimination of epoetin is uncertain, but may be largely by receptor-mediated uptake in the bone marrow and subsequent intracellular degradation.

Unwanted effects

- Nausea, vomiting, diarrhoea.
- Headache.
- Influenza-like symptoms early in treatment.
- Hypertension, which is dose-dependent and can be severe, leading to encephalopathy with seizures.
- Thrombosis of arteriovenous shunts for haemodialysis.
- Pure red cell aplasia (not affecting white cells or platelets) occurs rarely during subcutaneous administration in renal failure; this is usually associated with formation of antibodies to epoetin, necessitating discontinuation of treatment.

Therapeutic uses of epoetin

- Anaemia of end-stage renal disease. Other causes of anaemia should be excluded. Adequate iron stores are essential since erythropoiesis demands large amounts of iron. Intravenous iron supplements are often needed to maximise the response. Anaemia can be corrected in more than 90% of those treated, and treatment improves quality of life. Epoetin also modulates lipid metabolism, creating a less atherogenic plasma lipid profile, which may reduce the high cardiovascular mortality in renal failure. However, cardiovascular mortality and morbidity may be increased if the haemoglobin concentration is raised above 120 g/L.
- To increase red cell production prior to surgery. Autologous blood transfusion is becoming more popular to reduce the use of banked blood. Epoetin given twice weekly for 3 weeks before surgery can increase the number of units of blood that can be obtained.
- Anaemia associated with human immunodeficiency virus (HIV) infection or acquired immunodeficiency syndrome (AIDS).
- Anaemia associated with cytotoxic chemotherapy of nonmyeloid malignant disease (see Chapter 52). However, mortality may be increased if the haemoglobin concentration is raised beyond 120 g/L or epoetin is used before chemotherapy.
- Epoetin is sometimes abused by athletes to increase haematocrit and improve performance. This abuse is

---

> **Box 47.4** Causes of aplastic anaemia
>
> Drugs:
> - Cytotoxic agents
> - Chloramphenicol
> - Sulfonamides
> - Nonsteroidal antiinflammatory drugs
> - Gold salts
> - Carbimazole
> - Phenytoin
> - Carbamazepine
> - Phenothiazines
> - Chlorpropamide
>
> Radiation
> Infections (e.g. hepatitis, Epstein–Barr virus)
> Inherited (e.g. Fanconi anaemia)
> Malignant (e.g. myelodysplastic syndrome)

> **Box 47.5** More common causes of sideroblastic anaemia
>
> Congenital
> Acquired:
> - Myelodysplastic syndrome
> - Drugs and toxins:
>   - Isoniazid
>   - Chloramphenicol
>   - Alcoholism
>   - Lead poisoning

> **Box 47.6** Drugs causing haemolysis in glucose-6-phosphate dehydrogenase deficiency
>
> Antimalarials:
> - Primaquine
> - Pamaquine
>
> Analgesics:
> - Aspirin (high dose)
>
> Others:
> - Sulfonamides
> - Nalidixic acid
> - Dapsone

associated with an increased risk of arterial and venous thromboses.

DRUG TREATMENT IN OTHER ANAEMIAS

Certain other anaemias require specific drug therapy.

Aplastic anaemia

Failure of haematopoietic stem cell production has many causes, including certain drugs (Box 47.4). Drugs do not have a major role in treatment of aplastic anaemia. The anabolic steroid oxymetholone (see Chapter 46; available in the United Kingdom only on a named-patient basis) is sometimes used, but its effectiveness is unpredictable. Antilymphocyte globulin is helpful in some acquired aplastic anaemias, and is sometimes used in combination with ciclosporin (see Chapter 38).

Sideroblastic anaemia

This can also be caused by drugs (Box 47.5). It is characterised by accumulation of iron in the mitochondria of erythroblasts, which lie in a ring around the nucleus. Staining for iron reveals the characteristic ring sideroblasts. Pyridoxine supplements can increase the haemoglobin concentration in idiopathic acquired and hereditary forms of the disorder. They can also be useful for reversible sideroblastic anaemia associated with pregnancy, haemolysis, alcohol dependence or during treatment with the antituberculous drug isoniazid (see Chapter 51).

Autoimmune haemolytic anaemia

This can respond to immunosuppression with corticosteroids (see Chapter 44).

β-Thalassaemia major

This is a genetic disorder of haemoglobin synthesis with a hyperplastic bone marrow and refractory anaemia. Blood transfusions or excessive iron supplements lead to iron overload, with damage to the liver, heart and pancreas. Iron overload can be prevented with infusions of desferrioxamine mesilate (see Chapter 53), together with vitamin C, which enhances iron excretion. The oral iron chelators, deferiprone or deferasirox, are used when desferrioxamine is poorly tolerated or contraindicated.

Sickle cell anaemia

This inherited disorder occurs when more than 80% of the haemoglobin is HbS; fetal haemoglobin (HbF) forms the remainder. Hydroxycarbamide (see Chapter 52) reduces the frequency and severity of sickle cell crises. It raises the HbF concentration and also reduces the number of young red cells, which are those most likely to adhere to endothelium and occlude blood vessels.

DRUGS AS A CAUSE OF ANAEMIA

- Iron deficiency: Especially drugs causing bleeding from the upper gut – for example, nonsteroidal antiinflammatory drugs (NSAIDs).
- Aplastic anaemia: See Box 47.4.
- Sideroblastic anaemia: See Box 47.5.
- Haemolysis in glucose-6-phosphate dehydrogenase (G6PD) deficiency: See Box 47.6. G6PD is involved in generating reduced glutathione, which protects red cells against oxidative stresses. Oxidant drugs produce haemolysis in GP6D-deficient individuals, who are usually male (see Chapter 53).

NEUTROPENIA

Leucocytes are part of the first line of defence against pathogens. They include phagocytic cells (neutrophils,

> **Box 47.7** **Causes of neutropenia**
>
> Inherited:
>   Congenital agranulocytosis
>   Cyclical neutropenia
> Acquired:
>   Viral infection (e.g. hepatitis, influenza, rubella,
>   infectious mononucleosis)
>   Bacterial infection
>   Radiotherapy
>   Drugs, especially cytotoxic drugs, carbimazole
>   Autoimmune neutropenia
>   Hypersplenism
>   Marrow infiltration

monocytes and eosinophils) and nonphagocytic cells (lymphocytes and basophils). In addition to their role in acute inflammation, all these cells participate in regulation of cellular and humoral immunity through the production of cytokines. A reduction in the number of circulating neutrophils (neutropenia) in particular increases the risk of serious infection. There are several causes of neutropenia (Box 47.7). Neutropenia does not give rise to symptoms, but predisposes to infection, especially if the neutrophil count falls below 0.5×10^9/L.

DRUGS FOR NEUTROPENIA

Granulocyte colony-stimulating factors

Granulocyte colony-stimulating factors are produced by many cells, such as endothelial cells, monocytes and fibroblasts, and stimulate the maturation of pluripotent stem cells in the bone marrow. Granulocyte colony-stimulating factor (G-CSF) is produced by recombinant DNA technology. Therapeutic agents include:

- filgrastim (recombinant human G-CSF);
- lenograstim (glycosylated recombinant human G-CSF);
- pegfilgrastim (pegylated filgrastim).

    G-CSF is glycosylated in its natural state, but this does not seem to be a prerequisite for effectiveness. A transient fall in circulating neutrophils occurs within minutes of the injection, followed a few hours later by a substantial rise.

Pharmacokinetics

Granulocyte colony-stimulating factors are given by prolonged intravenous infusion or subcutaneous infusion or injection. Daily injections of filgrastim or lenograstim are given until there is an adequate neutrophil response. Pegfilgrastim has a longer duration of action than filgrastim, and is only given once after chemotherapy. Filgrastim and lenograstim are eliminated both by the kidney and by neutrophil uptake. Pegfilgrastim is not eliminated by the kidney, and has a prolonged effect in neutropenia, since few neutrophils are available to contribute to its elimination.

Unwanted effects

- Musculoskeletal or bone pain.
- Headache.
- Fever.
- Fatigue.

- Anorexia, nausea, vomiting, diarrhoea.
- Myeloproliferative disorders with long-term treatment.
- Osteoporosis with long-term treatment.

THERAPEUTIC USE OF COLONY-STIMULATING FACTORS

The use of these drugs remains controversial in many indications.

Congenital neutropenia

Survival is prolonged by G-CSF, which reduces life-threatening infection, but 10% of people develop acute myeloid leukaemia as a result of treatment.

Chemotherapy-induced neutropenia

The duration of neutropenia may be reduced, with a limitation of associated sepsis. However, with many chemotherapy regimens, there is no evidence that long-term survival is improved by G-CSF, and with some regimens, the risk of acute myeloid leukaemia may be increased. G-CSF treatment is therefore reserved for those regimens that have greater than 20% historical risk of febrile neutropenia. It is also used when chemotherapy has previously been associated with a febrile neutropenic episode and the drug dosage cannot be reduced for subsequent courses.

Mobilisation of progenitor cells into peripheral blood for harvesting prior to bone marrow transplantation

The white blood cell count rises 7–12 days after treatment and is accompanied by an increase in haematopoietic stem cells, which are collected via a cell-separation machine. G-CSF use can be followed by the chemokine receptor antagonist plerixafor, which mobilises haematopoietic stem cells into peripheral blood.

SELF-ASSESSMENT

True/false questions

1. Dietary iron is transported in the blood mostly bound to ferritin.
2. Pernicious anaemia is caused by reduced vitamin B_{12} absorption.
3. In vitamin B_{12} deficiency treatment is rarely required for more than 3 months.
4. The blood film in pernicious anaemia shows microcytosis.
5. Both vitamin B_{12} and folate are essential for DNA synthesis.
6. Folic acid cannot be given orally.
7. Phenytoin can cause folate deficiency.
8. Erythropoietin reduces apoptosis of red blood cell progenitors.
9. Filgrastim is a recombinant form of erythropoietin.
10. Plerixafor is a chemokine antagonist.

One-best-answer (OBA) questions

1. Identify the *correct* statement concerning the properties of erythropoietin.
   A. Erythropoietin is mainly synthesised by the adrenal glands.
   B. Erythropoietin can correct anaemia in end-stage renal disease.
   C. Erythropoietin is an effective anaemia treatment, even if iron levels are low.
   D. Use of erythropoietin improves athletic performance with no adverse effects.
   E. Erythropoietin can be given orally.
2. Identify the *incorrect* statement concerning the usage and properties of folic acid and its metabolites.
   A. Tetrahydrofolate is involved in the synthesis of the nucleotide bases in DNA.
   B. Folic acid is often given with hydroxocobalamin.
   C. Folate is absorbed in the stomach.
   D. Tetrahydrofolic acid is given rather than folic acid to correct the folate deficiency caused by methotrexate.
   E. Folic acid in pregnancy reduces the risk of neural tube defects.

Case-based questions

A 40-year-old woman complained to her GP of fatigue and heavy menstrual periods lasting 7 days and occurring every 28 days. Her GP noted that she was pallid; her haemoglobin level was 67 g/L and mean cell volume (MCV) was 61 fL (normal MCV is 76–96 fL). Other blood measurements of platelets and white cell counts were unremarkable.

1. How do you interpret these data and what were the possible reasons?
2. What biochemical tests could have helped the diagnosis?
3. The tests confirmed iron-deficiency anaemia. What pharmaceutical preparation should have been given?
4. Several iron formulations were tried, as the woman felt unwell taking ferrous sulfate. What unwanted effects might she have experienced?
5. Where was the iron absorbed?
6. After 2 months of oral iron therapy, the haemoglobin value was 80 g/L. Was this a sufficient response?
7. The woman was intolerant of oral iron. What could have been the reasons for the poor response?
8. What alternative treatment could have been administered?
   With the new treatment regimen, her haemoglobin rose to 115 g/L over 2–3 weeks.

ANSWERS

True/false answers

1. **False.** Iron is transported in the blood bound to transferrin and stored in tissues as ferritin and haemosiderin.
2. **True.** Autoimmune loss of gastric parietal cells reduces production of intrinsic factor, which is needed for vitamin B_{12} absorption in the distal ileum.
3. **False.** In pernicious anaemia vitamin B_{12} is given (as hydroxocobalamin) by intramuscular injection every 2–3 months for life.

4. **False.** Macrocytes (enlarged red cells) are found in the blood in pernicious anaemia.
5. **True.** Folate is necessary for synthesis of purines and pyrimidines, and vitamin B_{12} is a cofactor in their synthesis.
6. **False.** Folic acid is given orally each day for up to 4 months to replenish stores.
7. **True.** Some anticonvulsant drugs including phenytoin, primidone, carbamazepine and valproate, and other drugs including the oral hypoglycaemic drug metformin, sulfasalazine (used in inflammatory bowel disease) and oral contraceptives, can interfere with folate metabolism.
8. **True.** Erythropoietin increases survival of erythroid progenitor cells in the bone marrow.
9. **False.** Filgrastim is a recombinant form of granulocyte colony-stimulating factor (G-CSF), which promotes formation of neutrophils and other granulocytes in the bone marrow.
10. **True.** Plerixafor is an antagonist of the CXCR4 chemokine receptor and is used with a recombinant G-CSF to mobilise stem cells for harvesting.

One-best-answer (OBA) answers

1. **Answer B** is correct.
   A. Incorrect. The kidneys are the main site of erythropoietin production.
   B. **Correct.** Anaemia due to renal disease is commonly treated with erythropoietin.
   C. Incorrect. Adequate iron stores are necessary for erythropoietin to be successful.
   D. Incorrect. Erythropoietin may enhance performance by increasing haematocrit, but with an increased risk of thrombosis.
   E. Incorrect. It is a glycoprotein that can be given by intravenous or subcutaneous routes.
2. **Answer C** is the incorrect statement.
   A. Correct. Tetrahydrofolate is a folic acid metabolite utilised in the synthesis of the purine and pyrimidine bases in DNA.
   B. Correct. Neurological damage can be caused if folic acid is given alone when both folate and vitamin B_{12} are deficient.
   C. **Incorrect.** Folate is absorbed in the proximal jejunum, and absorption is deficient in coeliac disease.
   D. Correct. Methotrexate inhibits the synthesis of tetrahydrofolate by dihydrofolate reductase. Synthetic tetrahydrofolate (folinic acid) bypasses this block.
   E. Correct. Folic acid is given prophylactically in pregnancy, and in higher amounts if there is a history of a neural tube defect in a previous pregnancy.

Case-based answers

1. The haemoglobin concentration (67 g/L) is below normal for a nonpregnant woman (115 g/L), indicating anaemia. The MCV (61 fL) is also low. A common cause of low MCV is iron-deficiency anaemia, which is common in menstruating women. Another cause is gastrointestinal bleeding, including haemorrhoids.
2. Serum ferritin would be low and total iron-binding capacity elevated.

3. Oral ferrous salts (e.g. ferrous sulfate), the form most easily absorbed.
4. Gastrointestinal distension and loose bowel movements are common.
5. Iron is absorbed from the duodenum and upper jejunum.
6. The rise in haemoglobin was insufficient; it should be about 10 g/L each week.
7. Poor response could be due to poor adherence to treatment, continued bleeding or malabsorption.
8. Alternative treatment could have been slow intravenous injection or infusion of iron sucrose or iron dextran.

FURTHER READING

Bennett, C.L., Djulbegovic, B., Norris, L.B., et al., 2013. Colony-stimulating factors for febrile neutropenia during cancer therapy. N. Engl. J. Med. 368, 1131–1139.

Camaschella, C., 2015. Iron-deficiency anemia. N. Engl. J. Med. 372, 1832–1843.

Cappellini, M.D., Fiorelli, G., 2008. Glucose-6-phosphate dehydrogenase deficiency. N. Engl. J. Med. 371, 64–74.

Hunt, A., Harrington, D., Robinson, S., 2014. Vitamin B$_{12}$ deficiency. Br. Med. J. 349, g5226.

Kaushansky, K., 2006. Lineage-specific hematopoietic growth factors. N. Engl. J. Med. 354, 2034–2046.

Macdougall, I.C., Eckardt, K.-U., 2006. Novel strategies for stimulating erythropoiesis and potential new treatments for anaemia. Lancet 368, 947–953.

Compendium: drugs used to treat anaemias and neutropenia

Drug	Characteristics
Drugs used in iron-deficiency anaemia	
Iron	
Oral formulations	
Ferrous sulphate Ferrous fumarate Ferrous gluconate Polysaccharide–iron complex Sodium feredetate	These oral formulations have only marginal differences in the efficiency of iron absorption. Dosage is adjusted to provide similar content of elemental iron (100–200 mg daily) for treatment, with lower doses for prophylaxis. Can be given with folic acid in pregnancy
Parenteral formulations	
Parenteral iron is used when oral iron is unsuccessful due to poor adherence, tolerance or absorption.	
Iron carboxymaltose	Ferric hydroxide core stabilised by a carbohydrate shell. Given by slow intravenous injection or infusion
Iron dextran	A complex of ferric hydroxide with dextran containing 5% iron. Given by slow intravenous injection or infusion
Iron isomaltoside 1000	Ferric hydroxide complexed with carbohydrate. Given by slow intravenous injection or infusion
Iron sucrose	A complex of ferric hydroxide with sucrose containing 2% iron. Given by slow intravenous injection or infusion
Drugs used in megaloblastic anaemias	
Cyanocobalamin	Metabolised to cobalamin and incorporated into vitamin B$_{12}$. Given orally, or by intramuscular injection at monthly intervals
Folic acid	Metabolised to tetrahydrofolate. Folate deficiency responds to a short course of treatment. Given orally, often with hydroxocobalamin
Hydroxocobalamin	Hydroxocobalamin has replaced cyanocobalamin as the drug of choice in the United Kingdom. Given by intramuscular injection at 3-month intervals
Drugs used in hypoplastic, haemolytic and renal anaemias	
Darbepoetin alpha	Long-acting recombinant form of renal erythropoietin. Used for anaemia associated with chronic renal disease and anaemia in adults receiving chemotherapy for nonmyeloid malignancies. Given by intravenous injection (half-life 20 h) or subcutaneously (30–90 h)
Epoetin alpha, beta and zeta	Used for anaemia associated with chronic renal disease, to increase autologous blood in healthy people and for anaemia in adults receiving chemotherapy for malignancies. Given by intravenous or subcutaneous injection. Half-life: 4–6 h

Compendium: drugs used to treat anaemias and neutropenia (cont'd)

Drug	Characteristics
Methoxy polyethylene glycol-epoetin beta	Long-acting, pegylated version of epoetin beta. Used for anaemia associated with chronic renal disease; given by intravenous or subcutaneous injection. Half-life: 140 h
Oxymetholone	Used for 3–6 months for treatment of aplastic anaemia. Given orally. Half-life: 9 h

Treatment of iron overload

Drug	Characteristics
Deferasirox	Given orally for iron overload in thalassaemia major, for people requiring frequent blood transfusions and those intolerant to desferrioxamine. Half-life: 8–16 h
Deferiprone	Given orally for iron overload in thalassaemia major and for people intolerant to desferrioxamine. Half-life: 1.5 h
Desferrioxamine mesilate (deferoxamine mesilate)	Chelating agent used for iron overload in thalassaemia major (or aluminium overload in people undergoing dialysis), and for haemochromatosis in people in whom repeated venesection is contraindicated. Given by subcutaneous infusion. Half-life: 6 h

Drugs used in neutropenia

All drugs are recombinant colony-stimulating factors given parenterally; for specialist use only.

Drug	Characteristics
Filgrastim	Unglycosylated recombinant human granulocyte colony-stimulating factor (G-CSF). Used for neutropenia, following cytotoxic chemotherapy of malignancy, and for severe congenital neutropenia. Given by subcutaneous injection or intravenous infusion. Half-life: 3.5 h
Lenograstim	Glycosylated recombinant human G-CSF. Used for reduction in the duration of neutropenia, for example following cytotoxic chemotherapy of malignancy. Given by subcutaneous injection or intravenous infusion. Half-life: 1–3 h
Pegfilgrastim	Long-acting pegylated derivative of filgrastim. Used for neutropenia, for example following cytotoxic chemotherapy of malignancy. Given by subcutaneous injection. Half-life: 15–80 h
Plerixafor	Chemokine receptor (CXCR4) antagonist. Used with G-CSF to improve mobilisation and yield of stem cells for transplantation. Given by subcutaneous injection. Half-life: 3–5 h

48

Lipid disorders

LIPIDS AND LIPOPROTEINS

Lipids have many functions such as energy storage in adipose tissue (triglycerides), intracellular signalling (various intracellular messengers and extracellular mediators linked to G protein-coupled receptors, and steroid hormones synthesised from cholesterol) and as the main structural component of cell membranes (glycerophospholipids, sphingomyelin and cholesterol). Lipid and lipoprotein metabolism is complex and the following account is a very brief summary, sufficient to establish the mechanism of action of drugs used to correct lipid abnormalities.

CHOLESTEROL AND TRIGLYCERIDES

About 75% of cholesterol is synthesised in the body. Of this, 10% of daily production of cholesterol is by the liver and 15% in the intestines, with the rest synthesised in the adrenal glands and reproductive organs. About 25% of the daily supply of cholesterol is from the diet, mainly in the consumption of eggs, cheese, meat or fish. The synthesis of cholesterol from acetyl CoA involves several enzymes, but the rate-limiting step is the conversion of 3-hydroxy-3-methylglutaryl-coenzyme A (HMG-CoA) to mevalonate that is catalysed by HMG-CoA reductase. The cellular supply of cholesterol is maintained at a steady level by regulation of HMG-CoA reductase activity. Intracellular cholesterol is a feedback inhibitor of HMG-CoA reductase activity, suppresses gene expression to reduce synthesis of the enzyme and induces rapid proteolytic degradation of the enzyme.

Cholesterol leaves hepatocytes either by transport into the circulation as cholesteryl esters (cholesterol complexed with fatty acid; discussed later) or by secretion into the bile after incorporation into bile salt micelles (Figs 48.1 and 48.2). Virtually all of the cholesterol secreted in bile is reabsorbed and taken up by the liver, which also retains about 50% of cholesterol that is not incorporated into bile salts.

Triglycerides (fatty acids esterified with glycerol) comprise over 95% of dietary fat, and can also be synthesised from intermediary metabolites formed in the liver from excess carbohydrate in the diet. Triglycerides are stored in adipose tissue, from where they can be mobilised as nonesterified free fatty acids to act as an energy substrate during periods of fasting.

LIPOPROTEINS

Lipids (triglycerides and esters of cholesterol) have low water solubility and circulate in plasma encased in a coat of apolipoproteins within a phospholipid monolayer. Together, these create lipoproteins that are water-soluble and which make the triglycerides and cholesteryl esters transportable. The lipoproteins can be differentiated according to the triglyceride/cholesterol ratio they carry, their apolipoprotein (apo) constituents and their density (Table 48.1). They are usually classified according to their density into very-low-density (VLDL), low-density (LDL), intermediate-density (IDL) and high-density (HDL) lipoproteins and chylomicrons. There are specific cell-surface receptors for processing different apolipoproteins, and these determine where and how

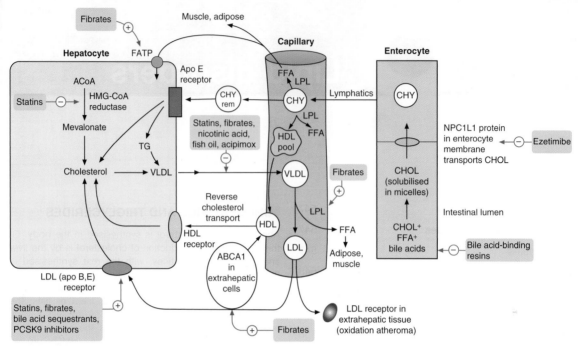

Fig. 48.1 Major pathways in lipoprotein formation and metabolism. Dietary lipids including cholesterol (CHOL) and free fatty acids (FFA) in the gut are emulsified by bile acids and transported within chylomicrons (CHY) to the liver. They are then circulated as cholesterol and triglycerides (TG) to tissues in very-low-density lipoproteins (VLDL), where endothelial lipoprotein lipase (LPL) liberates FFA in adipose and muscle for storage or metabolism. The resulting low-density lipoproteins (LDL) are returned to hepatocytes via LDL receptors, or taken up by LDL receptors in extrahepatic tissues, where they are oxidised and contribute to atherogenesis. The high-density lipoprotein (HDL) pool (nascent HDL) is derived from the chylomicrons following the action of LPL, and the reverse cholesterol pathway returns HDL to the liver via HDL receptors. Lipid-lowering drugs and their principal targets are shown with red arrows. *ABCA1,* ATP-binding cassette transporter A1 (also known as cholesterol efflux regulatory protein, CERP); *ACoA,* acetyl coenzyme A; *Apo,* apolipoprotein; *CHY rem,* chylomicron remnant; *FATP,* fatty acid transport protein; *HMG-CoA reductase,* 3-hydroxyl-3-methylglutaryl-coenzyme A reductase.

Table 48.1 Apolipoprotein and lipid composition of major lipoproteins and their sources

Lipoprotein	Major associated apolipoproteins	Cholesterol (%)	Triglycerides (%)	Source
Chylomicrons	Apo A/apo B/apo B$_{48}$/apo C/apo E	3	90	Intestine
VLDL	Apo C/apo B$_{100}$/apo E	20	50	Liver
LDL	Apo B$_{100}$	50	7	VLDL
HDL	Apo A	40	6	Chylomicrons, VLDL, liver, intestine

HDL, High-density lipoproteins; *LDL,* low-density lipoproteins; *VLDL,* very-low-density lipoproteins.

particular fractions of circulating cholesterol and triglyceride will be handled (see Table 48.1). In healthy individuals, about 70% of plasma cholesterol is carried by LDL and 20% by HDL. The least-dense and largest-diameter lipoproteins, known as chylomicrons, are exclusively concerned with the transport of dietary lipid from the intestine to the liver. Their low density and large size reflect their high content of triglycerides (see Table 48.1), and they are almost completely removed from blood after a 12 hours fast. VLDL carries about 60% of plasma triglyceride in the fasting state. The ratio of cholesterol to triglyceride carried is greatest in the HDL fraction.

Microsomal triglyceride transfer protein (MTP) has a central role in assembly of apo B48 on chylomicrons and apo B100 on VLDL, IDL and LDL (see Table 48.1).

PROCESSING OF LIPIDS ABSORBED FROM THE GUT

Cholesterol and free fatty acids are solubilised by bile acids in the gut lumen to facilitate absorption into enterocytes (see Fig. 48.1). Soluble cholesterol is transported into the

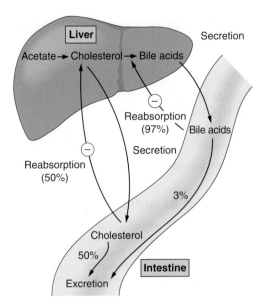

Fig. 48.2 Enterohepatic cycling of cholesterol and bile acids. Bile acids are secreted via the bile duct into the duodenum, where they aid in dietary lipid absorption, and are then returned to the liver by the portal circulation. A circled minus sign indicates a negative-feedback effect. Percentages are in relation to the amount excreted in bile.

enterocyte from the intestinal lumen by a specific lipid transmembrane transporter called Nieman-Pick C1-like 1 protein (NPC1L1). Triglyceride absorption does not require a specific transporter. Cholesterol and triglycerides are then incorporated into chylomicrons within enterocytes (see Table 48.1). Chylomicrons pass into the lymphatic system and then into the circulation. The apo C-II in chylomicrons activates endothelial lipoprotein lipase, which hydrolyses triglycerides to free fatty acids (see Table 48.1). Free fatty acids are utilised by muscle and liver as an energy source or stored as triglycerides in adipose tissue. After removal of triglycerides from the chylomicrons, the remaining surface lipoprotein and lipid fractions leave the particles to enter the HDL pool as 'nascent HDL' (see Fig. 48.1). The cholesterol-rich chylomicron remnants are removed from the circulation by hepatocytes, a process mediated by apolipoprotein E (apo E) receptors.

PLASMA TRANSPORT AND LIVER PROCESSING OF LIPIDS

Cholesterol (as cholesteryl esters) is transported to tissues by VLDL and LDL and from tissues to the liver by HDL. A high plasma concentration of LDL is associated with atheromatous disease.

Triglycerides in the liver that are surplus to synthetic and oxidative requirements, along with some cholesterol, are released into the circulation as the apo-B rich VLDL. Apo

C-II on the surface of VLDL activates endothelial lipoprotein lipase to break down triglycerides into free fatty acids and glycerol, leaving cholesterol-rich IDL, which retains apo-B (not shown in Fig. 48.1). IDL is either cleared by the liver or hepatic lipase releases free fatty acids from the remaining triglycerides, which generates LDL. LDL is the most cholesterol-rich lipoprotein (see Table 48.1). Up to 75% of LDL is removed from the circulation by uptake into liver cells via apo-B and hepatic LDL receptors. Hepatic LDL receptors are degraded by the enzyme proprotein convertase subtilisin/kexin type 9 (PCSK9), which plays a major role in cholesterol homeostasis. The circulating concentration of LDL rises if there is either excess production of LDL or deficient LDL receptor numbers on the liver.

The remainder of the LDL cholesterol is taken up by peripheral LDL receptors and non-LDL scavenger receptors, particularly on monocytes and macrophages. These cells express LDL receptors when they need cholesterol. When plasma LDL rises, scavenger-receptor-mediated uptake of cholesterol will increase. Circulating LDL-rich monocytes migrate into the subendothelial space of arterial walls, where they undergo a series of changes to become macrophages. LDL particles can cross the endothelium of arterial walls and in the presence of necrotic cell debris and free radicals in the endothelium, the LDL becomes oxidised. Macrophages take up more oxidised LDL by phagocytosis and form foam cells, which create lipid-rich deposits that are the precursor of atheromatous plaques (discussed later).

The size of LDL particles varies from large and buoyant to small and dense. Small dense LDL is especially rich in cholesterol and is particularly atherogenic because it binds less efficiently to hepatic LDL receptors and is therefore exposed to scavenger receptors for longer. The production of small dense LDL is increased in metabolic disturbance such as hypertriglyceridaemia and insulin resistance.

HDL carries cholesterol mobilised from peripheral tissues (and particularly oxidised cholesterol derivatives), and transports it to other cells that require cholesterol and to the liver where it is cleared (reverse cholesterol transport). The efflux of cholesterol from peripheral tissues is mediated by ATP-binding cassette transporter A1 (ABCA1), which combines with apo A-I to form nascent HDL. Free cholesterol in nascent HDL is esterified by the enzyme lecithin-cholesterol acyltransferase (LCAT) to create mature HDL. HDL is believed to protect against atheroma by this reverse cholesterol transport from peripheral tissues to the liver. The enzyme cholesterol ester transfer protein (CETP) can transfer cholesterol from HDL to VLDL in exchange for triglycerides. The extent of this exchange depends on the concentration of circulating triglycerides.

Atherogenic patterns of circulating lipoproteins can result from the following:

- high dietary intake of saturated fat.
- primary (inherited) disorders of enzymes or receptors involved in lipid metabolism. Most inherited hyperlipidaemias are polygenic, but an important inherited defect is familial hypercholesterolaemia (FH), a single recessive gene disorder that affects 1 in 500 of the population, who have reduced synthesis of LDL receptors.
- secondary lipid disorders, when hyperlipidaemia results from diseases that affect lipid metabolism – for example, liver disease, nephrotic syndrome, hypothyroidism.

FORMATION OF ATHEROMA

Abnormalities of plasma lipoprotein metabolism produce excessive concentrations of circulating cholesterol and/or triglyceride. Their clinical importance lies in their relationship to the production of atheroma (mainly raised plasma LDL cholesterol with a contribution from triglycerides) and pancreatitis (plasma triglycerides >12 mmol/L).

Atheroma is focal thickening of the intima of arteries, produced by a combination of cells, elements of connective tissue, lipids and debris. Atheromatous plaques preferentially affect parts of the arterial tree where there is turbulent blood flow, such as branch points. Turbulence leads to endothelial dysfunction and inhibits production of the vasodilator molecule nitric oxide. Endothelial dysfunction is also promoted by atherogenic factors such as smoking, diabetes mellitus or hypertension. The endothelium expresses adhesion molecules and produces proinflammatory cytokines and chemokines, which attract monocytes and some T-lymphocytes that penetrate the arterial wall and accumulate in the subendothelial tissue.

LDL in lipid-rich monocytes and excess free LDL in the arterial wall undergo enzymatic and free radical oxidation of the cholesterol component to produce a cytotoxic and chemotactic lipid that can further activate the endothelium. Monocytes differentiate into macrophages under the influence of endothelial cytokines, and the macrophages take up more oxidised LDL via scavenger receptors. The cholesterol accumulates as droplets in the cytosol, creating lipid-rich foam cells. Foam cells initiate fatty streaks that are the precursor of atheroma. T-cells in the developing atheromatous lesion recognise lipid antigens and release cytokines that attract further inflammatory cells and initiate a T-helper cell type 1 inflammatory response (see Chapter 38). Macrophage cytokines recruit smooth muscle cells that migrate from the media into the inflammatory lesion and also stimulate production of an extracellular fibrous matrix. A collagen-rich cap forms over the subendothelial plaque. The extent of the inflammatory response determines whether the cap becomes fibrous and stable, or is destabilised by infiltration of inflammatory cells that make the cap prone to rupture or surface erosion with subsequent thrombus formation. Plaque destabilisation underlies the development of acute coronary syndromes and many cases of ischaemic stroke (see Chapters 5 and 9).

DRUGS FOR HYPERLIPIDAEMIAS

3-HYDROXY-3-METHYLGLUTARYL-COENZYME A REDUCTASE INHIBITORS ('STATINS')

atorvastatin, pravastatin, rosuvastatin, simvastatin

Mechanism of action and effects

HMG-CoA reductase inhibitors competitively inhibit the enzyme that catalyses the rate-limiting step in the synthesis of cholesterol (see Fig. 48.1). Their most important action is in the liver, where the fall in hepatic cholesterol levels produces a compensatory upregulation in the number of LDL receptors on hepatocytes, with increased clearance of circulating LDL cholesterol. In the liver, the cholesterol is reprocessed to form bile salts. The extent of the reduction in plasma LDL cholesterol ranges from 25% to 55%, depending on the specific statin and the dose (Table 48.2). Short-acting statins, such as simvastatin, are most effective for reducing LDL cholesterol when taken at night, which is the time when most cholesterol synthesis occurs. Statins also reduce the circulating concentration of VLDL by stimulating lipoprotein lipase, and therefore reduce circulating triglycerides. A modest increase in HDL cholesterol is usually seen, due to increased synthesis of the constituent apo A1. This is a result of the activation of the peroxisome proliferator-activated receptor α (PPAR-α; see the section on fibrates later in this chapter).

Statins have several other potentially beneficial actions on the atherothrombotic process, which are unrelated to their ability to reduce plasma lipids (Box 48.1). There is increasing evidence that some of these may contribute significantly to the beneficial actions of statins in reducing clinical events in people with atherothrombotic disease.

Pharmacokinetics

Simvastatin is a prodrug activated by first-pass hepatic metabolism to a hydroxyacid metabolite, which has a half-life

Table 48.2 Average reduction in low-density lipoprotein cholesterol by statins					
Daily dose	**5 mg**	**10 mg**	**20 mg**	**40 mg**	**80 mg**
Atorvastatin	—	37%	43%	49%	55%
Fluvastatin	—	—	21%	27%	33%
Pravastatin	—	20%	24%	29%	—
Rosuvastatin	38%	43%	48%	53%	—
Simvastatin	—	27%	32%	37%	42%

Data from NICE Clinical Guideline 181 (July 2014; http://www.nice.org.uk/guidance/cg181), which classifies statins by their ability to reduce LDL cholesterol as high intensity (>40% reduction), medium intensity (31–40% reduction) or low intensity (20–30% reduction).

of 1–2 hours. Pravastatin is a hydrophilic drug eliminated mainly by the kidneys; its half-life is 1–2 hours. Atorvastatin undergoes first-pass metabolism, in part to active derivatives, and has a very long half-life of over 30 hours. Rosuvastatin is eliminated mainly in the bile and has a half-life of 20 hours.

Unwanted effects

- Gastrointestinal upset, including nausea, vomiting, abdominal pain, flatulence and diarrhoea.
- Central nervous system effects, such as dizziness, blurred vision and headache.
- Transient disturbance of liver function tests and, rarely, hepatitis.
- Myalgia (muscle pain) or myositis (muscle inflammation) and rarely rhabdomyolysis. In some people there is a raised serum creatine kinase concentration suggesting muscle damage, but no muscle symptoms. The mechanism of the myopathy remains uncertain, but it is likely that some people have minor metabolic abnormalities in their striated muscle that makes the muscle more susceptible to reduction of its fat substrate. There is an increased risk of muscle problems when a statin is used in combination with a fibrate, nicotinic acid, fusidic acid, ciclosporin and several other drugs (see Chapter 38).

SPECIFIC CHOLESTEROL ABSORPTION INHIBITOR

ezetimibe

Mechanism of action

Ezetimibe acts at the brush border of the small intestinal mucosa to inhibit the NPC1L1 transporter and reduce cholesterol absorption from the gut by about 50%. It has no effect on the absorption of triglycerides, bile acids or fat-soluble vitamins. Given alone, ezetimibe reduces plasma total cholesterol by about 15% and LDL cholesterol by about 20%. When taken with a low dose of statin, the combination is as effective as three doublings of the statin dose in reducing plasma total cholesterol.

Pharmacokinetics

Ezetimibe undergoes enterohepatic circulation, which gives it a long half-life of about 22 hours.

Unwanted effects

- Diarrhoea, abdominal pain.
- Headache.
- Angioedema.

BILE ACID-BINDING (ANION-EXCHANGE) RESINS

colesevelam, colestipol, colestyramine

Mechanism of action

Bile acids are synthesised from cholesterol in the liver and are secreted into the duodenum to aid absorption of dietary fat. They are then reabsorbed in the terminal ileum and returned to the liver in the portal circulation (see Fig. 48.2). Bile acid-binding resins are insoluble, nonabsorbable polymers that bind bile salts in the gut and prevent enterohepatic circulation of bile acids.

The size of the hepatic bile acid pool is tightly regulated via binding of bile salts to the farnesoid X receptor (FXR), a gene regulator. Depletion of intrahepatic bile acids releases FXR to stimulate conversion of cholesterol to bile acids. This reduces intrahepatic cholesterol, which promotes compensatory upregulation of hepatic LDL receptors in order to replenish liver cholesterol. LDL cholesterol is then cleared more rapidly from plasma, with a fall in circulating LDL levels of 15–20%. Reduced binding of bile acids to FXR also produces a small rise in plasma triglycerides through inhibition of lipoprotein lipase and also a small rise in HDL cholesterol.

Unwanted effects

- Unpalatability. Sachets containing several grams of powder have to be taken, usually mixed with food. The taste and texture limit acceptability and for this reason resins are no longer widely used.
- Constipation or, occasionally, diarrhoea.
- Interference with the absorption of certain acidic drugs – for example, digoxin, warfarin and levothyroxine. These drugs should be given at least 1 hour before or 4 hours after taking a resin.

FIBRATES

ciprofibrate, fenofibrate

Mechanism of action

The main mechanism of fibrate drugs is activation of gene transcription factors known as PPARs, particularly PPAR-α, which regulate the expression of genes that control lipoprotein metabolism. Fibrates are related to thiazolidinediones, and their PPAR-mediated actions are described in Chapter 40. PPAR-α is expressed in several tissues, including the liver, heart and kidney. There are several consequences of PPAR-α activation, which reduce circulating LDL cholesterol and triglycerides and increase HDL cholesterol:

- increased free fatty acid uptake by the liver due to induction of the fatty acid transporter protein in the cell membrane. In the liver, fatty acids are esterified as a result of increased acyl-CoA synthase activity. The esterified fatty acids are less available for hepatic triglyceride synthesis.
- increased lipoprotein lipase activity, which enhances the clearance of triglycerides from lipoproteins in the plasma (see Fig. 48.1).
- formation of larger, more buoyant LDL with increased affinity for its receptors, thus removing it more readily from the circulation.
- increased plasma HDL because of enhanced apo AI production and increased ABCA1 activity.

Pharmacokinetics

Fenofibrate is a prodrug that undergoes complete first-pass metabolism to the active form. Excretion is primarily by the kidney with a half-life of 20 hours. Ciprofibrate is metabolised in the liver and has a very long half-life of more than 2 days.

Unwanted effects

- Gastrointestinal upset.
- Rash or pruritus.
- Dizziness, headache.
- Increased lithogenicity of bile theoretically increases the risk of gallstones, but this has not been a problem with the clinical uses of these drugs.
- Myalgia and myositis are uncommon, unless there is impaired renal function or the fibrate is used in combination with a statin.
- Drug interactions include inhibition of the effect of warfarin (see Chapter 11).

NICOTINIC ACID AND DERIVATIVES

Examples

nicotinic acid (niacin), acipimox

Mechanism of action

Nicotinic acid is a B vitamin which has effects on lipids at pharmacological doses. It inhibits hepatic diacylglycerol acyltransferase-2, which is a key enzyme for triglyceride synthesis. As a result, hepatic apo B degradation is enhanced and the hepatic secretion of VLDL and LDL is reduced. Nicotinic acid also acts at specific niacin receptors (NIACR) in the skin, which may contribute to the flushing caused by the drug. Nicotinic acid reduces circulating triglycerides by up to 35% and LDL cholesterol modestly by up to 15%. HDL cholesterol is increased by up to 25% as a result of reduced hepatic uptake of the HDL molecule. A decrease in the activity of hepatic lipase also shifts the distribution of HDL subfractions, with a predominant elevation of HDL$_2$, which has greater protective effect than the HDL$_3$ subfraction. Acipimox is a synthetic derivative of nicotinic acid that is longer-acting but less effective for lowering LDL cholesterol.

Pharmacokinetics

Nicotinic acid undergoes hepatic metabolism, with the generation of metabolites thought to be responsible for the hepatotoxicity that can occur with high doses.

Unwanted effects

Nicotinic acid is often poorly tolerated, but unwanted effects can be reduced by increasing the dosage gradually.

- Cutaneous vasodilation is particularly troublesome and causes flushing and itching. The action of nicotinic acid on niacin receptors in the skin increases the production of prostaglandin (PG) D$_2$ and PGE$_2$, which cause the flushing. The flushing can be reduced by taking a small dose of aspirin 30 minutes before nicotinic acid.
- Abdominal pain, dyspepsia and diarrhoea.
- Hepatotoxicity.
- Headache.
- Exacerbation of gout.

OMEGA-3 FATTY ACIDS

Omega-3 fatty acids are long-chain polyunsaturated acids such as α-linolenic acid, which is found in plants, and eicosapentaenoic acid (EPA) and docosahexaenoic acid (DHA), which are found in high quantities in oily fish such as mackerel and sardines. Although there is little conclusive evidence that they reduce the risk of cardiovascular disease, they have several potential cardioprotective effects:

- PPAR-α activation (see the section on fibrates later in this chapter), with reduction in plasma triglyceride.
- reduction of plasma fibrinogen, decreasing thrombogenesis.
- they substitute for arachidonic acid membrane phospholipids, resulting in increased production of the prostanoid thromboxane A$_3$ in platelets. This has a lower ability to induce platelet aggregation, compared with the thromboxane A$_2$ formed from arachidonic acid (see Chapter 11).
- membrane stabilisation in heart muscle, with reduced susceptibility to ventricular arrhythmias and sudden cardiac death.

Unwanted effects

- Gastrointestinal upset with nausea, belching, diarrhoea or constipation.
- Prolonged bleeding time.

PROPROTEIN CONVERTASE SUBTILISIN/ KEXIN TYPE 9 INHIBITORS

Examples

evolocumab, alirocumab

Mechanism of action

PCSK9 inhibitors are monoclonal antibodies that inhibit the enzyme proprotein convertase subtilisin/kexin type 9 and prevent it from degrading LDL receptors on the surface of liver cells. The increased LDL receptor expression reduces circulating LDL cholesterol by 45–70%.

Pharmacokinetics

Evolocumab and alirocumab are injected subcutaneously every 2 weeks. Metabolism is by proteolysis, with very long half-lives of about 11–20 days.

Unwanted effects

- Nasopharyngitis.
- Arthralgia, back pain.
- Injection site pain.
- Rash.

MANAGEMENT OF HYPERLIPIDAEMIAS

Cardiovascular disease is the major risk associated with raised plasma LDL cholesterol. The relationship with raised LDL cholesterol is strongest for coronary atherosclerosis and peripheral vascular atherosclerosis, and to a lesser extent for cerebrovascular disease and atherothrombotic stroke. HDL cholesterol is protective against atherosclerosis, and HDL cholesterol less than 1.0 mmol/L is associated with an exponential increase in the risk of atheromatous disease. The ratio of total cholesterol to HDL cholesterol provides a much more sensitive indicator of the relative risk of developing cardiovascular disease than total cholesterol alone. While a high ratio of total cholesterol to HDL cholesterol predicts the relative risk of cardiovascular disease, the absolute risk (i.e. the overall number of individuals in the population who will develop disease in a particular time period) will be determined by the coexistence of other risk factors (discussed later).

Raised plasma triglycerides are an independent predictor of the risk of atherosclerosis, but less so than raised plasma cholesterol. Nevertheless, when raised triglycerides coexist with an atherogenic cholesterol profile, the overall risk is enhanced. A markedly raised plasma triglyceride concentration (>12 mmol/L) confers an increased risk of acute pancreatitis. Isolated hypertriglyceridaemia should be treated intensively for this reason alone.

Secondary causes of hyperlipidaemia, such as diabetes mellitus, hypothyroidism and nephrotic syndrome, should be excluded or treated before embarking on other aspects of management.

Lipid lowering for primary prevention of cardiovascular disease

Atherothrombotic disease has a multifactorial aetiology, and any strategy for primary prevention must consider all relevant treatable factors. Drug treatment of hyperlipidaemia for primary prevention should only be considered if there is a sufficiently high absolute risk of disease, and should not be based on the cholesterol level alone. Important factors to consider in risk management include the following.

- Smoking: Smoking doubles the risk of coronary artery disease, while stopping smoking reduces the risk close to that of someone who has never smoked in 3–5 years (see Chapter 5).
- Physical activity: A physically active lifestyle reduces the risk of myocardial infarction by up to 50% compared with a sedentary lifestyle.
- Maintaining ideal body weight: Obesity increases the risk of myocardial infarction by up to 50%.
- Mild-to-moderate alcohol consumption: A modest alcohol intake (see Chapter 54) can reduce the risk of myocardial infarction by about one-third. A high alcohol intake increases blood pressure, and thus increases cardiovascular risk.
- Treating hypertension (see Chapter 6): Although this is more effective for the prevention of stroke, it also reduces the risk of myocardial infarction, especially in older people.
- Control of diabetes mellitus: There is conflicting evidence on whether close control of plasma glucose reduces vascular events, but the risk of ischaemic heart disease in diabetes mellitus is at least twice that of people without diabetes mellitus. In people aged over 40 years with diabetes mellitus, intensive management of coexistent risk factors should be undertaken.
- Modifying the diet: Dietary management should be advised for all people with hypercholesterolaemia, with a reduction in saturated fat intake (saturated fat decreases hepatic LDL receptors) and an increase in monounsaturated fats (which increases hepatic LDL cholesterol receptors). Eating a diet containing fresh fruit and vegetables reduces oxidation of LDL, and therefore makes it less atherogenic.

When lipid-lowering treatment is considered, the goal is to reduce the plasma cholesterol. LDL cholesterol is a powerful predictor of future cardiovascular disease, especially in young people. The greatest risk is present when there is FH, a dominantly inherited genetic defect that predisposes to premature coronary heart disease, even in the absence of other risk factors. Heterozygous FH is associated with reduced LDL receptors on liver cells, and the total serum cholesterol is usually greater than 7.5 mmol/L in adult life. Lipid-lowering therapy in heterozygous FH, usually with a statin, should normally begin before the age of 10 years, with the goal of reducing plasma LDL cholesterol by 50%. Homozygous FH is a condition with LDL receptor activity of less than 2%, very high circulating LDL cholesterol and atherothrombotic disease arising in the second or third decade of life. Most drugs are ineffective for reducing plasma cholesterol in homozygous FH, and treatment is usually by LDL apheresis using an extracorporeal circulation to remove LDL cholesterol. The drug lomitapide, which inhibits MTP and reduces apo secretion and LDL formation, is a recent option for treating homozygous FH either used alone, with a statin or with apheresis.

For other forms of multigenic and acquired hypercholesterolaemia, the risk of cardiovascular disease should first be estimated using risk tables that assess the contribution of the total cholesterol:HDL ratio, systolic blood pressure, smoking, family history and other risk factors such as rheumatoid arthritis and socioeconomic deprivation (such as QRISK in the United Kingdom). The question exercising the minds of health economists is not whether treatment is effective, but when it becomes cost-effective. As part of a multiple risk factor intervention strategy, drug therapy for raised LDL cholesterol has a role for those at higher absolute risk, usually because several other risk factors coexist or there is a history of premature coronary artery disease in a first-degree relative. In the United Kingdom, lipid-lowering drugs are recommended if the predicted 10-year cardiovascular disease risk (a combination of coronary heart disease and stroke risk) is greater than 10%. There is no target cholesterol recommendation for primary prevention, except for those with FH for whom a 50% reduction in LDL cholesterol is recommended. For other people, using a dose of statin that has been shown to reduce cardiovascular events is recommended, regardless of the achieved reduction in plasma LDL cholesterol.

The ability of cholesterol-lowering drugs (and particularly statins) to prevent ischaemic heart disease has been demonstrated in many trials. Reducing plasma total cholesterol by 25–30% (with a reduction in LDL cholesterol of 30–35%) with a statin reduces the subsequent risk of myocardial infarction or vascular death by about 30%.

Secondary prevention of cardiovascular disease

Once cardiovascular disease is clinically apparent, the subsequent risk of death from vascular events is increased compared with the general population. Clinical evidence of vascular disease confers much greater absolute risk of a further event than a similar, or even higher, plasma cholesterol concentration in those without coronary artery disease. A recent episode of acute coronary syndrome confers the highest risk. At slightly lower absolute risk are those with stable angina pectoris, peripheral vascular disease or ischaemic stroke. Reduction of even 'normal' plasma cholesterol concentrations in people with established vascular disease reduces the subsequent risk of both fatal and nonfatal cardiovascular events.

Current evidence supports the use of statins as first-line therapy. Trials with fibrates have shown less marked benefit, unless the major lipid abnormality is low HDL cholesterol (see also Chapter 5). The target cholesterol concentration is total cholesterol below 4.0 mmol/L (LDL cholesterol <2.0 mmol/L). When this is not achieved with a statin alone, then combinations of drugs, such as a statin with ezetimibe or a fibrate, may be used, although there is little evidence of improved clinical outcomes. There is also the option of adding a PCSK9 inhibitor to a statin, which can produce a marked reduction in LDL cholesterol. There is evidence that the combination reduces the risk of subsequent myocardial infarction and cardiovascular death. The use of omega-3 fatty acids after myocardial infarction may have a modest cardioprotective effect, which may not entirely relate to their effects on plasma lipids.

Lowering plasma cholesterol for secondary prevention of coronary artery disease should be only one aspect of a comprehensive strategy for improving prognosis (see Chapter 5).

Mechanisms of prevention of coronary events by lipid-lowering drugs

There is a close relationship between the degree of LDL cholesterol reduction and the reduced risk of coronary events,

especially when it is achieved with a statin. Overall there is a 20% reduction in risk for every 1.0 mmol/L reduction in plasma total cholesterol concentration. Reducing plasma cholesterol probably stabilises existing atheromatous plaques by preventing lipid accumulation in their core, and therefore reduces the risk of plaque rupture. Statins prevent the growth of existing coronary artery plaques and reduce the formation of new plaques. High doses of a statin may even produce some regression of existing plaque. An antiinflammatory effect of statins may be important, measured by a reduction in plasma high-sensitivity C-reactive protein (CRP). Other actions of statins, such as reduction in thrombogenicity of blood and inhibition of smooth muscle proliferation in atheromatous plaques, may contribute to the clinical benefit, but their roles remain speculative.

Although there is less evidence that lipid-lowering drugs other than statins have the same ability to reduce cardiovascular events, it is widely accepted that lowering LDL cholesterol should provide some protection against atheroma however it is achieved.

Management of hypertriglyceridaemia

When triglycerides are markedly raised, control of diabetes mellitus, weight loss and reduction of alcohol intake should be considered when appropriate. When drug therapy is necessary, modest hypertriglyceridaemia in association with hypercholesterolaemia will usually respond to a statin. Extremely high plasma triglyceride concentrations usually respond well to a fibrate or to nicotinic acid. Combination therapy with a statin and a fibrate may be necessary in some high-risk individuals to achieve an acceptable lipid profile.

SELF-ASSESSMENT

True/false questions

1. The risk of coronary disease is strongly related to the plasma triglyceride concentration.
2. Genetic factors contribute to the development of hypercholesterolaemia.
3. Anion-exchange resins enhance the absorption of bile acids from the gut.
4. Statins inhibit HMG-CoA reductase.
5. Decreased hepatic cholesterol synthesis results in increased numbers of HDL receptors.
6. Pravastatin lowers plasma LDL cholesterol by about 10%.
7. Co-administration of statins and fibrates has no greater effect than giving each drug separately.
8. Ezetimibe blocks cholesterol absorption in the intestinal mucosa.
9. Fenofibrate inhibits lipoprotein lipase by activating PPAR-α.
10. Nicotinic acid reduces triglyceride synthesis in the liver.
11. Skin flushing is a common unwanted effect of nicotinic acid.
12. Arachidonic acid is an omega-3 fatty acid.

13. Alirocumab is a monoclonal antibody that blocks LDL receptors.

One-best-answer (OBA) questions

1. Identify the *most accurate* statement concerning lipids and cardiovascular disease.
   A. A high total plasma cholesterol/HDL cholesterol ratio reduces cardiovascular risk.
   B. VLDL has a greater percentage of cholesterol than HDL.
   C. The outer coat of lipoproteins is a phospholipid bilayer.
   D. Reducing dietary saturated fat reduces coronary disease risk.
   E. Even moderate alcohol consumption increases the risk of myocardial infarction.
2. Identify the *inaccurate* statement concerning the actions of statins.
   A. Statins alter smooth muscle proliferation in atherosclerotic plaques.
   B. Statins may cause myalgia.
   C. Statins reduce plasma CRP.
   D. Statins suppress lipoprotein lipase activity.
   E. Statins decrease plasma HDL concentrations.

Case-based questions

A 58-year-old man recovered from an anterior myocardial infarction. His fasting plasma cholesterol was 7.8 mmol/L. You want to reduce his risk of a further myocardial infarction by lowering his cholesterol.
1. What advice should be offered?
2. What drug should be recommended and why?
3. What reduction in plasma cholesterol should be aimed for, and when should a response be expected?
4. What unwanted effects should be looked out for?

ANSWERS

True/false answers

1. **False.** Cardiovascular risk is most closely associated with high LDL cholesterol, which leads to lipid peroxidation and formation of foam cells in atheromatous plaque. Triglyceridaemia is a secondary risk factor.
2. **True.** The best understood genetic risk is FH, in which a recessive disorder causes low LDL receptor expression and predisposes to premature coronary disease.
3. **False.** The anion-exchange resins sequester bile acids in the gut, decreasing the absorption of dietary cholesterol. They also increase incorporation of hepatic cholesterol into bile acids, leading to further loss of cholesterol in bile secretions into the gut.
4. **True.** HMG-CoA reductase is the rate-limiting enzyme for cholesterol synthesis in the liver.
5. **False.** Reducing cholesterol synthesis in the liver results in increased LDL receptor expression and hence increased LDL clearance from the plasma.
6. **False.** Statins reduce plasma LDL cholesterol by 25–55%, depending on the drug and the dose (see Table 48.2).
7. **False.** Statins and fibrates act mainly by different mechanisms, and their co-administration can help achieve target plasma cholesterol concentrations, although the additional benefit on clinical outcomes is unclear.
8. **True.** Ezetimibe reduces cholesterol absorption by blocking the intestinal NPC1L1 cholesterol transporter.
9. **False.** Fibrates activate PPAR-α, but this increases lipoprotein lipase activity and clears triglycerides from the plasma.
10. **True.** Nicotinic acid inhibits triglyceride synthesis by diacylglycerol acyltransferase-2 in the liver, hence reducing production of VLDL and LDL.
11. **True.** Nicotinic acid may cause skin flushing by stimulating PG synthesis, and it can be reduced by a nonsteroidal antiinflammatory drug (NSAID).
12. **False.** Arachidonic acid is an omega-6 fatty acid and the precursor of prothrombotic thromboxane A_2. Omega-3 fatty acids include EPA and DHA found in fish oils, which may have cardioprotective effects.
13. **False.** Alirocumab prevents the degradation of LDL receptors on hepatocytes by inhibiting PCSK9; the enhanced expression of LDL receptors clears up to 70% of LDL cholesterol from the circulation.

One-best-answer (OBA) answers

1. **Answer D** is correct.
   A. Incorrect. A low ratio of total cholesterol to HDL cholesterol is associated with lower cardiovascular risk.
   B. Incorrect. VLDL carries a greater load of triglycerides, so the proportion of cholesterol is lower in VLDL (20%) than in HDL (40%).
   C. Incorrect. The lipoprotein coat is a phospholipid monolayer, in which apolipoproteins are embedded, and provides a lipophilic interior for the transport of triglycerides.
   D. **Correct.** High dietary intake of saturated fat is associated with coronary disease, with other risk factors such as obesity, diabetes mellitus, smoking and family history also playing important roles.
   E. Incorrect. Moderate alcohol consumption reduces myocardial infarction risk by about 30%.
2. **Answer E** is the inaccurate statement.
   A. Correct. The effect on smooth muscle proliferation may improve plaque stability.
   B. Correct. Statins can cause muscle pain and, rarely, rhabdomyolysis.
   C. Correct. The reduced plasma CRP reflects an antiinflammatory action of statins.
   D. Correct. This action on lipoprotein lipase reduces plasma triglycerides.
   E. **Incorrect.** Statins increase plasma HDL concentration by 5–15%.

Case-based answers

1. General advice would include a low-fat diet, exercise and stopping smoking. Concomitant risk factors including obesity, diabetes mellitus and hypertension should be investigated.
2. A statin would be recommended as the first-choice drug in preventing cardiovascular events. Statins are of proven benefit based on data from many studies, and they are well tolerated.

3. The response would depend upon the chosen statin, its dosage and additional lifestyle changes, but the recommended targets are a total cholesterol concentration less than 4 mmol/L and LDL cholesterol less than 2 mmol/L. Several weeks of treatment may be required to achieve this reduction.

4. Gastrointestinal upsets are common. The use of statins is not recommended in people with hypothyroidism or liver disease. Thyroid and liver function tests should be performed. The patient should be advised to report unexplained muscle pain.

FURTHER READING

Baber, U., Toto, R.D., de Lemos, J., 2007. Statins and cardiovascular risk reduction in patients with chronic kidney disease and end-stage renal failure. Am. Heart J. 153, 471–477.

Cholesterol Treatment Trialists' (CTT) Collaboration, 2015. Efficacy and safety of LDL-lowering therapy among men and women: meta-analysis of individual data from 174,000 participants in 27 randomised trials. Lancet 385, 1397–1405.

Cholesterol Treatment Trialists' (CTT) Collaboration, 2012. The effects of lowering LDL cholesterol with statin therapy in people at low risk of vascular disease: meta-analysis of individual data from 27 randomised trials. Lancet 380, 581–590.

Collins, R., Reith, C., Emberson, J., et al., 2016. Interpretation of the evidence for the efficacy and safety of statin therapy. Lancet 388, 2532–2561.

Desai, C.S., Martin, S.S., Blumenthal, R.S., 2014. Non-cardiovascular effects associated with statins. Br. Med. J. 349, g3743.

Gutierrez, J., Ramirez, G., Rundek, T., et al., 2012. Statin therapy in the prevention of recurrent cardiovascular events: a sex-based meta-analysis. Arch. Intern. Med. 172, 909–919.

Kwak, S.M., Nyung, S.-K., Lee, Y.J., et al., 2012. Efficacy of omega-3 fatty acid supplements (eicosapentaenoic acid and docasahexaenoic acids) in the secondary prevention of cardiovascular disease: a meta-analysis of randomized, double-blind, placebo-controlled trials. Arch. Intern. Med. 172, 686–694.

Ridker, P., 2014. Lipids and cardiovascular disease 1. LDL cholesterol: controversies and future therapeutic directions. Lancet 384, 607–617.

US Preventive Services Task Force, 2016. Statin use for the primary prevention of cardiovascular disease in adults. JAMA 316, 1997–2007.

Compendium: drugs used to treat hyperlipidaemias

Drug	Characteristics
HMG-CoA reductase inhibitors ('statins')	
Statins are first-line drugs for lowering LDL cholesterol. Used in symptomatic cardiovascular disease and in asymptomatic people at increased cardiovascular risk. Given orally.	
Atorvastatin	High-intensity statin. Used for primary hypercholesterolaemia, heterozygous familial hypercholesterolaemia or mixed hyperlipidaemia. Half-life: 32–36 h
Fluvastatin	Low- to medium-intensity statin. Used as adjunct to diet in primary hypercholesterolaemia and mixed hyperlipidaemias and for prophylaxis of coronary atherosclerosis. Half-life: 2–3 h
Pravastatin	Low-intensity statin. Used as adjunct to diet in primary hypercholesterolaemia and for prophylaxis of coronary atherosclerosis. Mainly renal excretion. Half-life: 1–2 h
Rosuvastatin	High-intensity statin. Used in primary hypercholesterolaemia, mixed dyslipidaemia and homozygous familial hypercholesterolaemia. Minimal hepatic metabolism. Half-life: 20 h
Simvastatin	Low- to medium-intensity statin. Prodrug converted rapidly to active analogue. Used as an adjunct to diet in primary hypercholesterolaemia and mixed hyperlipidaemias, and for prophylaxis of coronary atherosclerosis. Half-life: 2 h
Drugs that sequester bile acids	
Bile acid sequestrants act within the gut to reduce bile acid reabsorption; they reduce plasma LDL cholesterol but can aggravate hypertriglyceridaemia. Given orally.	
Colesevelam	A lipid-lowering polymer; used for primary hypercholesterolaemia as an adjunct to dietary measures, given alone or with a statin; improves glycaemic control in type 2 diabetes in adults
Colestipol	Anion-exchange resin that binds bile acids. Used for hyperlipidaemias not responding to diet and other measures
Colestyramine	Anion-exchange resin that binds bile acids. Used for hyperlipidaemias, and for primary hypercholesterolaemia in men aged 35–59, and to treat pruritus associated with biliary obstruction

Compendium: drugs used to treat hyperlipidaemias (cont'd)

Drug	Characteristics
Specific inhibitors of cholesterol absorption	
Ezetimibe	Prodrug converted to active drug in liver and intestine. Inhibits the intestinal cholesterol transporter NPC1L1. Used as adjunct to dietary measures, and a statin in primary and homozygous familial hypercholesterolaemia. Given orally. Half-life: 22 h
Fibrates	
Act mainly by reducing serum triglycerides with variable effects on LDL cholesterol; used as first-line treatment for hypertriglyceridaemia, or in people intolerant of statins. Given orally.	
Bezafibrate	Used as adjunct to lifestyle measures in mixed hyperlipidaemia if statin is contraindicated or not tolerated, or in severe hypertriglyceridaemia. Half-life: 1–2 h
Ciprofibrate	Used as adjunct to lifestyle measures in mixed hyperlipidaemia if statin is contraindicated or not tolerated, or in severe hypertriglyceridaemia. Half-life: 38–86 h
Fenofibrate	Prodrug of fenofibric acid. Used in mixed hyperlipidaemia if statin contraindicated or not tolerated, or in severe hypertriglyceridaemia; also as adjunct to statin in mixed hyperlipidaemia in people at high cardiovascular risk. Half-life: 20 h
Gemfibrozil	Used as adjunct to lifestyle measures in mixed hyperlipidaemia or primary hypercholesterolaemia if statin is contraindicated or not tolerated, or in severe hypertriglyceridaemia; also used in primary prevention of cardiovascular disease in men with hyperlipidaemias. Half-life: 1–2 h
Nicotinic acid and derivatives	
Used in combination with statins or as monotherapy in patients intolerant to statins. Given orally.	
Acipimox	Less effective for hypertriglyceridaemias than nicotinic acid, with fewer unwanted effects. Half-life: 1–2 h
Nicotinic acid (niacin)	Reduces both cholesterol and triglycerides, but use limited by prostaglandin-mediated vasodilation. Half-life: 0.5 h
PCSK9 inhibitors	
Alirocumab	Monoclonal antibody; prevents proprotein convertase subtilisin/kexin type 9 (PCSK9) degrading LDL receptors on hepatocytes. Given subcutaneously. Half-life: 12–20 days
Evolocumab	Monoclonal antibody; prevents PCSK9 degrading LDL receptors on hepatocytes. Given subcutaneously. Half-life: 11–17 days
Other treatments	
Omega-3 acid ethyl esters	Used orally as adjunct for treating hypertriglyceridaemia, but little evidence for effectiveness in reducing risk of cardiovascular disease
Lomitapide	Inhibitor of microsomal triglyceride transfer protein (MTP); reduces lipoprotein secretion and circulating lipids. Specialist use for treatment of homozygous familial hypercholesterolaemia. Given orally. Half-life: 29 h

HMG-CoA reductase, 3-hydroxyl-3-methylglutaryl-coenzyme A reductase; *LDL*, low-density lipoprotein; *NPC1L1*, Niemann-Pick C1-like protein 1; *PCSK9*, proprotein convertase subtilisin/kexin type 9.

10

The skin and eyes

49 Skin disorders

VEHICLES FOR TOPICAL SKIN APPLICATIONS

Topical treatment of skin disease reduces the risk of systemic unwanted effects, but adherence may be adversely affected by inconvenience or problems using the preparation. Vehicles that carry the drug for topical application have different properties, and choosing an appropriate vehicle for the condition to be treated is important. In addition, the effectiveness of a topical drug depends on its ability to penetrate the epidermis, which is influenced by the vehicle or base in which the drug is carried. Ageing skin absorbs drugs more readily, and hydration aids drug penetration. Four types of vehicle are used:

- *ointments*, which are greases such as white or yellow soft paraffin. They are more occlusive on the skin than creams, and this keeps the skin hydrated and enhances drug absorption. Preservatives are not needed. Suspension of a fine powder in an ointment creates a paste which will stay where it is placed on the skin. The main use

of pastes is to apply noxious chemicals that should be confined to one area of the skin.
- *creams*, which are emulsions of water with grease that have an emollient and cooling effect. They are less greasy than ointments and are absorbed more quickly into the skin. Preservatives are used to prevent growth of bacteria and fungi, and these can lead to allergic contact dermatitis.
- *lotions*, which are watery suspensions. They are less messy for use on wet areas and hairy skin, and they have a drying and cooling effect on the skin.
- *gels*, which have a high water content and carry suspensions of insoluble drugs. The gelling agents aid drug absorption, and they can be particularly useful for application to the face or scalp.

ATOPIC AND CONTACT DERMATITIS

Dermatitis is a term used to describe eczematous inflammation of the skin. It has a significant underlying genetic predisposition, but is triggered by external factors.

ATOPIC ECZEMA (ATOPIC DERMATITIS)

Atopic eczema affects 15–30% of children and up to 10% of adults. The majority of cases begin in the first 5 years of life, and there is an association with the other atopic disorders, asthma and hay fever. The pathogenesis of atopic eczema is determined by a combination of genetic and environmental factors. Mutations in the gene that codes for filaggrin (a protein that binds to keratin in epithelial cells) lead to impairment of the barrier function of the skin, which may allow increased exposure to irritants and allergens. In atopic individuals, circulating mononuclear cells have a reduced ability to produce interferon γ, which normally inhibits both IgE production and the proliferation of T-helper type 2 (Th2) lymphocytes. Allergens can then trigger IgE-mediated sensitisation, with increased eosinophils in the peripheral blood and a raised plasma IgE concentration (see Chapter 39). In affected skin, keratinocytes produce cytokines that stimulate eosinophil activation and adhesion to vascular walls. The consequence of these processes is that both Th2-cells and eosinophils proliferate in the eczematous lesions.

Exposure to microbial antigens in early life promotes the normal Th1-cell dominance and suppresses the development of Th2-cells. It is possible that the increasing use of antibacterial drugs in childhood may partially explain the rise in atopic dermatitis.

Affected skin is erythematous with oedema, weeping and vesicles in the acute stages. In the chronic stage, the permeability barrier function of the skin is impaired, resulting in increased transepidermal water loss. The skin becomes scaly and extremely dry, and scratching produces excoriation and thickening (lichenification) of the skin, often affecting the flexures.

CONTACT DERMATITIS

There are two main triggers:

- An external agent producing direct irritation (irritant contact dermatitis), usually affecting the hands and caused by surgical gloves, sweating, frequent handwashing or use of antiseptics such as chlorhexidine.
- Immunological sensitisation involving a delayed hypersensitivity response (allergic contact dermatitis; see Chapter 39). Once the skin has been sensitised, the potential for further reaction persists indefinitely. Sensitisation can arise in response to the topical application of drugs.

OTHER TYPES OF DERMATITIS

These include nummular (discoid) eczema, photosensitive dermatitis, stasis dermatitis (due to venous hypertension in the legs) and seborrhoeic dermatitis (in the mesolabial folds and scalp).

TREATMENT OF ATOPIC ECZEMA

- Emollients (substances that soften the skin) are a fundamental part of treatment. They leave an occlusive layer that seals the surface of the skin and reduces water loss; the addition of humectants (hygroscopic substances) such as urea and glycerol can further enhance water retention. Ointments are the most effective emollients, but are greasy and not well accepted by most people. Creams are more cosmetically acceptable, but aqueous cream (once widely used) should be avoided, as it weakens the epidermal barrier.
- Avoidance of irritants, such as soaps, detergents, alcohols and astringents.
- Identification of allergens and their subsequent elimination.
- Topical corticosteroid ointment (see Chapter 44) applied once daily is effective when an emollient is insufficient. A burst of 5–7 days of treatment with a potent corticosteroid such as betamethasone valerate (Box 49.1) can gain control, but the antiinflammatory effect diminishes

with prolonged regular use (tachyphylaxis). Potent corticosteroid should not be applied to the face or genitals, because of the risk of skin thinning. In these areas, a mild corticosteroid such as hydrocortisone should be used. Emollients are used to maintain control after short-term use of a corticosteroid, although a potent topical corticosteroid applied 2 days/week can prevent relapse.

- Topical calcineurin inhibitors, such as tacrolimus (see Chapter 38), directly or indirectly reduce activation of many of the inflammatory cells involved in the pathogenesis of the dermatitic lesions, including T-cells, dendritic cells, mast cells and keratinocytes. Local burning is the major unwanted effect, and there is a theoretical increased risk of skin cancer. Tacrolimus is as effective as a potent corticosteroid for moderate to severe eczema.
- Sedative antihistamines (see Chapter 39) taken at night assist sleep, although they have little effect on itching.
- Immunosuppressant therapy with azathioprine or ciclosporin (see Chapter 38) is used for treatment-resistant eczema. The main limitation is rapid relapse when treatment is stopped.
- Phototherapy with narrow-band ultraviolet B (UVB) radiation can be helpful but increases the future risk of skin cancer.
- Cotton or silk fitted clothing is often advocated to reduce scratching, although there is little evidence of benefit, and paste bandages on the limbs can be useful to occlude excoriated areas.
- Systemic antibacterial drugs are given for secondary infection. Antistaphylococcal agents are often helpful if the skin lesions are poorly controlled with other treatments.

TREATMENT OF CONTACT DERMATITIS

- Provision of a barrier to an irritant (e.g. wearing gloves or removing an allergen) may be sufficient.
- Mild topical corticosteroid ointment (see Box 49.1).
- Potassium permanganate soaks can help to dry up exudative lesions.

PSORIASIS

Psoriatic skin lesions are produced by a very rapid proliferation of epidermal keratinocytes. Cell turnover time is decreased from about 40 days to as little as 3–4 days, which prevents adequate cell maturation. Instead of producing a normal keratinous surface layer, the skin thickens (acanthosis) in ridges, with increased numbers of acanthocytes forming a silvery scale with dilated upper dermal capillaries. The dermis and epidermis are also infiltrated by neutrophils, lymphocytes, macrophages and dendritic antigen-presenting cells.

There is a genetic component to psoriasis, which interacts with unknown environmental factors to produce an autoimmune reaction in the dermis. Psoriasis can be provoked or exacerbated by several drugs, including lithium, chloroquine, hydroxychloroquine, β-adrenoceptor antagonists, nonsteroidal antiinflammatory drugs (NSAIDs) and angiotensin-converting enzyme inhibitors.

The pathogenesis of psoriasis begins with antigen-presenting cells in the dermis, which mature and migrate

Box 49.1	Potency of topical corticosteroids
Mild	Hydrocortisone
Moderately potent	Clobetasone butyrate
Potent	Betamethasone valerate
	Hydrocortisone butyrate
Very potent	Clobetasol propionate

to regional lymph nodes where they activate T-cells. T-cells then proliferate and enter the circulation and extravasate into the skin at sites of inflammation, assisted by local chemokine production. In the dermis a Th1-cell immune response triggers secretion of cytokines such as interferon γ, tumour necrosis factor (TNF) α, and interleukins (IL)-2, IL-8, IL-12, IL-17 and IL-23. These cytokines stimulate cell proliferation and impair maturation of keratinocytes, and produce the vascular changes in the skin.

Chronic plaque psoriasis (psoriasis vulgaris) accounts for 90% of cases. Plaques are most often found on the elbows, knees, shins, sacrum, genitalia and scalp. Various subtypes of psoriasis present with different clinical manifestations, such as guttate psoriasis and pustular psoriasis. Inflammatory arthritis occurs in up to 25% of people with psoriasis (see Chapter 30).

DRUGS FOR TREATMENT OF PSORIASIS

There are several treatments for the skin lesions, both topical and systemic, but none produce long-term remission.

Topical therapy

Emollients

These reduce scaling and itching and may be sufficient in mild psoriasis (see the previous section on atopic dermatitis). They can also be used with a keratolytic.

Keratolytics

Keratolytics such as salicylic acid break down keratin and soften skin, which improves penetration of other treatments. Salicylic acid ointment is most frequently used.

Vitamin D analogues

Vitamin D regulates epidermal proliferation and differentiation. It also has immunosuppressant properties. Vitamin D analogues (e.g. calcipotriol, calcitriol) are clean and simple to apply, and are particularly useful for chronic plaque psoriasis, although complete clearing of the plaques is unusual. Calcipotriol should be avoided on the face and in flexures, where it often causes irritation. Calcitriol is better tolerated in sensitive areas, but short-term use of a mild or moderately potent topical corticosteroid (see Box 49.1) is usually preferred for treatment of these sites. Excessive use of vitamin D analogues can lead to hypercalcaemia, but this is not a problem at recommended dosages. The ease of use of vitamin D analogues makes them a popular choice if a keratolytic is insufficient, but short remissions necessitate continuous treatment.

Topical retinoid

Retinoids are discussed more fully under systemic treatments. Tazarotene gel can be applied to plaque psoriasis and has minimal systemic absorption. Unlike other retinoids, tazarotene is selective for retinoic acid receptor (RAR) proteins, with no affinity for retinoid X receptors (RXR; discussed later). This may reduce unwanted effects, which are mainly local irritation of healthy skin with pruritus. Tazarotene should be avoided for 1 month before conception, because of potential teratogenic effects.

Topical calcineurin inhibitors

These are infrequently used for psoriasis, but may be helpful to avoid prolonged use of topical corticosteroid. They include tacrolimus, as noted previously with the treatment of atopic eczema.

Dithranol

Dithranol is an anthracene derivative that impairs DNA replication and decreases cell division and is effective for healing psoriatic plaques. In the hospital (or when attending outpatient treatment), it is applied in a stiff paste to the plaque so that the dithranol does not burn normal skin, and is left in contact with the plaque for 24 hours. At home, dithranol is used as a cream that is applied to the plaque for 30 minutes and then washed off. The oxidation products of dithranol stain the skin brown, leaving discoloration of healed areas for a few days. They also stain clothes and bedding a mauve colour that will not wash out. Since dithranol irritates normal skin, it should not be used in flexures.

Coal tar preparations

Crude coal tar is a mixture of a large number of phenols, hydrocarbons and heterocyclic compounds that have a cytostatic action. It enhances the healing effect of UVB radiation on psoriatic lesions. The main disadvantages are messiness and modest efficacy when used alone. More refined tar preparations have greater acceptability, but are even less effective.

Phototherapy

Ultraviolet light produces improvement in psoriasis by inhibiting DNA synthesis and depleting intraepidermal T-cells. It should not be used on individuals with very fair skin who are prone to sunburn. Narrow-band UVB (311–313 nm) given 2–3 times a week for 15–30 treatments once a year as needed produces a useful response in 80% of cases of mild to moderate chronic plaque psoriasis. Long-wavelength UVA (320–400 nm) requires more specialised equipment and prior administration of an oral psoralen as a photosensitising drug (a process called photochemotherapy or psoralen and ultraviolet A [PUVA] therapy). Psoralen probably intercalates between pyrimidine base pairs in the DNA helix and inhibits cell replication. Psoralen can produce nausea and headache acutely. The long-term risks of phototherapy, but especially PUVA, include accelerated skin ageing and an increased incidence of skin cancer. PUVA is more effective than treatment with UVB and is used for severe, resistant psoriasis, but systemic treatments are increasingly preferred.

Topical corticosteroid preparations

These should be used sparingly on limited areas, since unwanted effects can be troublesome (see Chapter 44). Withdrawal of a high-potency corticosteroid (see Box 49.1) can produce a rebound exacerbation and even generalised pustular psoriasis.

Systemic treatments

Systemic treatment is used for the more severe forms of psoriasis.

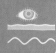

Methotrexate

This is a very effective treatment at low dosages for resistant and widespread psoriasis. Its main actions are cytostatic and immunosuppressant (see Chapter 38). Either oral or intramuscular treatment is used once a week. Bone marrow depression and hepatotoxicity with liver fibrosis are the main complications; blood counts and serum procollagen III, to identify liver toxicity, must be checked every 3 months.

Retinoids

This term covers vitamin A (retinol) and therapeutically useful synthetic vitamin A derivatives, such as acitretin. Given orally, they are antiinflammatory and cytostatic. Vitamin A, and its metabolites all-*trans*-retinoic acid and 9-*cis*-retinoic acid, are involved in epithelial cell growth and differentiation. Retinoids enter cells by endocytosis and interact with two forms of retinoic acid nuclear receptor, RARs and RXRs, which are related to steroid/thyroid hormone receptors (see Chapter 1). The retinoid–receptor complex initiates gene transcription and affects cell growth and differentiation by modulation of growth factors and their receptors. The response of psoriatic lesions is delayed by up to 2 months. Unwanted effects are almost universal, dose-dependent and reversible. These include dry lips and nasal mucosa, dryness of the skin with localised peeling over the digits, and transient thinning of hair. Longer-term problems include ossification of ligaments and increased plasma triglycerides and cholesterol. There is a high risk of teratogenesis, and women must use adequate contraception during treatment, and stop treatment for 3 years before conception.

Ciclosporin

Ciclosporin (see Chapter 38) is highly effective in psoriasis at lower doses than those required for prevention of allograft rejection. Improvement is seen within 2 weeks, but remissions are usually short-lived.

Biologic agents

Adalimumab (given by subcutaneous injection) or infliximab (via intravenous infusion; see Chapter 30) are therapies that block TNFα and are highly effective in treatment-resistant psoriasis and for psoriatic arthropathy. Infliximab produces the more rapid response, sometimes within 3 weeks. Ustekinumab (by subcutaneous injection) is an inhibitor of IL-12 and IL-23 that has similar efficacy to infliximab.

PDE4 inhibitor

Apremilast is a PDE4 inhibitor that downregulates the inflammatory response by reducing TNFα and some interleukins. It is usually considered when other systemic therapy is unsuccessful or poorly tolerated. It is effective for chronic plaque psoriasis and psoriatic arthropathy. Unwanted effects include diarrhoea, nausea and headache.

Fumaric acid esters

This is an oral treatment (unlicensed in the United Kingdom) for severe psoriasis that probably works by promoting a Th2-cell response in place of the Th1-dominant response found in psoriasis. This results from inhibition of nuclear factor κB (NF-κB), which enhances T-cell apoptosis. Fumaric acid is poorly absorbed from the gut and is therefore given as an ester that is rapidly hydrolysed after absorption to the active derivative dimethylfumarate. Unwanted effects include gastrointestinal upset in more than two-thirds of people, and flushing in one-third, but these usually subside with continued treatment. Improvement of psoriasis can take 6–8 weeks.

CHOICE OF TREATMENT FOR PSORIASIS

Topical treatments are preferred, with phototherapy or systemic treatments used when topical treatment is inadequate. Combinations of treatments are often more effective than a single agent, and continued treatment is usually necessary to avoid relapse. Stress can aggravate psoriasis, and smoking and alcohol should be reduced.

For less severe chronic plaque psoriasis, topical vitamin D (or analogues) is often combined with short-term use of a mild or moderately potent topical corticosteroid (1–2 weeks a month, especially for sensitive areas) as first-line treatment. The combination produces a response within 2–4 weeks. If topical corticosteroid is needed continuously, a topical calcineurin inhibitor should be considered as an alternative. An emollient containing urea or salicylic acid can reduce plaque thickness and scale, which will improve absorption of other topical drugs. Dithranol is as effective as vitamin D analogues, but is less easily applied and less well tolerated.

In more severe psoriasis, a vitamin D analogue and topical corticosteroid can be used together with phototherapy, or with systemic agents to allow doses of systemic drugs to be reduced. Conventional systemic therapy with methotrexate, acitretin or ciclosporin is used first. Biologic agents are usually reserved for failure to respond to these drugs. Narrowband UVB can also be used in combination with acitretin or biological therapies.

ACNE VULGARIS

Acne is very common in adolescence. While it often regresses in the late teens or early twenties, half of all those affected continue to experience symptoms into adult life. Acne affects areas of skin with large numbers of sebaceous glands, especially the face, neck, back and chest. Acne has a genetic background, which determines the rate of sebum production, particularly in response to androgens. Androgens are produced at puberty and induce hypertrophy of sebaceous glands, and the excess secretion rate in predisposed individuals triggers the acne. Acne can also be produced by systemic corticosteroids or anabolic steroids (see Chapter 46). In women, it can be a manifestation of polycystic ovary syndrome (see Chapter 43). Smoking and a diet high in dairy products or with a high glycaemic load increase the risk of acne.

Increased production of sebum in response to androgenic stimulation distends the pilosebaceous duct. Proliferation of keratinocytes causes hyperkeratosis at the mouth of the hair follicle, which blocks the duct, producing a small closed papule (comedo) called a whitehead. If the duct then opens, compacted follicular cells and oxidized melanin at the tip give comedones the appearance of a blackhead. Sebum promotes growth of a resident anaerobic bacterium on the skin, *Propionibacterium acnes*, which degrades triglycerides in sebum to free fatty acids and glycerol. *P. acnes* also releases chemotactic factors and inflammatory mediators. The combination of released mediators with the irritant free fatty acids produces inflammatory lesions (papules, pustules and nodules) which can coalesce to form multilocular cysts. These inflammatory lesions can scar, leaving permanent disfigurement.

Mild acne is confined to the face and consists of papules and pustules with few inflammatory lesions. Moderate acne usually also involves the trunk and has increased numbers of inflammatory lesions. Severe acne presents with nodules and cysts, which are usually widespread.

DRUGS FOR TREATMENT OF ACNE

There are several effective treatments for acne. The choice will depend on the nature of the lesions and their severity. Topical treatments do not influence the rate of production of sebum.

Topical treatments

- *Retinoids* (such as isotretinoin, adapalene) are vitamin A derivatives with a keratolytic action that unblocks the pilosebaceous follicles and allows the flow of sebum to extrude the plug (comedolytic action). Some retinoids also have an antiinflammatory action. The cellular basis of these actions is similar to that of acitretin (discussed further in the section on psoriasis). Topical retinoids can cause erythema and scaling, which can be minimised by starting with a low concentration. Adapalene is an extensively modified retinoid that has a faster onset of action than isotretinoin and produces less skin irritation.
- *Azelaic acid* has an antibacterial action against *P. acnes* and is effective against bacteria that have become resistant to erythromycin and tetracycline. It also inhibits the division of keratinocytes, which may reduce follicular plugging and prevent the development of comedones. The most frequent unwanted effects are local burning, scaling or itching, while hypopigmentation can be a problem with darker skin.
- *Benzoyl peroxide* has antibacterial activity against *P. acnes* by generating reactive oxygen species in the follicle and also has weak antiinflammatory and keratolytic actions. It is usually used when inflammatory lesions are present. Benzoyl peroxide produces scaling and skin irritation, especially with higher concentrations, although this may be transient. It can bleach clothing and hair, and degrades isotretinoin (but not adapalene), which should be applied separately.
- *Topical antibacterials*, for example clindamycin and erythromycin (see Chapter 51), are less effective than oral antibacterials but have fewer unwanted effects. They have weak antiinflammatory and comedolytic action in addition to their direct action against *P. acnes*. Bacterial resistance arises with regular use, so topical antibiotics should be used in combination with benzoyl peroxide or a topical retinoid to improve antibacterial penetration into lesions, as well as for their synergistic actions on the lesions. Topical antibacterials should ideally not be used for more than 12 weeks.

Systemic treatments

- *Oral antibacterials* (especially lymecycline and doxycycline) have an antibacterial action against *P. acnes* and also an antiinflammatory action and are used for inflammatory acne (papules/pustules). Treatment should be given for no longer than 12 weeks, and they should be combined with a topical retinoid or benzoyl peroxide to improve efficacy. Ciprofloxacin and trimethoprim (see Chapter 51) can also be used, but widespread resistance to tetracycline and erythromycin make these less suitable choices.
- *Hormonal therapies* such as ethinyloestradiol or the antiandrogen cyproterone acetate (see Chapter 46) are useful in women with moderate or severe acne. They are given in combination with a nonandrogenic progestogen (such as norgestimate or desogestrel) as a combined oral hormonal contraceptive (see Chapter 45). They reduce sebum flow by 40%, but improvement can take 3–6 months. Progestogen-only contraceptives can exacerbate acne.
- *Isotretinoin* is used orally in severe acne and gives an almost 100% probability of complete remission. High doses can produce prolonged remission. Unwanted effects include dry lips, nose and eyes; increased plasma triglycerides; and less commonly, myalgia. Teratogenesis is a problem and, although the half-life of the metabolites is less than 2 days, conception should be avoided during treatment and for 1 month after stopping treatment.

CHOICE OF TREATMENT FOR ACNE

Initially, management of noninflammatory comedones should be with topical treatment. Topical retinoids are increasingly used for all but severe acne or as maintenance treatment, with azelaic acid as an alternative option. For early inflammatory lesions a topical antibacterial or benzoyl peroxide are also recommended, either as single agents or in combination. Oral antibiotics are used for moderately severe acne, with oestrogen or antiandrogen therapy (as combined oral hormonal contraceptives) being alternatives for women. Systemic treatment with isotretinoin is used for severe unresponsive acne, but is also an option for moderately severe acne. The most common reason for treatment failure is probably nonadherence to the recommended regimen.

SELF-ASSESSMENT

True/false questions

1. Atopic dermatitis is the most common form of dermatitis.
2. Oral corticosteroids are the mainstay of treatment of atopic dermatitis.
3. Oral antihistamines reduce itching in atopic dermatitis.
4. Th2-lymphocytes are the dominant immune cells in psoriasis.
5. Immunosuppressant drugs are contraindicated in severe psoriasis.
6. Retinoids reduce cell growth and differentiation.
7. Severe inflammatory acne should be treated with topical or systemic antibacterials.
8. Antibacterial drug resistance in *Propionibacterium acnes* is rare.

One-best-answer (OBA) question

Choose the *accurate* statement about psoriasis and its treatment.
A. Psoriasis may be improved by atenolol.
B. Psoriasis may be exacerbated by exposure to sunshine.
C. Methotrexate has few unwanted effects in the treatment of psoriasis.
D. Calcipotriol is a vitamin D analogue applied topically for psoriasis.
E. Ustekinumab is a monoclonal antibody directed against TNFα.

Case-based questions

A 7-year-old girl with a history of atopic asthma developed a red, scaly and dry rash in her knee and elbow flexures, and on her arms and cheeks. The rash was extremely itchy, and she was scratching the affected areas, causing excoriation and weeping. Her mother had had atopic dermatitis when she was young.
1. What was the possible diagnosis?
2. What treatments should be tried initially?
3. What other factors should be considered?

ANSWERS

True/false answers

1. **True.** Atopic dermatitis is an inflammatory condition with a familial tendency.
2. **False.** Corticosteroids are used topically in atopic dermatitis for up to 4 weeks.
3. **True.** A sedative antihistamine (e.g. promethazine) may be of value, although direct effects on itching are limited.
4. **False.** Psoriasis is thought to be driven mainly by Th1-lymphocytes, with production of TNFα, interleukin (IL)-12 and IL-23.
5. **False.** The immunosuppressants ciclosporin or methotrexate can be used in severe psoriasis resistant to other drugs.
6. **True.** Oral retinoids such as vitamin A and its derivatives reduce cell growth and can be used in psoriasis, but may be teratogenic. Oral and topical retinoids are also useful in acne.

7. **True.** A topical retinoid is used together with oral or topical antibacterials; suitable topical antibacterials are erythromycin and clindamycin.
8. **False.** Resistance of *P. acnes* to antibacterials is increasing, including cross-resistance to erythromycin and clindamycin; when possible, drugs with an antibacterial action should be used, such as benzoyl peroxide or azelaic acid.

One-best-answer (OBA) answer

Answer D is correct.
A. Incorrect. β-Adrenoceptor antagonists and other drugs including NSAIDs and angiotensin converting enzyme (ACE) inhibitors can exacerbate psoriasis.
B. Incorrect. Regular short exposures to sunlight or ultraviolet light benefit psoriasis by increasing production of vitamin D and slowing skin cell proliferation.
C. Incorrect. Methotrexate can produce bone marrow depression and hepatoxicity, and regular monitoring is required.
D. **Correct.** Calcipotriol is a topical vitamin D analogue with beneficial actions in psoriasis, including inhibition of T-cell proliferation and cytokine release.
E. Incorrect. Ustekinumab is an inhibitor of IL-12 and IL-23 and is used in drug-resistant psoriasis; modulators of TNFα (e.g. infliximab, etanercept) are also used.

Case-based answers

1. Atopic dermatitis is possible because of the appearance of the rash, the child's atopy, and her mother's history of the condition.
2. Initial management approaches should include good skin hygiene with regular bathing (but avoiding soaps), and the use of emollients in bath water and applied topically to moisturise the skin. Drug treatments should include short courses of topical hydrocortisone, and a topical antihistamine or oral sedative antihistamine if the itch is severe, although there is no consensus that antihistamines are beneficial. Topical doxepin may also help reduce itch.
3. Contributory factors such as allergies to food and other allergens, psychological factors, and removal of irritants and allergens should be assessed. Severe acute exacerbations may require rigorous topical measures and antibacterial treatment.

FURTHER READING

Bieber, T., 2008. Atopic dermatitis. N. Engl. J. Med. 358, 1483–1494.

Brown, S., Reynolds, N.J., 2006. Atopic and non-atopic eczema. Br. Med. J. 332, 584–588.

Dawson, A.L., Dellavalle, R.P., 2013. Acne vulgaris. Br. Med. J. 346, f2634.

Jabba-Lopez, Z.K., Wu, K.P.C., Reynolds, N.J., 2014. Newer agents for psoriasis in adults. Br. Med. J. 349, g4026.

Menter, A., Griffiths, C.E.M., 2007. Psoriasis 2. Current and future management of psoriasis. Lancet 370, 272–284.

Naldi, L., Rebora, A., 2009. Seborrheic dermatitis. N. Engl. J. Med. 60, 387–396.

Wasserbauer, N., Ballow, M., 2009. Atopic dermatitis. Am. J. Med. 122, 121–125.

Compendium: drugs used in the treatment of skin disorders

Drug	Characteristics
Corticosteroids	
Given topically for inflammatory skin conditions. See Chapter 44 for further details.	
Alclometasone dipropionate	Synthetic corticosteroid used for inflammatory skin disorders such as eczemas
Beclometasone dipropionate	Use restricted to severe conditions, such as eczema unresponsive to less potent drugs, and psoriasis. Metabolised to active monopropionate (half-life: 0.5 h)
Betamethasone esters	Potent. Use restricted to severe conditions, such as eczema unresponsive to less potent drugs, and psoriasis
Clobetasol propionate	High potency. Use restricted to short-term treatment of severe resistant conditions, such as eczema unresponsive to less potent drugs, and psoriasis
Clobetasone butyrate	Moderately potent. Used for eczema and dermatitis of all types and for maintenance between courses of more potent corticosteroids
Diflucortolone valerate	Use restricted to severe conditions, such as eczema unresponsive to less potent drugs, and for psoriasis
Fludroxycortide	Used for inflammatory skin disorders such as eczema
Fluocinolone acetonide	Used for inflammatory skin disorders such as eczema, and psoriasis
Fluocinonide	Use restricted to severe conditions, such as eczema unresponsive to less potent drugs, and for psoriasis
Fluocortolone	Use restricted to severe conditions, such as eczema unresponsive to less potent drugs, and for psoriasis
Fluticasone propionate	Used for severe inflammatory skin disorders such as eczema unresponsive to less potent corticosteroids
Hydrocortisone	Low potency. Used for mild inflammatory skin disorders such as eczema and nappy rash. Can be used for perioral inflammatory lesions
Hydrocortisone butyrate	Potent. Use of the butyrate ester is restricted to severe conditions, such as eczema unresponsive to less potent drugs, and for psoriasis
Mometasone furoate	Used for severe inflammatory skin disorders such as eczema unresponsive to less potent corticosteroids, and for psoriasis
Triamcinolone acetonide	Used for severe inflammatory skin conditions, such as eczema unresponsive to less potent drugs, and psoriasis
Drugs for eczema and/or seborrhoeic dermatitis	
Given topically. Topical corticosteroids may also be given.	
Ichthammol	A sulfonated shale oil. Used for chronic lichenified eczema
Pimecrolimus	Calcineurin inhibitor (see Chapter 38). Used for short-term treatment of mild to moderate atopic eczema when topical corticosteroids cannot be used, and for short-term treatment of facial, flexural or genital psoriasis in patients unresponsive to, or intolerant of, other topical therapy
Tacrolimus	Calcineurin inhibitor (see Chapter 38). Used for moderate to severe atopic eczema unresponsive to other treatment
Drugs for psoriasis	
Acitretin	Retinoid. Given orally for severe, extensive and resistant psoriasis. Half-life: 50 h
Calcipotriol (calcipotriene)	Vitamin D analogue. Used topically for plaque psoriasis
Calcitriol	Vitamin D analogue (see Chapter 42). Used topically for mild to moderate plaque psoriasis
Ciclosporin	Calcineurin inhibitor (see Chapter 38). Given orally for short-term treatment of severe atopic dermatitis and severe psoriasis. Half-life: 27 h
Coal tar	Contains polycyclic aromatic hydrocarbons; applied topically for chronic atopic eczema
Dithranol (anthralin)	Applied topically for subacute and chronic plaque psoriasis
Fumaric acid esters	Given orally for severe psoriasis. Not licensed in the United Kingdom

Compendium: drugs used in the treatment of skin disorders (cont'd)

Drug	Characteristics
Methotrexate	Folate antagonist used in the treatment of severe uncontrolled psoriasis, rheumatoid arthritis (see Chapter 30) and malignant disease (see Chapter 52). Given orally or by intravenous or intramuscular injection. Half-life: 8–10 h
Salicylic acid	Used with coal tar and dithranol preparations as a keratolytic in scaly psoriasis. Applied topically. See Chapter 29
Tacalcitol	Vitamin D_3 analogue (1,24-dihydroxy-vit D_3). Used topically for plaque psoriasis
Tazarotene	Retinoid. Applied topically for mild to moderate plaque psoriasis
Ustekinumab	Antibody directed against IL-12 and IL-23. Given by subcutaneous injection for moderate to severe psoriasis resistant to other therapy. Half-life: 15–32 days

Drugs for acne and rosacea

In addition to the topical preparations listed here, antibiotics such as clindamycin, doxycycline, erythromycin, minocycline, oxytetracycline, tetracycline and trimethoprim (see Chapter 51) can be used in the treatment of acne.

Drug	Characteristics
Adapalene	Retinoid-like drug with keratolytic action. Used topically for mild to moderate acne
Azelaic acid	Anticomedonal and antibacterial actions. Used topically for acne and rosacea
Benzoyl peroxide	Powerful oxidising agent with antibacterial activity. Used topically for acne
Co-cyprindiol	Coformulation of cyproterone acetate (see Chapter 46) and ethinylestradiol (see Chapter 45). Used for the treatment of severe acne unresponsive to antibiotics and for hirsutism in women
Isotretinoin	Retinoid (13-*cis*-retinoic acid); an isomer of tretinoin. Used topically for mild to moderate acne. Applied topically, or given orally (half-life: 10-20 h)
Tretinoin	Retinoid (all-*trans*-retinoic acid). Used topically for mild to moderate acne

Preparations for warts and calluses

Preparations not suitable for application to face or anogenital areas

All compounds used topically to produce localised tissue destruction.

Drug	Characteristics
Formaldehyde	Used for warts, particularly plantar warts
Glutaraldehyde	Used for warts, particularly plantar warts
Salicylic acid	Used for plantar and mosaic warts, corns, verrucas and calluses
Silver nitrate	Used for warts, verrucas, umbilical granulomas and overgranulation tissue

Preparations suitable for application to anogenital areas

Used topically.

Drug	Characteristics
Imiquimod	Licensed for external keratinised or nonkeratinised anogenital warts; also licensed for the treatment of superficial basal cell carcinoma and actinic keratosis
Podophyllum (podophyllotoxin)	Used for soft, nonkeratinised external anogenital warts

50

The eye

• •

Vision depends upon the eye converting light that falls on the retina into an electrical signal to be carried to the brain through the optic nerve. The eye must focus objects sharply on the retina, with innate refraction provided mainly by the cornea. To adjust the innate focus of the eye, the ciliary muscle alters the shape of the lens, allowing accommodation to objects at different distances. The iris determines the size of the pupil and the amount of light entering the eye. The autonomic nervous system innervates both the ciliary muscles and the iris.

Accommodation

Accommodation is determined by the ciliary muscle, which is a circular (constrictor) smooth muscle that is attached to the lens by suspensory ligaments. The ciliary muscle has only parasympathetic innervation (mediated by acetylcholine acting through muscarinic receptors; see Chapter 4). In the absence of parasympathetic stimulation, the ciliary muscle remains relaxed and exerts radial tension on the suspensory ligaments. This pulls on the lens capsule, which flattens the lens and adjusts visual acuity for distant vision. When the ciliary muscle contracts in response to parasympathetic stimulation, this reduces tension on the suspensory ligaments, and the capsule of the lens is relaxed. The lens then becomes shorter and fatter and accommodates for viewing near objects.

Drugs that are agonists at muscarinic receptors produce ciliary muscle contraction and adjust the lens for viewing near objects, blurring distant vision. Drugs that are antagonists at muscarinic receptors prevent ciliary muscle contraction and adjust the lens for viewing distant objects, with blurring of near vision. This state is called cycloplegia (Fig. 50.1).

Pupil size

The diameter of the pupil is determined by the relative tone in the two smooth muscle layers of the iris. The circular (constrictor) muscle is the more powerful and is under the control of parasympathetic nervous innervation (mediated by acetylcholine acting through muscarinic receptors). The radial (dilator) muscle is sympathetically innervated (mediated by noradrenaline acting on α_1-adrenoceptors).

The light reflex is the primary determinant of pupil size, with increased light causing the pupil to constrict and reduce the amount of light that reaches the retina. Pupillary constriction also accompanies accommodation for near vision. This increases the depth of focus and therefore reduces the amount of accommodation needed to focus the image on the retina.

■ Pupillary constriction is known as miosis and is caused by contraction of the circular muscle of the iris. Miosis can be produced by muscarinic receptor agonists.
■ Dilation of the pupil is called mydriasis and is caused by contraction of the radial muscle of the iris. Mydriasis can be produced either by muscarinic receptor antagonists (which paralyse the circular muscle leaving unopposed action of the radial muscle) or by α_1-adrenoceptor agonists (which contract the radial muscle).

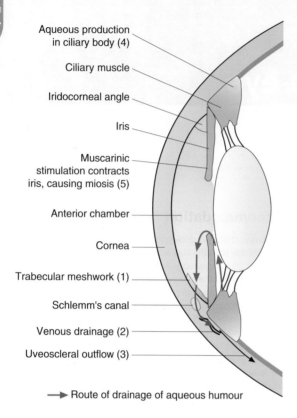

Aqueous production in ciliary body (4)

Ciliary muscle

Iridocorneal angle

Iris

Muscarinic stimulation contracts iris, causing miosis (5)

Anterior chamber

Cornea

Trabecular meshwork (1)

Schlemm's canal

Venous drainage (2)

Uveoscleral outflow (3)

➤ Route of drainage of aqueous humour

Fig. 50.1 **The route of drainage of aqueous humour from the eye and the sites of action of drugs used in the treatment of glaucoma.** The mechanisms by which some drugs benefit glaucoma are still uncertain but are thought to include the following: (a) in angle-closure glaucoma, muscarinic agonists (e.g. pilocarpine) facilitate aqueous humour drainage (1, 2) by constricting the iris (5), which widens the iridocorneal angle; (b) carbonic anhydrase inhibitors (e.g. acetazolamide) decrease aqueous humour production (4); (c) β-adrenoceptor antagonists (e.g. timolol) reduce aqueous humour production (4) and increase drainage (1); (d) selective α_2-adrenoceptor agonists (e.g. brimonidine) decrease aqueous humour production (4); (e) prostaglandin $F_{2\alpha}$ analogues (e.g. latanoprost) enhance aqueous humour outflow (1, 2, 3) and may improve ocular blood flow.

Dilation of the pupil also has the effect of moving the iris toward the cornea and narrowing the anterior angle between the iris and the cornea. This can reduce aqueous humour outflow through Schlemm's canal.

Drainage of aqueous humour

The space between the cornea at the front of the eye and the iris is the anterior chamber, and that between the iris and the lens is the posterior chamber (see Fig. 50.1). Both are filled with a clear liquid known as aqueous humour. Aqueous humour is constantly secreted into the posterior chamber by the epithelium of the ciliary body. It then flows via the cleft between the anterior surface of the lens and the iris, through the pupil to the anterior chamber. Most aqueous humour leaves the eye through the trabecular meshwork that drains via Schlemm's canal into the episcleral veins (see Fig. 50.1). About 10% of the aqueous humour drains through the sclera (uveoscleral outflow).

Pressure within the eye is maintained by a balance between the production of aqueous humour and its drainage. Intraocular pressure rises if drainage of the aqueous humour is impaired. High intraocular pressure can damage retinal ganglion cells, and is one of the factors that leads to progressive loss of vision in the disease known as glaucoma.

Production of aqueous humour is influenced by innervation from the sympathetic nervous system. It is reduced by α_2-adrenoceptor stimulation of the ciliary body and increased by β_2-adrenoceptor stimulation. If the anterior chamber of the eye is abnormally shallow, there will be a narrow anterior-chamber angle between the iris and cornea (iridocorneal angle; see Fig. 50.1). Dilation of the pupil with thickening of the circular muscle narrows the angle further and can impede drainage of aqueous humour through the trabecular meshwork. This can produce an acute rise in pressure in the eye. Conversely, constriction of the circular muscle of the iris makes the pupil smaller and moves the iris away from the trabecular meshwork, widening the anterior angle and facilitating aqueous humour drainage. Uveoscleral flow is enhanced by prostaglandins.

TOPICAL APPLICATION OF DRUGS TO THE EYE

Drugs applied in solution or as an ointment to the anterior surface of the eye can penetrate to the anterior chamber and the ciliary muscle, principally through the cornea. There is little diffusion from the surface of the eye to the more posterior structures. The high water content of the cornea makes lipid solubility less important for adequate penetration of a drug than is the case for transdermal drug delivery, but formulation of the carrier is important to avoid irritation of the conjunctiva.

Systemic absorption of the drug following topical application to the surface of the eye can occur either via conjunctival vessels or from the nasal mucosa after drainage of the excess drug through the tear ducts. Topical administration of drugs in solution to the eye can therefore produce systemic effects. Drainage through the tear ducts can be reduced by shutting the eye for at least 1 minute after putting in drops and by compressing the nasolacrimal duct at the medial corner of the eye with a finger. Both eye drops and ointments are usually administered into the pocket which can be formed by gently pulling the lower eyelid downward (the lower fornix).

Microbial contamination is a potential problem once eye preparations have been opened. Multiple-application containers have preservative added to reduce the risk, but it is not advisable to use any eye preparation more than a month after it has been opened. Preparations free of preservatives reduce the risk of intolerance and allergy to the preservative.

GLAUCOMA

Glaucoma is a group of disorders characterised by loss of retinal ganglion cells and is a form of optic neuropathy. In many cases the intraocular pressure is raised, and ischaemia of the optic nerve head may be the cause. However, when ocular hypertension is detected, only a small proportion of those affected will develop glaucoma. In up to 50% of cases of glaucoma the pressure in the anterior chamber of the eye is normal, and retinal cell loss is related to poor support of the ganglion cells by the collagenous lamina cribrosa or vascular factors such as ischaemia of the optic nerve head. This reduces the ability of the optic nerve head to withstand the stress imposed by the normal pressure in the eye.

The diagnosis of glaucoma requires the presence of both structural and functional changes in the eye. Evidence of optic disc damage is found with deepening and widening of the depression or cup of the optic disc. Progressive visual defects occur, initially as scotomas (blind spots) in the peripheral visual field. These scotomas enlarge, resulting in tunnel vision and finally total blindness. Glaucoma is the second most common cause of visual impairment in the United Kingdom.

There are two forms of glaucoma:

- **Open-angle glaucoma** is caused by obstruction to aqueous humour outflow through the trabecular meshwork as a result of injury or death of meshwork cells. It can be associated with raised or normal intraocular pressure.
- **Angle-closure glaucoma** is less common, and results from the iris physically obstructing the drainage angle and therefore the trabecular meshwork. This usually arises when there is a shallow anterior chamber, such as occurs in long-sighted (myopic) individuals. The condition is usually chronic and asymptomatic, with a risk of acute attacks of high intraocular pressure with pain and sudden visual loss.

DRUGS FOR GLAUCOMA

β-Adrenoceptor antagonists

betaxolol, timolol

β-Adrenoceptor antagonists reduce the formation of aqueous humour by the ciliary body. They have no effect on accommodation or pupil size. Systemic absorption can produce the typical unwanted effects associated with these compounds, particularly bronchospasm, bradycardia and worsening of uncontrolled heart failure. The contraindications for topical use in the eye are the same as those for oral use. Timolol is a nonselective β-adrenoceptor antagonist, whereas betaxolol is β_1-adrenoceptor selective, but they have similar efficacy in the eye.

Sympathomimetics

apraclonidine

Apraclonidine and brimonidine are selective α_2-adrenoceptor agonists that reduce aqueous humour production. They can cause dry mouth, gastrointestinal disturbances, taste disturbances and headache. Allergy to brimonidine is common.

Carbonic anhydrase inhibitors

acetazolamide, brinzolamide, dorzolamide

The intracellular mechanism of action of carbonic anhydrase inhibitors is discussed in Chapter 14. Carbonic anhydrase in the eye is responsible for about 70% of the Na^+ that enters the anterior chamber, which is accompanied by water to maintain isotonicity. Therefore the enzyme plays a key role in aqueous humour production, and its inhibition reduces aqueous humour production.

Acetazolamide is taken orally. Dorzolamide and brinzolamide are topical preparations for the eye, with fewer systemic unwanted effects (see Chapter 14); their duration of action in the eye is 6–12 hours.

Prostaglandin analogues

latanoprost, travoprost

These drugs are analogues of prostaglandin $F_{2\alpha}$. Their efficacy in glaucoma may result from increased uveoscleral outflow of aqueous humour. This may be in part due to a reduction in collagen in the uveal meshwork. Prostaglandin analogues also increase blood flow to the optic nerve, and this may contribute to neuroprotection in the retina. The reduction in intraocular pressure is greater than that achieved by β-adrenoceptor antagonists. The major disadvantage of prostaglandin analogues is an increase in brown pigmentation of the iris and increased growth of eyelashes. A rare complication in people who have no lens in the eye (aphakia) is the development of cystoid macular oedema, which responds to treatment with nonsteroidal antiinflammatory drugs. The prostaglandin analogues have a long duration of action of 1–2 days, well in excess of their much shorter half-lives.

Miotic drugs (muscarinic agonists)

pilocarpine

Pilocarpine is a muscarinic receptor agonist that contracts the circular sphincter muscle of the iris to produce miosis and opens up the drainage channels in the anterior chamber of the eye. The miotic effect lasts for about 4 hours, but more prolonged miosis can be achieved by the use of a gel delivery system. It can be used for angle-closure glaucoma, but is not a treatment of choice, since there is a risk of ciliary muscle spasm, which produces blurred vision and an ache over the eye (especially in younger people).

TREATMENT OF GLAUCOMA

In open-angle glaucoma, reducing intraocular pressure (the only modifiable risk factor) can slow the rate of disease progression sufficiently to prevent significant visual impairment. However, many cases present with established visual loss. The target pressure reduction is individually determined. Treatment of ocular hypertension without evidence of visual loss may prevent the onset of glaucoma.

In primary open-angle glaucoma, a topical prostaglandin analogue is the treatment of choice, because of the relative lack of ocular unwanted effects. If this produces an inadequate reduction in intraocular pressure, then combined use with a topical β-adrenoceptor antagonist can give an additive effect. Fixed combination formulations are frequently used to improve adherence. If these agents cannot be used, then the choice of a second-line drug lies between a topical carbonic anhydrase inhibitor or a sympathomimetic. Surgery may also be considered at this point. Laser burns applied to the trabecular meshwork (trabeculoplasty) can produce an increase in aqueous humour outflow, but drug treatment may still be required. Drainage surgery (trabeculectomy) is an alternative primary treatment and can often bring about long-term pressure control. The therapeutic challenge is to develop neuroprotective drugs to retard neuronal apoptosis in the retina.

Angle-closure glaucoma is treated by laser peripheral iridotomy or surgical peripheral iridectomy to provide a channel for aqueous humour to flow through the iris. If drug therapy is required after surgery, then topical treatment with a prostaglandin analogue or a β-adrenoceptor antagonist can be used.

MYDRIATIC AND CYCLOPLEGIC DRUGS

ANTIMUSCARINICS (MUSCARINIC RECEPTOR ANTAGONISTS)

phenylephrine

Antimuscarinic drugs are both mydriatic (dilating the pupil) and cycloplegic (paralysing the ciliary muscle).

- Tropicamide is weak and short-acting (about 4–6 hours), which makes it useful for dilating the pupil for fundal examination.
- Cyclopentolate is longer-acting (up to 24 hours) and has a rapid onset of action.
- Homatropine and atropine have actions up to 3 and 7 days, respectively.

The longer-acting compounds are used to prevent adhesions (posterior synechiae) in anterior uveitis (often in combination with phenylephrine). Dark irises are more resistant to pupillary dilation with these drugs, as the pigments adsorb the drug.

The degree of cycloplegia will depend on the dose of drug; small doses produce pupil dilation, but diffusion is insufficient to reach the ciliary muscle. UK law does not specifically prohibit driving after pupil dilation, but many people find that their vision is impaired for several hours. Care must be taken when using these drugs in individuals

predisposed to acute angle-closure glaucoma (discussed previously). Local irritation in the eye is the most common unwanted effect, but systemic effects occasionally occur in children or the elderly (see Chapter 4).

SYMPATHOMIMETICS

atropine, cyclopentolate, homatropine, tropicamide

Phenylephrine is a relatively selective α_1-adrenoceptor agonist that stimulates the radial muscle of the iris and produces mydriasis (pupil dilation) within 60–90 minutes of application, lasting 5–7 hours. It does not affect the ciliary muscle, and therefore does not affect accommodation. The main use when given alone is to create mydriasis for diagnostic procedures. It is a vasoconstrictor, and can decrease vascular congestion of the conjunctiva and oedema of the eyelid in allergic conjunctivitis. It is often combined with an antihistamine in over-the-counter preparations. It can also be given together with muscarinic receptor antagonist drugs such as tropicamide to produce preoperative pupil dilation for procedures such as cataract surgery. Local irritation is the most common unwanted effect, although systemic vasoconstriction with hypertension or coronary artery spasm can occur if high doses are used.

OTHER TOPICAL APPLICATIONS FOR THE EYE

Several other drugs are used topically in the eye.

ANTIBACTERIAL AGENTS

Antibacterial agents (see Chapter 51) are given topically for local infections such as blepharitis, conjunctivitis or trachoma (caused by chlamydial infection). Aqueous solutions are diluted rapidly or flushed away by lacrimation and should initially be used every 1–2 hours; ointments are often given for longer action, especially at night. Examples of broad-spectrum antibacterial agents for topical use are gentamicin, chloramphenicol, ciprofloxacin, fusidic acid and (for trachoma) azithromycin. Cefuroxime can be injected into the anterior chamber of the eye for prophylaxis of endophthalmitis after cataract surgery.

ANTIVIRAL AGENTS

Topical aciclovir is used for herpes simplex infection, which causes dendritic corneal ulcers (see also Chapter 51).

CORTICOSTEROIDS

Local inflammatory conditions of the anterior part of the eye, such as uveitis and scleritis, are treated with topical corticosteroids – for example, dexamethasone or prednisolone (see Chapter 44). Care must be taken to exclude a viral dendritic ulcer and glaucoma before using them, since these conditions can be exacerbated by corticosteroids. Prolonged use of corticosteroids can lead to thinning of the sclera or cornea, or formation of a 'steroid cataract'.

ANTIALLERGIC AGENTS

Several subsets of ocular allergy have been described. The most common are immunoglobulin (Ig) E mediated, such as seasonal allergic conjunctivitis, perennial allergic conjunctivitis and vernal conjunctivitis, which affects children and young adults, especially in warm climates. Non-IgE (T-cell)-mediated allergies include some forms of vernal conjunctivitis, contact blepharoconjunctivitis and atopic keratoconjunctivitis. Symptoms include itching and redness, tearing, and in severe forms visual disturbance.

Topical antihistamines are widely used for allergic conjunctivitis. First-generation drugs such as antazoline can cause a burning sensation in the eye and in over-the-counter formulations are usually given in combination with the sympathomimetic xylometazoline to reduce redness of the eye and oedema. Second-generation drugs such as levocabastine are longer-acting and better tolerated (see Chapter 39). Oral antihistamines are effective and may be preferred if there are also symptoms from allergic rhinitis. Topical mast cell stabilisers such as sodium cromoglicate or nedocromil (see Chapter 12) are generally less effective than antihistamines and must be given for up to 2 weeks before symptoms are relieved. The nonsteroidal antiinflammatory drug diclofenac is sometimes used topically for seasonal allergic conjunctivitis. Topical corticosteroids are used for the non-IgE-mediated forms of ocular allergy.

LOCAL ANAESTHETICS

Oxybuprocaine or lidocaine eye drops (see Chapter 18) provide surface anaesthesia for measurements of pressure in the anterior chamber (tonometry). For minor surgical procedures, such as removal of cataracts, tetracaine gives more profound anaesthesia and may be combined with injection of a small amount of lidocaine into the anterior chamber.

NONSTEROIDAL ANTIINFLAMMATORY DRUGS

Diclofenac, flurbiprofen and ketorolac (see Chapter 29) can be applied topically for pain following surgery or laser treatment in the eye.

DRY EYE SYNDROME

Tears are a complex layered fluid. The hydrophobic outer surface layer is secreted by meibomian glands. The aqueous middle layer is secreted by the lacrimal glands; it contains antibodies for control of infectious agents and also acts as an osmotic regulator. The hydrophilic inner layer is produced by conjunctival goblet cells. Dry eye syndrome can be associated with Sjögren syndrome, in which there is an autoimmune response directed against the lacrimal glands, or occur independently, but in both types the underlying mechanism is usually chronic inflammation of the ocular surface mediated by T-cells. It results in discomfort (dryness, grittiness), blurred vision, photophobia and potentially damage to the surface of the eye. In some people it can paradoxically be associated with periods of excess tears after a period of very dry eyes.

Medication such as antihistamines, oral hormonal contraceptives and β-adrenoceptor antagonists can decrease tear production, and should be withdrawn. The most common treatment is with artificial tear substitutes such as hypromellose (hydroxypropyl-methylcellulose), but it may need to be reapplied every hour. The surface mucin in the eye is often abnormal when there is tear deficiency, and the mucolytic agent acetylcysteine is then effective when added to hypromellose. Carbomers, synthetic high-molecular-weight polymers of acrylic acid, cling better to the surface of the eye than hypromellose and need less frequent application. They may be particularly useful when applied before sleep. Local corticosteroid is used for short periods to treat inflammation resulting from the lack of tears. Severe keratitis in dry eye syndrome can be treated with ciclosporin eye drops, which improve tear production after 3–6 months of regular use.

AGE-RELATED MACULAR DEGENERATION

Age-related macular degeneration (ARMD) is the main cause of irreversible visual loss in the Western world. About half of cases have a defect in the complement factor H gene, and a further 30% have another identified genetic predisposition. These genetic defects may predispose to chronic inflammation in the retina and oxidative damage specifically to macular cells. Smoking and obesity are additinal powerful risk factors. There are two main types of ARMD:

- Dry (nonexudative) ARMD involves hypertrophic changes in the retinal pigment epithelium under the macula leading to pigmentary deposits, and also formation of yellow deposits of extracellular debris called drusen.
- Wet (exudative) ARMD shows similar changes to dry ARMD, but with additional development of new blood vessels (choroidal neovascularisation) under the macula, which leak blood and protein.

About 85% of cases present with early ARMD, which then can develop into either late wet ARMD or late dry ARMD. Dry ARMD is associated with minor visual disturbance and is currently untreatable. By contrast, wet ARMD produces severe visual loss in 70% of eyes within 2 years. Retinal hypoxia promotes synthesis of vascular endothelial growth factor (VEGF-A) by retinal pigment epithelial cells. VEGF-A is an angiogenic protein that induces growth of new blood vessels and increases vascular permeability. Uncontrolled expression of VEGF-A appears to contribute to the pathogenesis of wet ARMD.

TREATMENT OF AGE-RELATED MACULAR DEGENERATION

Treatment is only available for wet ARMD. Options include:

- High-dose combinations of antioxidants lutein, zeaxanthin and vitamins C and E with copper and zinc may retard the

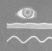

progression of ARMD, although the evidence is equivocal. Advice should be given on stopping smoking.

- Intravitreal injection of a VEGF-A inhibitor such as the monoclonal antibody ranibizumab or the recombinant fusion protein aflibercet. Treatment of early exudative ARMD with VEGF-A inhibitors significantly improves visual acuity in about 30% of eyes, with some improvement in a further 45%, compared with no treatment.
- Laser photocoagulation of neovascular tissue is now less commonly used, as it is less effective than VEGF-A inhibitors.
- Photodynamic therapy using the photosensitising agent verteporfin. Verteporfin is infused intravenously and activated in the eye by nonthermal red light, producing cytotoxic derivatives. This injures vascular endothelial cells and leads to vessel thrombosis in the laser-activated choroidal neovascular membrane. Photodynamic therapy is less effective than anti-VEGF-A therapy and is now only used for a small number of cases.

DIABETIC RETINOPATHY

Diabetic retinopathy is caused by damage to the retinal microcirculation that occurs in the presence of prolonged hyperglycaemia, and is exacerbated by other conditions that cause vascular damage, such as hypertension.

There are two types of retinopathy:

- Nonproliferative diabetic retinopathy (NPDR) with micro-aneurysms, blot haemorrhages and cotton wool spots, which initially spares the macula (background retinopathy). This type of retinopathy does not affect visual acuity.
- Proliferative diabetic retinopathy (PDR) is the response to capillary occlusion which causes retinal ischaemia. Formation of fragile new blood vessels (neovascularisation) that grow out of retinal capillaries into the vitreous is promoted by several angiogenic factors, including VEGF-A. Vision can be impaired by the new blood vessels producing preretinal or vitreous haemorrhage or retinal detachment.

VEGF-A also promotes increased vascular permeability, and localised damage to the retina, especially the macula, can result from breakdown of the blood–retina barrier, causing diabetic macular oedema. Diabetic macular oedema can arise at any stage of retinopathy.

TREATMENT OF DIABETIC RETINOPATHY

Background diabetic retinopathy does not require specific treatment, but progression to proliferative retinopathy can be reduced by control of blood glucose, blood pressure reduction, and lowering of low density lipoprotein (LDL) cholesterol and triglycerides. More advanced forms of retinopathy require treatment to preserve sight.

- Panretinal laser photocoagulation is still the mainstay of treatment for PDR and is continued until there is regression of new vessels. Focal laser treatment may be appropriate for focal macular oedema.
- Intravitreal corticosteroid injections with fluocinolone or dexamethasone are effective for diabetic macular oedema, but increase the risk of ocular hypertension and cataracts. Sustained-release formulations avoid the need for repeated injections.

- Intravitreal injection of an anti-VEGF-A agent (see the previous section on ARMD) is effective for both diabetic macular oedema and PDR, but requires repeated injections over several years. It is the preferred treatment for diffuse macular oedema and can be combined with laser photocoagulation.

SELF-ASSESSMENT

True/false questions

1. The production of aqueous humour is enhanced in glaucoma.
2. Brimonidine reduces aqueous humour secretion and causes mydriasis.
3. Stimulation of β-adrenoceptors in the ciliary body reduces aqueous humour production.
4. Tropicamide should be avoided in people with glaucoma.
5. Accommodation of the lens is controlled by the sympathetic autonomic nervous system.
6. Cocaine causes mydriasis when administered topically to the eye.
7. Cyclopentolate is a short-acting mydriatic drug used for fundal examination.
8. Pilocarpine causes accommodation for near vision.
9. Dry (nonexudative) age-related macular degeneration (ARMD) produces severe visual loss.
10. Ranibizumab may be given by intravitreal injection in wet ARMD.

Extended-matching-item questions

Match each statement (1–4) with the appropriate drug from options A–H.
A. Atropine
B. Phenylephrine
C. Pilocarpine
D. Ranibizumab
E. Tetracaine
F. Timolol
G. Tropicamide
H. Verteporfin

1. An antagonist of receptors in the ciliary body that will reduce aqueous production in glaucoma but with no effect on pupil size.
2. A drug that dilates the pupil without affecting accommodation or production of aqueous humour.
3. A relatively short-acting drug that will dilate the pupil and is weakly cycloplegic.
4. A photosensitiser used in photodynamic therapy of ARMD.

Case-based questions

During a routine eye examination, the optician noted a raised intraocular pressure with optic nerve changes in a 56-year-old woman. Further tests revealed she had open-angle (simple) glaucoma.
1. What is the most common cause of open-angle glaucoma?
2. What drugs could be used for this condition?
3. What precautions should be taken when using these drugs?

ANSWERS

True/false answers

1. **False.** Glaucoma is due to reduced outflow of aqueous humour, resulting from obstruction of the trabecular meshwork or closure of the anterior angle, not due to altered synthesis of aqueous humour.
2. **False.** The selective action of brimonidine on α_2-adrenoceptors reduces aqueous humour production in the ciliary body but does not cause mydriasis or reduce the anterior angle.
3. **False.** Aqueous humour production in the ciliary body is reduced by antagonists of β-adrenoceptors, such as timolol.
4. **True.** Tropicamide blocks muscarinic receptors in the circular muscle of the iris, causing mydriasis, which narrows the anterior angle and may reduce aqueous drainage in angle-closure glaucoma.
5. **False.** The ciliary muscle of the lens is innervated only by parasympathetic autonomic nerves, with muscarinic receptor stimulation causing ciliary muscle contraction and accommodation for near vision.
6. **True.** Formerly used as a local anaesthetic, cocaine causes mydriasis by preventing reuptake of released noradrenaline, which contracts the iris radial muscle.
7. **False.** Cyclopentolate acts for 12–24 hours; tropicamide acts for about 4 hours and is therefore more useful for fundal examination.
8. **True.** Pilocarpine is a muscarinic receptor agonist; it contracts the ciliary muscle, causing the lens to accommodate for near vision, and the iris circular muscle, causing miosis.
9. **False.** Dry ARMD causes only minor visual disturbance. Wet (exudative) ARMD produces severe visual loss in 70% of eyes within 2 years.
10. **True.** Ranibizumab is a VEGF-A inhibitor that reduces angiogenesis, and hence neovascularisation in wet ARMD.

Extended-matching-item answers

1. **Answer F**. Timolol is a β-adrenoceptor antagonist and reduces aqueous production but does not affect the pupil size, which is controlled by muscarinic and α_1-adrenergic receptors on the iris circular and radial muscles, respectively.
2. **Answer B**. Phenylephrine will dilate the pupil by α_1-adrenoceptor stimulation of the iris, but not the ciliary muscle (muscarinic receptors).
3. **Answer G**. Tropicamide is a relatively short-acting muscarinic receptor antagonist with only a weak blocking action on muscarinic receptors on the ciliary muscle.
4. **Answer H**. Verteporfin is a photosensitising agent for photodynamic therapy of some patients with wet ARMD, although this treatment has been largely superseded by VEGF inhibitors.

Case-based answers

1. The most common cause of open-angle glaucoma is reduced drainage of aqueous humour through the trabecular meshwork into Schlemm's canal and the episcleral veins.
2. β-Adrenoceptor antagonists or prostaglandin analogues are the first drugs of choice for open-angle glaucoma. α_2-Adrenoceptor agonists, carbonic anhydrase inhibitors or muscarinic agonists could also be used.
3. Avoid β-adrenoceptor antagonists in asthma, bradycardia, heart block and heart failure. Avoid prostaglandin analogues in pregnancy and asthma. Avoid α_2-adrenoceptor agonists in severe cardiovascular disease. Avoid carbonic anhydrase inhibitors in pregnancy; they can cause hypokalaemia and electrolyte imbalance. Avoid muscarinic receptor agonists in conjunctival or corneal damage, cardiac disease and asthma.

FURTHER READING

Antionetti, D.A., Klein, R., Gardner, T.W., 2012. Diabetic retinopathy. N. Engl. J. Med. 366, 1227–1239.

Chakravarthy, U., Evans, J., Rosenfeld, P.J., 2010. Age-related macular degeneration. Br. Med. J. 340, c981.

Das, A., Stroud, S., Mehta, A., et al., 2015. New treatments for diabetic retinopathy. Diabetes Obes. Metab. 17, 219–230.

King, A., Azuara-Blanco, A., Tuulonen, A., 2013. Glaucoma. BMJ. 346, f3518.

Leonardi, A., Bogacka, E., Faquert, J.L., et al., 2012. Ocular allergy: recognizing and diagnosing hypersensitivity disorders of the ocular surface. Allergy 67, 1327–1337.

Quigley, H.A., 2011. Glaucoma. Lancet 377, 1362–1377.

Compendium: drugs used in the eye

Drug	Characteristics
Treatment of infections	
Antibacterials	
Mostly topical (eye drops or ointments), but systemic treatment may be necessary in some cases (see Chapter 51).	
Azithromycin	Macrolide. Used for purulent bacterial conjunctivitis and trachomatous conjunctivitis
Cefuroxime	Given by intracameral injection to prevent endophthalmitis after cataract surgery

Compendium: drugs used in the eye (cont'd)

Drug	Characteristics
Chloramphenicol	Broad-spectrum antibacterial. Drug of choice for superficial eye infections
Ciprofloxacin	Quinolone; broad-spectrum antibacterial. Used for a wide range of infections, including *Pseudomonas aeruginosa*; also used for corneal ulcers
Fusidic acid	Used for staphylococcal infections
Gentamicin	Aminoglycoside; broad-spectrum antibacterial. Used for a wide range of infections, including *P. aeruginosa*
Levofloxacin	Quinolone; broad-spectrum antibacterial. Active against Gram-positive and especially Gram-negative organisms
Moxifloxacin	Quinolone; broad-spectrum antibacterial. Used for a wide range of infections
Neomycin	Aminoglycoside; broad-spectrum antibacterial. Used for a wide range of infections
Ofloxacin	Quinolone; broad-spectrum antibacterial. Used for a wide range of infections, including *P. aeruginosa*
Polymyxin B	Used for Gram-negative organisms, including *P. aeruginosa*
Propamidine isetionate	Specialist use in treatment of the rare but sight-threatening condition *Acanthamoeba keratitis*
Tobramycin	Aminoglycoside; broad-spectrum antibacterial. Used for a wide range of infections, including *P. aeruginosa*

Antivirals

Drug	Characteristics
Aciclovir	Used for local treatment of herpes simplex infections (see Chapter 51)
Ganciclovir	Used as slow-release implants inserted surgically for sight-threatening cytomegalovirus retinitis (see Chapter 51)

Treatment of inflammation

Corticosteroids

The drugs below are used locally for short-term treatment of inflammation. Oral corticosteroids (see Chapter 44) are given for anterior segment inflammation.

Drug	Characteristics
Betamethasone sodium phosphate	Available in coformulations with neomycin
Dexamethasone	Also given as intravitreal implant for treatment of macular oedema following branch retinal vein occlusion
Fluorometholone	Only used topically
Loteprednol etabonate	Only used topically
Prednisolone	Used topically
Rimexolone	Only used topically

Other antiinflammatory preparations

Many are histamine H1 receptor antagonists, given topically (see also Chapter 39). Nonsteroidal antiinflammatory drugs, including diclofenac, flurbiprofen and ketorolac (see Chapter 29), are used as eye drops for short-term inflammation and pain associated with ocular surgery and laser therapy.

Drug	Characteristics
Antazoline	Histamine H_1 receptor antagonist. Used for allergic conjunctivitis, in combination with xylometazoline (an α-adrenergic agonist)
Azelastine hydrochloride	Histamine H_1 receptor antagonist. Used for allergic conjunctivitis
Emedastine	Histamine H_1 receptor antagonist. Used for seasonal allergic conjunctivitis
Epinastine hydrochloride	Histamine H_1 receptor antagonist. Used for seasonal allergic conjunctivitis
Ketotifen	Antihistamine and mast cell stabiliser. Used for seasonal allergic conjunctivitis
Lodoxamide	Mast cell stabiliser. Used for allergic conjunctivitis, including seasonal allergic conjunctivitis

Compendium: drugs used in the eye (cont'd)

Drug	Characteristics
Nedocromil sodium	Mast cell stabiliser. Used for allergic conjunctivitis, including seasonal allergic conjunctivitis
Olopatadine	Antihistamine and mast cell stabiliser. Used for allergic conjunctivitis, including seasonal allergic conjunctivitis
Sodium cromoglicate	Mast cell stabiliser. Used for allergic conjunctivitis, including seasonal allergic conjunctivitis

Mydriatics and cycloplegics

Given topically.

Drug	Characteristics
Atropine	Long-acting antimuscarinic (up to 7 days). Used for refraction procedures in children and for anterior uveitis
Cyclopentolate	Intermediate-acting antimuscarinic (up to 24 h). Used for refraction procedures in children
Homatropine	Long-acting antimuscarinic (up to 3 days). Used for treatment of anterior segment inflammation
Phenylephrine hydrochloride	Sympathomimetic α_1-selective adrenoceptor agonist. Used for mydriasis in diagnostic or therapeutic procedures
Tropicamide	Short-acting antimuscarinic (3–6 h). Used to facilitate examination of the fundus

Local anaesthetics

Given topically for pain during ocular procedures. See Chapter 18.

Drug	Characteristics
Lidocaine hydrochloride	Also used for eyelid surgery
Oxybuprocaine (benoxinate)	Widely used
Proxymetacaine hydrochloride	Causes less initial stinging and is useful for children
Tetracaine hydrochloride	Widely used. Produces more profound anaesthesia and is suitable for removing corneal sutures

Treatment of glaucoma

β-Adrenoceptor antagonists

Given topically for primary open-angle glaucoma.

Drug	Characteristics
Betaxolol	Selective β_1-adrenoceptor antagonist
Carteolol hydrochloride	Nonselective β-adrenoceptor antagonist
Levobunolol hydrochloride	Nonselective β-adrenoceptor antagonist
Timolol	Nonselective β-adrenoceptor antagonist

Miotics

Drug	Characteristics
Pilocarpine	Muscarinic receptor agonist. Used in the treatment of primary angle-closure glaucoma and in some secondary glaucomas

Sympathomimetics

Drug	Characteristics
Apraclonidine	Selective α_2-adrenoceptor agonist. Used short term to delay laser treatment or surgery in glaucoma poorly controlled by other therapy; also used after anterior segment laser surgery
Brimonidine	Selective α_2-adrenoceptor agonist. Used alone for open-angle glaucoma or ocular hypertension when β-adrenoceptor antagonists are inappropriate, or as adjunctive therapy if other antiglaucoma therapy is ineffective

Carbonic anhydrase inhibitors

Drug	Characteristics
Acetazolamide	Used for open-angle, and secondary and preoperative angle-closure glaucoma. Given orally or by intravenous injection as an adjunct to other treatments; not recommended for long-term use. Half-life: 6–9 h

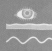

Compendium: drugs used in the eye (cont'd)

Drug	Characteristics
Brinzolamide	Used topically alone or in combination with a β-adrenoceptor antagonist for ocular hypertension and open-angle glaucoma if β-adrenoceptor antagonists are inappropriate or ineffective; can also be used as an adjunct to a prostaglandin analogue
Dorzolamide	Used topically alone or in combination with a β-adrenoceptor antagonist for ocular hypertension and open-angle glaucoma if β-adrenoceptor antagonists are inappropriate or ineffective

Prostaglandin analogues

Used topically to reduce ocular pressure in ocular hypertension and open-angle glaucoma.

Bimatoprost	Prostamide analogue of prostaglandin (PG)F$_{2\alpha}$. Used alone or as adjunctive therapy
Latanoprost	Synthetic analogue of PGF$_{2\alpha}$. Also available as coformulation with timolol
Tafluprost	Fluorinated analogue of PGF$_{2\alpha}$; prodrug hydrolysed to tafluprost acid. Preservative-free to reduce irritation
Travoprost	Synthetic analogue of PGF$_{2\alpha}$; prodrug hydrolysed to active travoprost acid

Drugs for neovascular (wet) ARMD

Specialist use only.

Aflibercept	VEGF inhibitor. Given by intravitreal injection for wet ARMD, and for macular oedema secondary to central retinal vein occlusion, and for diabetic macular oedema
Pegaptanib sodium	Pegylated antagonist of VEGF. Given by intravitreal injection for wet ARMD, but not recommended
Ranibizumab	VEGF inhibitor. Given by intravitreal injection for wet ARMD, for diabetic macular oedema, for macular oedema secondary to branch or central retinal vein occlusion, and for choroidal neovascularisation secondary to pathologic myopia. Can be given concomitantly with laser photocoagulation
Verteporfin	Photosensitising agent used intravenously in the photodynamic treatment of some patients with wet ARMD. Half-life: 5–6 h

Drugs for tear deficiency (dry eye)

All given topically as eye drops or ointments. Oral pilocarpine can also be used.

Acetylcysteine	Mucolytic
Hypromellose	Hydroxypropyl-methylcellulose. May need hourly application. Often used with acetylcysteine
Carbomers	Cross-linked polymers of acrylic acid. Longer-acting than hypromellose
Other drugs for tear deficiency, and ocular lubricants	Include macrogols (polyethylene glycols), polyvinyl alcohol, carmellose, hydroxyethylcellulose, soft or liquid paraffin, soybean oil, sodium hyaluronate solution, and sodium chloride solution

ARMD, Age-related macular degeneration; *VEGF*, vascular endothelial growth factor.

11

Chemotherapy

11

Chemotherapy

Chemotherapy of infections

● ●

Antimicrobial drugs are chemical substances of natural or synthetic origin that suppress the growth of, or destroy, micro-organisms including bacteria, fungi, helminths, protozoa and viruses. The term *antibiotic* is widely used but should be reserved for those antimicrobial drugs that are themselves derived from micro-organisms. The term *antimicrobial* or the more specific terms *antibacterial, antifungal, antihelminthic, antiprotozoal* and *antiviral* are used in this book.

Effective antimicrobial drugs have certain key attributes. To minimise unwanted effects in humans, most are designed to act selectively on processes that are distinctive or unique to the target pathogen. They must also be able to penetrate human tissues to reach the site of infection. Micro-organisms can acquire resistance to various antimicrobial drugs and will then be less affected by them, so there is a continuing effort to discover and develop antimicrobial drugs that avoid or overcome the evolving mechanisms of resistance.

BACTERIAL INFECTIONS

CLASSIFICATION OF ANTIBACTERIAL DRUGS

Antibacterial drugs can be classified in several overlapping ways.

Firstly, they can be *bacteriostatic* or *bactericidal*. This categorisation depends largely on the concentration of drug that can be achieved safely in plasma without causing significant toxicity in the person who takes the drug. Bacteriostatic antibacterials inhibit bacterial growth but do not destroy the bacteria at plasma concentrations that are safe for humans; inhibition of bacterial growth instead allows natural immune mechanisms to eliminate the bacteria. Such drugs will be less effective in immunocompromised individuals or when the bacteria are dormant and not dividing. In contrast, bactericidal antibacterials kill bacteria at plasma concentrations safe for humans, but immune mechanisms still play a role in the final elimination of the bacteria. Some bactericidal drugs are more effective when bacterial cells are actively dividing, and may therefore be less effective if taken together with a bacteriostatic drug. For antibacterials to be bactericidal, they must be present at adequate concentration; too low a concentration may render them only bacteriostatic.

Secondly, antibacterials can be grouped according to their *mechanisms of action* (Fig. 51.1):

■ inhibition of the synthesis of bacterial cell wall peptidoglycans or activation of enzymes that disrupt the cell wall (e.g. β-lactams).
■ increased permeability of the bacterial cell phospholipid membrane, leading to leakage of intracellular contents (e.g. polymyxins).
■ impaired bacterial ribosome function, producing a reversible inhibition of protein synthesis (e.g. aminoglycosides, macrolides). Such drugs can show selectivity because bacterial 70S ribosomes differ structurally from the 80S ribosomes in humans.
■ selective block of bacterial metabolic pathways (e.g. trimethoprim).
■ interference with replication of bacterial DNA or RNA (e.g. quinolones).

Thirdly, antibacterials may be classified according to whether their *spectrum of activity* against bacteria is limited (narrow-spectrum drugs) or extensive (broad-spectrum drugs).

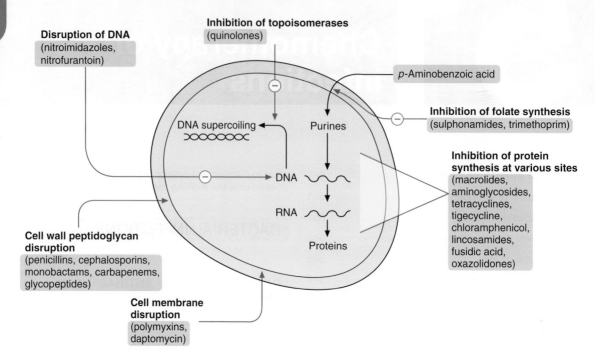

Fig. 51.1 Mechanisms of action of the main classes of antibacterial drugs. See text for mechanisms of action of antibacterial drugs used in tuberculosis.

Finally, antibacterials can be classified by *chemical structure*. In the following text, the antimicrobial drugs are grouped according to their mechanism of action and then by their chemical structure. Cross-referencing to other methods of classification may be necessary. The drug compendium at the end of the chapter is aligned with the *British National Formulary*.

ANTIMICROBIAL RESISTANCE

Antimicrobial resistance is the ability of microbes to grow in the presence of a drug that would normally kill them or limit their growth. Resistance to antibacterial drugs can be intrinsic to the bacterium (innate resistance) or can be acquired by modification of its genetic structure (acquired resistance).

Resistance is a major problem in treating infections with bacteria and also for many protozoa (e.g. malaria) and viruses (e.g. human immunodeficiency virus [HIV]), but is less significant in fungal infections (unless the person is immunocompromised).

ANTIBACTERIAL DRUG RESISTANCE

There are four general processes by which a bacterium can acquire resistance to antibacterial drugs (Fig. 51.2):

- modification of the bacterium such that it produces enzymes that inactivate the drug; examples are β-lactamase enzymes, which inactivate some penicillins, and acetylating enzymes, which can inactivate aminoglycosides,
- modification of the bacterium so that penetration of the drug is reduced; an example is the absence of the membrane protein D2 porin in resistant *Pseudomonas*

aeruginosa, which prevents penetration of the β-lactam antibacterial imipenem,
- acquisition of efflux pumps that remove the antibacterial drug from the cell faster than it can enter; an example is quinolone efflux pumps in *Staphylococcus aureus*,
- structural change in the target molecule for the antibacterial drug; examples are mutated penicillin-binding proteins in resistant enterococci that have a low affinity for binding of cephalosporins and mutated dihydrofolate reductase that is not inhibited by trimethoprim (see Fig. 51.4).

The major mechanisms by which bacteria develop an acquired resistance to antibacterial drugs are spontaneous mutation, conjugation, transduction and transformation.

Spontaneous mutation

In this process, a single-step genetic mutation in a bacterial population leads to resistant organisms that selectively survive and grow while sensitive bacteria are killed by an antibacterial drug. This is termed *vertical evolution*.

The other three mechanisms involve acquisition from other resistant organisms of genetic material that confers resistance. This is termed *horizontal evolution*.

Conjugation

Direct cell-to-cell contact is a way of exchanging genetic material that confers antibacterial resistance. It usually involves the transfer of self-replicating circular fragments of DNA (plasmids), which can contain multiple resistance genes. A transposon (a DNA sequence that can change its relative position within the genome) may facilitate transfer of

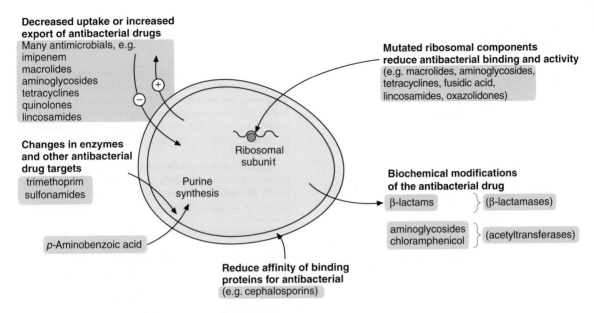

Fig. 51.2 Mechanisms of bacterial resistance to antibacterial drugs. Bacterial resistance to individual antibacterial drugs may arise from multiple mechanisms. These include modifications to the target molecule that reduce drug binding, enhanced cellular export or reduced uptake of the drug and changes in biochemical pathways that modify the drug molecule or bypass its actions.

sections of DNA from one organism to another by jumping to plasmid DNA. Transfer of the plasmid occurs via a connecting structure called a *pilus*. The plasmid can remain outside the genome of the bacterium or can be incorporated into it, when it is more stable but less transmissible. Conjugation is by far the most important source of extrinsic DNA transfer between bacteria.

Transduction

Bacteria are susceptible to infection by viruses known as *bacteriophages*. During replication of the bacteriophages, the host bacterial cell's DNA (containing resistance genes) may be replicated along with bacteriophage DNA and taken into the virus. The phage carrying the resistance genes can then infect other bacterial cells and spread resistance. This method of acquired resistance is rare.

Transformation

Uptake of DNA from dead bacteria by live bacteria can spread resistance genes.

ANTIBACTERIAL DRUGS

The antibacterial drugs in this section are grouped by their mechanism of action and then by their chemical structure.

Drugs affecting the cell wall: β-lactam antibacterials

The drugs in this class all have a β-lactam ring, which must be intact for them to be active (Fig. 51.3). The β-lactam antibacterials include penicillins, cephalosporins, monobactams and carbapenems. Some are susceptible to attack by bacterial β-lactamases, also known as penicillinases, that split the β-lactam ring, but others have structural modifications that confer resistance to β-lactamase inactivation.

Mechanism of action of β-lactam antibacterials

Beta-lactam antibacterials bind to several penicillin-binding proteins in bacteria. Some of these proteins are transpeptidases, which are required for cross-linking of the peptidoglycan layer of the cell wall surrounding certain bacteria and are essential for their survival. Inhibition of transpeptidase activity by β-lactam antibacterials prevents the bacterium from synthesising an intact cell wall when it divides. The transmembrane osmotic gradient then leads to swelling, rupture and death of the bacterium.

Some bacterial cells also contain enzymes that cause cell lysis when activated. The binding of β-lactam antibacterials to other specific penicillin-binding proteins within bacteria reduces the production of natural inhibitors of lysis-inducing enzymes, promoting lysis of the bacterial cell wall.

Penicillins

penicillins: benzylpenicillin, phenoxymethylpenicillin
aminopenicillins: amoxicillin, ampicillin, flucloxacillin
ureidopenicillins: piperacillin
amidinopenicillin: pivmecillinam
carboxypenicillin: ticarcillin

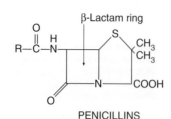

PENICILLINS

CEPHALOSPORINS

CARBAPENEMS

MONOBACTAMS

CLAVULANIC ACID

Fig. 51.3 **The structural backbones of some β-lactam antibacterial drugs.** The β-lactamase inhibitor clavulanic acid is also shown.

Spectrum of activity

Penicillins consist of a thiazolidine ring connected to a β-lactam ring, to which is attached a side chain that determines many of the antibacterial and pharmacological characteristics of particular penicillins (see Fig. 51.3 and Table 51.1).

Benzylpenicillin (penicillin G) and phenoxymethylpenicillin (penicillin V) are active against many aerobic Gram-positive bacteria, a more limited range of Gram-negative bacteria (e.g. cocci – gonococci and meningococci) and many anaerobic

micro-organisms. Gram-negative bacilli are not sensitive to these drugs. Benzylpenicillin and phenoxymethylpenicillin are effective only against organisms that do not produce β-lactamases (see below).

Flucloxacillin has an acyl side chain attached to the β-lactam ring, which prevents access of β-lactamase to the ring and makes the drug resistant to inactivation by the enzyme. Flucloxacillin is generally less effective than benzylpenicillin against bacteria that do not produce β-lactamase and is usually reserved for treating β-lactamase-producing staphylococci.

Ampicillin and amoxicillin are aminopenicillins that have an extended spectrum of activity to include many Gram-negative bacilli. However, they are less effective than benzylpenicillin against Gram-positive cocci. Both drugs are inactivated by β-lactamase.

Other extended-spectrum penicillins include ureidopenicillins (e.g. piperacillin), which are active against *P. aeruginosa*, and amidinopenicillins (e.g. pivmecillinam), which are active mainly against Gram-negative bacteria. Carboxypenicillins (e.g. ticarcillin) are not widely used but have activity against *Pseudomonas* species, *Proteus* species and *Bacteroides fragilis*.

Clavulanic acid is a potent inhibitor of several β-lactamases. It is structurally related to the β-lactam antibiotics, although it has little intrinsic antibacterial activity (see Fig. 51.3). It is available in combined formulations with penicillins that are destroyed by β-lactamase, such as amoxicillin (as co-amoxiclav) or ticarcillin (see Table 51.1); the combination drugs can be used to treat infections caused by some β-lactamase-producing organisms that would otherwise be resistant to the antibacterial. Tazobactam has similar properties to clavulanic acid and is used in combination with piperacillin.

Resistance

Resistance to penicillins is most often due to the production of β-lactamases that hydrolyse the β-lactam ring (see Fig. 51.3). There are hundreds of β-lactamases, many of which are closely related to penicillin-binding proteins, but some are structurally different metalloenzymes. The β-lactamases produced by various organisms have widely differing spectra of activity. Some bacteria, particularly *S. aureus*, release extracellular β-lactamases. In Gram-negative bacteria the β-lactamases are located between the inner and outer cell membranes in the periplasmic space. Extended-spectrum β-lactamases (ESBLs) are β-lactamases that also hydrolyse extended-spectrum 'third-generation' cephalosporins, such as cefotaxime and ceftriaxone, and monobactams such as aztreonam (see below). ESBLs are most often produced by enterobacteria. The genetic information for β-lactamase production is often encoded in a plasmid, and this may be transferred to other bacteria by conjugation. By contrast, the broader-spectrum β-lactamases are often encoded by chromosomal genes.

An alternative type of penicillin resistance occurs in gonococci and in meticillin-resistant *S. aureus* (MRSA), which develop mutated penicillin-binding proteins that do not bind β-lactam antibacterials. Meticillin has now been discontinued but the name MRSA is still used.

Pharmacokinetics

Only about one third of an oral dose of benzylpenicillin (penicillin G) is absorbed; the rest is destroyed by acid in the stomach, so benzylpenicillin is restricted to intramuscular

Table 51.1 Examples of penicillins and their properties

	GRAM-POSITIVE STAINING			GRAM-NEGATIVE STAINING		
	Streptococci	*Staphylococcus aureus*		Enterobacteriaceae (coliforms)	*Pseudomonas aeruginosa*	*Bacteroides fragilis*
		β-Lactamase negative	*β-Lactamase positive*			
Benzylpenicillin/ phenoxymethylpenicillin	+	+	0	0	0	++
Broader spectrum						
Amoxicillin/ampicillin	+	+	0[a]	++	0	0
Beta-lactamase-resistant						
Flucloxacillin	+	+	+[b]	0	0	0
Antipseudomonal						
Ticarcillin	+	+	0[c]	+	+	+/0
Piperacillin	+	+	0[c]	+	+	+/0

[a]Can be used combined with a β-lactamase inhibitor, e.g. amoxicillin plus clavulanic acid (co-amoxiclav). [b]Resistance is increasing. [c]Ticarcillin available only with clavulanic acid. Piperacillin is combined with the β-lactamase inhibitor tazobactam.
+, Active; +/0, variable activity; 0, inactive or poor activity.

or intravenous administration. The phenoxymethyl derivative (penicillin V) is more acid-stable and better absorbed from the gut; it has a similar spectrum of activity as benzylpenicillin but is generally less active. Flucloxacillin and amoxicillin are rapidly and almost completely absorbed from the gut, but ampicillin is incompletely absorbed. These drugs can also be given intramuscularly or intravenously. Penicillins are widely distributed through the body, although transport across the meninges is poor unless they are acutely inflamed (e.g. in meningitis). The half-lives of most penicillins are short (typically 1–2 hours) because they are rapidly eliminated by the kidney, mainly by active secretion at the proximal tubule. The amidinopenicillin pivmecillinam is a pro-drug for oral use, which is hydrolysed to mecillinam. The carboxypenicillin ticarcillin is available only in combination with clavulanic acid, which inhibits β-lactamase, for intravenous use. The ureidopenicillin piperacillin is given intravenously in combination with the β-lactamase inhibitor tazobactam.

Unwanted effects

Penicillins are normally well tolerated and have a high therapeutic index.

- Nausea, vomiting.
- Allergic reactions in 1–10% of exposed individuals. Penicillins and their breakdown products bind to proteins and act as haptens, stimulating the production of antibodies that mediate the allergic response (see Chapters 38 and 53). Manifestations of allergy to penicillins include fever, vasculitis, serum sickness, exfoliative dermatitis, Stevens–Johnson syndrome and anaphylactic shock. Cross-allergenicity is widespread among various penicillins and to a lesser extent with cephalosporins.
- Aminopenicillins (e.g. amoxicillin) frequently produce a nonallergic maculopapular rash in people with glandular fever. This does not recur if another type of penicillin is given.

- Reversible neutropenia and eosinophilia with prolonged high doses.
- Encephalopathy with excessively high concentrations of penicillin in the cerebrospinal fluid (CSF). This occurs in severe renal failure or after inadvertent intrathecal injection (which should never be given).
- Diarrhoea or *Clostridium difficile*-related colitis as a result of disturbance of normal colonic flora, especially with broad-spectrum penicillins.
- Cholestatic jaundice, especially with flucloxacillin or clavulanic acid.

Cephalosporins

Examples

first generation: cefadroxil, cefalexin
second generation: cefaclor, cefuroxime
third generation: cefotaxime, cefixime, ceftazidime, ceftriaxone

Spectrum of activity

Like penicillins, cephalosporins have a β-lactam group, but this is fused to a dihydrothiazine ring, which makes cephalosporins more resistant to hydrolysis by β-lactamases (see Fig. 51.3). Cephalosporins are often classified by generations, the members within each generation sharing similar antibacterial activity. Successive generations tend to have increased activity against Gram-negative bacilli, usually at the expense of Gram-positive activity, and an increased ability to cross the blood–brain barrier (Table 51.2).

- First-generation cephalosporins (e.g. cefadroxil or cefalexin) have activity against staphylococci and most streptococci but not enterococci.
- Second-generation cephalosporins (e.g. cefuroxime) have additional activity against some Gram-negative

Table 51.2 Examples of β-lactams other than penicillins and their spectra of activity

	Staphylococcus aureus	Haemophilus influenzae	Enterobacteriaceae (coliforms)	Pseudomonas aeruginosa	Bacteroides fragilis	Ability to cross blood–brain barrier	Resistance to β-lactamase
Cephalosporins							
First generation							
Cefadroxil/cefradine (oral)	+	0	+/0	0	0	+/0	+
Cefalexin (oral)	+	0	+/0	0	0	+/0	+
Second generation							
Cefuroxime axetil (oral)	+	+	+	0	+	+	+
Cefuroxime (parenteral)	+	+	+	0	+	+	+
Third generation							
Cefixime (oral)	0	+	+	0	0	+	+
Cefotaxime (parenteral)	+	+	+	0	+	+	+
Ceftazidime (parenteral)	0	0	+	+	0	+/0[a]	+
Monobactams							
Aztreonam	0	+	0	+	+	+	+/0
Carbapenems							
Imipenem	+	+	+	+	+	+	+

[a]Some cephalosporins penetrate better into the CNS in the presence of inflamed meninges.
This table is a general guide to selected drugs and susceptibilities of organisms can vary widely.
Staphylococcus aureus is a Gram-positive-staining organism. Other illustrative bacteria are Gram-negative-staining.

bacteria, such as *Haemophilus influenzae* and *Neisseria gonorrhoeae*. They are able to penetrate the blood–brain barrier.

■ Third-generation cephalosporins have improved β-lactamase stability and are able to penetrate the CSF in useful quantities. They also have greater Gram-negative activity than the other two generations. Cefixime includes *Proteus* and *Klebsiella* species within its spectrum, but it has no activity against staphylococci (see Table 51.2). Ceftazidime has good activity against *Pseudomonas* species.

Resistance

The later generations of cephalosporins are more resistant to β-lactamase hydrolysis of the β-lactam ring than the earlier generations (see Table 51.2). However, ESBLs can be acquired by *Escherichia coli* and other enterobacteria, which confers resistance to third-generation cephalosporins.

Pharmacokinetics

First-generation oral cephalosporins are well absorbed from the gut. Several second- and third-generation drugs (e.g. cefuroxime and cefotaxime) are acid-labile and must be given by a parenteral route. Cefuroxime has been formulated as a pro-drug for oral use (cefuroxime axetil). Most cephalosporins are excreted primarily by the kidney and have short half-lives (<3 hours), but cefixime is mainly eliminated by biliary excretion. Ceftriaxone has a longer half-life (6–9 hours), probably as a result of extensive plasma protein binding.

Unwanted effects

■ Nausea, vomiting, abdominal discomfort.
■ Headache.
■ Rashes, including erythema multiforme and toxic epidermal necrolysis.
■ Cephalosporins can produce allergic reactions similar to those observed with the penicillins. Fewer than 10% of people who are allergic to penicillins show cross-allergy to cephalosporins, but a history of a serious reaction to penicillins precludes the use of cephalosporins.
■ Diarrhoea or *C. difficile*-related colitis can be caused by disturbance of normal bowel flora. This is more common with oral cephalosporins and is more frequent than with many other antimicrobials.

Monobactams

aztreonam

Aztreonam is a β-lactam antibacterial related to the penicillins but with a single ring structure ('monocyclic β-lactam') (see Fig. 51.3). It has little cross-allergenicity with the penicillins and has been successfully given to people with proven penicillin allergy. Its spectrum of activity is limited to Gram-negative bacteria, including *P. aeruginosa*, *Neisseria meningitidis*, *N. gonorrhoeae* and *H. influenzae*, with no activity against Gram-positive bacteria or anaerobes. Aztreonam is given intramuscularly or intravenously and is resistant to most β-lactamases. However, ESBLs that confer resistance to aztreonam can be acquired by *E. coli* and other

enterobacteria. Aztreonam is excreted by the kidney and has a half-life of about 1.7 hours. Unwanted effects are similar to those of other β-lactam antibacterials.

Carbapenems

ertapenem, imipenem, meropenem

Imipenem is a β-lactam drug with an extremely broad spectrum of bactericidal activity. It has potent activity against Gram-positive cocci, including some β-lactamase-producing pneumococci (see Table 51.2), Gram-negative bacilli – including *P. aeruginosa*, *Neisseria suppurans* and *Bacteroides* species – and also many anaerobic bacteria. Imipenem can penetrate the blood–brain barrier and is resistant to β-lactamases. Narrow-spectrum resistance to imipenem in *P. aeruginosa* occurs from a mutation that results in loss of a specific cell membrane uptake pathway.

Meropenem and ertapenem are structurally related and have broad spectra of activity against Gram-positive and Gram-negative bacteria, but ertapenem is inactive against *Pseudomonas* species. Imipenem, meropenem and ertapenem are given intravenously; imipenem can also be given by deep intramuscular injection. Imipenem is rapidly hydrolysed by dihydropeptidases in the kidney so is always given in combination with the dihydropeptidase inhibitor cilastatin. Meropenem and ertapenem are not inactivated by the renal dihydropeptidase and can be given alone.

Carbapenems are mainly excreted by the kidney and have short half-lives (1–5 hours). Unwanted effects are similar to those of other β-lactam antibacterials except for neurotoxicity with seizures, which is more common with imipenem than with other carbapenems.

Other drugs affecting the cell wall

Glycopeptides

teicoplanin, telavancin, vancomycin

Mechanism of action

Vancomycin, teicoplanin and telavancin are high-molecular-weight glycopeptide compounds that inhibit bacterial cell wall synthesis by preventing the linking of peptidoglycan constituents (see Fig. 51.1). Telavancin additionally disrupts cell membrane permeability. Glycopeptides are bactericidal.

Spectrum of activity

The glycopeptides are active only against Gram-positive bacteria, particularly meticillin-resistant staphylococci. They do not penetrate the cell wall of Gram-negative bacteria. They are usually reserved for the treatment of serious Gram-positive bacterial infection or for bacterial endocarditis that is not responding to other treatments. Telavancin is licensed for hospital-acquired pneumonia caused by MRSA in adults. Vancomycin given orally is also effective against *C. difficile*, which colonises the colon when the normal gut flora is disturbed by other antibacterial drugs, causing diarrhoea and colitis. Metronidazole (see below) is preferred for this indication, but resistance to metronidazole is increasingly common.

Resistance

Acquired resistance to vancomycin, teicoplanin and telavancin is uncommon. In *S. aureus* it arises as a result of a multi-step genetic acquisition of a thickened peptidoglycan cell wall. This traps the drug and prevents it reaching its target on the cytoplasmic membrane. For other bacteria, plasmid-mediated resistance involves incorporation of D-lactate into the cell wall in place of D-alanine. This modification prevents binding of the glycopeptide.

Pharmacokinetics

The glycopeptides are poorly absorbed orally and are given by intravenous infusion for systemic infection. Teicoplanin can also be given by intramuscular injection. Oral vancomycin is used only for treating *C. difficile*-related colitis. Glycopeptides are mainly excreted by the kidney; vancomycin and telavancin have much shorter half-lives (5–11 hours) than teicoplanin (32–176 hours).

Unwanted effects

Dose adjustment based on monitoring of the trough plasma concentrations of vancomycin and teicoplanin may reduce the risk of toxic effects.

- Nephrotoxicity, which may be enhanced if used in combination with an aminoglycoside. Telavancin has a higher risk of nephrotoxicity than vancomycin.
- Thrombophlebitis at the site of infusion.
- Rashes, including Stevens–Johnson syndrome and toxic epidermal necrolysis. Rapid intravenous injection of glycopeptides may produce upper body flushing, the 'red man' syndrome.
- Blood disorders, including neutropenia, thrombocytopenia.
- Ototoxicity is uncommon. It usually starts with tinnitus.
- Nausea and diarrhoea. Telavancin may produce taste disturbances (dysgeusia).
- Fungal infections are common with telavancin.

Daptomycin
Mechanism of action

Daptomycin is a cyclic lipopeptide antibacterial with a unique mode of action. It binds to the cell wall of Gram-positive bacteria and creates transmembrane channels that allow leakage of intracellular ions, destroying the membrane potential across the cell.

Spectrum of activity

Daptomycin does not penetrate the membrane of Gram-negative bacteria. It is bactericidal against a similar spectrum of organisms as vancomycin and is used to treat complicated skin and soft tissue infections.

Resistance

Resistance may occur when the bacterial membrane structure changes to prevent binding of the drug.

Pharmacokinetics

Daptomycin is given intravenously and eliminated unchanged by the kidneys, with a half-life of about 8 hours.

Unwanted effects

- Gastrointestinal upset.
- Injection-site reactions.

Polymyxins

colistimethate sodium

Mechanism of action

Polymyxins bind to the cell wall of susceptible bacteria and alter the permeability of the outer and inner membranes to K+ and Na+ ions. The cell's osmotic barrier is lost and the bacteria are killed by lysis (see Fig. 51.1).

Spectrum of activity

Polymyxins have bactericidal action against Gram-negative bacteria, including *Pseudomonas* species, but are inactive against Gram-positive bacteria.

Resistance

Acquired resistance is rare.

Pharmacokinetics

Colistimethate sodium is very poorly absorbed from the gut and is usually given by inhalation or topically to the skin. Penetration into joint spaces and the CSF is poor. It is excreted unchanged by the kidneys and has a half-life of 4–8 hours. It is occasionally given by mouth for bowel sterilisation.

Unwanted effects

Substantial toxicity limits the systemic administration of polymyxins.

- Nephrotoxicity with dose-related reversible renal impairment.
- Neurotoxicity produces dizziness, confusion, and circumoral and peripheral paraesthesias. Rarely, neuromuscular blockade produces respiratory paralysis with apnoea.
- Bronchospasm or sore throat after inhalation.
- Local irritation at the injection site.

Drugs affecting bacterial DNA
Quinolones (fluoroquinolones)

ciprofloxacin, moxifloxacin, norfloxacin

Mechanism of action

Quinolones inhibit replication of bacterial DNA by blocking the ligase domain of bacterial DNA gyrase (topoisomerase

II); some also inhibit topoisomerase IV. These enzymes relax DNA supercoils and enable DNA replication and repair (see Fig. 51.1). The effect of quinolones is bactericidal.

Spectrum of activity

Ciprofloxacin has a broad spectrum of activity and is active against many micro-organisms resistant to penicillins, cephalosporins and aminoglycosides. Its spectrum includes Gram-positive bacteria, but it has only moderate activity against *Streptococcus pneumoniae* and *Enterococcus faecalis*. It is active against most Gram-negative bacteria, including *H. influenzae*, *P. aeruginosa*, *N. gonorrhoeae* and *Enterobacter* and *Campylobacter* species. Its spectrum extends to chlamydia and some mycobacteria but not anaerobes.

Moxifloxacin has a broad spectrum of activity against Gram-positive and Gram-negative bacteria but is inactive against *P. aeruginosa*. It has greater activity than ciprofloxacin against pneumococci. Norfloxacin is mainly useful for urinary tract pathogens.

Resistance

Resistance to quinolones is relatively uncommon but can arise from mutations that alter key sites in DNA topoisomerase II or IV and reduce quinolone binding to the enzymes or that produce alterations in proteins that bind to topoisomerase II and protect it from the action of quinolones. Increased active efflux of the drugs from the cell can also occur (see Fig. 51.2).

Pharmacokinetics

Oral absorption of ciprofloxacin is variable but adequate. Intravenous formulations of some quinolones are available, including ciprofloxacin and moxifloxacin. Ciprofloxacin is widely distributed but CSF penetration is poor unless there is meningeal inflammation. Ciprofloxacin and norfloxacin are eliminated mainly by the kidney and have short half-lives (3–4 hours). Moxifloxacin is well absorbed from the gut; it is metabolised in the liver and has a longer half-life (12 hours).

Unwanted effects

- Nausea, vomiting, abdominal pain, diarrhoea.
- CNS effects: dizziness, headache, tremor, seizures (especially in persons with a history of epilepsy).
- Ear pain, tinnitus.
- Rashes.
- Pain and inflammation in tendons, occasionally with tendon rupture (especially in the elderly or with concomitant use of corticosteroids).
- Moxifloxacin prolongs the Q–T interval on the electrocardiogram (ECG) and predisposes to ventricular arrhythmias. The risk is greater if it is used in combination with other proarrhythmic drugs (see Chapter 8).
- Drug interactions: inhibition of hepatic cytochrome P450 by ciprofloxacin and norfloxacin increases the plasma concentrations of theophylline (see Chapter 12), warfarin (see Chapter 11) and ciclosporin (see Chapter 38), which can produce toxicity. Moxifloxacin is not metabolised by cytochrome P450 and does not cause these interactions. The absorption of quinolones from the gut is decreased by oral iron salts.

Metronidazole and tinidazole

Mechanism of action

Metronidazole and tinidazole are nitroimidazoles; they are bactericidal only after they have been converted to an intermediate transient toxic metabolite, which inhibits bacterial DNA synthesis and degrades existing DNA. Only some anaerobes and some protozoa contain the oxidoreductase enzyme, which converts these drugs to their toxic derivatives; they are not produced in human cells or in aerobic bacteria. These drugs are equally active against dividing and nondividing cells.

Spectrum of activity

Metronidazole and tinidazole are active mainly against anaerobic bacteria and protozoa, including *B. fragilis*, *Clostridium* species, *Gardnerella vaginalis* and *Giardia lamblia*. Metronidazole is an important drug for treating *C. difficile*-related colitis caused by use of broad-spectrum antimicrobials. Metronidazole or tinidazole are important constituents of the triple or quadruple therapy used for eliminating *Helicobacter pylori* (see Chapter 33). They are also amoebicidal, with activity against *Entamoeba histolytica*.

Resistance

Acquired resistance is becoming more common. For example, in some countries a significant percentage of strains of *H. pylori* are resistant to metronidazole, as are some strains of *C. difficile*. Resistance results most commonly from reduced uptake of the drug and the development of altered oxidoreductases that convert metronidazole less efficiently to its active product. Resistance to tinidazole is less common.

Pharmacokinetics

Metronidazole is well absorbed orally and can also be given intravenously or by rectal suppositories. Metronidazole penetrates well into body fluids, including vaginal and pleural fluids and the CSF, and it can cross the placenta. Tinidazole is given orally and distributes into tissues including the brain. Metronidazole and tinidazole are eliminated mainly by metabolism in the liver and have half-lives of 6–9 hours and 12–14 hours, respectively.

Unwanted effects

- Nausea, vomiting, metallic taste, decreased appetite.
- Intolerance to alcohol can occur by a mechanism similar to the disulfiram reaction (see Chapter 54).
- Rashes.

Nitrofurantoin

Mechanism of action

Nitrofurantoin is activated inside bacteria by reduction via the flavoprotein nitrofurantoin reductase to unstable metabolites, which disrupt ribosomal RNA, DNA and other intracellular components. It is bactericidal, especially to bacteria present in acid urine.

Spectrum of activity

Nitrofurantoin is active against most Gram-positive cocci and *E. coli*. *Pseudomonas* species are naturally resistant, as are many *Proteus* species. Its use is confined to infections of the lower urinary tract.

Resistance

Chromosomal resistance occurs, but is uncommon and due to reduced nitrofurantoin reductase activity.

Pharmacokinetics

Nitrofurantoin is well absorbed from the gut. Its half-life in plasma is very short (<1 hour) and therapeutic plasma concentrations are not achieved. It is excreted largely unchanged in the urine, giving urinary concentrations high enough to treat lower urinary tract infections, but the low tissue concentrations are inadequate for the treatment of acute pyelonephritis.

Unwanted effects

- Gastrointestinal upset is common, including anorexia, nausea and vomiting.
- Pulmonary toxicity with long-term use produces acute allergic pneumonitis or chronic interstitial fibrosis.
- Hepatotoxicity (rare).
- Peripheral neuropathy.

Drugs affecting bacterial protein synthesis

Macrolides

azithromycin, clarithromycin, erythromycin, telithromycin

Mechanism of action

Macrolides interfere with bacterial protein synthesis by binding reversibly to the 50S subunit of the bacterial ribosome, where they inhibit peptidyl transferase activity and block translocation of the aminoacyl-transfer RNA (tRNA) from the A site to the P site, preventing elongation of the polypeptide chain. The action is primarily bacteriostatic (see Fig. 51.1).

Spectrum of activity

Erythromycin has a similar spectrum of activity to broad-spectrum penicillins and is often used for treating individuals who are allergic to penicillin. It is effective against Gram-positive bacteria and gut anaerobes but has poor activity against *H. influenzae*. It is also used for infections by *Legionella*, *Mycoplasma*, *Chlamydia*, *Mycobacterium* and *Campylobacter* species and for *Bordetella pertussis*. Although erythromycin is primarily bacteriostatic, it is bactericidal at high concentrations for some Gram-positive species, such as group A streptococci and pneumococci.

Azithromycin has less activity than erythromycin against Gram-positive bacteria but enhanced activity against *H. influenzae*. Clarithromycin has slightly greater activity than erythromycin and is also used as part of the multi-drug treatment of *H. pylori* (see Chapter 33). Telithromycin is a derivative of erythromycin active against penicillin- and erythromycin-resistant *S. pneumoniae*.

Resistance

Bacteria become resistant to macrolides by protective methylation or mutation of their ribosomal targets, by activation of efflux pumps that export the drugs and by drug inactivation.

Pharmacokinetics

Erythromycin is destroyed at acid pH and is therefore given orally as an enteric-coated tablet or an acid-stable pro-drug (erythromycin ethyl succinate); it can also be administered intravenously. Clarithromycin is acid-stable and well absorbed from the gut. Both erythromycin and clarithromycin are metabolised in the liver with short half-lives (1–3 hours). Azithromycin is poorly absorbed from the gut and can be given orally or intravenously. It is widely distributed and released slowly from the tissues and then excreted unchanged in the bile; it has a long half-life of about 2 days. Telithromycin is well absorbed from the gut and metabolised in the liver, with a half-life of 10 hours.

Unwanted effects

- Epigastric discomfort, nausea, vomiting and diarrhoea are common with the oral preparation of erythromycin. Other macrolides are better tolerated.
- Rashes.
- Cholestatic jaundice with erythromycin, usually if treatment is continued for more than 2 weeks.
- Prolongation of the Q–T interval on the ECG, with a predisposition to ventricular arrhythmias (see Chapter 8).
- Drug interactions: erythromycin, clarithromycin and telithromycin inhibit P450 drug-metabolising enzymes (CYP3A4, CYP2D6) and can increase the plasma concentration of other drugs metabolised by these enzymes, including carbamazepine (see Chapter 23), ciclosporin (see Chapter 38) and simvastatin (see Chapter 48).

Aminoglycosides

gentamicin, netilmicin, streptomycin, tobramycin

Mechanism of action

Aminoglycosides inhibit protein synthesis in bacteria by binding irreversibly to the 30S ribosomal subunit (see Fig. 51.1). This inhibits transfer of aminoacyl-tRNA to the peptidyl site, causing premature termination of the peptide chain; it also increases the frequency of misreading of mRNA. Aminoglycosides may also damage bacterial cell membranes, causing leakage of intracellular contents. They are bactericidal. While aminoglycosides share common properties, they have some important differences that can be exploited in particular clinical circumstances, as described below.

Spectrum of activity

Aminoglycosides are active against many Gram-negative bacteria (including *Pseudomonas* species) and some Gram-positive bacteria. They are inactive against anaerobes, which are unable to take up the drugs. Aminoglycosides are particularly useful for serious Gram-negative infections, when they have a synergistic action with drugs that disrupt cell-wall synthesis (e.g. penicillins). Gentamicin is the most widely used aminoglycoside. Streptomycin is used occasionally as a component of the drug regimen to treat *Mycobacterium tuberculosis* (see below).

Resistance

Resistance to aminoglycosides is transferred by plasmids and is an increasing problem. It can occur by several mechanisms, the most frequent being the production of transferase enzymes that acetylate, phosphorylate or adenylylate aminoglycosides in the bacterial periplasmic space, with poor uptake of the modified drug (see Fig. 51.2). Netilmicin is less susceptible to these enzymes and is effective against many gentamicin-resistant bacteria. Changes in lipopolysaccharide phenotype can also reduce drug penetration. Such resistance can be overcome by the co-administration of antibacterials that disrupt cell-wall synthesis, such as penicillins. Changes in a number of bacterial ribosomal proteins can reduce drug binding and antibacterial effectiveness, particularly for streptomycin.

Pharmacokinetics

Aminoglycosides are poorly absorbed from the gut and are only given parenterally. They are rapidly excreted by the kidney and have short half-lives (1–4 hours). They do not cross the blood–brain barrier but do cross the placenta. Blood concentrations of aminoglycosides should always be measured to guide dosing. With multiple daily doses, the peak plasma concentration (measured 1 hour after dosing) is important to ensure bactericidal efficacy, and the trough concentration (immediately before the next dose) should be low enough to minimise the risk of toxic effects due to drug accumulation. Once-daily dosage regimens for aminoglycosides are increasingly used and are no more toxic than multiple daily dosages.

Tobramycin is available in powder form for inhalation and in a preservative-free solution for administration by nebuliser for the management of bronchiectasis (including cystic fibrosis) if the respiratory tract is colonised by *P. aeruginosa*.

Unwanted effects

Most unwanted effects of aminoglycosides are dose-related and many are reversible; they are most closely related to high trough concentrations of the drug or to total drug exposure.

- Ototoxicity can lead to both vestibular and auditory dysfunction. Prolonged treatment or high plasma drug concentrations lead to accumulation of the aminoglycoside in the inner ear, resulting in disturbances of balance or deafness that are often irreversible. Mutations in the human gene encoding mitochondrial 12S ribosomal RNA predispose to ototoxicity. Older age, pre-existing hearing problems, renal insufficiency and use of loop diuretics are also risk factors. Netilmicin causes less ototoxicity than the other aminoglycosides.
- Renal damage occurs through retention of aminoglycosides in the proximal tubular cells of the kidney. It is usually reversible and is manifest initially by a defect in the concentrating ability of the kidney, with mild proteinuria followed by a reduction in the glomerular filtration rate.

- Acute neuromuscular blockade can occur, usually if the aminoglycoside is used with anaesthetic drugs (see Chapter 17), and aminoglycosides can enhance the effects of other neuromuscular-blocking drugs (see Chapter 27). This action is the result of inhibition of pre-junctional acetylcholine release and also reduced postsynaptic sensitivity. It is reversed by intravenous Ca^{2+} salts.

Tetracyclines

Examples

doxycycline, minocycline, oxytetracycline

Mechanism of action

Tetracyclines enter bacteria mainly by an active uptake mechanism that is not found in human cells. They are bacteriostatic and inhibit protein synthesis by binding reversibly to the 30S subunit of bacterial ribosomes, inhibiting the binding of aminoacyl-tRNAs.

Spectrum of activity

Tetracyclines have a broad spectrum of activity against many Gram-positive and Gram-negative bacteria and in infections caused by rickettsiae, amoebae, *Chlamydia psittaci*, *Chlamydia trachomatis*, *Coxiella burnetii*, *Vibrio cholerae* and *Mycoplasma*, *Legionella* and *Brucella* species. They are useful in acne (see Chapter 49). Minocycline is active against *N. meningitidis*, unlike other tetracyclines.

Resistance

Resistance is carried by plasmids. Mechanisms include increased export of the tetracycline drug from the bacterium, modification of the drug by bacterial enzymes or decreased binding of the drug to the bacterial 30S ribosomal subunit; this last may be due to changes in ribosomal RNA structure or to protection of the ribosomal binding site by bacterial proteins (see Fig. 51.2). Resistance to the tetracyclines develops slowly, but in the United Kingdom it is now widespread among most Gram-positive and several Gram-negative bacteria. Micro-organisms that have developed resistance to one tetracycline frequently display resistance to the others.

Pharmacokinetics

Tetracyclines are incompletely absorbed from the gut, particularly if taken with food. Absorption of oxytetracycline is further impaired by milk, antacids (see Chapter 33), iron and increased intestinal pH. Tetracyclines bind to divalent and trivalent cations, forming inactive chelates (see Chapter 56). The tetracyclines diffuse reasonably well into sputum, urine, and peritoneal and pleural fluid; they cross the placenta but penetrate the CSF poorly.

Tetracyclines are concentrated in the liver and are to some extent excreted via the bile into the small intestine, from where they are partially reabsorbed. Drug concentrations in the bile may be three to five times higher than in the plasma. Tetracyclines are mainly eliminated unchanged in the urine with the exception of doxycycline, which is largely eliminated in the bile. All of the tetracyclines have half-lives within the range 8–22 hours.

Unwanted effects

- Nausea, vomiting, epigastric discomfort and diarrhoea.
- In children, tetracyclines produce permanent yellow–brown discoloration of growing teeth by chelating with Ca^{2+}; they can also cause dental hypoplasia. Tetracyclines should be avoided during the latter half of pregnancy and in children during the first 12 years of life.
- Antianabolic effects can occur in human cells from inhibition of protein synthesis (not seen with doxycycline or minocycline). If there is pre-existing impairment of renal function, it can lead to uraemia.
- Idiopathic intracranial hypertension, with headache and visual disturbances.

Tigecycline

Mechanism of action

Tigecycline is a glycylcycline with structural similarities to the tetracyclines and also binds to the 30S subunit of bacterial ribosomes to impair protein synthesis.

Spectrum of activity

Tigecycline has a broad spectrum of activity against Gram-positive and Gram-negative bacteria, including some anaerobes. It is used for complicated skin and soft tissue infections and for complicated abdominal infections caused by resistant bacteria. Tigecycline is active against MRSA, vancomycin-resistant enterococci, *Proteus* species and *P. aeruginosa*.

Resistance

Tigecycline is less susceptible than tetracyclines to bacterial resistance caused by ribosomal mutation and ribosomal protection proteins, but resistance occurs due to modification of the drug by bacterial enzymes and increased efflux pump activity.

Pharmacokinetics

Tigecycline is given intravenously and is well distributed in tissues; it is not known whether it crosses the blood–brain barrier. It is excreted largely unchanged in the bile and urine and has a very long half-life (about 27–42 hours).

Unwanted effects

The most common unwanted effects are similar to those of tetracyclines.

Chloramphenicol

Mechanism of action

Chloramphenicol inhibits protein synthesis in bacteria by binding irreversibly to the 50S subunit of bacterial ribosomes (see Fig. 51.1), where it blocks peptide chain elongation by inhibiting peptidyl transferase activity. The effect is mainly bacteriostatic but can be bactericidal in some bacteria.

Spectrum of activity

Chloramphenicol is a broad-spectrum antibacterial, active against many Gram-positive cocci (both aerobic and anaerobic) and Gram-negative bacteria. The sensitivities of all these bacteria are variable, but the drug has a bactericidal effect on *E. coli*, *Staphylococcus pneumoniae*, *H. influenzae*, *N. meningitidis*, *B. pertussis*, *V. cholerae* and *Salmonella*, *Shigella* and *Bacteroides* species. It is bacteriostatic for some streptococci and staphylococci.

Because of its toxicity, chloramphenicol is reserved for life-threatening infections, particularly with *H. influenzae* or *Salmonella typhi*. It is also used topically to treat conjunctivitis (see Chapter 50).

Resistance

Resistance is transferred by plasmids and most commonly involves the production of acetyltransferases that acetylate the drug, preventing it from binding to the ribosome. The acetyltransferases are produced by many Gram-negative bacteria but can also be induced in Gram-positive bacteria. Resistant bacteria may also show reduced uptake of the drug or mutation of the 50S ribosomal subunit.

Pharmacokinetics

Chloramphenicol is well absorbed orally and can also be given intravenously. It is widely distributed, including into the CSF and the biliary tree; it crosses the placenta and is present in breast milk. Chloramphenicol is metabolised in the liver and has a half-life of 1.5–4 hours.

Unwanted effects

- The most important unwanted effect of systemic use is bone marrow toxicity. Reversible anaemia, thrombocytopenia or neutropenia can occur, particularly in those receiving high or prolonged dosing. Aplastic anaemia is rare but usually fatal.
- Peripheral neuritis, optic neuritis, headache.
- Rashes.
- Blurred vision and transient burning or stinging sensations when used as eye-drops.
- Premature infants and babies less than 2 weeks old have immature glucuronyl transferase and reduced drug elimination. Chloramphenicol can accumulate in neonates, causing the 'grey baby syndrome'. Initial symptoms include vomiting and cyanosis, followed by hypothermia, vasomotor collapse and an ashen grey discoloration of the skin. There is a high mortality.
- Drug interactions: chloramphenicol inhibits the cytochrome P450 isoforms CYP2C19 and CYP3A4, increasing the plasma concentrations of other drugs including coumarin anticoagulants and clopidogrel (see Chapter 11) and phenytoin (see Chapter 23).

Lincosamides

clindamycin

Mechanism of action

Clindamycin acts on the 50S subunit of bacterial ribosomes to inhibit protein synthesis in a similar manner to the macrolide antibacterials.

Spectrum of activity

Clindamycin is active against Gram-positive cocci, including streptococci and penicillin-resistant staphylococci and also against many anaerobes, especially *Bacteroides fragilis*. It is used for staphylococcal bone infection such as osteomyelitis and sometimes for soft tissue infections.

Resistance

Resistance develops by modification of the 50S ribosomal binding site, increased drug efflux and drug modification. Cross-resistance may occur with macrolide antibacterials.

Pharmacokinetics

Clindamycin is well absorbed orally. Widely distributed, it crosses the placenta and appears in breast milk but not in the CSF. It is eliminated largely by hepatic metabolism and has a half-life of 2–3 hours.

Unwanted effects

- Nausea, vomiting, abdominal discomfort, diarrhoea and rarely *C. difficile*-related colitis.
- Rashes.
- Jaundice and abnormal liver function tests.
- Neutropenia, thrombocytopenia.

Fusidic acid

Mechanism of action

Fusidic acid is a steroid compound that inhibits bacterial protein synthesis. It inhibits elongation of the peptide chain by interacting with elongation factor G (EF-G) in the ribosome.

Spectrum of activity

Fusidic acid is a narrow-spectrum antibacterial mainly active against Gram-positive bacteria. It is most commonly used to treat penicillin-resistant *S. aureus*, especially in cases of osteomyelitis. It is bactericidal.

Resistance

Resistance occurs and involves chromosomal mutations in ribosomal EF-G that reduce drug binding. Resistance develops rapidly when fusidic acid is used alone, so it is usually given in combination with another drug.

Pharmacokinetics

Oral absorption is complete but an intravenous formulation is available. Distribution into synovial fluid and soft tissues is good, and the drug concentrates in bone. Fusidic acid is metabolised in the liver and excreted in bile; it has a half-life of 9 hours.

Unwanted effects

- Thrombophlebitis with intravenous infusions.
- Cholestatic jaundice.
- Drowsiness, dizziness.
- Nausea, vomiting.

Oxazolidinones

Linezolid

Mechanism of action

The oxazolidinones are active against nonreplicating bacteria. They have a unique mechanism of action, binding to a 23S ribosomal RNA in the 50S ribosomal subunit and preventing the initiation of protein synthesis, unlike many other antibacterials that inhibit chain elongation.

Spectrum of activity

Linezolid is active against a range of Gram-positive organisms, including MRSA and vancomycin-resistant *Enterococcus faecium*.

Resistance

Resistance is due to point mutations in the 23S ribosomal RNA target for the drug and to changes in ribosomal proteins. This can develop with prolonged treatment or with inadequate doses.

Pharmacokinetics

Linezolid is well absorbed orally and distributes widely, including into the CSF. It is mainly metabolised in the liver and has a half-life of 5–7 hours.

Unwanted effects

- Headache.
- Fungal infections, candidiasis.
- Nausea, vomiting, taste disturbances, diarrhoea.
- Myelosuppression with anaemia, neutropenia and thrombocytopenia.
- Optic neuropathy with prolonged use (over 28 days).
- Hepatotoxicity (abnormal liver function tests).
- Linezolid is a weak nonselective monoamine oxidase inhibitor, and dietary restriction of tyramine is advisable (see Chapter 22).

Drugs affecting bacterial metabolism

Sulfonamides

sulfadiazine, sulfamethoxazole

The therapeutic importance of the sulfonamides has diminished because of the spread of resistance; there are now only a few nonetheless important situations in which they are first-choice antibacterial drugs. Sulfamethoxazole is used only in combination with the dihydrofolate reductase inhibitor trimethoprim, as co-trimoxazole (see below).

Mechanism of action

Folate is essential for cell growth and is used to manufacture thymidine and also purines for incorporation into DNA. Unlike humans, who obtain folate from the diet, bacteria cannot utilise pre-formed folate and must synthesise it from *p*-aminobenzoic acid (PABA). Sulfonamides are structurally similar to PABA and inhibit dihydropteroate synthetase in the synthetic pathway for folic acid (Fig. 51.4).

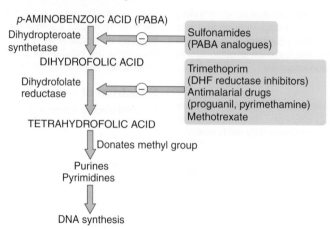

The Folic Acid Pathway:

Fig. 51.4 **Sites of action of sulfonamides and dihydrofolate (DHF) reductase inhibitors in the folic acid pathway.**
Selective inhibitors of bacterial, plasmodial and human DHF reductase isozymes are used respectively as antibacterial (trimethoprim), antimalarial (proguanil, pyrimethamine) and anticancer (methotrexate) drugs (see Chapter 52).

Spectrum of activity

Sulfonamides have a bacteriostatic action against a wide range of Gram-positive and Gram-negative bacteria and are also active against *Toxoplasma*, *Chlamydia* and *Nocardia* species. Because of the frequency of resistance in many of these micro-organisms, sulfonamides are given as sole therapy only for the treatment of nocardiosis or toxoplasmosis.

Resistance

Resistance is common and occurs through the production of a mutated dihydropteroate synthetase with reduced affinity for sulphonamide binding (see Figs 51.2 and 51.4). Resistance is transmitted among Gram-negative bacteria by plasmids. Resistance in *S. aureus* occurs as a result of excessive synthesis of PABA. Some resistant bacteria have reduced uptake of sulphonamides.

Pharmacokinetics

Sulfonamides are well absorbed orally. They are widely distributed and cross the blood–brain barrier and placenta. A topical formulation of sulfadiazine is available for treatment of burns.

Sulfonamides are metabolised in the liver initially by acetylation, which shows genetic polymorphism. The acetylated products have no antibacterial action but retain a risk of toxicity, particularly in slow acetylators. The parent drugs and their *N*-acetyl metabolites are excreted by the kidney. Most sulfonamides have half-lives of about 12 hours.

Unwanted effects

- Nausea, vomiting, and diarrhoea.
- Rashes, including toxic epidermal necrolysis and Stevens–Johnson syndrome.
- Haemolysis in individuals with glucose-6-phosphate dehydrogenase deficiency (see Chapters 47 and 53).
- Neutropenia, thrombocytopenia.

- Sulfonamides should not be used in the last trimester of pregnancy or in neonates because the drug competes for bilirubin-binding sites on albumin; this can raise the concentration of unconjugated bilirubin and increases the risk of kernicterus.

Trimethoprim

Trimethoprim can be used alone or, less commonly, is combined with the sulfonamide sulfamethoxazole as co-trimoxazole.

Mechanism of action

Trimethoprim inhibits dihydrofolate reductase, which converts dihydrofolate to tetrahydrofolate (see Fig. 51.4). The bacterial enzyme is inhibited at much lower concentrations of trimethoprim than its mammalian counterpart. The combination of trimethoprim with sulfamethoxazole (as co-trimoxazole) acts synergistically to prevent folate synthesis by bacteria. However, resistance to the sulfamethoxazole component and the incidence of unwanted effects limit the value of this combination.

Spectrum of activity

Trimethoprim has broad-spectrum bacteriostatic activity against Gram-positive and Gram-negative bacteria. In many urinary and respiratory tract infections trimethoprim alone gives results similar to the combination with sulfamethoxazole. Co-trimoxazole is effective against the protozoan *Pneumocystis jirovecii*, which causes pneumonia in people with acquired immunodeficiency syndrome (AIDS) or other immunodeficiencies, and this is now its major indication (see below).

Resistance

Resistance to trimethoprim is common and occurs in a variety of ways, including the production of mutated dihydrofolate reductase, which is insensitive to the drug.

Pharmacokinetics

Trimethoprim is well absorbed from the gut and most is eliminated unchanged by the kidney; it has a half-life of 9–17 hours. Co-trimoxazole is available for intravenous use.

Unwanted effects

- Nausea, vomiting, diarrhoea and sore mouth, all of which are usually mild.
- Rashes.
- Bone marrow depression.
- Folate deficiency, leading to megaloblastic changes in the bone marrow, is rare except in people with depleted folate stores.

Drugs used for tuberculosis

Tuberculosis is usually treated with a multi-drug regimen because of the rapid development of resistance. Some drugs used to treat mycobacterial infections also have other clinical uses.

Rifamycins

rifabutin, rifampicin, rifaximin

Mechanism of action and spectrum of activity

Rifamycins inhibit bacterial DNA-dependent RNA polymerase and prevent the initiation of mRNA transcription, particularly in mycobacteria. They have a bactericidal action. Rifampicin (rifampin) has a broad spectrum of activity and is used in combination with other drugs for the treatment of mycobacterial infections (*M. tuberculosis* and *Mycobacterium leprae*), brucellosis, *Legionella* infections, serious staphylococcal infections and endocarditis. In the United Kingdom, rifampicin is considered an essential drug for the treatment of tuberculosis. Rifampicin is also used for prophylaxis against meningococcal meningitis and *H. influenzae* type B infection. Rifabutin is used for the treatment of tuberculosis and for prophylaxis against infection with *Mycobacterium avium* complex (which most commonly occurs in people infected with HIV) and other mycobacterial infections. Rifaximin is a nonabsorbable rifamycin used to treat traveller's diarrhoea (see Chapter 35).

Resistance

Resistance to rifamycins develops rapidly, which limits the wider use of rifampicin and rifabutin as antibacterial drugs other than as part of combination treatment for tuberculosis. Resistance to the rifamycins arises from genetic mutation of the bacterial DNA-dependent RNA polymerase.

Pharmacokinetics

Oral absorption of rifampicin is good; an intravenous formulation of rifampicin and oral formulations combined with other antituberculosis drugs are available. The bioavailability of rifabutin is low (20%) compared with rifampicin. Rifampicin and rifabutin are metabolised in the liver and have half-lives of 1–6 hours and 35–40 hours, respectively. Oral bioavailability of rifaximin is less than 1%.

Unwanted effects

- Nausea and anorexia.
- Diarrhoea and antibiotic-associated colitis with rifampicin.
- Hepatotoxicity, usually producing only a transient rise in plasma transaminases but occasionally more severe; regular monitoring is recommended.
- Rifampicin and rifabutin may cause orange discoloration of tears, sweat and urine.
- Leucopenia, thrombocytopenia or anaemia with rifabutin.
- Influenza-like symptoms (myalgia, pyrexia), respiratory symptoms, renal failure, shock, disseminated intravascular coagulation and acute haemolytic anaemia.
- Drug interactions of rifamycins: induction of cytochrome P450 isoenzymes (including CYP2C9, CYP3A4) and other drug-metabolising enzymes in the liver (see Chapter 2) can reduce plasma concentrations of oestrogen in those taking oral contraceptives (see Chapter 45) and of many other drugs including warfarin (see Chapter 11), phenytoin (see Chapter 23) and sulphonylureas (see Chapter 40).

Isoniazid
Mechanism of action

Isoniazid is an important and specific drug for the treatment of *M. tuberculosis*. It is a pro-drug activated by catalase–peroxidase activity within the mycobacteria. The active product inhibits enzymes involved in the synthesis of long-chain mycolic acids, which are unique to the cell wall of mycobacteria, and also inhibits enzymes required for nucleic acid synthesis. Isoniazid is bactericidal against dividing mycobacteria, but bacteriostatic on resting mycobacteria. In the United Kingdom it is considered an essential drug, along with rifampicin, for the treatment of tuberculosis.

Resistance

Resistance occurs rapidly if isoniazid is used alone. It is due to mutations that reduce the activity of the catalase-peroxidase and related enzymes responsible for activation of the pro-drug. Resistance is currently uncommon in developed countries but can be troublesome in developing countries.

Pharmacokinetics

Oral absorption of isoniazid is good but is reduced by food. Intravenous and intramuscular formulations are also available. Isoniazid is metabolised by acetylation in the liver, which is subject to genetic polymorphism. Rapid acetylators show extensive first-pass metabolism; their plasma isoniazid concentrations are half of those in slow acetylators. The half-life is 0.5–2 hours in rapid acetylators and 2–6.5 hours in slow acetylators.

Unwanted effects

- Nausea, vomiting, constipation, dry mouth.
- Peripheral neuropathy with high doses. This can be prevented by prophylactic use of oral pyridoxine supplements in people at high risk – for example, those with diabetes, alcoholism, chronic renal failure, malnutrition

or HIV infection. Neuropathy is more common in slow acetylators.

- Hepatitis is rare, but regular monitoring with liver function tests is recommended.
- Rashes.
- Systemic lupus erythematosus-like syndrome. Positive antinuclear antibodies are found in 20% of people during long-term treatment, but fewer develop symptoms.

Pyrazinamide

Mechanism of action

Pyrazinamide is a pro-drug converted to pyrazinoic acid by pyrazinamidase, an enzyme found in *M. tuberculosis*. In acid conditions, liberated pyrazinoic acid re-enters *M. tuberculosis* cells and is trapped owing to the weak efflux activity of this mycobacterial species for the compound. The antimycobacterial mechanism of pyrazinoic acid is unclear, but it may inactivate a key enzyme in fatty acid synthesis; also altered membrane potential due to low intracellular pH may disrupt other cellular pathways. Pyrazinamide is unusual among antibacterial drugs by being selectively bactericidal for dormant *M. tuberculosis* cells and less active in dividing cells.

Resistance

Resistance results from mutations in the gene that codes for pyrazinamidase. It develops rapidly if pyrazinamide is used as a sole treatment for tuberculosis.

Pharmacokinetics

Oral absorption of pyrazinamide is good and it crosses inflamed meninges, so it is active in tuberculous meningitis. Metabolism occurs in the liver; it has a long half-life (9–10 hours).

Unwanted effects

- Hepatotoxicity: a rise in plasma bilirubin usually requires cessation of treatment; regular monitoring is recommended.
- Nausea and vomiting.
- Arthralgia.
- Sideroblastic anaemia.

Ethambutol

Mechanism of action

Ethambutol probably functions as an arabinose analogue and inhibits arabinosyl transferase, resulting in impaired synthesis of the mycobacterial cell wall. Ethambutol is primarily bacteriostatic. It is effective against *M. tuberculosis* and several other mycobacteria, including *M. avium* complex.

Resistance

Resistance may be due to gene mutations that reduce the binding of ethambutol to arabinosyl transferase. It develops slowly but is common during prolonged treatment of tuberculosis if ethambutol is used alone.

Pharmacokinetics

Oral absorption of ethambutol is good; it distributes into the brain and across the placenta. It is mainly eliminated unchanged by the kidney. The half-life is long (10–15 hours).

Unwanted effects

- Visual disturbances: optic neuritis produces initial red-green colour blindness, then reduced visual acuity; these effects are dose-related but usually reversible.
- Peripheral neuritis.
- Hyperuricaemia, gout.
- Nephrotoxicity.

Other drugs used in the treatment of tuberculosis

Other antituberculosis drugs can be used as second-line treatments in multi-drug-resistant disease. These include *para*-aminosalicylic acid, bedaquiline, capreomycin, cycloserine, delamanid and streptomycin (see the drug compendium at the end of this chapter). Newer macrolides (azithromycin, clarithromycin), quinolones (moxifloxacin) and the aminoglycoside amikacin are also used. Drugs used in countries other than the United Kingdom include thiacetazone and protionamide.

Drugs used for leprosy

The drugs recommended for the treatment of leprosy, which is caused by *M. leprae*, are rifampicin (see above), dapsone and clofazimine.

Dapsone

Mechanism of action and use

Dapsone is a sulphone related to the sulfonamides and acts similarly by inhibiting folate synthesis by dihydropteroate synthase. It is the most active drug against *M. leprae*. Dapsone is also used to treat *Pneumocystis* pneumonia and dermatitis herpetiformis.

Resistance

Resistance can develop, as for sulfonamides (see above).

Pharmacokinetics

Dapsone is well absorbed from the gut and widely distributed. It is metabolised in the liver and undergoes enterohepatic cycling. It has a long half-life (10–80 hours).

Unwanted effects

- Blood disorders: haemolysis and methaemoglobinaemia (see Chapter 53). These are rare at the doses used for the treatment of leprosy, but the risk is higher in people with glucose-6-phosphate dehydrogenase deficiency.
- 'Dapsone syndrome': rash, fever and eosinophilia may occur after 3–6 weeks of treatment, leading to exfoliative dermatitis, hepatitis and psychosis if treatment is not stopped.
- Neuropathy.
- Anorexia, nausea, vomiting.
- Skin hypersensitivity reactions.

Clofazimine

Mechanism of action and use

Clofazimine is an iminophenazine dye that interferes with guanine bases during mycobacterial DNA replication. It is used as a second-line drug in the event of dapsone intolerance in people with leprosy. It is given orally.

Pharmacokinetics

Clofazimine has a variable oral bioavailability and is eliminated slowly in the bile. It has a very long half-life (70 days) and can accumulate in the body.

Unwanted effects

- Gastrointestinal upset (common), abdominal pain.
- Brownish-black discoloration of the skin, hair, faeces and body fluids is very common. Discoloration of soft contact lenses may also occur.
- Acne, rash, pruritus, photosensitivity.
- Corneal pigmentation, dimmed vision.

PRINCIPLES OF ANTIBACTERIAL THERAPY

Antibacterial therapy is widely misused, which encourages the selection of resistant organisms. In particular, the use of antibacterials for viral illnesses such as the common cold or sore throat is to be discouraged. The following guidelines outline the principles that should be considered in the choice of a safe and effective antibacterial therapy.

Empirical treatment

Most antibacterial therapy is started without prior identification of the organism and its antibacterial drug sensitivities. Such treatment should be guided by the clinical diagnosis and knowledge of the most common pathogenic bacteria responsible for the infection to be treated. Local information about patterns of antibacterial resistance is an important consideration.

Spectrum of antibacterial activity

A drug with a narrow spectrum of activity should be used in preference to a broad-spectrum drug whenever possible. The unnecessary use of broad-spectrum antibacterials encourages the development of resistant bacteria. This can present problems for the person treated owing to the selection of resistant pathogens or colonisation by resistant bacteria from the environment. For the community, the selection of resistant pathogens can create problems by rendering standard antibacterial therapy less reliable. Broad-spectrum antibacterial cover is sometimes appropriate – for example, in a seriously ill person when the infecting bacterium is unknown and a variety of bacteria could be causing the condition being treated.

Combination therapy

Treatment with more than one antibacterial drug should not be used routinely. It may, however, be valuable to provide broad-spectrum cover in serious illness when the organism is unknown, for example the combination of cefotaxime and metronidazole to cover aerobic and anaerobic organisms in suspected Gram-negative septicaemia. When resistance is likely to develop readily to the first-choice drug during prolonged treatment, the use of combination therapy can minimise that risk – for example, in the treatment of infective endocarditis or tuberculosis.

Bactericidal versus bacteriostatic drugs

In some situations, bactericidal drugs are preferred to bacteriostatic drugs – for example, for the treatment of infective endocarditis (when bacteria divide infrequently) or when the person being treated is immunocompromised (and host defences are ineffective for assisting eradication). In most other situations the choice is not important.

Site of infection

This may determine the choice of drug; for example, some antibacterials achieve only low concentrations in the biliary tree, urine, bone or CSF.

Mode of administration

Oral therapy is usually preferred to parenteral treatment. Exceptions include the treatment of serious infections for which reliable plasma drug concentrations are essential, when the drug is available only in parenteral formulation, or when gastrointestinal absorption may be unreliable – for example, after abdominal surgery.

Duration of therapy

This should be as short as is compatible with adequate treatment of the infection. The decision is often arbitrary – for example, 7–10 days in many infections. Some infections can be effectively treated over much shorter periods; for example, courses of 1–3 days are usually adequate for uncomplicated lower urinary tract infections in women. There is evidence that the conventional longer courses of treatment for many other infections may be unnecessary. For a few infections, long periods of treatment may be essential to eliminate semi-dormant organisms or those in 'privileged sites' where antibacterial drug penetration is poor. Examples include infective endocarditis, osteomyelitis and tuberculosis. Some antibacterials produce a 'post-antibiotic effect', in which there is delayed regrowth of surviving bacteria following exposure to the drug. This is most marked with aminoglycosides such as gentamicin, but it also occurs with other drugs, including β-lactam antibacterials.

Chemoprophylaxis

The use of chemoprophylaxis to prevent infection is important in many situations. Common examples include prevention of meningococcal meningitis, *H. influenzae* type B infection or pertussis in close contacts of an infected person, and pre-operative prophylaxis before many surgical procedures. More prolonged prophylaxis is used to prevent pneumococcal infection after splenectomy or in people with sickle cell disease.

TREATMENT OF SELECTED BACTERIAL INFECTIONS

This section is not intended to be comprehensive. It outlines the approach to antibacterial therapy in several common bacterial infections. The choice of antibacterial drug for these infections will depend on factors such as local patterns of bacterial resistance or the risk of *C. difficile* infection, which make universal recommendations impossible.

Upper respiratory tract infections

Most upper respiratory tract infections are caused by viruses, producing symptoms of the common cold. Symptomatic treatment is all that should be offered, with an antihistamine (e.g. chlorphenamine; see Chapter 39) or an antimuscarinic spray (e.g. ipratropium; see Chapter 12) to reduce rhinorrhoea and sneezing. An α-adrenoceptor agonist (e.g. xylometazoline) given orally or nasally can reduce nasal congestion, but prolonged use can provoke a rebound effect (rhinitis medicamentosa) (see Chapter 39). A nonsteroidal anti-inflammatory drug (NSAID; see Chapter 29) can be used to reduce associated headache and malaise. Antibacterial drugs are widely prescribed for upper respiratory tract symptoms but have no benefit.

Sinusitis and otitis media

Sinusitis and otitis media accompany catarrhal conditions in childhood and frequently follow an upper respiratory tract infection. Sinusitis produces headache, facial pain, fever and purulent rhinorrhoea. A nasal decongestant such as an α-adrenoceptor agonist can be helpful, in conjunction with an analgesic. An antibacterial is often not beneficial in acute sinusitis unless there is marked facial swelling and pain or failure to resolve after 7 days. The most common infecting organisms are *H. influenzae* (which often produces β-lactamase), *S. pneumoniae* and *Moraxella catarrhalis.* Suitable antibacterial drugs include amoxicillin (or amoxicillin with clavulanic acid if there is no improvement after 48 hours), doxycycline and clarithromycin. Chronic sinusitis usually requires correction of an anatomical obstruction in the nose.

Otitis media is very common in childhood. When associated with an effusion in the middle ear, increased pressure causes pain and perforation of the eardrum. The organisms responsible are similar to those causing acute sinusitis. In more than 80% of affected children, the condition is self-limiting over 2–3 days without treatment. An antibacterial such as amoxicillin or clarithromycin should be used if symptoms have not resolved after 72 hours or if there are systemic symptoms. Surgery is occasionally necessary for recurrent infections.

Lower respiratory tract infections

Acute bronchitis

This is characterised by new-onset, often productive cough without evidence of pneumonia. It is usually caused by a viral infection and the cough often takes 2–4 weeks to resolve without treatment. Antibacterial treatment is inappropriate and does not alter the course of the illness. Even if there is underlying chronic obstructive airways disease, the evidence for benefit from antibacterial drugs is small, although they may slightly shorten the duration of symptoms. In such cases *S. pneumoniae* (pneumococcus), *H. influenzae* or *M. catarrhalis* are commonly found in the sputum, but these micro-organisms are often isolated in remissions as well. If an antibacterial drug is used, treatment for 5 days with amoxicillin, doxycycline or clarithromycin will be effective against the most likely pathogens. Co-amoxiclav (amoxicillin with clavulanic acid) can be used for resistant *H. influenzae.*

Pneumonia

Primary community-acquired pneumonia is most commonly caused by *S. pneumoniae* and less commonly by *H. influenzae* and staphylococci. 'Atypical' micro-organisms – such as *Legionella* species, *Mycoplasma pneumoniae* or *Chlamydia pneumonia* – can also cause pneumonia. Appropriate antibacterial treatment will be dictated by the most likely infecting agent.

Amoxicillin is the treatment of choice if pneumococcus is suspected. For people who are penicillin-allergic, clarithromycin will cover the most likely micro-organisms, including 'atypical' ones. Oral amoxicillin combined with clarithromycin is often used for community-acquired pneumonia requiring admission of the person to hospital. Doxycycline is increasingly used as an alternative oral treatment because of a lower risk of *C. difficile*-related colitis. Severe community-acquired pneumonia (defined by the CURB-65 score; Table 51.3) is usually treated with intravenous therapy comprising benzylpenicillin with intravenous clarithromycin or doxycycline. Co-amoxiclav is often used in place of benzylpenicillin for life-threatening pneumonia or when Gram-negative organisms are suspected to cover β-lactamase-producing organisms. A quinolone with activity against pneumococci, such as moxifloxacin, would be an alternative choice. Adjunctive treatment of pneumonia may include supplemental oxygen via a face mask, pain relief for pleurisy and ensuring adequate hydration.

Secondary pneumonias occur in patients with other concurrent diseases, often during a stay in hospital (nosocomial or hospital-acquired pneumonia). A wide range of pathogens may be involved and parenteral drug treatment is usually necessary. A cephalosporin (e.g. cefuroxime) or co-amoxiclav is often used for early-onset infections or an antipseudomonal penicillin (e.g. piperacillin with tazobactam) or ciprofloxacin for late-onset infection. An aminoglycoside such as gentamicin can be added for severe infection where *P. aeruginosa* is suspected.

Table 51.3 CURB-65 score for predicting mortality in community-acquired pneumonia
Confusion of new onset (abbreviated mental test score ≤8/10)
Blood **u**rea nitrogen >7 mmol/L (>19 mg/dL)
Respiratory rate ≥30 breaths per minute
Blood pressure: systolic <90 mm Hg or diastolic ≤60 mm Hg
Age ≥**65** years
Each risk factor scores one point. Mortality at 30 days is predicted by total score: zero, mortality 0.7%; score 1–2, 3.1%; score 3, 17%; score 4, 41.5% and score 5, 57%.

Chronic lung sepsis

This encompasses lung abscess, empyema and bronchiectasis. The pathogens in lung abscesses vary according to the immune status of the individual. Ideally, treatment should be directed by isolation and sensitivity testing of the bacteria. Empyema requires drainage and then specific antibacterial therapy directed at the cultured pathogen. Bronchiectasis is most frequently associated with colonisation by *H. influenzae*, and less often *Pseudomonas* species or *S. pneumoniae*. A quinolone such as moxifloxacin or a macrolide such as azithromycin are suitable empirical treatment choices. Increasing use is being made of inhaled nebulised antibacterial drugs, such as tobramycin, to treat frequent exacerbations. Adjunctive treatment with bronchodilators, mucolytics and physiotherapy may be useful (see also cystic fibrosis, Chapter 13).

Urinary tract infections

Urinary tract infections are more common in women than men because of the shorter female urethra. Infections can occur in structurally normal urinary tracts or in association with a structural genitourinary abnormality that impairs drainage of urine or acts as a focus for infection, such as a stone in the kidney or bladder. An indwelling urinary catheter is often associated with bacterial colonisation of the urine that is almost impossible to eradicate but often does not cause any symptoms.

The most frequent bacterial cause of urinary tract infection is *E. coli*. Hospital-acquired infections are often caused by *Klebsiella*, *Enterobacter* and *Serratia* species or by *P. aeruginosa*, because these organisms can be selected as resistant bacteria following antibacterial usage. *Proteus mirabilis* is often found if there are stones in the urinary tract. Less commonly, staphylococci, especially *Staphylococcus saprophyticus*, are responsible.

Uncomplicated urinary tract infection is confined to the bladder (cystitis) and in women can be treated by a short course (3 days) of an aminopenicillin such as amoxicillin. Alternative drugs include a first-generation cephalosporin (e.g. cefalexin), trimethoprim and nitrofurantoin. A quinolone such as ciprofloxacin can be useful for *P. aeruginosa* infections. Men should be treated for longer (usually 7 days).

Complicated urinary tract infections also involve the kidney (pyelonephritis), or the prostate in males, and require longer courses of treatment. For pyelonephritis, initial intravenous therapy is usually started with broad-spectrum drugs such as aztreonam, ciprofloxacin or cefuroxime, sometimes with an initial dose of gentamicin; treatment is usually continued for 10–14 days. For acute prostatitis, oral treatment with trimethoprim or ciprofloxacin for at least 4 weeks is recommended.

Treatment of infection with an indwelling urinary catheter is recommended only if there are systemic symptoms of infection, such as fever or rigors.

Long-term antibacterial prophylaxis against urinary tract infections may be necessary to prevent recurrent infection if there are underlying urinary tract abnormalities. Suitable drugs, usually given at low dosage, include trimethoprim, nitrofurantoin and cefalexin.

Gastrointestinal infection

In the United Kingdom, infectious diarrhoea is usually caused by viruses and is self-limiting. However, gastroenteritis (a syndrome that includes nausea, vomiting, diarrhoea and abdominal discomfort) can result from ingestion of bacterial pathogens.

'Food poisoning' of bacterial origin can occur from ingestion of a pre-formed bacterial toxin (e.g. from *Clostridium botulinum* or *S. aureus*), with onset of symptoms usually within hours, or it can be caused by ingested bacteria infecting the bowel. Severe bacterial infection of the large intestine can cause dysentery, an inflammatory disorder often associated with fever, abdominal pain, and blood and pus in the faeces. The most common cause of bacterial diarrhoea (especially in children in developing countries) is *E. coli*, which produces powerful enterotoxins. In other circumstances, *Salmonella* species, *Campylobacter* species, *V. cholerae*, *Shigella* species or various other organisms are responsible.

If diarrhoea is severe, fluid replacement is often necessary. Antibacterial treatment is not usually recommended even if bacterial infection is suspected unless there are systemic symptoms such as fever, rigors and hypotension. Ciprofloxacin and clarithromycin are effective for *Campylobacter* enteritis and shigellosis. *Salmonella* infections can be treated with ciprofloxacin unless *S. typhi* is suspected, when cefotaxime is preferred.

Antibacterial drugs can cause diarrhoea due to alteration of bowel flora; it usually resolves rapidly when the drug is withdrawn. However, if it is complicated by colonisation with *C. difficile*, oral metronidazole, vancomycin or fidaxomicin will be necessary to eliminate the pathogen.

Biliary tract infection

Acute cholecystitis and cholangitis are often caused by *E. coli* and most often occur if there is biliary obstruction. Supportive treatment with fluid and electrolyte replacement is usually required. Antibacterial therapy with a cephalosporin, ciprofloxacin or gentamicin is usually effective. Combination therapy is recommended if the infection is severe; alternatively, a ureidopenicillin such as piperacillin with tazobactam can be given alone. Treatment is usually given for 7–10 days.

Osteomyelitis

Infection of bone produces necrotic tissue and generates an avascular privileged site for bacteria that antibacterial drugs penetrate to only a limited extent. Organisms involved include *S. aureus*, which adheres readily to bone matrix, various streptococci, *Serratia* species, *P. aeruginosa* and enteric Gram-negative rods.

Early antibacterial treatment is essential and surgical intervention may be necessary to remove necrotic tissue. The choice of drug depends on the suspected organisms. First-line treatment is often with flucloxacillin or clindamycin; if a prosthesis is present or the infection is severe, the drug should be combined with fusidic acid or rifampicin for the first 2 weeks. Amoxicillin or cefuroxime is usually used if *H. influenzae* is identified, or vancomycin for MRSA. Acute infections are treated with intravenous antimicrobials for 6 weeks, but chronic infections are treated for at least 12 weeks. If long-term therapy is necessary for chronic refractory osteomyelitis, an oral quinolone such as ciprofloxacin can be substituted.

Septic arthritis

The most common organism is *S. aureus*; less frequently streptococci are found. The standard treatment is with flucloxacillin or clindamycin for individuals who are penicillin-allergic. Vancomycin is used for MRSA. Treatment should be continued for 4–6 weeks.

Cellulitis

This usually complicates a wound, ulcer or dermatosis. In most cases the infecting organisms are *S. aureus* or streptococci. Treatment is usually with a β-lactam antibacterial that is active against β-lactamase-producing *S. aureus*. Flucloxacillin is normally used. Clarithromycin or clindamycin is used for individuals who are penicillin-allergic.

Septicaemia

Septicaemia is a bacterial infection involving the bloodstream and can present with fever or, if more severe, result in circulatory collapse from vasodilation, capillary leak and impaired myocardial contractility. Gram-positive organisms are a more frequent cause than Gram-negative organisms, with about 60% of infections arising from respiratory, intra-abdominal and urinary tract sources. Septicaemia is a medical emergency requiring intensive fluid replacement, plasma volume expansion and electrolyte correction. Noradrenaline (norepinephrine) or other vasopressors may be used to support the blood pressure (see Chapter 4). There have been many advances in our understanding of the pathogenesis of sepsis and the associated immune activation but our ability to manage the complications of sepsis has been little improved. Adrenal insufficiency is common in severe sepsis and treatment with low-dose hydrocortisone may reduce the duration of shock.

If the source of the infection is not clinically apparent, empirical antibacterial therapy is given to cover as wide a range of potential infecting organisms as possible. The prognosis is much worse if first-line drugs are ineffective. Suitable treatment would be with an antipseudomonal penicillin such as piperacillin with tazobactam or a broad-spectrum cephalosporin (e.g. cefotaxime, or ceftazidime if pseudomonal infection is suspected). A carbapenem such as meropenem or imipenem (with cilastatin) can be used if the infection was hospital-acquired. Metronidazole is added if anaerobic infection is suspected, or vancomycin if MRSA is suspected.

Immunocompromised and neutropenic individuals are at particularly high risk from septicaemia. A combination of gentamicin with a broad-spectrum penicillin, cephalosporin, piperacillin with tazobactam or meropenem can be given. Metronidazole is usually added if anaerobic infection is suspected; flucloxacillin or vancomycin is added if Gram-positive infection is suspected. Failure to respond to such triple therapy within 48 hours may indicate a fungal infection, for which amphotericin (see below) can be added.

Infective endocarditis

The majority of cases of infective endocarditis are caused by bacterial pathogens, most commonly oral streptococci, followed by enterococci, *S. aureus* and coagulase-negative staphylococci. Endocarditis usually arises on the endothelial surface of a pre-existing heart defect (e.g. valvular heart defect, ventricular septal defect) or on a prosthetic heart valve. It arises when micro-organisms enter the bloodstream and become established on the endocardium, where they may adhere to pre-existing fibrin–platelet vegetations. Bacteria enter the blood during dental procedures, vigorous teeth cleaning or some surgical procedures.

Untreated infection can destroy the infected heart valve and produce severe haemodynamic disturbance. Systemic complications can also arise from embolisation of vegetation from the valve, from bacteraemia, or through immune complexes that form in response to the infection.

When infection is suspected, blood cultures must be taken and empirical antimicrobial treatment started. Prior to identification of the organism, treatment is usually started with intravenous flucloxacillin or benzylpenicillin combined with low-dose gentamicin. If the organism is sensitive to penicillin, the benzylpenicillin is continued for 4 weeks and the gentamicin stopped after 2 weeks. Vancomycin and rifampicin are substituted for the penicillin in people with penicillin allergy when there is infection on a prosthetic heart valve or if MRSA is suspected.

Antibacterial prophylaxis is no longer recommended prior to procedures such as dental treatment, since there is no good evidence that it prevents endocarditis.

Meningitis

Bacterial meningitis is a medical emergency. The most likely organism depends on the age of the person (Table 51.4). Empirical selection of therapy is usually necessary and treatment should be started at the first suspicion of bacterial meningitis. A single dose of benzylpenicillin can be given if the person is outside hospital, but cefotaxime (with the addition of amoxicillin for those over 50 years old) is the preferred treatment in hospital. Chloramphenicol is an option for those who have an allergy to both penicillin and cephalosporins. Treatment is given for 7 days for meningococcus and 10 days for *H. influenzae* or pneumococcus. Rifampicin is given for 2–4 days before hospital discharge if the meningitis was caused by meningococcus or *H. influenzae*. Close contacts of people with meningococcal or *H. influenzae* type B meningitis are usually given rifampicin as prophylaxis against infection.

Dexamethasone should be considered immediately and no later than 12 hours after starting the antibacterial. This reduces the frequency of neurological complications.

Table 51.4 Organisms commonly causing bacterial meningitis

Age	Organism
<1 month	Group B streptococci
1 month to 4 years	*Haemophilus influenzae*
>4 years to young adult	*Neisseria meningitidis* (meningococcus)
Older adults	*Streptococcus pneumoniae* (pneumococcus)

Tuberculosis

M. tuberculosis readily develops resistance to single-drug therapy. Three or four drugs are used for the first 2 months ('initial phase') to rapidly reduce the bacterial population prior to information on bacterial sensitivities becoming available, following which treatment is continued with two drugs for a further 4 months ('continuation phase') to achieve a cure. In some cases, more prolonged treatment may be necessary, especially for tuberculous meningitis or resistant mycobacteria.

A standard regimen in the United Kingdom includes rifampicin, isoniazid, ethambutol and pyrazinamide for the initial phase (or until bacterial sensitivities are known), followed by rifampicin and isoniazid (preferably in a combination preparation) for the continuation phase. More prolonged treatment is sometimes necessary for cavitating lung disease or slow clearance of bacteria from the sputum. Ethambutol is not used to treat young children because of the difficulty in monitoring for eye toxicity.

Streptomycin is used in some countries in the initial phase of treatment or if resistance to isoniazid is known. Thiacetazone is often used with isoniazid and initially streptomycin in countries that cannot afford rifampicin. Adherence to the treatment regimen can be a major problem in the treatment of tuberculosis; combination tablets are often used to maximise adherence. In developed countries, directly observed treatment (DOT) has been instituted to improve adherence. This can result in major improvements in mycobacterial eradication rates.

Multi-drug-resistant tuberculosis (with resistance to at least rifampicin and isoniazid) is becoming more common, and new treatment strategies are needed to deal with emerging strains of *M. tuberculosis*. There are also increasing problems with the treatment of tuberculosis in people with HIV infection. This reflects the propensity for interactions among the antiretroviral drugs and antituberculous therapy as well as overlapping unwanted effects.

FUNGAL INFECTIONS

Fungi (including yeasts) usually infect skin or superficial mucous membranes but less commonly can involve internal organs. Most fungal infections occur because of an underlying defect in host immunity. Fungi grow more readily in immunocompromised individuals or following the suppression of normal flora by antibacterials. Good hygiene and the avoidance of sources of infection are important complementary approaches to the use of antifungal drugs.

Compared with antibacterial drugs, fewer drugs have been developed that have activity against fungi, and many of these are toxic to humans. A simplified outline of the mechanisms of action of antifungal drugs is shown in Fig. 51.5.

ANTIFUNGAL DRUGS

Drugs that impair membrane barrier function

Polyenes

Examples

amphotericin, nystatin

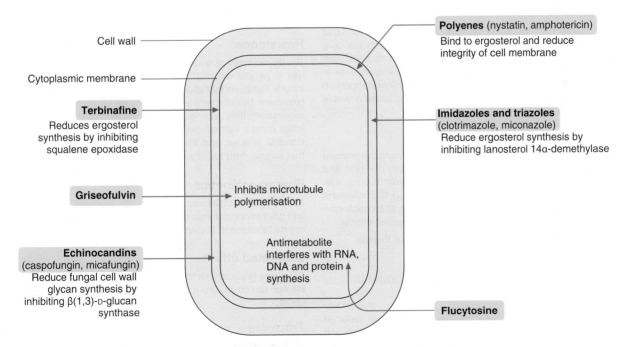

Fig. 51.5 **Sites of action of antifungal drugs.** Polyenes, imidazoles, triazoles and terbinafine target the synthesis or function of ergosterol, which is found in fungal cell membranes in place of cholesterol; the echinofungins inhibit fungal cell wall synthesis and griseofulvin impairs the polymerisation of fungal microtubules.

Mechanism of action

Polyenes bind to ergosterol in the cell membrane of fungi and form aqueous pores that promote leakage of intracellular ions and disrupt active transport mechanisms dependent on membrane potential. They can be fungistatic or fungicidal.

Spectrum of activity

Nystatin is particularly effective for infections with *Candida* species. Amphotericin is active against all common fungi that cause systemic infection (*Candida*, *Aspergillus*, *Mucor* and *Cryptococcus* species).

Resistance

Acquired resistance to polyene antifungals is rare but can occur in immunosuppressed people. Fungi develop mutations that enhance synthetic pathways for alternative sterols that replace ergosterol within the cell membrane and are unaffected by polyenes.

Pharmacokinetics

Nystatin is too toxic for systemic use and is not absorbed from the gastrointestinal tract. It is therefore used topically for *Candida albicans* infections – for example, as creams for skin infection, as vaginal pessaries or orally for buccal and bowel infections.

Amphotericin is poorly absorbed from the gut and is given intravenously for the treatment of serious systemic fungal infections. Amphotericin binds to steroids in human tissues and is released slowly and eliminated via the biliary tract and kidneys. It has a very long half-life (about 2 days).

Lipid delivery vehicles for amphotericin have been developed to reduce its nephrotoxicity. These formulations alter drug distribution and help to concentrate the drug at the site of infection, with the lipid component probably being cleared from the blood by mononuclear phagocytes. Lipid formulations include liposomal spheres (in which the drug is dissolved in phospholipid membrane vesicles) and lipid complexes (in which the phospholipid components exist in ribbons interspersed with amphotericin). A colloidal dispersion of lipid discs incorporating amphotericin is no longer available in the United Kingdom.

Unwanted effects

Nystatin is virtually free of both toxic and allergic unwanted effects when used topically. Used buccally for oral and perioral infection, it can cause nausea. Host toxicity with amphotericin is due to binding of the drug to cholesterol rather than ergosterol. Intravenous infusion of amphotericin is commonly associated with several unwanted effects.

- Fever and rigors during the first week of therapy.
- Anorexia, nausea, vomiting, diarrhoea.
- Headache, muscle and joint pain.
- Anaphylaxis, which makes a test dose advisable.
- Anaemia.
- Dose-related nephrotoxicity, which is the major limiting factor in treatment. It presents with reduced glomerular filtration rate and produces hypokalaemia and hypomagnesaemia through tubular leakage of K^+ and Mg^{2+}. Lipid formulations substantially reduce the risk of nephrotoxicity and are particularly useful to treat people with pre-existing renal impairment.

- Arrhythmias.
- Hearing loss, diplopia, convulsions, peripheral neuropathy.

Drugs that inhibit cell wall synthesis

Imidazoles

clotrimazole, econazole, miconazole

Mechanism of action

The imidazoles inhibit lanosterol 14α-demethylase, a form of cytochrome P450 that participates in the conversion of lanosterol to ergosterol. Reduced ergosterol synthesis alters fungal cell membrane fluidity, reduces the activity of membrane-associated enzymes and increases cell-wall permeability. Accumulation of ergosterol precursors in the cell causes growth arrest.

Spectrum of activity

Imidazoles are generally used in topical formulations for superficial fungal infections, for example of the mouth, skin and vagina. They are active against a wide variety of filamentous fungi including many *Candida* species, but they are less active against *Candida krusei*. Clotrimazole, econazole amd miconazole are used for vaginal candidiasis and for dermatophyte infections such as ringworm (tinea); the causative fungi of the latter vary geographically but generally are *Trichophyton*, *Microsporon* or *Epidermophyton* species. Miconazole is also used topically for oral infections and can be given orally for intestinal infections as it is poorly absorbed from the gut.

Resistance

The development of resistance is rare except during long-term use in people with AIDS. The mechanisms of resistance include mutations that alter the structure of the target enzyme, lanosterol 14α-demethylase, or increase its transcriptional expression; they also include the development of active efflux pumps that remove drug from the cell, especially in *Candida* species, and the generation of bypass pathways that reduce drug toxicity.

Pharmacokinetics

Absorption of imidazoles from the skin, mucosal surfaces and gastrointestinal tract is poor, but the absorbed fractions are metabolised in the liver with half-lives of 8–30 hours.

Unwanted effects

These are unusual with topical formulations, although local irritation can occur. Oral miconazole can cause gastrointestinal upset.

Triazoles

fluconazole, itraconazole, voriconazole

Mechanism of action and spectrum of activity

The triazoles have a similar mechanism of action and spectrum of activity to the imidazoles (see above). Fluconazole is used for candidiasis and for cryptococcal infection. Itraconazole is used for mucocutaneous candidiasis and for dermatophyte infections, such as pityriasis versicolor (caused by an organism known as *Malassezia furfur* or *Pityosporum orbiculare*) and tinea corporis or pedis (ringworms). Voriconazole is an 'extended-spectrum' triazole used for invasive aspergillosis, and serious infections caused by *Scedosporium* species, *Fusarium* species, or invasive fluconazole-resistant *C. krusei* and *Candida glabrata*.

Resistance

As with imidazoles, the development of resistance to triazoles is uncommon except during long-term use in people with AIDS. Resistance to fluconazole is more prevalent than for the other triazoles. The mechanisms of resistance are also similar to those of the imidazoles, including enhanced drug efflux and target enzyme modifications.

Pharmacokinetics

Oral absorption of triazoles is good. Formulations are also available for intravenous use. The triazoles are metabolised in the liver and have long half-lives (6–35 hours). Fluconazole penetrates well into the CSF, which is useful for the treatment of cryptococcal meningitis.

Unwanted effects

- Nausea, abdominal pain and diarrhoea.
- Headache, dizziness.
- Photosensitivity with voriconazole.
- Abnormalities of liver function and, occasionally, hepatitis or cholestasis. These are more common during prolonged treatment with itraconazole. Monitoring of liver function during systemic treatment is essential.
- Increased risk of heart failure with itraconazole. The mechanism of its negative inotropic effect is not known.
- Rashes, including Stevens–Johnson syndrome.

Terbinafine

Mechanism of action and use

Terbinafine is an allylamine compound that inhibits squalene epoxidase, the enzyme that converts squalene to ergosterol in the cell wall. The drug therefore impairs fungal cell wall synthesis, and the intracellular accumulation of squalene is probably cytotoxic (see Fig. 51.5). It is used topically for the treatment of dermatophyte infections of the nails and systemically for ringworm infections.

Resistance

Resistance is rare, particularly in dermatophyte infections, but may occur owing to enhanced efflux pump activity or mutations in squalene epoxidase.

Pharmacokinetics

Terbinafine penetrates well into the stratum corneum and hair follicles after topical use. After oral administration, it is metabolised in the liver and has a long half-life (11–17 hours).

Unwanted effects

These are unlikely with topical use of the drug, but oral use may cause:

- nausea, taste disturbance, anorexia, abdominal discomfort and diarrhea,
- headache,
- rashes, which are occasionally severe,
- fatigue, myalgia, arthralgia.

Echinocandins

anidulafungin, caspofungin, micafungin

Mechanism of action

Echinocandins target the glucans that are found in fungal cell walls but not in human cells (see Fig. 51.5). They inhibit the fungal enzyme β(1,3)-D-glucan synthase and prevent production of the main structural polymer in the fungal cell wall. Echinocandins are used to treat invasive candidiasis; caspofungin is also used as a second-line drug in invasive aspergillosis.

Resistance

This is uncommon at present, but in *Candida* species resistance can occur from mutations encoding structural changes in the glucan synthase target enzyme, which no longer binds the drug, and from enhanced activity of efflux pumps.

Pharmacokinetics

Oral absorption of echinocandins is limited and they are given only by intravenous infusion. They have high affinity for plasma proteins and their distribution into the CSF is poor. Elimination is by hepatic metabolism or slow spontaneous degradation with very long half-lives up to 40–50 hours.

Unwanted effects

- Nausea, vomiting, abdominal pain, diarrhoea.
- Dyspnoea.
- Flushing, fever.
- Headache.
- Rashes.
- Hypokalaemia, hypomagnesaemia.
- Hepatobiliary disturbance.

Drugs that inhibit macromolecule synthesis

Flucytosine

Mechanism of action and use

Flucytosine is converted to 5-fluorouracil (5-FU) selectively in fungal cells by cytosine deaminase. 5-FU is an antimetabolite that competes with uracil for incorporation into fungal RNA; it is metabolised to compounds that inhibit enzymes involved in DNA synthesis (see Fig. 51.5).

Flucytosine is active only against yeasts such as *Candida*, *Aspergillus* and *Cryptococcus* species. For systemic infections including refractory invasive candidiasis and cryptococcal meningitis, it is used in combination with amphotericin.

Resistance

Intrinsic resistance of some yeast strains to flucytosine is due to impaired uptake of the drug. Acquired resistance arises readily from mutations that produce a deficiency of cytosine deaminase or through excessive synthesis of uracil, which competes with the drug.

Pharmacokinetics

Flucytosine is available only for intravenous use. It is mainly eliminated unchanged in the urine and has a short half-life (3 hours).

Unwanted effects

- Nausea, abdominal pain, diarrhoea.
- Rashes.
- Bone marrow suppression.

Drugs that interact with microtubules

Griseofulvin

Mechanism of action and use

Griseofulvin binds persistently to keratin in skin and nails and makes them resistant to dermatophyte infection. It inhibits dermatophyte mitosis by impairing the polymerisation of microtubule protein (see Fig. 51.5). Griseofulvin is orally active against dermatophytes such as *Microsporum*, *Epidermophyton* and *Trichophyton* species; it is not used topically. Although effective for refractory or widespread dermatophyte infections, it has been largely superseded by newer antifungals, particularly for nail infections. It remains the drug of choice for trichophyton infections in children.

Resistance

Intrinsic resistance to griseofulvin is related to greater energy-dependent export of the drug from the fungal cell.

Pharmacokinetics

Griseofulvin shows variable absorption from the gut. It is selectively concentrated in skin and nail beds; only low concentrations are found in plasma. Elimination of the unbound fraction is by hepatic metabolism and the half-life is long (10–21 hours).

Unwanted effects

- Nausea, vomiting, diarrhoea.
- Headache.
- Skin rashes, urticaria.

TREATMENT OF SPECIFIC FUNGAL INFECTIONS

Aspergillus

Aspergillus species can cause an invasive fungal infection that most commonly affects the lung. However, in immunocompromised individuals it can invade more widely and infect the heart, brain, sinuses and skin. The treatment of choice is voriconazole, which is more effective and less toxic than amphotericin. If this fails, itraconazole can be used. Caspofungin, or another echinocandin, is reserved for infections that have failed to respond to standard treatments or for those people who cannot tolerate the other drugs.

Candida

Amphotericin or nystatin is often used for oral candidiasis. If there is oropharyngeal disease that is refractory to topical treatment, an absorbed drug such as fluconazole or itraconazole is used orally. Vulvovaginal infection is treated with cream and pessaries; imidazole drugs such as clotrimazole are usually the first choice. Nystatin is an alternative for vulvovaginal candidiasis, but it stains clothing yellow. For recurrent vulvovaginal infections, oral fluconazole or itraconazole should be taken once a week for 6 months. Superficial candidal infections of the skin are treated topically with cream, usually containing an imidazole. Terbinafine or nystatin can also be used topically.

Invasive candidiasis occurs mainly as a hospital-acquired infection, particularly in people who have had abdominal surgery, parenteral nutrition, multiple antibacterial drugs or central vascular lines. *Candida albicans* is still the single most common organism, but *C. krusei*, *C. glabrata* and *Candida parapsilosis* are increasingly common. Amphotericin is the treatment of choice, sometimes combined with fluconazole. Caspofungin is an alternative.

Cryptococcus

Infection with *Cryptococcus* species usually occurs in people who are immunocompromised. It can cause life-threatening meningitis and is treated with intravenous amphotericin together with flucytosine. Fluconazole is an alternative and can also be given orally for prophylaxis against relapse.

Skin and nail infections

Topical therapy is usually suitable for infections with most dermatophytes. Fungal infection of the scalp (tinea capitis), body (tinea corporis), groin (tinea cruris), hand (tinea manuum), foot (tinea pedis) or nail (tinea unguium) will respond to most azoles. Griseofulvin is usually reserved for treatment of scalp infections. Nail infection usually requires systemic treatment with terbinafine or itraconazole.

Pityriasis versicolor can be treated topically or orally with itraconazole or with oral fluconazole.

Prophylaxis in immunocompromised individuals

Individuals who are immunocompromised are at greater risk of fungal infection. Prophylaxis is often given with oral fluconazole, since this has better oral absorption than most azoles.

VIRAL INFECTIONS

Viruses are small infective particles consisting of either DNA or RNA inside a protein coating (capsule), which in some viruses may be further surrounded by a lipoprotein coating. The proteins can have antigenic properties. Viruses lack any inherent metabolic machinery and must use the host's metabolic processes to replicate. Viruses access host cells after binding to recognition sites that are endogenous receptors for normal cellular constituents – for example, adrenoceptors, cytokine receptors, glycoproteins and so on (Fig. 51.6). Drugs that interfere with host cell-membrane cytokine receptors, such as chemokine (C-C motif) receptor 5 (CCR5) (see below) and surface glycoproteins will inhibit viral entry into host cells and interrupt virus replication.

The host will normally eliminate the virus by killing the infected cell. Cytotoxic T-lymphocytes recognise the viral surface proteins that are expressed by infected cells. The host can also produce antibodies that bind to and inactivate virus particles extracellularly. Vaccination is designed to generate this response.

Because viruses utilise the host's metabolic processes, it is difficult to damage the virus without also damaging the host. Importantly, antiviral drugs are effective only while the virus is replicating, so the earlier they are given in the course of the infection the more likely they are to be effective. An

outline of the replication of RNA and DNA viruses is shown in Fig. 51.7 (see also Fig. 51.6). Since the replicative mechanisms involved may be distinctive to one type of virus, some antiviral drugs are specific for a particular class of virus.

New antiviral drugs are being introduced into clinical practice at an increasing rate. Drugs are available to treat infection by RNA viruses (e.g. HIV, hepatitis C and influenza viruses) and DNA viruses (e.g. herpesviruses, cytomegalovirus and hepatitis B virus). Most of these drugs work by disturbing various steps in the replicative pathways of the virus. Because of the development of resistance and the variability in viral sensitivity to drugs, it is sometimes necessary to use drug combinations that target different processes in the virus replication.

Resistance to antiviral drugs occurs readily. This relates to the high rate of natural occurrence of mutations in the viral genome and production of quasi-species of the virus. Viral polymerases have a high inherent error rate (especially RNA viruses), and viruses tolerate a large number of nucleoside mutations without losing their infectivity. Normally the large variety of viral quasi-species will be dominated by the variant most selected for survival; therefore use of an antiviral drug will select for growth of resistant variants.

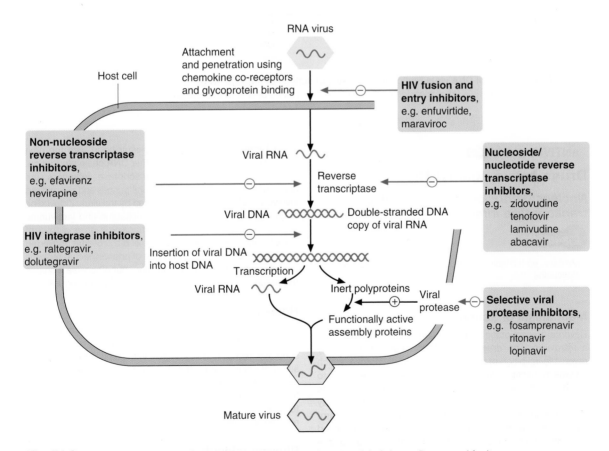

Fig. 51.6 Principles of RNA virus replication and sites of action of antiviral drugs. Drugs used for human immunodeficiency virus (HIV) infection are nucleoside/nucleotide inhibitors of HIV reverse transcriptase, or target other HIV proteins (integrase, protease) or the entry of HIV into host cells.

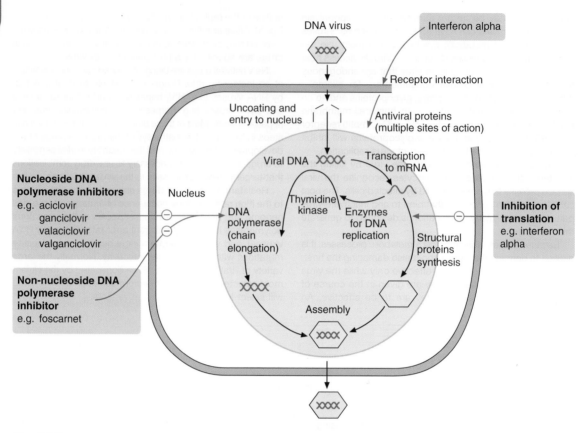

Fig. 51.7 **Principles of DNA virus replication and sites of actions of antiviral drugs.** Drugs used for infection with herpes viruses and cytomegalovirus are nucleoside or non-nucleoside inhibitors of viral DNA polymerase.

ANTIVIRAL DRUGS

Drugs active against HIV

Nucleoside/nucleotide HIV reverse transcriptase inhibitors

abacavir, emtricitabine, lamivudine, tenofovir disoproxil, zidovudine

Mechanism of action

Reverse transcriptase inhibitors are active against HIV, a retrovirus. The drugs inhibit RNA virus replication by reversible inhibition of viral HIV reverse transcriptase, which reverse transcribes viral RNA into DNA for insertion into the host DNA sequence (see Fig. 51.6). The nucleos(t)ide reverse transcriptase inhibitors (NRTIs) are activated by phosphorylation in two steps to the 5′-triphosphate form by cellular kinases. Inhibition of viral replication is achieved by competitive binding of the activated drug to the enzyme–template–primer complex in place of the natural 5′-deoxynucleoside triphosphates. The drugs lack the 3′-hydroxyl group on the deoxyribose moiety required for

normal formation of a phosphodiester bond with the next nucleotide, so they terminate further DNA chain elongation.

The nucleoside reverse transcriptase inhibitors are analogues of precursors of the natural purines and pyrimidines involved in DNA transcription initiated by the virus. Zidovudine is an analogue of thymidine, emtricitabine and lamivudine are analogues of cytidine, and abacavir is an analogue of deoxyguanosine. Tenofovir disoproxil is a pro-drug converted to tenofovir, a nucleotide analogue of adenosine that requires only diphosphorylation for activation, but otherwise it shares the mechanism of action of the nucleoside analogues.

Resistance

Resistant quasi-species emerge within weeks or months by mutations affecting the drug-binding site on reverse transcriptase, resulting in an increase in the affinity for the natural substrate compared with the drug. A second mechanism of resistance is enhanced excision of the incorporated drug from the DNA chain by pyrophosphorolysis, allowing elongation to continue normally. Because of the rapid development of resistance, multiple drug therapy is used to treat HIV infection.

Pharmacokinetics

These drugs are almost completely absorbed from the gut. Elimination of abacavir and zidovudine is mainly by hepatic metabolism and the half-lives are short (1–2 hours). Emtricitabine, lamivudine and tenofovir are mainly eliminated unchanged by the kidney, with half-lives in the range 1–17 hours.

Unwanted effects

These are often so severe that they lead to withdrawal of therapy. They are probably related to inhibition of host mitochondrial enzymes, with impaired generation of intracellular adenosine triphosphate (ATP) leading to multiple organ disorders.

- Neutropenia and anaemia are the most frequent unwanted effects (usually occurring in individuals with advanced AIDS).
- Nausea, vomiting, diarrhoea, abdominal pain.
- Headache, insomnia.
- Myalgia or myositis, especially with high doses.
- Severe, potentially life-threatening hepatomegaly with steatosis and lactic acidosis.
- Pancreatitis.
- Lipodystrophy syndrome with fat redistribution (loss of subcutaneous fat, buffalo hump, breast enlargement), insulin resistance and dyslipidaemia; this may be due to inhibition of regulatory proteins in adipocytes.

Non-nucleoside HIV reverse transcriptase inhibitors

efavirenz, nevirapine, rilpivirine

Mechanism of action and resistance

The non-nucleoside reverse transcriptase inhibitors (NNRTIs) bind directly to HIV-1 reverse transcriptase at a hydrophobic site remote from the enzyme's active site to produce a conformational change that prevents substrate binding. They have greater antiviral activity than nucleoside analogue inhibitors and are better tolerated. Resistance emerges rapidly by single point mutations in reverse transcriptase that reduce binding or access of the drugs to the hydrophobic binding site unless they are used in combination with at least two other antiretroviral drugs.

Pharmacokinetics

Oral absorption of nevirapine and rilpivirine is good, while that of efavirenz is variable and incomplete. They are metabolised by hepatic CYP3A4 and 'CYP3A4 and CYP2B6 and also induce these enzymes' also induce these enzymes. They have very long half-lives of about 2 days.

Unwanted effects

- Rashes (severe in 10%), especially with nevirapine.
- Nausea, vomiting, abdominal pain, diarrhoea.
- Headache, drowsiness, fatigue.
- Depression and psychiatric disturbances with efavirenz and rilpivirine.
- Hepatotoxicity with nevirapine, which can cause potentially fatal fulminant hepatitis.
- Multiple interactions with drugs metabolised by hepatic CYP3A4 and CTP2B6, including HIV protease inhibitors, antifungal drugs and proton pump inhibitors.

HIV protease inhibitors

atazanavir, darunavir, fosamprenavir, indinavir, lopinavir, ritonavir

Mechanism of action

In HIV infection there are some steps in viral replication that differ from the mRNA translation processes in host cells. In the virus, RNA is translated into inert precursor polyproteins rather than the functional proteins that are the products of host cells. Viral HIV-1 protease cleaves these precursor polyproteins to the structural proteins and enzymes required by the virus for budding from the host membrane (see Fig. 51.6). HIV protease inhibitors block the active site of the viral protease and cause the production of defective virus particles that are less infectious. They do not affect virus activity in host cells that are already infected.

Resistance

Resistance occurs by mutations affecting the amino acid sequence of the HIV protease target. Multiple mutations are required for high-level resistance, but over one-third of the amino acid residues in HIV protease can be changed without diminishing viral capacity for replication. High plasma drug concentrations delay the onset of resistance, as does the combination of a protease inhibitor with two reverse transcriptase inhibitors. Sequential use of more than one protease inhibitor encourages high-level resistance.

Pharmacokinetics

Oral absorption varies between the protease inhibitors. All are metabolised by, and inhibit, CYP3A4 in the liver. They have half-lives in the range 2–10 hours.

Unwanted effects

- Nausea, vomiting, abdominal pain, diarrhoea.
- Lipodystrophy syndrome (see nucleoside HIV reverse transcriptase inhibitors).
- Hepatic dysfunction.
- Nephrolithiasis with indinavir.
- Pancreatitis.
- Circumoral and peripheral paraesthesiae with ritonavir.
- Drug interactions (see Chapter 56): inhibition of the cytochrome P450 enzyme CYP3A4 can enhance the unwanted effects of protease inhibitors; the concurrent use of inducers of CYP3A4 can lower plasma concentrations of the protease inhibitor and encourage viral resistance. Conversely, inhibition of CYP3A4 by a low dose of ritonavir can increase the clinical effect of other protease inhibitors (boosted protease inhibition), a useful action that allows less frequent dosing with the other drug. Ritonavir also inhibits the metabolism of drugs such as warfarin (see Chapter 11) and carbamazepine (see Chapter 23). The use of protease inhibitors with simvastatin (see Chapter 48) should be avoided because of an increased risk of myopathy.

HIV fusion–entry inhibitor

enfuvirtide

Mechanism of action

To enter a host cell, HIV fuses with the host cell membrane. This fusion is facilitated by a conformational change in a viral glycoprotein, gp41, in the viral cell membrane. Enfuvirtide is a 36-amino-acid peptidomimetic that binds to the gp41 glycoprotein and prevents the conformational change, blocking HIV fusion and entry into host cells. Enfuvirtide is used when there is resistance or intolerance to other antiretroviral drugs.

Resistance

This occurs by gene mutation that modifies the gp41 glycoprotein target of the drug.

Pharmacokinetics

Enfuvirtide is given twice daily by subcutaneous injection. It is metabolised by hydrolysis to its constituent amino acids and has a half-life of 4 hours.

Unwanted effects

- Injection-site reactions.
- Hypersensitivity reactions: rash, fever, nausea, vomiting, chills, rigors, low blood pressure, respiratory distress, glomerulonephritis, and raised liver enzymes.
- Pancreatitis, gastro-oesophageal reflux disease, anorexia, weight loss.
- Peripheral neuropathy, tremor, anxiety, nightmares, vertigo.
- Diabetes mellitus.

Chemokine (C-C motif) receptor 5 co-receptor antagonist

maraviroc

Mechanism of action

CCR5 is a receptor for several chemokines, including RANTES (regulated upon activation, normal T-cell expressed and secreted) and macrophage inflammatory proteins MIP-1α and MIP-1β. It is expressed on many cells, including T cells, macrophages, dendritic cells and microglia. CCR5 also acts as a viral co-receptor that facilitates entry of HIV into the cell. Some HIV strains use other chemokine receptors such as CCR4, or both CCR4 and CCR5, to access cells. HIV strains which use CCR5 are predominant early in the infection. Maraviroc selectively binds to CCR5 and prevents interaction with CCR5-tropic strains of HIV, inhibiting their entry into the cell. It has no effect on viruses that use CCR4 or are dual-tropic for CCR4 and CCR5. Maraviroc is used in combination with other antiretroviral drugs for individuals who have already received other antiretroviral treatment. Resistance is uncommon but may arise from changes in the viral envelope glycoproteins that interact with CCR5.

Pharmacokinetics

Maraviroc is only partially absorbed from the gut. It is metabolised in the liver and has a long half-life (14–18 hours).

Unwanted effects

- Nausea, diarrhoea, abdominal pain, anorexia, malaise.
- Upper respiratory tract infections, cough.
- Rashes.
- Depression, insomnia, headache.

HIV integrase inhibitors

elvitegravir, dolutegravir, raltegravir

Mechanism of action

Once inside a host cell, HIV integrates its DNA into the host genome by the action of a specific viral integrase. Elvitegravir, dolutegravir and raltegravir inhibit the integrase and prevent DNA strand transfer from the viral genome. They are used in combination with other antiretroviral drugs, particularly for viral strains resistant to other drugs. Elvitegravir is available only in a combination formulation with two NRTIs (emtricitabine and tenofovir disoproxil) or cobicistat, which has no intrinsic antiretroviral activity but boosts the activity of elvitegravir by inhibiting its breakdown by hepatic CYP3A4.

Resistance

This arises from mutations in the viral integrase drug target and currently occurs most commonly to raltegravir. Resistance to one integrase inhibitor confers cross-resistance to other integrase inhibitors.

Pharmacokinetics

The integrase inhibitors are well absorbed from the gut. They are excreted in the bile after glucuronide conjugation and unchanged in the urine. They have half-lives of 9–14 hours.

Unwanted effects

- Nausea, vomiting, diarrhoea, abdominal pain.
- Headache, dizziness, insomnia, abnormal dreams.
- Rashes, sometimes with fever, arthralgia, myalgia, angioedema and hepatitis.

Drugs for herpesvirus and cytomegalovirus infections

Nucleoside inhibitors of viral DNA polymerase

aciclovir, ganciclovir, valaciclovir, valganciclovir

Mechanism of action

Aciclovir and ganciclovir are guanosine analogues that are active against many DNA viruses by inhibiting the synthesis of viral DNA (see Fig. 51.7). They are activated by phosphorylation to a monophosphate by viral thymidine kinase; this initial dependence on a viral enzyme prevents cytotoxic effects in human cells. The monophosphorylated drug is then converted to a triphosphate by host intracellular kinases. The triphosphate derivatives of aciclovir and ganciclovir are potent inhibitors of viral DNA polymerase; this terminates viral DNA synthesis and thus inhibits viral replication (see Fig. 51.7).

Spectrum of activity

Aciclovir is most active against herpesviruses (both simplex and zoster). It is active against cytomegalovirus (CMV) only at high doses. Ganciclovir is also active against herpesviruses and has much greater activity than aciclovir against CMV, possibly because it is a better substrate for the CMV protein kinase which activates it.

Resistance

Viral mutants arise that are deficient in thymidine kinase or have alterations in viral DNA polymerase. Thymidine kinase-deficient mutants of herpesvirus usually develop in immunocompromised individuals – for example, those with AIDS or after bone marrow transplantation, when resistance rates average 5–10%.

Pharmacokinetics

Aciclovir can be given orally, intravenously or topically to the skin or eye. Absorption from the gut is poor. The drug is widely distributed, but concentrations in the CSF are low compared with those in plasma. Most is eliminated by the kidneys, and the half-life is 3 hours. Valaciclovir is an ester pro-drug of aciclovir with higher oral bioavailability.

Ganciclovir is given intravenously for acute infections since it is poorly absorbed from the gut; it penetrates into the CSF moderately well. It is eliminated by the kidney and has a half-life of 4 hours. Valganciclovir is an ester pro-drug of ganciclovir with better oral absorption.

Unwanted effects

Most unwanted effects occur with intravenous use and are much more frequent with ganciclovir than with aciclovir.

- Severe local phlebitis at an infusion site.
- Nausea, vomiting, abdominal pain, diarrhoea.
- Rashes, including photosensitivity.
- Headache, dizziness, confusion, convulsions.
- Nephrotoxicity is caused by crystallisation of aciclovir in the kidney. It can be limited by a high fluid intake.
- Bone marrow suppression is the most frequent serious unwanted effect with ganciclovir, with neutropenia occurring in up to 40% of people and thrombocytopenia less frequently.

Non-nucleoside inhibitors of viral DNA polymerase

foscarnet sodium

Mechanism of action

Foscarnet is an inorganic pyrophosphate compound that binds to the pyrophosphate-binding sites of viral DNA polymerase, inhibiting its role in DNA chain elongation. Affinity for the viral DNA polymerase is a hundred times greater than for the host cell DNA polymerase. Foscarnet does not rely on intracellular activation for its antiviral activities (see Fig. 51.7). It inhibits replication of CMV and herpes simplex virus.

Pharmacokinetics

Because foscarnet is a highly polar molecule, it is given only intravenously. Foscarnet is eliminated by the kidneys and has a half-life of about 5 hours.

Unwanted effects

- Nausea, vomiting, diarrhoea.
- Neutropenia.
- Headache, tremor, dizziness, mood disturbances.
- Nephrotoxicity, causing a rise in plasma creatinine; good hydration reduces kidney damage.

Drugs for treating hepatitis viruses

Drugs for treating hepatitis B and C virus infections include nucleoside/nucleotide analogues (entecavir, lamivudine, ribavirin, tenofovir disoproxil), protease inhibitors (bocepravir, telaprevir and others), inhibitors of other viral proteins (such as daclatasvir), and the cytokine interferon alpha. Ribavirin is also used to treat respiratory syncytial virus (RSV). Drug treatment of hepatitis virus infection is discussed in Chapter 36.

Drugs for treating influenza virus

M₂ ion channel inhibitors

amantadine

Amantadine is active only against influenza A and inhibits the transmembrane M_2 ion channel, which permits H^+ entry into the viral particle. This is required for uncoating of the virus once it has penetrated the host cell, so viral replication is inhibited. Amantadine is no longer recommended for influenza A; its use in Parkinson's disease is discussed in Chapter 24.

Neuraminidase inhibitors

oseltamivir, zanamivir

Mechanism of action

Influenza viruses carry two surface glycoproteins, a haemagglutinin and a neuraminidase. The haemagglutinin mediates entry of the virus into the host cell. Neuraminidase cleaves cellular-receptor sialic acid residues, to which newly formed viruses are attached as they bud from the infected cell. The released virions can then infect new cells. Neuraminidase inhibitors inhibit the neuraminidases of both influenza A and B and are effective against isolates resistant to amantadine.

Pharmacokinetics

Zanamivir is administered by inhalation; only 2% of the inhaled drug is absorbed; it is then excreted unchanged with a half-life of 2–5 hours. Oseltamivir is a more lipophilic molecule that is taken orally and is converted by hepatic esterases to the active oseltamivir carboxylate, which is excreted by the kidneys and has a half-life of 6–10 hours.

Unwanted effects

- Gastrointestinal disturbance with oseltamivir.
- Headache, fatigue, insomnia, dizziness with oseltamivir.
- Bronchospasm with inhaled zanamivir.

Immunomodulators

Interferon alpha

Interferon alpha is most often used in the treatment of chronic hepatitis B infection and is discussed in Chapter 36. Other clinical uses of interferon alpha include the treatment of:

- condylomata acuminata,
- AIDS-related Kaposi's sarcoma,
- hairy cell leukaemia,
- recurrent or metastatic renal cell carcinoma (see Chapter 52).

Palivizumab

Mechanism of action and use

Palivizumab is a humanised monoclonal antibody with potent neutralising and fusion-inhibiting activity against respiratory syncytial virus (RSV). RSV is a common cause of mild respiratory illness in infants but can produce more severe illness in premature infants or those with congenital heart disease or bronchopulmonary dysplasia. Palivizumab reduces the ability of RSV to replicate and infect cells by binding to an antigenic site on the surface of the virus particle. It can be given to at-risk children under the age of 2 years prior to commencement of the RSV season (October to April in the northern hemisphere) and monthly thereafter.

Pharmacokinetics

Palivizumab is given intramuscularly into the anterolateral aspect of the thigh. The routes of elimination are unknown; it has a very long half-life of about 20 days.

Unwanted effects

- Fever.
- Injection-site reactions.

TREATMENT OF SPECIFIC VIRAL INFECTIONS

HIV infection

Multi-drug therapy is essential for the treatment of HIV infection because of the rapid emergence of resistant strains. The most frequently used treatment regimens include two nucleoside analogue reverse transcriptase inhibitors (e.g. tenofovir with emtricitabine or abacavir with lamivudine) combined with either a protease inhibitor (e.g. atazanavir, darunavir or raltegravir) or a non-nucleoside reverse transcriptase inhibitor (e.g. efavirenz). A low dose of ritonavir is often added to the protease inhibitor (boosted protease therapy) to prolong its action by inhibiting its breakdown by CYP3A4 and simplify the dosing regimen. Such combinations are referred to as *highly active antiretroviral therapy* (HAART). HAART involves complex regimens that require adherence by the individual and careful assessment of the progress of viral suppression. Key principles include the following:

- Combination drug treatment should be started before substantial immunodeficiency is present. The goal is to suppress the virus before resistant mutants emerge or irreversible immune damage occurs. The optimal time to start treatment is not known but it should definitely be started when the CD4$^+$ T-lymphocyte count falls below 200×10^6/L. If this stage is missed, treatment is given when symptoms arise as a result of HIV infection.
- When resistance occurs, modification of drug therapy should involve the addition or change of at least two drugs. Resistance of the HIV virus persists indefinitely. However, if toxicity limits the tolerability of one drug, a single substitution of a similar drug is a reasonable option.
- Optimal treatment should reduce the viral load to below detectable limits and achieve a rise in CD4$^+$ lymphocyte count. This may take 6 months of optimal therapy.
- Failure to achieve full suppression of viral load should prompt a change in therapy if adherence is believed to be good. Poor adherence with therapy is likely to encourage the development of drug resistance (see above) and thus treatment failure. Drug therapy is ideally guided by patterns of resistance in the virus.
- The optimal duration of treatment is unclear, but withdrawal even when the CD4$^+$ T-cell count rises is probably associated with less favourable long-term outcomes.

Prophylaxis after accidental exposure to HIV may be required. The regimen depends on the level of risk: two drugs are often used for moderate-risk exposures or three drugs if the risk is high.

Varicella zoster virus infections

Varicella zoster virus (VZV) is a herpesvirus responsible for both chickenpox and shingles (herpes zoster). Shingles arises from reactivation of the virus, which lies dormant in a dorsal root ganglion after the primary chickenpox infection. Chickenpox is rarely treated with antiviral therapy, although the use of oral aciclovir reduces lesion formation and results in quicker healing.

Herpes zoster is most commonly found in the elderly and in immunosuppressed people. The rash is often preceded by pain for 1–4 days. Complications of infection occur in 15–20% of people who develop herpes zoster and include meningoencephalitis, motor nerve paralysis, ocular complications and post-herpetic neuralgia. Oral antiviral drug therapy reduces pain and accelerates healing. It must be given while the virus is still replicating and therefore started within 72 hours of the onset of the rash. Oral aciclovir or valaciclovir are often used and are particularly indicated for those aged over 50 years (who are at greater risk of complications), for ophthalmic infections or in immunosuppressed people. The use of aciclovir has little effect on the risk of developing post-herpetic neuralgia but does reduce the risk of motor nerve damage. Corticosteroids such as prednisolone used as an adjunctive treatment to antiviral therapy reduce pain and produce more rapid healing of lesions but do not prevent the development of post-herpetic neuralgia. Analgesics are often required in the early phases of zoster, and post-herpetic neuralgia may require specific therapy (see Chapter 19).

Herpes simplex virus infections

Herpes simplex virus exists in two forms: type 1 produces either oral or genital ulceration and type 2 produces genital ulceration. Oral herpes simplex infection will respond to early topical application of aciclovir. Primary genital herpes produces multiple painful lesions and responds to oral aciclovir or valaciclovir given for 7–10 days. Recurrent lesions occur from reactivation of latent virus in the dorsal root ganglia, producing symptoms that are usually less severe than with primary episodes. After initial therapy with aciclovir or valaciclovir for up to 3 days, continuous suppressive therapy can be given to prevent further relapses.

Cytomegalovirus infection

CMV infection is common and usually produces mild symptoms. However, it can be devastating in immunosuppressed individuals. Troublesome complications in this group include retinitis (which can threaten sight), gastrointestinal manifestations (including oesophagitis, gastritis, cholecystitis or colitis), pneumonia and CNS involvement.

Intravenous ganciclovir is the treatment of choice for severe manifestations of CMV infection. Foscarnet can be used as an alternative to ganciclovir. For CMV retinitis, oral valganciclovir is used both for treatment and to prevent relapse. Oral valganciclovir or valaciclovir are given for the prevention of CMV infection, especially in renal transplant and bone marrow transplant recipients in whom CMV pneumonia is a major potential complication. Combined therapy with ganciclovir and CMV immunoglobulin may be more effective than ganciclovir alone for treatment of pneumonia in this situation.

Influenza

The use of a neuraminidase inhibitor, such as zanamivir or oseltamivir, reduces the duration of uncomplicated influenza by about 1 day. Treatment must be started within 48 hours of the onset of an influenza-like illness. People who are at greater risk of complications of influenza include those with chronic respiratory disease, significant cardiovascular disease, chronic renal disease, diabetes mellitus or those who are immunocompromised. However, there is little evidence that these drugs prevent the complications of influenza. Neuraminidase inhibitors are also effective for the prevention of influenza during an epidemic, reducing the likelihood of developing the illness by 70–90%. They should be considered for high-risk individuals who have not been vaccinated and who can be treated within 48 hours of contact with someone who has an influenza-like illness. Such prophylaxis is not a substitute for an effective vaccination campaign.

Viral hepatitis

This is discussed in Chapter 36.

Respiratory syncytial virus

RSV most commonly causes respiratory infections in children under 2 years old. It causes bronchiolitis and increased airway reactivity with wheezing. Treatment is usually symptomatic, but severe infection is sometimes treated with ribavirin. Palivizumab is given to prevent serious lower respiratory tract disease from RSV in children under 2 years old who are at high risk of complications.

PROTOZOAL INFECTIONS

MALARIA

Five species of the protozoan *Plasmodium* produce malaria in humans: *P. vivax*, *P. ovale* (two subspecies), *P. knowlesi*, *P. malariae* and *P. falciparum*. The motile infective forms of the parasite, sporozoites, are generated by repeated division of oocysts in the body of the infected female *Anopheles* mosquito (the vector) and transferred in the mosquito's saliva into the host's circulation during a blood meal (only female mosquitoes feed on blood). The parasite is rapidly sequestered in the host's liver and matures to tissue schizonts, which divide asexually to form merozoites (Fig. 51.8). When the pre-erythrocytic (liver) cycle is complete after 5–16 days, 10,000–40,000 merozoites escape into the blood and invade erythrocytes. *P. vivax* and *P. ovale* may continue to multiply in the liver, but *P. malariae*, *P. knowlesi* and *P. falciparum* do not.

Merozoites released from the liver then undergo the erythrocytic cycle, multiplying asexually in erythrocytes and using haemoglobin as the main source of nutrition. Infected erythrocytes rupture (haemolyse) and release merozoites to invade other erythrocytes. Some merozoites in the plasma differentiate into male and female gametocytes. A mosquito biting an infected individual ingests gametocytes, which then go through a sexual development cycle in the mosquito to form sporozoites.

Release of merozoites from erythrocytes every 2 or 3 days causes repeated bouts of tertian or quartan fever in humans. Premonitory clinical symptoms of malaria include chills; nausea, vomiting and headache are common. A fever follows, and the attack concludes with sweating. *Plasmodium falciparum* produces the most severe symptoms (malignant tertian malaria) because high levels of parasitaemia cause agglutination of red cells, which produces capillary thrombosis, especially in the brain, leading to cerebral malaria.

Because *P. vivax* and *P. ovale* can continue to multiply in the liver as hypnozoites, they form a reservoir of parasites that are difficult to eradicate and can emerge to produce relapses months or years after the initial infection. Drugs that treat only the erythrocytic phase will not produce a radical cure (elimination of all parasites), and relapsing infection can occur. Although *P. falciparum*, *P. malariae* and *P. knowlesi* do not have persistent liver forms, disease can recrudesce if parasites are not completely eliminated from the blood.

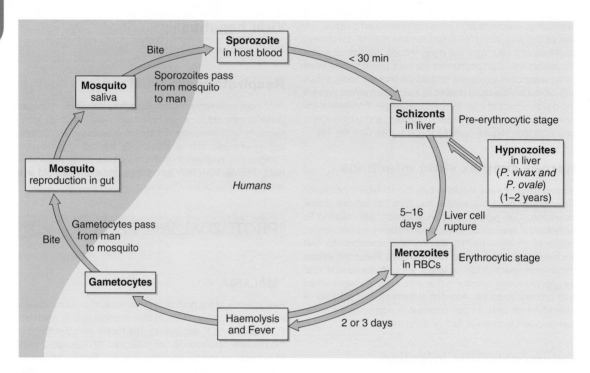

Fig. 51.8 **Life-cycle of the malarial parasite.** Most antimalarial drugs kill the *Plasmodium* parasites that cause repeated cycles of red blood cell (RBC) lysis and fever (erythrocytic stage). Primaquine kills parasites of *P. vivax* and *P. ovale* (hypnozoites) dormant in the liver (pre-erythrocytic stage).

Antimalarial drugs

Chloroquine

Mechanism of action and resistance

Chloroquine is a 4-aminoquinoline compound that interferes with the haem detoxification pathway in malarial parasites. Toxic haem monomers from plasmodial digestion of haemoglobin within infected erythrocytes are normally polymerised into inert biocrystals of haemozoin. Chloroquine, a basic drug, becomes trapped by the low pH within the digestive vacuoles of the parasite and is further concentrated 100-fold by binding to haematin, a stable dimer of haem. This prevents the further polymerisation of haem monomers, the accumulation of which increases membrane permeability and kills the parasite.

Chloroquine (and its close relative hydroxychloroquine) also possesses slow-onset antiinflammatory activity, which is useful in the treatment of rheumatoid arthritis (see Chapter 30).

Resistance of *P. falciparum* to chloroquine is very common, particularly in Southeast Asia, and is due to increased expression of a putative efflux transporter in the digestive vacuole membrane. It also confers cross-resistance to mefloquine (see below).

Pharmacokinetics

Chloroquine is completely absorbed from the gut or can be given intravenously. It is selectively concentrated in melanin-containing tissues – for example, the retina of the eye and in the liver, spleen and kidney. Approximately half is converted in the liver to active metabolites and the rest is excreted unchanged by the kidney. The half-life is very long during chronic dosing; an initial half-life of up to 6 days is followed by a slow phase of tissue elimination with a half-life of greater than 1 month.

Unwanted effects

- Nausea, vomiting, diarrhoea and abdominal pain.
- Cardiovascular depression after intravenous use, with hypotension and heart block.
- Seizures.
- Tinnitus and deafness.
- Retinopathy with cumulative doses, producing retinal pigmentation and visual field defects. Visual function should be monitored.
- Rashes, pruritus, hair loss and skin depigmentation.

Mefloquine

Mechanism of action and resistance

Mefloquine is a 4-aminoquinoline compound and may have a similar mode of action to that of chloroquine. Resistance to mefloquine is less common but increasing; it arises from increased activity of the same efflux transporter.

Pharmacokinetics

Mefloquine is well absorbed from the gut and has a high affinity for lung, liver and lymphoid tissue. Extensive metabolism occurs in the liver, but the elimination half-life is very long (2–4 weeks).

Unwanted effects

- CNS effects: dizziness, vertigo, headache, sleep disorders. Less commonly, severe neuropsychiatric disturbances can occur, including nightmares, anxiety, depression, auditory and visual hallucinations and suicidal ideation. Mefloquine should be discontinued if neuropsychiatric symptoms appear, and it should not be given to people with a previous history of psychiatric disorder.
- Gastrointestinal effects, similar to those seen with chloroquine.
- Myalgia, arthralgia.
- Chest pain, tachycardia, hypotension.

Primaquine

Mechanism of action

Unlike the structurally related drugs chloroquine and mefloquine, primaquine affects only the exoerythrocytic parasite. It enters the parasite in the liver and may act by inhibiting mitochondrial respiration. It is used after treatment with chloroquine or mefloquine, to eradicate *P. vivax* or *P. ovale* from the liver (a radical cure).

Pharmacokinetics

Primaquine is completely absorbed from the gut and rapidly metabolised in the liver, producing active compounds. The half-life is 4–10 hours.

Unwanted effects

- Intravascular haemolysis in people with glucose-6-phosphate dehydrogenase (G6PD) deficiency (see Chapter 47). G6PD activity in erythrocytes produces reduced nicotinamide adenine dinucleotide phosphate (NADPH), which keeps glutathione in the reduced state, thereby maintaining cell wall integrity and preventing haemolysis (see Chapter 53). G6PD activity should be checked before treatment with primaquine is initiated.
- Gastrointestinal effects similar to those seen with chloroquine.

Quinine

Mechanism of action and resistance

The antimalarial properties of quinine, derived from the bark of the cinchona tree, have been known for centuries. It is similar to chloroquine in its mechanism of action. The mechanism of resistance to quinine is unclear but has been associated with changes in three transporter proteins. Quinine resistance is relatively rare, enabling the use of quinine with other drugs in the treatment of acute drug-resistant malaria.

Pharmacokinetics

Quinine is well absorbed from the gut but can also be given by intravenous infusion. Metabolism in the liver is extensive, and the half-life is about 6 hours in healthy people, becoming much longer in those with severe malaria.

Unwanted effects

- 'Cinchonism': tinnitus, headache, nausea, flushing, visual disturbances with vertigo and, if severe, hearing loss.
- Stimulation of insulin secretion, producing hypoglycaemia.
- Bradycardias, heart block or ventricular tachycardia, most often with intravenous loading doses.

Pyrimethamine with sulfadoxine

Mechanism of action and resistance

Pyrimethamine selectively inhibits the plasmodial form of dihydrofolate reductase, reducing the production of folic acid required for nucleic acid synthesis in the malarial parasite (see Fig. 51.4). Because of the widespread emergence of resistance, pyrimethamine should be given only in combination with the sulfonamide sulfadoxine. It is used to treat acute malaria (with other drugs) but not for prophylaxis. Resistance to sulfadoxine and pyrimethamine arises from changes in their respective targets, dihydroperoate synthetase and dihydrofolate reductase.

Pharmacokinetics

Pyrimethamine is well absorbed from the gut and undergoes extensive hepatic metabolism. Its half-life is approximately 2–6 days.

Unwanted effects

Pyrimethamine is usually well tolerated; occasional effects are

- photosensitive rashes,
- insomnia,
- megaloblastic anaemia, due to inhibition of human folate metabolism with high doses.

Proguanil

Mechanism of action and resistance

Proguanil inhibits plasmodial dihydrofolate reductase (see Fig. 51.4) mainly through cycloguanil, its active metabolite, which inhibits folate production in both pre-erythrocytic and erythrocytic parasites. It is often used for malarial prophylaxis alone or in combination with chloroquine. It can also be used in the prophylaxis and treatment of *P. falciparum* in combination with atovaquone (see below). Resistance is caused by changes in the plasmodial dihydrofolate reductase.

Pharmacokinetics

Absorption of proguanil from the gut is good and extensive metabolism occurs in the liver to cycloguanil, its potent active derivative. Cycloguanil has a short half-life (2 hours), but its plasma profile reflects its slow formation from proguanil (12–24 hours).

Unwanted effects

- Mouth ulcers.
- Epigastric discomfort, diarrhoea.

Artemether with lumefantrine

Mechanism of action and resistance

Artemether is a semi-synthetic derivative of artemisinin extracted from the herb *Artemisia annua*. It is activated by complexing with iron in the haem ingested by the malarial parasite. The resulting compound produces carbon-centred free radicals and reactive oxygen species that disrupt Ca^{2+} transport and other cellular functions in the parasite. It is used with lumefantrine, which may work by inhibiting the haem detoxification pathway in the parasite. The combination reduces the emergence of resistance, but monotherapy with artemisinin derivatives in some countries has generated plasmodial resistance, arising in part owing to increased efflux transporter activity.

Pharmacokinetics

Artemether is well absorbed from the gut and rapidly hydrolysed to an active metabolite that has a short half-life of 2–3 hours. Lumefantrine absorption from the gut is greatly enhanced by a high-fat meal; it undergoes hepatic metabolism and has a half-life of 2–6 days.

Unwanted effects

- Abdominal pain, nausea, anorexia, diarrhoea.
- Headache, dizziness, sleep disturbance, fatigue.

Treatment of malaria

Chemotherapy of malaria falls into three categories:

- rapid-acting blood schizonticides (to kill schizonts in acute malaria): chloroquine, mefloquine, quinine, artemether with lumefantrine,
- slow-acting blood schizonticides (to suppress blood infections): pyrimethamine with sulfadoxine, proguanil (alone or with atovaquone),
- tissue schizonticide (to eliminate liver parasites): primaquine.

The recommended drug to use within each category depends on the type of parasite and the pattern of resistance where the infection was acquired. If the infecting organism is unknown, it is assumed to be *P. falciparum*, which carries the greatest risk. The latest drug recommendations should be obtained from tropical disease advisory centres.

Following are examples for current recommended treatments for acute attacks of high- and low-risk malaria.

For *P. falciparum*, chloroquine and mefloquine resistance is common. Oral quinine (or intravenous quinine for serious infections) for 5–7 days is followed by pyrimethamine with sulfadoxine for 7 days or by doxycycline or clindamycin (see antibacterials, discussed above) if the plasmodia are resistant to sulfadoxine. Alternatively, proguanil with atovaquone or artemether with lumefantrine are used for 3 days.

For benign malaria, chloroquine is taken for 3 days. For *P. vivax* and *P. ovale,* primaquine is then taken for 14 days to destroy hepatic parasites.

Prophylaxis against malaria

The recommendations for prophylaxis depend on patterns of resistance in the area to be visited. Chloroquine or proguanil is often recommended for areas where resistance is low. For many areas a combination of both drugs is desirable. Mefloquine, doxycycline or proguanil with atovaquone are recommended in some areas where there is a high risk of chloroquine-resistant malaria. Prophylaxis must also take into account the unwanted effects of the drugs and other factors such as pregnancy and renal or hepatic impairment. Prophylaxis must be started 1 week before travel (or 2–3 weeks for mefloquine, or 1–2 days for proguanil with atovaquone or for doxycycline) and continued for 4 weeks after leaving a malarial area (or 1 week for proguanil with atovaquone) to protect against infection acquired immediately prior to departure.

OTHER PROTOZOAL INFECTIONS

Details of the natural history of other protozoal infections are not given in this book. Important drugs available in the United Kingdom for these conditions are discussed later. An outline of therapeutic uses is given in Table 51.5.

Atovaquone

Mechanism of action and uses

Atovaquone acts on cytochrome proteins in the inner mitochondrial membrane. It inhibits mitochondrial electron transport required for pyrimidine synthesis and is selective for protozoa that cannot utilise pre-formed pyrimidines.

Atovaquone is used as a second-line drug for the treatment of *P. jirovecii* and *Toxoplasma gondii* infections. It is also active against *Plasmodium* species (used in combination with

Table 51.5 Selected protozoan infections and antiprotozoal drugs

Protozoa	Disease	Drug examples
Plasmodium species	Malaria	Chloroquine, mefloquine, primaquine, quinine, proguanil, pyrimethamine with sulfadoxine, atovaquone, artemether with lumefantrine
Entamoeba histolytica	Amoebic dysentery	Diloxanide, metronidazole, tinidazole,
Trichomonas vaginalis	Vaginitis	Metronidazole, tinidazole
Giardia lamblia	Gastrointestinal dysfunction	Metronidazole, tinidazole, mepacrine
Leishmania species	Cutaneous or visceral (kala-azar) leishmaniasis	Stibogluconate, pentamidine, amphotericin
Trypanosoma species	Trypanosomiasis (sleeping sickness), Chagas' disease	Suramin,[a] nifurtimax,[a] benznidazole,[a] eflornithine, pentamidine, melarsoprol[a]
Toxoplasma gondii	Encephalomyelitis, toxoplasmosis	Pyrimethamine plus sulfadiazine, trimetrexate[a]
Pneumocystis jirovecii	Pneumocystis pneumonia	Co-trimoxazole, pentamidine, atovaquone, trimetrexate[a]

[a]Not available or used in the United Kingdom for protozoal infection.

the folate inhibitor proguanil), *E. histolytica* and *Trichomonas vaginalis.*

Pharmacokinetics

Oral absorption of atovaquone is poor. The absorbed fraction is excreted in the urine and bile, which results in enterohepatic cycling, giving it a long half-life of about 1–3 days.

Unwanted effects

- Diarrhoea, nausea, vomiting.
- Rashes.
- Headache, insomnia.
- Neutropenia.

Pentamidine

Mechanism of action and uses

Pentamidine isetionate undergoes rapid active uptake into the protozoal cell, where it binds avidly to transfer RNA and inhibits the ribosomal synthesis of protein, with additional actions on the synthesis of nucleic acids and phospholipids.

Pentamidine is used in *Pneumocystis jirovecii* pneumonia, leishmaniasis and trypanosomiasis. It is cytotoxic to *P. jirovecii* in the nonreplicating state; because of its toxicity, however, it is usually reserved for people who are intolerant of co-trimoxazole.

Pharmacokinetics

Pentamidine is given intravenously or inhaled as an aerosol for *P. jirovecii* pneumonia. It can be given by deep intramuscular injection for leishmaniasis or trypanosomiasis. Pentamidine is metabolised in the liver and has a very long half-life (10–14 days).

Unwanted effects

- Inhaled pentamidine produces bronchial irritation with cough and bronchospasm.
- Intravenous pentamidine is nephrotoxic, and can produce irreversible hypoglycaemia and life-threatening arrhythmias such as ventricular tachycardia. It can also cause injection-site reactions, dizziness, severe hypotension, syncope, rash, gastrointestinal disturbances, abnormal liver function tests and acute renal failure.

Sodium stibogluconate

Mechanism of action and use

Sodium stibogluconate is an organic antimony derivative. Its mechanism is unclear but it may act by binding to thiol groups in the parasite and inhibiting the formation of high-energy phosphates (ATP and guanosine triphosphate [GTP]). It is used to treat visceral leishmaniasis.

Pharmacokinetics

Sodium stibogluconate must be given parenterally, either by intramuscular injection or by slow intravenous infusion. It is eliminated by the kidneys and has a half-life of 6 hours.

Unwanted effects

- Anorexia, nausea, vomiting, abdominal pain, diarrhoea.
- Headache.

- Lethargy.
- Myalgia, arthralgia.
- Cough and substernal pain during intravenous infusion.

Diloxanide furoate

Mechanism of action and use

The mechanism of action of diloxanide furoate is unknown. It is used to treat chronic amoebiasis in asymptomatic individuals who are excreting cysts of *E. histolytica* in the stool. Acute infection is treated with metronidazole or tinidazole (see Table 51.5).

Pharmacokinetics

Diloxanide furoate is given orally and is hydrolysed in the gut to diloxanide and furoic acid; 90% of the diloxanide is then absorbed and rapidly conjugated in the liver. The unabsorbed fraction of diloxanide may contribute to the drug's effectiveness in amoebic dysentery.

Unwanted effects

- Flatulence, anorexia, nausea and diarrhoea.
- Urticaria, pruritus.

HELMINTHIC INFECTIONS

Details of the natural history of helminthic infections are not given here, but an outline of the more commonly encountered conditions and drug treatments is given in Table 51.6. Drugs specifically for helminthic infections are discussed below.

ANTIHELMINTHIC DRUGS

Ivermectin

Mechanism of action and use

Ivermectin is an avermectin compound used to treat filariasis (especially onchocerciasis, for which it is the drug of choice), hookworm and *Strongyloides stercoralis* infection. It inhibits influx of Cl^- ions via an action on glutamate-gated membrane ion channels, producing muscle hyperpolarisation and paralysis of the filariae. Treatment with a single dose reduces microfilarial levels for several months and can be repeated every 6–12 months if necessary. It is unlicensed in the United Kingdom but available on a 'named patient' basis.

Pharmacokinetics

Ivermectin is well absorbed from the gut and excreted mainly in the faeces. It undergoes some hepatic metabolism and has a long half-life (18 hours).

Unwanted effects

- Burning sensation on the skin, itching.

Diethylcarbamazine

Mechanism of action and use

Diethylcarbamazine is a piperazine derivative and a first-line treatment for filariasis. Its mechanism of action is not well

Table 51.6 Helminth infections

Helminth	Common name	Drug examples
Enterobius vermicularis	Threadworm	Mebendazole, piperazine[a]
Ascaris lumbricoides	Roundworm	Mebendazole, levamisole, piperazine[a]
Toxocara canis	Dog roundworm	Tiabendazole, diethylcarbamazine
Taenia species	Tapeworm	Niclosamide, praziquantel
Ancylostoma species, *Necator* species	Hookworm	Mebendazole, albendazole
Microfilariae (e.g. *Loa loa*, *Wuchereria bancrofti*, *Brugia malayi*)		Diethylcarbamazine, ivermectin
Strongyloides stercoralis		Iver mectin, albendazole
Echinococcus granulosa	Hydatid disease	Albendazole

[a]Not currently available in the United Kingdom; some others are available only on a 'named patient' basis (see text).

understood. It may inhibit arachidonic acid metabolism in the filariae and also triggers exposure of antigens on the surface coat, rendering the parasites more susceptible to immune attack by antibody-mediated phagocytosis. Treatment is usually required for 2–3 weeks to eliminate the microfilariae. Diethylcarbamazine is not licensed in the United Kingdom but is available on a 'named patient' basis.

Pharmacokinetics

Oral absorption is good, and approximately half the drug is metabolised in the liver; the rest is excreted unchanged by the kidneys. The half-life is 12–14 hours.

Unwanted effects

Most problems are caused by release of antigens from dying filariae. The onset is about 2 hours after dosing and is almost diagnostic of the disease. The reaction is occasionally severe and life-threatening. The reaction includes:

- fever,
- headache,
- nausea,
- muscle and joint pains,
- itching,
- postural hypotension.

Benzimidazoles

albendazole, mebendazole, tiabendazole

Mechanism of action and uses

The benzimidazoles all bind selectively to tubulin in helminths, preventing its polymerisation into cytoskeletal microtubules and impairing parasite motility and other functions. Tiabendazole and albendazole also inhibit parasite-specific fumarate reductase, reducing energy production by the Krebs' cycle and impairing glucose uptake. The drugs are active against the adults, larvae and eggs. Tiabendazole and albendazole

are available in the United Kingdom only on a 'named patient' basis.

Uses include (see also Table 51.6):

- mebendazole: threadworm, roundworm, whipworm, hookworm,
- tiabendazole: *S. stercoralis*, hookworm (cutaneous larva migrans),
- albendazole: hydatid cysts, *S. stercoralis*, hookworm (including cutaneous larva migrans).

Pharmacokinetics

Oral absorption of tiabendazole is almost complete; metabolism in the liver is extensive and the half-life is very short (about 1 hour). The oral absorption of mebendazole and albendazole is poor (<10%); these drugs act principally within the gut.

Unwanted effects

- Gastrointestinal effects are common with tiabendazole and include abdominal pain, anorexia, nausea, vomiting and diarrhoea; they are less severe with the other drugs.
- Dizziness and drowsiness can occur with tiabendazole.

Piperazine

Mechanism of action and uses

Piperazine is given orally to treat threadworm and roundworm infections in some countries but is not currently available in the United Kingdom. It is a selective agonist of gamma-aminobutyric acid (GABA) receptors in helminths, an action that suppresses acetylcholine-mediated smooth muscle contractility, producing a reversible flaccid paralysis in the parasite.

Pharmacokinetics

Absorption of piperazine is rapid from the gut; 10–30% of the dose is eliminated unchanged in urine; few other pharmacokinetic data are available.

Unwanted effects

Gastrointestinal upset can occur.

Niclosamide

Mechanism of action and use

Niclosamide is given orally to treat tapeworm infection. It inhibits the generation of ATP by preventing phosphorylation of adenosine diphosphate (ADP) in mitochondria. It is ineffective against larval worms. Purgatives are usually given after niclosamide to remove viable ova from the gut. Niclosamide is available in the United Kingdom only on a 'named patient' basis.

Pharmacokinetics

Oral absorption is poor (up to 15%).

Unwanted effects

- Gastrointestinal upset, nausea, abdominal pain.
- Light-headedness.
- Pruritus.

Praziquantel

Mechanism of action and uses

Praziquantel is given orally to treat tapeworm infection and schistosomiasis. It is known to increase permeability of the cell membrane of sensitive helminths to Ca^{2+} ions, probably causing muscular contraction and paralysis and allowing expulsion or digestion of the parasite. It may also reduce cellular uptake of adenosine, which cannot be synthesised by the parasites. Praziquantel is available in the United Kingdom only on a 'named patient' basis.

Pharmacokinetics

Praziquantel is well absorbed from the gut but extensive first-pass metabolism limits its plasma concentrations. It has a plasma half-life of 1 hour.

Unwanted effects

- Dizziness, headache, lassitude.
- Gastrointestinal upset.

SELF-ASSESSMENT

True/false questions

1. Resistance to antibacterials may be due to mutations in bacterial ribosomes.
2. Benzylpenicillin has a short half-life as it is rapidly excreted by the kidneys.
3. Broad-spectrum penicillins can promote colonic infection with *C. difficile*.
4. Penicillins act by inhibiting peptidyl transferase activity.
5. The antipseudomonal penicillin ticarcillin is resistant to β-lactamase.
6. Cefotaxime is a third-generation cephalosporin.
7. Individuals who are allergic to penicillins are also allergic to cephalosporins.
8. Imipenem is rapidly metabolised in the kidney.
9. Meropenem is bacteriostatic at normal doses.
10. Ciprofloxacin is ineffective for *P. aeruginosa* infections in cystic fibrosis.
11. Moxifloxacin increases the toxicity of theophylline and warfarin.
12. Erythromycin commonly causes gastrointestinal disturbances.
13. Gentamicin has a low incidence of unwanted effects.
14. Gentamicin is not active when given orally.
15. Metronidazole can be used for eradicating *H. pylori*.
16. Antibacterials are effective for the majority of people with sore throat.
17. Tetracyclines should be avoided during pregnancy and in young children.
18. Vancomycin is active against β-lactamase-producing Gram-positive bacteria.
19. Rifampicin is a front-line drug for the treatment of tuberculosis.
20. Isoniazid is active against a wide range of bacteria.
21. Co-trimoxazole is the drug of choice for uncomplicated urinary tract infection.
22. Trimethoprim administration can result in folate deficiency.
23. Imidazoles and triazoles have the same mechanism of antifungal action.
24. The antifungal action of griseofulvin is due to inhibition of squalene epoxidase.
25. Amphotericin can be given in liposomal formulations.
26. Ivermectin is the drug of choice for onchocerciasis.

One-best-answer (OBA) questions

1. Choose the *most accurate* statement about HIV:
   A. Binding of HIV by the chemokine receptor CCR5 on the host cell membrane inhibits entry of the virus.
   B. Low doses of ritonavir reduce the activity of other protease inhibitors.
   C. Once resistance of HIV has developed, it persists indefinitely.
   D. Zidovudine acts in HIV by preventing viral entry to the host cells.
   E. The non-nucleoside reverse transcriptase inhibitors treat HIV by preventing insertion of the viral DNA into the host genome.
2. Identify the *least accurate* statement regarding the treatment of malaria:
   A. Primaquine kills parasites in the liver (hypnozoites) in *P. falciparum* infections.
   B. Chloroquine concentrates in infected erythrocytes and suppresses the erythrocytic stage of the malarial parasite's reproduction.
   C. In many areas prophylaxis against malaria requires the administration of two drugs.
   D. Primaquine can induce severe anaemia in people with glucose-6-phosphate dehydrogenase (G6PD) deficiency.
   E. Proguanil acts to inhibit malarial parasite folate production.

Case-based questions

Case 1

Mr J.W., age 40 years, lives at home and was previously healthy, but he saw his GP in August, 5 days after returning from a conference abroad, where he had stayed in a large hotel and indulged his passion for frequent whirlpool baths. He had characteristic symptoms of pneumonia, including pleuritic chest pain and the sudden development of fever and cough, producing yellow sputum. He was disorientated. Physical examinations and chest radiography supported the diagnosis.

1. Before the results of the microbiological test were available, what treatment would you have commenced and by what route of administration?
2. How do the drugs that you are proposing to give work?

Case 2

Mr R.H., age 80 years, had influenza and was admitted to hospital when he developed symptoms similar to those of Mr J.W. (see previous discussion) and became seriously ill. A chest radiograph showed multiple abscesses.

1. What treatment would you have commenced before microbiological results were available?
2. What antibacterial could be used if the organism was not treatable by β-lactamase-resistant penicillins?

Case 3

A 31-year-old man suffering from AIDS was admitted with shortness of breath, cough and generalised chest discomfort. Chest radiography revealed diffuse bilateral opacities and a blood gas analysis demonstrated an arterial partial oxygen pressure (P_aO_2) of 8.0 kPa (normal range 11.0–14.0 kPa). Sputum culture was uninformative. A bronchoalveolar lavage was performed and transbronchial biopsies taken.

1. What was the likely clinical diagnosis?
2. What microscopic investigation could have been useful and what might it have shown?
3. How could this man have been managed and what factors needed to be considered?
4. What drug treatment unrelated to the infection could have further exposed him to the increased risk of opportunistic infection?
5. What prophylactic treatment could be commenced?

Case 4

Twenty-four hours after attending a convention, a 36-year-old man became ill with a temperature, abdominal pain, vomiting and diarrhoea. Faeces were collected and inoculated onto culture plates with several different types of culture medium. Pale-coloured nonlactose-fermenting colonies were identified.

1. What organisms might have been causing this infection?
2. *Salmonella enteritidis* phage type 4 was eventually identified. How should this man be managed?
3. What was most likely to have caused this infection?

ANSWERS

True/false answers

1. **True.** Mutations affecting bacterial ribosomal RNA and proteins can reduce binding of antibacterials that inhibit protein synthesis, such as macrolides and tetracyclines. As well as target modification, other mechanisms of resistance to antimicrobial drugs include reduced uptake, increased export or biochemical modification of the drug and the development of alternative metabolic pathways to bypass its action.

2. **True.** Benzylpenicillin is actively secreted into the proximal tubule by the organic acid transporter OAT1 (see Table 2.1). This can be inhibited by probenecid or by other drugs that use the same secretory mechanism, such as aspirin.

3. **True.** Broad-spectrum penicillins may alter the balance of gut flora and allow overgrowth of pathogenic bacteria such as *C. difficile*, producing colitis.

4. **False.** Penicillins disrupt the synthesis of bacterial cell-wall peptidoglycans, not ribosomal synthesis of proteins.

5. **False.** Ticarcillin is broken down by β-lactamase, so it is given with the β-lactamase inhibitor clavulanic acid.

6. **True.** Cefotaxime is a third-generation cephalosporin that penetrates the CNS and is resistant to β-lactamases.

7. **False.** Only about 10% of penicillin-allergic individuals show cross-sensitivity to cephalosporins, but a history of severe allergic reaction to penicillin precludes use of cephalosporins.

8. **True.** Unlike other carbapenems, imipenem is rapidly metabolised by renal dihydropeptidase and is always given in combination with cilastatin, a dihyhdropeptidase inhibitor.

9. **False.** Like all β-lactam antibacterials given in correct doses, meropenem is bactericidal.

10. **False.** The quinolones have good activity against *Pseudomonas* species.

11. **False.** The quinolones ciprofloxacin and norfloxacin, but not moxifloxacin, inhibit hepatic cytochrome P450 and increase plasma concentrations of theophylline, warfarin and other drugs.

12. **True.** Erythromycin often causes nausea and diarrhoea. Azithromycin is better tolerated.

13. **False.** Gentamicin is nephrotoxic and ototoxic; its peak and trough plasma concentrations should be monitored.

14. **True.** Gentamicin is poorly absorbed from the gastrointestinal tract and is given only parenterally.

15. **True.** Metronidazole is commonly used in triple therapy with a proton pump inhibitor and other antibacterials to eliminate *H. pylori*.

16. **False.** Most sore throats are caused by viruses; those with bacterial causes usually resolve without antibacterials.

17. **True.** Tetracyclines can chelate with Ca^{2+} and form permanent yellow–brown deposits on developing teeth if given during pregnancy or to young children.

18. **True.** Vancomycin is reserved for MRSA and metronidazole-resistant *C. difficile*, which causes colitis.

19. **True.** Rifampicin is used in the United Kingdom in both the initiation and continuation phases of tuberculosis treatment in combination with other antituberculous drugs. It is a broad-spectrum antibacterial that is also used in other serious diseases caused by Gram-negative bacteria such as *Legionella* and mycobacteria and for MRSA.

20. **False.** Isoniazid is a highly selective inhibitor of the production of mycolic acids, which are unique to the cell wall of *Mycobacterium* species.
21. **False.** Uncomplicated urinary tract infections are usually treated with an aminopenicillin such as amoxicillin. Alternatives include a first-generation cephalosporin (e.g. cefalexin), trimethoprim and nitrofurantoin. Trimethroprim alone is usually preferred to co-trimoxazole in urinary tract infections owing to the lower risk of severe side effects compared with the combination drug.
22. **True.** Trimethoprim inhibits the synthesis of folate required for the production of nucleotides; folate deficiency can result in megaloblastic anaemia, which is preventable during long-term treatment by giving folinic acid.
23. **True.** Imidazoles and triazoles suppress ergosterol synthesis by inhibiting lanosterol 14α-demethylase; they also share a similar spectrum of antifungal activity.
24. **False.** Griseofulvin inhibits dermatophyte mitosis by impairing microtubule formation. Squalene epoxidase synthesises ergosterol and is the target of the antifungal terbinafine.
25. **True.** Lipid delivery vehicles such as liposomal formulations reduce the nephrotoxicity of amphotericin.
26. **True.** Ivermectin is the drug of choice for onchocerciasis (river blindness) and is also used for other helminth infectuons.

One-best-answer (OBA) answers

1. **Answer C** is the most accurate.
   A. Incorrect. Binding of HIV to the chemokine receptor CCR5 (and/or CCR4) facilitates its entry into host cells.
   B. Incorrect. Ritonavir inhibits breakdown of other protease inhibitors by CYP3A4 enzymes and is used to enhance their activity (boosted protease inhibition).
   C. **Correct.** When resistance of HIV arises, it persists indefinitely and drug treatment should be modified.
   D. Incorrect. Zidovudine is a nucleoside reverse transcriptase inhibitor and prevents the formation of DNA from viral RNA.
   E. Incorrect. The non-nucleoside inhibitors act directly on HIV reverse transcriptase to prevent formation of DNA from viral RNA. Insertion of viral DNA into the host genome is blocked by HIV integrase inhibitors such as elvitegravir.
2. **Answer A** is the least accurate.
   A. **Incorrect.** Only infections by *Plasmodium vivax* and *Plasmodium ovale* result in dormant parasites (hypnozoites) remaining in the liver; they require primaquine for their eradication.
   B. Correct. Chloroquine concentrates 100-fold in red cells and interferes with the ability of the parasite to detoxify digestion products of haemoglobin.
   C. Correct. In areas where resistance is a problem, prophylaxis with chloroquine plus proguanil or atovaquone plus either mefloquine, doxycycline or proguanil is recommended.
   D. Correct. Toxic metabolites of primaquine can induce haemolysis in people with G6PD deficiency.
   E. Correct. Proguanil inhibits dihydrofolate (DHF) reductase in plasmodia.

Case-based answers

Case 1

1. The most common cause of community-acquired infection is *S. pneumoniae*, but other 'atypical' organisms could be involved. In Mr J.W., who was previously well, a recent stay in a hotel abroad might indicate the involvement of *Legionella* species, which multiply in warm water – for example, in the tanks of air-conditioning systems. The incubation time is 5–10 days. Co-amoxiclav (amoxicillin and clavulanic acid) plus erythromycin or another macrolide should be given orally before the diagnosis is confirmed. If his condition is severe, rifampicin should also be given. The treatment should be reviewed as soon as the microbiology sensitivities are known.
2. Amoxicillin is bactericidal and acts by interfering with bacterial cell wall peptidoglycan synthesis. It also allows greater activity of enzymes that lyse bacterial cells. Clavulanic acid inhibits β-lactamase, thus extending the spectrum of activity of amoxicillin. Erythromycin inhibits bacterial protein synthesis by acting on the bacterial ribosome. Rifampicin inhibits DNA-dependent RNA polymerase in many Gram-positive bacteria (such as *Legionella*) and Gram-negative bacteria.

Case 2

1. *S. aureus* is a likely cause of acute pneumonia following an attack of influenza. Although the treatment must be guided by the sensitivity tests, most *S. aureus* strains are sensitive to flucloxacillin and this is the most appropriate antibiotic to start with. In the circumstances, it may be combined with fusidic acid or gentamicin. *S. aureus* commonly produces abscesses in the lungs. Pulmonary infection with *S. aureus* may also occur in people with cystic fibrosis. A Gram's stain of the sputum would demonstrate Gram-positive cocci in clusters, typical of staphylococci. The production of coagulase and DNase would identify the organism as *S. aureus*. Many different species of coagulase-negative staphylococci exist and are found as part of the normal skin flora. The coagulase-negative staphylococci are typical causes of prosthetic valve endocarditis, joint prostheses and infected venous catheters. Of concern is the prevalence of meticillin-resistant staphylococci (MRSA), which pose a threat to people who are frail or immunocompromised.
2. A range of other second-choice antibacterials effective against β-lactamase-producing *S. aureus* might be useful. For example, fusidic acid, gentamicin, a cephalosporin, a quinolone or erythromycin may be effective. There are increasing concerns about MRSA. Vancomycin, a bactericidal glycopeptide that inhibits cell-wall synthesis, is effective against some MRSA, or linezolid may be used if the glycopeptide is unsuitable.

Case 3

1. Clinically, the man is likely to have *Pneumocystis jirovecii* pneumonia (formerly known as *Pneumocystis carinii*

pneumonia, or PCP), which is the predominant respiratory illness in people with AIDS. The causative organism, which is a protozoan, is believed to be acquired at a young age and reactivates with waning immunity. The organism is endemic in the community and multiplies within the lungs, causing symptoms. There is often a seasonal prevalence of PCP. Symptoms can be scant and, if present, consist of breathlessness and cough. Induced sputum or bronchoalveolar lavage specimens should be sent to the laboratory for the detection of P. jirovecii and routine culture.

2. P. jirovecii can be detected in sputum or lavage by staining with methenamine silver stain for typical casts. It can also be detected by use of polymerase chain reaction (PCR)-based tests and on lung biopsy.

3. The treatment of choice is high-dose co-trimoxazole. Many people with AIDS have hypersensitivity reactions to sulphonamides and are taking multiple drug combinations. Alternative treatments for PCP are aerosolised or parenteral pentamidine, dapsone and trimethoprim, primaquine, etc.

4. Long-term treatment with corticosteroids or other immunosuppressants.

5. After an attack of PCP, a prophylactic regimen should be taken – for example, nebulised pentamidine or oral trimethoprim 3 days per week.

Case 4

1. *Salmonella*, *Shigella*, *Proteus* and *Pseudomonas* species are nonlactose-fermenting and produce pale-coloured colonies on this medium. All were contenders.

2. Antibacterials have no role to play in the management of the majority of cases of *Salmonella* gastroenteritis. Exceptions are when the gastroenteritis occurs in an individual who is immunocompromised or if there is evidence of systemic invasion. Ciprofloxacin would be the antibacterial of choice; it can be given orally and is cheaper than intravenous preparations. Dehydration and electrolyte imbalance should be corrected by fluid replacement. Control of the diarrhoea by antidiarrhoeal drugs is contraindicated because of the risk of inducing paralytic ileus and causing septicaemia.

3. Food poisoning, as this case would seem to involve from the history, is a notifiable condition and should be reported to the consultant in Communicable Disease Control. Because the man has attended a convention, it is possible that this is part of an outbreak and all persons attending the convention should be contacted to find out if they have been symptomatic and to collect faecal specimens for culture. Specimens of food, if still available, should also be collected for culture.

FURTHER READING

Antibacterial drugs

Bartlet, J.G., 2002. Antibiotic-associated diarrhoea. N. Engl. J. Med. 346, 334–339.

Cahill, T.J., Prendergast, B.D., 2016. Infective endocarditis. Lancet 387, 882–893.

Calhoun, J.H., Manring, M.M., 2005. Adult osteomyelitis. Infect. Dis. Clin. North Am. 19, 765–786.

Damodaran, S.E., Madhan, S., 2011. Televancin: a novel lipoglycopeptide antibiotic. J. Pharmacol. Pharmacother. 2, 135–137.

Dheda, K., Barry, C.E., Maartens, G., 2016. Tuberculosis. Lancet 387, 1211–1226.

Gotts, J.E., Matthay, M.A., 2016. Sepsis: pathophysiology and clinical management. Br. Med. J. 353, i1585.

Gruchella, R.S., Pirmohamed, M., 2006. Antibiotic allergy. N. Engl. J. Med. 354, 601–609.

Gupta, K., Trautner, B.W., 2013. Diagnosis and management of recurrent urinary tract infections in non-pregnant women. Br. Med. J. 346, f3140.

Hawkey, P.M., Livermore, D.M., 2012. Carbapenem antibiotics for serious infections. Br. Med. J. 344, e3236.

Hoagland, D.T., Lui, J., Lee, R.B., et al., 2016. New agents for the treatment of drug-resistant *Mycobacterium tuberculosis*. Adv. Drug Deliv. Rev. 102, 55–72.

Holmes, A.H., Moore, L.S.P., Sundsfjord, A., et al., 2016. Understanding the mechanisms and drivers of antimicrobial resistance. Lancet 387, 176–187.

Jacoby, G.A., Munoz-Price, L.S., 2005. The new β-lactamases. N. Engl. J. Med. 352, 380–391.

Mathews, C.J., Weston, V.C., Jones, A., et al., 2010. Bacterial septic arthritis in adults. Lancet 375, 846–855.

Phoenix, G., Das, S., Joshi, M., 2012. Diagnosis and management of cellulitis. Br. Med. J. 345, e4955.

Prina, E., Ranzani, O.T., Torres, A., 2015. Community-acquired pneumonia. Lancet 386, 1097–1108.

Ten Hacken, N.H., Kerstjens, H.A., 2011. Bronchiectasis. Br. Med. J. Clin. Evid.

Van de Beek, D., Broewer, M.C., Thwaites, G.E., et al., 2012. Advances in treatment of bacterial meningitis. Lancet 380, 1693–1702.

Venekamp, R.P., Sanders, S.L., Glasziou, P.P., et al., 2015. Antibiotics for acute otitis media in children. Cochrane Database Syst. Rev. (6), CD000219.

Antifungal drugs

Kanafani, Z.A., Perfect, J.R., 2008. Resistance to antifungal agents: mechanisms and clinical impact. Clin. Infect. Dis. 46, 120–128.

Martin-Lopez, J.E., 2015. Candidiasis (vulvovaginal). Br. Med. J. Clin. Evid. pii: 0815.

Moriarty, B., Hay, R., Morris-Jones, R., 2012. The diagnosis and management of tinea. Br. Med. J. 345, e4380.

Pankhurst, C.L., 2013. Candidiasis (oropharyngeal). Br. Med. J. Clin. Evid.

Patterson, T.F., 2005. Advances and challenges in management of invasive mycoses. Lancet 366, 1013–1025.

Pfaller, M.A., 2012. Antifungal drug resistance mechanisms, epidemiology, and consequences for treatment. Am. J. Med. 125 (Suppl.), S3–S13.

Antiviral drugs

Cortez, K.J., Maldarelli, F., 2011. Clinical management of HIV drug resistance. Viruses 3, 347–378.

Dunning, J., Baillie, J.K., Cao, B., et al., 2014. Antiviral combinations for severe influenza. Lancet Infect. Dis. 14, 1259–1270.

Esté, J.A., Telenti, A., 2007. HIV entry inhibitors. Lancet 370, 81–88.

Glezen, W.P., 2008. Prevention and treatment of seasonal influenza. N. Engl. J. Med. 359, 2579–2585.

Sauerbrei, A., 2016. Optimal management of genital herpes. Infect. Drug Res. 9, 129–141.

Volberding, P.A., Deeks, S.G., 2010. Antiretroviral therapy and management of HIV infection. Lancet 376, 49–62.

Wareham, D.W., Breuer, J., 2007. Herpes zoster. Br. Med. J. 334, 1211–1215.

Antiprotozoal drugs

Chelsea, M., Petri, W.A., 2013. Amoebic dysentery. Br. Med. J. Clin. Evid. 2013, 0918.

Davies, A.P., Chalmers, R.M., 2009. Cryptosporidiosis. Br. Med. J. 339, b4168.

Flannery, E.L., Chatterjee, A.K., Winzeler, E.A., 2013. Antimalarial drug discovery—approaches and progress towards new medicines. Nat. Rev. Microbiol. 11, 849–862.

Freedman, D.O., 2008. Malaria prevention in short-term travellers. N. Engl. J. Med. 359, 603–612.

Guidelines for the Treatment of Malaria, 2015. 3rd ed. World Health Organization, Geneva. Available from:: http://www.ncbi.nlm.nih.gov/books/NBK294440/.

Lalloo, D.G., Hill, D.R., 2008. Preventing malaria in travellers. Br. Med. J. 336, 1362–1366.

Montoya, J.G., Liessenfeld, O., 2004. Toxoplasmosis. Lancet 363, 1965–1977.

Petersen, I., Eastman, R., Lanze, M., 2011. Drug-resistant malaria: molecular mechanisms and implications for public health. FEBS Lett. 585, 1551–1562.

Antihelminthic drugs

Gray, D.J., Ross, A.G., Li, Y.-S., et al., 2011. Diagnosis and management of schistosomiasis. Br. Med. J. 342, d2651.

McManus, D.P., Gray, D.J., Zhang, W., et al., 2012. Diagnosis, treatment and management of echinococcus. Br. Med. J. 344, e3866.

Taman, A., Azab, M., 2014. Present-day anthelmintics and perspectives on future new targets. Parasitol. Res. 113, 2425–2433.

Compendium: drugs used for infections

Drug	Characteristics
Antibacterial drugs	
Penicillins	
All penicillins are β-lactam antibacterials that disrupt cell wall synthesis.	
Amoxicillin	Broad-spectrum aminopenicillin. Used for urinary tract infections, otitis media, sinusitis, bronchitis, uncomplicated community-acquired pneumonia, *Haemophilus influenzae* infections, invasive salmonellosis and listerial meningitis. Given orally, by intramuscular injection or by intravenous injection or infusion. Also given with clavulanic acid as co-amoxiclav. Half-life: 1 h
Ampicillin	Broad-spectrum aminopenicillin. Uses similar to amoxicillin. Given orally, by intramuscular injection, by intravenous injection or by infusion. Half-life: 1–2 h
Benzylpenicillin (penicillin G)	Used for throat infection, otitis media, streptococcal endocarditis, meningococcal disease, pneumonia and anthrax. Given by intramuscular injection, slow intravenous injection or infusion. Half-life: 0.5–1 h
Co-amoxiclav	See amoxicillin
Co-fluampicil	See flucloxacillin
Flucloxacillin (floxacillin)	Beta-lactamase-resistant aminopenicillin. Used for infections caused by β-lactamase-producing staphylococci. Given orally, by intramuscular injection or by intravenous injection or infusion. Also given combined with ampicillin as co-fluampicil. Half-life: 0.8–1.2 h
Phenoxymethyl penicillin (penicillin V)	Used for tonsillitis, otitis media, erysipelas, rheumatic fever and pneumococcal infection prophylaxis. Given orally. Half-life: 0.5 h
Piperacillin	Antipseudomonal ureidopenicillin. Used for infections of lower respiratory tract, urinary tract, abdomen and skin. Given by intravenous infusion; available only in combination with tazobactam (β-lactamase inhibitor). Half-life: 0.7–1.2 h
Pivmecillinam hydrochloride	Pro-drug rapidly hydrolysed to mecillinam. Antipseudomonal amidinopenicillin. Active against many Gram-negative bacteria including *Escherichia coli*, *Klebsiella*, *Enterobacter* and salmonellae. Used for urinary tract infections. Given orally. Half-life: 1–2 h (mecillinam)
Temocillin	Beta-lactamase-resistant carboxypenicillin. Used for infections caused by Gram-negative bacteria. Given by intramuscular or intravenous injection or by intravenous infusion. Half-life: 4–5 h
Ticarcillin	Antipseudomonal carboxypenicillin; also active against *Proteus* species. Given by intravenous infusion in combination with clavulanic acid. Half-life: 1 h

Compendium: drugs used for infections (cont'd)

Drug	Characteristics
Cephalosporins, carbapenems and other β-lactams	
All are β-lactam compounds that disrupt bacterial cell wall synthesis.	
Aztreonam	Monobactam. Active only against Gram-negative bacteria and used for infections by *P. aeruginosa*, *H. influenzae* and *Neisseria meningitides*. Given by deep intramuscular injection, by intravenous injection or by infusion. Half-life: 1.7 h
Cefaclor	Second-generation cephalosporin. Used for sensitive Gram-negative or Gram-positive infections of urinary tract (unresponsive to other drugs), respiratory tract and soft tissues and for otitis media and sinusitis. Given orally. Half-life: 0.5–1 h
Cefadroxil	First-generation cephalosporin. Uses similar to cefaclor. Given orally. Half-life: 1–2 h
Cefalexin	First-generation cephalosporin. Uses similar to cefaclor. Given orally. Half-life: 1 h
Cefixime	Third-generation cephalosporin. Uses similar to cefaclor but for acute infections only; also used for gonorrhoea. Given orally. Half-life: 2.5–3.8 h
Cefotaxime	Third-generation cephalosporin. Uses similar to cefaclor; also used for gonorrhoea, surgical prophylaxis, *Haemophilus epiglottitis* and meningitis. Given by deep intramuscular injection, or by intravenous injection (over 3–5 min) or infusion. Half-life: 0.9–1.3 h
Cefradine	First-generation cephalosporin. Uses similar to cefaclor; also used for surgical prophylaxis. Given orally, by deep intramuscular injection or by intravenous injection (over 3–5 min) or infusion. Half-life: 1.3 h
Ceftaroline fosamil	Pro-drug converted to ceftaroline. Fifth-generation cephalosporin; similar to cefotaxime but extended activity against Gram-positive bacteria including MRSA. Used for community-acquired pneumonia and complicated skin and soft-tissue infections. Given by intravenous infusion. Half-life: 2.5 h (ceftaroline)
Ceftazidime	Third-generation cephalosporin. Uses similar to cefaclor; also used for surgical prophylaxis. Given by deep intramuscular injection or by intravenous injection or infusion. Half-life: 1.8–2.2 h
Ceftriaxone	Third-generation cephalosporin. Uses similar to cefaclor; also used for surgical prophylaxis and prophylaxis of meningococcal meningitis. Given by deep intramuscular injection, or by intravenous injection or infusion. Half-life: 6–9 h
Cefuroxime	Second-generation cephalosporin. Uses similar to cefaclor; also used for surgical prophylaxis. Given orally (as cefuroxime axetil pro-drug), by deep intramuscular injection or by intravenous injection or infusion. Half-life: 1.2 h (cefuroxime)
Doripenem	Carbapenem. Broad-spectrum activity against both Gram-negative and Gram-positive organisms. Used for hospital-acquired pneumonias and for complicated intra-abdominal and urinary tract infections. Given by intravenous infusion. Half-life: 1 h
Ertapenem	Carbapenem. Broad-spectrum activity against both Gram-negative and Gram-positive organisms. Used for abdominal and acute gynaecological infections and for community-acquired pneumonia. Given by intravenous infusion. Half-life: 4.5 h
Imipenem (with cilastatin)	Carbapenem. Active against aerobic and anaerobic Gram-negative and Gram-positive organisms. Used for hospital-acquired septicaemia and for surgical prophylaxis. Always given with cilastatin (to inhibit renal dihydropeptidase) by deep intramuscular injection or intravenous infusion. Half-life: 1 h
Meropenem	Carbapenem. Used for aerobic and anaerobic Gram-negative and Gram-positive infections. Given by intravenous injection or intravenous infusion. Half-life: 1 h
Beta-lactamase inhibitors	
Given with some β-lactam antibacterial drugs susceptible to hydrolysis by β-lactamase (penicillinase).	
Clavulanic acid	Given in combination with amoxicillin (co-amoxiclav) or ticarcillin. Half-life: 1 h
Tazobactam	Given in combination with piperacillin. Half-life: 0.7–1.5 h

Compendium: drugs used for infections (cont'd)

Drug	Characteristics
Quinolones	
Quinolones are bactericidal drugs that inhibit DNA replication and repair by actions on DNA gyrases and topoisomerases.	
Ciprofloxacin	Active against Gram-positive and especially Gram-negative organisms, including *Salmonella*, *Shigella*, *Campylobacter*, *Neisseria* and *Pseudomonas* species. Used for respiratory (not pneumococcal pneumonia), urinary and gastrointestinal tract infections, chronic prostatitis, gonorrhoea and septicaemia. Given orally or by intravenous infusion. Half-life: 3–4 h
Levofloxacin	Similar activity to ciprofloxacin but more active against pneumococci. Used for acute sinusitis, acute exacerbations of chronic bronchitis, and community-acquired pneumonia when first-line treatment is contraindicated or ineffective. Given orally or as an intravenous infusion. Half-life: 6–8 h
Moxifloxacin	Similar activity to ciprofloxacin but more active against pneumococci and inactive against *P. aeruginosa* or MRSA. Used for treatment of sinusitis, community-acquired pneumonia, exacerbations of chronic bronchitis, pelvic inflammatory disease or complicated skin and soft-tissue infections unresponsive to other antibacterials. Given orally. Half-life: 12 h
Nalidixic acid	Used in uncomplicated urinary tract infections. Given orally. Half-life: 1.5 h
Norfloxacin	Used in uncomplicated urinary tract infections. Given orally. Half-life: 3 h
Ofloxacin	Used for infections of urinary tract and lower respiratory tract and for gonorrhoea, nongonococcal urethritis and cervicitis. Given orally or as intravenous infusion. Half-life: 6–7 h
Macrolides	
Macrolides inhibit protein synthesis by binding to the 50S ribosomal subunit. Their antibacterial spectrum is similar to that of penicillins; they are used as alternatives in penicillin-allergic patients.	
Azithromycin	Used for respiratory tract infections, otitis media, skin and soft tissue infections, uncomplicated chlamydial infections, nongonococcal urethritis and moderate typhoid due to multiple antibacterial-resistant organisms. Given orally. Half-life: 40–60 h
Clarithromycin	Used for respiratory tract infections, otitis media, mild to moderate skin and soft tissue infections and for *Helicobacter pylori* eradication. Given orally or by intravenous infusion. Half-life (3 h) increases at high doses (9 h)
Erythromycin	Used for *Campylobacter* enteritis, pneumonia, Legionnaires' disease, syphilis, nongonococcal urethritis, chronic prostatitis, diphtheria and whooping cough prophylaxis and for acne vulgaris and rosacea. Given orally or by intravenous infusion. Half-life: 1–1.5 h
Spiramycin	Used on a 'named patient' basis for toxoplasmosis. Half-life: 6–8 h
Telithromycin	Ketolide derivative of erythromycin. Used for community-acquired pneumonia, bronchitis, sinusitis, β-haemolytic streptococcal pharyngitis, or tonsillitis when β-lactams are inappropriate. Given orally. Half-life: 10 h
Aminoglycosides	
Aminoglycosides inhibit protein synthesis by binding irreversibly to the 30S ribosomal subunit. They are bactericidal drugs active against Gram-negative and Gram-positive organisms. Gentamicin is the aminoglycoside of choice in the United Kingdom and is used for serious infections.	
Amikacin	Used for serious Gram-negative infections resistant to gentamicin. Given by intramuscular injection, slow intravenous injection or intravenous infusion. Half-life: 2 h
Gentamicin	Used for septicaemia and neonatal sepsis, CNS infections (including meningitis), biliary tract infections, acute pyelonephritis and prostatitis, endocarditis, pneumonia in hospital and as adjunct in listerial meningitis; given by intramuscular injection, slow intravenous injection, intravenous infusion or by intrathecal injection. Half-life: 1–4 h
Neomycin	Toxicity restricts use to skin infections and for bowel sterilisation before surgery. Given orally. Half-life: 2 h
Tobramycin	Uses similar to those of gentamicin. Given by intramuscular injection, slow intravenous injection or intravenous infusion. Half-life: 2–3 h

Compendium: drugs used for infections (cont'd)

Drug	Characteristics

Tetracyclines

Tetracyclines are broad-spectrum antibacterials that inhibit protein synthesis by binding to the 30S ribosomal subunit. Use is limited by increasing resistance but they remain drugs of choice for infections caused by Chlamydia *(trachoma, psittacosis, salpingitis, urethritis and lymphogranuloma venereum),* Rickettsiae *(including Q-fever),* Brucella *and the spirochaete* Borrelia burgdorferi *(Lyme disease); also used in mycoplasmal infections, refractory periodontal disease, chronic bronchitis exacerbations, and for leptospirosis in penicillin hypersensitivity. All except tigecycline are given orally.*

Drug	Characteristics
Demeclocycline	Main uses given previously. Half-life: 10–15 h
Doxycycline	Main uses given previously; also for chronic prostatitis, sinusitis, syphilis, pelvic inflammatory disease, anthrax, malaria, rosacea and acne vulgaris; also used with quinine in the treatment of malaria. Half-life: 18–22 h
Lymecycline	Main uses given previously. Half-life: 8–10 h
Minocycline	Broader spectrum than other tetracyclines. Main uses given previously; also used for acne vulgaris. Half-life: 12–16 h
Oxytetracycline	Main uses given previously; also used for acne vulgaris and rosacea. Half-life: 9 h
Tetracycline	Main uses given previously; also used for acne vulgaris and rosacea. Half-life: 9 h
Tigecycline	Glycylcycline structurally related to tetracyclines, with similar unwanted effects. Used for complicated intra-abdominal, skin or soft tissue infections. Given by intravenous infusion. Half-life: 27–42 h

Sulfonamides and trimethoprim

Sulfonamide antibacterials and trimethoprim are inhibitors of folate synthesis. Their importance has declined owing to increasing resistance and the availability of better alternatives.

Drug	Characteristics
Sulfadiazine	Sulfonamide. Used for prevention of rheumatic fever recurrence. Given orally or by intravenous infusion; silver sulfadiazine cream is available for topical use. Half-life: 7–12 h
Sulfamethoxazole	Sulfonamide. Used only in combination with trimethoprim (as co-trimoxazole) for *Pneumocystis jirovecii* (where it is the drug of choice), toxoplasmosis, nocardiasis and for other susceptible acute infections. Given orally or by intravenous infusion. Half-life: 6–20 h
Trimethoprim	Dihydrofolate reductase inhibitor. Used with sulfamethoxazole (as co-trimoxazole), and alone for urinary tract infections and bronchitis (when it is given orally). Half-life: 9–17 h

Other antibacterial drugs

Drug	Characteristics
Chloramphenicol	Bacteriostatic antibiotic; protein synthesis inhibitor acting at 50S ribosomal subunit. Potent but toxic broad-spectrum activity. Systemic use limited to life-threatening infections, especially *H. influenzae* and typhoid fever. Given orally or intravenously; also used topically for eye and ear infections. Half-life: 1.5–4 h
Clindamycin	Lincosamide; mechanism similar to that of macrolides. Because of toxicity, use limited to staphylococcal bone and joint infections and for peritonitis; also used for MRSA in bronchiectasis, bone and joint infections and for skin and soft-tissue infections. Given orally, by deep intramuscular injection or by intravenous infusion. Half-life: 2–3 h
Colistin (colistimethate sodium)	Polymyxin; bactericidal by solubilising bacterial cell membrane. Used for infections by Gram-negative organisms, including *P. aeruginosa*. Given orally (for bowel sterilisation only), by intravenous injection or infusion or in cystic fibrosis by inhalation (nebuliser). Half-life: 4–8 h
Daptomycin	Lipopeptide; bactericidal action by disruption of cell membrane function. Used for complicated skin and soft tissue infections by Gram-positive bacteria. Given by intravenous infusion. Half-life: 8–9 h
Fidaxomicin	Macrocyclic drug; inhibits bacterial RNA polymerase. Very low oral absorption and narrow spectrum against Gram-positive bacteria, especially clostridia. Used for *Clostridium difficile* infection. Given orally. Half-life: 8–10 h
Fosfomycin	Phosphonic acid; inhibits peptidoglycan synthesis. Used for acute osteomyelitis, complicated urinary-tract infections, hospital-acquired lower respiratory-tract infections and bacterial meningitis when first-line treatments are inappropriate or ineffective. Half-life: 2–4 h
Fusidic acid (sodium fusidate)	Steroid; inhibits bacterial protein synthesis. Narrow-spectrum antibacterial. Use restricted to penicillin-resistant staphylococcal infections. Given orally or by intravenous infusion. Half-life: 9 h

Compendium: drugs used for infections (cont'd)

Drug	Characteristics
Linezolid	Oxazolidinone; inhibits initiation of bacterial protein synthesis. Used for pneumonia and complicated skin and soft tissue infections caused by Gram-positive organisms. Given orally or by intravenous infusion. Half-life: 5–7 h
Methenamine	Heterocyclic compound that degrades to formaldehyde and ammonia. Used for prophylaxis and long-term treatment of lower urinary tract infections. Given orally as enteric-coated formulation. Half-life: 4 h
Metronidazole	Nitroimidazole; disrupts microbial DNA in anaerobic bacteria. Used for surgical and gynaecological sepsis, antibiotic-associated colitis and eradication of *H. pylori*. Given orally, rectally or by intravenous infusion. Half-life: 6–9 h
Nitrofurantoin	Active metabolites disrupt bacterial DNA, RNA and ribosomal and other proteins. Given orally for urinary tract infections. Half-life: 0.3–1 h
Rifaximin	Nonabsorbable rifamycin compound; inhibits bacterial RNA synthesis. Used for uncomplicated traveller's diarrhoea. Given orally
Teicoplanin	Glycopeptide inhibitor of bacterial cell wall synthesis. Used for Gram-positive infections, including endocarditis, peritonitis, and for prophylaxis in orthopaedic surgery. Given by intramuscular injection, intravenous injection or infusion. Half-life: 32–176 h
Telavancin	Glycopeptide; inhibits bacterial cell wall synthesis and disrupts cell membranes. Used for hospital-acquired pneumonia in adults caused by MRSA when other antibacterials are unsuitable. Given by intravenous infusion. Half-life: 8 h
Tinidazole	Nitroimidazole; actions and uses similar to those of metronidazole. Given orally. Half-life: 12–14 h
Vancomycin	Glycopeptide inhibitor of bacterial cell wall synthesis. Used for prophylaxis and treatment of endocarditis and other serious Gram-positive cocci infections and for *C. difficile*-related colitis. Given orally (for colitis) or by intravenous infusion. Half-life: 5–11 h

Drugs for tuberculosis

Tuberculosis is typically treated in the United Kingdom with a combination of isoniazid, rifampicin, pyrazinamide and ethambutol in the initial phase (2 months) and with isoniazid and rifampicin in the continuation phase (4 months). Longer treatment and other drugs may be needed if resistance or nonrespiratory complications occur and in immunocompromised patients. Other indications for these drugs are also listed.

p-Aminosalicylic acid (4-aminosalicylate)	Used in combination with other antituberculous drugs when resistance to first-line drugs occurs. Given orally. Half-life: 5–10 h
Bedaquiline	Quinolone, but with novel action to inhibit the proton pump for mycobacterial ATP synthase. Used for pulmonary tuberculosis in combination with other drugs when resistance to first-line drugs occurs. Given orally. Half-life: 2–8 months
Capreomycin	Protein synthesis inhibitor. Used in combination with other drugs when resistance to first-line drugs occurs. Given by deep intramuscular injection. Half-life: approximately 12 h
Cycloserine	Amino acid analogue; inhibits cell wall synthesis. Used in combination with other drugs when resistance to first-line drugs occurs. Given orally. Half-life: 4–30 h
Delamanid	Novel inhibitor of the synthesis of mycolic acids in *M. tuberculosis* cell wall. Used for pulmonary tuberculosis in combination with other drugs when resistance to first-line drugs occurs. Given orally. Half-life: 32–38 h
Ethambutol hydrochloride	Arabinose analogue; inhibits mycobacterial cell wall synthesis. First-line drug (initial phase only) included in regimen if resistance to isoniazid is suspected. Given orally. Half-life: 10–15 h
Isoniazid	Pro-drug; active product inhibits mycolic acid synthesis. First-line antituberculous drug. Given orally or by intramuscular or intravenous injection. Half-life: 0.5–2 h (rapid acetylators), 2–6.5 h (slow acetylators)
Pyrazinamide	Pro-drug of pyrazinoic acid, which lowers mycobacterial pH and inhibits fatty acid synthesis. First-line drug (initial phase only), particularly useful in tuberculous meningitis. Given orally. Half-life: 9–10 h
Rifabutin	Rifamycin compound; inhibits DNA-dependent RNA polymerase. Used for prophylaxis against *Mycobacterium avium* complex infections and for treatment of nontuberculous mycobacterial disease and pulmonary tuberculosis. Given orally. Half-life: 35–40 h

Compendium: drugs used for infections (cont'd)

Drug	Characteristics
Rifampicin (rifampin)	Rifamycin compound; inhibits DNA-dependent RNA polymerase. Key first-line antituberculous drug; also used for brucellosis, Legionnaires' disease, leprosy and serious staphylococcal infections. Given orally or by intravenous infusion. Half-life: 1–6 h
Streptomycin	Aminoglycoside; inhibits protein synthesis at 30S ribosomal subunit. Use is mainly restricted to resistant organisms (also used as adjunct in treatment of brucellosis). Given by deep intramuscular injection. Half-life: 2–3 h

Drugs used in leprosy

These drugs are recommended for leprosy, often used in combination. Other drugs including ofloxacin, minocycline and clarithromycin are less active.

Clofazimine	Dye that disrupts DNA function. Second-line drug for leprosy. Given orally. Half-life: 70 days
Dapsone	Sulfone; inhibits folate synthesis. Key front-line drug for leprosy. Given orally. Half-life: 10–80 h
Rifampicin	See drugs for tuberculosis discussed previously

Antifungal agents

Antifungals include polyenes, imidazoles, triazoles, echinocandins and other drugs. Polyenes interact with ergosterol to form pores in fungal cell membranes. Triazoles and imidazoles inhibit fungal synthesis of ergosterol, and echinocandins inhibit synthesis of glucans in fungal cell walls.

Amorolfine	Morpholine; depletes ergosterol in fungal cell membranes by inhibiting D14 reductase and D7–D8 isomerase. Used for fungal infections of skin and nails, applied as a cream or nail lacquer. Negligible absorption
Amphotericin	Polyene. Active against most fungi. Given by intravenous infusion for systemic infections. Half-life: 1–14 days
Anidulafungin	Echinocandin. Used in invasive candidiasis. Given by intravenous infusion. Half-life: 40–50 h
Caspofungin	Echinocandin. Used for invasive aspergillosis unresponsive to amphotericin or itraconazole and for invasive candidiasis. Given by intravenous infusion. Half-life: 40–50 h
Clotrimazole	Imidazole. Used topically for fungal skin infections and vaginal candidiasis. Applied as a cream, powder or spray. Minimal absorption
Econazole nitrate	Imidazole. Used for fungal skin infections and vaginal candidiasis; applied as a cream. Negligible absorption
Fluconazole	Triazole. Used for local and systemic fungal infections, including fungal meningitis. Given orally or by intravenous infusion. Half-life: 30 h
Flucytosine	Antimetabolite; partly converted to 5-fluorouracil. Used for systemic fungal infections in combination with amphotericin or fluconazole. Given by intravenous infusion. Half-life: 3 h
Griseofulvin	Microtubule inhibitor. Used for widespread or intractable dermatophyte infections of the skin, scalp and nails where topical treatment has been ineffective. Given orally. Half-life: 10–21 h
Itraconazole	Triazole. Used for numerous local and systemic fungal infections. Given orally. Half-life: 20 h
Ketoconazole	Imidazole. Used topically for skin and vaginal infections; oral use no longer recommended for systemic mycoses
Micafungin	Echinocandin. Used to treat invasive candidiasis and to prevent candidiasis in patients with neutropenia. Given by intravenous infusion. Half-life: 10–17 h
Miconazole	Imidazole. Used topically for oral skin and vaginal infections or orally for intestinal infections. Half-life: 20–25 h
Nystatin	Polyene. Used principally for *Candida albicans* infections of skin and mucous membranes. Given topically; not absorbed from skin or gut
Posaconazole	Triazole. Used in invasive infections unresponsive to amphotericin or other suitable treatments. Given orally. Half-life: 35 h
Terbinafine	Allylamine; inhibits squalene epoxidase in fungal cell membranes. Drug of choice for fungal nail infections; also used for ringworm infection. Given orally or topically. Half-life: 11–17 h
Tioconazole	Imidazole. Used for fungal nail infections. Applied as a solution; negligible absorption
Voriconazole	Triazole. Used for invasive aspergillosis and other serious fungal infections. Given orally or by intravenous infusion. Half-life: 6 h

Compendium: drugs used for infections (cont'd)

Drug	Characteristics
Antiviral agents	
Reverse transcriptase inhibitors	
These reverse transcriptase (RT) inhibitors are nucleoside/nucleotide analogues or non-nucleoside drugs used for treatment of HIV infection in combination with other antiretroviral drugs; other indications are listed under individual drugs.	
Abacavir	Nucleoside RT inhibitor. Given orally. Half-life: 1.5 h
Didanosine	Nucleoside RT inhibitor. Given orally. Half-life: 0.6–1.4 h
Efavirenz	Non-nucleoside RT inhibitor. Given orally. Half-life: 40–70 h
Emtricitabine	Nucleoside RT inhibitor. Given orally. Half-life: 10–40 h
Etravirine	Non-nucleoside RT inhibitor. Used in regimens containing a boosted protease inhibitor for HIV infection resistant to other non-nucleoside reverse transcriptase inhibitors and protease inhibitors. Given orally. Half-life: 30–40 h
Lamivudine	Nucleoside RT inhibitor; also used for chronic hepatitis B with evidence of viral replication. Given orally. Half-life: 5–16 h
Nevirapine	Non-nucleoside RT inhibitor; used in advanced disease in combination with at least two other drugs. Given orally. Half-life: 25–30 h
Rilpivirine	Non-nucleoside RT inhibitor. Given orally. Half-life: 45 h
Stavudine	Nucleoside RT inhibitor. Given orally. Half-life: 1–1.6 h
Tenofovir disoproxil	Pro-drug of tenofovir, a nucleotide RT inhibitor. Given orally. Half-life: 17 h
Zidovudine	Nucleoside RT inhibitor. The first anti-HIV drug to be introduced; also used for prevention of maternal–fetal HIV transmission. Given orally or by intravenous infusion. Half-life: 1 h
HIV protease inhibitors	
Protease inhibitors are used for treatment of HIV infection in combination with other antiretroviral drugs.	
Atazanavir	Used in individuals treated previously with other antiretroviral drugs. Given orally. Half-life: 7 h
Darunavir	Used in combination with other antiretroviral drugs. Given orally. Half-life: 15 h
Fosamprenavir	Phosphate ester pro-drug converted to amprenavir in gut mucosa. Used in individuals treated previously with other antiretroviral drugs. Given orally. Half-life: 8 h (amprenavir)
Indinavir	Used in combination with nucleoside RT inhibitors. Given orally. Half-life: 2 h
Lopinavir (with ritonavir)	Lopinavir available only in combination with ritonavir. Given orally. Half-life: 5–6 h (lopinavir)
Ritonavir	Low doses increase effects of several other protease inhibitors by blocking their metabolism by CYP3A4. Used for progressive and advanced HIV infection in combination with nucleoside reverse transcriptase inhibitors and protease inhibitors. Given orally. Half-life: 3–5 h
Saquinavir	The first HIV protease inhibitor to be introduced. Given orally. Half-life: 5–7 h
Tipranavir	Used for HIV infection resistant to other protease inhibitors and in those treated previously with other antiretroviral drugs. Given orally. Half-life: 6 h
Viral DNA polymerase inhibitors	
Nucleoside analogue and non-nucleoside drugs that inhibit viral DNA polymerase; used in herpes simplex, varicella zoster and cytomegalovirus (CMV) infections.	
Aciclovir	Used for herpes simplex and varicella zoster infections. Given orally, topically or by intravenous infusion. Half-life: 3 h
Famciclovir	Pro-drug converted to penciclovir. Used for treatment of herpes zoster, acute genital herpes simplex and suppression of recurrent genital herpes infections. Given orally. Half-life: 2 h (penciclovir)
Foscarnet	Used for CMV retinitis in people with AIDS and for mucocutaneous herpes simplex infections unresponsive to aciclovir in immunocompromised people. Given by intravenous infusion. Half-life: 3–7 h

Compendium: drugs used for infections (cont'd)

Drug	Characteristics
Ganciclovir	Related to acyclovir but more active against CMV. Used for life-threatening or sight-threatening CMV infections in immunocompromised people only. Given by intravenous infusion. Half-life: 4 h
Inosine pranobex	Used for mucocutaneous herpes simplex, genital warts and subacute sclerosing panencephalitis. Given orally. Half-life: <1 h
Valaciclovir	Ester pro-drug of aciclovir; uses similar to those of aciclovir. Given orally. Half-life: 3 h (aciclovir)
Valganciclovir	Ester pro-drug of ganciclovir. Used for CMV retinitis in people with AIDS and for prevention of CMV infection following transplantation from an infected donor. Given orally. Half-life: 4 h (ganciclovir)

Other antivirals

For drugs used in viral hepatitis, see Chapter 36.

Amantadine	M_2 ion channel inhibitor. Licensed for prophylaxis and treatment of influenza A but no longer recommended; used in Parkinson's disease (see Chapter 24). Given orally. Half-life: 10–15 h
Cobicistat	Pharmacokinetic inhibitor of CYP3A4. Used to boost antiviral activity of elvitegravir in combination with emtricitabine and tenofovir disoproxil. Given orally. Half-life: 3–4 h
Dolutegravir	HIV integrase inhibitor. Used for HIV infection in combination with other antiretroviral drugs. Given orally. Half-life: 14 h
Elvitegravir	HIV integrase inhibitor. Available only in combination with the NRTIs emtricitabine and tenofovir disoproxil and the pharmacokinetic booster cobicistat. Given orally. Half-life: 9–14 h
Enfuvirtide	HIV fusion inhibitor. Used with other antiretroviral drugs for resistant HIV infection or in people intolerant to other drugs. Given by subcutaneous injection. Half-life: 4 h
Idoxuridine	Phosphorylated metabolite that impairs viral DNA transcription. Used rarely for topical infections with herpes simplex and herpes zoster
Maraviroc	Chemokine co-receptor CCR5 antagonist. Used with other antiretroviral drugs for treatment of resistant HIV infection. Given orally. Half-life: 14–18 h
Oseltamivir	Neuraminidase inhibitor; activated in liver. Used to treat influenza in at-risk people if started within 48 h of onset of symptoms. Given orally. Half-life: 6–10 h
Palivizumab	Monoclonal antibody against respiratory syncytial virus (RSV) antigen. Used for prevention of serious lower respiratory tract infection by RSV in neonates and children under 2 years. Given by intramuscular injection. Half-life: 20 days
Raltegravir	HIV integrase inhibitor. Used for the treatment of HIV infection resistant to other antiretroviral drugs. Given orally. Half-life: 9 h
Ribavirin (tribavirin)	Used by inhalation for severe RSV bronchiolitis in infants and children; also given orally in permutations with other drugs (interferon alpha, peginterferon alpha, sofosbuvir, protease inhibitors) for chronic hepatitis C infection (see Chapter 36). Half-life: 7–21 days
Zanamivir	Neuraminidase inhibitor. Used to treat influenza in at-risk subjects if started within 48 h of onset of symptoms. Given by inhalation. Half-life: 2–5 h

Antiprotozoal drugs

Antimalarials

Artemether with lumefantrine	Used for the treatment of acute uncomplicated *falciparum* malaria. Given orally. Half-life: 2–3 h (artemether), 2–6 days (lumefantrine)
Atovaquone	Used with proguanil for the prophylaxis or treatment of *falciparum* malaria; also used for mild to moderate pneumocystis pneumonia. Given orally. Half-life: 1–3 days
Chloroquine	Used for chemoprophylaxis and treatment of malaria and also for rheumatoid arthritis and lupus erythematosus. Given orally or by intravenous infusion. Half-life: 30–60 days
Mefloquine	Used for chemoprophylaxis and treatment of uncomplicated *falciparum* and chloroquine-resistant *vivax* malaria. Given orally. Half-life: 15–33 days
Piperaquine with artenimol	Licensed for acute treatment of uncomplicated *falciparum* malaria, but not currently recommended. Given orally. Half-life: 22 days (piperaquine), 1 h (artenimol)

Compendium: drugs used for infections (cont'd)

Drug	Characteristics
Primaquine	Used only for eradication of liver stages of vivax and ovale malaria. Given orally. Half-life: 4–10 h
Proguanil	Folate inhibitor; pro-drug of cycloguanil. Used for chemoprophylaxis of malaria. Given orally (alone or with atovaquone). Half-life: 12–24 h (proguanil), 2 h (cycloguanil)
Pyrimethamine	Folate inhibitor. Used for malaria treatment only in combination with sulfadoxine (as Fansidar). Given orally. Half-life: 2–6 h
Quinine	Used for treatment but not prophylaxis of malaria. Given orally or by intravenous infusion. Half-life: 6–47 h
Sulfadoxine	Sulfonamide. Used only in combination with pyrimethamine (as Fansidar) for treatment of *P. falciparum* malaria. Given orally. Half-life: 10 days

Other antiprotozoals

Drug	Characteristics
Diloxanide furoate	Used for amoebiasis and drug of choice for asymptomatic *E. histolytica* infections. Given orally
Eflornithine	Ornithine decarboxylase inhibitor. Given intravenously for trypanosomiasis (sleeping sickness); also used topically for hirsutism. Half-life: 8 h
Mepacrine (quinacrine)	Used for giardiasis; also used for discoid lupus erythematosus. Given orally
Metronidazole	Antibacterial and amoebicidal drug. Used for intestinal and extra-intestinal amoebiasis and for urogenital trichomoniasis and giardiasis. Given orally. Half-life: 6–9 h
Pentamidine isetionate	Used for pneumocystis pneumonia, leishmaniasis and trypanosomiasis. Given by inhalation (nebuliser), by deep intramuscular injection or by intravenous infusion. Half-life: 10–14 days
Sodium stibogluconate	Pentavalent antimony compound. Used for leishmaniasis. Given by intramuscular injection or slow intravenous infusion. Half-life: 6 h
Tinidazole	Antibacterial and antiprotozoal drug. Uses similarly to metronidazole. Given orally. Half-life: 12–14 h

Antihelminthic drugs

Drug	Characteristics
Albendazole	Used on a 'named patient' basis either alone or as an adjunct to surgery for echinococcal infections and for cutaneous hookworm larval infections. Given orally. Half-life: 8–12 h
Diethylcarbamazine	First-line drug for use against filariae. Given orally. Half-life: 12–14 h
Ivermectin	Used on a 'named patient' basis as the drug of choice for onchocerciasis; also used for cutaneous hookworm larval infections and for chronic *Strongyloides* infections. Given orally. Half-life: 18 h
Levamisole	Used on a 'named patient' basis as the drug of choice for *Ascaris lumbricoides* infection. Given orally. Half-life 4–6 h
Mebendazole	Used for threadworm, roundworm, whipworm and hookworm infections. Given orally. Half-life: 3–9 h
Niclosamide	Used on a 'named patient' basis for tapeworm infections. Given orally; not used in the United States
Piperazine	Used for threadworm and roundworm infections, but not currently available in the United Kingdom. Given orally. Half-life: >24 h
Praziquantel	Used on a 'named patient' basis for tapeworm infections and bilharziasis. Given orally. Half-life: 1 h
Tiabendazole	Used on a 'named patient' basis as the drug of choice for *Strongyloides* infection; also for cutaneous hookworm larval infections; Given orally. Half-life: 1.2 h

CMV, cytomegalovirus; *HBV*, hepatitis B virus; *HCV*, hepatitis C virus; *HIV*, human immunodeficiency virus; *MRSA*, meticillin-resistant *Staphylococcus aureus*; *RSV*, respiratory syncytial virus; *RT*, reverse transcriptase.

52 Chemotherapy of malignancy

Approximately 20–25% of people in the Western world die from cancer. Surgery and radiotherapy are valuable for treating localised cancers but are less effective in prolonging life once the tumour has spread to produce metastases. The introduction of cytotoxic chemotherapy to kill rapidly proliferating neoplastic cells has had a major impact on the treatment of malignant disease, especially diffuse tumours. Successful treatment of cancer frequently involves a multidisciplinary approach, which also includes psychological and social support.

A wide range of different drugs to treat cancer has been introduced into clinical practice since the 1970s, with a variety of mechanisms and sites of action within cancer cells. Although the drugs differ in their specific cellular targets, the majority rely on the rapid rate of growth and division of cancer cells to provide a degree of selectivity between normal and malignant tissue. Recent developments in molecular biology are resulting in the discovery of new potential targets for drug action and a resurgence of cytotoxic drug development. The ability of molecular biological approaches to define the mechanisms of cell–cell communication, apoptosis and angiogenesis will undoubtedly prove a major stimulus for the production of new drugs with greater selectivity for cancer cells. In addition, there is growing understanding of the potential for immunotherapy in the treatment of cancer.

There are a number of in vivo animal tests for detecting antineoplastic activity, but these frequently over-predict the likely effectiveness of a compound in clinical use. This occurs because the animal tumours used as models have a much higher proportion of vulnerable cells undergoing division (a higher growth fraction) than human tumours. A placebo-controlled clinical trial in humans of a new antineoplastic drug given as sole treatment is now unethical if an effective drug is already available. The efficacy of any new drug is therefore usually assessed by adding it to the best available current therapy. A successful new drug would have to show a clinically significant benefit above that of the optimal current treatment. As a result, many recent advances in cancer chemotherapy have arisen from the more effective use of existing drugs by optimising drug combinations and regimens and by minimising toxicity rather than through the introduction of novel compounds.

Cytotoxic drugs share a number of generic properties and characteristics, both beneficial and adverse, which will be discussed first. The major classes of drug will then be discussed, with information on mechanisms of action and general toxic effects.

MOLECULAR ORIGINS OF CANCER

Cancers develop as a result of abnormalities in the control of cell function. Normal cells are regulated by numerous external factors that control their growth and death. These include growth factors, cytokines and hormones that activate or suppress the genes controlling cell division. Most cancers probably arise from multiple genetic mutations in a cell, with sequential gene defects resulting in progressive changes through initial metaplastic and dysplastic phases, then progressing to invasive and ultimately metastatic cancer.

About 85% of cancers arise from exposure to environmental factors such as viruses, radiation and chemicals, with inherited genetic mutations accounting for the remainder. The environmental factors produce DNA damage, which in the normal cell can be repaired before the cell completes its cycle of division. A second protective mechanism is apoptosis (programmed cell death) of severely damaged cells. Cancer may arise by various mechanisms that influence gene expression and cell-cycle control. These include the following:

- inactivation of tumour suppressor genes or changes in microRNA genes (encoding RNA molecules which regulate gene expression) will promote unregulated cell proliferation,
- inactivation of genes that repair DNA.
- activation of proto-oncogenes to growth-promoting oncogenes: proto-oncogenes are normal gene sequences that control cell proliferation and differentiation. If they are activated to oncogenes as a result of chromosomal rearrangement, gene mutations or gene amplification, tumour development will ensue. Products of oncogene activation include growth factor receptor-associated tyrosine kinases and other intracellular signalling transducers, nuclear transcription factors, chromatin remodellers and apoptosis regulators. Gene mutations that activate oncogenes allow cell growth in the absence of stimulation by an external regulator.
- suppression of apoptosis: cells with damage to genetic material that inactivates tumour suppressor genes fail to undergo programmed cell death.

Defective function of the tumour suppressor protein p53 may be a factor in preventing DNA repair, reducing apoptosis and permitting uncontrolled cell proliferation in more than 50% of tumours. Activation of telomerase and lengthening of chromosomal telomeres may also be important. Telomeres

are the regions at the ends of chromosomes; their progressive shortening as healthy cells divide eventually arrests further cell division as the cell becomes senescent. In cancer cells, telomerase activation and chromosomal recombination can protect or extend the telomeres, immortalising the cell for continued growth and division. Growth factors such as vascular endothelial growth factor (VEGF) secreted by cancer cells promote angiogenesis and increase blood supply to the tumour. Other secreted factors can impede the host's immune response to the cancer cells. Genetic changes in cancer cells can give rise to metabolic changes or the expression of transporters, such as P-glycoprotein, that confer resistance to chemotherapy.

ANTINEOPLASTIC DRUGS

MECHANISMS OF ACTION

The majority of antineoplastic drugs act on the process of DNA synthesis within the cancer cell, as summarised in Fig. 52.1. Selectivity of these drugs for cancer cells compared with normal tissues is determined by the rate of DNA synthesis and cell division. Resting cells in the G_0 phase are resistant to many antineoplastic drugs (Fig. 52.2). *Cell cycle-specific antineoplastic drugs*, such as the antimetabolites, work effectively only when the cells are in the appropriate phase of the cell cycle at the time of treatment. *Noncell cycle-specific antineoplastic drugs*, such as the alkylating drugs, nitrosoureas and cisplatin, have a 'hit-and-run' action on DNA, and it is not critical when the cell is exposed because the drug effect becomes apparent when the cells attempt to divide.

The sensitivity of a cancer to treatment depends on its growth fraction, which is the fraction of cells undergoing mitosis at any given time. In Burkitt's lymphoma, almost 100% of neoplastic cells are undergoing division simultaneously, and they are very sensitive to chemotherapy, showing a dramatic response to a single dose of cyclophosphamide. In contrast, the growth fraction in a carcinoma of the colon is less than 5% of cells, resulting in its relative resistance to chemotherapy. However, metastases from colonic carcinoma deposited in the liver and elsewhere initially have a high growth fraction and are more sensitive to anticancer drugs.

The following have been shown using in vitro cancer cell lines and other approaches.

- Essentially complete eradication of tumour cells is necessary to prevent regrowth.
- Antineoplastic drugs produce a proportional cell kill; in other words, a proportion such as 95% of the cells present may be eliminated during a single course of treatment. Consequently, multiple treatments may be necessary to eradicate the cancer, with successive treatments producing an exponential decrease in the number of viable cancer cells remaining.
- Efficacy of chemotherapy with cell cycle-specific drugs in vitro is increased if treatment is timed to coincide with the appropriate phase of cell division within the cell population.

In vivo, the immune system probably contributes to the final removal of residual malignant cells; however, most

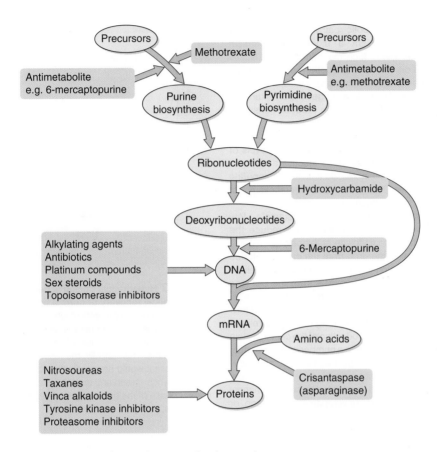

Fig. 52.1 Molecular sites of action of the main groups of anticancer drugs.

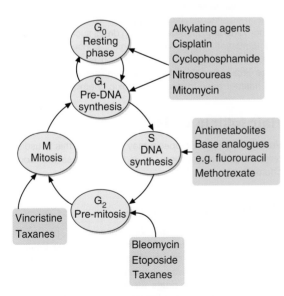

Fig. 52.2 Sites of action of key examples of cell cycle-specific anticancer drugs.

antineoplastic drugs compromise immunoresponsiveness by killing proliferating immune cells, which will reduce this removal process. The periodicity of doses is probably less critical in vivo because cancer cell cycles are not synchronised within the target cell population between treatments. In clinical practice, dose intervals are often established to allow recovery of healthy cells from toxic effects of the treatment. Therefore, while these concepts apply to in vivo cancer treatment, risk–benefit considerations may change with successive treatments and preclude complete eradication of the tumour.

RESISTANCE

Resistance to chemotherapeutic drugs may develop in a number of ways, many of which are analogous to the mechanisms that generate the resistance of pathogenic microbes to antimicrobial drugs (see Chapter 51). These are explained later in the text for individual drugs, but include a number of general mechanisms.

■ Reduced drug uptake. For example, the folate synthesis inhibitor methotrexate enters cells by the high-affinity transport system (the reduced folate carrier) for tetrahydrofolic acid (THF), and downregulation of the transporter in cancer cells limits the uptake of methotrexate and confers resistance to the drug.

- Use of alternative metabolic pathways and salvage mechanisms to circumvent a blocked biochemical process in cancer cells. Such mechanisms are usually drug-specific. For example, induction of asparagine synthesis in cells exposed to crisantaspase (asparaginase).
- Mutation of intracellular drug targets. For example, production of topoisomerase II with reduced sensitivity to the inhibitory effects of anthracyclines.
- Increased inactivation of the drug compound within the cancer cell. For example, high intracellular levels of glutathione S-transferase isozymes inactivate cisplatin and alkylating drugs, and increased activity of thiopurine S-methyltransferase increases the metabolism of mercaptopurine and tioguanine.
- Reduced activation of prodrugs. For example, low intracellular levels of deoxycytidine kinase reduce the activation of cytarabine (cytosine arabinoside).
- Increased removal of the drug from the cancer cell due to increased expression of protein carriers for the elimination of complex foreign chemicals from the cell (see Fig. 2.2), including a number of cytotoxic compounds. There are several such proteins (see Table 2.1), including P-glycoprotein and the multi-drug resistance-related proteins (MRPs). Increased production of the carrier protein confers multi-drug resistance to a number of compounds, including vinca alkaloids, etoposide, taxanes, anthracyclines, dactinomycin, mitomycin C and mitoxantrone. Because some carriers can be inhibited by calcium channel blockers (such as nifedipine or verapamil), ciclosporin, or tamoxifen, these drugs may be added to cytotoxic drug regimens to prevent resistance.

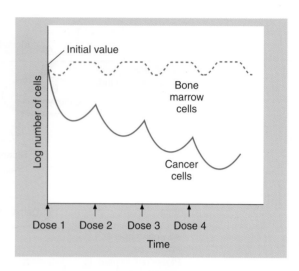

Fig. 52.3 Hypothetical dosing schedule of anticancer drugs to allow recovery of normal tissues. At least 10^9 tumour cells are usually present when tumours are first detectable. The malignant cells show a greater proportional kill than normal cells because a larger fraction is in division at any given time. Theoretically, the response of the malignant cells to dose 2 would be greater than for dose 1 if cell cycles became synchronised and dose 2 were given during the correct phase of the growth cycle. A typical dose interval is 3–4 weeks.

UNWANTED EFFECTS

Cytotoxic antineoplastic drugs are among the most toxic compounds given to humans. Many have a therapeutic index of approximately 1, as the therapeutic dose is essentially the same as the toxic dose. Because drug action is usually greater in tissues with a high growth fraction, a number of normal, rapidly dividing nonmalignant tissues are also affected, including bone marrow, gut mucosa and hair follicles. In addition to effects that occur in all rapidly dividing tissues, some chemotherapeutic drugs have specific toxic effects on other tissues, such as cardiotoxicity (particularly with anthracycline drugs) and ototoxicity (with platinum compounds). Many chemotherapeutic drugs are hepatotoxic or nephrotoxic. Dosage regimens are usually designed so that normal tissues, especially bone marrow and gut, can recover between doses (Fig. 52.3). Appropriate measures may be required to reduce potentially harmful exposure of healthcare staff who handle cytotoxic drugs.

Gastrointestinal tract

Mucosal cells have a rapid turnover. Toxicity can produce anorexia, mucosal ulceration or diarrhoea. A sore mouth (oral mucositis) is most common with fluorouracil, methotrexate and the anthracyclines. Nausea, vomiting, diarrhoea and loss of appetite are common, especially with alkylating drugs and cisplatin; this may limit an individual's ability to tolerate an optimal dosage regimen (see Chapter 32).

Bone marrow

Myelosuppression is a serious consequence of treatment and can lead to severe neutropenia, thrombocytopenia and sometimes anaemia. It often occurs 7–10 days after a cycle of chemotherapy but is delayed with drugs such as melphalan and lomustine. These haematological consequences may limit the drug dosage that the person is able to tolerate. There is a high risk of both infection (neutropenic sepsis) and haemorrhage following cytotoxic chemotherapy.

Hair follicle cells

Partial or complete alopecia may occur, but this is usually temporary. Scalp cooling can reduce hair loss with some chemotherapy agents.

Reproductive organs

Both sexes are affected and sterility can result, particularly after therapy with cyclophosphamide or cytarabine. Because of the mechanisms of action of cytotoxic drugs, most have teratogenic activity. Pregnant women should not be exposed to cytotoxic drugs for treatment or as members of the healthcare team. Alkylating agents or procarbazine can cause permanent male infertility. Drugs that mimic or affect the activity of sex hormones are frequently used for the treatment of breast or prostate cancer; these inevitably produce adverse effects on sexual function.

Growing tissues in children

Of particular concern in children is the possibility that intensive cytotoxic chemotherapy can impair growth. Children treated with cytotoxic drugs for malignancy also have an increased risk (approximately 10%) of developing a second malignancy, which is often leukaemia.

Extravasation of intravenous drug

If anticancer drugs leak from a vein into the surrounding tissues, they can cause severe local tissue necrosis.

Tumour lysis syndrome

Rapid breakdown of malignant cells and the release of their intracellular contents can produce hyperuricaemia (from breakdown of nucleic acids), hyperkalaemia, hyperphosphataemia and hypocalcaemia (due to precipitation of calcium phosphate), with consequent renal damage or arrhythmias. The syndrome is most common with treatment of non-Hodgkin's lymphoma, Burkitt's lymphoma and acute leukaemias. Tumour lysis syndrome can be ameliorated by good hydration (>2.5 L/day) and by use of allopurinol (a xanthine oxidase inhibitor) to reduce production of uric acid, or in those at high risk, rasburicase (recombinant urate oxidase) to enhance uric acid breakdown (see Chapter 31).

Peripheral neuropathy

Pain, tingling, numbness and cold sensations may occur in the hands and feet due to damage to sensory nerves, although motor and autonomic nerves can also be affected. Chemotherapy-induced peripheral neuropathy occurs most commonly with vinca alkaloids, taxanes and platinum compounds. It is progressive and may be irreversible.

DRUG COMBINATIONS

It is common practice to treat many cancers with a combination of different antineoplastic drugs simultaneously. Potential combinations of drugs are investigated using in vitro and in vivo experiments before they are subjected to clinical evaluation in humans. The most successful combinations are those that show synergistic activity on cancer cells, rather than a simple additive effect, while showing no increase in their systemic toxicity. Criteria for selecting ideal combinations are as follows:

- each drug should have a different site and mechanism of action within the cancer cell; this will increase efficacy while reducing the likelihood of resistance.
- each drug should have a different site for any organ-specific toxicity; some common toxicity is almost inevitable because nearly all drugs affect tissues with a high growth fraction.
- each drug should be an active antineoplastic drug in its own right; a second drug would not be given simply to increase the formation of an active metabolite of the first, although sometimes drugs are given to reduce the development of toxicity or resistance to another drug.

SPECIFIC ANTINEOPLASTIC DRUGS

The drug compendium at the end of this chapter outlines the licensed uses of individual drugs and notes any unusual or limiting toxicity.

DRUGS AFFECTING NUCLEIC ACID FUNCTION

Alkylating drugs

Examples

busulfan, chlorambucil, cyclophosphamide, melphalan

Mechanism of action and uses

Sulphur mustard gases were used as chemical warfare agents in World War I, their name deriving from their distinctive odour. These gases caused bone marrow suppression in addition to the respiratory toxicity for which they were developed. Replacement of the divalent sulfur atom by trivalent nitrogen allowed the introduction of a complex side chain, which resulted in a range of more stable, nonvolatile nitrogen mustard compounds that could be given therapeutically under controlled conditions. The side chain of alkylating drugs undergoes a metabolic activation step that involves loss of part of the molecule (e.g. the Cl is lost from $-CH_2CH_2Cl$) and yields a highly reactive product that binds to DNA or proteins. Many alkylating drugs are bifunctional (i.e. have two reactive groups). The reactive alkylating group(s) in the molecule may be

- nitrogen mustard: $N-CH_2CH_2Cl$ (with Cl being the leaving group); for example, carmustine (BCNU), chlorambucil, cyclophosphamide, ifosfamide, lomustine (CCNU), melphalan;
- sulfonate ester: $-CH_2OSO_2CH_3$ (with SO_2CH_3 being the leaving group); for example, busulfan, treosulfan;
- nitrosourea: $-NNO$; for example, carmustine, lomustine;
- cyclic nitrogen derivative (ethylenimines); for example, thiotepa.

Covalent binding of nitrogen mustards, sulfonate esters and cyclic nitrogen compounds to DNA prevents DNA replication and mRNA transcription. Covalent binding of nitrosoureas to proteins blocks DNA repair processes and other cellular functions.

When alkylating drugs bind to DNA nucleotides, such as to guanine, the alkylated nucleotide may either be repaired, in which case the cell survives, or it may interfere with DNA replication by:

- being misread,
- undergoing further metabolism via ring opening,
- cross-linking to another guanine molecule via a second reactive group (with bifunctional drugs).

Because of the covalent nature of the product, these effects are not cell cycle-specific (see Fig. 52.2). Alkylating agents are used to treat a wide variety of leukaemias, lymphomas and solid tumours.

Pharmacokinetics

The pharmacokinetic characteristics of the alkylating drugs depend on the nature of the reactive group(s) and the third nonreactive substituent on the N atom. Cyclophosphamide is an orally active pro-drug that is activated to two toxic metabolites, acrolein and phosphoramide mustard. Ifosfamide metabolism is similar to that of cyclophosphamide, and toxic metabolites of both cyclophosphamide and ifosfamide are excreted in the urine. Melphalan and chlorambucil, which have an aromatic substituent, undergo rapid metabolism. Most alkylating agents have half-lives of less than 6 hours, but the duration of action on DNA is very long.

Unwanted effects

- Alkylating drugs are highly cytotoxic and cause bone marrow suppression and neutropenia. Amifostine is used to reduce the severity of neutropenia induced by cyclophosphamide or cisplatin (see cisplatin, below). It is a pro-drug that is metabolised in neutrophils by alkaline phosphatase to a free thiol metabolite that binds to the reactive metabolites of these cytotoxic drugs.
- Fertility is reduced through impaired gametogenesis.
- Long-term use of alkylating drugs can cause the development of acute myeloid leukaemia, especially if combined with radiotherapy.
- Busulfan, carmustine and treosulfan can cause pulmonary fibrosis.
- Busulfan and treosulfan commonly cause skin pigmentation.
- Cyclophosphamide and ifosfamide cause bladder toxicity with haemorrhagic cystitis due to the formation of acrolein; it can be prevented by prior treatment with mesna (mercaptoethane sulfonic acid; see Chapter 53), which detoxifies acrolein in the bladder. Bladder cancer can develop years after cyclophosphamide therapy; it is not known if this is prevented by mesna.

Cytotoxic antibiotics

anthracyclines: doxorubicin, epirubicin
other antibiotics: bleomycin, dactinomycin, mitomycin, mitoxantrone

Mechanisms of action and uses

The cytotoxic antibiotics have diverse chemical structures.

- The anthracyclines are all quinone-containing planar four-ringed structures that contain an amino sugar group.
- Mitoxantrone is an anthracycline derivative with a three-ringed planar quinone structure and amino-containing side chains, and mitomycin is a nonplanar tricyclic quinone.
- Bleomycin and dactinomycin are complex peptide or glycopeptide derivatives.

Cytotoxic antibiotics have several possible mechanisms of action.

- Intercalation: this is shown particularly by the anthracyclines, with the planar ring system intercalating between DNA bases and the amino sugar part binding to the deoxyribose phosphate groups. Intercalation blocks reading of the DNA template during replication and transcription and prevents the action of topoisomerase II, the enzyme that relaxes DNA supercoils by creating double-stranded breaks.
- Histone eviction: doxorubicin and other anthracyclines displace histone proteins from the chromatin structure, disrupting the processes that detect and repair damaged DNA.
- Free radical attack: metabolism of the drugs gives rise to superoxide and hydroxyl radicals and hydrogen peroxide, which cause DNA damage and cytotoxicity.
- Membrane effects: interference with membrane function can occur either directly or via oxidative damage by free radicals.

In general, the mechanisms of action are not cell cycle-specific, although some members of the class show greatest activity at certain phases of the cycle – for example, S phase (doxorubicin, mitoxantrone), G_1 and early S phase (mitomycin) and G_2 phase and mitosis (bleomycin).

Cytotoxic antibiotics have a wide spectrum of activity and are used to treat several leukaemias and lymphomas as well as some solid tumours.

Pharmacokinetics

The cytotoxic antibiotics are poorly absorbed from the gut and are given intravenously. They are eliminated by metabolism and some have very long half-lives (mostly 12 hours or longer).

Unwanted effects

Many of these drugs have radiomimetic properties. They should not be used at the same time as radiotherapy, since toxicity can be greatly increased.

- General cytotoxicity.
- Doxorubicin, epirubicin and mitoxantrone produce dose-related, irreversible myocardial damage leading to cardiomyopathy due to free radical formation and oxidative stress as well as nuclear cytotoxicity. The cardiomyopathy may not become apparent until several years after treatment. Liposomal formulations of doxorubicin and longer infusion times may reduce the cardiac toxicity, as does concurrent infusion of the iron chelator dexrazoxane.
- Painful skin eruptions with liposomal doxorubicin.
- Bleomycin often causes skin pigmentation.
- Bleomycin and mitomycin produce dose-related pulmonary fibrosis.
- Tissue extravasation during infusion of anthracyclines produces severe necrosis, which can be minimised by subsequent intravenous infusion of dexrazoxane.

Platinum compounds

carboplatin, cisplatin, oxaliplatin

Mechanism of action and uses

The platinum drugs generate a reactive complex that creates cross-links between guanine nucleotides within the same

DNA strand or bridging complementary strands of DNA and also between DNA and proteins. The result is similar to the effect of alkylating drugs by blocking replication and transcription. Cisplatin and carboplatin are used for ovarian and lung tumours. Cisplatin is also used for several other solid tumours. Oxaliplatin is used with fluorouracil for advanced colorectal cancer.

Pharmacokinetics

These drugs are given by intravenous infusion and are mainly excreted by the kidney as platinum compounds. Cisplatin and oxaliplatin have very long half-lives (24–60 hours), largely owing to extensive protein binding.

Unwanted effects

- Severe nausea, vomiting, anorexia and diarrhoea.
- Nephrotoxicity with irreversible renal impairment; hydration is important to minimise the risk.
- Hypokalaemia, hypomagnesaemia.
- Ototoxicity with hearing loss and tinnitus.
- Visual disturbances.
- Peripheral neuropathy (especially with oxaliplatin).
- Myelosuppression (more marked for carboplatin).

Most effects are more marked for cisplatin than for carboplatin. Amifostine (see above) is used to reduce the severity of cisplatin-induced neutropenia in advanced ovarian cancer. It also reduces the nephrotoxicity of cisplatin.

Antimetabolites

Folic acid antagonists

methotrexate

Mechanism of action and uses

An astute clinical observation that the administration of folic acid to children with leukaemia exacerbated their condition led to the development of methotrexate, a folate antagonist. This represented an important landmark in cancer chemotherapy.

Folic acid in its reduced form, tetrahydrofolic acid (THF), is an important biochemical intermediate. It is essential for reactions that involve the addition of a single carbon atom, such as the introduction of the methyl group into thymidylate and the synthesis of the purine ring system. During such reactions, THF is oxidised to dihydrofolic acid (DHF), which must be reduced back to THF by dihydrofolate reductase before it can accept a further one-carbon group and be reused.

Methotrexate has a very high affinity for mammalian dihydrofolate reductase and inhibits its active site. This blocks purine and thymidylate synthesis and inhibits the synthesis of DNA, RNA and protein. It may show selectivity for cancer cells because these rely more on de novo synthesis of purines and pyrimidines, whereas normal tissues use salvage pathways that reutilise preformed purines and pyrimidines to a greater extent. Methotrexate is specific for S phase and slows G_1 to S phase.

Methotrexate is given for acute lymphoblastic leukaemia, non-Hodgkin's lymphomas and various solid tumours. It is also used as an immunosuppressant at lower doses in nonmalignant conditions such as inflammatory joint diseases and psoriasis. The mechanism of its immunosuppressant effect differs from its anticancer actions (see Chapter 38).

Pharmacokinetics

Methotrexate is well absorbed from the gut but can also be given intravenously or intrathecally. It is eliminated by renal excretion.

Unwanted effects

- Toxicity to normal, rapidly dividing tissues, especially the bone marrow.
- Hepatotoxicity can follow chronic therapy as an immunosuppressant (see Chapter 38).

Toxicity is increased in the presence of reduced renal excretion, and methotrexate should be avoided if there is significant renal impairment. Folinic acid (leucovorin) is frequently administered shortly after high-dose methotrexate to reduce mucositis and myelosuppression. Nonsteroidal antiinflammatory drugs such as aspirin can reduce the renal excretion of methotrexate and increase its toxicity.

Base analogue antimetabolites

purine antagonists: fludarabine, gemcitabine, mercaptopurine, tioguanine
pyrimidine antagonists: capecitabine, cytarabine, fluorouracil, raltitrexed, tegafur

Mechanism of action and uses

A number of useful chemotherapeutic drugs have been produced by simple modifications to the structures of normal purine and pyrimidine bases (Fig. 52.4). These act in a number of ways to interfere with DNA synthesis, typically following intracellular phosphorylation and the incorporation of the triphosphate product into DNA or RNA. Detailed mechanisms are given for each drug in the compendium at the end of this chapter. Base analogue antimetabolites are used for a wide variety of leukaemias, lymphomas and solid tumours.

Pharmacokinetics

Base analogues are mainly absorbed and metabolised by the pathways involved in absorption and metabolism of the corresponding unmodified base. Oral absorption is often erratic and most of these drugs are given intravenously. The urine is a minor route of elimination (up to 1% of the parent drug) and most half-lives are in the range 1–8 hours. Tegafur is a pro-drug of fluorouracil given in combination with gimeracil, which inhibits the breakdown of fluorouracil, and oteracil, which reduces its gastric toxicity.

Unwanted effects

- Typical cytotoxic effects are common; myelosuppression, in particular, can be severe and prolonged after cladribine, cytarabine, fludarabine and tioguanine.
- Drug interaction: allopurinol (see Chapter 31) interferes with the metabolism of 6-mercaptopurine; the dose should be reduced if these drugs are used concurrently.

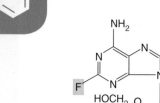

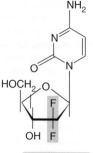

Fludarabine (F replaces
H of adenosine and ribose
is replaced by arabose)

Fluorouracil
(F replaces H
of uracil)

Gemcitabine
(F replaces H and
OH on ribose ring)

6-Mercaptopurine
(sulfur substitute
in purine)

Fig. 52.4 **The structures of some antimetabolite drugs, illustrating their similarity to normal bases and nucleotides.** The structural changes are highlighted.

MITOTIC INHIBITORS

Vinca alkaloids

vinblastine, vincristine, vindesine, vinorelbine

Mechanism of action and uses

The vinca alkaloids are complex natural chemicals isolated from the periwinkle plant (*Vinca rosea*). Vinca alkaloids bind to tubulin; they inhibit polymerisation and therefore assembly of microtubules, thus producing M-phase arrest of mitosis. Because microtubules are essential for numerous other cellular functions – including maintenance of cell shape, motility and transport between organelles – the vinca alkaloids also affect the nonmitotic cell cycle.

Vinca alkaloids are used to treat various lymphomas and acute leukaemias. They are also effective in some solid tumours.

Pharmacokinetics

Vinca alkaloids are usually given intravenously. Elimination is largely by metabolism with little renal excretion. They have very long half-lives.

Unwanted effects

The spectrum of unwanted effects differs among various drugs despite their close structural similarities.

- General cytotoxicity. Myelosuppression is dose-limiting for vinblastine, vindesine and vinorelbine but unusual with vincristine.
- Neurotoxicity, usually a sensory neuropathy, is dose-limiting with vincristine. It causes peripheral paraesthesiae, loss of tendon reflexes, abdominal pain and constipation. Motor weakness and autonomic neuropathy occasionally accompany the sensory neuropathy.

- Severe tissue damage if the drugs extravasate from the infusion site.

Camptothecin analogues (topoisomerase I inhibitors)

irinotecan, topotecan

Mechanism of action and uses

These drugs are semi-synthetic derivatives of a cytotoxic alkaloid isolated from the Chinese tree *Camptotheca acuminata*. The drugs inhibit topoisomerase I, which is important in DNA transcription and translation. The enzyme relieves the torsional strain in DNA by producing single-strand breaks that, under normal cell conditions, are then religated. The drugs bind to the DNA–topoisomerase I complex and prevent religation. Although this binding is readily reversible, the consequences are irreversible because cell death occurs when a double-strand break is produced at the DNA replication fork during S phase. Inhibition of DNA repair increases the sensitivity of the cell to ionising radiation.

Irinotecan is given as second-line treatment for metastatic colorectal cancer. Topotecan is used for lung, cervical or ovarian cancer.

Pharmacokinetics

They are large complex molecules that are given by intravenous infusion and eliminated mainly by hepatic metabolism.

Unwanted effects

- General cytotoxicity, with dose-limiting myelosuppression.
- Neutropenia.
- Severe diarrhoea: cholinergic stimulation produces early diarrhoea, but other toxicity can result in delayed onset of diarrhoea.

Epipodophyllotoxins (topoisomerase II inhibitors)

etoposide

Mechanism of action and uses

Etoposide is a synthetic derivative of a compound extracted from the mandrake root (*Podophyllum peltatum*). It is active during the G_2 phase and binds to the complex of DNA and topoisomerase II, an enzyme that regulates DNA supercoiling by introducing double-stranded breaks. The etoposide-bound complex inhibits DNA replication by preventing religation of the DNA and leads to cell apoptosis.

Etoposide is used for small-cell lung carcinoma, lymphomas and testicular cancer.

Pharmacokinetics

Etoposide can be given orally or intravenously. Elimination is largely by metabolism.

Unwanted effects

- General cytotoxicity.
- Severe tissue damage if the drug extravasates from the infusion site.

Taxanes

docetaxel, paclitaxel

Mechanism of action and uses

The drugs used clinically are produced from taxane, a diterpenoid extracted from the bark of the Pacific yew tree (*Taxus brevifolia*). Taxanes promote the assembly of microtubules but inhibit their depolymerisation, leading to the formation of stable and nonfunctional microtubular bundles in the cell. They bind to a different site to that targeted by vinca alkaloids. The cell is inhibited during the G_2 and M phases of the cell cycle. Taxanes are also radiosensitisers, since cells in the G_2 and M phases are more sensitive to radiation.

Taxanes are used to treat ovarian, breast and prostate cancer and a variety of other solid tumours.

Pharmacokinetics

Taxanes are given intravenously because of poor oral absorption. They are extensively metabolised in the liver and have half-lives of 10–20 hours.

Unwanted effects

- General cytotoxicity.
- Severe hypersensitivity reactions can occur, with hypotension, angioedema and bronchospasm. Routine premedication with histamine (H_1 and H_2) receptor antagonists (see Chapters 33 and 39) combined with a corticosteroid (see Chapter 44) is recommended for paclitaxel and premedication with a corticosteroid for docetaxel.

- Neutropenia is dose-limiting.
- Arthralgia/myalgia syndrome.
- Paclitaxel causes peripheral sensory neuropathy, with motor neuropathy at high dosages.
- Docetaxel causes persistent leg oedema due to fluid retention.

DRUGS AFFECTING TYROSINE KINASES AND OTHER PROTEIN KINASES

The products of activated oncogenes include various cell-surface receptors; these activate a range of intracellular tyrosine kinases that autophosphorylate the receptor (see Chapter 1). There are about 20 families of receptors, including VEGF receptors, of which there are three types: (1) the human epidermal growth factor (EGF) receptors HER1, HER2, HER3 and HER4; (2) platelet-derived growth factor (PDGF) receptors; and (3) fibroblast growth factor (FGF) receptors. Autophosphorylation of the receptor triggers a series of intracellular pathways that stimulate the proliferation of cancer cells and block apoptosis.

Drugs acting on these processes can be subdivided into monoclonal antibodies that block the growth factor receptor on the cell surface and small organic molecules that act on the receptor-associated tyrosine kinase or on other intracellular kinases involved in the signalling pathways that control cell division, gene transcription, motility and apoptosis. The latter include Bruton's tyrosine kinase (BTK), Janus-associated tyrosine kinases (JAK), phosphoinositide 3-kinases, mechanistic (mammalian) target of rapamycin (mTOR) and B-raf kinase.

Tyrosine kinase receptor inhibitors

bevacizumab, cetuximab, trastuzumab

Mechanism of action and uses

Bevacizumab is a monoclonal antibody that inhibits VEGF receptor tyrosine kinase and reduces tumour angiogenesis. It is given by intravenous infusion as part of the first-line treatment of metastatic colorectal cancer, lung cancer and renal cell carcinoma. Unwanted effects include mucocutaneous bleeding, gastrointestinal perforation and impaired wound healing.

Cetuximab is a monoclonal antibody that binds to the extracellular domain of the EGF receptor HER1 and blocks ligand-induced activation of tyrosine kinase. It is given by intravenous infusion in cases of colorectal tumour expressing epidermal growth factor receptor (EGFR) and in combination with radiotherapy for locally advanced squamous cell cancer of the head and neck. Unwanted effects may occur with the infusion, including chills, fever and hypersensitivity reactions. Severe keratitis leading to blindness has also been reported.

Trastuzumab is a monoclonal antibody used for metastatic breast cancer when the tumour overexpresses HER2 receptors. It binds to HER2 and prevents activation of tyrosine kinase. Unwanted effects may occur with the infusion, including chills, fever and hypersensitivity reactions. Cardiotoxicity occurs if trastuzumab is used with anthracyclines, leading to heart failure.

Inhibitors of tyrosine kinases and other protein kinases

dasatinib, erlotinib, imatinib, sorafenib, sunitinib

These drugs represent a growing group of small-molecule compounds that block the intracellular activity of tyrosine kinases, preventing transduction of signals from a variety of tyrosine kinase-linked receptors or inhibiting other intracellular protein kinases; some have multiple kinase targets (see drug compendium at the end of this chapter for details). The drugs inhibit cell proliferation and enhance apoptosis.

- Dasatinib inhibits multiple tyrosine kinases, including those associated with VEGF and PDGF receptor families and with Bcr-Abl the product of fusion between Abelson murine leukemia viral oncogene homolog 1. Bcr-Abl is a constitutively-expressed hybrid protein produced by fusion of the breakpoint cluster region protein (Bcr) and the Abelson murine leukemia viral oncogene homolog 1 (Abl) genes. It is constitutively expressed in leukaemias associated with the Philadelphia chromosome. Dasatinib is used for chronic myeloid leukaemia and acute lymphoblastic leukaemia.
- Erlotinib inhibits signalling by the EGF receptor HER1. It is used to treat lung and pancreatic cancers.
- Imatinib inhibits signals from the PDGF receptor family and Bcr-Abl. It is used to treat chronic myeloid leukaemia, acute lymphoblastic leukaemia and a variety of rare tumours.
- Sunitinib and sorafenib inhibit signalling by several receptor tyrosine kinases, including the VEGF and PDGF receptor families. They are used to treat renal cell carcinoma; sunitinib is also used for gastrointestinal stromal tumours and sorafenib also for hepatocellular cancer.

Pharmacokinetics

These drugs are generally well absorbed from the gut and most are metabolised in the liver, sometimes to active metabolites. The half-lives range from a few hours to several days.

Unwanted effects

- Cytotoxic effects.
- Gastrointestinal upset.
- Dizziness, headache, insomnia.
- Oedema with dasatinib and imatinib.

PROTEASOME INHIBITORS

bortezomib

Mechanism of action

Proteasomes are large cellular complexes that degrade proteins. Damaged, misfolded or unneeded proteins are labelled by enzymatic conjugation with ubiquitin, an 8.5-kDa protein; the ubiquitinated complex is then destroyed in the proteasome by proteolysis. Bortezomib is a boron-containing peptide that inhibits the catalytic site of the 26S proteasome. This probably reduces the degradation of pro-apoptotic proteins such as p53, leading to programmed cell death. Multiple myeloma cells are particularly sensitive to proteasome inhibition.

Pharmacokinetics

Bortezomib is given intravenously. It is metabolised in the liver and has a half-life of 9–15 hours.

Unwanted effects

- Gastrointestinal disturbances (nausea, vomiting, diarrhoea, anorexia).
- Cytotoxic effects.
- Peripheral neuropathy, fatigue.
- Visual and auditory disturbances.
- Mood disorders (anxiety), dizziness, hallucinations.
- Pyrexia.
- Postural hypotension, vertigo, syncope.

HORMONAL AGENTS

Some drugs used in cancer therapy suppress cell division by actions at intracellular steroid receptors or by influencing the metabolism of steroidal hormones; examples include corticosteroids and drugs that control the division of cells sensitive to sex hormones. Cancers that arise from cell lines possessing steroid receptors that promote their growth and cell division are frequently susceptible to inhibitory steroids.

Glucocorticoids

Glucocorticoids (see Chapter 44) suppress lymphocyte mitosis and are used to treat leukaemia and lymphoma; they are also helpful in reducing oedema around a tumour.

Oestrogens

Oestrogens such as ethinylestradiol (see drug compendium at end of this chapter and also Chapter 45) suppress prostate cancer cells, both locally and in metastases, and provide symptomatic improvement; gynaecomastia is a common unwanted effect.

Progestogens

Progestogens such as medroxyprogesterone acetate (see drug compendium in this chapter and Chapter 45) suppress endometrial cancer cells and kidney cancer metastases.

Oestrogen receptor antagonists

Breast cancer can be suppressed by oestrogen receptor antagonists such as tamoxifen. Tamoxifen is active orally and binds competitively to oestrogen receptors. It shows both oestrogenic effects (on bone) and antioestrogenic effects (on breast tissue). Tamoxifen inhibits oestrogen-regulated genes and reduces the secretion of growth factors by tumour cells.

Tumour cells are affected mainly in the G_2 phase of the cell cycle. Tamoxifen is extensively metabolised in the liver and has active metabolites with long half-lives; therefore several weeks of treatment are necessary to achieve steady-state concentrations. Unwanted effects include hot flushes and amenorrhoea in premenopausal women and vaginal bleeding in postmenopausal women. Tamoxifen inhibits CYP3A4 and thus reduces the metabolism of other enzyme substrates, such as warfarin.

Aromatase inhibitors

Aromatase is the enzyme that converts androgens to oestrogens. Inhibitors of aromatase may be nonsteroidal (e.g. anastrazole and letrozole) or steroids (e.g. exemestane). They reduce oestrogen production in postmenopausal women, who produce oestrogen mainly from androstenedione and testosterone in many tissues such as adipose tissue, skin, muscle and liver. Aromatase is also present in the cells of two-thirds of breast cancers. Aromatase inhibitors are used in post-menopausal women to treat breast cancers that are oestrogen-dependent.

Androgen receptor antagonists

These drugs (e.g. flutamide; see drug compendium in this chapter and Chapter 46) suppress prostate cancer cells.

Gonadorelin analogues

Gonadorelin is synthetic gonadotrophin-releasing hormone (GnRH) (see drug compendium in this chapter and Chapter 43). Gonadorelin analogues (e.g. buserelin) suppress prostate cancer cells.

MISCELLANEOUS ANTICANCER DRUGS

There are many other anticancer drugs with a wide variety of mechanisms of action. Further details (including therapeutic uses and serious adverse effects) are given in the drug compendium at the end of this chapter.

Mechanisms of action and uses

Numerous biochemical sites and mechanisms other than those described previously for the major drug groups have been identified as targets for anticancer drugs. Actions of miscellaneous drugs include the following:

- Removal of asparagine required for protein synthesis (crisantaspase).
- Inhibition of incorporation of thymidine and adenine into DNA (procarbazine).
- Inhibition of adenosine deaminase, which causes a buildup of deoxyadenosine triphosphate (dATP), inhibiting the formation of other deoxyribonucleotide triphosphates (pentostatin).
- Inhibition of reduction of ribonucleotides to deoxyribonucleotides (hydroxycarbamide).
- Inhibition of DNA repair by an alkylating action, especially on thiol groups (dacarbazine and temozolomide).

- Superoxide production, causing DNA backbone cleavage and cell apoptosis (trabectedin).
- Increased cell differentiation and inhibition of proliferation by action on retinoic acid receptors (RAR) and retinoid X receptors (RXR) (bexarotene, tretinoin) (see Chapter 49).
- Inhibition of the hedgehog signalling pathway of basal epidermal cell proliferation by blockade of the 'smoothened' (SMO) GPCR-like receptor (vesmodegib).
- Photodynamic activation in superficial tumours by laser light to produce cytotoxic oxygen free radicals (porfimer sodium, temoporfin).
- Inhibition of angiogenesis with a soluble decoy receptor for VEGF (aflibercept).
- Immunomodulation by inhibition of tumour necrosis factor α and other pro-inflammatory chemokines and inhibition of angiogenesis (lenalidomide, pomalidomide and thalidomide).
- Activation of cytotoxic killer cells (see Chapter 38); interleukin-2 (aldesleukin) is a recombinant T-lymphocyte cytokine.
- Monoclonal antibodies: several monoclonal antibodies have been developed that have anticancer activity. For example:
  - Alemtuzumab, an anti-CD52 antibody, and the anti-CD20 antibodies obinutuzumab and ofatumumab, which produce lysis of B-lymphocytes in treatment-resistant or rapidly relapsing chronic lymphocytic leukaemia.
  - Rituximab, an anti-CD20 antibody, which produces lysis of B-lymphocytes in chemotherapy-resistant advanced follicular lymphoma (see also Chapter 49).
  - Catumaxomab, a trifunctional molecule that binds to the epithelial cell adhesion molecule (EpCAM) on epithelial tumour cells, to CD3 on T-lymphocytes and to Fc receptors on several accessory cells such as macrophages, natural killer cells or dendritic cells; it cross-links the cells and triggers an immune reaction against the cancer cell.
  - Ipilimumab, which binds to cytotoxic T-lymphocyte antigen 4 (CTLA-4), an inhibitory immune checkpoint receptor; the drug blocks CTLA-4 and enhances cytotoxic T-cell activity. It is used to treat metastatic melanoma.

CLINICAL USES OF ANTINEOPLASTIC DRUGS

Different forms of cancer vary in their sensitivity to chemotherapy. The most responsive include lymphomas, leukaemias, choriocarcinoma and testicular carcinoma, while solid tumours such as sarcomas, adrenocortical and squamous cell bronchial carcinomas generally have a poor response. An intermediate response is shown by other cancers – for example, those of the bowel, bladder, head and neck, small-cell bronchogenic tumours and hormone-related cancers (breast, ovary, endometrium and prostate). In addition, the sensitivity of an individual tumour can change during treatment with antineoplastic drugs because of the development of resistance.

Chemotherapy can be used alone to treat cancer or in combination with surgery or with radiation (chemoradiation). Chemotherapy may be given as a curative or a palliative treatment or to reduce the risk of relapse after tumour removal. *Adjuvant chemotherapy* refers specifically to treatment following a surgical procedure that appears to have removed all tumour, with the intention of preventing relapse from occult disease. Neoadjuvant chemotherapy is given before surgery to reduce tumour size.

Chemotherapy is supplemented in many cancer types by the use of orally effective small-molecule inhibitors, which often require the presence of a particular gene mutation in the target molecule for effect (see later sections). These are excellent examples of the increasing personalization of cancer treatments, and such drugs have converted some solid cancers from rapidly fatal conditions to diseases that can remain well controlled or radiologically resolved, sometimes for many years.

A major new development in systemic therapy over recent years is immunotherapy, which targets the cancer by immune attack. Examples of drugs that have become mainstream treatments are a vaccine in advanced prostate cancer and the immunostimulatory antibody ipilimumab in melanoma.

ANTICANCER DRUG THERAPY FOR SPECIFIC MALIGNANCIES

The following discussion selects some important cancers and outlines the role of chemotherapeutic drugs in their management. The choice of specific regimens is a complex process involving an assessment of the patient's frailty and prognosis, his or her wishes, and the drug's toxicity. Clinical trials are producing a continuing flow of improved therapeutic options, and this is a field of medicine that changes rapidly.

OESOPHAGEAL CANCER

Oesophageal cancer usually presents with advanced disease, with 50% being unresectable or having radiological metastases at presentation. Two common forms are recognized: squamous cell carcinoma, which is more common in older smokers, and adenocarcinoma, which accounts for 75% of cases in the United Kingdom and is associated with gastro-oesophageal reflux, obesity and Barrett's metaplasia. For squamous cell cancers, if the disease is localized, chemoradiation followed by surgical resection or radical chemoradiation is used. Combination chemotherapy with epirubicin, oxaliplatin, and capecitabine, or with epirubicin, cisplatin and fluorouracil are typical chemotherapy regimens. They are also used for unresectable cancers. The identification of a HER2/neu mutation in some oesophageal cancers predicts responses to additional chemotherapy with trastuzumab.

GASTRIC CANCER

Surgery alone can be curative for early disease (although 80% of tumours recur locally or with metastases after resection), but 65% present with more advanced, unresectable disease. For individuals considered suitable for radical surgical resection, neoadjuvant and adjuvant chemotherapy using a combination of epirubicin, oxaliplatin and capecitabine improves survival. Fluorouracil or capecitabine combined with cisplatin can be palliative in advanced disease (response rate of 65%). Approximately 15% of tumours are HER-2

positive, and cisplatin, with either capecitabine or fluorouracil and trastuzumab can be considered for palliative treatment. VEGFR-2-positive tumours show some response to the targeted antibody ramucirumab.

PANCREATIC CANCER

Most pancreatic cancers present late, and 5-year survival is low because of metastatic progression. For operable tumours (15–20% of all pancreatic cancers), surgery followed by adjuvant chemotherapy with gemcitabine or fluorouracil is the treatment of choice. For inoperable locally advanced tumours, chemoradiation with capecitabine is used. Metastatic disease can be treated with a combination of fluorouracil with oxaliplatin and irinotecan.

COLORECTAL CANCER

Surgery is the mainstay of treatment for people with colorectal cancer without metastatic disease. If there is a high risk of relapse (Duke's grade C or some grade B), a combination of oxaliplatin with fluorouracil or capecitabine improves survival by 10–15%. Pre-operative chemoradiation reduces metastatic spread and, for rectal cancer, reduces local recurrence. Once a person has survived for 5 years, life expectancy is similar to that of the general population.

In advanced and metastatic colorectal cancer, the fluoropyrimidines fluorouracil or capecitabine, with or without oxaliplatin or irinotecan, improve survival and quality of life. The EGFR-targeted monoclonal antibodies cetuximab or panitumumab can be added to oxaliplatin or irinotecan-containing regimens in V-Ki-ras2 Kirsten rat sarcoma viral oncogene homolog (KRAS) wild-type colorectal tumours, leading to increased response rates. Bevacizumab, a monoclonal antibody targeting VEGF, can also enhance the effect of standard chemotherapy irrespective of KRAS status, and is now widely used in combination with chemotherapy.

LUNG CANCER

There are four principal types of lung cancer. Nonsmall-cell cancers (adenocarcinoma, squamous cell cancer and large-cell cancer) account for about three-quarters of cases, with small-cell cancer responsible for the remainder.

For nonsmall-cell lung cancer, superficial lesions are amenable to several treatments, including photodynamic therapy with porfimer sodium. Surgical resection can be curative in the early stages. Neoadjuvant or adjuvant chemotherapy with cisplatin combined with one of several other drugs improves survival if the tumour is resectable. Radiotherapy or chemoradiotherapy is used after surgery when the tumour is not fully resectable or for palliation of metastases. Chemotherapy has a limited place for advanced or recurrent disease and is mainly palliative. The current gold standard is the combination of a platinum compound (carboplatin or cisplatin) with one of several newer-generation drugs (docetaxel, paclitaxel, vinorelbine, gemcitabine).

About 15% of nonsmall-cell lung cancers, mainly adenocarcinomas, carry an activating mutation in the EGFR gene. These tumours are responsive to treatment with tyrosine kinase inhibitors such as erlotinib and gefitinib, which have maintained remissions for years in some cases. Other treatment targets have been identified, such as the cMET/anaplastic lymphoma kinase (ALK) translocation, which accounts for about 20% of nonsquamous cell carcinomas and can be treated with crizotinib.

Small-cell lung cancer is more sensitive to chemotherapy and has an initial response rate of 60–70%, with complete remission in 20–30% of cases. Examples of regimens are cisplatin combined with etoposide or cyclophosphamide with doxorubicin and vincristine. Radiotherapy is also given for limited-stage disease. Topotecan can be considered for relapsed disease.

MELANOMA

Survival in melanoma is related to tumour thickness, with 5-year survival falling from more than 95% with superficial tumours to less than 50% survival if the depth is greater than 4 mm. Wide surgical excision is the treatment of choice. Postsurgical adjuvant chemotherapy does not improve survival or disease-free outcome. Interferon alpha was the first drug shown to increase disease-free survival, but it has only a small impact (3–5%) on overall survival.

The management of advanced (inoperable) disease is determined by the presence or absence of a mutation in the *BRAF* gene (mutation V600E). Tumours with this mutation (40–50%) can be treated with vemurafenib, a B-Raf tyrosine kinase inhibitor, with initial disease control in about 80% of cases. However the effect is sometimes short-lived, with a median progression-free survival of 6 months. This appears to be mainly due to the unmasking of mutations in other signalling networks. To overcome this, combination with dabrafenib – an inhibitor of MEK protein, another intracellular signalling protein – is used. Tumours with a *BRAF* wild-type gene or that progress after B-Raf inhibition can be treated with the immunotherapeutic antibody ipilimumab, which produces responses over 5 years in just over 20% of cases. Chemotherapy with dacarbazine, temozolamide or the vinca alkaloids (vincristine or vinblastine) produces tumour responses in 10–20% of people, but without any clear effect on survival. Combination chemotherapy increases toxicity with no improvement in response.

RENAL CANCER

Nephrectomy is the treatment of choice for early-stage renal cancer. However, up to one-third of people have metastases at the time of diagnosis. Prior to the introduction of tyrosine kinase inhibitors for the treatment of advanced disease, interferon alpha was commonly used, with response rates in the region of 10–15%. In people with significant primary tumours and metastatic disease of modest volume, cytoreductive nephrectomy, radiofrequency ablation or tumour embolisation was generally offered and improves survival, with a small proportion of metastases spontaneously regressing after surgery. With the advent of more active systemic agents, the role of nephrectomy in the presence of metastatic disease is less clear. The majority of people with renal cell cancer have the clear cell variant, which is associated with high expression of VEGF. Agents that target this pathway are effective in the treatment of metastatic disease.

- Drugs – such as sorafenib, sunitinib or pazopanib – that inhibit multiple intracellular tyrosine kinases are used as the first-line treatment for advanced disease. They produce high responses rates, with an average duration of response of around 1 year.
- Both the mTOR inhibitor everolimus and the VEGF-targeted tyrosine kinase inhibitors axitinib or pazopanib are used after failure of first-line therapy. By sequencing first-, second- and sometimes third-line treatment for advanced kidney cancer, the disease can now be controlled for several years.
- Immunotherapy with interferon alpha combined with bevacizumab or aldesleukin (interleukin-2) produces responses in about 15% of cases. The toxicity of treatment can be high, but for a small proportion of those treated an extremely durable response can be achieved. More recently a peptide vaccine has been shown to have encouraging effects on survival in those vaccinated at progression after first-line treatment with sunitinib or sorafenib.

BLADDER CANCER

Superficial bladder tumours are removed surgically, but recurrence rates are high. Intravesical immunotherapy with bacillus Calmette–Guérin (BCG) vaccine is used to limit recurrence in superficial disease. For more advanced disease, neoadjuvant chemotherapy with gemcitabine and cisplatin improves survival. A bladder-sparing approach using transurethral resection followed by concurrent chemotherapy (cisplatin, methotrexate and vinblastine) and irradiation has given promising results for those who do not want cystectomy.

PROSTATE CANCER

Treatment is largely determined by the extent of spread of the cancer and there are several options.

- 'Watchful waiting' for localised disease confined to the prostate. This is usually used for individuals with a life expectancy of less than 10 years, since many tumours do not progress in this time.
- Radical prostatectomy for localised disease, usually in men under 70 years, in whom the risk of subsequent metastases is reduced from 25% to 15%. Impotence is a common sequel, occurring in 35–60% of cases.
- Radiotherapy for localised disease or locally advanced disease in older men. Impotence follows therapy in 40–60% of cases.
- Interstitial implantation of radioactive pellets for localised disease or locally advanced disease (brachytherapy). This can be combined with external radiotherapy for intermediate- or high-risk localized disease.
- Hormonal therapy for lymph node involvement or distant metastases. Prostate cancer is hormone-dependent for growth. Androgen deprivation therapy can be achieved by GnRH analogues such as leuprolide or goserelin (see Chapter 43). Tumour flare reactions are prevented by the use of antiandrogen therapy (e.g. with flutamide or cyproterone acetate; see Chapter 46) for the first few weeks to block adrenal androgen activity. Androgen deprivation therapy is combined with radiotherapy for intermediate- or high-risk localized disease,
- Resistant disease can be treated by chemotherapy with drugs such as docetaxel and cabazitaxel. Response rates of about 50% can be achieved. Painful metastatic deposits

can be treated with radiotherapy or with strontium-89, which is taken up by sclerotic metastases.

■ A new class of hormonal therapies has shown promising activity in advanced prostate cancer. Abiraterone is a 17-α hydroxylase inhibitor that prevents extra-testicular synthesis of androgens (see Chapter 46). It has low toxicity and increases survival when used either before or after chemotherapy for tumours that have become resistant to castration levels of testosterone inhibition. New androgen receptor antagonists with enhanced potency, such as enzalutamide (see Chapter 46), also increase survival in people with castration-resistant disease.

TESTICULAR CANCER

Testicular tumours are either seminomas or nonseminomatous germ cell tumours, depending on the tissue of origin. Cure rates are now greater than 95%. For *seminomas*, treatment choices include:

■ orchidectomy then follow-up for recurrence or chemotherapy with carboplatin if the recurrence risk is high.
■ for locally advanced disease, surgery is followed by radiotherapy, perhaps combined with carboplatin.
■ for metastatic disease, chemotherapy with bleomycin, etoposide and cisplatin (BEP) is one example of the combinations used. If the tumour recurs, treatment with paclitaxel, ifosfamide and cisplatin is one option. High-dose chemotherapy can be combined with stem cell transplant.

For *nonseminomatous* germ cell tumours, treatment choices include orchidectomy for early disease, which may be followed by chemotherapy with a regimen containing cisplatin. For more advanced or recurrent disease, combination chemotherapy with BEP produces an 85% complete remission rate when combined with surgery.

OVARIAN CANCER

Initial surgery for ovarian cancer is followed by chemotherapy for all disease that is not localised to the ovary (which occurs in 80% of cases). About 70% of these women respond to chemotherapy, with complete remission in 10–20%. Carboplatin or cisplatin with paclitaxel is often used. Liposomal doxorubicin, radiotherapy and bevacizumab are among the options for more advanced disease.

CERVICAL CANCER

Surgery or radiotherapy is the mainstay for local disease, but chemoradiation is used if there are poor prognostic predictors or in the case of advanced disease. Cisplatin is most frequently used and improves survival by 30%. For recurrent disease, the combination of cisplatin and paclitaxel has a small advantage over cisplatin alone.

ENDOMETRIAL CANCER

Surgery is the usual initial treatment for endometrial cancer. Adjuvant radiotherapy is given to the pelvis, and radiotherapy is also used for extrauterine metastases. Disseminated disease can be treated by hormone therapy with progestogens, but responses are poor (less than one-third of those treated) and depend on the presence of progesterone receptors on the tumour cells. Adjuvant chemotherapy with drugs such as carboplatin plus paclitaxel has a palliative role in advanced disease.

BREAST CANCER

Breast-conserving surgery is the treatment of choice for very early disease and for oestrogen receptor-positive tumours; it is usually followed by local radiotherapy. The risk of invasive recurrence is low; if this occurs, it is treated by mastectomy followed by chemotherapy. Chemotherapy or hormonal therapy is used for larger locally invasive tumours or distant spread, or as neoadjuvant treatment for recurrence.

Determination of the hormone receptor status of the tumour is an important guide to the most appropriate hormonal therapy or chemotherapy.

Oestrogen receptor-positive tumours

About 80% of tumours express the oestrogen receptor. For *premenopausal* women with oestrogen receptor-positive tumours:

■ tamoxifen remains the cornerstone of treatment, with or without chemotherapy. Aromatase inhibitors are ineffective before the menopause.
■ tamoxifen can be combined with ovarian ablation using a GnRH analogue such as goserelin.

In early disease, hormonal treatment is usually given for 10 years. Tamoxifen reduces breast cancer mortality by more than 30%, with continuing benefit after stopping treatment for 15 years. The 10–20% of women whose tumour becomes unresponsive to one hormonal treatment may still respond to the use of an alternative class of drug.

Options for adjuvant hormonal therapy for *postmenopausal* women with oestrogen receptor-positive tumours include the following:

■ nonsteroidal aromatase inhibitors such as anastrazole or letrozole or the steroidal aromatase inhibitor exemestane; these are more effective than tamoxifen. They can also be used as neoadjuvant therapy to reduce the extent of surgical resection. It is important to monitor bone density with the use of these drugs.
■ antioestrogen therapy (e.g. with tamoxifen) is considered second-line treatment for hormone-responsive cancer. If tamoxifen is used, switching to an aromatase inhibitor after 5 years further improves disease-free survival.
■ the selective oestrogen receptor downregulator (SERD) fulvestrant is an alternative second-line treatment for locally advanced or metastatic disease.
■ progestogens such as megestrol acetate are used as a third-line treatment.
■ GnRH analogues such as goserelin (see Chapter 43) are a fourth-line treatment.

Advanced disease can be also treated with hormonal therapy. If resistance develops, the combination of everolimus and exemestane may control the disease.

Box 52.1 **Simplified classification of acute myeloid leukaemias**

Acute myeloid leukaemia
Acute myeloblastic leukaemia
Acute promyelocytic leukaemia
Acute myelomonocytic leukaemia
Acute monocytic/monoblastic leukaemia
Acute erythroleukaemia
Acute megakaryoblastic leukaemia

Oestrogen receptor-negative tumours

Chemotherapy (treatment that does not involve hormonal manipulation) is used for oestrogen receptor-negative tumours, HER2-positive tumours, and younger women (especially under 35 years but also up to 70 years of age) or for hormonally unresponsive disease. Various regimens are used, such as doxorubicin or epirubicin with cyclophosphamide, combined with docetaxel for node-positive disease, which produces response rates of up to 40%.

Trastuzumab can be used for cancers that express HER2. After 1 year of treatment, it reduces early recurrence and improves survival by 35%.

ACUTE MYELOID LEUKAEMIAS

The acute myeloid leukaemias are a heterogeneous group of disorders (Box 52.1) that are differentiated on morphological grounds. Acute myeloid leukaemia is responsible for up to 15% of childhood leukaemias and is the commonest leukaemia of adult life. Complications usually result from bone marrow failure, and the management of serious infection or bleeding are important issues in supportive care. The risk of infection is amplified by chemotherapy. The initial aim of chemotherapy is to reduce 'blast' cells in the marrow to below 5% of the total cell population (remission) with induction therapy and then to eradicate the leukaemic cells with consolidation therapy, usually involving at least two or three cycles of additional treatment.

Intravenous chemotherapy with two or more drugs is used in the induction phase to reduce the development of resistance. A typical regimen consists of daunorubicin with cytarabine, which produces remission in 65–70% of individuals under 60 years of age; older people have a less favourable response. Consolidation is achieved with further courses of similar therapy for three to four cycles. Haematopoietic stem cell transplantation may be considered after remission is achieved. In children, treatment for the central nervous system is also given with intrathecal methotrexate. Salvage treatment is used for failure to enter remission or for relapse, with high-dose cytarabine alone or combined with fludarabine.

For acute promyelocytic leukaemia, the best initial response is obtained with tretinoin (all-*trans* retinoic acid), a vitamin A derivative (see Chapter 49) and consolidation is achieved by the addition of an anthracycline such as idarubicin or daunorubicin.

ACUTE LYMPHOBLASTIC LEUKAEMIA

Acute lymphoblastic leukaemia is most common in children under 10 years of age, with a few cases occurring after age 40 years. Supportive therapy is similar to that for acute myeloid leukaemia. Entry into a treatment trial of new therapeutic regimens will usually be offered, as the treatment of this type of leukaemia is rapidly advancing.

Remission induction (eradication of 99% of leukaemic cell burden) is typically achieved with combinations of three or more drugs. In children, vincristine and prednisolone or dexamethasone with crisantaspase, doxorubicin or daunorubicin is often used. Four or more drugs are used for children with high-risk disease and for most adults. Cyclophosphamide is often used for T-cell leukaemias, and imatinib or dasatinib added if the cells are Philadelphia chromosome-positive. Consolidation therapy is initially implemented with at least two multidrug intensification modules, using various combinations of a corticosteroid with vincristine, crisantaspase, methotrexate and mercaptopurine. Continuation therapy is used after the first 5 months with mercaptopurine and methotrexate for at least 2 years. Eradication of cranial disease is important, using intrathecal methotrexate, cytarabine and hydrocortisone; cranial irradiation is less commonly used. Selective use of haematopoietic stem cell transplantation can further improve outcome.

The results of treatment in childhood are excellent, with about 80% survival at 5 years, compared with 40% if the disease occurs in adult life.

CHRONIC MYELOID LEUKAEMIA

Chronic myeloid leukaemia occurs in all age groups but is rare in children. Most disease follows an initial chronic course lasting 3–4 years, with subsequent transformation to an accelerated phase, when survival is just 3–6 months. Imatinib is standard treatment for the chronic phase and achieves cytogenetic remission in up to 87% of people. Nilotinib or dasatinib are options after the failure of imatinib. Interferon alpha, usually given with cytarabine or hydroxycarbamide, is an alternative for those who do not tolerate imatinib. In younger people, allogeneic stem cell transplantation is the treatment of choice after failed chemotherapy.

For advanced disease with blast crisis, combination chemotherapy can be considered, such as the regimen used for acute myeloid leukaemia or acute lymphoblastic leukaemia, depending on the type of transformation.

CHRONIC LYMPHOCYTIC LEUKAEMIA

Chronic lymphocytic leukaemia is predominantly a disease of the elderly. Cure is unusual and median survival is 5–8 years, but treatment is given to control symptoms due to the disease. Therefore treatment may not be necessary if the disease is causing few problems, but oral chlorambucil, often combined with prednisolone, can be given for up to 6 months to regress the disease. Transformation of the disease to a more aggressive form can occur after several years, with increasing disease bulk, lymphoma-related symptoms or bone marrow failure. Fludarabine, cyclophosphamide and rituximab are used for individuals who are fit enough to tolerate more intensive treatment, as the combination produces a more prolonged remission. For those who are not fit enough for intensive chemotherapy, either chlorambucil or bendamustine can be given, perhaps with the addition of rituximab, with the goal of reducing leukaemic cells in the marrow to below 30%.

MALIGNANT LYMPHOMAS

The malignant lymphomas are a diverse group of disorders comprising Hodgkin's lymphoma and a variety of non-Hodgkin's lymphomas, which are classified by histopathological and cytochemical techniques. Low-grade non-Hodgkin's lymphomas are managed in a similar way to chronic lymphocytic leukaemia and have a similar prognosis. Non-Hodgkin's lymphomas of intermediate grade are curable in about 40% of cases, using courses of combination chemotherapy with cyclophosphamide, doxorubicin, vincristine and prednisolone ('CHOP' therapy – an acronym based on the generic and proprietary names of the drugs). Rituximab may improve survival when added to standard chemotherapy, and radiotherapy is sometimes used as adjunctive treatment or for relapsed disease. More frequent intensive therapy is required for high-grade, aggressive non-Hodgkin's lymphomas.

For Hodgkin's lymphoma, radiotherapy is curative if the tumour is localised; combination chemotherapy is the usual approach for more extensive disease. The most frequently used regimen is doxorubicin, bleomycin, vinblastine and dacarbazine (ABVD).

MULTIPLE MYELOMA

Multiple myeloma is mainly a disorder of the elderly. Treatment is aimed at suppressing the monoclonal protein in the blood. Supportive therapy is often required to treat hypercalcaemia, renal impairment and infection. A bisphosphonate is often given together with chemotherapy to prevent hypercalcaemia. Rehydration and analgesia for bone pain are often required. Radiotherapy may be used to treat localized areas of disease for pain control, lytic bone lesions or fractures.

Autologous stem cell transplantation is increasingly used as primary therapy after intensive chemotherapy and can produce 30–50% complete remission. Induction chemotherapy is with either two or three drugs, using regimens such as dexamethasone in combination with cyclophosphamide, bortezomib, thalidomide or lenalidomide.

For individuals who are not eligible for transplantation, chemotherapy is usually with oral melphalan and prednisolone combined with either thalidomide or bortezomib. This reduces the myeloma protein in blood by more than 50% in half of those treated. Median survival with this treatment is 3 years.

SELF-ASSESSMENT

True/false questions

1. Cancer cells are not subject to the normal feedback mechanisms that restrict cell multiplication.
2. Cells resting in G_0 phase are most susceptible to antineoplastic drugs.

3. Adverse effects of anticancer drugs include secondary carcinogenesis.
4. Alkylating agents interfere with normal DNA synthesis.
5. Methotrexate competitively inhibits deoxythymidylate kinase.
6. Folinic acid (leucovorin) reverses the action of methotrexate.
7. Fluorouracil is a purine antagonist.
8. The effects of cytotoxic antibiotics are due to their intercalation between DNA bases.
9. Most base analogue antimetabolites are pro-drugs activated by dephosphorylation.
10. Vinca alkaloids and taxanes share a common mechanism of action.
11. Tyrosine kinase inhibitors block signalling by growth factors.
12. Tamoxifen blocks oestrogen receptors on bone cells, causing osteoporosis.

One-best-answer (OBA) question

1. How does irinotecan act as an antineoplastic drug?
   A. It alkylates base pairs and blocks DNA polymerase.
   B. It blocks conversion of ribonucleotide to deoxyribonucleotide.
   C. It inhibits depolymerisation of microtubules.
   D. It inhibits folic acid-dependent thymidine formation.
   E. It prevents religation of DNA, leaving strand breaks.

Case-based questions

1. What are the criteria for combination chemotherapy of cancer? How well do the following treatment regimens meet the criteria?
   A. Acute lymphoblastic leukaemia (initial phase for induction of remission): intravenous vincristine, subcutaneous crisantaspase (asparaginase) and oral prednisolone.
   B. Non-Hodgkin's lymphoma: cyclophosphamide, doxorubicin, vincristine and prednisolone (CHOP regimen).
   C. Testicular teratoma in an adult: intravenous etoposide, bleomycin and cisplatin.
2. Why are doses of some anticancer drugs corrected to body surface area rather than weight? Does the use of surface area correction result in higher or lower doses for children compared with simple correction for body weight? Taking the example in Table 52.1 of an adult male (body weight 72.1 kg) given 100 mg of a drug, what doses would a 1-year-old child weighing 9.9 kg be given if corrected for body weight or for surface area?

ANSWERS

True/false answers

1. **True.** Dysfunction in the mechanisms that normally regulate cell multiplication is a characteristic of cancer cells.
2. **False.** Although some anticancer drugs affect the resting phase, cancer cells are typically most susceptible when they are actively dividing; the sensitivity of a tumour therefore depends on its growth fraction.

Table 52.1 Examples of body weights and surface areas in children and adults

Age (years)	Body weight (kg)	Height (m)	Body surface area (m²)
Children			
0.5	7.4	0.658	0.350
1.0	9.9	0.747	0.434
3	14.5	0.96	0.613
6	21.5	1.168	0.835
Adults			
Male	72.1	1.753	1.874
Female	60.3	1.676	1.681

3. **True.** Secondary cancers can occur, such as bladder cancer with cyclophosphamide (due to urinary excretion of toxic metabolites) and lymphoma with alkylating agents.
4. **True.** The alkylated bases produce various effects on DNA function, including misreading.
5. **False.** Methotrexate inhibits dihydrofolate reductase, a key enzyme in the folate pathway required for synthesis of purines and thymidine.
6. **True.** Leucovorin is used to rescue normal tissues when given after methotrexate; methotrexate has a preferential effect on cancer cells, and giving leucovorin 24 hours afterwards overcomes its unwanted actions in normal tissues such as bone marrow and gut mucosa.
7. **False.** Fluorouracil is a pyrimidine analogue (fluorinated uracil).
8. **True.** Along with DNA intercalation, shown particularly by anthracyclines, cytotoxic antibiotics such as bleomycin also generate superoxide and hydrogen peroxide that cleave DNA.
9. **False.** Many base analogues such as cytarabine and gemcitabine are activated by intracellular phosphorylation to triphosphate derivatives, which are incorporated into DNA.
10. **False.** Vinca alkaloids prevent mitosis by inducing microtubule disassembly, whereas taxanes inhibit mitosis by promoting formation of stable but nonfunctional microtubules.
11. **True.** Drugs such as dasatinib, erlotinib and imatinib inhibit the receptor tyrosine kinase families associated with growth factors including EGF, VEGF and PDGF; some also block kinases in downstream signalling pathways.
12. **False.** Tamoxifen is a selective oestrogen receptor modulator (SERM) that blocks oestrogen receptors on breast cancer cells but is an agonist at oestrogen receptors on bone cells, preventing osteoporosis.

One-best-answer (OBA) answer

1. **Answer E** is correct. Topoisomerase I unwinds DNA by creating single-strand breaks that are then religated; irinotecan inhibits topoisomerase I and prevents DNA transcription and replication. Answer A is the mechanism of action of alkylating agents (such as cyclophosphamide), and answer B is that of the ribonucleotide reductase inhibitor hydroxycarbamide. Prevention of microtubule depolymerisation (answer C) is the mechanism of taxanes such as docetaxel, while the folate antagonist methotrexate impairs the synthesis of thymidine and purines (answer D).

Case-based answers

1. The criteria for combination therapy in cancer treatment are as follows:
   - Each drug should have a different target within the cell; this increases cell kill and decreases drug resistance.
   - Each drug should show different unwanted effects; ideally this will produce additive efficacy but not toxicity and hence an increase in therapeutic index.
   - Each drug should be active as a single agent; the ethics of clinical trials means that new drugs are not usually tested for this criterion in clinical studies.

   The sites of action and side effects of the drugs in each regimen are shown in Table 52.2. All three regimens use drugs with different mechanisms of action (meeting the first criterion), although regimen C is targeted only at DNA function. Regimen B contains three drugs that produce bone marrow toxicity, contravening the second criterion, and this will need careful monitoring during therapy. For each drug regimen, the third criterion can be assumed to be met because all the agents are well-used drugs.

2. Because many of the drugs used in cancer therapy are toxic at therapeutic doses, it is important to tailor the dosage to the individual. Children have a higher cardiac output and greater hepatic and renal blood flows than adults on a body-weight basis. The elimination of drugs therefore tends to be faster in children than in adults and proportionally higher doses are necessary to give the same blood levels. Hepatic and renal blood flows are related to body weight to the power of approximately 0.7. Since body surface area is also proportional to body weight to the power of 0.7, it is usual to correct the drug doses by surface area to take better account of the rate of elimination. Surface area is calculated from a nomogram, or estimated using the approximation that it correlates with $weight^{0.7}$ or by using the more accurate Du Bois equation:

$$\text{Surface area} = 71.84 \times \text{weight}^{0.425} \times \text{height}^{0.725}$$

where surface area is in metres squared, weight is in kilograms and height is in metres. In the example, the adult male (body weight 72.1 kg) is given 100 mg of a drug. Simple correction for body weight of the 1-year-old child (9.9 kg) would suggest 13.7 mg (= 100 mg × 9.9 kg/72.1 kg) is the appropriate dose. However, using the surface area values in Table 52.1 (derived from the Du Bois formula), the dose would be 100 mg × 0.434 m²/1.874 m² = 23.2 mg. An approximation using surface area estimated as $weight^{0.7}$ gives a dose of 100 mg × $9.9^{0.7}$/$72.1^{0.7}$ = 24.9 mg, close to that obtained using the Du Bois formula. These results appear counterintuitive if children are assumed to be 'more sensitive' to drugs.

Table 52.2 Mechanisms of action and toxic effects of three treatment regimens

	Mechanism of action	Principal toxicity
(A) Acute lymphoblastic leukaemia		
Vincristine	Binds to tubulin/metaphase arrest	Bone marrow suppression, peripheral neuropathy
Crisantaspase	Depletes asparagine in blood	Decreased clotting factors, albumin and insulin
Prednisolone	Reduces DNA transcription of cytokines	Glucocorticoid actions
(B) Non-Hodgkin's lymphoma (CHOP regimen)		
Cyclophosphamide	Alkylates DNA	Bone marrow suppression, nausea/vomiting
Doxorubicin	Intercalation into DNA, oxygen free radicals	Bone marrow suppression, cardiotoxicity
Vincristine	Binds to tubulin/metaphase arrest	Bone marrow suppression, peripheral neuropathy
Prednisolone	Reduces DNA transcription of cytokines	Glucocorticoid actions
(C) Testicular teratoma		
Etoposide	Increases DNA cleavage by topoisomerase II	Bone marrow suppression, nausea, alopecia
Bleomycin	Oxidative damage to DNA	Pulmonary fibrosis
Cisplatin	Cross-links DNA	Nausea, bone marrow suppression, nephrotoxicity, ototoxicity

FURTHER READING

Drugs and drug action

Ciardiello, F., Tortora, G., 2008. EGFR antagonists in cancer treatment. N. Engl. J. Med. 358, 1160–1174.

Coate, L., Cuffe, S., Horgan, A., et al., 2010. Germline genetic variation, cancer outcome, and pharmacogenetics. J. Clin. Oncol. 28, 4029–4037.

Croce, C.M., 2008. Oncogenes and cancer. N. Engl. J. Med. 358, 502–511.

Grisold, W., Cavaletti, G., Windebank, A.J., 2012. Peripheral neuropathies from chemotherapeutics and targeted agents: diagnosis, treatment, and prevention. Neuro Oncol. 14 (4), 45–54.

Jayson, G.C., Kerbel, R., Ellis, L.M., et al., 2016. Antiangiogenic therapy in oncology: current status and future directions. Lancet 388, 518–529.

Kong, Y.W., Ferland-McCollough, D., Jackson, T.J., et al., 2012. MicroRNAs in cancer management. Lancet Oncol. 13, e249–e258.

Li, W., Zhang, H., Assaraf, Y.G., et al., 2016. Overcoming ABC transporter-mediated multidrug resistance: molecular mechanisms and novel therapeutic drug strategies. Drug Resist. Updat. 27, 14–29.

McLornan, D.P., List, A., Mufti, G.J., 2014. Applying synthetic lethality for the selective targeting of cancer. N. Engl. J. Med. 371, 1725–1735.

Sun, Y., Ma, L., 2015. The emerging molecular machinery and therapeutic targets of metastasis. Trends Pharmacol. Sci. 36, 349–359.

Torgovnick, A., Schumacher, B., 2015. DNA repair mechanisms in cancer development and therapy. Front. Genet. 6, 157.

Wilson, P.M., Danenberg, P.V., Johnston, P.G., et al., 2014. Standing the test of time: targeting thymidylate biosynthesis in cancer therapy. Nat. Rev. Clin. Oncol. 11, 282–298.

Gastrointestinal cancer

Brenner, H., Kloor, M., Pox, C.P., 2014. Colorectal cancer. Lancet 383, 1490–1502.

Kamisawa, T., Wood, L.D., Itoi, T., et al., 2016. Pancreatic cancer. Lancet 388, 73–85.

Rustgi, A.K., El-Serag, H.B., 2014. Esophageal carcinoma. N. Engl. J. Med. 371, 2499–2509.

van Cutsem, E., Sagaert, X., Topal, B., et al., 2016. Gastric Cancer. Lancet 388, 2654–2664.

Lung cancer

Hissch, F.R., Suda, K., Wiens, J., et al., 2016. New and emerging targeted treatments in advanced non-small-cell lung cancer. Lancet 388, 1012–1024.

Tan, W.L., Jain, A., Takano, A., et al., 2016. Novel therapeutic targets on the horizon for lung cancer. Lancet Oncol. 17, e347–e362.

Van Meerbeeck, J.P., Fennell, D.A., De Ruysscher, D.K., 2011. Small-cell lung cancer. Lancet 378, 1741–1755.

Urogenital cancer

Attard, G., Parker, C., Eeles, R.A., et al., 2016. Prostate cancer. Lancet 387, 70–82.

Capitanio, U., Montorsi, F., 2016. Renal cancer. Lancet 387, 894–906.

Jayson, G.C., Kohn, E.C., Kitchener, H.C., et al., 2014. Ovarian cancer. Lancet 384, 1376–1388.

Kamat, A.M., Hahn, N.M., Efstathiou, J.A., et al., 2016. Bladder cancer. Lancet 388, 2796–2810.

Morice, P., Leary, A., Creutzberg, C., et al., 2016. Endometrial cancer. Lancet 387, 1094–1108.

Petignat, P., Roy, M., 2007. Diagnosis and management of cervical cancer. Br. Med. J. 335, 765–768.

Rajpert-De Meyts, E., McGlynn, K.A., Okamoto, K., et al., 2016. Testicular germ cell tumours. Lancet 387, 1762–1774.

Breast cancer

Benson, J.R., Jatoi, I., Keisch, M., et al., 2009. Early breast cancer. Lancet 373, 1463–1479.

Yeo, B., Turner, N.C., Jones, A., 2014. Medical management of breast cancer. Br. Med. J. 348, g3608.

Melanoma

Eggermont, A.M., Spatz, A., Robert, C., 2014. Cutaneous melanoma. Lancet 383, 816–827.

Johnson, D.B., Sosman, J.A., 2015. Therapeutic advances and treatment options for metastatic melanoma. JAMA Oncol. 1, 380–386.

Acute leukaemias

Döhner, H., Weisdorf, D.J., Bloomfield, C.D., 2015. Acute myeloid leukemia. N. Engl. J. Med. 373, 1136–1152.

Hunger, S.P., Mullighan, C.G., 2015. Acute lymphoblastic leukemia in children. N. Engl. J. Med. 373, 1541–1552.

Chronic leukaemias

Apperley, J.F., 2015. Chronic myeloid leukaemia. Lancet 385, 1447–1459.

Routledge, D.J.M., Bloor, A.J.C., 2016. Recent advances in therapy of chronic lymphocytic leukaemia. Br. J. Haematol. 174, 351–367.

Lymphomas

Armitage, J.O., 2010. Early-stage Hodgkin's lymphoma. N. Engl. J. Med. 363, 653–662.

Shankland, K.R., Armitage, J.O., Hancock, B.W., 2012. Non-Hodgkin lymphoma. Lancet 380, 848–857.

Townsend, W., Linch, D., 2012. Hodgkin's lymphoma in adults. Lancet 380, 836–847.

Multiple myeloma

Palumbo, A., Anderson, K.A., 2011. Multiple myeloma. N. Engl. J. Med. 364, 1046–1060.

Röllig, C., Knop, S., Bornhäuser, M., 2015. Multiple myeloma. Lancet 385, 2197–2208.

Compendium: drugs used in the treatment of cancer

Drug	Characteristics
Unwanted effects that are severe and dose-limiting or not shared by other drugs in the same class are listed under characteristics; for general unwanted effects of drug class, see text.	
Drugs that affect nucleic acid function	
Alkylating agents	
Widely used drugs; act by damaging DNA and thereby interfering with cell division.	
Bendamustine	Used for treatment of chronic lymphocytic leukaemia, non-Hodgkin's lymphoma and multiple myeloma. Risk of teratogenesis. Given intravenously. Half-life: 0.5 h
Busulfan	Mainly used for effects on the bone marrow (e.g. chronic myeloid leukaemia). Risk of myelosuppression and irreversible bone marrow aplasia; rarely pulmonary fibrosis. Given orally or by intravenous infusion. Half-life: 2–3 h
Carmustine (BCNU)	Alkylates DNA and the nitroso function inactivates DNA repair. Used for multiple myeloma, lymphoma and brain tumours. Risk of renal damage and progressive pulmonary fibrosis. Given intravenously. Half-life: 0.5 h
Chlorambucil	Used mainly in lymphocytic leukaemia, non-Hodgkin's lymphoma and Hodgkin's disease. Risk of vomiting. Given orally. Half-life: 1–2 h
Cyclophosphamide	Widely used for leukaemias, lymphomas and solid tumours. Risk of haemorrhagic cystitis (mesna is antidote). Given orally or by intravenous injection. Half-life: 4–10 h
Estramustine	Oestrogen molecule linked to a nitrogen mustard group; acts as alkylating agent, especially on microtubule proteins, and increases circulating oestrogen levels. Used for prostate cancer. Given orally. Half-life: 20–24 h
Ifosfamide	Uses similar to cyclophosphamide. Risk of cystitis (see mesna antidote). Given by intravenous injection. Half-life: 4–15 h
Lomustine (CCNU)	Similar to carmustine. Mainly used for Hodgkin's disease and some solid tumours. Risk of permanent bone marrow damage. Given orally. Half-life: 1–5 h
Melphalan	Used mainly for multiple myeloma, ovarian adenocarcinoma, advanced breast cancer and neuroblastoma. Given orally or by intravenous injection. Half-life: 1.5 h
Thiotepa	Used for bladder cancer. Given by intravesicular injection. Half-life: 1.5–4 h
Treosulfan	High oral bioavailability; nonenzymatic degradation (1–2 h) Used mainly for ovarian cancer. Risk of allergic alveolitis and pulmonary fibrosis. Given orally or by intravenous injection. Half-life: 1–2 h

Compendium: drugs used in the treatment of cancer (cont'd)

Drug	Characteristics
Cytotoxic antibiotics	
Widely used drugs; many act as radiomimetics and should be avoided if treatment includes radiotherapy.	
Bleomycin	Used for testicular cancer, lymphomas and squamous cell carcinoma. Risk of dermatological effects and progressive pulmonary fibrosis. Given intravenously or intramuscularly. Half-life: 2–4 h
Dactinomycin (actinomycin D)	Mainly used for paediatric solid tumours. Risk of bone marrow toxicity, gastrointestinal toxicity. Given intravenously. Half-life: 36 h
Daunorubicin	Anthracycline. Used for acute leukaemias and AIDS-related Kaposi's sarcoma. Risk of bone marrow toxicity. Given intravenously. Half-life: 24–48 h. Liposomal formulation available (half-life: 5 h)
Doxorubicin	Anthracycline. Widely used for leukaemias, lymphomas and a variety of solid tumours. Risk of myelosuppression, cardiotoxicity. Given intravenously. Liposomal formulation available. Half-life: 2–10 h
Epirubicin	Anthracycline. Uses are similar to doxorubicin. Risk of myelosuppression; less cardiotoxic than doxorubicin. Given intravenously. Half-life: 11–69 h
Idarubicin	Anthracycline. Used mainly for acute leukaemias and advanced breast cancer unresponsive to first-line treatments. Risk of myelosuppression. Given orally or intravenously. Half-life: 12–35 h
Mitomycin	Mainly used for upper gastrointestinal and breast cancers and by bladder instillation for superficial bladder tumours. Risk of myelosuppression, nephrotoxicity, lung fibrosis. Given intravenously. Half-life: 0.5–1.5 h
Mitoxantrone	Anthracenedione. Used to treat metastatic breast cancer, non-Hodgkin's lymphoma and nonlymphocytic leukaemia. Risk of myelosuppression, cardiotoxicity. Given by intravenous infusion. Highly variable half-life (4–220 h)
Pixantrone	Used as fifth-line monotherapy for refractory or multiply relapsed aggressive non-Hodgkin's B-cell lymphomas. Given intravenously. Half-life: 15–45 h
Platinum compounds	
Carboplatin	Active form produced by interaction with water. Used for ovarian cancer and some other solid tumours. Risk of myelosuppression; nausea and vomiting (less than with cisplatin). Given by intravenous injection. Half-life: 1.5 h
Cisplatin	Active form produced by interaction with water; used for solid tumours such as ovarian cancer, metastatic seminoma and testicular teratoma. Risk of nausea and vomiting, nephrotoxicity, myelosuppression, ototoxicity. Given by intravenous injection. Half-life: 24–60 h
Oxaliplatin	Used for metastatic colorectal cancer. Risk of neurotoxicity. Given intravenously. Half-life: 27 h
Antimetabolites	
Incorporated into nucleic acids or combine irreversibly with cellular enzymes essential for normal cell division.	
Azacitadine	Pyrimidine analogue; inhibits DNA methyltransferase. Used in the treatment of myelodysplastic syndromes, chronic myelomonocytic leukaemia and acute myeloid leukaemia in adults. Given by subcutaneous injection. Half-life: <1 h
Capecitabine	Fluoropyrimidine pro-drug rapidly hydrolysed to fluorouracil. Used as monotherapy for metastatic colorectal cancer. Given orally
Cladribine	Purine analogue; the triphosphate is incorporated into DNA and blocks DNA polymerase and DNA ligase. Used for hairy cell leukaemia. Risk of myelosuppression, neurotoxicity. Given by intravenous infusion. Half-life: 7 h
Clofarabine	Purine analogue; phosphorylated form inhibits ribonucleotide reductase and DNA polymerase, terminating DNA chain elongation. Used for acute lymphoblastic leukaemia in refractory or relapsed disease in people aged 1–21 years. Given by intravenous infusion. Half-life: 5 h
Cytarabine (cytosine arabinoside)	Pyrimidine analogue; triphosphate incorporated into DNA and blocks DNA polymerase and DNA ligase; mostly active in S phase. Used for inducing remission in acute myeloblastic leukaemia. Risk of myelosuppression. Given intravenously, subcutaneously or intrathecally. Half-life: 1–3 h
Decitabine	Mechanism similar to that of azacitadine. Used for newly diagnosed acute myeloid leukaemia in people over 65 years who are not candidates for standard induction chemotherapy. Risk of anaemia, thrombocytopaenia. Given by intravenous infusion

Compendium: drugs used in the treatment of cancer (cont'd)

Drug	Characteristics
Fludarabine phosphate	Prodrug of fludarabine, a purine analogue; the triphosphate is incorporated into DNA and blocks DNA polymerase and DNA ligase; mostly active in S phase. Used for B-cell chronic lymphocytic leukaemia. Risk of myelosuppression. Given orally or by intravenous injection or infusion. Half-life: 7–20 h
Fluorouracil	Fluorinated pyrimidine analogue (fluoropyrimidine); phosphorylated derivatives are incorporated into DNA and RNA and inhibit thymidylate synthase; some selectivity for G_2 and S phases. Used for cancers of the gastrointestinal tract and malignant and pre-malignant skin lesions. Relatively low toxicity. Given topically or by intravenous injection or infusion or intra-arterial infusion. Half-life: 0.25 h
Gemcitabine	Purine analogue; triphosphate incorporated into DNA and blocks elongation and promotes apoptosis; specific for S phase. Used for palliative treatment of nonsmall-cell lung and pancreatic cancer. Limited toxicity. Given intravenously. Half-life: <0.5 h
Mercaptopurine	Sulphur-substituted purine; the monophosphate inhibits de novo purine synthesis; triphosphate incorporated into DNA and/or RNA, giving cytotoxicity; specific for S phase. Limited toxicity. Used for maintenance therapy for acute leukaemias; also used in inflammatory bowel disease. Given orally. Half-life: 1–1.5 h
Methotrexate	Folate analogue, inhibits dihydrofolate reductase. Used for maintenance therapy for childhood acute lymphoblastic leukaemia, choriocarcinoma, non-Hodgkin's lymphoma and some solid tumours; also used for rheumatoid arthritis and psoriasis. Risk of myelosuppression (folinic acid is antidote). Given orally, intravenously, intramuscularly or intrathecally. Half-life: <12 h
Nelarabine	Purine analogue; triphosphate selectively inhibits DNA synthesis in T cells. Used for T-cell acute lymphoblastic leukaemia and T-cell lymphoblastic lymphoma in relapsing disease or those refractory to previous regimens. High risk of neurotoxicity. Given by intravenous infusion. Half-life: 0.5 h
Pemetrexed	Substituted purine compound; inhibits dihydrofolate reductase, thymidylate synthase and other folate-dependent enzymes. Used with cisplatin for malignant pleural mesothelioma. Given by intravenous infusion. Half-life: 3.5 h
Raltitrexed	Folate analogue; used for palliation of metastatic colon cancer when fluorouracil cannot be used. Risk of myelosuppression. Given intravenously. Half-life: 10–12 days
Tegafur (with gimeracil and oteracil)	Prodrug of fluorouracil (a fluoropyrimidine). Used with gimeracil (which enhances fluorouracil activity by blocking its breakdown) and oteracil (which reduces fluorouracil toxicity in gut). Given orally with cisplatin in advanced gastric cancer
Tioguanine	Tioguanine metabolites inhibit de novo purine synthesis and purine nucleotide interconversions and are incorporated into DNA; active in G_1 and S phases. Used for acute leukaemia and chronic myeloid leukaemia. Risk of myelosuppression. Given orally. Half-life: 3–6 h

Mitotic inhibitors

Vinca alkaloids and taxanes inhibit mitotic cell division by actions on microtubules. Inhibitors of topoisomerase I and II interfere with DNA replication during cell division.

Vinca alkaloids

Vinca alkaloids inhibit assembly of microtubules in mitosis; used for a variety of cancers.

Vinblastine	Used for acute leukaemias, lymphomas and nonsolid tumours (e.g. breast and lung). Risk of myelosuppression. Given by intravenous injection. Half-life: 20–80 h
Vincristine	Used for acute leukaemias, lymphomas and nonsolid tumours (e.g. breast and lung). Risk of peripheral and autonomic neuropathy. Given by intravenous injection. Half-life: 85 h
Vindesine	Used for acute leukaemias, lymphomas and nonsolid tumours (e.g. breast and lung). Risk of myelosuppression. Given by intravenous injection. Half-life: 25 h
Vinflunine	Used for advanced or metastatic transitional cell carcinoma of the urothelial tract after failure of a platinum-containing regimen. Risk of myelosuppression. Given intravenously. Half-life: 40 h
Vinorelbine	Semisynthetic vinca alkaloid made from vinblastine. Used for advanced breast and nonsmall-cell lung cancer. Risk of myelosuppression. Given intravenously. Half-life: 28–44 h

Compendium: drugs used in the treatment of cancer (cont'd)

Drug	Characteristics
Topoisomerase I inhibitors	
Topoisomerase I is involved in maintaining the structure of DNA during transcription and replication.	
Irinotecan	Used for metastatic colorectal cancer. Risk of myelosuppression, gastrointestinal effects. Given by intravenous infusion. Half-life: 6 h
Topotecan	Used for metastatic ovarian cancer when first-line treatment has failed. Risk of myelosuppression, gastrointestinal effects. Given by intravenous infusion. Half-life: 2–3 h
Topoisomerase II inhibitor	
Topoisomerase II is involved in the breaking and religating of DNA strands during cell division.	
Etoposide	Used for small-cell carcinoma of the bronchus, lymphomas and testicular cancer. Risk of myelosuppression, alopecia. Given orally or by slow intravenous infusion. Half-life: 4–8 h
Taxanes	
Taxanes inhibit microtubule depolymerisation and prevent mitosis.	
Cabazitaxel	Used with a corticosteroid for hormone-refractory metastatic prostate cancer in people previously treated with docetaxel; high risk of hypersensitivity reactions. Given by intravenous infusion. Half-life: 95 h
Docetaxel	Used for advanced or metastatic anthracycline-resistant breast cancer. Risk of hypersensitivity reactions; myelosuppression; peripheral neuropathy; fluid retention. Given by intravenous infusion. Half-life: 11 h
Paclitaxel	Used for advanced ovarian cancer and as secondary treatment for breast and nonsmall-cell lung cancer. Risk of hypersensitivity reactions, myelosuppression, peripheral neuropathy. Given by intravenous infusion. Half-life: 19 h
Drugs that affect function of tyrosine kinases and other protein kinases.	
Tyrosine kinase receptor inhibitors	
Bevacizumab	VEGF receptor-inhibiting antibody. Used as part of first-line treatment of metastatic colorectal cancer. Risk of mucocutaneous bleeding and arterial thromboembolism. Given by intravenous infusion. Half-life: approximately 20 days
Cetuximab	EGF receptor HER1 antibody. Used for metastatic colorectal cancer expressing EGFR. Risk of hypersensitivity reactions (rash, airway obstruction). Given by intravenous infusion. Half-life: approximately 100 days
Pertuzumab	Inhibits dimerization of HER2 with other EGF receptors. Used in advanced HER2-positive breast cancer in combination with other drugs. Given intravenously. Half-life: 18 days
Panitumumab	EGF receptor HER1 antibody. Used for metastatic colorectal cancer. Risk of severe skin reactions. Given by intravenous infusion. Half-life: 7.5 days
Trastuzumab	EGF receptor HER2 antibody; causes cell-cycle arrest. Used for HER2-positive metastatic breast cancer. Risk of cardiotoxicity, especially if used with anthracyclines (see above). Given by intravenous infusion. Half-life: 25 days
Inhibitors of tyrosine kinases and other protein kinases	
Inhibit tyrosine kinases associated with enzymes for growth factors (e.g. EGF, PDGF, VEGF) or other protein kinases associated with cell growth and apoptosis (e.g. mTOR, BRAF, Bcr-Abl).	
Afatinib	Inhibits EGFR and HER2 tyrosine kinases. Used for metastatic nonsmall cell lung cancer with activating EGFR mutations. Risk of ocular adverse reactions. Given orally. Half-life: 37 h
Axitinib	Inhibits VEGF and PDGF tyrosine kinases. Used for advanced renal cell carcinoma following failure of previous treatment with sunitinib or a cytokine (aldesleukin or interferon alfa). Given orally. Half-life: 3–6 h
Bosutinib	Inhibits Bcr-Abl tyrosine kinase. Used for unresponsive Philadelphia chromosome-positive chronic myeloid leukaemia. Given orally. Half-life: 20–25 h
Cabozantib	Multiple protein kinase inhibitor. Used for unresectable locally advanced or metastatic medullary thyroid carcinoma. Risk of fatigue. Given orally. Half-life: 55 h
Crizotinib	Inhibits a constitutive fusion product of ALK. Used for ALK-positive advanced nonsmall cell lung cancer. Risk of cardiac failure. Given orally. Half-life: 42 h

Compendium: drugs used in the treatment of cancer (cont'd)

Drug	Characteristics
Dabrafenib	B-Raf kinase inhibitor; causes apoptosis. Used as monotherapy for unresectable or metastatic melanoma with a BRAF V600 mutation. Risk of ocular adverse reactions. Given orally. Half-life: 8 h
Dasatinib	Multiple tyrosine kinase inhibitor. Used for chronic myeloid leukaemia in those resistant to or intolerant of imatinib. Risk of pulmonary arterial hypertension. Given orally. Half-life: 3–5 h
Erlotinib	Selective inhibitor of EGF receptor HER1 tyrosine kinase. Used for advanced or malignant small-cell lung cancer after failure of previous therapy. Risk of gastrointestinal effects. Given orally. Half-life: 36 h
Everolimus	Protein kinase (mTOR) inhibitor. Used for advanced renal cell carcinoma, neuroendocrine pancreatic tumours, giant cell astrocytoma, and HER2-negative advanced breast cancer. Risk of hypersensitivity reactions, Q–T interval prolongation. Given orally. Half-life: 30 h
Gefitinib	EGFR tyrosine kinase inhibitor; used for advanced or metastatic nonsmall-cell lung cancer with activating mutations of EGFR. Risk of interstitial lung disease, hepatotoxicity. Given orally. Half-life: 41 h
Ibrutinib	Inhibits BTK; reduces B-cell migration and survival. Used for mantle cell lymphoma, Waldenström's macroglobulinaemia and for chronic lymphocytic leukaemia. Risk of CYP3A4 drug interactions. Given orally. Half-life: 4–6 h
Idelasib	Inhibits phosphoinositide 3-kinase; inhibits cell growth and induces apoptosis. Used with rituximab for chronic lymphocytic leukaemia. Risk of hepatotoxicity and infections. Given orally. Half-life: 8 h
Imatinib	PDGF receptor inhibitor. Used for newly diagnosed chronic myeloid leukaemia (under special circumstances). Risk of gastrointestinal effects. Given orally. Half-life: 40 h
Lapatinib	Dual EGF (HER1) and HER2 receptor tyrosine kinase inhibitor. Used for advanced or metastatic HER2-positive breast cancer. Risk of pulmonary toxicity, hepatotoxicity. Given orally. Half-life: 24 h
Nilotinib	Multiple tyrosine kinase inhibitor. Used for chronic myeloid leukaemia. Risk of myelosuppression, Q–T interval prolongation. Given orally. Half-life: 17 h
Nintedanib	Tyrosine kinase inhibitor; blocks VEGF, PDGF and FGF receptors. Used with docetaxel in advanced nonsmall-cell lung cancer. Given orally. Half-life: 10–15 h
Pazopanib	Inhibitor of multiple tyrosine kinases, including VEGF receptor family and PDGF receptors. Used for advanced renal cell carcinoma. Risk of hepatotoxicity, hypertension, cardiac dysfunction. Given orally. Half-life: 31 h
Ponatinib	Inhibits Bcr-Abl tyrosine kinase. Used for chronic myeloid leukaemia and Philadelphia chromosome-positive acute lymphoblastic leukaemia in people with the T315I mutation. Risk of vascular occlusion. Given orally
Regorafenib	Inhibits multiple tyrosine kinase activities, including VEGF receptor tyrosine kinase. Used for metastatic colorectal cancer and gastrointestinal stromal tumours in patients unresponsive or intolerant of previous treatment. Given orally. Half-life: 20–30 h
Ruxolitinib	Inhibits Janus-associated tyrosine kinases JAK1 and JAK2. Used in myelofibrosis and polycythaemia vera. Given orally. Half-life: 3 h
Sorafenib	Inhibits VEGF and PDGF receptor tyrosine kinases and other kinases. Used for advanced renal cell carcinoma. Risk of gastrointestinal effects. Given orally. Half-life: 25–48 h
Sunitinib	Inhibits VEGF and PDGF receptor tyrosine kinases. Used for malignant gastrointestinal stromal tumours. Risk of gastrointestinal effects. Given orally. Half-life: 40–60 h
Temsirolimus	Prodrug of sirolimus; inhibits protein kinase mTOR. Used for advanced renal cell carcinoma and for relapsed or refractory mantle cell lymphoma. Risk of life-threatening hypersensitivity reactions. Given by intravenous infusion. Half-life: 73 h (sirolimus)
Vandetanib	Inhibitor of multiple tyrosine kinase receptors, including VEGF and HER1. Used for aggressive and symptomatic medullary thyroid cancer. Risk of Q–T interval prolongation, encephalopathy, skin reactions. Given orally. Half-life: 19 days
Vemurafenib	B-Raf kinase inhibitor; causes apoptosis in melanoma cells. Used for BRAF V600 mutation-positive unresectable or metastatic melanoma. Risk of Q–T interval prolongation, skin reactions, photosensitivity. Given orally. Half-life: 52 h

Compendium: drugs used in the treatment of cancer (cont'd)

Drug	Characteristics
Proteasome inhibitor	
Bortezomib	Boron-containing peptide that inhibits the proteasome. Used for progressive multiple myeloma. Risk of nausea, vomiting and diarrhoea. Given by intravenous injection. Half-life: 15 h
Drugs for breast cancer	
See also miscellaneous anticancer drugs listed below.	
Anastrozole	Nonsteroidal aromatase inhibitor. Used as adjunct for oestrogen receptor-positive early breast cancer and for advanced metastatic breast cancer in postmenopausal women. Risk of hot flushes, vaginal bleeding, gastrointestinal effects. Given orally. Half-life: 40–50 h
Eribulin	Inhibits growth of microtubules and blocks mitosis. Used for metastatic breast cancer unresponsive to other drugs. Risk of myelosuppression, peripheral neuropathy and Q–T interval prolongation. Given intravenously. Half-life: 40 h
Exemestane	Irreversible steroid inhibitor of aromatase. Used for advanced breast cancer in postmenopausal women in whom antioestrogen therapy has failed. Risk of hot flushes and gastrointestinal effects. Given orally. Half-life: 24 h
Fulvestrant	SERD. Used for oestrogen receptor-positive breast tumours. Risk of hot flushes, gastrointestinal effects. Given by deep intramuscular depot injection. Half-life: 40 days
Letrozole	Nonsteroidal aromatase inhibitor. Used for advanced metastatic breast cancer unresponsive to other antioestrogens in postmenopausal women. Risk of hot flushes, gastrointestinal effects. Given orally. Half-life: 2 days
Tamoxifen	Nonsteroidal antioestrogen. Used for oestrogen receptor-positive breast cancer. Risk of exacerbated pain from bone metastases. Given orally. Half-life: 7–14 days
Toremifene	Nonsteroidal oestrogen receptor antagonist. Used for hormone-dependent metastatic breast cancer in postmenopausal women. Risk of hot flushes; vaginal bleeding/discharge and numerous other effects. Given orally. Half-life: 5 days
Trastuzumab	Used for metastatic breast cancer; see above.
Drugs for prostate cancer	
See also miscellaneous anticancer drugs listed below.	
Bicalutamide	Antiandrogen. Used for advanced prostate cancer to cover the 'flare' associated with administration of gonadorelin analogues. Risk of hot flushes, pruritus, gynaecomastia, rare serious hepatic and cardiovascular effects. Given orally. Half-life: 7–10 days
Buserelin	Gonadorelin analogue. Used for advanced prostate cancer. Risk of tumour 'flare' leading to spinal cord compression, ureteric obstruction and bone pain. Given by subcutaneous injection for 7 days and then intranasally. Half-life: 1–1.5 h
Cyproterone acetate	Antioestrogen. Used for prostate cancer and to cover 'flare' of gonadorelin analogues. Unwanted effects similar to those of bicalutamide. Given orally. Half-life: 2 days
Degarelix	Gonadotrophin-releasing hormone inhibitor. Used to treat advanced hormone-dependent prostate cancer. Unlike gonadorelin analogues (see Chapter 43), does not induce a testosterone surge or tumour flare. Risk of Q–T interval prolongation. Given by subcutaneous injection. Half-life: 23–61 days
Flutamide	Antiandrogen; similar to bicalutamide. Used for advanced prostate cancer and to cover 'flare' of gonadorelin analogues. Given orally. Half-life: 8 h
Goserelin	Gonadorelin analogue; similar to buserelin. Used for prostate cancer and advanced breast cancer. Given by subcutaneous implant into anterior abdominal wall. Half-life: 4 h
Leuprorelin acetate (leuprolide)	Gonadorelin analogue; similar to buserelin. Used for advanced prostate cancer. Given by subcutaneous or intramuscular injection. Half-life: 3–4 h
Triptorelin	Gonadorelin analogue; similar to buserelin. Used for advanced prostate cancer (and endometriosis). Given by intramuscular injection

655 Chemotherapy of malignancy

Compendium: drugs used in the treatment of cancer (cont'd)

Drug	Characteristics
Miscellaneous anticancer drugs	

The following drugs directly affect the cancer; other drugs used in the management of cancer (e.g. antiemetics) are described in the appropriate chapters.

Drug	Characteristics
Aflibercept	Soluble decoy receptor that traps VEGF and prevents binding to receptors; reduces angiogenesis. Used in combination with other drugs in metastatic colorectal cancer resistant to other drugs. Given intravenously; also intravitreal preparation used for age-related macular degeneration. Half-life: 6 days
Aldesleukin (interleukin-2)	Recombinant interleukin-2. Use restricted to metastatic renal cell carcinoma. Risk of pulmonary oedema, hypotension, and bone marrow, hepatic, renal, thyroid and CNS toxicity. Given by subcutaneous injection. Half-life: 3–12 h
Alemtuzumab	Antibody against CD52 antigen; causes lysis of B-lymphocytes. Used for chronic lymphocytic leukaemia unresponsive to an alkylating agent. Risk of cytokine release syndrome (characterised by severe dyspnoea). Given by intravenous infusion. Half-life: 1–14 days
Arsenic trioxide	Mechanism of action not defined. Used for acute promyelocytic leukaemia unresponsive to other treatment. Risk of leucocyte activation syndrome. Given by intravenous infusion
Bacillus Calmette–Guérin (BCG)	Immunostimulant that produces a nonspecific, localised immune reaction with histocyte and leucocyte infiltration. Used for bladder carcinoma. Given by bladder instillation
Bexarotene	RXR agonist. Used for cutaneous T-cell lymphoma. Risk of leucopenia. Given orally. Half-life: 7 h
Crisantaspase (asparaginase)	Bacterial enzyme that depletes circulating L-asparagine required by tumour cells. Used for acute lymphoblastic leukaemia. Risk of anaphylaxis, CNS depression, hyperglycaemia. Given by intramuscular or subcutaneous injection. Half-life: 7–13 days
Catumaxomab	Antibody to EpCAM and CD3. Used for malignant ascites associated with EpCAM-positive carcinomas. Risk of fever, vomiting. Given by intraperitoneal infusion. Half-life: 2 days
Dacarbazine	Prodrug of active alkylating agent. Used for metastatic melanoma and soft tissue sarcomas. Risk of myelosuppression, intense nausea and vomiting. Given intravenously. Half-life: 5 h
Diethylstilbestrol	Oestrogen; inhibits hypothalamic–pituitary axis by negative feedback. Used rarely for prostate cancer or breast cancer. Given orally. Half-life: 2–3 days
Hydroxycarbamide (hydroxyurea)	Inhibits conversion of ribonucleotides to deoxyribonucleotides by ribonucleotide reductase. Used for chronic myeloid leukaemia. Given orally. Half-life: 2–6 h
Interferon alfa	Cytokine; used for certain lymphomas and solid tumours. Risk of nausea, lethargy, ocular effects, depression, myelosuppression and cerebrovascular, liver and kidney problems. Given by subcutaneous or intravenous injection. Half-life: 3–4 h
Ipilimumab	Antibody that potentiates T cells by blocking inhibitory signals from CTLA-4. Used for metastatic melanoma. Risk of fatal immune-mediated adverse reactions, particularly gastrointestinal, due to T-cell activation. Given by intravenous infusion. Half-life: 15 days
Lenalidomide	Immunomodulator and antiangiogenic actions similar to those of thalidomide. Used in multiple myeloma unresponsive to other therapies. Risk of thromboembolism, severe neutropenia, teratogenesis. Given orally. Half-life: 3 h
Medroxyprogesterone acetate	Progestogen. Used for endometrial and breast cancer, rarely for prostate and renal cancer. Given orally or by deep intramuscular injection. Half-life: 30–50 days
Megestrol acetate	Progestogen. Used for endometrial and breast cancer. Given orally. Half-life: 15–20 h
Mitotane	Mechanism of action unknown. Used for advanced or inoperable adrenocortical carcinoma. Risk of gastrointestinal and CNS disturbances; toxic to adrenal cortex, producing hypercortisolism. Given orally. Half-life: 0.5–6 months
Norethisterone (norethindrone)	Progestogen. Used for endometrial cancer and also for renal and breast cancer. Given orally. Half-life: 5–12 h
Obinutuzumab	Anti-CD20 antibody; inhibits B-cell activation. Used for chronic lymphocytic leukaemia in patients for whom fludarabine is unsuitable. Risk of hepatitis B reactivation. Given intravenously. Half-life: 28 days
Ofatumumab	Anti-CD20 antibody; inhibits B-cell activation. Used in chronic lymphocytic leukaemia in patients refractory to fludarabine and alemtuzumab. Risk of pneumonia. Given intravenously. Half-life: 14 days

Compendium: drugs used in the treatment of cancer (cont'd)

Drug	Characteristics
Pentostatin	Adenosine deaminase inhibitor. Used for hairy cell leukaemia. Risk of myelosuppression, immunosuppression. Given intravenously. Half-life: 3–15 h
Pomalidomide	Immunomodulator and antiangiogenic actions; similar to thalidomide. Used with dexamethasone for multiple myeloma unresponsive to other treatments. Given orally. Half-life: 8 h
Porfimer sodium	Porphyrin oligomer; accumulates in tumour and is activated by laser light. Used in photodynamic treatment of small-cell lung cancer and for oesophageal cancer. Risk of photosensitivity. Given by intravenous injection. Half-life: 40–50 h
Prednisolone	Glucocorticoid (see Chapter 44). Used for marked antitumour effect in acute lymphoblastic leukaemia, Hodgkin's disease and non-Hodgkin's lymphoma; also used in palliative care. Given orally, topically and by intramuscular injection. Half-life: 2–4 h
Procarbazine	Cytotoxic mechanism unclear, but inhibits incorporation of adenosine and thymidine into DNA. Used in Hodgkin's disease. Ingestion with alcohol may produce a disulfiram-like effect. Given orally. Half-life: 0.1 h
Rituximab	Anti-CD20 antibody that lyses B-lymphocytes. Used for chemotherapy-resistant advanced follicular lymphoma. Risk of cytokine release syndrome (fever, chills, nausea, allergic reactions, severe dyspnoea). Given by intravenous infusion. Half-life: 19–32 days
Temoporfin	Porphyrin-derived photosensitiser; accumulates in tumour and is activated by laser light. Used in photodynamic treatment of small-cell lung cancer and for oesophageal cancer. Risk of photosensitivity. Given by intravenous injection. Half-life: 40–50 h
Temozolomide	Analogue of dacarbazine converted to same active product. Used as second-line treatment for malignant glioma. Given orally. Half-life: 2 h
Thalidomide	Immunomodulator with antiangiogenic action. Used with an alkylating drug and a corticosteroid in multiple myeloma. Risk of thromboembolism, peripheral neuropathy, teratogenesis. Given orally. Half-life: 5–7 h
Trabectedin	Inhibits an oncogene transcription factor. Used for advanced soft tissue sarcoma and with doxorubicin for ovarian cancer. Risk of hepatotoxicity, myelosuppression. Given intravenously. Half-life: 180 days
Tretinoin (all-*trans*-retinoic acid)	Retinoid RAR and RXR agonist. Used for remission of acute promyelocytic leukaemia. Highly teratogenic. Given orally. Half-life: 1–2 h
Vismodegib	Competitive antagonist of cell-surface SMO ('smoothened') receptor; inhibits signalling via hedgehog pathway. Used in basal cell carcinoma. Risk of severe birth defects. Given orally. Half-life: 4 days

Antidotes

Chemoprotectants are used to reduce the toxicity of one or more anticancer drugs.

Drug	Characteristics
Amifostine	Rapidly converted to active product that detoxifies reactive metabolites of platinum and alkylating agents and scavenges free radicals. Used before cytotoxic treatment to reduce risk of neutropenia-related infection and to reduce cisplatin nephrotoxicity. Risk of hypotension. Given by intravenous infusion. Half-life: 0.2 h
Dexrazoxane	Iron chelator; protects against anthracycline-induced free radical damage. Used for anthracycline-induced extravasation. Given by intravenous infusion. Half-life: 2–4 h
Folinic acid (leucovorin) and levofolinate	Given 24 h after methotrexate to speed recovery from myelosuppression. Given orally or by intramuscular or intravenous injection. Half-life: 0.75 h
Mesna (mercaptoethane sulphonic acid)	Used orally before cyclophosphamide or ifosfamide treatment or intravenously afterwards to prevent urothelial toxicity from acrolein metabolite. Half-life: 1 h
Oteracil	Given with tegafur (and gimeracil). Poorly absorbed from gut, where it reduces gut toxicity by inhibiting production of fluorouracil
Palifermin	Human keratinocyte growth factor; acts on epithelial cells to aid cellular defences. Used for oral mucositis during treatment of haematological malignancies. Given intravenously. Half-life: 3–5 h

BTK, *Bruton's tyrosine kinase*; CTLA-4, *cytotoxic T-lymphocyte antigen 4*; EGF, *epidermal growth factor*; EGFR, *epidermal growth factor receptor*; EpCAM, *epithelial cell adhesion molecule*; FGF, *fibroblast growth factor*; mTOR, *mammalian target of rapamycin*; PDGF, *platelet-derived growth factor*; RAR, *retinoic acid receptor*; RXR, *retinoid X receptors*; SERD, *selective oestrogen receptor downregulator*; VEGF, *vascular endothelial growth factor*.

12

General features:
drug toxicity and prescribing

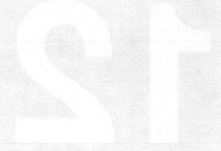

12

General features: drug toxicity and prescribing

53

Drug toxicity and overdose

Most therapeutic drugs produce their beneficial response by altering human homeostatic mechanisms; only antimicrobial agents and parasiticides are designed to produce a therapeutic response without direct action on human metabolic or physiological processes. Some therapeutic agents, for example atropine (belladonna), tubocurarine (curare), ergot alkaloids (causing St. Anthony's fire), digoxin (digitalis) and dicoumarol (causing haemorrhagic disease in cattle), have pharmacological properties that were first recognised as a result of either accidental or intentional poisonings. It is hardly surprising that all drugs are capable of producing adverse effects if the dosage is high enough. One type of relationship between a potentially beneficial

drug and a poison was recognised five centuries ago when Paracelsus stated, 'All things are toxic and it is only the dose which makes something a poison.'

Some of the medicines prescribed today were first used as relatively crude plant extracts – for example, digitalis glycosides and opium extracts. It was the identification and isolation of the active chemical entities that allowed the dose and purity of the active ingredient to be controlled sufficiently to optimise the ratio between benefit and risk. In this respect, the current vogue for poorly characterised herbal remedies could be considered to represent a backward step.

Drug toxicity can develop at normal therapeutic doses of a drug or as a result of an acute overdose. In some cases, toxicity occurs in the majority of treated individuals because of the nature of the drug (e.g. cytotoxic agents used for cancer chemotherapy), but significant toxicity is rare with the majority of commonly prescribed drugs when used at recommended dosages. There is considerable interindividual variability in both the nature and severity of adverse reactions, and toxicity can be reduced by taking into account factors that are known to increase susceptibility, such as age, concurrent disease or body weight, when selecting both the drug and the dosage. Genetic factors may also be taken into account for some drugs (see Chapters 1 and 2). Usually a reduction in dosage or a change of drug during chronic treatment will reduce the severity of adverse effects (but see the discussion on immunological mechanisms later in this chapter).

Toxicity following an acute overdose usually produces predictable adverse reactions, which may be life-threatening and/or prejudice long-term health. Rapid treatment is then required, and this may be aimed at preventing further drug absorption, increasing drug elimination/inactivation and managing the adverse effects produced.

This chapter is therefore divided into two main sections:

- Drug toxicity and adverse effects, which discusses mechanisms of adverse effects produced both during normal drug therapy and after an overdose;
- Self-poisoning and drug overdose, which is concerned with the management of intentional or accidental drug overdose.

DRUG TOXICITY AND ADVERSE EFFECTS

There is no consistent use of terminology in describing effects of drugs that were not intended when the drug was prescribed. Adverse effects of a drug are those that can occur when the drug is used at therapeutic doses; these have also been referred to as collateral effects. Drug toxicity is more commonly applied to effects that occur at supratherapeutic doses. This section provides a framework for classifying adverse and toxic effects of drugs, which are referred to in the individual drug monographs as unwanted effects. The term *side effect* is a widely used alternative, although more strictly it refers to unwanted effects that are unrelated to the principal mechanism of action of the drug.

The beneficial effects of a drug in one situation (e.g. the antidiarrhoeal effect of opioids) may be an adverse effect in other circumstances (e.g. constipation, when an opioid is used for pain relief). Therefore even classification of the nature of effect into beneficial or adverse may depend on the condition being treated. The adverse effects caused by different drugs are listed in the British National Formulary (BNF; www.evidence.nhs.uk), and it is apparent that for most drugs, potential adverse effects are more numerous than beneficial properties. It is important to remember that such lists are not always exhaustive, and prescribers should be alert to both predicted and unexpected reactions to medicines. The prescriber should consider the risk–benefit ratio for each individual and the suitability of alternative drugs and/or treatments, and people who are prescribed drugs should be informed of the risk–benefit balance inherent in their treatment (see Chapter 55). The patient information leaflet (PIL) included with the dispensed medicine represents a useful but not complete way of providing such advice. Prescribers should also be aware of the risks of adverse and toxic effects arising from drug interactions.

It should be appreciated that all drugs are associated with some risk of adverse effects and toxicity, although both the severity and incidence differ widely among drugs. In general, the acceptability of a risk of an unwanted effect is related to the severity of the disease being treated; for example, serious idiosyncratic reactions with incidences of 1 in 10,000 have led to the withdrawal of some nonsteroidal antiinflammatory drugs (NSAIDs), whereas some cancer chemotherapeutic agents can cause significant toxicity in nearly all individuals.

A useful indication of the safety margin available for a drug is given by the therapeutic index (TI):

$$\text{Therapeutic index} = \frac{\text{Dose resulting in toxicity}}{\text{Dose giving therapeutic response}}$$

Drugs such as diazepam have a TI of about 50, and it is difficult for even the most inept doctor to cause serious toxicity with diazepam. In contrast, digoxin has a TI of only about 2, and for such drugs toxicity may be precipitated by relatively small changes in dosage regimen or in the clearance of the drug from the body. The TI relates to serious toxicity and does not indicate the potential for minor adverse effects, which may inconvenience the person enough for him or her to stop treatment but are not considered to represent drug toxicity.

TYPES OF UNWANTED EFFECT

Adverse drug reactions (ADRs) are usually divided into two main types:

■ Type A ('augmented'): These effects are usually dose-related and largely predictable from the known pharmacological and biochemical effects of the drug or its metabolites.

■ Type B ('bizarre'): These effects are not obviously dose-related and are idiosyncratic and unpredictable; they are often immunological in nature.

This classification makes no allowance for time-dependency of some adverse events, or for the underlying susceptibility of the individual. Other classifications of adverse reactions have been described, such as continuing (type C), delayed (type D), end-of-use (type E), failure of therapy (type F) or genetic/genomic (type G). These classifications are not mutually exclusive, and classification of an adverse event along multiple axes, such as dose-relatedness, time-relatedness and susceptibility, may be more meaningful.

PHARMACOLOGICAL TOXICITY

In 'pharmacological toxicity', the toxic reaction is a predictable extension of the known pharmacology of the drug at its site(s) of action (Table 53.1), and should be recognised readily when monitoring the individual's response to treatment. There are numerous examples in this book where the adverse effect is really an excessive therapeutic action.

For many drug effects, the response increases with increase in dose, with low subtherapeutic doses giving an inadequate response, therapeutic doses giving the desired response, but very high doses giving an excessive response that can be regarded as a form of toxicity (response 1 in Fig. 53.1). A good example is warfarin (see Chapter 11), inadequate doses of which are associated with a lack of the desired antithrombotic effect, while at excessive doses there is a risk of haemorrhage due to excessive anticoagulation. This has given rise to the concept of a 'therapeutic window', which is a range of doses or blood/plasma concentrations within which most individuals should show a beneficial response with minimal risk of adverse effects (illustrated by response 1 in Fig. 53.1). The concept is particularly valuable in the interpretation of measurements of drug concentrations in plasma, which can be used to monitor adherence to treatment and to assess likely response (Table 53.2).

In many other cases, the toxic reaction may be unrelated to the primary therapeutic effect (Table 53.3), and caused by a secondary effect that is not the primary aim of the treatment given (response 2 in Fig. 53.1). This toxicity will often be present to a limited extent in some people at appropriate therapeutic doses.

Table 53.1 Examples of drugs with adverse effects related to their primary therapeutic properties

Drug	Adverse effect
Acetylcholinesterase inhibitors	Muscle weakness
β-Adrenoceptor antagonists	Heart block when used as an antiarrhythmic
Insulin	Hypoglycaemia
General anaesthetics	Medullary depression
Loop diuretics	Hypokalaemia
Warfarin	Haemorrhage

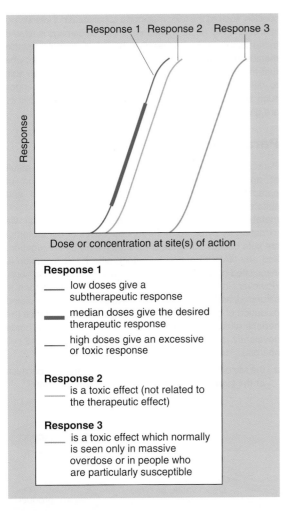

Response 1

_____ low doses give a subtherapeutic response

▬▬▬ median doses give the desired therapeutic response

_____ high doses give an excessive or toxic response

Response 2

_____ is a toxic effect (not related to the therapeutic effect)

Response 3

_____ is a toxic effect which normally is seen only in massive overdose or in people who are particularly susceptible

Fig. 53.1 **Dose–response relationships in relation to toxicity.** Response 1 is the primary therapeutic effect, the magnitude of which increases with dose from subtherapeutic through therapeutic to potentially toxic. Response 2 is an undesired effect seen at a dose only slightly greater than those producing the therapeutic effect. Response 3 is an adverse effect normally seen only in overdose.

The separation of therapeutic and toxic dose–response curves is a measure of the TI. If these are very close (e.g. responses 1 and 2 in Fig. 53.1), then there is a low safety margin (low TI), and most individuals will show some degree of toxicity at normal therapeutic doses – for example, myelo-suppression with cytotoxic anticancer drugs. For drugs with high TIs (e.g. responses 1 and 3 in Fig. 53.1), toxicity would not be seen at normal doses; for example a β-adrenoceptor antagonist would be very unlikely to cause myocardial depres-sion and heart failure in people with normal left ventricular function. However, the toxic effect may occur in individuals who are unusually sensitive because of their genetics or their physical condition; for example, standard doses of a β-adrenoceptor antagonist can precipitate heart failure in people with preexisting impaired left ventricular function.

Pharmacological toxicity is the most common cause of adverse effects. Such toxicity can be minimised by an

Table 53.3 Examples of drugs with adverse effects not related to their primary therapeutic use

Drug	Adverse effects
β-Adrenoceptor agonists	Increase in heart rate when used in asthma
β-Adrenoceptor antagonists	Reduction in heart rate when used for hypertension
Aminoglycosides	Deafness
Anticancer drugs	Myelosuppression
Anticonvulsants	Sedation when used for epilepsy
Antipsychotics	Dystonias or parkinsonism
Corticosteroids	Glaucoma
Drugs for Parkinson's disease	Hallucinations and confusion
Opioid analgesics	Respiratory depression
Paracetamol	Liver failure
Statins	Rhabdomyolysis
Thalidomide	Birth defects
Thiazides	Glucose intolerance

Table 53.2 Examples of therapeutic windows based on plasma concentrations

Drug	Therapeutic concentration range (typical values)		Toxic response
	Minimum	**Maximum**[a]	
Aspirin (analgesia) (µg/mL)	20	300	Tinnitus, metabolic acidosis
Carbamazepine (µg/mL)	4	10	Drowsiness, visual disturbances
Digitoxin (ng/mL)	15	30	Bradycardia, nausea
Digoxin (ng/mL)	0.8	3	Bradycardia, nausea
Gentamicin (µg/mL)	2	12	Ototoxicity, renal toxicity
Phenytoin (µg/mL)	10	20	Nystagmus, lethargy
Theophylline (µg/m)	10	20	Tremor, nervousness

[a]The maximum concentration may be limited by toxicity related to the primary therapeutic response (e.g. carbamazepine) or to an unrelated effect (e.g. gentamicin).

assessment of the risk–benefit balance for the individual to be treated. This should take into account factors that may influence both pharmacokinetics and target-organ sensitivity, including age, physiological status (e.g. renal function), concurrent medication, disease processes, environmental factors (e.g. smoking), and so on.

Because of the predictable nature of pharmacological toxicity, it is usual for some treatments to be co-prescribed with drugs that will reduce the possibility of toxic effects; examples include antiemetics given with cancer chemotherapy, vitamin B_6 given with isoniazid, and leucovorin (folinic acid) given after high-dose methotrexate.

BIOCHEMICAL TOXICITY

In 'biochemical toxicity', the toxicity or tissue damage is caused by an interaction of the drug or an active metabolite with cell components, especially macromolecules such as structural proteins and enzymes. A generalised scheme is given in Fig. 53.2. For most licensed drugs, this form of toxicity is identified and characterised during preclinical studies in animals and monitored in clinical trials (see Chapter 3), for example by measuring changes in serum levels of liver or muscle enzymes.

In some situations, an understanding of the mechanism of toxicity has allowed the development of appropriate treatments or antidotes. An example is the key observation that the thiol (–SH) group of the endogenous tripeptide glutathione can prevent cell damage caused by highly reactive chemical species, such as the toxic metabolite of paracetamol (discussed later and in Fig. 53.3). The nature of the cell damage is related to the stability of the toxic reactive chemical; extremely unstable metabolites may bind covalently to and inactivate the enzyme that forms them, whereas more stable species may be able to diffuse to a distant site (e.g. DNA) and initiate changes such as cancer. Important examples of biochemical toxicity are given in the following sections.

Paracetamol

Paracetamol-induced hepatotoxicity represents the result of an imbalance between metabolic detoxification of paracetamol via conjugation with glucuronic acid and sulfate, and metabolic activation to an unstable toxic metabolite (*N*-acetyl-*p*-benzoquinone imine [NAPQI]) via oxidation by cytochrome P450. Low doses of paracetamol are safe because they are eliminated mainly by conjugation, and any NAPQI created by cytochrome P450 oxidation is inactivated by a cytoprotective pathway involving glutathione. However, in overdose, the sulfate conjugation reaction is saturated, and there is increased cytochrome P450-mediated oxidation of paracetamol to NAPQI (see Fig. 53.3). Once the hepatic glutathione is depleted, this toxic metabolite binds covalently to proteins and causes oxidative stress and cell necrosis. This biochemical mechanism explains:

- the site of toxicity (centrilobular necrosis in the liver because of the large amounts of cytochrome P450 present);

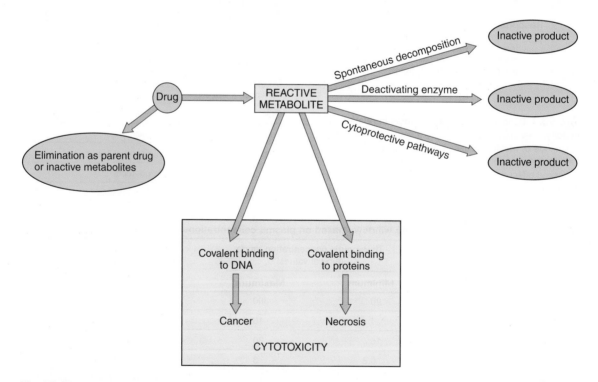

Fig. 53.2 **Metabolism and cytotoxicity.** In this scheme, the propensity of the reactive metabolite of a cytotoxic drug to cause adverse biochemical effects on cellular DNA and proteins depends on the balance between formation of the reactive metabolite from the parent drug, and the rate of elimination of both the reactive metabolite and the parent drug by alternative metabolic routes. Therapeutic interventions are aimed at either increasing elimination of the parent drug or enhancing cytoprotective pathways to reduce the cytotoxic effects.

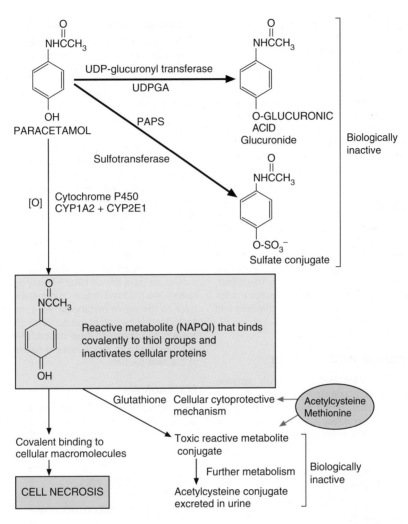

Fig. 53.3 **Pathways of paracetamol metabolism.** In overdose, the concentrations of 3′-phosphoadenosine 5′-phosphosulphate (PAPS; for sulfation) and glutathione (for cytoprotection) are depleted, and extensive macromolecular binding leads to hepatocellular necrosis. *N*-Acetylcysteine and methionine replenish glutathione to conjugate the toxic metabolite. *NAPQI, N*-Acetyl-*p*-benzoquinone imine; *UDPGA,* uridine diphosphate glucuronic acid.

- the increased toxicity seen in individuals treated with inducers of cytochrome P450 (especially alcohol-related induction of CYP2E1);
- the increased toxicity seen in individuals with low hepatic stores of glutathione due to poor nutrition;
- the successful treatment of paracetamol overdose with acetylcysteine or methionine, which provide an additional source of thiol groups for inactivation of NAPQI (see the discussion of the treatment of specific drug poisonings later in the chapter).

Cyclophosphamide

Cyclophosphamide is an anticancer drug. Its highly toxic metabolites bind to DNA as part of their mechanism of action, but they are eliminated in the urine and cause haemorrhagic cystitis due to cell damage in the bladder

(see Chapter 52). This adverse effect can be prevented by prior treatment with mesna (mercaptoethane sulfonic acid), which possesses both a thiol group for cytoprotection and a highly polar sulphonic acid group, and results in high renal excretion and delivery of this cytoprotective molecule to the bladder epithelium. Mesna is usually given either orally 2 hours before the cyclophosphamide or intravenously at the same time to cover the period of maximum urinary excretion of toxic cyclophosphamide metabolites. It is not known whether mesna also protects against bladder cancer, which can arise about 10–20 years after initial treatment with cyclophosphamide.

Isoniazid

Isoniazid, which is used for the treatment of tuberculosis (see Chapter 51), causes hepatitis in about 0.5% of treated individuals. This is believed to result from the formation of a reactive metabolite, *N*-acetylhydrazine, which is produced by acetylation followed by oxidative metabolism. The biochemical basis for the susceptibility of some individuals to the hepatotoxic metabolite is not known. Fast acetylators (see Chapter 2) form more *N*-acetylhydrazine than slow acetylators but, unexpectedly, they are not more sensitive to isoniazid hepatotoxicity. Susceptibility may be related to the balance between further activation of *N*-acetylhydrazine (by oxidation) and its detoxification (by further acetylation); if this is so, then fast acetylators may produce more active metabolite but also inactivate it more rapidly.

Spironolactone

Spironolactone (see Chapter 14) is oxidised by cytochrome P450. The metabolite formed in the testes binds to and destroys testicular cytochrome P450; this causes a decrease in the metabolism of progesterone to testosterone, a step which is also catalysed by a cytochrome P450. This effect, combined with an antiandrogenic action at receptor sites (pharmacological toxicity), can result in gynaecomastia and decreased libido.

Aromatic amines and nitrites

Aromatic amines, such as the antileprosy drug dapsone and some antimalarials (e.g. primaquine), are oxidised in the liver to active metabolites, which are released into the circulation, where they can affect erythrocytes, causing methaemoglobinaemia and/or haemolysis.

Methaemoglobinaemia

In the erythrocyte, the active metabolite interacts with molecular oxygen (O_2), which then oxidises haemoglobin (Fe^{2+}) to methaemoglobin (Fe^{3+}) and also oxidises the active metabolite itself (Fig. 53.4A). Because of the large amounts of haemoglobin compared with the amount of drug given, this would be inconsequential, were it not for the fact that the oxidised active metabolite can be recycled back to the active metabolite by reduction with nicotinamide adenine dinucleotide phosphate (reduced NADPH) in the erythrocyte. Consequently, each molecule of the metabolite undergoes repeated redox cycling and is able to oxidise many molecules of haemoglobin. NADPH is formed during the metabolism of glucose 6-phosphate by glucose-6-phosphate dehydrogenase (G6PD; see Fig. 53.4A). The activity of G6PD, and hence the amounts of NADPH, are determined genetically. There is a high incidence of G6PD deficiency in people of African ancestry, and this incidence is very high in those of Mediterranean ancestry, such as Kurdish people. Such individuals have limited NADPH reserves and a low ability to reduce the oxidised active drug metabolite (see Fig. 53.4A) back to the active metabolite. As a consequence, there is limited redox cycling of the active drug metabolite and they are less susceptible to drug-induced methaemoglobinaemia, but they are more susceptible to haemolysis (as discussed in the next section).

Haemolysis

This arises from an increase in erythrocyte membrane permeability associated with accumulation of oxidised glutathione (GS–SG in Fig. 53.4B) in the erythrocyte. Oxidised

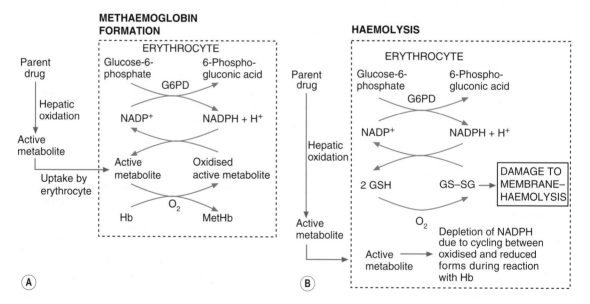

Fig. 53.4 **Mechanisms of methaemoglobinaemia and haemolysis.** In methaemoglobinamia **(A)**, the active drug metabolite oxidises haemoglobin (Hb) to methaemoglobin (MetHb). The oxidised active metabolite is repeatedly recycled to the active metabolite by reduced nicotinamide adenine dinucleotide phosphate (NADPH) generated by glucose-6-phosphate dehydrogenase (G6PD). In **(B)**, the depletion of NADPH as a result of methaemoglobinaemia depletes levels of the reduced glutathione (GSH) necessary for maintaining erythrocyte cell membrane integrity; the build-up of oxidised glutathione dimers (GS–SG) causes membrane damage and haemolysis. The active metabolite may also react directly with glutathione to lower GSH concentrations.

glutathione accumulates because redox cycling of the drug metabolite linked to the formation of methaemoglobin (see Fig. 53.4A; along with the previous discussion) results in depletion of NADPH, which is the cofactor essential for maintaining glutathione in the reduced state. Individuals with G6PD deficiency are very susceptible to haemolysis caused by aromatic amines and nitrites, because the low endogenous levels of NADPH are depleted rapidly and oxidised glutathione cannot then be reduced. Given the geographical distribution of G6PD deficiency, it is ironic that the amino groups associated with this form of toxicity are often present in drugs used to treat tropical infections (such as primaquine for the treatment of malaria; see Chapter 51 and Box 47.6).

IMMUNOLOGICAL TOXICITY

Immunological toxicity is frequently referred to as 'drug allergy' and is the form of toxicity with which people may be most familiar (e.g. penicillin allergy). Immunological mechanisms are implicated in a number of common adverse effects, such as rashes and fever, but may also be involved in organ-directed toxicity. The term *allergy* may not be strictly correct for all forms of immunologically mediated toxicity, but it is probably better than 'hypersensitivity', which has also been used to describe an elevated sensitivity to any mechanism or effect.

Low-molecular-weight compounds (<1100 Da) are not able to elicit an allergic response directly but can do so after the compound, or a metabolite, has formed a stable or covalent bond with a macromolecule. Covalent binding to a normal protein produces a hapten–protein conjugate that is recognised as foreign by the immune system and can act as an antigen (Fig. 53.5).

Immunologically mediated toxicity can show a wide range of characteristics:

- Toxicity is unrelated to dose. Once the antibody has been produced, even very small amounts of antigen can trigger a reaction.
- There is normally a lag of at least 3 days between initial exposure and the development of symptoms; however, the first dose of a subsequent treatment may give an immediate reaction.
- Cross-reactivity is possible among different compounds that share the same antigenic determinant or structural component involved in antibody recognition, such as the penicilloyl group of the penicillin family.
- The incidence varies widely among different drugs – for example, from about 1 in 10,000 people for phenylbutazone-induced agranulocytosis to 1 in 20 for ampicillin-related skin rashes.
- The response is idiosyncratic but genetically controlled. Individual responsiveness cannot be predicted, but individuals who have a history of atopic disease are more likely to develop a 'drug allergy'.

The effects produced may be subdivided into the classic four types of allergic reaction, of which types and 1 and 4 are the most common (see Chapter 38).

- *Type 1: immediate or anaphylactic reactions.* These are mediated via IgE antibodies attached to the surface of basophils and mast cells; the synthesis and release of numerous mediators (e.g. histamine, prostanoids and leukotrienes) produces effects that include urticaria, bronchoconstriction, hypotension, oedema and shock. A skin-prick challenge test usually produces an acute inflammatory response. Examples of drugs having this type of effect are penicillins and peptide drugs, such as crisantaspase (asparaginase).
- *Type 2: cytotoxic reactions.* The antigen is formed by the drug binding to a cell membrane; subsequent interaction of this antigen with circulating IgG, IgM or IgA antibodies activates complement and initiates cell lysis. Depending on the carrier cell to which the drug is bound, cell lysis can result in thrombocytopenia (e.g. cephalosporins, quinine), neutropenia (e.g. metronidazole) or haemolytic anaemia (e.g. penicillins, rifampicin and possibly methyldopa).
- *Type 3: immune-complex reactions.* The antigen–antibody interaction occurs in serum, and the complex formed is deposited on endothelial cells, basement membranes and so on, to initiate a more localised inflammatory reaction, such as arteritis or nephritis. Examples include serum sickness (urticaria, angioedema, fever) with penicillins, lupus erythematosus-like syndrome with hydralazine and procainamide (especially in slow acetylators) and possibly NSAID-related nephropathy.
- *Type 4: cell-mediated delayed-type reactions.* Reaction to the eliciting exposure is delayed. The reactions occur mostly in skin through the formation of an antigen between the drug (hapten) and skin proteins. This is followed by an infiltration of sensitised T-lymphocytes, which recognise the antigen and release cytokines to produce local inflammation, oedema and irritation (e.g. contact dermatitis).

In addition to true immunologically mediated toxicity, as described previously, there are examples of 'pseudoallergic' reactions, such as aspirin-intolerant asthma, which shows many of the characteristics listed previously (e.g. induction of asthma only in susceptible individuals), but for which a true immunological basis has not been demonstrated. In aspirin intolerance, cross-sensitivity with other NSAIDs in fact suggests a common pharmacological mechanism based on cyclo-oxygenase inhibition (see Chapter 29).

It has been estimated that drug allergy accounts for about 10% of ADRs but that severe reactions are rare. For example, only about 5 in 10,000 individuals develop an anaphylactic reaction to penicillins, but about a half of these are sufficiently serious to warrant hospital treatment (see Chapter 39). However, given the large numbers of people taking drugs such as penicillins, drug allergy is an important source of iatrogenic morbidity.

THE YELLOW CARD SCHEME

Reporting suspected ADRs is an important part of pharmacosurveillance (see Chapter 3). Healthcare professionals in the United Kingdom should report suspected ADR to the Medicines and Healthcare Products Regulatory Agency (MHRA) using the Yellow Card scheme. Reports can be made online (www.mhra.gov.uk/yellowcard), or by post using the cards included in the print editions of the BNF, BNF for Children and Nurse Prescribers Formulary. It is not necessary to be certain about the relationship with the drug to report a suspected ADR, and reporting an ADR does not breach patient confidentiality. The MHRA is particularly interested in receiving Yellow Card reports when suspected ADRs are

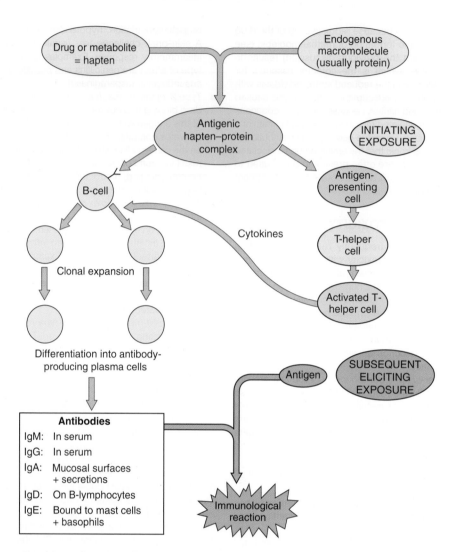

Fig. 53.5 **Mechanisms of drug allergy.** The drug or drug metabolite binds as a hapten to an endogenous macromolecule. The initial exposure produces an antigenic hapten–protein complex, which results in the production of antibodies via B-cell clonal expansion and differentiation, regulated by cytokines from activated T-helper cells. The eliciting exposure occurs later (usually at least 3 days later, during which time therapy may or may not be continuing); antigen–antibody interaction then exposes a complement-binding site, which triggers the reaction. The nature of the immunological reaction depends on the nature of the antibody and/or localisation of the antigen. Treatment is with immunosuppressant drugs (see Chapter 38).

serious, are delayed, appear in children or older people or are associated with new drugs or applications (Box 53.1). The minimum information which must be completed on a Yellow Card are:

- at least one piece of patient information, which can be any of: age, sex, weight, initials, height, or a local identification number;
- name(s) of suspect drug(s) thought to have caused the ADR;
- brief description of the ADR;
- contact details of the reporter.

Currently about 20,000 Yellow Card reports are made each year, with about 10% from members of the general public. The MHRA publishes details of Yellow Card reports in Drug Analysis Prints. Known ADRs are listed in the BNF and in greater detail in the summary of product characteristics available for most drugs in the electronic Medicines Compendium (www.medicines.org.uk).

SELF-POISONING AND DRUG OVERDOSE

Self-poisoning can be either accidental or deliberate. Approximately 200,000 episodes are recorded in hospital each year in England and Wales, although many more are managed in the community. Accidental poisoning is common

Important categories of suspected adverse drug reactions requiring Yellow Card reporting to the Medicines and Healthcare Products Regulatory Agency

- ADRs to black triangle (▼) products (new drugs being intensively monitored to confirm their risk–benefit profile)
- ADRs to new combinations of drugs, new routes of administration, or new indications for established drugs
- Serious ADRs with established medicines (fatal, life-threatening, disabling, incapacitating, congenital abnormality, requiring or extending hospitalisation)
- ADRs in children
- ADRs in elderly people
- Delayed drug effects
- Congenital anomalies
- ADRs to herbal remedies

ADR, Adverse drug reactions; *MHRA,* Medicines and Healthcare Products Regulatory Agency (www.mhra.gov.uk).

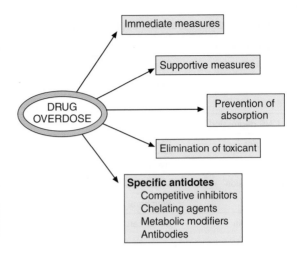

Fig. 53.6 Principles underlying the management of drug overdose.

in children under 5 years of age, when it often involves household products as well as medicines. A second peak of self-poisoning occurs in the teens and early twenties, when it is more frequent in females. The incidence then progressively falls with increasing age. Most deliberate self-poisoning represents 'parasuicide' or attention-seeking behaviour. Deaths from intentional self-poisoning and accidental overdose still average about 3000 each year in England and Wales, with about two-thirds being male, especially in the age group 30–49 years. Heroin and morphine overdoses are the most common single cause of death from drug overdose, accounting for almost 25% of the total. True suicide attempts account for about 1000 deaths a year, occurring most frequently in those over 45 years. It is important to recognise that at any age the severity of poisoning bears little relationship to suicidal intent.

The drugs most frequently used for intentional self-poisoning are benzodiazepines, analgesics and antidepressants, often taken together with alcohol. It is important to attempt to identify the cause of the poisoning, because it may determine the most suitable treatment. However, it should be remembered that information from the person about which drug was taken, the amount taken and the time of overdosing is frequently unreliable. TICTAC (www.tictac.org.uk) is a computerised database which enables registered users to identify tablets and capsules, and can be helpful in determining what has been taken.

MANAGEMENT PRINCIPLES

The emergency treatment of poisoning is described in the BNF. Additional sources of information include the United Kingdom National Poisons Information Service (www.npis.org) and its computer database TOXBASE (www.toxbase.co.uk), which has information on household products and industrial and agricultural chemicals as well as drugs, and is available to registered users.

The management of drug overdose outlined in the following sections has a number of principal aims (Fig. 53.6).

MANAGING ADVERSE EFFECTS

Immediate measures

There are certain immediate measures required when someone presents with a possible drug overdose or poisoning:

- Remove the person from contact with the poison if appropriate (e.g. gases, corrosives).
- Assess vital signs (i.e. pulse, respiration and pupil size) and inspect the person for injury.
- Ensure a clear airway. If breathing but unconscious, place in the coma position.
- Obtain a clear history, if possible.
- Preserve any evidence (e.g. bottles, written notes, etc.).

Supportive measures

Examples of unwanted effects seen in drug overdose are shown in Table 53.4. A number of the effects will require supportive measures (Fig. 53.7).

Cardiac or respiratory arrest

This may result from a toxic effect of the drug on the heart, from depression of the respiratory centre or from metabolic disturbance. Assisted ventilation, ranging from mouth-to-mouth or Ambu-bag inflation to the use of a ventilator, may be required. In some circumstances, recovery is possible even after prolonged resuscitation.

Hypotension

Low blood pressure is common in severe poisoning with central nervous system (CNS) depressants. A systolic blood pressure below 70 mm Hg can cause irreversible brain damage, but any degree of low blood pressure should be treated if accompanied by poor tissue perfusion or low urine output. Depression of the vasomotor centre can cause arterial dilation and peripheral venous pooling, producing a low central venous pressure (CVP). The CVP should be

Table 53.4 Complications of acute poisonings

Complication	Cause	Examples of poisons
Cardiac arrest	Direct cardiotoxicity	Many
	Hypoxia	
	Electrolyte/metabolic disturbance	
CNS depression		Many
Seizures	Direct neurotoxicity	Tricyclic antidepressants, theophylline
	Hypoxia	Many
Hypotension	Myocardial depression	β-Adrenoceptor antagonists, tricyclic antidepressants
	Peripheral vasodilation	Many
Arrhythmia	Direct cardiotoxicity	β-Adrenoceptor antagonists, tricyclic antidepressants, verapamil, digoxin
	Hypoxia	Many
	Electrolyte/metabolic disturbance	Many
Renal failure	Hypotension	Many
	Rhabdomyolysis	Opioids, hypnotics, ethanol, carbon monoxide
	Direct nephrotoxicity	Paracetamol, heavy metals
Hepatic failure	Direct hepatotoxicity	Paracetamol, carbon tetrachloride
Respiratory depression	Direct neurotoxicity	Sedatives, hypnotics, opioids

CNS, Central nervous system.

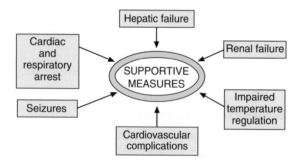

Fig. 53.7 Main effects of overdose requiring supportive measures.

raised to 10–15 cm H$_2$O (measured from the midaxillary line) by intravenous infusion of a crystalloid solution, such as 0.9% saline. A vasoconstrictor such as noradrenaline (norepinephrine; see Chapter 4) is rarely required. If hypotension occurs in association with a normal or raised CVP, this suggests myocardial depression. A positive inotropic drug such as the β$_1$-adrenoceptor agonist dobutamine (see Chapter 7) should then be used.

Arrhythmias

Disturbances of cardiac rhythm are most common during poisoning with tricyclic antidepressants, certain antipsychotics and some antihistamines. They should only be treated if severe. Ventricular arrhythmias causing hypotension often

require intervention, but caution should be exercised if there is a long Q–T interval on the electrocardiogram, since the tachycardia often fails to respond to standard antiarrhythmic drugs. It is essential to correct metabolic derangements that predispose to arrhythmias – for example, hypothermia, hypoxia, hypercapnia, hypokalaemia, hyperkalaemia and acidosis. If there is widening of the QRS complex after overdose of a tricyclic antidepressant, then intravenous sodium bicarbonate should be given to reduce the risk of serious arrhythmias.

Seizures

These may be caused by a treatable underlying cause such as hypoxia, hypoglycaemia or hypocalcaemia, or they may be a direct toxic effect of the drug on neuronal function. The treatment of choice is lorazepam or diazepam intravenously, or rectal diazepam if the intravenous route is unavailable (see Chapter 20). Artificial ventilation with neuromuscular blockade (see Chapter 27) is used if the seizures cannot be controlled.

Renal failure

Kidney damage is usually a consequence of prolonged hypotension. Other causes include a direct nephrotoxic effect of the drug and renal damage produced by the products of toxic muscle necrosis (rhabdomyolysis).

Hepatic failure

This usually results from the direct toxic effects of specific agents, such as paracetamol.

Impaired temperature regulation

Hypothermia is common, and can be caused by depression of the metabolic rate with reduced heat production and by increased heat loss from cutaneous vasodilation. It is common with phenothiazine antipsychotics and barbiturates, but is seen with any prolonged coma. Rewarming, preferably by wrapping in a 'space blanket', reduces the risk of serious ventricular arrhythmias. By contrast, CNS stimulants such as ecstasy and other CNS stimulants can produce hyperthermia, as can aspirin, which uncouples cellular oxidative phosphorylation.

REDUCING TOXICITY

The adverse effects can be reduced by:

- minimising further drug absorption;
- maximising drug elimination;
- negating effects with antidotes, etc.

Prevention of absorption of poisons

There are two principal methods of preventing further absorption of the drug: gastric aspiration/lavage and activated charcoal. However, gastric aspiration and lavage, or inducing emesis with an irritant such as ipecacuanha, are not recommended, since they have little effect on drug absorption and increase the risk of aspiration of gastric contents.

Activated charcoal

This formulation of charcoal has a large adsorbent area and is given as a suspension in water. Activated charcoal adsorbs or binds the drug, and retains it in the gastrointestinal lumen. Not all drugs are adsorbed onto charcoal (Table 53.5). About 10 g of charcoal is required for every 1 g of poison, which makes it impractical for poisons that are usually ingested in large quantities. For suitable drugs, an initial dose of 50 g of charcoal for adults can prevent absorption if given within 1 hour of drug ingestion (later after poisoning with modified-release preparations, or drugs with antimuscarinic properties that delay gastric emptying). Charcoal should not be given to drowsy or comatose persons because of the risk of aspiration into the lungs. Constipation is the major unwanted effect of charcoal; charcoal should not be given in the absence of bowel sounds, because of the risk of bowel obstruction.

Elimination of poisons

There are three principal methods of enhancing elimination of the drug: activated charcoal, renal elimination and haemodialysis/haemoperfusion.

Activated charcoal

Repeated administration of 50 g of activated charcoal every 4 hours for up to 24–36 hours achieves further retention of the adsorbed drug in the small intestine. The drug is continuously being transferred in both directions across the gut wall, with the concentration gradient normally favouring net absorption, owing to the high concentration free in the solution within the gut lumen. If drug in the bowel is bound onto the charcoal, this lowers the free concentration and can result in net transfer from the body into the gut and thereby enhance elimination of the compound. Repeated-dose activated charcoal is useful for overdose with phenobarbital, carbamazepine, dapsone, quinine and theophylline.

Renal elimination

Altering urine pH, while maintaining normal urine flow, can be effective in increasing the renal elimination of drugs that are weak electrolytes. Modification of urine pH to increase the extent of ionisation of the drug will reduce reabsorption from the renal tubule (see Chapter 2). Weak acids, such as salicylates, are excreted more readily when urine is alkalinised (alkaline diuresis, achieved by giving sodium bicarbonate).

Forced diuresis with intravenous infusion of large quantities of fluid was advocated in the past for drugs or toxic metabolites that are mostly eliminated unchanged by the kidney. However, serious disturbances of fluid or electrolyte balance can occur, and therefore it is no longer recommended.

Haemodialysis

This is reserved for the most severely poisoned individuals. The technique is only successful if a large proportion of the body burden of the drug is retained in the plasma and available for removal (i.e. the drug has a low apparent volume of distribution). Haemodialysis relies on diffusion of the drug from the blood across a semipermeable membrane into the dialysis fluid; it is used for salicylates, phenobarbital, methanol, ethylene glycol, sodium valproate and lithium.

Specific antidotes

Antidotes are available for only a minority of the drugs commonly involved in poisoning cases. Some examples are given in the following sections.

Table 53.5 Drug adsorption onto activated charcoal

Drugs/compounds not adsorbed	Drugs/compounds adsorbed
Acids	Aspirin
Alkalis	Benzodiazepines
Cyanide	Carbamazepine
DDT (insecticide)	Calcium channel blockers
Ethanol	Dapsone
Ethylene glycol (antifreeze)	Digoxin
Ferrous salts	Ecstasy (MDMA)
Lead	Paraquat (herbicide)
Lithium	Phenobarbital
Mercury	Quinine
Methanol	Theophylline
Organic solvents	Tricyclic antidepressants

MDMA, Methylenedioxymetamfetamine.

Competitive receptor antagonists

- Atropine acts at muscarinic receptors to block the parasympathetic effects of excess acetylcholine caused when organophosphate insecticides irreversibly inhibit acetylcholinesterase. It is given by intravenous or intramuscular injection.
- Naloxone acts at opioid receptors to reverse the effects of opioid analgesics. Its short half-life, compared with those of most opioids, means that repeated injections or preferably an infusion is usually needed. Naloxone can precipitate acute withdrawal in someone who is dependent on opioids.
- Flumazenil is an antagonist of benzodiazepine action on γ-aminobutyric acid type A (GABA$_A$) receptors. It is given intravenously, but is rarely needed for the treatment of intentional benzodiazepine overdose, because fatalities are uncommon with this class of drug. Flumazenil can cause seizures in benzodiazepine-dependent individuals. It is used to reverse the effects of benzodiazepines when toxicity occurs in people with chronic liver disease.

Chelating agents

Chelating agents act by forming a complex with the drug or chemical, thereby reducing its free (active) concentration:

- desferrioxamine mesilate for iron salts, given by intravenous infusion;
- dicobalt edetate for cyanide, given by intravenous injection;
- sodium calcium edetate for lead, given by intravenous infusion;
- sodium nitrite, together with sodium thiosulfate, for cyanide, with both given by intravenous injection.

Compounds that affect drug metabolism

- Fomepizole (available by special order) is a competitive inhibitor of alcohol dehydrogenase given by intravenous injection as the treatment of choice in methanol or ethylene glycol poisoning; it blocks the formation of their toxic metabolites formaldehyde and glycoaldehyde, respectively. Alternatively, with caution, their formation can be slowed with oral or intravenous ethanol, which is a preferential substrate for alcohol dehyrogenase with less toxic metabolites.
- Acetylcysteine provides a substrate for conjugation of the cytotoxic metabolite of paracetamol (NAPQI), when the natural conjugating ligand, glutathione, is depleted (discussed later).

Antibodies

Digoxin can be neutralised in severe poisoning by specific antibody fragments. The antibodies are raised in sheep and cleaved to remove the antigenic crystalline (Fc) portion of the molecule while retaining the specific antigen-binding fragment (Fab).

SOME COMMON SPECIFIC POISONINGS

PARACETAMOL

Paracetamol overdose can be fatal, with about 150 deaths occurring each year in England and Wales. Metabolism of paracetamol takes place in the liver, mainly producing nontoxic conjugates (see Fig. 53.3). A small amount is oxidised by the cytochrome P450 system to the reactive intermediate NAPQI, which is normally inactivated by conjugation with the thiol group of glutathione. When hepatic glutathione is depleted by paracetamol overdose, oxidative stress coupled with NAPQI-mediated denaturation of proteins produces hepatic necrosis. Similar processes in the kidney can cause renal tubular necrosis.

In the first 24 hours there are few symptoms, apart from nausea, vomiting, abdominal pain and sweating, which usually resolve. Liver damage begins within 24 hours of a large overdose, producing right upper quadrant pain and tenderness. Jaundice is apparent by 36–48 hours, and liver damage is maximal by 3–4 days. Severe liver failure, requiring transplantation for survival, can ensue. The most sensitive measures of liver damage are the prothrombin time, or the international normalised ratio (INR), and the plasma unconjugated bilirubin. Renal failure is seen in about a quarter of cases with severe liver damage.

Activated charcoal in large doses is recommended within 2 hours of a potentially serious paracetamol overdose. Because antidotes are most effective when given early, blood should be analysed for paracetamol if there is any suspicion of poisoning. Blood should be taken at 4 hours or more after the suspected overdose. Earlier sampling is not informative because a low plasma level at that time could reflect incomplete absorption of a large overdose, rather than ingestion of a small overdose. Antidotes used in paracetamol poisoning, such as acetylcysteine and methionine, are used to replace glutathione as a thiol donor in the liver; glutathione itself is not used, because it cannot enter liver cells from the blood.

Intravenous acetylcysteine is the preferred treatment for potentially serious poisoning, and should be started prior to the analysis of a plasma paracetamol concentration. Treatment started within 8 hours of ingestion of paracetamol avoids serious hepatotoxicity. Methionine can be given orally if acetylcysteine is not available, but not with or after activated charcoal, because methionine can compete with paracetamol for adsorption. Methionine should not be used if there is vomiting, or started more than 10–12 hours after ingestion of paracetamol, since the efficacy of methionine in late poisoning is unknown.

A graph is available (Fig. 53.8) to indicate the risk of liver damage for a given plasma paracetamol concentration related to the time after ingestion. Treatment is necessary if potentially toxic paracetamol concentrations are detected above the treatment line. After 15 hours, plasma concentrations must be interpreted by extrapolation of the graph. However, after a staggered overdose or when the time of the overdose is unknown, the plasma concentration is uninterpretable and treatment should always be given. Treatment used to be confined to the first 15 hours after overdose, but the risk of death can be reduced even when the antidote is delayed for up to 4 days in the presence of liver damage.

SALICYLATES

Salicylate poisoning is now uncommon in the United Kingdom. Aspirin is hydrolysed rapidly to salicylic acid after absorption, but further metabolism by conjugation with glycine

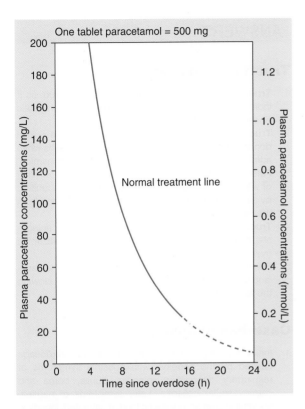

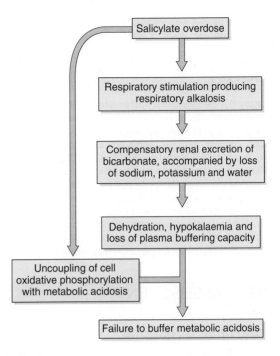

Fig. 53.9 The metabolic consequences of salicylate overdose.

Fig. 53.8 Paracetamol plasma concentration and time since overdose. Individuals with paracetamol plasma concentrations above the normal treatment line require intravenous acetylcholine (or oral methionine).

is rate-limited. Symptoms of toxicity are nausea, vomiting, abdominal pain, tinnitus, deafness, hyperventilation and sweating. Agitation frequently occurs in adults, but children become comatose. The chain of metabolic events produced by aspirin is shown in Fig. 53.9.

Activated charcoal is recommended for reducing absorption if given early. Correction of fluid, electrolyte and acid–base balance is fundamental to successful management; a fluid deficit of 3–4 L is not unusual in severe poisoning. Forced alkaline diuresis is no longer advocated to enhance salicylate elimination (discussed previously); simple alkalinisation of the urine with 1.26% oral sodium bicarbonate solution to raise the pH above 7.5 is effective and safer. Haemodialysis is the treatment of choice in severe poisoning, especially if there is severe metabolic acidosis.

TRICYCLIC ANTIDEPRESSANTS

Approximately 400 deaths per year occur in England and Wales from overdose with tricyclic antidepressants. The antimuscarinic effects of tricyclic antidepressants delay gastric emptying, and oral activated charcoal is used routinely for up to 4 hours after the overdose. Drowsiness and confusion are followed by seizures and coma in more severe poisoning. Cardiac depression can produce hypotension. Serious arrhythmias, such as ventricular tachycardia, can

occur, and ECG monitoring is recommended for at least 24 hours. If there is widening of the QRS complex on the ECG, then intravenous infusion of sodium bicarbonate can prevent or treat arrhythmias. Antiarrhythmic drugs should usually be avoided.

OPIOID ANALGESICS

The triad of signs characteristic of opioid overdose are:

- respiratory depression;
- pinpoint pupils;
- impaired consciousness.

They can be reversed rapidly by administration of naloxone (see Chapter 19), which is a competitive antagonist at opioid μ-receptors. After an initial intravenous bolus dose of naloxone, it is often necessary to give repeated boluses or a continuous infusion, because the half-life of naloxone is very short compared with those of most opioids. In poisoning with buprenorphine, the effect of naloxone is often incomplete, and assisted ventilation may also be needed. Acute poisoning with organophosphorus insecticides can produce signs that are similar to those with opioids, but naloxone will have no effect.

BETA-ADRENOCEPTOR ANTAGONISTS

Poisoning by β-adrenoceptor antagonists usually presents with bradycardia and hypotension. More severe effects, including coma and convulsions, can occur with some drugs in this class. Treatment of the bradycardia is with intravenous atropine, which may increase the blood pressure. Cardiogenic shock that does not respond to atropine should initially be treated with intravenous glucagon, which has a positive inotropic effect. A temporary cardiac pacemaker may be necessary.

ECSTASY

Ecstasy (3,4-methylenedioxymetamfetamine, MDMA) toxicity is characterised by tachycardia, hyperreflexia, hyperpyrexia and initial hypertension followed by hypotension. In severe cases, delirium, seizures, coma and cardiac dysrhythmias may occur. MDMA is metabolised by CYP2D6, and genetic differences in this enzyme may result in wide interindividual differences in susceptibility to the toxic effects of MDMA. Some people may present with hyponatraemia, possibly as a result of drinking excessive water as a precaution to prevent dehydration. Treatments include activated charcoal, but only for up to 2 hours postingestion, since MDMA is absorbed rapidly, and diazepam for agitation or seizures.

SELF-ASSESSMENT

True/false questions

1. The therapeutic index (TI) is the ratio between the dose of a drug that results in significant toxicity and the dose that provides a therapeutic response.
2. Mesna reduces the cytotoxic effects of cyclophosphamide on the bladder.
3. Acidification of the urine (acid diuresis) enhances excretion of aspirin.
4. Flumazenil is a GABA$_A$ receptor antagonist.
5. Fomepizole accelerates the breakdown of methanol.

Case-based questions

A 70-year-old man with a history of depressive illness and alcohol abuse was prescribed a compound analgesic containing 30 mg codeine phosphate and 500 mg paracetamol (co-codamol 30/500) for back pain. Eight hours after collecting his prescription, he was seen as an emergency by his GP, who considered the man had taken an overdose and admitted him to hospital.

1. What features might be seen soon after the overdose and during the subsequent 24–48 hours?
2. Outline suitable pharmacological treatments that should be undertaken.
3. Would co-dydramol have been a safer alternative to prescribe?

ANSWERS

True/false answers

1. **True.** A high TI is a desirable property of a drug, as it indicates that significant toxicity is unlikely at therapeutic doses.
2. **True.** Mesna (mercaptoethane sulfonic acid) is a thiol donor which protects against haemorrhagic cystitis when administered with the cytotoxic drug cyclophosphamide.
3. **False.** Acidification of the urine would enhance excretion of weak bases. Weak acids such as aspirin are ionised by alkalinisation of the urine, so less is reabsorbed from the renal tubule.
4. **True.** Flumazenil is a competitive GABA$_A$ receptor antagonist that can be given intravenously in benzodiazepine overdose.
5. **False.** Fomepizole inhibits the metabolism of methanol (and ethylene glycol) by alcohol dehydrogenase, slowing the formation of toxic metabolites.

Case-based answers

1. Initial features would be those of opioid overdosage caused by the codeine, with possible symptoms of respiratory depression, pinpoint pupils, coma and cardiovascular collapse. Later symptoms of nausea, abdominal pain and sweating (and, if untreated, jaundice) are due to liver damage caused by the toxic metabolite of paracetamol.
2. Naloxone is a rapid reversible antagonist of opioids at μ-, κ- and δ-receptors. It has a short half-life and may have to be given repeatedly. Acetylcysteine conjugates with the hepatotoxic metabolite of paracetamol (NAPQI) and is most effective when given early after an overdosage; the risk of liver damage is related to the time of ingestion before treatment and the plasma paracetamol concentrations. Chronic alcohol consumption would increase the toxic effects of codeine and paracetamol; alcohol enhances the central depressant actions of the opioid and also induces cytochrome P450 enzymes, increasing formation of NAPQI and causing toxicity at lower paracetamol doses. The toxicity of paracetamol would also be increased by other cytochrome P450-inducing drugs.
3. Codydramol contains paracetamol with the opioid dihydrocodeine and is likely to produce similar unwanted effects to co-codamol in overdose.

FURTHER READING

Adam, J., Pichler, W.J., Yerly, D., 2011. Delayed hypersensitivity: models of T-cell stimulation. Br. J. Clin. Pharmacol. 71, 701–707.

Ardern-Jones, M.R., Friedmann, P.S., 2011. Skin manifestations of drug allergy. Br. J. Clin. Pharmacol. 71, 672–683.

Aronson, J.K., 2009. Medication errors: definitions and classification. Br. J. Clin. Pharmacol. 67, 599–604.

Boyer, E.W., 2012. Management of opioid analgesic overdose. N. Engl. J. Med. 367, 146–155.

Buckley, N.A., Dawson, A.H., Isbister, G.K., 2016. Treatments for paracetamol poisoning. Br. Med. J. 353, i2579.

Frew, A., 2011. General principles of investigating and managing drug allergy. Br. J. Clin. Pharmacol. 71, 642–646.

Sivilotti, M.L.A., 2016. Flumazenil, naloxone and the 'coma cocktail'. Br. J. Clin. Pharmacol. 81, 428–436.

Thong, B.Y., Tan, T.C., 2011. Epidemiology and risk factors for drug allergy. Br. J. Clin. Pharmacol. 71, 684–700.

Compendium: drugs used to treat drug toxicity and drug overdose, and drugs used to treat toxicity due to environmental chemicals

Drug	Characteristics
Drugs used to treat drug toxicity and drug overdose	
Acetylcysteine	N-Acetylated amino acid. Used for paracetamol overdose. Given by intravenous infusion. Half-life: 5–6 h
Charcoal activated	Adsorbent. Taken as oral suspension for a range of drug overdoses (see Table 53.5); adsorbs drug within gut and reduces its absorption
Ethanol	Can be used with caution for methanol or ethylene glycol poisoning
Fomepizole	Alcohol dehydrogenase inhibitor. Given by intravenous injection for methanol or ethylene glycol poisoning; blocks formation of toxic metabolites formaldehyde and glycoaldehyde, respectively. Half-life: variable. Ethanol can also be used, with caution
Flumazenil	γ-Aminobutyric acid type A (GABA$_A$) receptor antagonist. Used for benzodiazepine overdose. Given intravenously. Half-life: 40–80 min
Methionine	Amino acid. Used for paracetamol overdose. Given orally
Naloxone	Opioid antagonist with rapid onset and short duration of action. Used to treat opioid overdose. Given by injection. Half-life: 1–1.5 h
Drugs used to treat toxicity due to environmental chemicals	
Iron poisoning/overload	
Desferrioxamine (deferoxamine) mesilate	Chelating agent. Given by continuous intravenous infusion. Half-life: 6 h. See also Chapter 47
Cyanide poisoning	
Dicobalt edetate	Chelating agent. Given by intravenous injection
Hydroxocobalamin	Binds cyanide to form cyanocobalamin. Given by intravenous injection. Half-life: 26 h
Sodium nitrite	Used with sodium thiosulphate. Given by intravenous injection
Sodium thiosulphate	Converts cyanide to thiocyanate. Given by intravenous injection with sodium nitrite
Heavy metals	
Dimercaprol	Forms complexes with heavy metals. Largely superseded by other chelating agents. Given by intramuscular injection. Half-life: 4 h
Sodium calcium edetate	Chelating agent. Used for poisoning by various metals, especially lead. Given by intravenous infusion
Organophosphate pesticides	
Atropine sulphate	Muscarinic antagonist; reduces cholinergic effects of organophosphates. Also used in overdose with β-adrenoceptor antagonists. Given intravenously. Half-life: 2–5 h
Pralidoxime	Reactivates acetylcholinesterase (see Chapters 4 and 27). Given by slow intravenous injection. Half-life: 1 h

54 Substance abuse and dependence

Substance abuse is characterised by compulsive drug-seeking and drug-taking behaviour and an inability to control intake (addiction); there may also be symptoms of withdrawal when the drug becomes unavailable (dependence).

Dependence-inducing drugs are mind-modifying (psychotropic) substances. They may be taken recreationally, initially because of the pleasurable effect they produce, but later to avoid unpleasant withdrawal symptoms. Dependence produces different degrees of need for the drug, from mild desire to an intense craving. In other cases, the drug is initially prescribed to treat a medical problem.

THE BIOLOGICAL BASIS OF DEPENDENCE

The mechanisms of drug dependence are relatively poorly understood, but involve complex dysfunctional adaptations of the neurocircuits in the brain that subserve physiological motivation and reward processes. The mesocorticolimbic dopaminergic reward pathway is central to these processes, and depending upon the particular stimulus and the functional status of the individual, its activation can result in a spectrum of responses from slight mood elevation to intense pleasure or euphoria. Stimulation of the mesocorticolimbic reward pathway can result from a plethora of factors – for example, food intake, sexual activity and the controlled and occasional use of lifestyle drugs such as alcohol and nicotine.

THE MESOCORTICOLIMBIC REWARD PATHWAYS

The mesocorticolimbic reward pathway consists of several structures:

- the ventral tegmental area, which projects to the nucleus accumbens via the medial forebrain bundle;
- the nucleus accumbens (involved in motivation);
- the amygdala (mediates association of reward with cues and negative reinforcement);
- the hippocampus (associated with memory and learning);
- the prefrontal cortex (involved in regulation of limbic reward systems and executive function such as self-control, salience attribution and awareness).

The reward pathway is activated by impulses arising in the ventral tegmental area, which are relayed through the medial forebrain bundle, via the nucleus accumbens, to the prefrontal cortex (Fig. 54.1). Activation of the ventral tegmental area results in dopamine release in the nucleus accumbens. Occasional and limited administration of most drugs of abuse causes release of dopamine either directly in the nucleus accumbens (e.g. cannabinoids, alcohol) or as a consequence of neural activity in the ventral tegmental area (e.g. cocaine, amfetamines), while opioids appear to cause dopamine release at both sites. Key cells in the nucleus accumbens are the medium spiny neurons that selectively express either dopamine D_1 receptors, stimulation of which increases intracellular cAMP, or dopamine D_2 receptors, stimulation of which reduces cAMP generation. Changes in the balance of D_1 and D_2 receptor signalling within the nucleus accumbens may initiate processes that result in drug dependence, because with repeated use the drug-related dopamine release becomes essential to maintain a 'normal' level of activity in the pathway. Other neurotransmitters are also important, including glutamate acting at AMPA and NMDA receptors. Alterations in AMPA receptor subunit structure that enhance cell permeability to Ca^{2+} ions increase the efficiency of transmission and are implicated in long-term potentiation of synaptic strength. Chronic exposure of the mesocorticolimbic system to dependence-inducing drugs eventually leads to neuroadaptive changes. Upregulation of intraneuronal cAMP in D1-type medium spiny cells causes expression of transcription factors including cAMP response element-binding protein (CREB), NF-κB and ΔFosB. In animal models ΔFosB activity is both necessary and sufficient for neuroplastic changes in response to dependence-inducing drugs. These changes may be mediated by gene transcription of brain-derived neurotrophic factor (BDNF), which can regulate the number of dendrites on various neurons. Changes in the reward and

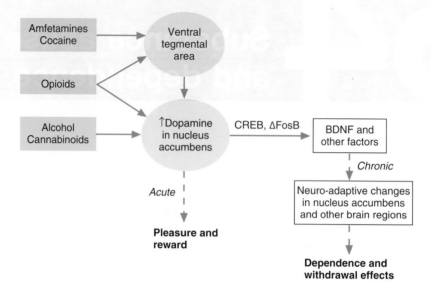

Fig. 54.1 The role of dopamine in reward pathways in the mesocorticolimbic system and the effects of drugs that cause dependence. The diagram illustrates only a small part of the complex mechanisms involved in the processes of reward and the ways that drugs can lead to dependence. Dopaminergic neurons in the ventral tegmental area release dopamine at the nucleus accumbens, increasing cAMP in medium spiny neurons and other cells via dopamine D_1 receptors. Drugs of abuse potential such as alcohol, amfetamines, cannabinoids, cocaine and opioids increase dopamine in the nucleus accumbens by acting locally on dopaminergic, glutamatergic, GABAergic, enkephalinergic and other pathways, or indirectly via the ventral tegmental area, or at both sites; the increased dopamine in the nucleus accumbens provides the pleasurable and rewarding effects of the drug. Persistent and excessive dopamine generation with chronic drug use causes gene transcriptional changes mediated by cAMP response element-binding protein and other transcription factors, including ΔFosB. Transcription of brain-derived neurotrophic factor (BDNF) and other growth factors causes neuroadaptive changes in the mesocorticolimbic reward pathway and in other brain regions including the dorsal striatum, amygdala, hippocampus and frontal cortex. These neuroplastic changes are believed to underlie the dependence and withdrawal effects of the drugs. *cAMP,* Cyclic adenosine monophosphate; *CREB,* cAMP response element-binding protein; *DA,* dopamine; *DYN,* dynorphin; *GABA,* γ-aminobutyric acid; *GLU,* glutamate.

other pathways may therefore become neurally 'imprinted', even if the causative drug is stopped for long periods, which might explain the vulnerability to relapse after detoxification. There are probably genetic and epigenetic influences on the neurochemical events involved in the reward pathways that also increase susceptibility to addiction.

Neuroplastic changes triggered by drugs occur in many structures associated with the mesocorticolimbic pathway, such as the dorsal striatum (a region implicated in habits, routines and conditioned responses), the amygdala, the hippocampus and the prefrontal cortex. Drug craving is influenced by the amygdala, particularly the anxiety and negative affect involved in acute withdrawal. Conditioned responses provide powerful cues to drug-taking in specific social circumstances, and this conditioning is reinforced by aspects of the drug-taking process. Eventually, becoming conditioned to fear drug withdrawal effects that can be relieved by the drug may lead to any source of stress or frustration becoming a cue for drug use. Dependence is associated with recruitment of stress systems in the brain on drug withdrawal, with an elevation of corticotropin-releasing hormone (CRH) and noradrenaline, and suppression of the antistress neuropeptide Y.

In contrast, physical dependence on a drug is unrelated to activity in the mesocorticolimbic system and arises from excessive noradrenergic output from the locus coeruleus, a

Box 54.1	Common drugs of abuse

Psychomotor stimulants
- Cocaine
- Amfetamines and derivatives
- Nicotine

Psychotomimetic agents
- Hallucinogens (e.g. LSD, mescaline, psilocybin)
- Cannabis and synthetic cannabinoids
- Dissociative anaesthetics (e.g. ketamine, PCP)

Central nervous system depressants
- Alcohol (ethanol)
- Benzodiazepines
- γ-Hydroxybutyric acid (GHB)
- Inhaled solvents
- Opioids (see Chapter 19)

Novel psychoactive substances (NPS)
- Numerous synthetic derivatives of amfetamines, cannabis, cathinones and opioids

structure in the base of the brain that is involved in arousal and vigilance.

This chapter covers drugs that are encountered in clinical practice primarily because of their abuse, such as ecstasy and cannabis, or because of their potential to cause dependence, such as nicotine and ethanol (Box 54.1).

DRUGS OF ABUSE

PSYCHOMOTOR STIMULANTS

Several drugs that have central stimulant properties are abused and produce dependence. Those more commonly encountered are considered here.

Cocaine

Cocaine is an alkaloid obtained from the leaves of the coca plant and is usually taken as the hydrochloride salt. 'Crack' cocaine contains the free base form in relative low purity and is named after the crackling sound produced when it is smoked.

Mechanism of action and effects

The psychomotor effects of cocaine are due to inhibition of reuptake transporters for monoamines in presynaptic nerve terminals, particularly the dopamine reuptake transporter (DAT), and to a lesser extent the noradrenaline transporter (NET) and the serotonin transporter (SERT). This in turn may activate opioid systems in the brain, with upregulation of μ-receptors (see Chapter 19). Increased dopaminergic activity in the reward pathway promotes dependence. Changes in various pituitary neuroendocrine functions occur with more prolonged use; in particular, the release of corticotropin and luteinising hormone (LH) are enhanced. Tolerance to the psychomotor effects of cocaine is limited.

Effects of cocaine include:

- intense euphoria.
- alertness and wakefulness.
- increased confidence and strength.
- heightened sexual feelings.
- indifference to concerns and cares.
- anxiety, paranoia, restlessness and tactile hallucinations, especially with habitual use.
- severe psychological, but not physical, dependence, brought about by the reinforcing effect of the rapid onset and brief duration of action; this develops particularly rapidly with 'crack' cocaine.
- tolerance, which occurs rapidly, requiring escalating doses to achieve the same effect.
- despondency and despair rapidly following withdrawal (the 'crash' or 'come down'). After chronic use, withdrawal can produce a dysphoric mood with fatigue, vivid dreams, insomnia, exhaustion, increased appetite and either psychomotor retardation or agitation, irritability and aggressive and stereotyped behaviour.
- toxic paranoid psychosis, with delusions of great stamina, occurs with chronic use.
- in overdose, excessive catecholamine concentrations produce convulsions, hypertension, cardiac rhythm disturbances and hyperthermia (due to excessive muscle activity and reduced heat loss); if severe, death can occur from respiratory depression and circulatory collapse. The cardiovascular toxicity can be treated with combined α- and β-adrenoceptor blockade, and seizures by intravenous diazepam.
- cocaine snuff produces necrosis of the nasal septum through its indirect vasoconstrictor action, mediated by noradrenaline at vascular α_1-adrenoceptors.
- exposure *in utero* leads to impaired brain development and other teratogenic effects.

Pharmacokinetics

Cocaine, as the hydrochloride salt, is used orally, intranasally (cocaine snuff) or by intravenous injection; the intravenous route gives an intense and rapid onset of effect. 'Crack' cocaine is prepared by mixing cocaine hydrochloride with sodium bicarbonate or ammonia and water, then heating to volatilise the free base. The product is a relatively low-purity form of the free base, but when smoked, it produces intense effects similar to intravenous use. Cocaine is metabolised by plasma and liver esterases, and its half-life is very short.

Management of cocaine dependence

There are no recognised drug treatments for cocaine dependence. Prolonged behavioural treatments remain the main approach. Tricyclic antidepressants (especially desipramine) are sometimes advocated for the severe depression that can occur on withdrawal.

Amfetamine and derivatives

Amfetamine, dexamfetamine, metamfetamine and 3,4-methylenedioxymetamfetamine (MDMA, 'ecstasy') have little medical value. Dexamfetamine is sometimes used as a treatment for attention deficit hyperactivity disorder (ADHD; see Chapter 22).

Mechanism of action and effects

Amfetamine and related drugs have indirect sympathomimetic effects, releasing monoamines from central nervous system (CNS) neurons (see Chapter 4). They are taken up into presynaptic nerve terminals, where they block vesicular uptake of dopamine, serotonin and noradrenaline by the vesicular monoamine transporters (VMATs), increasing their concentrations in the cytoplasm. This induces release of the monoamines into the synapse by reversing the respective reuptake transporters for dopamine (DAT), serotonin (SERT) and noradrenaline (NET) in the neuronal membrane. CNS stimulation by amfetamine is most marked in the reticular formation, although it also occurs in many other areas of the brain, including the reward pathway. The D-isomer (dexamfetamine) is twice as potent as the L-isomer of amfetamine in its central stimulant activity. Effects of amfetamine include:

- euphoria, similar to that experienced with cocaine; this is particularly intense after intravenous use.
- increased self-confidence, reduced fatigue and increased alertness for repetitive tasks.
- anorexia.
- irritability, agitation.
- psychotic behaviour during repeated use over a few days or with acute intoxication, causing hallucinations, delusions of grandiosity, paranoia and aggressive behaviour and repetitive actions.
- acute intoxication causing hyperthermia, panic, tremor, confusion, hallucinations and aggressiveness.

- peripheral sympathomimetic effects leading to hypertension (sometimes with cerebral haemorrhage) and cardiac arrhythmias.
- tolerance develops rapidly to some of the central effects of amfetamines, such as anorexia, presumably through central monoamine depletion; tolerance to the euphoric effects and motor stimulation is slower.
- withdrawal leads to prolonged sleep, followed by fatigue, depression and increased appetite; other symptoms include anxiety, craving, headaches, restlessness and vivid dreams.

MDMA (ecstasy) is more selective than amfetamine for serotonin release, and produces euphoria similar to that of amfetamine but with less stimulant activity. Direct agonist activity at serotonin 5-HT$_1$ or 5-HT$_2$ receptors may contribute to its effects, including release of oxytocin associated with the euphoric action. Disturbance of thermoregulatory homeostasis occurs, leading to a syndrome resembling heat stroke with hyperthermia and dehydration, usually after exertion in hot environments. Stimulation of antidiuretic hormone (ADH) release can cause thirst and water retention with subsequent water intoxication and hyponatraemia. The toxic effects of MDMA include cardiac arrhythmias, seizures, muscle damage and severe metabolic acidosis, which may be fatal. The long-term toxicity may include memory impairment, anxiety or depression. Most use is intermittent, and dependence on MDMA is unusual, although cravings can occur with regular use.

Pharmacokinetics

Although amfetamine is sometimes used intravenously or via nasal inhalation, absorption from the gut is rapid and complete. Amfetamine readily crosses the blood–brain barrier. About half is excreted unchanged in the urine, and the rest is metabolised in the liver. Amfetamine is a basic drug and its half-life varies according to urine flow and pH; at low urine pH, greater ionisation of amfetamine increases its excretion, whereas at high urine pH the half-life is longer because of greater reabsorption of the nonionised drug in the renal tubule. Metabolites of amfetamine are believed to contribute to the psychotic effects seen with long-term use.

Ecstasy is usually taken orally. It undergoes hepatic metabolism via CYP2D6, and polymorphism of this enzyme may explain some of the serious intoxication that occurs with the drug, although the half-life does not differ much between poor and extensive metabolisers (about 5 hours in both).

Management of amfetamine dependence

There are no recognised treatments for amfetamine dependence, which relies on behavioural therapies.

Cathinone stimulants

Mechanism of action

Cathinone and cathine are derived from the khat plant, which is used recreationally by people in the Arabian peninsula and Horn of Africa. They probably stimulate release of monoamines from neuronal vesicles and inhibit their reuptake. Their psychoactive and physical effects are relatively weak but resemble those of amfetamines. They are used intranasally or buccally, although they can be injected, smoked or taken rectally.

Pharmacokinetics

Cathinones are metabolised in the liver, but there is little information about their pharmacokinetics. They have short half-lives in animal studies.

Nicotine and tobacco

Mechanism of action

Over 300 chemical compounds are present in tobacco smoke, but the actions of nicotine are central to the addictive pharmacological effects of smoking. Nicotine has dose-related peripheral actions. At low doses, stimulation of aortic and carotid chemoreceptors enhances sympathetic nervous system activity, and at higher doses there is direct stimulation of the nicotinic N$_1$ receptors in autonomic ganglia (see Chapter 4). At even higher doses, nicotine acts as a ganglion-blocking agent. Initial stimulation of autonomic nervous tissue is therefore followed by depression. Effects on the CNS are mediated by presynaptic nicotinic receptors that are structurally distinct from those in the periphery. Stimulation of CNS nicotinic receptors increases neuronal permeability to Na$^+$ or Ca^{2+} and enhances the release of glutamate, which promotes dopamine release. With prolonged use nicotine inhibits the release of γ-aminobutyric acid (GABA). Nicotinic receptors are found in the mesocortical and mesocorticolimbic dopaminergic systems, in projections from the ventral forebrain to the cortex that mediate arousal, and in hippocampal projections where stimulation enhances learning and short-term memory. Tolerance to the CNS effects of nicotine is rapid due to receptor desensitisation.

Effects of nicotine and tobacco

Tobacco components, including nicotine, have effects on a number of organ systems.

Respiratory effects

The lungs are the first area to be in contact with the chemical components of tobacco smoke and are also exposed to particles and gases. Tars and other irritants, rather than nicotine, are responsible for the chronic damage to the lungs.

- An increase in blood carboxyhaemoglobin concentration (from carbon monoxide in tobacco smoke) decreases oxygen-carrying capacity. This may be important in ischaemic heart disease, increasing the chance of provoking angina.
- Increased mucus secretion, with reduced activity of bronchial cilia and consequent decreased clearance of lung secretions, leads to chronic bronchitis.
- Progressive destruction of the supporting tissue in the bronchioles produces emphysema and chronic obstructive pulmonary disease (COPD). Smoking is the major cause of this condition in Western societies.
- The risk of lung cancer is increased to about 20 times that of a nonsmoker. Inhalation of tobacco smoke is a major contributory factor and explains the greater risk in cigarette smokers. Giving up smoking reduces the risk progressively over about 10 years of abstinence. The constituent of tobacco smoke responsible for altering DNA structure and initiating the cancer process remains controversial, but the relationship between smoking and lung cancer has been confirmed by numerous epidemiological studies.

Cardiovascular effects

- Stimulation of the autonomic nervous system and sensory receptors in the heart increases heart rate, blood pressure and cardiac output.
- The risk of cardiovascular disease is increased by smoking cigarettes, but not by pipe and cigar smoking, and it occurs at a younger age. The overall risk of death from coronary artery disease is doubled in smokers compared with nonsmokers, and the magnitude of the effect is related to the numbers of cigarettes smoked. Peripheral vascular disease and stroke are also increased. Even passive smokers have an excess risk of vascular disease of 25%. The major reason for the excess of events is accelerated formation of atheromatous plaques and enhanced platelet aggregability. The risk of vascular disease falls over the first 3–5 years after stopping smoking to a level close to that of people who have never smoked.

Psychological effects

The psychological effects of smoking are substantial, as indicated by the difficulties experienced by those attempting to quit.

- Decreased appetite, with weight gain on stopping smoking.
- Emotional dependence on nicotine and the physical act of smoking is powerful. Physical withdrawal is less marked than psychological withdrawal but includes restlessness, irritability, anxiety, depression, difficulty concentrating, sleep disturbance and increased appetite.

Other effects

Nicotine and smoking have a number of other effects.

- Peptic ulceration is twice as common in smokers.
- Smoking is a risk factor for osteoporosis.
- Smoking in pregnancy, especially during the second half, has several effects. The most important are an increased risk of a low-birth-weight child and increased perinatal mortality. The vasoconstrictor effects of nicotine are responsible. Physical and mental development are slowed in children born to mothers who smoked during pregnancy.
- Smoking induces several hepatic cytochrome P450 isoenzymes and increases the clearance of CYP1A2 substrates such as theophylline (see Chapter 12) and imipramine (see Chapter 22).

Pharmacokinetics of nicotine

Nicotine can be absorbed from the mouth in its nonionised form, which is found in the less acidic environment of cigar and pipe tobacco smoke. Cigarette smoke, which is acidic, ionises nicotine, which can only be absorbed in significant amounts from the lungs. About 10% of the nicotine from a cigarette is absorbed, but at a faster rate than from cigars or a pipe, owing to the larger surface area of the lungs, and results in a higher but less prolonged peak plasma concentration. Nicotine can also be absorbed transdermally. It is metabolised in the liver; the major metabolite, cotinine, has a much longer half-life (about 10–40 hours) than nicotine (0.5–2 hours), and its concentration in plasma, saliva or urine can be used as a monitor of smoking behaviour.

Dependence on and withdrawal from nicotine

Withdrawal is often difficult to achieve unless motivation is high. Smokers should be supported by counselling about the health benefits of quitting and advice on overcoming problems such as weight gain. Behavioural therapy as an aid to quitting has a success rate of 20% at 1 year. Pharmacotherapy is often used to reduce the intensity of withdrawal symptoms.

Nicotine-replacement therapy

Smokers usually adjust their smoking habit to maintain plasma nicotine concentrations just above a threshold that averts withdrawal symptoms. The plasma concentration falls rapidly within 1–2 hours of the last cigarette, and rather more slowly after smoking a cigar or pipe. The resultant craving for nicotine can be reduced by nicotine replacement, delivered via transdermal patches, sublingual tablets, chewing gum, an inhaler (with most absorption occurring in the mouth) or a nasal spray. E-cigarettes may also help smokers quit smoking. They use a battery-operated heating element to deliver a chemical-filled aerosol that may include flavourings, colourings and other chemicals, but there is controversy over the potential health risks associated with their use. The delivery method for nicotine determines the rate at which plasma nicotine concentrations increase, and is most rapid after the nasal spray. The individual can choose the most appropriate vehicle for his or her needs and preferences. Established cardiovascular disease is a caution for, but not a contraindication to, nicotine-replacement therapy. Behavioural therapy enhances the success rate achieved by nicotine-replacement therapy. The use of nicotine-replacement therapy delivered by a patch doubles the chance of achieving abstinence. Increasing emphasis is now also placed on the benefits of reducing the numbers of cigarettes used by smokers unable or unwilling to quit completely. Combining a nicotine patch with a short-acting form of nicotine delivery is more successful than using a patch alone.

Bupropion

Bupropion is an atypical antidepressant. It is a weak inhibitor of neuronal reuptake of noradrenaline and dopamine, and probably works by enhancing mesocorticolimbic dopaminergic activity; it also has nicotine receptor antagonist activity. Most antidepressants are ineffective for smoking cessation, but the use of bupropion gives smoking cessation rates equal to nicotine-replacement therapy using a patch. Treatment should be started 1–2 weeks before a 'quit date'. Used together with nicotine-replacement therapy, bupropion produces a modest increase in the chance of stopping. An additional benefit is that smokers who use bupropion as an aid to quitting are less likely to gain weight. It is given as a modified-release formulation and has a long half-life (24 hours). Elimination is by hepatic metabolism, which also generates active metabolites. Unwanted effects include anxiety, headache, insomnia and dry mouth. There is an increased risk of epileptic seizures, and bupropion should be avoided if there is a past history of seizures. Nortriptyline is probably as effective as bupropion for smoking cessation.

Varenicline

This is a partial agonist at nicotine receptors, with high selectivity for the CNS receptor subtype involved in addiction. It produces about 30–45% of the response expected from nicotine, and blocks the effect of added nicotine. The modest release of dopamine reduces craving and nicotine withdrawal symptoms. Treatment should be started 1–2 weeks before a 'quit date', and combined with behavioural support. Success rates are greater than for nicotine delivered by a patch or with bupropion. Varenicline is excreted unchanged by the kidney and has a half-life of 24 hours. Unwanted effects include gastrointestinal disturbances, dry mouth, headache, dizziness, drowsiness and sleep disturbance. Depression with suicidal thoughts has also been reported, but the validity of the association is unclear.

PSYCHOTOMIMETIC AGENTS

Hallucinogens

Lysergic acid diethylamide (LSD), psilocybin ('magic mush-rooms'), mescaline (from peyote cactus) and dimethyltryptamine (DMT) from ayahuasca (a South American herbal drink) are adrenergic hallucinogens that have structural similarities to monoamine neurotransmitters. LSD is the most potent hallucinogen.

Mechanism of action and effects

The actions of hallucinogens on the brain are probably related to postsynaptic 5-HT$_2$ receptor stimulation in the cerebral cortex and locus coeruleus, a region of the midbrain that receives sensory signals. LSD also produces presynaptic 5-HT$_{1A}$ receptor blockade in the dorsal raphe neurons, inhibiting firing of neuronal projections to the forebrain. Tolerance to LSD occurs rapidly, and appears to be related to downregulation of these receptors. The actions of LSD, psilocybin and mescaline are similar, and they share several properties, including cross-tolerance.

- Visual hallucinations are frequent, especially with high doses, and auditory acuity is accentuated. There may be an overlap of sensory impressions such that music is 'seen' or colours 'heard' (synaesthesia), which can produce severe anxiety. Time appears to pass slowly. Emotions are altered, with either elation or depression, and rapid mood swings can occur. The overall experience can produce a good or a bad 'trip', and can vary in the same individual on different occasions.
- Serious psychotic reactions occasionally occur, and long-term psychotic disorders can be precipitated. The other unpleasant persistent effect in some individuals is 'flashback', seeing bright flashes, or halos or trails attached to moving objects.
- Physical consequences of CNS stimulation include dizziness, weakness, drowsiness and paraesthesiae.
- Excessive sympathetic nervous system stimulation with large doses produces nausea, salivation, lacrimation, dizziness, mydriasis, tremor, hyperthermia, tachycardia and hypertension.
- Tolerance can occur within 5 days.
- Emotional dependence is frequent, but physical dependence is not seen.

Pharmacokinetics

Oral absorption of these drugs is good. Physical effects begin after about 20 minutes, but psychoactive effects are delayed for 2–4 hours and then last up to 12 hours. DMT has a rapid onset of hallucinogenic action, within 15–30 minutes, but the duration is only 1–2 hours. Elimination is by hepatic metabolism, and the half-lives are short.

Cannabis

Cannabis can be smoked as marijuana, which consists of dried leaves or flowers of the *Cannabis sativa* (hemp) plant, or as a resin extracted from the leaves of the plant and then dried, known as hashish. Solvent extraction of the resin produces cannabis oil, which can be added to tobacco. The hallucinogenic effects of cannabis are much less marked than those of the aminergic hallucinogens such as LSD.

Mechanism of action and effects

The constituent compounds (cannabinoids) interact with specific CB1 receptors in the brain. These receptors are coupled to G$_i$ proteins that reduce intracellular cAMP production, and inhibit cell membrane Ca^{2+} and K$^+$ channels. The natural ligands are the arachidonic acid derivatives anandamide, 2-arachidonylglycerol and noladin ether. CB1 receptors are found in greatest density in areas of the brain involved in cognition and pain recognition (cerebral cortex), memory (hippocampus), reward (mesocorticolimbic system) and motor coordination (substantia nigra and cerebellum).

- The psychomotor effects result largely from tetrahydrocan-nabinol (THC) and one of its metabolites, 11-hydroxy-THC, which produce euphoria, heightened intensity of sensations, and relaxation. Occasionally panic reactions, hallucinations and depersonalisation can occur. Psychotic reactions are rare except in predisposed individuals, but the use of cannabis increases the risk of developing schizophrenia. Recent memory is markedly impaired, and complex mental tests are executed less well, although the user may perceive that their performance is enhanced. Motor incoordination may affect driving ability.
- Effects on the cardiovascular system include tachycardia and increased systolic blood pressure with a postural fall.
- The tars inhaled during chronic use of cannabis predispose to heart disease, chronic bronchitis and lung cancer.
- THC has an antiemetic action (see Chapter 32), which may be useful during cancer chemotherapy (see Chapter 52).
- Cannabinoids have analgesic effects that are used by some people with multiple sclerosis to control neuropathic pain.
- Tolerance to the psychomotor effects of cannabis occurs with regular use, and there is evidence of dependence.

Pharmacokinetics

Metabolism of THC is extensive, with some active metabolites being produced. The high lipid solubility of THC means that absorption from the lung or gut is high; it is rapidly metabolised with a half-life of only 1.5 hours. The psychomotor effects last for 2–3 hours after inhalation.

Dissociative anaesthetics

Phencyclidine (PCP) and ketamine differ from adrenergic hallucinogens in their mode of action. Both drugs were developed as anaesthetics, but PCP was withdrawn because of severe adverse effects (hallucinations, mania, delirium and disorientation).

Mechanism of action and effects

Both drugs block the excitatory effects of glutamate at glutamate *N*-methyl-D-aspartate (NMDA) receptors. These receptors are abundant in the cortex, basal ganglia and sensory pathways of the CNS. PCP also releases dopamine from nerve terminals in a manner similar to amfetamine. The term dissociative anaesthetic refers to the feelings of detachment (dissociation) from the environment and self that are produced by the drugs. These are not true hallucinations.

- Acute effects include euphoria, decreased inhibition, a feeling of immense power, analgesia, altered perception of time and space, and depersonalisation. Ketamine creates a 'mellow, colourful wonderworld'.
- Catatonic rigidity can occur, followed by ataxia and slurring of speech.
- Adverse experiences include confusion, restlessness, disorientation and impaired judgement. Irritability, paranoia, depression and anxiety are also common. Psychotic reactions are precipitated in susceptible people.
- Ketamine can produce near-death experiences.
- Persistent abuse of PCP leads to memory loss, speech and thought difficulties, and depression that persist for months after the last use.
- Tolerance is unusual, but psychological dependence occurs.

Pharmacokinetics

PCP is rapidly absorbed from the gut, nose or lungs after smoking. Effects are seen within minutes of ingestion and usually last 4–6 hours. It is a weak base that is excreted in the urine. It is also excreted into the stomach, and reabsorbed by the small intestine. The half-life is variable and can be up to 2 days. Ketamine is abused intravenously. It is metabolised in the liver and has a short half-life (see Chapter 17).

CENTRAL NERVOUS SYSTEM DEPRESSANTS

Alcohol (ethyl alcohol, ethanol)

Mechanism of action and effects

Alcohol has multiple actions on the CNS. Nonspecific actions such as increased fluidity of neuronal cell membranes (cf. general anaesthetics) may be important by reducing Ca^{2+} flux across the cell membrane, but several other actions have been described (Box 54.2). Overall, alcohol facilitates central inhibitory neurotransmission, particularly enhancing the effects of GABA, and therefore it is a general CNS depressant. After acute alcohol intake there is an initial depression of inhibitory neurons, particularly in the mesocorticolimbic system, which produces a sense of relaxation, but this is followed by progressive depression of all CNS functions. Mental processes that are modified by education, training and previous experience are affected first, while relatively 'mechanical' tasks are less impaired. Despite subjective impressions, there is no increase in mental or physical capabilities, unless anxiety has previously reduced performance. All effects are closely related to blood alcohol concentration (Table 54.1). In people who regularly use large amounts of alcohol, tolerance is seen to many of its psychological effects.

Alcohol increases dopamine release in the nucleus accumbens indirectly by activating presynaptic GABA receptors that actually inhibit GABA release. This is explained by the different alpha subunits on the presynaptic receptors that are sensitive to alcohol, whereas the postsynaptic receptors are not. Long-term use of alcohol produces long-lasting adaptive changes in the NMDA receptor that enhance their function. Opioid and serotonin receptor stimulation is also involved in the reinforcing effects of alcohol on the brain.

Alcohol intake is usually measured in units; in the United Kingdom, one unit is equivalent to 8 g (or 10 mL) of pure alcohol (Box 54.3).

Other effects of alcohol

Alcohol has a range of effects on many body systems.

Cardiovascular effects

- A modest alcohol intake may have protective effects on the circulation by inhibiting platelet aggregation and

---

Box 54.2 Possible mechanisms of action of alcohol

- Activation of $GABA_A$ receptors
- Inhibition of glutamate NMDA receptors
- Activation of serotonin and opioid receptors
- Inhibition of monoamine oxidase B in neurons
- Inhibition of Na^+/K^+-ATPase in neuronal membranes
- Increased neuronal adenylyl cyclase activity
- Decreased intracellular phosphatidylinositol system activity, leading to reduced Ca^{2+} availability

---

Table 54.1 The effects of alcohol at various plasma concentrations

Plasma concentration (mg/100 mL)	Effects
30	Mild euphoria owing to suppression of social inhibitory pathways in the cortex; the individual is more talkative and emotionally labile with loss of self-control; the risk of accidental injury is increased
80	Delayed reactions and reduced comprehension; memory impairment; the risk of serious injury in a road accident is more than doubled (80 mg/100 mL is the legal limit for driving in the United Kingdom)
100–200	Speech becomes slurred and motor coordination is impaired
>300	Often produces loss of consciousness
>400	Frequently fatal as a result of respiratory and vasomotor centre depression

increasing high-density lipoprotein cholesterol. The form in which the alcohol is taken is probably not important. The extent of this beneficial effect is probably greatest at 1 unit per day and is lost when intake exceeds 3–4 units per day.

- Higher intake of alcohol has pressor effects that raise blood pressure, possibly through increased vascular sensitivity to catecholamines. This increases the risk of coronary artery disease and stroke.
- Cardiac arrhythmias can be provoked by high alcohol intake, particularly atrial fibrillation. This can occur after an alcoholic binge ('holiday heart' syndrome), or following more chronic abuse (see Chapter 8).
- Alcoholic cardiomyopathy is a dilated cardiomyopathy that is only partially reversible with abstinence, and can lead to heart failure. An average intake of 10 units of alcohol daily for 8–10 years can produce this condition.

Liver

- Hypoglycaemia occurs as a consequence of the metabolism of alcohol in the liver. The metabolic process generates excess protons, which enhance the conversion of glucose, via pyruvate, to lactate and predisposes to lactic acidosis. People with a high alcohol intake often have a low-carbohydrate diet, which compounds hypoglycaemia. Hypoglycaemia tends to occur several hours after heavy alcohol intake and can contribute to seizures on alcohol withdrawal.
- The lactic acidosis created by alcohol metabolism in the liver impairs the renal excretion of uric acid, which predisposes to gout.
- Lactic acidosis also facilitates the synthesis of saturated fatty acids, which accumulate in the liver, leading to a fatty liver, possibly with altered liver function. Plasma triglycerides are also increased.
- Alcoholic hepatitis is usually a consequence of short-term heavy alcohol abuse. It can be fatal.
- Cirrhosis of the liver occurs with prolonged alcohol abuse, but individual susceptibility varies widely. On average, consumption of more than 8 units per day for at least 10 years is required for cirrhosis to occur in men. About two-thirds of this amount creates the same risk for women. Established cirrhosis reduces the first-pass metabolism and clearance of drugs eliminated by the liver (see Chapter 56).
- Chronic high intake of alcohol induces hepatic drug-metabolising enzymes, especially CYP2E1, which decreases the effectiveness of some therapeutic drugs (e.g. warfarin, phenytoin and carbamazepine).

Other gastrointestinal consequences

- Erosive gastritis can occur as a result of stimulation of gastric secretions.
- Pancreatitis is probably caused by raised triglycerides or by pancreatic duct obstruction by proteinaceous secretions induced by alcohol.

Sexual function

- Sexual desire is often increased by alcohol, but the ability to sustain penile erection is reduced, possibly because of the vasodilator actions of alcohol.
- Direct damage to the Leydig cells of the testis reduces the circulating testosterone, leading to reduced libido, infertility and a loss of the male distribution of body hair. Altered steroid metabolism in the liver leads to an increase in circulating oestrone in males, which causes gynaecomastia.

Neuropsychiatric effects

- A combination of alcohol toxicity with deficiencies of vitamin B_6 and thiamine in the diet of alcoholics predisposes to peripheral neuropathy and dementia. Specific midbrain damage can result and produces the syndromes of Wernicke's encephalopathy and Korsakoff's psychosis. This is a particular risk during acute withdrawal in people dependent on alcohol because of the high metabolic demand for thiamine.
- Alcohol has anticonvulsant properties and withdrawal predisposes to seizures, even in individuals without a history of epilepsy.
- Alcohol can disturb sleep patterns, with decreased rapid eye movement (REM) sleep and increased stage 4 sleep during intoxication. Withdrawal increases REM sleep, with associated nightmares (see Chapter 20).
- Dose-related memory impairment can be caused by suppressed hippocampal function.
- Subdural haematoma is more common after head injury in heavy drinkers, perhaps as a consequence of cerebral atrophy.
- Depression or anxiety states are more common in heavy drinkers.

Carcinogenesis and teratogenesis

- Cancers of the mouth, oesophagus and liver are more common with heavy alcohol use. Colon and breast cancer may also be increased.
- The fetal alcohol syndrome is believed to be caused by the effects of alcohol on neuronal adhesion molecules that regulate neuronal migration. Heavy maternal drinking during pregnancy leads to impaired learning and memory in the child. Genetic factors may be involved in the susceptibility of the fetus to these problems.

Pharmacokinetics

Although ethanol is absorbed from the stomach, the majority is absorbed from the small intestine, due to its larger surface area. High concentrations of alcohol (above 20%) and large volumes inhibit gastric emptying and delay absorption, as do foods high in fat or carbohydrate. Therefore peak blood alcohol concentrations depend on the amount and concentration

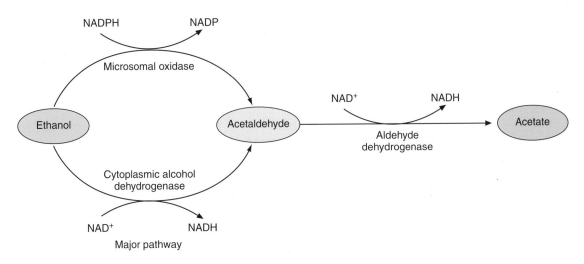

Fig. 54.2 **The metabolism of alcohol.** Alcohol dehydrogenase is responsible for 80–90% of the metabolism of ethanol. The microsomal oxidase is a minor pathway dependent on CYP2E1, the activity of which is increased by enzyme inducers such as alcohol itself. NAD^+, nicotinamide adenine dinucleotide (oxidised); NADH, nicotinamide adenine dinucleotide (reduced); NADP, nicotinamide adenine dinucleotide phosphate.

of the alcohol and on whether or not it was taken with food. Following absorption, alcohol undergoes substantial first-pass metabolism in the liver. The extent of first-pass metabolism of alcohol is related to the speed of absorption; thus with slower absorption, such as when alcohol is taken with food, less alcohol will reach the systemic circulation. Distribution of alcohol is fairly uniform, and the ready passage across the blood–brain barrier and high cerebral blood flow ensure rapid access to the CNS. The effects on the brain are more marked when the concentration is rising, indicating a degree of acute tolerance. Metabolism occurs mainly in the liver (Fig. 54.2), more than 90% being oxidised, mainly by alcohol dehydrogenase, while the rest is removed unchanged in expired air (in direct proportion to the blood concentration, which is the basis of the alcohol breath test) or in the urine. Alcohol metabolism shows saturation kinetics due to the limited supply of nicotine adenine nucleotide (NAD^+), which is the cofactor for the oxidative process. The maximum rate of alcohol metabolism averages 8 g/hour (or 1 unit/hour). The initial metabolic reaction mediated by alcohol dehydrogenase produces acetaldehyde, which is subsequently metabolised by aldehyde dehydrogenase to acetic acid (see Fig. 54.2). Genetic variability in alcohol and aldehyde dehydrogenases occurs among ethnic groups, leading to different capacities for alcohol or aldehyde metabolism. Accumulation of acetaldehyde in the circulation is responsible for many of the unpleasant effects of a hangover. Small amounts of alcohol are metabolised via the microsomal ethanol oxidising system (CYP2E1), the activity of which is increased by enzyme inducers such as alcohol itself (which does not affect the activity of alcohol dehydrogenase; see Chapter 36).

Some drugs, such as metronidazole (see Chapter 51), inhibit aldehyde dehydrogenase, leading to acetaldehyde accumulation if alcohol is taken with them. Typical 'hangover' effects of flushing, sweating, headache and nausea then occur after even small amounts of alcohol.

Alcohol abuse and dependence

There are no reliable estimates of the number of people in the United Kingdom with alcohol-related problems, although it has been suggested that 1–2% of the population are affected. The distribution curve for alcohol consumption is continuous but skewed at higher alcohol intakes. The risk of alcohol-related problems rises with the average alcohol intake. There is no 'safe' level of alcohol intake, but hazardous drinking is defined as a level or pattern of alcohol intake that will probably eventually cause harm. It applies to anyone drinking more than the recommended limits of 14 units per week. Harmful drinking is at a level that is already causing damage to physical or mental health. Dependent drinking is identified by features common to all drug dependence.

Up to 30% of hospital admissions are for alcohol-related problems, although the contribution of heavy drinking is often unrecognised. Screening for alcohol abuse can be carried out by obtaining a complete history of alcohol intake and using either the Alcohol Use Disorders Identification Test (AUDIT) or the Fast Alcohol Screening Test (FAST; Box 54.4). Abnormal measurements of both the mean corpuscular volume (MCV) of red cells (which is raised with increasing alcohol intake because of an effect of alcohol on the cell membrane) and the liver enzyme γ-glutamyl transpeptidase (γGT) will identify about 75% of people with an alcohol problem.

Psychological dependence on alcohol is common, but physical dependence also occurs. Withdrawal symptoms occur 6–24 hours after the last drink in dependent persons. If mild, these are related to autonomic hyperactivity and include anxiety, agitation, tremor, sweating, anorexia, nausea and retching. Convulsions can occur through neuronal excitation. Insomnia, tachycardia and hypertension are common with more severe withdrawal reactions. The most severe form of withdrawal is *delirium tremens*, with confusion, paranoia and visual and tactile hallucinations. Delirium tremens can cause death from respiratory and cardiovascular collapse.

1. Men: How often do you have *eight* or more drinks on one occasion?
   Women: How often do you have *six* or more drinks on one occasion?

   Never (0)   Less than monthly (1)   Monthly (2)   Weekly (3)   Daily (or almost daily) (4)

2. How often during the last year have you been unable to remember what happened the night before because you had been drinking?

   Never (0)   Less than monthly (1)   Monthly (2)   Weekly (3)   Daily (or almost daily) (4)

3. How often during the last year have you failed to do what was normally expected of you because of drinking?

   Never (0)   Less than monthly (1)   Monthly (2)   Weekly (3)   Daily (or almost daily) (4)

4. In the last year has a relative or friend, or a doctor or other health worker, been concerned about your drinking or suggested you cut down?

   No (0)   Yes, on one occasion (2)   Yes, on more than one occasion (4)

[a]One drink = ½ pint of beer or 1 glass of wine or 1 single spirits. On question 1, if the answer is Never (score = 0), then the patient is not misusing alcohol. If the answer is Weekly (3) or Daily/Almost daily (4), then the patient is a hazardous, harmful or dependent drinker. If the answer is Less than monthly (1) or Monthly (2), then questions 2, 3 and 4 should be considered. If the aggregate score is 3 or more for questions 1–4, out of the possible total of 16, the patient is misusing alcohol. Based on Hodgson et al. 2002. The FAST Alcohol Screening Test. *Alcohol Alcoholism*. 37, 61–66.

If an individual is drinking excessively, controlled drinking may be an option. However, if there is alcohol dependence or alcohol-related problems, then abstinence is usually preferable.

Controlled detoxification is usually undertaken with a sedative agent, such as a benzodiazepine (see Chapter 20), to attenuate withdrawal symptoms. Chlordiazepoxide or diazepam is usually used, decreasing the dose over 7–10 days. Clonidine (a presynaptic α_2-adrenoceptor agonist at the vasomotor centre in the brain; see Chapter 6) can be useful, by reducing the excessive sympathetic stimulation that accompanies withdrawal. β-Adrenoceptor antagonists (see Chapter 5) may be helpful for the same reason. Multivitamin preparations containing an adequate amount of thiamine should be given intravenously for acute withdrawal and orally for 1 month to prevent Wernicke's encephalopathy. Relapse is common after withdrawal from alcohol.

Three drugs are licensed in the United Kingdom to assist in the management of chronic alcohol dependence. Acamprosate can be used to reduce the craving for alcohol. It may activate $GABA_A$ receptors and block glutamate NMDA receptors, although several other contributory effects have been suggested. It has few unwanted effects and is nonaddictive. Nalmefene is a selective opioid antagonist that is licensed for reducing alcohol consumption by reducing the reinforcing effects of alcohol on the mesocorticolimbic system. Naltrexone, a long-acting opioid receptor antagonist, can also reduce the craving associated with alcohol withdrawal, but is not licensed for this indication in the United Kingdom. Disulfiram, an inhibitor of acetaldehyde dehydrogenase, causes unpleasant hangover symptoms after small amounts of alcohol. Given alone, or with psychosocial rehabilitation, it can help to maintain abstinence. Other potential agents to reduce the urge to drink include ondansetron (see Chapter 32), topiramate and gabapentin (see Chapter 23).

Gamma-hydroxybutyric acid

Mechanism of action and effects

γ-Hydroxybutyric acid (GHB) was originally introduced as a general anaesthetic, but is now used illegally as an intoxicant,

a 'date rape' drug or by athletes to improve performance. Its precursors γ-butyl-lactone (GBL) and 1,4-butanediol are also abused. GHB acts as an agonist at a specific inhibitory GHB receptor in the cortex and hippocampus of the brain, and also as an agonist at $GABA_B$ receptors, which mediate its sedative effects. GHB receptor activation stimulates dopamine release. GHB receptor stimulation also increases growth hormone release, which is the basis of its abuse by athletes and bodybuilders. In a similar manner to alcohol, GHB produces euphoria, increased libido and increased sociability. At high doses it produces nausea, dizziness, drowsiness, agitation, visual disturbances, amnesia and coma. Both psychological and physical dependence occur. Withdrawal can be treated with baclofen (see Chapter 24).

Pharmacokinetics

GHB is usually taken orally and occasionally intravenously. It has low oral bioavailability, is metabolised in the liver and has a short half-life of 30 minutes. The clinical effect lasts for 1.5–3 hours, and longer if taken with alcohol.

Inhaled solvents

Various organic solvents are abused as recreational drugs. Examples include butane, toluene and diethyl ether. Inhalation via a plastic bag held over the mouth or from an open container produces rapid intoxication, resembling that produced by alcohol. These compounds probably act in a similar way to volatile general anaesthetics (see Chapter 17). Death can occur from asphyxiation during inhalation, while long-term use produces brain damage by increasing neuronal apoptosis.

NEW PSYCHOACTIVE SUBSTANCES

In recent years there has been an explosion in the number of new psychoactive substances (NPS, also known as 'designer' drugs and formerly as 'legal highs'), including some linked to the deaths of recreational users. NPS include synthetic compounds based mostly upon the chemical structures of older drug groups such as amfetamines, ecstasy, cannabis, cathinones and opioids. Many do not have formal drug names and are known instead by a variety of chemical or street names. NPS include:

- Psychotomimetics: Derivatives of lysergic acid, mescaline, tryptamines (such as DMT), benzofurans, phenethylamines, and others.
- Synthetic cannabinoids, many with greater potency at cannabinoid CB1 receptors than the main active compound in cannabis (THC).
- Stimulants: Derivatives of cathinones (mephedrone, methylone and flephedrone); numerous amfetamine derivatives.
- Sedatives: Methylated and fluorinated derivatives of fentanyl and other opioids; benzodiazepine derivatives.
- Dissociatives: Derivatives of PCP and ketamine; methoxetamine (MXE) is more potent and has a longer duration of action than ketamine.

NPS are developed in clandestine laboratories and sold in the 'grey market' to evade legal restrictions on controlled drugs, but because they cannot be marketed legally for human consumption, they may be sold ostensibly as incense, bath salts, plant food or room freshener. They are used recreationally, mainly by young people, for their psychoactive properties, many of which are poorly understood. NPS may be harmful, as they have not undergone testing on animals or humans and there is little information available on their effects. The Psychoactive Substances Act (2016) prohibits the production, distribution, sale and supply of all psychoactive substances in the United Kingdom, with exemptions for those in everyday use such as alcohol, caffeine, prescription medicines and drugs already controlled under the Misuse of Drugs Act (1971).

CONTROLLED DRUGS

The UK Misuse of Drugs Act (1971) defines the classes of controlled drugs and lays down the criminal penalties for offences, including possession, sale, offering to supply or providing premises for the production or supply of controlled drugs. The act also licenses controlled drugs such as opioids for medical use. There are three main classes of controlled substance:

- Class A: Includes heroin, cocaine, MDMA (ecstasy), metamfetamine, LSD, DMT and psilocybin mushrooms
- Class B: Includes amfetamines, cannabis, codeine, ketamine, MXE and methylphenidate
- Class C: Includes γ-hydroxybutyrate (GHB), benzodiazepines and anabolic steroids

Penalties vary for offences involving substances in each class. Drugs in class B that are formulated for injection become class A substances. Individual drugs can be reclassified based on advice from the Advisory Council on the Misuse of Drugs (ACMD).

SELF-ASSESSMENT

True/false questions

1. Cocaine causes mydriasis by inhibiting the reuptake of noradrenaline into nerve terminals.
2. 'Crack' cocaine is the free-base form of cocaine.
3. Cocaine use has little damaging effect on the cardiovascular system.
4. Tolerance to the euphoric and anorexic effects of cocaine develops rapidly.
5. MDMA (ecstasy) blocks the release of serotonin (5-HT) from nerve endings.
6. MDMA causes hyperthermia and dehydration.
7. The effects of MXE are similar to those of ketamine.
8. Amfetamines are used to treat ADHD.
9. Cannabis impairs driving ability.
10. The euphoria caused by cannabis lasts for 24 hours.
11. THC, the main active ingredient of cannabis, causes nausea and vomiting.
12. Cannabis acts on specific receptors in the brain.
13. Nicotine causes tachycardia and reduced gut motility.
14. Tolerance to the effects of nicotine develops slowly.
15. Varenicline is a partial agonist of nicotine receptors in the CNS.
16. Cotinine has a long half-life and can be measured in serum to determine smoking habits.
17. Nicotine patches given alone are the optimum method for someone giving up smoking.
18. A physical withdrawal symptom does not occur when giving up smoking.
19. Alcohol is initially metabolised in the liver to acetaldehyde.
20. Chronic intake of alcohol induces hepatic drug-metabolising enzymes.
21. Even moderate alcohol intake increases the incidence of cardiovascular disease.
22. Some individuals have a genetically determined low ability to metabolise alcohol.
23. Disulfiram produces acute sensitivity to alcohol by blocking its conversion to acetaldehyde.
24. Acamprosate, which is used to encourage abstinence, acts on alcohol metabolism in a similar way to disulfiram.
25. The symptoms of alcohol withdrawal (detoxification) cannot be controlled by pharmacological means.
26. Alcohol can cause a macrocytosis.
27. Alcohol enhances secretion of ADH.
28. Plasma levels of γGT are depressed with heavy alcohol intake.
29. Cathinone derivatives in the khat plant produce sedation.
30. GHB may be abused by athletes.

ANSWERS

True/false answers

1. **True.** Cocaine blocks monoamine reuptake; in the eye, the resulting increase in noradrenaline causes mydriasis by contraction of radial pupillary muscles.
2. **True.** Unlike the salt form of cocaine, the free base can be illicitly smoked.
3. **False.** Acute effects include cardiac arrhythmias, and chronic use can lead to heart failure.
4. **True.** Tolerance develops to euphoria and appetite suppression in only a few days.
5. **False.** MDMA (ecstasy) increases release of serotonin and other monoamines by preventing their uptake into synaptic vesicles and promoting their release from the

cytoplasm into the synapse. It may also be an agonist at serotonin receptors.

6. **True.** Malignant hyperthermia resembling heat stroke and dehydration is observed in some individuals after ingesting MDMA.

7. **True.** MXE is a class B controlled drug with dissociative effects resembling those of ketamine, but it has greater potency and longer duration.

8. **True.** Amfetamines can be used to treat ADHD (but not an approved use in United Kingdom).

9. **True.** Cannabis impairs driving ability and the performance of complex mental tasks, and may give rise to psychotic reactions in predisposed individuals.

10. **False.** The euphoric effects last only 2–3 hours.

11. **False.** The related cannabinoid, nabilone, is used to inhibit nausea and vomiting in patients taking cytotoxic drugs.

12. **True.** Cannabis acts on cannabinoid receptors CB1 in the brain and periphery. The natural ligands for these receptors include anandamide. Synthetic cannabinoids may have greater affinity for CB1 receptors than THC found in cannabis.

13. **True.** These effects are caused by stimulation of nicotinic N_1 receptors in autonomic ganglia.

14. **False.** Tolerance to nicotine develops rapidly.

15. **True.** Varenicline reduces tobacco cravings by partial agonism at CNS nicotinic receptors, and it partially blocks the additional effect of nicotine if tobacco is smoked.

16. **True.** Cotinine is an inactive nicotine metabolite with a half-life of 10–40 hours; it can be measured in saliva, serum or urine.

17. **False.** Nicotine-replacement therapy should be supplemented with counselling.

18. **False.** Irritability, sleep disturbances and reduced psychomotor test performance occur on giving up smoking.

19. **True.** Alcohol is mainly metabolised to acetaldehyde (by alcohol dehydrogenase) and then to acetic acid (by aldehyde dehydrogenase).

20. **True.** The induction of CYP2E1 by alcohol can decrease the effectiveness of some drugs such as warfarin and phenytoin.

21. **False.** Moderate alcohol intake (below 3–4 units per day for men) has cardiovascular protective effects.

22. **True.** Some individuals have a genetically determined variant of alcohol dehydrogenase that has a reduced capacity to metabolise alcohol. Its incidence is low in white people but higher in people from some Far Eastern countries.

23. **False.** Disulfiram blocks conversion of acetaldehyde to acetic acid by aldehyde dehydrogenase; the accumulation of acetaldehyde causes sickness, headache and hangover symptoms, following even a small amount of alcohol intake.

24. **False.** Acamprosate acts to reduce the craving for alcohol, not by inhibiting its metabolism, although its precise mechanism of action is unclear.

25. **False.** Benzodiazepines can attenuate withdrawal symptoms, but there is a risk of dependence to these agents.

26. **True.** Alcohol intake is a common cause of macrocytosis (increased red cell volume) in the absence of anaemia.

27. **False.** The diuresis resulting from alcohol intake is partly caused by inhibition of release of ADH.

28. **False.** Plasma γGT is elevated in heavy alcohol intake.

29. **False.** Cathinone and its derivatives have amfetamine-like properties and cause wakefulness and insomnia.

30. **True.** GHB has sedative activity but also increases growth hormone release, which is the basis of its abuse by athletes and bodybuilders.

FURTHER READING

Benowitz, N.L., 2010. Nicotine addiction. N. Engl. J. Med. 362, 2295–2303.

Castaneto, M.S., Gorelick, D.A., Desrosiers, N.A., et al., 2014. Synthetic cannabinoids: epidemiology, pharmacodynamics, and clinical implications. Drug Alcohol Depend. 144, 12–41.

Connor, J.P., Haber, P.S., Hall, W.D., 2016. Alcohol use disorders. Lancet 387, 988–998.

Day, E., Copello, A., Hull, M., 2015. Assessment and management of alcohol use disorders. Br. Med. J. 350, h715.

Dunlap, B., Cifu, A.S., 2016. Clinical management of opioid use disorder. J. Am. Med. Assoc. 316, 338–339.

Hartmann-Boyce, J., Aveyard, P., 2016. Drugs for smoking cessation. Br. Med. J. 352, i571.

Johnson, B.A., 2010. Medication treatment of different types of alcoholism. Am. J. Psychiatry 167, 630–639.

Kjellgren, A., Jonsson, K., 2013. Methoxetamine (MXE): a phenomenological study of experiences induced by a "legal high" from the internet. J. Psychoact. Drugs. 45, 276–286.

Moore, T.H.M., Zammit, S., Lingford-Hughes, A., et al., 2007. Cannabis use and risk of psychotic or affective mental health outcomes: a systematic review. Lancet 370, 319–328.

Reuter, P., Pardo, B., 2016. Can new psychoactive substances be regulated effectively? An assessment of the British Psychoactive Substances Bill. Addiction 112 (1), 25–31. doi:10.1111/add.13439.

Robison, A.J., Nestler, E.J., 2011. Transcriptional and epigenetic mechanisms of addiction. Nat. Rev. Neurosci. 12, 623–637.

Schuckit, M.A., 2014. Recognition and management of withdrawal delirium (delirium tremens). N. Engl. J. Med. 371, 2109–2113.

Schuckit, M.A., 2016. Treatment of opioid-use disorders. N. Engl. J. Med. 375, 357–368.

Volkow, N.D., Koob, G.F., McLellan, A.T., 2016. Neurobiologic advances from the brain disease model of addiction. N. Engl. J. Med. 374, 363–371.

Winstock, A.R., Mitcheson, L., 2012. New recreational drugs and the primary care approach to patients who use them. Br. Med. J. 344, e288.

Zwar, N.A., Mendelsohn, C.P., Richmond, R.L., 2014. Supporting smoking cessation. Br. Med. J. 348, f7535.

Compendium: drugs of abuse and drugs used to treat drug dependence

Drug	Characteristics
Drugs of abuse	
Alcohol (ethyl alcohol, ethanol)	Intoxicant. Oxidation by alcohol dehydrogenase is saturated at normal alcohol intakes; zero-order kinetics (approximately 8 g/h)
Amfetamine	Dexamfetamine is active form, sometimes used for treatment of hyperactivity in children (especially in United States). Numerous amfetamine derivatives are abused recreationally. Half-life: 8–10 h
Anabolic steroids	Anabolic steroids such as nandrolone are abused by athletes and bodybuilders. See Chapter 46
Benzodiazepines	See Chapter 20
Betel nut	Seed of the *Areca* palm from Indian subcontinent, SE Asia and Pacific region. Betel nut contains arecoline, arecaidine and guvacine alkaloids and is chewed for CNS stimulant effect, sometimes with tobacco. Carcinogenic with or without tobacco
Cannabis (Δ-9-tetrahydro-cannabinol, THC)	Delta-9-tetrahydrocannabinol is the main active constituent; the 11-hydroxy metabolite is also active. Half-life: 1.5 h
Cathinone stimulants (khat)	Cathinone and cathine found in khat plant; amfetamine-like actions. Numerous cathinone derivatives are abused recreationally. Half-life: 1.5 h
Cocaine	Stimulant. Limited use as a local anaesthetic. Abuse involves nonoral routes (mostly nasal or inhalation). Half-life: 1–1.5 h
Dimethyltryptamine (DMT)	Psychotomimetic tryptamine compound, related to serotonin (5-HT), psilocybin (4-PO-DMT) and psilocin (4-HO-DMT). Found in a South American vine used in ayahuasca drink
'Ecstasy' (3,4-methylenedioxy-metamfetamine; MDMA)	Stimulant. The amfetamine analogue (MDA) and ethylamfetamine analogue (MDE, 'Eve') show similar properties. Numerous derivatives and analogues also abused recreationally. Half-life: 4–6 h
γ-Hydroxybutyric acid (GHB)	Sedative. Abused recreationally for euphoric and aphrodisiac effects; also abused by athletes due to enhanced growth hormone release. Half-life: 0.5–1 h
Lysergic acid diethylamide (LSD)	Hallucinogen. Low dependence potential. Many lysergic acid derivatives are also abused. Half-life: 5 h
Ketamine	Dissociative anaesthetic. See Chapter 17
Mescaline	Hallucinogen derived from peyote cactus; numerous derivatives also developed. Half-life: 6 h
Metamfetamine	Stimulant. Half-life: 10–12 h
Methlyphenidate	Given orally for attention deficit hyperactivity disorder (ADHD) and narcolepsy (see Chapter 22); used intranasally by recreational abusers. Half-life: 3 h
Methoxetamine (MXE)	Ketamine analogue; sedative, euphoric and dissociative effects are of longer duration (2–4 h) than with ketamine (1–2 h)
Modafinil	Atypical dopamine uptake inhibitor; promotes wakefulness. Used for ADHD (see Chapter 22), and also recreationally and for fatigue. Half-life: 15 h
Nicotine	Exposure to nicotine can be assessed by measuring cotinine in saliva, blood or urine. Half-life (nicotine): 0.5–2 h. Half-life (cotinine): 10–40 h. For nicotine replacement therapy, see below
Novel psychoactive substances (NPS; 'legal highs')	Wide variety of compounds, usually derivatives of amfetamines, ecstasy, lysergic acid, cannabinoids, cathinone and opioids
Opioids	See Chapter 19
Phencyclidine (PCP)	Dissociative anaesthetic. Half-life: 7–50 h
Psilocybin	Found in *Psylocybe* ('magic') mushrooms; prodrug converted in minutes to active hallucinogen psilocin. Half-life: (psilocin) 1–2 hours

Compendium: drugs of abuse and drugs used to treat drug dependence (cont'd)

Drug	Characteristics
Drugs used to treat drug dependence	
Cigarette smoking	
Bupropion	Atypical antidepressant. Used as an adjunct to smoking cessation. Given orally. Half-life: 24 h
Nicotine	Nicotine replacement therapy. Used as an adjunct to smoking cessation. Given sublingually as chewing gum, transdermally as a patch, or by inhaler or nasal spray. Peak plasma concentrations reached at 4–5 min (nasal spray), 15 min (inhalation), 15–30 min (gum) or 2–12 h (patch)
Varenicline	Partial agonist of CNS nicotine receptors. Used as an adjunct to smoking cessation. Given orally. Half-life: 24 h
Alcohol dependence	
The drugs below are used as adjuncts to psychosocial support.	
Acamprosate calcium	Used for the maintenance of abstinence. Given orally. Half-life: 20–33 h
Disulfiram	Acetaldehyde dehydrogenase inhibitor. Used in the treatment of chronic alcohol dependence when acamprosate or naltrexone are not suitable. Given orally. Half-life: 60–120 h
Nalmefene	Opioid receptor antagonist. Used in chronic alcohol dependence. Given orally. Half-life: 6–16 h. See also naltrexone, below
Opioid dependence	
Opioid dependence is discussed in Chapter 19.	
Buprenorphine	Used as an adjunct to treatment of dependence. See Chapter 19
Lofexidine	Used for management of symptoms of withdrawal. See Chapter 19
Methadone	Used as an adjunct to treatment of dependence. See Chapter 19
Naltrexone	Opioid receptor antagonist. Used to prevent relapse in detoxified formerly opioid-dependent individuals (see Chapter 19); also unlicensed use in alcohol dependence. Given orally. Half-life: 4 h

• •

About 80% of drug prescribing occurs in general practice (primary medical care). On average, men visit their general practitioners three to four times each year and women visit five times, and about two-thirds of these consultations end with the issuing of a prescription. Prescribing is particularly frequent for elderly people, who are likely to continue treatment for long periods of time and to receive prescriptions for multiple drugs concomitantly (polypharmacy). For these reasons, regular review of prescribed treatment should take place to determine whether it is still appropriate or necessary, and to ensure that important drug interactions and unwanted effects are not overlooked. Some drugs also require regular monitoring to determine efficacy (e.g. warfarin, antihypertensive drugs), blood concentrations (e.g. lithium) or biochemical effects (e.g. amiodarone, thiazide diuretics).

DUTIES OF THE PRESCRIBER

There are certain legal requirements that must be met when a medicine is prescribed. The information to be recorded is:

- the name of the person for whom the drug is prescribed (surname and initial) and address; in the case of children up to 12 years, the person's age must be specified.
- drug name (without abbreviation).
- dose.
- route of administration (usually given on the manufacturer's product information rather than the prescription).
- frequency of administration (with minimum dose-interval for preparations to be taken 'as required').

- either the quantity to be supplied or the duration of therapy.
- the prescriber's name, address and signature.
- the date.

GENERIC PRESCRIBING

In most situations the generic name of a drug (usually the international nonproprietary name [INN]) is preferred to the proprietary name (a 'brand' or trade name approved for use by a specific pharmaceutical company). Different pharmaceutical companies may market the same generic drug under different proprietary names, often with variations in formulation or dose, and the proprietary name(s) for the drug may also vary between countries. Another advantage is that the generic name may indicate the nature of the drug. For example, all β-adrenoceptor antagonist drug names end with -olol, such as atenolol, bisoprolol and metoprolol, but the proprietary names for these drugs (e.g. Tenormin, Cardicor and Lopresor) give little idea of the active ingredient. Another problem with proprietary names is that they rarely give any indication when there is more than one active ingredient; for example, Tenoret contains both atenolol and chlortalidone. The generic names for many compound preparations have this indicated by the term 'co-'; for example, co-tenidone is the generic equivalent of Tenoret.

Another advantage of generic prescribing is that pharmacists can dispense any product that meets the necessary specifications, rather than having to buy in a specific brand. This helps simplify stock holding and avoids unnecessary delays when dispensing. However, different generic preparations of the same drug may differ in the tablet size, colour or scoring, as well as brand name. Therefore it is important to inform the person taking the drug if a different brand is dispensed.

Generic prescribing is sometimes cheaper than prescribing by trade name, although the difference depends on pack size and other commercial factors and is sometimes marginal. It is likely that economic arguments and the increasing use of electronic prescribing systems have contributed to an increasing tendency for doctors to prescribe by generic name in recent years.

One potential hazard of generic prescribing involves drugs with a narrow therapeutic index. Stringent controls have largely eliminated the problem of variations in bioavailability from different brands, except for some modified-release formulations of drugs such as those for lithium or theophylline. Different release characteristics from the formulation can influence the plasma concentration profile of the drug and affect efficacy and toxicity, and in these situations prescribing by brand is recommended. Examples are modified-release formulations of lithium salts and some antiepileptic drugs.

DOSAGE

The total exposure to a medicine during a course of treatment is related to the size of the individual dose, its frequency of administration and the duration of therapy. The route of administration may also be important.

Dose

This is an essential item on all prescriptions and should be written in grams (g), milligrams (mg), or micrograms (which should not be abbreviated). Quantities of less than 1 g should be written in milligrams (e.g. 400 mg, rather than 0.4 g), and quantities less than 1 mg should be written in micrograms (e.g. 500 micrograms, rather than 0.5 mg), because μg is easily mistaken for mg when handwritten. For fluid doses, ml or mL is acceptable. Decimal points should be avoided wherever possible, but if unavoidable, a zero should precede the decimal point when there is no figure (e.g. 0.5 mL, not .5 mL).

Frequency and times of administration

Sometimes drugs are taken on one occasion only, while others must be given on a regular basis, in which case the frequency or times of administration should be specified. Such directions were traditionally given using a range of Latin acronyms and abbreviations, such as *b.d.* (for *bis die*), meaning 'twice daily'; some Latin acronyms remain in use and are listed in the British National Formulary (BNF), but the English equivalents (without abbreviation) are preferred (Table 55.1).

The route of administration

The route should be identified if there is any possibility of confusion. Abbreviations for routes of administration are widely accepted, including *p.o.*, oral; *i.v.*, intravenous; *i.m.*, intramuscular; *s.c.*, subcutaneous; and *p.r.*, rectal. Others, such as intrathecal, must not be abbreviated, because of the potential seriousness of inappropriate administration; for example, deaths have been caused by inappropriate intrathecal administration of vincristine. Confusion can arise with intravenous administration of drugs since there are numerous methods for delivery: drugs can be given by direct injection (either as a bolus or by slow injection) into a vein, or they can be infused, for example through the side arm of a continuously running intravenous drip, via a motor-driven pump or by addition to the intravenous infusion fluid reservoir. It is particularly important when prescribing drugs for intravenous administration to make clear the precise intentions.

The quantity to be supplied or the duration of therapy

Duration of therapy can be specified in a number of ways. Most general practice and outpatient prescriptions specify

Table 55.1 Acronyms and abbreviations for the timing and frequency of dosing in prescriptions[a]

Acronym/ abbreviation	Latin term	English equivalent
a.c.	ante cibum	Before food
b.d. (or *b.i.d.*)	bis (in) die	Twice daily
nocte		At night
o.d.	omni die	Every day
o.m.	omni mane	Every morning
o.n.	omni nocte	Every night
p.c.	post cibum	After food
p.r.n.	pro re nata	When required
q.d.s.	quater die sumendum	4 times daily
q.q.h.	quarta quaque hora	Every 4 hours
stat.	statim	Immediately
t.d.s.	ter die sumendum	3 times daily
t.i.d.	ter in die	3 times daily

[a]The Latin acronyms and abbreviations listed in the table remain acceptable but the English equivalents (without abbreviation) are preferred.

the amount to be dispensed (e.g. the total number of tablets or capsules). The duration of therapy will then be determined by the amount dispensed and the frequency of dosing. When the medicine is to be administered by a health professional or by a caregiver in a sheltered environment, the duration can be specified on the prescription sheet. Alternatively, it can be written on the prescription to be dispensed by a pharmacist. Medicines are now dispensed in original packs, with tablets individually packed by the pharmaceutical company. Specifying the duration of therapy is essential in the case of controlled drugs (see Chapter 54), such as opioids, for which there is a legal requirement that the total amount to be dispensed must be written in both figures and words.

OTHER ITEMS ON A PRESCRIPTION

Other essential items on prescriptions include the prescriber's signature and the address of his or her place of work. The latter is effectively waived for hospital prescriptions, since it is assumed that the prescriber is based at the hospital in question. The prescription must be dated. Computer-issued prescriptions are now almost universal in primary care. The specific requirements for these are essentially similar to those outlined previously. Use of computer-issued prescriptions avoids handwriting problems and assists in record-keeping and in data collection and analysis.

ADHERENCE, CONCORDANCE AND COMPLIANCE

The term 'compliance' describes the extent to which a person takes his or her medicine, but other terms such as adherence or concordance are now preferred, because they emphasise the partnership between the person and health professions in the process of taking medicines, rather than simply following instructions. It is frequently assumed that once a prescription has been given, the recipient will automatically follow the prescriber's instructions. However, there is abundant evidence that this is often not the case. Indeed, many prescriptions are not even taken to the pharmacist for dispensing; this may be because of cost or because the prescriber failed to discuss the 'hidden agenda' for which the presenting complaint was an excuse to see the doctor. In addition, a very substantial proportion of medicines collected are not taken in the manner intended.

The degree of adherence is affected by many factors, which include the duration of treatment. Fewer than 50% of people adhere fully during long-term therapy, such as that for high blood pressure or psychotic illness. There is increasing evidence that adherence to prescribed therapy can determine the outcome of treatment. For example, in treating hypertension, the control of blood pressure is substantially less good when adherence falls below 80% of prescribed doses.

The frequency of dosing has a major influence on adherence. Few people like taking their medicines with them to school or work. Therefore adherence with twice-daily regimens tends to be much better than that for more frequent administration. There is a further improvement in the extent of adherence with once-daily rather than twice-daily dosing. The formulation of a drug may also affect adherence; for example, young children and older people may be unable to operate metered dose inhalers for respiratory disease properly.

Unwanted effects can also reduce the likelihood of a person complying with therapy, but at times this can be turned to an advantage. For example, giving the entire dose of a tricyclic antidepressant at night means that the sedation it produces can be used to aid sleep. Giving the person advanced warning of likely unwanted effects such as dry mouth with this compound may earn the person's trust and encourage continuation of the therapy.

A proportion of nonadherence is caused by people forgetting whether or not they have taken their medicine on a particular day. The use of calendar packs or prepacked dispensing boxes can be helpful in this situation.

An individual's health beliefs are also particularly important. Adherence can be improved by involving the person in monitoring his or her disease and its control by therapy – for example, home monitoring of blood pressure, blood glucose checking in diabetes mellitus or peak flow measurements by people with asthma. Supplying accurate information about medicines can improve the level of satisfaction, and satisfied people are more likely to take their medicines.

INFORMING PEOPLE ABOUT THEIR MEDICINES

It is almost incredible to think that at one time doctors were reluctant to allow the name of a medicine to be shown on the container in which it was dispensed. However, paternalistic attitudes among the medical profession have been slow to disappear. Several surveys carried out in the early 1980s showed that most people felt that neither doctors nor pharmacists gave sufficient explanations about medicines. People are particularly keen to know:

- the name of the medicine;
- the purposes of treatment;
- when, how and for how long to take their medicine;
- what to do if a dose is missed;
- unwanted effects and what to do about these;
- any necessary precautions to take, such as possible effects on driving;
- any problems with alcohol or with other drugs.

Pharmaceutical manufacturers produce a printed leaflet about each medicine (patient information leaflet [PIL]), which is included in the original pack. These can also be viewed online, along with the highly detailed Summary of Product Characteristics (SPC), within the electronic Medicines Compendium (eMC; www.medicines.org/uk/emc). However, leaflets are complementary to, and not a substitute for, discussion with the medical practitioner, pharmacist, practice nurse, and so on. The Internet provides an increasingly rich source of information for people about their medicines and the variety of treatments available for their condition(s). However, advertising and the lack of peer review of most patient-orientated websites means that, in many cases, information the individual may have acquired before they first see their doctor may be incorrect and/or misunderstood.

RATIONAL PRESCRIBING

A definition of good prescribing has been proposed that encompasses four goals. These are to:

- maximise effectiveness;
- minimise harms;
- avoid wasting healthcare resources;
- respect the person's autonomy.

Irrational prescribing can take several forms, such as use of antibacterial drugs for viral infections, statin therapy for someone with late-stage malignancy, using expensive drugs when there are equally effective cheaper alternatives, using too high a drug dose in renal or hepatic impairment or under-dosage with an appropriate drug.

The standards against which rational prescribing can be judged will depend on locally or nationally agreed treatment protocols, or an agreed list of therapeutic alternatives. Ideally, prescribing should follow evidence-based guidelines, but it is often necessary to extrapolate these guidelines to situations not covered by the evidence. In the absence of evidence from clinical trials, it may be appropriate to use consensus guidelines produced by experts, and derived from a relevant evidence base.

Drugs are typically classified based on a shared mechanism of action, but drugs within a single class often show quantitative or qualitative differences. There has been considerable debate about whether it is reasonable to extrapolate a 'class effect' from a clinical study with one drug to others within the same class. Class effects may be related to clinical outcome (such as death or risk of stroke), effects on surrogate endpoints (such as reduction in blood pressure) or specific unwanted effects. Many consensus guidelines assume that drug efficacy is related to a class effect when there is a large body of information about several drugs in a class that suggests similar outcomes.

The sequence of events leading to a rational prescription involves initially making a diagnosis and determining prognosis. This may not always be possible, and it may be necessary to substitute differential diagnoses and rank these in order of probability and importance of treatment. The goal of treatment must then be determined. This may be curative, symptom relief, prevention or occasionally an aid to the diagnostic process. The prescriber should decide whether any treatment is necessary and, if so, should then select an appropriate first choice. The process is completed by monitoring the outcome and reaching a decision to stop, modify or continue treatment.

Assuming that the choice of drug is appropriate for the condition that the prescriber believes he or she is treating, there will be several further considerations involved in individualising drug treatment.

- Is this drug licensed for use in this condition? If not, prescribing may still be appropriate, but the prescriber should be familiar with the evidence to support the use of the drug.
- How does the drug compare with available alternatives in relation to published evidence of efficacy, safety, convenience and cost?
- Does the individual have co-existing conditions that will compromise the efficacy of the drug?
- Are there comorbidities that might benefit from the use of this treatment or an alternative option?
- Are any other drugs being taken that might adversely interact with your choice?
- Are there any absolute contraindications to using the drug in this individual?
- Are there relative contraindications to use in this individual, including comorbidities or common unwanted effects?
- Has the individual suffered previous adverse drug events that should make you cautious about using this particular drug?

The sequence of events in rational prescribing is also described in the prescribing competence framework devised by NICE and the Royal Pharmaceutical Society to support the education, training and clinical governance of medical and nonmedical prescribers; the 10 dimensions of the framework are shown in Box 55.1. Aspects of prescribing that ensure safe and effective outcomes of drug treatment are covered by dimensions 1–6 (Consultation). Wider issues concerning the duty of healthcare professionals to prescribe within legal and regulatory frameworks are covered by dimensions 7–10 (Prescribing governance).

PRESCRIBING SAFETY ASSESSMENT

Good understanding of clinical pharmacology is essential but not sufficient to become a safe and effective prescriber. Prescribing is a key component of undergraduate and postgraduate medical education reflected in many aspects of General Medical Council (GMC) publications, including 'Tomorrow's Doctors' (2009) and 'Good Practice in Prescribing and Managing Medicines and Devices' (2013; both available at

> **Box 55.1** The ten dimensions of the prescribing competency framework[a]
>
> **Consultation:**
> 1. Assess the patient (including drug history, differential diagnosis and investigations)
> 2. Consider the options (including nonpharmacological options, risks, co-morbidities, patient factors, adherence and drug resistance)
> 3. Reach a shared decision (with patients and/or carers)
> 4. Prescribe (with awareness of benefits, risks, unwanted effects, interactions, contraindications and cautions)
> 5. Provide information (with clear advice on actions if concerns arise)
> 6. Monitor and review (establishing, maintaining and adapting a management plan, and monitoring effectiveness and adverse reactions)
>
> **Prescribing governance:**
> 7. Prescribe safely (recognising self-limitations, risks and benefits, and reporting prescribing errors)
> 8. Prescribe professionally (based on the interests of the patient and with knowledge of the appropriate legal and regulatory frameworks)
> 9. Improve prescribing practice (using appropriate reflection, feedback and prescribing analysis tools)
> 10. Prescribe as part of a team (based on relationships with other healthcare professionals)
>
> [a]Adapted from: Royal Pharmaceutical Society and NICE. A competency framework for all prescribers. www.rpharms.com/unsecure-support-resources/prescribing-competency-framework.asp. July 2016.

> **Box 55.2** The eight domains of the UK prescribing safety assessment[a]
>
> - Prescribing (80 marks)
> - Prescription review (32 marks)
> - Planning management (16 marks)
> - Providing information (12 marks)
> - Calculation skills (16 marks)
> - Adverse drug reactions (16 marks)
> - Drug monitoring (16 marks)
> - Data interpretation (12 marks)
>
> [a]The PSA comprises 60 questions totalling 200 marks across the eight domains.

www.gmc-uk.org). Concerns about the quality of teaching of prescribing have nevertheless arisen in the United Kingdom. Several studies have demonstrated the extent and types of poor prescribing practice within the National Health Service (NHS), and the majority of UK medical students and new graduates lack confidence in their prescribing education and postgraduate skills. This may be due in part to a relative decline in the numbers of clinical pharmacologists as a medical specialty in recent years.

These factors contributed to the development of a national assessment of undergraduate prescribing skills by the UK Medical Schools Council (MSC) and the clinical section of the British Pharmacological Society (BPS). The prescribing safety assessment (PSA) was piloted in 2012 and has the primary aim of improving patient safety. In its present form, it is an invigilated online assessment taken by all UK medical students in their final year of study. A pass in the PSA is valid for 2 years. Depending on medical school, a student who fails the PSA in his or her final year either may not be able to graduate or may be required to pass the PSA at a further attempt during Foundation training.

The PSA consists of 60 questions across eight domains worth a total of 200 marks (Box 55.2), to be completed normally within 2 hours. Most questions are case-based and aligned with the clinical areas of medicine, surgery, elderly care, paediatrics, psychiatry, obstetrics and gynaecology, and general practice. Open access to the BNF and BNF for Children (www.evidence.nhs.uk) is provided to students sitting the PSA.

Further information on the PSA is available online (https://prescribingsafetyassessment.ac.uk/), including full details on question types, sample questions and practice papers.

Other online resources for e-learning of prescribing, such as the SCRIPT Safe Prescriber Toolkit (www.safeprescriber.org), may also be used by medical schools. The Further Reading section that follows includes a selection of texts and workbooks tailored to help medical students prepare for the PSA and for their careers as safe and effective prescribers.

FURTHER READING

General prescribing

Aronson, J.K., 2012. Balanced prescribing: principles and challenges. Br. J. Clin. Pharmacol. 74, 566–572.

Ashcroft, D.M., Lewis, P.J., Tully, M.P., et al., 2015. Prevalence, nature, severity and risk factors for prescribing errors in hospital inpatients: prospective study in 20 UK hospitals. Drug Saf. 38, 833–843.

Bond, C., Blenkinsopp, A., Raynor, D.K., 2012. Prescribing and partnership with patients. Br. J. Clin. Pharmacol. 74, 581–588.

Burnier, M., 2006. Medication adherence and persistence as the cornerstone of effective antihypertensive therapy. Am. J. Hypertens. 19, 1190–1196.

Davis, T., 2011. Paediatric prescribing errors. Arch. Dis. Child. 96, 489–491.

Heaton, A., Webb, D.J., Maxwell, S.R.J., 2008. Undergraduate preparation for prescribing: the views of 2413 UK medical students and recent graduates. Br. J. Clin. Pharmacol. 66, 128–134.

Maxwell, S.R.J., Cameron, I.T., Webb, D.J., 2015. Prescribing safety: ensuring that new graduates are prepared. Lancet 385, 579–581.

Maxwell, S., Mucklow, J., 2012. e-Learning initiatives to support prescribing. Br. J. Clin. Pharmacol. 74, 621–631.

Osterberg, L., Blaschke, T., 2005. Adherence to medication. N. Engl. J. Med. 353, 487–497.

Rissman, R., Dubois, E.A., Franson, K.L., et al., 2012. Concept-based learning of personalized prescribing. Br. J. Clin. Pharmacol. 74, 589–596.

Ross, S., Maxwell, S., 2012. Prescribing and the core curriculum for tomorrow's doctors: BPS curriculum in clinical pharmacology and prescribing for medical students. Br. J. Clin. Pharmacol. 74, 644–661.

Santaguida, P.L., Helfand, M., Raina, P., 2005. Challenges in systematic reviews that evaluate drug efficacy. Ann. Intern. Med. 142, 1066–1072.

Shah, R.R., Shah, D.R., 2012. Personalized medicine: is it a pharmacogenetic mirage? Br. J. Clin. Pharmacol. 74, 698–721.

Spinewine, A., Schmader, K.E., Barber, N., et al., 2007. Appropriate prescribing in elderly people: how well can it be measured and optimized? Lancet 370, 173–184.

Thomas, S.H.L., Yates, L.M., 2012. Prescribing without evidence–pregnancy. Br. J. Clin. Pharmacol. 74, 691–697.

Preparation for the prescribing safety assessment (PSA)

Baker, E., Burrage, D., Lonsdale, D., et al., 2014. Prescribing Scenarios at a Glance. Wiley-Blackwell, Chichester. ISBN-13: 978-1118570869.

Brown, W., Loudon, K., Fisher, J., et al., 2014. Pass the PSA. Churchill Livingstone, Edinburgh. ISBN-13: 978-0702055188.

Choudhry, M., Fuggle, N.R., Iqbal, A., 2016. Get ahead! The Prescribing Safety Assessment. CRC Press, Boca Raton, FL, USA. ISBN-13: 978-1498719063.

Norton, D., Hamilton, E., Norton, N., et al., 2014. Prescribing Skills Workbook. JP Medical Publishing Ltd, London. ISBN-13: 978-1907816864.

Qureshi, Z., Maxwell, S. (Eds.), 2014. The Unofficial Guide to Prescribing. Churchill Livingstone, Edinburgh. ISBN-13: 978-0702055201.

Ross, S., 2014. Prescribing at a Glance. Wiley-Blackwell, Chichester, West Sussex, UK; Malden, MA. ISBN-13: 978-1118257319.

Savickas, V., Kayyali, R.Q., 2013. Student Success in the Prescribing Safety Assessment (PSA) (Masterpass). CRC Press, Boca Raton, FL, USA. ISBN-13: 978-1846199783.

56 Drug therapy in special situations

PRESCRIBING IN PREGNANCY

Guidelines for prescribing during pregnancy are set out in the British National Formulary (BNF; www.evidence.nhs.uk). Pregnancy can be associated with medical problems that require treatment, and pregnant women may also require continued treatment for chronic conditions not related to the pregnancy, such as diabetes, depression, epilepsy and hypertension. Many drugs cross the placenta, and exposure of the fetus to any unnecessary drug is undesirable, particularly in the first trimester between the 3rd and 11th weeks of pregnancy, because of the risk of teratogenicity. In the second and third trimesters, drugs may affect the growth or functional development of the fetus, whereas drugs given at full term may influence labour or affect the neonate after delivery. The magnitude of the potential problem is illustrated by the fact that about 50% of women take prescribed medication during pregnancy, although this occurs most often late in pregnancy, and an unrecorded proportion will take over-the-counter medications, including herbal and homeopathic remedies.

Unequivocal teratogenic activity of drugs in humans is limited to a relatively small number of compounds, but their effects are irreversible and affect the whole life of the offspring. In the United States, drugs are assessed for risk in pregnancy by the FDA, based on evidence from animal and human studies. From 1979 to 2015, the risk was expressed in lettered categories, ranging from A (no evidence in human studies) to D (positive evidence), with category X comprising known teratogens; a similar system operates in Australia. In the UK, the BNF identifies drugs which may have harmful effects in pregnancy and indicates the trimester(s) of risk. Evidence of risk in pregnancy is currently lacking for up to 40% of licensed drugs.

The potential catastrophic consequences of the administration of a teratogenic drug were highlighted by the thalidomide tragedy in the 1960s. Thalidomide was introduced as a sedative and hypnotic, and used for the treatment of pregnancy-associated morning sickness. Following its introduction there was a dramatic increase in the incidence of phocomelia (abnormal or absent development of limb buds). The drug was banned once the association was recognised, and this resulted in the incidence of phocomelia decreasing to previous levels (Fig. 56.1). The teratogenic potential of thalidomide in humans is extremely high (affecting 30% of fetuses exposed to the drug in the first trimester), but it was not detected in animal testing because the drug is not teratogenic in rodents, and teratogenic effects are seen in rabbits only at 100-fold higher doses than in humans or other primates. This observation resulted in the legal requirement for two or more animal species in preclinical teratogenicity testing. The thalidomide tragedy led to a significant reduction in the proportion of women taking any prescription drug during pregnancy, particularly in the first trimester. Thalidomide continues in use as a treatment for multiple myeloma and for leprosy; the drug should never be given to women with childbearing potential.

The list of drugs known to be teratogenic is relatively short but includes thalidomide, many anticonvulsants, some chemotherapeutic drugs (e.g. alkylating agents and

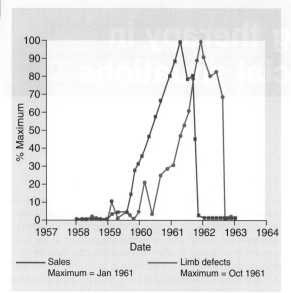

Fig. 56.1 Sales of thalidomide and the incidence of phocomelia. Thalidomide sales and phocomelia incidence are each expressed as a percentage of the reported maximum.

antimetabolites), warfarin, androgens, danazol, diethylstilbestrol (DES), lithium and retinoids (Table 56.1). Because of their long half-lives, some retinoids can result in teratogenesis, even if treatment for the mother is stopped several weeks before pregnancy occurs. Although teratogenesis is commonly thought of in terms of structural defects or dysfunctional growth in utero, it also refers to long-term functional deficits. For example, maternal consumption of alcohol during pregnancy may cause behavioural and cognitive abnormalities in childhood, despite the birth of a seemingly unaffected infant. Some drugs may exhibit a long latency period. DES, which was given during pregnancy between the 1940s and early 1970s in the mistaken belief that it reduced the risk of miscarriage, resulted in abnormalities in the offspring when they reached adulthood, including hypogonadism in males and vaginal adenocarcinoma in females.

In addition to known teratogens, a much larger number of drugs should be avoided or used with caution in pregnancy because of their potential to produce detrimental effects in the fetus. Examples include warfarin-induced anticoagulation (see Chapter 11), which may cause the abnormalities associated with fetal warfarin syndrome and predispose mothers to cerebral haemorrhage during delivery; in contrast, heparin is an effective anticoagulant in the mother and does not cross the placenta. Nonsteroidal antiinflammatory drugs (NSAIDs; see Chapter 29) can produce premature closure of the ductus arteriosus before delivery. Adverse effects produced at therapeutic doses, such as tachycardia with tricyclic antidepressants and growth restriction with corticosteroids, may also affect the fetus or neonate.

Whenever a drug is given to a pregnant woman, or a woman who has childbearing potential, an assessment should be made, taking into account any risk to the fetus balanced against the benefit to the mother and any risk associated with not treating the mother. For example, treatment with

anticonvulsants or antimalarials may be essential for the mother, despite the possible risk to the fetus/neonate. The risk to the fetus/neonate should be minimised whenever possible by selecting the drug with the least potential for teratogenicity, by prescribing the lowest effective dose and minimising the use of multiple drugs. Absence of evidence of teratogenicity does not imply that a risk does not exist, and little information is available on teratogenic risk for many drugs. Drugs which have been used extensively in pregnancy and appear to be safe should nevertheless be preferred to new or untried drugs. The BNF provides detailed information on potential adverse drug effects on the fetus and neonate, and guidance is also available from the UK Teratology Information Service (www.uktis.org).

PHARMACOKINETICS IN PREGNANCY

The placenta provides a potential barrier to the transfer of macromolecules such as heparin from the maternal circulation, but essentially all low-molecular-weight drugs can cross the placenta. Lipid-soluble drugs cross the placenta most readily, but hydrophilic drugs also will equilibrate with the fetal circulation over time. Limited drug metabolism can occur in the placenta, which may restrict fetal exposure of some drugs. Irrespective of direct exposure to the drug, the fetus may be affected by a drug that constricts placental blood vessels, impairing gas and nutrient exchange; or that causes uterine hypertonia, resulting in anoxic injury; or that alters maternal physiology in other ways, such as by causing hypotension.

The fetal liver and kidneys have only modest abilities to eliminate drugs, so drugs that reach the fetal circulation are usually cleared by the maternal routes of elimination. The fetus therefore represents a slowly equilibrating maternal compartment, with transfer across the placenta being determined by the concentration gradient between fetal and maternal circulations.

Maternal pharmacokinetics are affected by a number of physiological changes, especially in late pregnancy. Compared with nonpregnant women, these include:

- increased drug metabolism, due to hepatic blood flow that increases by up to 60%, and increased hepatocyte expression of cytochrome P450 isoenzymes including CYP2C9, CYP2D6 and CYP3A4, although some others, such as CYP2C19, are reduced;
- increased renal perfusion and glomerular filtration rate (GFR), enhancing the excretion of hydrophilic drugs and drug metabolites;
- increased plasma volume, resulting in reduced concentrations of albumin and other plasma proteins and potentially decreased protein binding of many drugs.

These changes mean that maternal drug concentrations are often lower than those in a nonpregnant woman given the same dose, so drug doses may need to be increased in pregnancy to compensate. Decisions on changes in drug dosage are nevertheless hampered by the lack of detailed pharmacokinetic information in pregnancy for most relevant drugs.

DRUGS AND BREASTFEEDING

Almost any compound present in the maternal circulation will enter breast milk and be ingested by the suckling baby.

Table 56.1 Examples of drug-induced teratogenicity and fetal/neonatal toxicity

Therapeutic drug	Teratogenic and adverse effects in fetus and neonate
ACE inhibitors	Affect fetal and neonatal blood pressure control and renal function; oligohydramnios
Alcohol	Fetal alcohol syndrome; growth restriction (see Chapter 54)
Aminoglycosides	Auditory or vestibular nerve damage
Amiodarone	Neonatal goitre
Androgens	Virilisation of female fetus
Anticancer drugs	Carcinogenic and teratogenic effects (also avoid before pregnancy)
Barbiturates	Fetal abnormalities; withdrawal effects in neonates
Benzodiazepines	Withdrawal effects in neonates
β-Adrenoceptor antagonists	Intrauterine growth restriction, neonatal hypoglycaemia and bradycardia
Carbamazepine	Neural tube defects
Carbimazole	Neonatal goitre
Corticosteroids	Intrauterine growth suppression (with prolonged treatment)
Dapsone	Neonatal haemolysis and methaemoglobinaemia
Diethylstilbestrol	Hypogonadism in male offspring and vaginal cancer in female offspring
Fibrinolytics	Premature separation of placenta in first 18 weeks
Finasteride	Genital abnormalities in male fetus
Lamotrigine	Teratogenicity
Leflunomide	Teratogenic in animals; effective contraception necessary for at least 2 years after end of treatment for women and 3 months for men
Lithium salts	Teratogenicity; cardiac abnormalities
NSAIDs	Premature closure of ductus arteriosus; pulmonary hypertension
Opioids	Neonatal respiratory depression and risk of withdrawal syndrome if the mother is habituated
Oral anticoagulants	Malformations; fetal or neonatal haemorrhage
Oxcarbazepine	Neural tube defects
Phenytoin	Congenital malformations; risk of neonatal haemorrhage due to vitamin K deficiency
Primaquine	Neonatal haemolysis and methaemoglobinaemia
Retinoids and retinoid-like drugs	Teratogenic, craniofacial malformations; some have long half-lives and effective contraception is essential for prolonged periods after stopping treatment and before pregnancy
Ribavirin	Teratogenic in animals; effective contraception necessary for at least 6 months after treatment for both women and men
Statins	Decreased cholesterol synthesis affects fetal development
Sulphonamides	Neonatal haemolysis and methaemoglobinaemia
Sulphonylureas	Neonatal hypoglycaemia
Thiazide diuretics	Growth retardation; electrolyte disturbance
Valproate	Congenital malformations and developmental delay in offspring

See BNF for detailed advice. Manufacturers of most drugs advise that they should be taken in pregnancy only if the potential benefit outweighs the possible risk; many also recommend that prescribing to women of childbearing age should be carried out with pregnancy in mind and contraception should be adequate before, during and after treatment.
ACE, Angiotensin-converting enzyme; *NSAIDs,* nonsteroidal antiinflammatory drugs.

However, with a few exceptions there is little evidence that drug intake via breastfeeding is of concern because most drugs enter breast milk in quantities too small to affect the baby. In general, drugs licensed for use in children can be safely given to the nursing mother, whereas drugs known to have serious toxic effects in adults, or that affect lactation (such as bromocriptine) should be avoided, including:

- cytotoxic drugs that may interfere with cellular metabolism of the nursing infant (e.g. cyclophosphamide, ciclosporin, doxorubicin, methotrexate);
- drugs of abuse, for which adverse effects on the infant during breastfeeding have been reported (e.g. amfetamine, cocaine, heroin, marijuana);
- radioactive compounds that require temporary cessation of breastfeeding (e.g. radioiodine);
- drugs that have been associated with significant effects on some nursing infants; these should be given to nursing mothers only with close monitoring (e.g. acebutolol, atenolol, bromocriptine, aspirin, ergotamine, lithium, phenindione, phenobarbital, primidone).

The absence of safety information for many drugs in lactation means that only essential drugs should be given to mothers during breastfeeding. The reader should refer to the up-to-date information in the BNF for detailed advice. Information on drug compatibility with breastfeeding is also provided by the UK Drugs in Lactation Advisory Service (www.ukmi.nhs.uk/ukdilas).

PHARMACOKINETICS IN LACTATION

Several factors influence drug transfer from the maternal circulation into breast milk, including the characteristics of the milk, the physicochemical properties of the drug and the amount of drug in the maternal circulation. Water-soluble drugs diffuse from plasma into milk, and the concentration in breast milk is similar to the free fraction in the maternal plasma. Lipid-soluble compounds also diffuse into breast milk and may concentrate because of the high fat content in milk.

The effects of drugs in breast milk depend on the extent of absorption, distribution and elimination of the drug in the neonate or infant (discussed later). Drugs may also have different pharmacodynamic properties in neonates or infants, compared with older children and adults. If drugs are given during breastfeeding, compounds with short half-lives are preferred because they are less likely to accumulate in neonates, who have lower drug clearance. The World Health Organization (WHO) nevertheless recommends that the health and developmental benefits of breastfeeding are usually greater than any likely risk from drugs in breast milk.

PRESCRIBING FOR CHILDREN

Both the pharmacokinetics and responses to drugs may differ in the young compared with adults, and there are also differences between neonates (<1 month), infants (1–12 months) and children, because many metabolic and physiological processes are immature at birth and develop rapidly in the first months of life. Particular care is needed in prescribing drugs that may affect growing or maturing organ systems such as the bones, teeth and the reproductive

---

Box 56.1　Developmental changes in the young that may alter drug handling compared with adults

- Low production of gastric acid and erratic gastric emptying in first year of life.
- Smaller ratio of gut surface area to body mass, but greater gut permeability to larger molecules.
- Greater proportion of body fat and larger extracellular volume may alter the volumes of distribution of some drugs.
- Maturation of drug-metabolising enzyme pathways in the liver occurs at different rates over the first year.
- GFR and tubular secretion are relatively low in the first year of life.
- Lower populations and reduced function of some gut flora.

GFR, Glomerular filtration rate.

---

system. Box 56.1 shows some of the pharmacokinetic differences between the young and adults.

Although medicines should usually be used within the terms of the product licence, many drugs given to children have not undergone formal clinical evaluation in this age group and are not specifically licensed for paediatric use. It is recognised that 'off-label' prescribing may be necessary, and the UK Medicines Act (1968) does not prohibit such unlicensed use. Clinical trials are needed in the paediatric population, but such studies raise significant ethical issues. The BNF for Children (www.evidence.nhs.uk) gives specific guidance on prescribing for children in the UK, often based on expert opinion in the absence of trial evidence.

PHARMACOKINETICS IN NEONATES AND CHILDREN

In neonates, inefficient metabolism and renal clearance mean that lower doses of some drugs are needed even after allowing for body weight, and doses need to be calculated with special care. The processes of drug elimination are largely mature by a few weeks of age, after which drug clearance adjusted to body weight is similar to or higher than that in adults (discussed later). However, children may be more susceptible to effects on growing or maturing tissues and organs. Generalisations are difficult, and each drug needs to be considered in its own right.

Absorption

Slow rates of gastric emptying and intestinal transit may slow the rate of drug absorption in neonates, but total absorption of poorly absorbed drugs may eventually be more complete because of longer contact with the intestinal mucosa. In the neonate, gastric pH is neutral, and this can reduce the absorption of weak acids but increase the absorption of weak bases.

Distribution

Neonates and young children have a lower body fat content and higher total body water than adults; this influences the distribution of both lipid- and water-soluble drugs. Neonates have a lower plasma albumin concentration, and higher concentrations of free fatty acids and bilirubin which may compete with drugs for plasma protein-binding sites. The overall effect is reduced plasma protein binding, which may increase the proportion of drug able to cross the blood–brain barrier. Drugs that are strongly bound to albumin should not be used during neonatal jaundice, because the drugs may displace bilirubin (which is mostly in the unconjugated form) from protein-binding sites and increase the risk of kernicterus.

Metabolism

The drug-metabolising enzyme systems are immature in the neonatal liver, and first-pass metabolism and hepatic drug clearances are low, especially for substrates of CYP1A2, CYP3A4 and glucuronidation. The clearances of substrates for these enzymes are two- to sixfold lower in neonates compared with adults. However, drug clearance is often higher in young children than in adults, because of their higher relative liver mass and greater hepatic blood flow per kilogram of body weight.

Renal elimination

Renal function in the neonate and infant is much less developed than in children or adults. The GFR in the newborn is about 40% of the adult level, and tubular secretory processes are poorly developed. Elimination of drugs such as digoxin, gentamicin and penicillin will therefore be slower until about 6–8 months of age.

In children, the faster hepatic elimination means that doses of metabolised drugs need to be higher than in adults after correcting for the difference in body weight. Prescribed doses are most accurately judged by considering both age and body surface area. In children, body surface area is a better guide to appropriate drug dosage than body weight. It can be estimated from a nomogram or by using the Du Bois formula:

$$\text{Body surface area} = 71.84 \times \text{weight}^{0.425} \times \text{height}^{0.725},$$

where body surface area is in square metres, weight in kilograms and height in metres. The drug dose for a child can be then approximated as:

$$\frac{\text{Adult dose} \times \text{surface area of child (in m}^2)}{1.8},$$

where 1.8 m^2 is the average body surface area of a 70 kg adult.

In the BNF for Children, drug doses are given by body weight, body surface area or age range, as appropriate.

PRESCRIBING FOR OLDER PEOPLE

Older people (usually defined as those over 70 years old) comprise a heterogeneous group who show considerable variation in 'biological' age. Changes occur in both the pharmacodynamics and pharmacokinetics of drugs with increasing age.

The density or numbers of receptors may be reduced with age; for example, β-adrenoceptors decrease in number, reducing the response to agonist drugs. Older people are often more susceptible to the effects of sedatives, hypnotics and antipsychotic drugs, possibly because of changes in receptor numbers and/or reduced efficiency of the blood–brain barrier. They are also more susceptible to the unwanted effects of NSAIDs on the gut.

Altered structure and function of target organs can influence the effects of drugs in older people. For example, baroreceptor function is impaired, and vasodilator drugs are more likely to provoke postural hypotension. The high peripheral resistance and less distensible arterial tree found with increasing age also respond less well to arterial vasodilators.

These changes reflect the ageing process itself, but they are often complicated by the presence of chronic disease and co-morbidity. The risks of unwanted effects are higher in the elderly as a consequence of these changes. Significant numbers of hospital admissions in the elderly are due to adverse drug reactions (see Chapter 53), and the risk of adverse reactions and drug interactions is highly correlated with polypharmacy. For these reasons, it is usual to start drug treatment in the elderly with the smallest effective dose. Rational prescribers should also seek to minimise the numbers of drugs used, with clear explanations of usage instructions and regular review of drug regimens. The BNF has a section of advice on prescribing in the elderly.

PHARMACOKINETICS IN OLDER PEOPLE

Absorption and distribution

Drug absorption across the gut wall is not greatly affected by ageing, although bioavailability may be increased due to reduced first-pass metabolism. Older people tend to have a lower lean body mass and a relative increase in body fat compared with young adults. The apparent volume of distribution (V_d) of water-soluble drugs such as digoxin may therefore be lower in the elderly, and a smaller loading dose would be needed. Conversely, lipid-soluble drugs may be eliminated more slowly because of their increased V_d resulting from increased body fat.

Metabolism

The size of the liver and its blood flow decrease with age. Although enzyme activity per hepatocyte probably shows little change, the overall capacity for drug metabolism, particularly phase 1 metabolic reactions (see Chapter 2), is reduced. This is particularly important for lipid-soluble drugs, such as nifedipine or propranolol, which undergo extensive first-pass metabolism, because lower hepatic metabolism increases oral bioavailability and reduces systemic clearance, raising plasma drug concentrations.

Renal elimination

Increasing age is also associated with a progressive reduction in GFR, so the elimination of polar drugs and metabolites is slower. This can produce toxicity when renally eliminated drugs with a low therapeutic index are prescribed (e.g. lithium, digoxin or gentamicin). Creatinine clearance is used as an estimate of GFR, but reduced muscle mass in older people results in reduced creatinine production. Plasma creatinine in the elderly therefore frequently remains within the normal laboratory reference range, even when renal function is substantially reduced, because the decreased creatinine production balances its reduced elimination. The Cockcroft and Gault equation, which relates plasma creatinine to creatinine clearance, contains elements reflecting sex- and age-dependent differences in muscle mass.

Creatinine clearance (mL/min) for males equals

$$\frac{1.23 \times (140 - \text{age in years}) \times \text{weight (in kg)}}{\text{plasma creatinine } (\mu\text{mol} \cdot \text{L}^{-1})},$$

and for females it equals

$$\frac{1.04 \times (140 - \text{age in years}) \times \text{weight (in kg)}}{\text{plasma creatinine } (\mu\text{mol} \cdot \text{L}^{-1})}.$$

As an alternative, the estimated glomerular filtration rate (eGFR; discussed later) is used to approximate GFR.

PRESCRIBING IN RENAL FAILURE

Individuals with renal failure show increased responses to many drugs, especially when the drug or any active metabolites are eliminated in the urine. Dose adjustment depends on the extent of renal impairment and on the proportion of total drug clearance that is due to renal excretion. The eGFR is often reported with laboratory estimations of serum creatinine. This is a useful guide to renal function, but does not consider weight as a variable that affects GFR. Nevertheless, for most drugs that are excreted by the kidney, it is an adequate guide for dosage adjustment.

There are also pharmacodynamic changes in renal failure; for example, there are altered responses to drugs in people with uraemia, and drugs acting on the central nervous system in particular produce enhanced responses, possibly because of increased permeability of the blood–brain barrier.

The BNF gives advice on drug prescribing in those with renal impairment. Renal impairment may produce abnormal drug responses due to one or more of the following factors:

- failure to excrete the drug or its metabolites may produce toxicity;
- increased sensitivity, even if elimination is unaltered;
- unwanted effects being poorly tolerated in such individuals.

PHARMACOKINETICS IN RENAL FAILURE

The activity of approximately 80% of current drugs is not affected by impaired renal function, because they are eliminated predominantly by hepatic metabolism, but the kidneys provide the major route of elimination for water-soluble drugs and water-soluble metabolites (see Chapter 2). Renal elimination of drugs can be affected indirectly by abnormal renal perfusion, such as might occur in shock, or directly by changes in the kidney (e.g. renal tubular necrosis).

Accumulation of drugs or their metabolites due to reduced renal function may increase the risk of toxicity.

There are several other ways in which renal impairment may influence the handling of drugs.

- Metabolism in the liver can be impaired in people with uraemia.
- The kidney has important metabolic activities, such as the 1-α-hydroxylation of vitamin D and the degradation of insulin, both of which can be impaired in renal failure.
- The distribution of drugs can be affected by changes in fluid balance in renal failure, and also by altered plasma protein binding (discussed later). The circulating concentration of albumin is decreased in severe renal failure with proteinuria. In addition, retained endogenous metabolites, such as the tryptophan metabolite indican, may compete for drug-binding sites on plasma proteins. The increased concentrations of free drug can lead to an enhanced response or to its increased elimination by glomerular filtration or metabolism.
- Tissue binding of digoxin is reduced in renal failure, so a lower loading dose should be given to compensate for the reduced volume of distribution.

The elimination of drugs by the kidney is significantly impaired only when the GFR is reduced below 50 mL/minute. For some drugs, clinically important accumulation does not occur until much lower filtration rates. Changes in renal tubular secretion of drugs in renal disease are less well understood.

A reduction in dosage of renally eliminated drugs in renal failure is usually necessary only when the compound has a low therapeutic index. Maintenance dosage may be lowered either by reducing the dose or by extending the dose interval (see Chapter 2, equation 2.21). Loading doses do not usually require any modification. For the purposes of dosage adjustment in renal impairment, the BNF uses the classification of chronic kidney disease based on eGFR values (in mL/minute per 1.73 m^2):

- Stage 1 (normal): eGFR greater than 90 (with other evidence of kidney damage, such as proteinuria);
- Stage 2 (mild): eGFR 60–89 (with other evidence of kidney damage);
- Stage 3 (moderate): eGFR 30–59;
- Stage 4 (severe): eGFR 15–29;
- Stage 5 (established renal failure): eGFR less than 15.

For some drugs, only established renal failure (stage 5) needs to be considered (e.g. a reduction in dosage is recommended for ampicillin), while for other drugs even mild impairment (stage 2) may be important (e.g. dosage reduction is recommended for carboplatin, and cisplatin should be avoided).

A further important consideration is the avoidance of drugs that have toxic effects on the kidney. Use of these in renal impairment can sometimes produce an irreversible decline in renal function.

PRESCRIBING IN LIVER DISEASE

Changes in both drug responses and pharmacokinetics can occur in liver disease. The BNF lists six main potential problems in prescribing for individuals with liver disease:

- impaired drug metabolism;
- hypoproteinaemia;

- reduced blood coagulation;
- hepatic encephalopathy;
- fluid overload;
- hepatotoxic drugs.

The severity of the liver disease is important, as is whether the disease is decompensated and includes jaundice, hypoproteinaemia or encephalopathy. Many of the pharmacodynamic and pharmacokinetic changes in liver failure arise from decreased hepatic synthesis of proteins that perform essential functions within the hepatocyte, or which are released into the blood, such as albumin and clotting factors.

Central nervous system (CNS) depressant drugs such as morphine and chlorpromazine have an enhanced effect in people with liver failure. This is caused by increased sensitivity of neuronal tissue and can provoke encephalopathy in susceptible people. Benzodiazepines used during investigational procedures in individuals with liver failure can produce profound and long-lasting effects, which may require reversal by the administration of the benzodiazepine antagonist flumazenil.

Encephalopathy may be triggered by drugs that cause constipation (which increases the formation of potentially toxic metabolites, such as ammonia, by the intestinal bacteria). Diuretics that produce hypokalaemia can also precipitate hepatic encephalopathy in chronic liver disease. Therefore potassium-sparing diuretics such as spironolactone are usually preferred to diuretics such as furosemide.

The reduced ability to synthesise vitamin K-dependent clotting factors makes people with chronic liver disease prone to clotting problems; they would be very sensitive to anticoagulant drugs, which are clearly contraindicated.

People with preexisting liver disease are likely to be more susceptible to hepatotoxic drugs. This raises a problem for pain relief, since paracetamol is hepatotoxic at high doses, whereas NSAIDs can increase the risk of gastrointestinal bleeding and cause fluid retention, while opioids can precipitate encephalopathy. In practice, lower doses of paracetamol are usually given, taking care that the amounts do not exceed the reduced threshold for hepatotoxicity shown by such individuals (see Chapter 53).

PHARMACOKINETICS IN LIVER DISEASE

The rate of absorption of drugs from the gut lumen is not greatly affected in liver disease. Distribution of drugs may be affected if synthesis of albumin is reduced, resulting in a higher percentage of free drug in plasma and possibly a greater risk of toxicity; examples of highly protein-bound drugs are phenytoin and prednisolone. Free drug concentrations may also be increased by elevated plasma bilirubin, which can displace drugs such as lidocaine and propranolol from their plasma protein-binding sites.

The liver has characteristics that facilitate the rapid and extensive uptake and metabolism of lipid-soluble drugs (Fig. 56.2). These include:

- fenestrations in the endothelium, allowing ready access to extracellular fluid;
- rapid diffusion across the space of Disse (which is a matrix consisting primarily of type 4 collagen);
- a brush border on hepatocytes, allowing rapid uptake;
- high intracellular enzyme activity for both phase 1 and phase 2 metabolism.

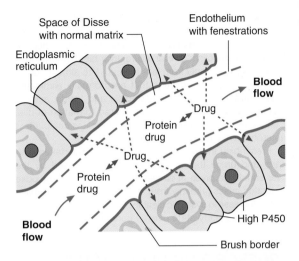

Fig. 56.2 Drug uptake from the sinusoid of a normal healthy liver.

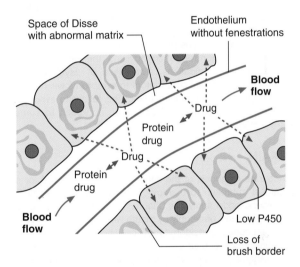

Fig. 56.3 Drug uptake from the sinusoid of a liver showing characteristic features of cirrhosis. The cirrhotic changes reduce the uptake and metabolism of drugs by hepatocytes.

Chronic liver disease can produce a number of changes that reduce the capacity of the liver to metabolise drugs (Fig. 56.3):

- fenestrations in the endothelium are lost;
- diffusion across the space of Disse may be reduced in fibrosis/cirrhosis as type 4 collagen is replaced by type 1 and type 3 collagen (which can form dense fibrils);
- the brush border on hepatocytes is lost;
- intracellular enzyme activity is reduced;
- intrahepatic vascular shunts may reduce the perfusion of hepatocytes.

Reduced hepatic elimination of drugs may result in a greater proportion of the drug or its metabolites being eliminated by other routes, such as the urine.

First-pass metabolism may be considerably reduced in conditions such as liver cirrhosis; the consequences are most apparent with drugs that normally undergo extensive hepatic first-pass metabolism. In liver failure, their bioavailability may increase considerably from less than 20% to almost 100%.

Biliary excretion of drugs that are normally eliminated unchanged in bile, such as rifampicin and fusidic acid, is impaired in conditions, causing impaired formation of bile. Reduced biliary elimination of drug metabolites could affect enterohepatic circulation (see Chapter 2).

Prescribing in liver disease should be undertaken with care, and drugs that are extensively metabolised by the liver should be given in smaller doses. The need for dose reduction arises primarily from an increase in bioavailability and a decrease in systemic clearance, both of which increase the average steady-state plasma concentration.

PRESCRIBING IN PALLIATIVE CARE

Symptom relief in palliative care often presents challenges to the prescriber, and the evidence to guide choice of treatments is often derived from experience rather than controlled trials. Palliative care services produce comprehensive guidelines for symptom control, often advising the use of drugs for unlicensed indications. Awareness of psychological, emotional and social contributors to symptoms will help to guide strategies for management. The following synopsis is not comprehensive, but covers an approach to some key symptoms.

PAIN

Accurate diagnosis of the cause of pain is essential for a rational approach to therapy. The principles of the WHO analgesic ladder apply (see Chapter 19). Analgesics should be given regularly, preferably by mouth with additional methods of pain control considered in all cases. These may include co-analgesics for neuropathic pain (see Chapter 19), surgery, radiotherapy, nerve blocks, transcutaneous electrical nerve stimulation (TENS), acupuncture and psychological support.

If a strong opioid is needed, then immediate-release morphine every 4 hours is preferred initially, increasing the dose by 30–50% every 2–3 days as required. When pain control is achieved, modified-release morphine every 12 hours can be used (giving the same total daily dose), with additional immediate-release morphine for breakthrough pain. Continuing pain despite persisting unwanted effects such as drowsiness suggests that the pain is not fully opioid-responsive. A laxative should always be given with a strong opioid.

Alternative opioids for palliative care include oxycodone or hydromorphone (which have a slightly different unwanted effect profile), diamorphine given by subcutaneous infusion (as its potency means it can be given in a smaller injection volume), methadone (particularly for neuropathic pain) or fentanyl (for transcutaneous use or in severe chronic kidney disease). Transdermal delivery of an opioid can be helpful if there is vomiting, intractable constipation or other unwanted effects in the presence of opioid-responsive pain. Care must be taken to give equivalent doses when changing from one opioid to another.

NAUSEA AND VOMITING

It is important to identify the cause if possible, since this will guide treatment. Drug therapy should always be considered as a cause of vomiting, and the responsible drug should be stopped or the dose reduced if possible. If drug therapy is required, then the choice will depend on the predominant contributory causes (see Chapter 32). Examples include dexamethasone for raised intracranial pressure, levomepromazine or benzodiazepines for anxiety, metoclopramide or prochlorperazine for drug-related vomiting, metoclopramide for gastric stasis, and metoclopramide, levomepromazine or cyclizine if the cause is not clear.

ANOREXIA/CACHEXIA/FATIGUE SYNDROME

This syndrome arises in terminal cancer, in heart failure and with chronic infection or inflammation. There is usually profound loss of weight and muscle bulk. It is often not possible to deal with causative factors, and management may include dexamethasone to suppress inflammation, methylphenidate or modafinil (see Chapter 22) for fatigue, in addition to encouraging exercise.

Constipation

Constipation may arise from drug therapy (e.g. opioids, antidepressants, antispasmodics, ondansetron), inactivity, dehydration, hypercalcaemia or concurrent disease. Adequate fluid intake is important, and if the underlying cause is not amenable to treatment, then symptomatic treatment should be given (see Chapter 35). Macrogols are usually used for opioid-induced constipation, although a stimulant such as senna may also be needed.

Breathlessness

Breathlessness is often multifactorial, and specific treatments may be successful. If there is no treatable cause, then nebulised saline can help to loosen secretions. Morphine, sometimes together with a benzodiazepine such as diazepam, can reduce the subjective sensation of breathlessness.

Hiccups

Hiccups can have a peripheral cause such as gastric distention, diaphragmatic irritation, liver enlargement or intrathoracic tumour. A variety of treatments have been advocated, indicating that all have limited efficacy. Options include metoclopramide, domperidone, a proton pump inhibitor, dexamethasone, baclofen and nifedipine. Central causes include raised intracranial pressure and uraemia, and treatment options include dexamathasone, levomepromazine, haloperidol and diazepam.

Use of a syringe driver

Near the end of life, drugs may need to be given by subcutaneous infusion via a small battery-powered pump.

Maintaining steady plasma drug concentrations may aid symptom control or give relief in someone who cannot swallow. Examples of drugs given by this route are:

- cyclizine, haloperidol or metoclopramide for vomiting;
- dexamethasone for neuropathic pain, raised intracranial pressure or vomiting;
- morphine, oxycodone or diamorphine for pain control;
- glycopyrronium to reduce respiratory secretions;
- hyoscine to relieve intestinal colic and to reduce secretions;
- levomepromazine for vomiting or as a sedative;
- midazolam for vomiting or seizures.

DRUG INTERACTIONS

Many people take more than one drug during a course of treatment because:

- combination therapy is preferable or necessary to produce an adequate effect or response; important examples are the chemotherapy of malignant disease and the treatment of hypertension.
- a single condition or pathology may give rise to a variety of symptoms that are controlled by different drugs.
- the person may have more than one condition or pathology, requiring treatment with drugs that are unrelated pharmacologically.

The term 'interaction' implies that the response to the combination of drugs is different to that which could be predicted from a simple aggregation of the effects of each drug given singly. Drug interactions may produce additive, synergistic or antagonist outcomes, and may be beneficial or potentially harmful because of altered clinical response or toxicity. Beneficial interactions are usually well characterised and have clear advantages – for example, combinations of anticancer drugs – and are the basis of prescribing recommendations. This section therefore focuses on adverse interactions, which are of greatest importance for drugs that have a narrow therapeutic index and for groups of people at increased risk, such as the elderly, who are the most likely to be taking several drugs concurrently. About 4% of hospital admissions in the UK are estimated to be caused by adverse drug interactions.

Interactions between drugs may arise at their common site of action (pharmacodynamics interactions) or from altered delivery of the drug to its site of action due to interference at sites of drug absorption, distribution, metabolism or excretion (pharmacokinetic interactions).

PHARMACODYNAMIC INTERACTIONS

Pharmacodynamic interactions are usually predictable based on the known mechanisms of action of the drugs. Interactions may relate to the principal site of action of the drug, or to secondary sites of action that are responsible for unwanted effects. In principle, drugs that are highly selective for a single site of action are less likely to produce pharmacodynamic interactions than drugs that show low selectivity. An example of a serious adverse synergistic interaction is between an angiotensin-converting enzyme (ACE) inhibitor, such as enalapril (see Chapter 6) and spironolactone (see Chapter 14); the ACE inhibitor reduces the production of aldosterone, thereby reducing the excretion of K^+, an effect which is exaggerated by the action of spironolactone, and the combination can cause potentially life-threatening hyperkalaemia.

PHARMACOKINETIC INTERACTIONS

Absorption

Co-administration of two drugs could give an interaction if one drug affects the rate or extent of absorption of the other drug, although such interactions are relatively uncommon in clinical practice. Changes in the rate of absorption (e.g. by increasing or decreasing gastric emptying or intestinal motility) will affect the peak concentration, but not usually the extent of absorption. Interactions affecting the extent of absorption may be more important; examples include the retention of drugs in the gut lumen (e.g. tetracycline antibiotics bind to divalent or trivalent metals, such as Ca^{2+} or Fe^{3+}, to form complexes that are not absorbed).

Distribution

Interactions affecting drug distribution may arise from competition for the nonspecific binding sites on plasma proteins, such as albumin (see Table 2.3). Drugs that bind to plasma proteins are usually more than 90% bound, but the low plasma concentration of most drugs compared with the concentrations of plasma proteins means that the availability of binding sites is rarely limiting and displacement by other drugs is uncommon. Interactions affecting plasma protein binding may be important when the displaced drug has a narrow therapeutic index, so that a change in free drug concentration increases the risk of drug toxicity.

Metabolism

Perhaps surprisingly, the simultaneous administration of two drugs that share a common pathway of metabolism rarely causes an interaction. This is because with therapeutic drug doses the plasma concentrations are usually far below the K_m values of drug-metabolising enzymes. The enzymes therefore do not become saturated, and first-order kinetics (see Chapter 2) still apply. An exception is the ingestion of ethanol in recreational doses that are orders of magnitude higher than those of most therapeutic drugs. The metabolism of ethanol by alcohol dehydrogenase is therefore saturated and follows zero-order kinetics. This allows ethanol to be used clinically to slow the metabolism by alcohol dehydrogenase of methanol or ethylene glycol, and reduce the generation of their highly toxic products (see Chapter 53).

Important interactions can occur, however, when one drug induces or inhibits the enzymes involved in the metabolism of another therapeutic drug; this is most commonly seen with drugs affecting the cytochrome P450 system because of the large number of P450 isoenzymes and their importance for the elimination of most drugs (Table 2.7). Induction or inhibition of hepatic enzymes can affect both systemic clearance and first-pass metabolism after oral dosage.

Enzyme inhibition occurs as soon as the inhibiting drug concentration is sufficiently high, and can occur after a single dose (e.g. cimetidine). Either one or both of the interacting drugs may be metabolised more slowly, resulting in higher plasma concentrations. In contrast, enzyme induction (e.g. by carbamazepine, phenytoin) requires a few days, as it results from gene transcription and protein translation of additional enzyme; the increased enzyme activity may then reduce the plasma concentrations of other drugs normally metabolised by that isoenzyme. This may decrease the clinical response to the affected compound, if it is an active drug, or it could increase the bioactivation of a prodrug to an active metabolite. When dosage with an enzyme-inducing drug is stopped, the enzyme activity usually declines over a period of 2–3 weeks. If the dosage of the second drug has been optimised for the drug combination, its plasma concentration may then increase markedly, giving a risk of toxicity. Most drugs that undergo cytochrome P450 metabolism are substrates for more than one P450 isoenzyme, and this reduces the risk of interactions. The risk is highest for drugs that are metabolised predominantly by a single P450 isoenzyme. The risk of interactions increases greatly when several drugs are taken concurrently.

Excretion

Each process involved in the renal elimination of drugs (glomerular filtration, pH-dependent reabsorption and renal tubular secretion) can be a site for drug interactions.

- Glomerular filtration depends on renal perfusion and only removes free drug (not protein-bound). In consequence, drugs affecting renal perfusion or plasma protein binding can give rise to interactions.
- pH-dependent reabsorption could be altered by drugs that affect urine pH, either directly or via metabolic effects; for example, the pH changes associated with aspirin overdose can affect the excretion of drugs taken concurrently.
- Renal tubular secretion can give rise to interactions when there is competition for the transporter system. Aspirin can interfere with the transport of both endogenous compounds (e.g. uric acid) and drugs (e.g. methotrexate).

The biliary excretion of drugs is not an important site for drug interactions, but the enterohepatic cycling of drugs can be affected by the co-administration of poorly absorbed broad-spectrum antibacterials, which affect the hydrolysis of drug conjugates in the lower bowel (Fig. 2.13).

The BNF has an extensive appendix listing pharmacodynamic and pharmacokinetic drug interactions. Many interactions are not clinically important, but significant interactions may require dose adjustment or drug substitution, or, if unavoidable, careful monitoring of plasma drug concentrations, biochemical markers or drug responses.

SELF-ASSESSMENT

True/false questions

1. The highest risk of teratogenicity is during the final trimester of pregnancy.
2. Drug doses may need to be increased in pregnancy.
3. After correction for body weight, drug doses in children are the same as for adults.
4. The bioavailability of lipid-soluble drugs is increased in the elderly.
5. Most drugs are not affected by impaired renal function.
6. Drugs that cause constipation can trigger encephalopathy in people with chronic liver disease.
7. Drugs that delay gastric emptying reduce the extent of absorption of other drugs.
8. Enzyme inducers can enhance clinical responses to prodrugs.

ANSWERS

True/false answers

1. **False.** The greatest risk of teratogenicity is during organogenesis in the first trimester.
2. **True.** While only the lowest effective doses of essential drugs should be used in pregnancy, these may need to be higher than in nonpregnant women, due to the increased volume of distribution and higher clearance.
3. **False.** Correction for body weight may underestimate drug doses in children due to their relatively high hepatic clearance; correction by body surface area is a better guide.
4. **True.** Lipid-soluble drugs are typically cleared by hepatic metabolism; lower hepatic blood flow in the elderly can reduce first-pass metabolism and increase oral bioavailability.
5. **True.** About 80% of drugs are eliminated by hepatic metabolism, so the plasma concentration of the parent drug is not affected by impaired renal function.
6. **True.** In chronic liver disease, constipation can increase the risk of encephalopathy from the generation of ammonia and other toxic products by the gut flora.
7. **False.** Delayed gastric emptying will slow the rate of absorption of most drugs and reduce their peak plasma concentrations, but the extent of absorption is not usually affected.
8. **True.** Bioconversion of a prodrug to its active derivative may be enhanced by an enzyme inducer.

FURTHER READING

Anderson, P.O., Manoguerra, A.S., Valdes, V., 2016. A review of adverse reactions in infants from medications in breastmilk. Clin. Pediatr. (Phila.) 55, 236–244.

Batchelor, H.K., Marriott, J.F., 2015. Formulations for children: problems and solutions. Br. J. Clin. Pharmacol. 79, 405–418.

Hubbard, R.E., O'Mahony, M.S., Woodhouse, K.W., 2013. Medication prescribing in frail older people. Eur. J. Clin. Pharmacol. 69, 319–326.

Jeong, H., 2010. Altered drug metabolism during pregnancy: hormonal regulation of drug-metabolizing enzymes. Expert Opin. Drug Metab. Toxicol. 6, 689–699.

Lees, J., Chan, A., 2011. Polypharmacy in elderly patients with cancer: clinical implications and management. Lancet Oncol. 12, 1249–1257.

Lewis, J.H., Stine, J.G., 2013. Review article: prescribing medications in patients with cirrhosis—a practical guide. Aliment. Pharmacol. Ther. 37, 1132–1156.

Mallet, L., Spinewine, A., Huang, A., 2007. Prescribing in elderly people 2. The challenge of managing drug interactions in elderly people. Lancet 370, 185–191.

Milton, J.C., Hall-Smith, I., Jackson, S.H.D., 2008. Prescribing for older people. Br. Med. J. 336, 606–609.

Pirmohamed, M., 2007. Prescribing in liver disease. Medicine (Baltimore) 35, 31–34.

Spinewine, A., Schmader, K.E., Barber, N., et al., 2007. Prescribing in elderly people 1. Appropriate prescribing in elderly people: How well can it be measured and optimised? Lancet 370, 173–184.

Starkey, E.S., Sammons, H.M., 2015. Practical pharmacokinetics: What do you really need to know? Arch. Dis. Child Educ. Pract. Ed. 100, 37–43.

Thomas, S.H.L., Yates, L.M., 2012. Prescribing without evidence—pregnancy. Br. J. Clin. Pharmacol. 74, 691–697.

Vargesson, N., 2015. Thalidomide-induced teratogenesis: history and mechanisms. Birth Defects Res. C Embryo Today 105, 140–156.

Verbeeck, R.K., Musuamba, F., 2009. Pharmacokinetics and dosage adjustment in patients with renal dysfunction. Eur. J. Clin. Pharmacol. 65, 757–773.

Index

Page numbers followed by "*f*" indicate figures, "*t*" indicate tables, and "*b*" indicate boxes.